CONSIDERATIONS FOR THE OLDER PATIENT, PEDIATRIC PATIENT, HOME

(continued on inside back cover)

CRITICAL CARE NURSING
A HOLISTIC APPROACH

SEVENTH EDITION

CRITICAL CARE NURSING

A HOLISTIC APPROACH

Carolyn M. Hudak, RN, PhD
Adult Nurse Practitioner
Denver, Colorado

Barbara M. Gallo, RN, MS, CNAA
Manager, High Tech Clinical Services
Visiting Nurse Association of Central Connecticut, Inc.
New Britain, Connecticut

Patricia Gonce Morton, RN, PhD
Associate Professor and Coordinator
Master's Program in Trauma/Critical Care Nursing
University of Maryland School of Nursing
Baltimore, Maryland

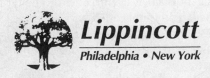

Lippincott
Philadelphia • New York

Acquisitions Editor: Susan M. Glover, RN, MSN
Developmental Editor: Eleanor Faven
Sponsoring Editor: Bridget Blatteau
Project Editor: Erika Kors
Senior Production Manager: Helen Ewan
Senior Production Coordinator: Nannette Winski
Design Coordinator: Doug Smock

7th Edition

9 8 7 6

Library of Congress Cataloging-in-Publications Data

Critical care nursing : a holistic approach / [edited by] Carolyn M.
   Hudak, Barbara M. Gallo, Patricia Gonce Morton. — 7th ed.
        p.   cm.
     Includes bibliographical references and index.
     ISBN 0-7817-9195-2 (alk. paper)
     1. Intensive care nursing.   2. Holistic nursing.   I. Hudak,
Carolyn M.   II. Gallo, Barbara M.   III. Morton, Patricia Gonce,
1952–   .
     [DNLM: 1. Critical Care—nurses' instruction.   2. Holistic
Nursing.   WY 154 C9328 1998]
RT120.I5C744   1998
610.73′61—dc21
DNLM/DLC
for Library of Congress   97-15951
                                                          CIP

Care has been taken to confirm the accuracy of the information presented and to describe generally accepted practices. However, the authors, editors, and publisher are not responsible for errors or omissions or for any consequences from application of the information in this book and make no warranty, express or implied, with respect to the contents of the publication.

The authors, editors and publisher have exerted every effort to ensure that drug selection and dosage set forth in this text are in accordance with current recommendations and practice at the time of publication. However, in view of ongoing research, changes in government regulations, and the constant flow of information relating to drug therapy and drug reactions, the reader is urged to check the package insert for each drug for any change in indications and dosage and for added warnings and precautions. This is particularly important when the recommended agent is a new or infrequently employed drug.

Some drugs and medical devices presented in this publication have Food and Drug Administration (FDA) clearance for limited use in restricted research settings. It is the responsibility of the health care provider to ascertain the FDA status of each drug or device planned for use in their clinical practice.

To Charlene A. Lark, RN, MSN, former Associate Director of Nursing, Denver General Health and Hospitals, who influenced, championed, and suffered through every edition of this book.

—Carolyn

To Joe D. Seagraves, a special friend.

—Bobbie

To my husband John, whose love, patience, and support made this project possible.

—Trish

Contributing Authors

M. SUE APPLE, RN, DNSc(C), CCRN
Cardiology Clinical Nurse Specialist
The Washington Hospital Center
Washington, DC
18: Common Cardiovascular Disorders

NANCY L. BARCZAK, RN, MS
Clinical Education Coordinator
University of Maryland Medical System
Baltimore, Maryland
27: Anatomy and Physiology of the Renal System

ANNE E. BELCHER, RN, PhD, FAAN
Associate Professor
Chair, Department of Acute and Long-Term Care
University of Maryland School of Nursing
Baltimore, Maryland
44: Anatomy and Physiology of the Hematological and
*   Immune Systems*
47: Common Immunological Disorders
*   Oncological Emergencies*

JULIE BENZ, RN, CNS, MS, CCRN
Critical Care Clinical Nurse Specialist
Lutheran Medical Center
Wheat Ridge, Colorado
19: Heart Failure

KATHRYN S. BIZEK, RN, MSN, CCRN, CS
Clinical Nurse Specialist
Medical/Cardiac Critical Care
Detroit Receiving Hospital and University Health Center
   and Associate Graduate Faculty
College of Nursing, Wayne State University
Detroit, Michigan
2: The Patient's Experience With Critical Illness

ELEANOR F. BOND, RN, PhD
Associate Professor
Biobehavioral Nursing and Health Systems
University of Washington School of Nursing
Seattle, Washington
37: Anatomy and Physiology of the Gastrointestinal
*   System*

SUSAN BONINI, RN, MSN
Clinical Nurse Educator
Medical Intensive Care Unit, Cardiac Critical Care Unit and
   Cardiology Services
University Hospital
Denver, Colorado
49: Hypoperfusion States

SEAN T. COLLINS, RNCS, MS, CNN, ANP
Western New England Renal and Transplant Associates
   and Nursing Faculty
College of Our Lady of the Elms
West Springfield, Massachusetts
30: Common Renal Disorders
*   Acute Renal Failure*

VICKI J. COOMBS, RN, MS, CCRN
Senior Research Nurse Coordinator
Interventional Cardiology
Johns Hopkins Hospital
Baltimore, Maryland
17: Patient Management: Cardiovascular System
*   Percutanous Transluminal Coronary*
*   Angioplasty and Percutaneous Balloon Valvuloplasty*

CHRISTINE M. CORCORAN, RN, MS, CCRN
Staff Nurse
Stanford University Hospital
Stanford, California
17: Patient Management: Cardiovascular System
*   Intra-Aortic Balloon Pump Counterpulsation*
*   Mechanical Circulatory Support*

ANDA CRAVEN, RN, MS, CNS
Fort Collins, Colorado
50: Trauma

JOCELYN A. FARRAR, RN, MS, CCRN
Instructor, Department of Acute and Long-Term Care
University of Maryland School of Nursing
Baltimore, Maryland
3: The Family's Experience With Critical Illness

JOHN E. FITZGERALD, DMD, PhD
Saint Joseph's College
University of Hartford
West Hartford, Connecticut
41: Anatomy and Physiology of the Endocrine System

MARY BETH FLYNN, RN, MS, CCRN
Clinical Nurse Educator
Surgical Intensive Care Unit, Burn Unit and Medical-Surgical
    Nursing Services
University Hospital
Denver, Colorado
49: Hypoperfusion States

MARTHA FOLEY, RN, BSN, CSPI
Certified Specialist in Poison Information
Rocky Mountain Poison Center
Denver, Colorado
52: Drug Overdose and Poisoning

BARBARA M. GALLO, RN, MS, CNAA
Manager, High Tech Clinical Services
Visiting Nurse Association of Central Connecticut, Inc.
New Britain, Connecticut
42: Patient Assessment: Endocrine System

CHRISTINE GRADY, RN, PhD
Assistant Director for Clinical Science
National Institute of Nursing Research
National Institutes of Health
Bethesda, Maryland
7: Ethical Issues in Critical Care
(The work of Christine Grady was done as part of her
    responsibilities for the U.S. Government)

TERESA HALLORAN, RN, MSN, CCRN
Clinical Care Services Director
Memorial Hospital
Bellville, Illinois
43: Common Endocrine Disorders

CAROLYN M. HUDAK, RN, PhD
Adult Nurse Practitioner
Denver, Colorado
25: Common Respiratory Disorders

KIMMITH M. JONES, RN, MS, CCRN
Faculty Associate, University of Maryland School of Nursing
Advanced Practice Nurse, Critical Care/Emergency Departments
Sinai Hospital of Baltimore
Baltimore, Maryland
47: Common Immunological Disorders
    Human Immunodeficiency Virus (HIV) Infection

KATHLEEN KEENAN, RN, MS, CCRN, NREMT-P
Formerly, Clinical Nurse Specialist
R Adams Cowley Shock Trauma Center
University of Maryland Medical System
Baltimore, Maryland
14: Interfacility Transport of the Critically Ill Patient

MARTHA M. KENNEDY, RN, MS, CCRN
Doctoral Student
University of Maryland School of Nursing
Baltimore, Maryland
16: Patient Assessment: Cardiovascular System
        Cardiac History and Physical Examination
23: Patient Assessment: Respiratory System
38: Patient Assessment: Gastrointestinal System
40: Common Gastrointestinal Disorders

SANDRA R. KEWMAN, RN, BSN, CCRN
Clinical Care Coordinator
Critical Care Medicine Unit
University of Michigan Health System
Ann Arbor, Michigan
4: Impact of the Critical Care Environment on the Patient

JAMES E. KOHL, RN, MS
Commander, Nurse Corps., US Navy
Bethesda, Maryland
48: Common Hematological Disorders
        Disseminated Intravascular Coagulation

JANICE C. KRUEGER, RN, MSN
Nephrology Clinical Nurse Specialist
Duke University Medical Center
Durham, North Carolina
30: Common Renal Disorders
        Acute Renal Failure

BARBARA KRUMBACH, RN, MS, CCRN
Professional Resources Educator
University Hospital
Denver, Colorado
17: Patient Management: Cardiovascular System
        Pharmacological Therapy, Cardiopulmonary
        Resuscitation

DEBORAH J. LAZZARA, RN, MS, CCRN
Clinical Nurse Specialist, Critical Care
Advocate Health Care
Christ Hospital and Medical Center
Oak Lawn, Illinois
5: Relieving Pain and Providing Comfort

CATHLEEN R. MAIOLATESI, RN, MS
Advanced Practice Nurse
Department of Gynecology and Obstetrics
Johns Hopkins Hospital
Baltimore, Maryland
11: The Critically Ill Pregnant Woman

MARGARET BOYLE MARCINEK, RN, MSN, EdD
Professor and Chair
Department of Nursing
California University of Pennsylvania
California, Pennsylvania
51: Burns

BARBARA McCOOL, RN, MS
Senior Scientist and Nurse Consultant
Food and Drug Administration
Office of Device Evaluation
Rockville, Maryland
  28: Patient Assessment: Renal System
  30: Common Renal Diseases

PATRICIA C. McMULLEN, CRNP, MS, JD
Associate Professor
Uniform Services
University of the Health Sciences
Graduate School of Nursing
  8: Legal Issues in Critical Care

JOHANNA L. MEEHAN, APRN, MSN, AOCN
Acute Care Nurse Practitioner
Bone Marrow Transplant Department
University of Connecticut Health Center
Farmington, Connecticut
  46: Organ and Hemopoietic Stem Cell Transplantation

MARILYNN MITCHELL, RN, MSN, CNRN, CRRN
Clinical Nurse Specialist
Methodist Hospital
Omaha, Nebraska
  31: Anatomy and Physiology of the Nervous System
  35: Common Neurological Disorders
  36: Spinal Cord Injury

PATRICIA A. MOLONEY-HARMON, RN, MS, CCRN
Advanced Practice Nurse
Children's Services
Sinai Hospital of Baltimore
Baltimore, Maryland
  10: The Critically Ill Pediatric Patient

PATRICIA GONCE MORTON, RN, PhD
Associate Professor and Coordinator
Master's Program in Trauma/Critical Care Nursing
University of Maryland School of Nursing
Baltimore, Maryland
  14: Interfacility Transport of the Critically Ill Patient
  15: Anatomy and Physiology of the Cardiovascular System
  *16: Patient Assessment: Cardiovascular System Cardiac
    History and Physical Examination Electrocardiographic
    Monitoring Dysrhythmias and the 12 Lead
    Electrocardiogram Effects of Serum Electrolyte
    Abnormalities on the Electrocardiogram*
  *17: Patient Management: Cardiovascular System
    Management of Dysrhythmias*
  19: Heart Failure
  20: Acute Myocardial Infarction
  22: Anatomy and Physiology of the Respiratory System
  23: Patient Assessment: Respiratory System

KATHLEEN S. OMAN, RN, PhD(C), CEN
Clinical Educator
Emergency Services
University Hospital
Denver, Colorado
  49: Hypoperfusion States

KAREN T. PARDUE, RN.C., MS
Assistant Professor
Department of Nursing
University of New England
Biddeford, Maine
  9: Rewards and Challenges of Critical Care Nursing

JOAN CHARTIER PRATT, RN, MS, CCRN
Staff Nurse
R Adams Cowley Shock Trauma Center
University of Maryland Medical System
Baltimore, Maryland
  39: Patient Management: Gastrointestinal System

BARBARA RESNICK, PhD, CRNP
Assistant Professor
University of Maryland School of Nursing
Baltimore, Maryland
and
Geriatric Nurse Practitioner
Roland Park Place
Baltimore, Maryland
  12: The Critically Ill Older Patient

CATHY ROSENTHAL-DICHTER, RN, MN, CCRN, FCCM
Doctoral Candidate and Teaching Assistant
University of Pennsylvania School of Nursing
Philadelphia, Pennsylvania
  10: The Critically Ill Pediatric Patient

LOIS SCHICK, RN, MN, MBA, CPAN, CAPA
Director Emergency Department, SurgiCare One, Clinical
    Decision Unit, Employee and Occupational Health
St. Joseph Hospital
Denver, Colorado
  13: The Postanesthesia Patient

RAE NADINE SMITH, RN, MS
Clinical Nurse Specialist
Medical Communicators and Associates, Inc.
Salt Lake City, Utah
  *17: Patient Management: Cardiovascular System
    Autologous Blood Transfusion*
  33: Patient Management: Nervous System

DEBRA L. SPUNT, RN, MS
Clinical Instructor
University of Maryland School of Nursing
Baltimore, Maryland
  *17: Patient Management: Cardiovascular System
    Cardiopulmonary Resuscitation*

MARY S. SWANSON, RN, MBA
Manager of Clinical Transplantation
Hartford Transplant Center
Hartford Hospital
Hartford, CT
  46: Organ and Hemopoietic Stem Cell Transplantation

PAULA TIMMERMAN, RN, MSN, AOCN
Oncology Clinical Nurse Specialist
Good Samaritan Hospital
Downers Grove, Illinois
   45: Patient Assessment: Hematological and Immune Systems
   48: Common Hematological Disorders
      Disorders of Red Blood Cells
      Disorders of White Blood Cells
      Disorders of Bone Marrow Failure
      Disorders of Hemostasis

TERRY L. TUCKER, RN, MS, CCRN, CEN
Critical Care Clinical Nurse Specialist
Veterans' Affairs Maryland Health Care System
Baltimore, Maryland
   16: Patient Assessment: Cardiovascular System
      Cardiac Laboratory Studies
      Cardiovascular Diagnostic Procedures

PHYLLIS A. URIBE, RN, BSN, CCRN
Trauma Education and Program Supervisor
Columbia Colorado Division
Columbia Swedish Medical Center
Englewood, Colorado
   32: Patient Assessment: Nervous System
   34: Head Injury

KATHRYN T. VON RUEDEN, RN, MS, CCRN, FCCM
Director of Clinical Research
Renaissance Technology Inc.
Newtown, Pennsylvania
   16: Patient Assessment: Cardiovascular System
      Hemodynamic Monitoring
   26: Adult Respiratory Distress Syndrome
   Collaborative Care Guides

ELIZABETH D. VOSSLER, APRN, MSN, FNP
Thoracic/Outpatient Transplant Coordinator
Hartford Transplant Associates
Hartford, Connecticut
   46: Organ and Hemopoietic Stem Cell Transplantation

BARBARA L. WEBER, RN, MS, CCRN, CVNS
Education Coordinator
Columbia Aurora Presbyterian Hospital
   and Columbia Aurora Regional Medical Center
Aurora, Colorado
   21: Cardiac Surgery

ROBERT H. WELTON, RN, MSN
Professional Development Coordinator
University of Maryland Medical Systems
Baltimore, Maryland
   30: Common Renal Disorders
      Fluid and Electrolyte Imbalances

DEBBIE FUNDERBURG WILMOTH, RN, BSN, CCRN
Clinician 3
Porter Medical Intensive Care Unit
University of Virginia Medical Center
Charlottesville, Virginia
   24: Patient Management: Respiratory System

MICHAEL L. WILLIAMS, RN, MSN, CCRN
Clinical Nurse Specialist—Thoracic Surgical Nursing
University of Michigan Health System
Doctoral Student
University of Michigan School of Nursing
Ann Arbor, Michigan
   1: Caring and Critical Thinking Within a Holistic Framework
   4: Impact of the Critical Care Environment on the Patient
   6: Patient and Family Education in a Changing Health Care
      Environment

KATHLEEN M. WRUK, RN, BSN, MHS
Managing Director
Rocky Mountain Poison and Drug Center
Denver, Colorado
   52: Drug Overdose and Poisoning

MARY ZORZANELLO, RN, MSN, CNN
Home Training Coordinator
Gambro Healthcare Services and Dialysis at Yale New Haven
New Haven, Connecticut
   29: Patient Management: Renal System

We would like to acknowledge and thank the following contributors to the previous edition:

   Patricia Barry, PhD, APRN, CS
   Karen D. Busch, RN, PhD
   Jacquelyn M. Clement, RN, PhD
   Sarah Dillian Cohn, MS, JD
   Lane D. Craddock, MD, FACP, FACC
   Crystal A. Cranor, RN, BSN, CCRN
   A. Gail Curry-Kane, RN, BS, ICP
   Barbara F. Fuller, RN, PhD
   Linda F. Hellstedt, RN, MSN, CCRN
   Eileen Brent Hemman, RN, MSN, CCRN
   Elisa J. Ignatious
   Diane Korte-Schwind, RN, MSN
   Joanne M. Krumberger, RN, MSN, CCRN
   Mary Kay Knight Macheca, RN, MSN(R), CDE
   Barbara C. Martin, RN.C, EdD
   Mary de Meneses, RN, EdD
   Joan D. Mersch, RN, MS
   Linda K. Ottoboni, RN, MS, CCRN
   Michele A. Parker, RN
   Suzanne M. Provenzano, RN, BSN, CCRN, CNRN
   Karen Robbins, RN, MS, CNN
   Carlena Robison
   Julie A. Shinn, RN, MA, FAAN, CCRN
   Janice Smith, RN, MS
   Marianne Stewart, RN, MSN, CCRN
   Roslyn Sykes, RN, PhD

List of Reviewers

JULIE BENZ, RN, CNS, MS, CCRN
Critical Care Clinical Nurse Specialist
Lutheran Medical Center
Wheat Ridge, Colorado

JANICE BOUNDY, RN, PhD
Associate Professor/Coordinator
St. Francis College of Nursing
Peoria, Illinois

BARBARA L. BULLOCK, RN, MSN, CCRN
Assistant Professor in Nursing
Houston Baptist University
Houston, Texas

JACQUELINE FOWLER BYERS, RN, PhD
Director
Quality Management
Orlando Regional Healthcare System
Orlando, Florida

MARC CELIA, RN, BSN, CCRN, NREMF-P
Staff Nurse
Surgical/Trauma Intensive Care
University of Pennsylvania Medical Center
Philadelphia, Pennsylvania

VICKI J. COOMBS, RN, MS, CCRN
Senior Research Nurse Coordinator
Interventional Cardiology
Johns Hopkins Hospital
Baltimore, Maryland

DEBORAH M. FROMAN, RN, MSN
ACLS Coordinator
University of Maryland Medical Systems
Baltimore, Maryland

MERLE R. KATAOKA-YAHIRO, RN, Dr.PH
Assistant Professor
School of Nursing
San Jose State University
San Jose, California

MARTHA M. KENNEDY, RN, MS, CCRN
Doctoral Student
University of Maryland School of Nursing
Baltimore, Maryland

CYNTHIA R. KING, RN, NP, MSN, CNA
Nurse Consultant
Special Care Consultants
and
Oncology Nurse Practitioner
Highland Hospital
Rochester, New York

JANICE C. KRUEGER, RN, MSN
Nephrology Clinical Nurse Specialist
Duke University Medical Center
Durham, North Carolina

DEITRA LEONARD LOWDERMILK, PhD, RNC
Clinical Professor
School of Nursing
University of North Carolina at Chapel Hill
Chapel Hill, North Carolina

STEVE MILLER, RN
formerly with
The Starzl Transplant Institute
Pittsburgh, Pennsylvania

JUDITH A. PAICE, RN, PhD, FAAN
Professor
College of Nursing
Rush University
and
Clinical Nurse Specialist, Pain Management
Department of Neurosurgery
Rush Medical Center
Chicago, Illinois

CHRIS PASERO, RN, BSN
Pain Management Consultant
Rocklin, California
and
Cofounder
American Society of Pain Management Nurses
Laguna Beach, California

DEBORAH POOL, RN, MS, CCRN
Instructor
Department of Nursing
Glendale Community College
Glendale, Arizona

VIRGINIA H. SECOR, RN, MSN
Instructor
Department of Adult and Elder Health
Nell Hodgson Woodruff School of Nursing
Emory University
Atlanta, Georgia

KATHLEEN RICE SIMPSON, MSN, RNC
Perinatal Clinical Nurse Specialist
St. John's Mercy Medical Center
St. Louis, Missouri

GAYLA SMITH, RN, MS, CCRN
Clinical Nurse Specialist
ICU/CCU/Telemetry
Western Medical Center
Santa Ana, California

SUSAN L. STACEY, RN, BSN
Nurse Manager
Pediatrics/PICU
Sacred Heart Medical Center
Spokane, Washington

ANGELA FRAWLEY TRIVANE, RN
Outpatient Surgery
Anne Arundel Medical Center
Annapolis, Maryland

KATHRYN T. VON RUEDEN, RN, MS, CCRN, FCCM
Director of Clinical Research
Renaissance Technology Inc.
Newtown, Pennsylvania

CHERYL WRAA, RN, BSN, CFRN
Clinical Resource Nurse, Flight Nurse
Life Flight
University of California, Davis Medical Center
Sacramento, California

Acknowledgments

This book could not have survived through seven editions without the help and support of many people. To our many colleagues who shared their expertise and became good friends along the way, we say a heartfelt thank you. Our publisher, Lippincott-Raven, has seen more than a few changes over the years, but their commitment to produce the finest book possible has never wavered. Our respect and gratitude to Eleanor Faven, Senior Developmental Editor, who introduced us to the concept of the developmental editor and made us wonder how we ever managed without one. Many thanks to Donna Hilton, RN, BSN, Vice President and Publisher, Nursing and Allied Health Publishing, and Susan Glover, RN, MSN, Senior Nursing Acquisitions Editor, who made us take a hard look at the book and came up with many cogent suggestions to improve it. Our appreciation also to Helen Ewan, Nannette Winski, and Erika Kors, who went the extra mile to smooth the production process for us.

We would like to acknowledge the efforts of Janice Muzynski, RN, MS, of Advocate Health Care in Chicago, for providing several recommendations for nurse contributors in that area. Joyce L. Fedeczko, MALS of Advocate's Health Sciences Library Network in Chicago provided timely support and critical input for our research needs.

Sincere appreciation to Sunni Kim, DDCS, Inc., and Kerry Damico, RN, Neuro Critical Care, University Hospital in Salt Lake City, for their valuable assistance in the preparation of the material on increased intracranial pressure in Chapter 33.

Carolyn, Bobbie, Tricia

Preface

We are humbled by the fact that our book, **Critical Care Nursing: A Holistic Approach**, has influenced and shaped the practice of critical care nursing for the past 25 years. When we published the first edition in 1973, we never dreamed that the text would be the mainstay of critical care nursing for an entire generation of nurses.

In addition to its widespread use in the United States, the text is an integral part of critical care nursing in many other countries. We are somewhat awed by the fact that the text was translated into Indonesian and Portuguese recently and will impact the care of critically ill patients half a world away. This knowledge has further increased our commitment to provide a book that is current, comprehensive, and practical.

Our primary goal for the seventh edition has been to reaffirm our standing as a classic, while we assist nurses in meeting the challenges of critical care nursing at the beginning of the twenty-first century. We want to promote excellence in the rapidly changing specialty of care of critically ill patients by offering a comprehensive knowledge base built on a holistic perspective. By blending theory and principles with the reality of clinical practice, the reader of this text will be able to manage critically ill patients with competence and confidence. If we can enable the reader to evolve to the level of nursing practice characterized by a focus on patient responses and to achieve a comfort level with technology so that technology becomes secondary to the patient—the true focus of critical care—we will have achieved our goal.

In preparing this seventh edition, we solicited reviews and feedback from both educators and clinicians in order to make this the best edition ever, tailored to the needs of students, educators, clinicians, and patients. To help us achieve this goal, over 50 recognized experts contributed to the text. Included in our distinguished group of contributors are staff nurses, clinical nurse specialists, and nurse educators all of whom are at the cutting edge of critical care nursing practice. In addition, we welcome as co-editor and co-author Patricia Gonce Morton, RN, PhD, an exceptionally qualified critical care nursing educator and practitioner.

We remain committed to our tradition of emphasizing the patient as the core of nursing practice. Information about pathophysiology, technology, procedures, and various interventions is intended to support the individual as the focus of care. To that end, many changes have been incorporated into the seventh edition.

ORGANIZATION

Critical Care Nursing: A Holistic Approach is organized into five parts. Part I, The Concepts of Holism Applied to Critical Care Nursing Practice, contains six chapters that set the foundation for the remainder of the text. Topics included here are caring, critical thinking, nursing process, the holistic framework, research, advocacy, the patient's and family's experience with critical illness (including stress, loss, and dying), the critical care environment, pain and comfort, and patient and family education.

Part II, Professional Practice Issues in Critical Care, includes three chapters of concern to the nursing profession. Ethical and legal issues are explored. A high point of Part II is a unique chapter describing the rewards and challenges of critical care nursing.

Part III, Special Populations in Critical Care, is new to the seventh edition. It offers valuable guidance when working with the pediatric patient, the pregnant woman, the older person, the postanesthesia patient, and the patient being transported between facilities.

Part IV, Critical Care Nursing: Alterations in Body Systems, is broken down into seven units. Each unit comprises separate chapters that develop care of the patient. Each unit begins with anatomy and physiology of the system, continues with patient assessment, general patient management, and common disorders. Selected disorders are addressed in separate chapters in each unit. New to this edition is a unit on the hematological and immune systems.

The text concludes with Part V, Multisystem Dysfunction. Chapters in this section include hypoperfusion states, trauma, burns, and drug overdose and poisoning.

Two appendices complete the textbook. An answer key to study questions is featured at the end of the book. It provides the reader not only with correct answers to the multiple choice questions but also with rationales for those answers. Algorithms to ACLS guidelines complete the appendices.

NEW CHAPTERS IN THIS EDITION

One of the purposes of a revised edition is to ensure that the content of every chapter reflects current information and the most recent developments in technology and health care. For this reason, 13 new chapters have been added to the seventh edition. These chapters include

> Chapter 1: Caring and Critical Thinking Within a Holistic Framework
> Chapter 5: Relieving Pain and Providing Comfort
> Chapter 9: Rewards and Challenges of Critical Care Nursing
> Chapter 10: The Critically Ill Pediatric Patient
> Chapter 11: The Critically Ill Pregnant Woman
> Chapter 14: Interfacility Transport of the Critically Ill Patient
> Chapter 18: Common Cardiovascular Disorders
> Chapter 44: Anatomy and Physiology of the Hematological and Immune Systems
> Chapter 45: Patient Assessment: Hematological and Immune Systems
> Chapter 46: Organ and Hemopoietic Stem Cell Transplantation
> Chapter 47: Common Immunological Disorders
> Chapter 48: Common Hematological Disorders
> Chapter 49: Hypoperfusion States

SPECIAL FEATURES

Another goal of the seventh edition is to include numerous pedagogical aids to help clarify important information for the reader. Display boxes, charts, tables, and illustrations are used extensively throughout the text to organize and summarize large amounts of special information for easy review and recall. The following are pedagogical aids providing emphasis to the content of the text.

List of Displays

We feel it is helpful for the reader to have easy access to the variety of displays appearing in the book. And so we have placed a list of prominent recurring displays inside the front and back covers and their facing page. A list of additional recurring displays is located after the Table of Contents. Information can be reviewed by studying the various displays.

Patients at Risk

To call attention to patients with worsening conditions or factors in their condition that put them at risk, a feature called *Red Flags* appears in this edition. *Red Flags* highlight risk factors, complications, and signs and symptoms. A special icon makes these factors stand out even more.

Clinical Applications

This feature includes displays called *Clinical Application* that help the reader understand and apply essential information to critical care nursing practice. *Clinical Application* displays include *Assessment Parameters, Diagnostic Studies, Drug Therapy*, and *Nursing Intervention Guidelines*.

Patient Care Studies

Where appropriate, *Patient Care Studies* have been included in chapters as an additional learning tool. These *Patient Care Studies*, under the title *Clinical Application*, provide an excellent focus for individual study, classroom discussion, or clinical conferences.

Collaborative Care Guides

Collaborative Care Guides replace many of the nursing care plans found in previous editions. *Collaborative Care Guides* are multidisciplinary in scope and are intended to reflect the contributions of various members of the health care team when caring for the critically ill patient. Working collaboratively with other members of the health care team is an essential responsibility of critical care nurses. It seems appropriate to use *Collaborative Care Guides* rather than traditional nursing care plans.

The Older Patient

As the number of older persons in the population increases, so does the number of critically ill patients who are older. Special attention should be directed to the needs of this segment of the population. Therefore, the text not only devotes an entire chapter (Chapter 12) to the needs of the older patient, but highlights their needs throughout the text in displays called *Considerations for the Older Patient*.

The Pediatric Patient

Although most critical care management is directed toward the adult, pediatric patients have special needs. Chapter 10 addresses pediatric needs. *Considerations for the Pediatric Patient* also give specific information about adaptations when caring for the child.

Home Care

Critical care nursing is practiced wherever there are critically ill patients. In today's world, critically ill patients are found not only in hospital intensive care units, but also in the home. *Considerations for Home Care* included in many chapters offer the reader guidelines for preparing patients and families for discharge as well as an overview of care provided in the home setting.

Patient Teaching

A helpful display, *Patient Teaching*, summarizes key points for teaching patients and families. These guides can be used to prepare patients for procedures, to assist patients in understanding their illness, and to explain postoperative or postprocedure activities.

Nursing Diagnoses and Collaborative Problems

Critical care nurses work both independently and collaboratively when caring for critically ill patients. To reflect this, selected chapters contain lists of nursing diagnoses that the nurse can treat independently. Additionally, collaborative problems are presented in which the nurse works with other members of the health care team in determining appropriate actions.

Clinical Research

Insights Into Clinical Research are highlighted in this edition to help the reader understand the importance of research-based practice. Each research summary provides an overview of a study relevant to the chapter contents. Through these reviews, the reader should gain an appreciation of the importance of research in nursing practice and be able to apply findings of research to practice.

Chapter Outlines and Objectives

Each chapter begins with an outline of the chapter and chapter objectives. These help orient the reader to chapter content and guide the reader to key concepts within each chapter. To reflect the higher level of responsibility in critical care nursing, the level of objectives has been carefully analyzed and raised to reflect critical thinking about chapter content.

Terminology

Readers of this book have had prerequisite courses including anatomy and physiology, nursing process, fundamentals of care, and nursing interventions. Regardless of this assumption, we have tried to define words when they are used and as units develop. Some terminology, when there is more than one term to be defined, is given in the displays within chapters.

References and Bibliographies

A list of current references cited in the chapter is given at the end of each chapter. In addition, the reader is given a bibliography to encourage further reading of key sources relevant to the chapter.

Testing Application

Clinical Applicability Challenges, divided into two sections, appear at the end of every chapter. The first section, *Self-Challenge: Critical Thinking* is intended to stimulate and help readers develop critical thinking skills. Classroom or clinical discussion of these problems can help learners explore alternatives and apply newly learned principles to the care of the critically ill patient. In addition, multiple choice *Study Questions* help readers test their grasp of the chapter content. Answers with rationales to the *Study Questions* appear in the Appendix.

Design and Color

Last but not least, the design and color of a book serve as pedagogical features when used selectively. With that in mind, an attractive design was developed to guide the reader's eyes to important information. A second color has been used carefully. As a result, much new art has been created for this edition.

◼ ANCILLARY PACKAGE

We have developed a special package, called **Instructional Resource Manual**, to accompany the seventh edition of **Critical Care Nursing: A Holistic Approach**. The all-inclusive resource manual will help the instructor with planning, reviewing, and testing and will supplement the student's learning. The resource manual comprises four parts: *Instructor's Manual, Student Review Tear Sheets, Transparency Masters*, and a *disk with test questions*.

The *Instructor's Resource Manual* has a variety of components to help the instructor prepare for effective teaching and application. *The Student Review Tear Sheets*, in a handy form, provide questions normally contained in a student study guide. Presenting this material in the resource manual means the student does not have to purchase a book in addition to the textbook. The instructor can tear out the sheets and copy them for review or testing. About 50 pieces of art, tables, or displays are included in the *Transparency Masters*. They are handy for the instructor who likes to use visual aids in class. NCLEX format is used for about 300 multiple choice test questions in the disk that accompanies the resource guide. By using the disk, instructors can customize and print their own test sheets. The format is easily accessible for any type of computer or software program.

Both instructors and students will benefit from the **Instructional Resource Manual**. This instructional package, complete in one unit, is new to the teaching and learning of critical care nursing. Combined with the additions, consistency of style, and current information in **Critical Care Nursing: A Holistic Approach**, we feel we are offering a package that will help the student establish a knowledge base and apply it clinically.

Carolyn M. Hudak, RN, PhD
Barbara M. Gallo, RN, MS, CNAA
Patricia Gonce Morton, RN, PhD

Contents in Brief

Contents

Additional Recurring Tables and Displays

OTHER RECURRING DISPLAYS

PART

I

*The Concepts
of Holism Applied
to Critical Care
Nursing Practice*

1

Caring and Critical Thinking Within a Holistic Framework

THE CARING FOCUS

CRITICAL THINKING AND THE NURSING PROCESS

A HOLISTIC FRAMEWORK
Physiological Survival and Adaptation

Psychological Adaptation
Social Interaction
Spirituality
Growth and Development
Family Processes
Culture and Ethnicity

RESEARCH-BASED PRACTICE

ADVOCACY

CONCLUSION

OBJECTIVES

Based on the content in this chapter, the reader should be able to:

- Analyze the importance of caring in critical care nursing practice.
- Construct instances of comingling critical thinking and the nursing process in the intensive care environment.
- Examine the concept of adaptation.
- Apply at least three models of nursing care to holism in the intensive care unit.
- Discuss the value of research in relation to critical care nursing.
- Propose opportunities for advocacy within the critical care environment.

Vision of the American Association of Critical-Care Nurses
A health care system driven by the needs of patients in which critical care nurses make their optimal contribution.

*L*ike all aspects of health care, critical care is undergoing rapid changes. The challenges facing the specialty of critical care nursing as the 21st century approaches are probably greater now than ever before. During these times of change, critical care nurses must maintain a focus on their primary mission—providing care to critically ill patients and their families and promoting a patient-driven system of health care.

Critical care nursing requires an ability to deal with crucial situations rapidly and with precision. Until recently, such care was limited to the traditional intensive care setting within a hospital. Critical care nursing, however, is no longer geographically defined. The American Association of Critical-Care Nurses, building on the American Nurses Association (ANA) Social Policy Statement, defines critical care nursing as the "specialty within nursing which deals specifically with human responses to life-threatening illness." This type of nursing care now occurs in acute care hospitals, subacute facilities, extended care facilities, and even in the home.

Historically, the care of the critically ill patient has been the focus of critical care nursing. Although the critically ill patient remains the raison d'être, there is a growing emphasis on caring for the family (and significant others) and fostering their role in helping the patient through the crises. Now family members of the critically ill patient are more likely to participate in the care of their loved one. As the health care system continues to change, family participation in care will evolve.

Today, more than ever, critical care nurses must be lifelong learners whose knowledge base helps them analyze information from multiple perspectives. To provide leadership for the 21st century, the critical care nurse is challenged to be comfortable with chaos and to view change as opportunity. The successful critical care nurse will influence patient care by functioning as a system thinker who is able to analyze situations from an organizational viewpoint rather than a personal perspective. Additionally, critical care nurses must be self-actualized—physically, emotionally, and spiritually strong—to meet the challenges of creating a patient-driven health care system.

Critical care nursing, like life itself, will continue to change and face new demands. Higher patient acuity, rapid technological advances, an increasingly older population, legal and ethical dilemmas, cost containment pressures, changes in care delivery systems, and a focus on outcome analyses are but a few of the challenges confronting critical care nursing. A caring focus, expert critical thinking, and research-based practice within a culturally sensitive, holistic framework are needed to meet these challenges.

■ THE CARING FOCUS

There is little dispute among nursing authorities that caring is the central focus of nursing. Leininger describes a strong link between *curing* (the major focus of medical care) and *caring* by health practitioners. "I hold [that caring] is the central concept and essence of nursing. Moreover, care is a vital factor for human growth, health maintenance, and survival. . . . Human caring and human relationships are closely interrelated. Human caring remains an essential dimension of professional work especially in dealing with life crises, health maintenance problems and changes in health practices."[1]

Watson portrays the "science of caring" as a balance of science and humanism: "Preservation of human care is a critical agenda for nursing and the health care system of today. . . . [N]ursing must achieve a delicate balance between scientific knowledge and humanistic practice behaviors."[2] Watson also addresses the close relationship between curing and caring. "Whereas curative factors aim at curing the patient of disease, carative factors aim at the caring process that helps the person attain (or maintain) health or die a peaceful death."[3] The philosophical foundation for the science of caring is composed of the following:

(1) the formation of a humanistic-altruistic system of values,
(2) the instillation of faith-hope, and
(3) the cultivation of sensitivity of one's self and to others[4]

Jourard vividly describes the nurse–patient relationship, caring, and the influence that they have on patient recovery. According to Jourard, the recovery of the patient depends to a great extent on the understanding that someone cares (Fig. 1–1). Caring by the nurse increases patient comfort, sense of self, and integrity. Lack of caring can actually have detrimental effects on the health and recovery of a patient. Human warmth, love, and responsive care are among the essentials in any recovery. The nurse is the professional who is most likely and able to provide these human aspects of care.[5] The essence of critical care nursing lies in the delicate balance of caring with critical thinking.

■ CRITICAL THINKING AND THE NURSING PROCESS

Critical thinking describes a process that is deliberate, analytical, and logical. It can be considered an umbrella term that includes the scientific process, the nursing process, diagnostic reasoning, and problem solving. The nursing process is a systematic framework for critical thinking in which the nurse seeks information, responds to clinical cues, and identifies and responds to issues affecting the patient's health. Clinical judgments are made after analysis of all available information. These judgments are the basis for formulating nursing diagnoses and statements about clinical problems, wellness, and strengths. Planning involves determining nursing interventions and expected outcomes. Interventions are specific guides, whereas outcomes clearly describe the patient or family behavior that will indicate achievement of goals.

Expected outcomes are used to evaluate the effectiveness of the interventions. The process is not complete until the interventions are effective and the problem is resolved. Reassessment, further planning, intervention, and reevaluation occur until the outcome is met.

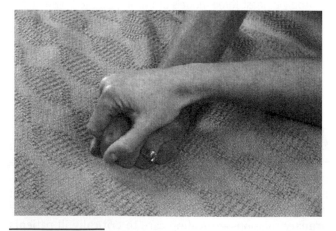

FIGURE 1-1
Touch conveys the message of caring. Sometimes a simple handclasp conveys more meaning than verbal communication. (Photo B. Proud.)

Steps in the Nursing Process

Assessment: Data are collected.
Diagnosis: Data are analyzed to identify health problems, strengths, resources.
Planning: A plan of action is developed that includes measurable outcomes and interventions.
Implementation: The plan is put into action.
Evaluation: The results are evaluated.

A HOLISTIC FRAMEWORK

Human beings cannot be reduced to their parts. Rather, an individual is the combination of his or her physiological, psychological, spiritual, and sociological being. Holism refers to this combination within individuals. Holistic nursing care involves providing nursing care while keeping the totality of the patient in mind. To provide a holistic perspective of care, nurses base their practice on physiological and psychosocial concepts and theories. Critical care nurses must have models for the following:

- Physiological survival and adaptation
- Psychological adaptation
- Social interaction

- Spirituality
- Growth and development
- Family processes
- Culture and ethnicity

These models are necessary for understanding and intervening on behalf of patients and their families.

The patient admitted to an intensive care unit (ICU) needs professional care directed not only at his or her pathophysiological problems, but also at the psychosocial, environmental, and family issues intertwined with the physical illness. Models of human and group behaviors are tools the critical care nurse uses, within the framework of the nursing process, to provide holistic nursing care.

Physiological Survival and Adaptation

The most basic of human needs are physiological, aimed at self-preservation or survival (Fig. 1–2). Fundamental human needs, although closely interrelated, have been arranged in order of dominance by Maslow's hierarchy.

When basic human needs are unmet, human beings seek to preserve their lives by directing all their energies toward those particular needs. For example, all the compensatory mechanisms of a person with inadequate cardiac output work to maintain the circulation of oxygen, thus meeting the most basic requirement for life. In this situation, energy

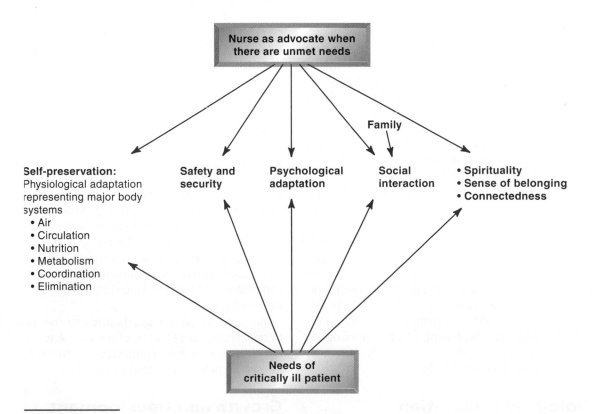

FIGURE 1-2

Basic human needs are aimed at survival. All of the critically ill patient's energies go into meeting these needs. After these needs are met, the patient can concentrate on higher levels of needs. The nurse helps the patient meet all these needs.

is directed away from less critical subsystems (such as gastrointestinal, integumentary, and renal) to help the organism through the physiological crisis. If the crisis is not stabilized, the subsystems eventually move from a compensatory state to a decompensatory state.

Although the need for a sense of security to allay anxiety is always present, it is not the most basic need. Instead, physiological needs, such as maintaining cardiac output, take priority.

A common model of physiological survival is the stress–adaptation framework. In this model, the individual makes immediate responses to stress. Adaptation is the change resulting from the individual's responses.

The patient attempts to cope with the environment in the following ways:

- Avoidance, in which one flees from the situation
- Counteraction, in which body defenses try to destroy the stressor, often at the expense of other systems
- Adaptation, in which one seeks to establish a compatible response to the stress and still retain a steady state

Although each person has physiological and psychological mechanisms that compensate for disequilibrium, there are situations in which the person cannot adapt without outside intervention. During these situations, the critical care nurse becomes the patient's advocate and fosters adaptation.

Nursing interventions are aimed at adaptation. By fostering responses that encourage physiologically and emotionally useful functioning, nurses enhance adaptation and aid the patient in reducing stress and conserving energy. Conversely, when nursing interventions or lack of them do not foster adaptation, the patient's energy is wasted, and a state of increased tension exists; that is, the patient has a diminished capacity to deal with a changing situation. Thus, stress is increased when a patient's energy is devoted to maladaptive functioning that perpetuates the disequilibrium, and stress is minimized when the patient expends energy that fosters adaptation to disequilibrium.

An example of maladaptation versus adaptation is seen when a patient with restrictive lung disease develops a lung infection resulting in increased $PaCO_2$ and decreased PaO_2. This patient cannot compensate because of restrictive lung disease; thus, the established pattern of breathing is maladaptive, perpetuating the problem of gas exchange. Adaptive nursing interventions involve helping the patient breathe more deeply and fostering the drainage of secretion either with breathing exercises or mechanical aids. Although energy is expended, it is spent usefully. By minimizing tension and stress and using adaptive nursing interventions, the patient is restored to a steady state with minimal stress to the rest of the body.

Psychological Adaptation

Psychological adaptation must be maintained along with physiological adaptation to obtain optimal health. An example of psychological adaptation versus maladaptation can be seen in a patient with chronic lung disease who has become ventilator dependent. This patient develops a level of security for ventilation and oxygenation that is often psychological. With ventilator weaning, the patient's anxiety causes tachypnea, greater anxiety, greater tachypnea and shortness of breath, and a vicious cycle begins. Adaptive nursing interventions focus on psychological coping, such as reassurance, presence, and allowing as much self-control as possible. Again, energy is expended, but it is directed at minimizing stress.

Social Interaction

Humans are social by nature—they work together, play together, establish families and households together. Interacting with other in individuals and groups is a necessary part of being human. Social interaction, if meaningful, can help in the recovery of critically ill patients.

Social isolation can be detrimental to well-being in all age groups. It can be particularly detrimental to the physical and psychological development of infants. For example, social isolation occurs when children with congenital heart disease are hospitalized for long periods of their lives. Some *fail to thrive*, while others have difficulty integrating into groups at school. Social isolation also occurs in the neonatal ICU in the form of failure to bond if parents are prohibited from frequent visitation and participation in care. Some studies have also shown the negative effects of social isolation on older individuals.

More studies have demonstrated the benefits of family interaction with patients. Clearly, social interaction with individuals who have meaning to the critically ill patient is therapeutic within the critical care environment. The critical care nurse can facilitate this social interaction and balance the patient's need for interaction with the potential detrimental effect of sensory overload (see Chapter 4).

Spirituality

Although individual beliefs about religion vary, spirituality exists within everyone. Spirituality is the belief that *I as an individual have a purpose in life—I am connected to others, and there is a reason for my existence.* In Maslow's framework, spirituality and "sense of belonging" can be considered synonymous. Spirituality, in many ways, is a compilation of emotions, values, and beliefs into the person we have become.

An understanding of spirituality that may prove helpful to critical care nurses is one of *connectedness*. Each person has a need to remain connected to others. Critical care nurses can help provide that connection.

Growth and Development

Another model well known to critical care nurses is Erikson's model of the developmental stages of psychosocial growth, which proposes eight stages through which individuals move as they age (see display). These stages are relative to chronological age but are not exact. Furthermore, an individual may fail to progress from one developmental step to another or return to a lower level of function when under stress.

Pediatric nurses rely heavily on developmental assessments to ensure that interventions are developmentally appropriate. For example, it is inappropriate to give a piece of a puzzle to a newborn, but it is appropriate to give puzzle pieces to a 6-year-old child because the older child knows something can be done with the puzzle. Although this model is somewhat harder to apply to adult stages, it remains helpful. For example, a middle-aged adult may be struggling with identity or intimacy issues, which can affect his or her motivation to engage actively in self-care. For the older adult, serious illness often prompts introspection and sharing of life achievements. In general, illness that threatens to undermine an earlier developmental achievement can have a profound effect on recovery.

Family Processes

Many perspectives exist in family processes. Many of these processes overlap or dovetail. Some have been adapted, expanded, or reformulated. Some theories and models describe family structure, functions, roles, power, communication, decision making, stress and coping. System models exist that provide a knowledge base for understanding that families have well developed patterns of behavior that they bring to their experience with critical illness. A broad understanding of family models, along with growing data on families experiencing a critical illness, can help critical care nurses give meaningful family care (see Chapter 3).

Culture and Ethnicity

Like other belief systems (spiritual, moral, ethical), cultural beliefs are integral to one's response to health concerns. Therefore, an understanding of cultural beliefs is an important part of nursing care of individuals, families, and groups. The ANA Position Statement on Cultural Diversity in Nursing Practice states, "Culture is one of the organizing concepts upon which nursing is based and defined."

Erikson's Eight Stages of Psychosocial Development

Trust versus mistrust	Infant
Autonomy versus doubt	Toddler
Initiative versus guilt	Preschool
Industry versus inferiority	Schoolage
Identity versus role confusion	Adolescent
Intimacy versus isolation	Young adult
Generativity versus adaptation	Middle adult
Integrity versus despair	Older adult

CLINICAL APPLICATION:
Nursing Intervention Guidelines
Culturally Sensitive Care

- Recognize your own cultural beliefs.
- Be open to different cultural perspectives.
- Learn about and experience the values of your own culture.
- Appreciate the cultural beliefs of others.
- Listen without imposing your own cultural beliefs on others.

Nurses have made great strides in developing knowledge and models for providing care that are sensitive to cultural beliefs and values. Nurses are also exploring cultural variations between and among cultural groups to develop culturally sensitive nursing interventions. Becoming culturally sensitive involves the applications listed in the accompanying display.

RESEARCH-BASED PRACTICE

Florence Nightingale has been credited with being the first nurse researcher. Through questioning, active data collection, and analysis, Nightingale was able to demonstrate the effectiveness of nursing interventions. Since Nightingale's time, the scientific method of inquiry has played an increasingly important role in critical care nursing.

Although nursing research was launched in Nightingale's time, only in the last several decades has significant progress been made in the development of a scientific base to support nursing practice. This progress has resulted in a shift toward research-based practice rather than practice rooted in tradition. A continued commitment to research is necessary so that critical care nurses can make optimal contributions to patient care. The focus of this research should help nurses understand the interaction of biobehavioral phenomena during health and illness. Future research endeavors must generate new knowledge, facilitate nursing decisions, and document the outcomes of nursing care.

All critical care nurses, regardless of their level of educational preparation, can contribute to nursing research. All critical care nurses have a responsibility to read current research literature and to apply the findings to clinical practice. Critical care nurses also can help build the scientific basis for nursing practice by participating in a research project through activities such as data collection. Nurses at the bedside are highly qualified to pose questions about nursing practice and to challenge the status quo, and critical care nurses with advanced degrees can provide leadership in research by serving as consultants and principal investigators for studies.

ADVOCACY

Critically ill patients often cannot cope effectively with all the physiological, psychological, and environmental problems of illness and the ICU (see Fig. 1–2). The nurse must help the patient do what he or she is unable to do alone, thus helping the patient to conserve energy. As an advocate for holistic care of critically ill patients and their families, the nurse contributes to the patient's physiological stability and to the patient's and family's psychological adaptation, effective coping, and spiritual comfort. Acting as a patient advocate means experiencing joy when patients recover and providing comfort when patients do not.

As a patient advocate, the nurse refrains from adding burdens that increase the patient's need to interact when such interaction does not foster adaptation. For example, the nurse will answer a patient's question about nearby equipment, knowing that energy spent in fearful suspense is less helpful than energy used to ask and listen. Likewise, the nurse may encourage the presence of a loved one, knowing that the energy the patient expends in persistently requesting a loved one to be present may not be as helpful as energy spent interacting with that person.

Critical care nurses foster security by decreasing physiological and emotional vulnerability. The feeling of security is lost or diminished whenever there is a decrease in the control of body functions. This can result from a wide range of events, such as fatigue from sleeplessness, difficulty breathing, paralysis, or restraint imposed by tubing or machinery. Regardless of the cause, the nurse intervenes to increase the patient's feeling of safety. This increased feeling of security is accomplished by using technical skill, assessment tools, medication, and interaction; providing assisted breathing with a respirator; encouraging breathing exercises; or staying with the patient during a time of anxiety or loneliness. Recognizing a patient's safety needs is an important element in the holistic approach to patient care. In addition, this consideration of the "whole" patient allows nurses to establish priorities as patient negotiators.

Negotiating for the patient is not without its hazards. Advocacy involves speaking on behalf of the patient, often as a minority voice and in the face of administrative, physician, or peer pressure. This kind of caring requires a great deal of energy on the part of the nurse. Therefore, to maintain emotional reserves, colleagues need to support one another and enhance one another's feelings of belonging and self-esteem.

CONCLUSION

The challenges facing both critical care nursing and health care in general are great. Critical care nurses should accept leadership in defining and refining the practice of critical care nursing. For instance, critical care nursing practice in the future will continue to change. The critical care nurse of the 21st century will continue to need expert critical thinking skills, clinical skills, and clinical leadership abilities. Through research and attention to various models of human behavior, critical care nurses will continue to provide outstanding nursing care to critically ill patients and their families.

Clinical Applicability Challenges

Self-Challenge: Critical Thinking

1. Choose a favorite model from among those discussed in the chapter. Debate its merits and applicability in caring for patients and families experiencing critical illness.

2. Explore the research basis of common critical care nursing interventions.

3. Evaluate the interventions within your critical care practice that promote caring.

REFERENCES

1. Leininger M: Forward. In Watson J (ed): Nursing: The Philosophy and Science of Caring, pp xii–xiii. Boulder, Colorado Associated University Press, 1985
2. Watson J: Nursing: The philosophy of Science of Caring, p xx. Boulder, Colorado Associated University Press, 1985
3. Watson J: Nursing: The philosophy of Science of Caring, p 7. Boulder, Colorado Associated University Press, 1985
4. Watson J: Nursing: The philosophy of Science of Caring, p 9. Boulder, Colorado Associated University Press, 1985
5. Jourard S: The Transparent Self: Self-Disclosure and Well-Being. Princeton, D Van Nostrand, 1964

BIBLIOGRAPHY

American Association of Critical-Care Nurses: The Nurse of the Future. Position Paper. Aliso Viejo, CA, The American Association of Critical-Care Nurses, 1993

Artinian NT: Selecting a model to guide family assessment. Dimensions of Critical Care Nursing 13(1):4, 1994

Fitzpatrick M: Leadership: Wherever patients and families are. Presidential Message at the National Teaching Institute. Anaheim, CA, American Association of Critical Care Nurses, May 1996

Redeker NS: Critical care nursing research: Opportunities and resources. American Journal of Critical Care 3(2):139, 1994

Vitrello J: The future is ours. Presidential Message at the National Teaching Institute. New Orleans, LA, American Association of Critical Care Nurses, May 1995

Zalumas J: Caring in Crisis: An Oral History of Critical Care Nursing. Philadelphia, University of Pennsylvania Press, 1995

2

The Patient's Experience With Critical Illness

PERCEPTION OF CRITICAL ILLNESS

STRESS

RESPONSE TO STRESS
Anxiety
    Causes of Anxiety
    Responses to Anxiety
Patterns of Adaptation

NURSING ASSESSMENT

NURSING INTERVENTIONS
Allowing Control
Transcultural Actions
Presencing and Reassurance
Cognitive Techniques
Guided Imagery and Relaxation Training
Deep Breathing

Music Therapy
Humor

LOSS AND RESPONSES TO LOSS

SPIRITUALITY AND HEALING

THE DYING PATIENT

OBJECTIVES

Based on the content in this chapter, the reader should be able to:

● Explore relationships among stress, response to illness, and anxiety.
● Construct nursing interventions to assist patients in their adaptation to critical illness.
● Compare and contrast techniques that the patient and family can learn in an effort to manage stress and anxiety.
● Describe phases of loss and specific nursing interventions for each phase.
● Develop nursing interventions that foster the ability of patients to draw strength from their personal spirituality.
● Determine personal strengths and weaknesses in dealing with dying patients and their families.

*T*he patient's experience in an intensive care unit (ICU) has lasting meaning for the patient and family members. Although actual painful memories are blurred by drugs and the mind's need to forget, attitudes that are highly charged with feelings about the nature of the experience survive. These attitudes shape the person's beliefs about nurses, physicians, health care, and the vulnerability of life itself.

This chapter describes specific measures that nurses use to support patients and their families through the stress of crisis and adaptation to illness, death, or return to health. An understanding and appreciation of the intricate relationships among mind, body, spirit, and the healing process will help the critical care nurse provide emotional support to the patient and family. It is the caring and emotional support from the nurse that will be remembered and valued. The chapter ends with a discussion of the dying patient.

◼ PERCEPTION OF CRITICAL ILLNESS

Admission to the ICU signals a threat to the life and well-being of all who are admitted. Critical care nurses perceive the unit as a place where fragile lives are vigilantly scrutinized, cared for, and preserved; however, patients and their families frequently perceive admission to critical care as a sign of impending death because of their own or others' experiences. Because of these distinct differences in perception of the meaning of critical care, miscommunication must be anticipated.

STRESS

Stress has been defined as a situation that exists when an organism is faced with any stimulus that causes a disequilibrium between psychological and physiological functioning. All hormone levels can be altered by stress. Extreme levels of stress damage human tissue and may interfere with adaptive response. If adaptive behaviors are effective, energy is freed and may be directed toward healing. If adaptive behaviors fail or are ineffective, however, the tension state is increased, as is the demand for energy. Thus, the original stress of illness looms larger (Fig. 2–1). Hans Selye has written extensively about stress.

RESPONSE TO STRESS

The characteristic problems of adapting to limitations enforced by illness can be understood by exploring the relationship between the physical and the sociopsychological response to the illness. There is an observable lag between the physical onset of illness and its emotional acknowledgment; that is, the patient experiences illness and disability physically before acknowledging them fully on an emotional level. Denial is an example of this lag. Likewise, after physical health has been stabilized, the patient still experiences concerns and fears related to acute illness. At this point, the patient is likely to resist independence and be reluctant to cooperate with increased expectations for activity and self-care. Preparation for return to health, acknowledgment of concerns about increased activity, and the reassurance of watchful eyes will help alleviate anxiety as the patient progresses.

If different patients' responses to illness could be plotted on a graph, they would show both common and unique points, just as electrocardiograms from different people show common characteristics and individual differences. The time and congruence between physical and sociopsychological responses vary, but the stages occur predictably. Like the electrical events of the heart, response to illness, both adaptive and maladaptive, can be anticipated.

The nurse has several responsibilities:

- Anticipate, assess, and monitor the response to illness.
- Recognize and support effective behaviors.
- Minimize and redirect ineffective behaviors.

Anxiety

CAUSES OF ANXIETY

Any stress that threatens one's sense of wholeness, containment, security, and control will cause anxiety. Illness is one such stress. A common cause of anxiety is a sense of isolation. Rarely is one lonelier than when in the midst of a socializing crowd of strangers. In such a situation, people attempt to include themselves, remove themselves, or emotionally distance themselves. The sick person surrounded by active and busy people is in a similar situation but with few resources available to reduce the sense of isolation. Hospital staff who ignore the presence of a patient, regardless of the patient's alertness, contribute to the patient's sense of isolation. Including the patient in conversations about treatment and providing a reassuring touch at frightening moments can reduce this sense of isolation.

Serious illness and the fear of dying also separate the patient from his or her family. The immediate development of

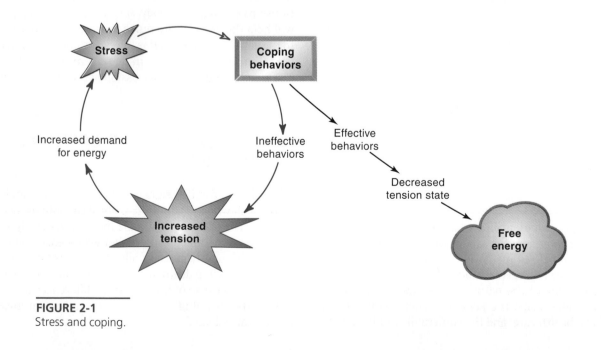

FIGURE 2-1
Stress and coping.

dependent and intimate relationships with strangers is required. The reassuring cliché, "You'll be all right," often meant to comfort, only reinforces the patient's sense of distance. It shuts off expression of fears and questions about what is to come next. The efficiency and activity that surround the patient increase the sense of separateness.

Another category of anxiety-provoking stimuli includes those that threaten the individual's security. Admission to the ICU dramatically confirms for the family and patient that their security on all levels is being severely threatened.

After the patient is admitted to the unit, the initial insecurity undoubtedly concerns life itself. Later, questions regarding such issues as length of hospitalization, return to work, financial implications, well-being of the family, and permanent limitations arise. The patient's insecurity continues and needs to be sensitively considered.

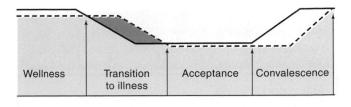

Wellness	Transition to illness	Acceptance	Convalescence

———— Level of physical well being
- - - - Degree of sociopsychological response

FIGURE 2-2
One pattern of responding (adaptation) to stress and illness.

Anxiety occurs when a person experiences the following:

- Threat of helplessness
- Loss of control
- Sense of loss of function and self-esteem
- Failure of former defenses
- Sense of isolation
- Fear of dying

RESPONSES TO ANXIETY

Physiological Responses

The physiological responses of rapid pulse rate, increased blood pressure, increased respirations, dilated pupils, dry mouth, and peripheral vasoconstriction may go undetected in a seemingly cool, calm, self-contained patient. These autonomic responses to anxiety are frequently the most reliable index of the degree of anxiety when behavioral and verbal responses are not congruent with the circumstances.

Sociopsychological Responses

Behavioral responses indicative of anxiety are often family based and culturally learned. They vary from quiet composure in the face of disaster to panic in the presence of an innocuous insect. Such extremes of control and panic use valuable energy. If this energy is not directed toward eliminating or adapting to the stressor, it only perpetuates the discomfort of the tension state. The goal of nursing care is always to promote physiological and emotional equilibrium.

Patterns of Adaptation

Figure 2–2 demonstrates one pattern of adapting to various stages of illness. The shaded area represents transition into illness and shows the disparity between actual health and the person's perception of his or her health. In this situation, there is denial. The acceptance phase demonstrates

that physical and mental well-being are congruent, whereas the convalescent phase shows that an emotional lag exists between physical and emotional well-being.

During stress, the patient regresses in an attempt to conserve energy. During times of acute exacerbation or heightened expectations or during any significant change, the initial response is regression to an earlier emotional position of safety. Weaning from a respirator, removal of monitor leads, increased activity, and reduction in medication often trigger anxiety and regression. This regression may even include a retreat into increased dependency, depression, and anger. At such times, the patient may find comfort in regressing to a state that has already been mastered. Behavior at this time may seem peculiar or irrational to the nurse. The regression is usually temporary and brief and can be used to identify the cause of anxiety. Nurses may become disappointed, anxious, or angry with the patient's regression and may want to retreat. It is more helpful, however, to acknowledge that regression is inevitable and to support the patient with intervention appropriate to earlier stages. The nurse helps the patient understand what is happening by explaining the emotional lag phenomenon.

▰▰▰ NURSING ASSESSMENT

Often it is not possible for the nurse simply to remove the stimulus that causes anxiety. In these circumstances, the nurse must assess the effectiveness of the patient's behaviors and either support them, help the patient modify them, or teach new behaviors. Frequently, levels of anxiety are so high that the anxious state becomes the stimulus that demands additional coping responses.

After assessing coping behaviors for effectiveness, the nurse has several choices:

- Support the behaviors.
- Help the patient modify behaviors.
- Teach new behavior.

Coping behaviors may be directed either toward eliminating the stress of illness or toward eliminating the anxiety state itself. The nurse must evaluate each behavior as to whether it helps restore a steady state. Behaviors that promote movement toward a steady state can then be supported and encouraged. The nurse may also need to help the patient modify or find substitutes for behaviors that are disruptive or threatening to homeostasis. At times, the nurse must introduce new behaviors to facilitate equilibrium and promote health.

NURSING INTERVENTIONS

Whenever possible, stress must be reduced or eliminated for critically ill patients. If this can be accomplished, the problem is quickly resolved, and the patient is returned to a state of equilibrium. Usually, however, the stress is not eliminated so easily, because many other stressors are introduced by attempts to remedy the original problem. If adaptive behaviors are effective, anxiety is reduced, and energy is directed toward rest and healing. A number of nursing interventions may be used to reduce anxiety and promote adaptation in critically ill patients. Often a combination of interventions is used.

Allowing Control

Nursing measures that reinforce a sense of control help increase the patient's autonomy and reduce the overpowering sense of loss of control. Providing order and predictability allows the patient to anticipate and prepare for what is to follow. Perhaps it creates only a mirage of control, but anticipatory guidance keeps the patient from being caught off-guard and allows the mustering of coping mechanisms.

Allowing small choices when the patient is willing and ready increases the patient's feeling of control over the environment. Would the patient prefer to lie on his or her right or left side? In which arm should the IV be placed? What height is preferred for the head of the bed? Does the patient want to cough now or in 20 minutes after pain med-

ication? Any decisions that afford the patient a certain amount of control and predictability are important. These small choices also may help the patient accept lack of control during procedures that involve little choice.

Transcultural Actions

Interventions for individual patients must be contextually based and culturally sensitive. Transcultural nursing refers to a formal area of study and practice that focuses on providing care that is compatible with individuals' cultural beliefs, values, and lifestyles. A cultural assessment will include the patient's usual response to illness, cultural norms, beliefs, and world views. Because individual responses and values may vary within the same culture, the patient should be recognized as an *individual* within the cultural context. Exploring the meaning of the critical event with the patient, family members, and significant others may give clues to the patient's perception of what is happening. Additionally, the nurse may ask if there is a particular ethnic or religious group with which the patient identifies and if there is anything the nurses may do to provide care that is sensitive to individual values or norms while the patient is hospitalized.

Presencing and Reassurance

Presence, or just "being there," can in itself be a meaningful strategy for the critically ill patient experiencing distress or anxiety. Presencing is the therapeutic use of self, adopting a caring attitude, and paying attention to one's needs. Reassurance can be provided to the patient in the form of presencing and touch. Reassurance can also be verbal. Verbal reassurance can be effective for patients if it provides realistic encouragement or clarifies misconceptions. Verbal reassurance is not valuable, however, if it prevents a patient from expressing his or her emotions or stifles the need for further dialogue. Reassurance is intended to reduce fear and anxiety and evoke a calmer, more passive response. It is best directed at patients expressing unrealistic or exaggerated fears.

Cognitive Techniques

Techniques that have evolved from cognitive theories of learning may help anxious patients and their families. They can be initiated by the patient and do not depend on complex insight or understanding of one's own psychological makeup. They can also be used to reduce anxiety in a way that avoids probing into the patient's personal life. Furthermore, the patient's friends and family members can be taught these techniques to help them and the patient reduce tension.

Internal Dialogue

Highly anxious people are most likely giving themselves messages that increase or perpetuate their anxiety. These messages are conveyed in one's continuously running "self-talk," or internal dialogue. The patient in the ICU may be silently saying things such as, "I can't stand it in here. I've got to get out." Another unexpressed thought might be, "I can't handle this pain." By asking the patient to share aloud what is going on in this internal dialogue, the nurse can bring to awareness the messages that are distracting the patient from rest and relaxation. Substitute messages should be suggested to the patient. It is important to ask the patient to substitute rather than delete messages because the internal dialogue is continuously operating and will not turn off, even if the patient wills it to do so. Therefore, asking the patient to substitute constructive, reassuring comments is more likely to help the patient significantly reduce the tension level. Comments such as, "I'll handle this pain just one minute at a time" or "I've been in tough spots before, and I am capable of making it through this one!" will automatically reduce anxiety and help the patient shape coping behaviors accordingly. Any message that enhances the patient's confidence, sense of control, and hope and that puts him or her in a positive, active role, rather than the passive role of victim, will increase the patient's sense of coping and well-being.

The nurse helps the patient develop self-dialogue messages that increase:

- Confidence
- Sense of control
- Ability to cope
- Optimism
- Hope

External Dialogue

A similar method can be applied to the patient's external conversation with other people. By simply requiring patients to speak accurately about themselves to others, the same goals can be accomplished. For example, patients who exclaim, "I can't do anything for myself!" should be asked to identify the things that they are able to do, such as lifting their own bodies, turning to one side, making a nurse feel good with a rewarding smile, or helping the family understand what is happening. Even the smallest movement in the weakest of patients should be acknowledged and claimed by the patient. This technique is useful in helping patients correct their own misconceptions of themselves

and the way others see them. This reduces patients' sense of helplessness and therefore their anxiety.

Cognitive Reappraisal

This technique asks the patient to identify a particular stressor and then modify his or her response to that stressor. In other words, the patient reframes his or her perception of the stressor in a more positive light so that the stimulus is no longer viewed as threatening. The patient is given permission to take personal control of responses to the stimulus. This technique may be combined with guided imagery and relaxation training.

Guided Imagery and Relaxation Training

These are two useful techniques that can be taught to the patient to help reduce tension. The nurse can encourage the patient to imagine either being in a very pleasant place or taking part in a very pleasant experience. The patient should be instructed to focus and linger on the sensations that are experienced. For example, asking the patient, "What colors do you see?" "What sounds are present?" "How does the air smell?" "How does your skin feel?" "Is there a breeze in the air?" helps increase the intensity of the fantasy and thereby promote relaxation through mental escape.

Guided imagery also can be used to help reduce unpleasant feelings of depression, anxiety, and hostility. Patients who must relearn life-sustaining tasks, such as walking and feeding themselves, can use imagery to prepare mentally to meet the challenge successfully. In these instances, patients should be taught to visualize themselves moving through the task and successfully completing it. If this method seems trivial or silly to the patients, they can be reminded that this method demands concentration and skill and is commonly used by athletes to improve their performance and to prepare themselves mentally before an important event.

The nurse can also use techniques that induce deep muscle relaxation to help the patient decrease anxiety. Deep muscle relaxation may reduce or eliminate the use of tranquilizing and sedating drugs. In *progressive relaxation*, the patient is first directed to find as comfortable a position as possible and then to take several deep breaths and let them out slowly. Next, the patient is asked to clench a fist or curl toes as tightly as possible, to hold the position for a few seconds, then to let go while focusing on the sensations of the releasing muscles. The patient should practice this technique, beginning with the toes and moving upward through other parts of the body—the feet, calves, thighs, abdomen, chest, and so on. This procedure is done slowly while the patient gives nonverbal signals (eg, lifting a finger) to indicate when each new muscle mass has reached a state of relaxation. Extra time and attention should be given to the back, shoulders, neck, scalp, and forehead, because many people experience physical tension in these areas.

Once a state of relaxation is achieved, the nurse can suggest that the patient fantasize or sleep as deeply as the patient chooses. The patient must be allowed to select and control the depth of relaxation and sleep, especially if the fear of death is prominent in the patient's mind. A moderately dark room and a soft voice will facilitate relaxation. Asking the patient to relax is frequently nonproductive compared with directing him to release a muscle mass actively, let go of tension, or imagine tension draining through the body and sinking deeply into the mattress. Again the patient is assisted to an active rather than passive role by the nurse's careful use of language.

Deep Breathing

When acutely anxious, the patient's breathing patterns may change, and the patient may hold his or her breath. This could be physically and psychologically detrimental. Teaching diaphragmatic breathing, also called abdominal breathing, to the patient may be useful as both a distraction and a coping mechanism. Diaphragmatic breathing can be taught easily and quickly in the preoperative patient or to a patient experiencing acute fear or anxiety. The patient may be asked to place a hand on the abdomen, inhale deeply through the nose, hold for a brief moment, and exhale through pursed lips. The goal is to have the patient push out his own hand to demonstrate the deep breath. The nurse may demonstrate the technique and perform it along with the patient, until the patient is comfortable with the technique and is in control. The mechanically ventilated patient may be able to modify this technique by concentrating on breathing and concentrate on pushing out the hand. Mechanically ventilated patients experiencing severe agitation may not be able to respond to this technique.

Music Therapy

Many nursing studies have demonstrated the use of music in the ICU to provide distraction and promote relaxation.[1] The patient is provided with a choice of specially recorded audiotapes and a set of headphones. Usually music sessions are 20 to 90 minutes long, once or twice daily. Music selections may vary by individual taste, but the most commonly used selections have a tempo of 60 to 70 beats; a simple, direct musical rhythm; and a low-pitched sound with primarily a string composition. Most patients prefer music that is familiar to them.[1]

Humor

A good *belly laugh* produces positive and psychological effects. Laughter can increase the level of endorphins, the body's natural pain killers, that are released into the bloodstream. Laughter can relieve tension and anxiety and relax muscles. The use of humor by nurses in critical care can help reduce procedural anxiety or provide distraction. Once again, the humor must be compatible with the context in which it is offered and with the individual's cultural perspective. Many nurses report using humor cautiously after they have established a rapport with the individual. Nurses also report that they are able to take cues from the patient and visitors regarding the appropriate use of humor. Patients have reported that nurses who have a good sense of humor are more approachable and easier to talk with. In an effort to incorporate the positive effects of humor into health care settings, some institutions have developed humor resource rooms or mobile humor carts. These provide patients with a variety of lighthearted reading materials, videotapes, and audiotapes. Also included on the cart may be games, puzzles, and magic tricks. Some nurses have created their own portable therapeutic humor kits. Use of humor by patients may help them reframe their anxiety and channel their energy toward feeling better.

■ LOSS AND RESPONSES TO LOSS

The threat of illness precipitates coping behaviors associated with loss. Patients must adjust to the loss of health or loss of a limb, a blow to self-concept, or a necessary change in lifestyle. Dying patients must adapt to the loss of life. All these events require a change—a loss of the familiar self-image and its replacement with an altered one. All losses include at least a temporary phase of lowered self-esteem. Regardless of the nature of the loss, the dynamics of grief present themselves in some form. The response to loss can be described in the following four phases: shock and disbelief, development of awareness, restitution, and resolution.

Each phase involves characteristic and predictable behaviors that fluctuate among the various phases in an unpredictable way. Through recognition and assessment of the behaviors and an understanding of their underlying dynamics, the nurse can plan interventions to support the healing process.

Shock and Disbelief

In the first stage of response to loss, patients demonstrate behaviors characteristic of denial. They fail to comprehend and experience the rational meaning and emotional impact of the diagnosis. Because the diagnosis has no emotional meaning, patients often fail to cooperate with precautionary measures. For example, patients may attempt to get out of bed against the physician's advice, or they may deviate from the prescribed diet and assert, "I am here for a rest!" Denial may go so far as to allow patients to project difficulties onto what is perceived as ill-functioning equipment, mistaken laboratory reports, or—more likely—the sheer incompetence of physicians and nurses.

When such blatant denial occurs, it is apparent that the problem is so anxiety provoking to the patient that it cannot be handled by the more sophisticated mental mechanisms of rational problem solving. The stressor is temporarily obliterated. This phase of denial may be the period during which the patient's resources, briefly blocked by the shock, can be regrouped for the battle ahead. Therefore, stripping away denial may render the patient helpless. Furthermore, although denial has its obvious hazards, it has been associated with higher rates of survival after myocardial infarctions.

NURSING INTERVENTIONS

The principle of intervention consists not of stripping away the defense of denial but of supporting the patient and acknowledging the situation through nursing care.

The nurse recognizes and accepts the patient's illness by watching the monitor or changing the dressings. In these ways, the nurse communicates acceptance of the patient through tone of voice, facial expression, and touch. The nurse must be able to reflect statements of denial back to the patient in a way that allows the patient to hear them—and eventually to examine their incongruity and apply reality—for example, by saying something such as, "In some ways you believe that having a heart attack will be helpful to you?" The nurse can also acknowledge the patient's difficulty in accepting restrictions by making comments such as, "It seems hard for you to stay in bed." By verbalizing what the patient is expressing, the nurse gently confronts behavior but does not cause anxiety and anger by reprimanding and judging. In this phase, the nurse supports denial by allowing for it but does not perpetuate it. Instead, the nurse acknowledges, accepts, and reflects the patient's new circumstance.

When the patient is in denial, the nurse demonstrates acceptance in several ways:

- Tone of voice
- Congruent facial expression
- Use of touch
- Use of reflection of inaccurate statements
- Avoiding joking with patient about serious issues

Development of Awareness

In this second stage of grief, the patient's behavior is characteristically associated with anger and guilt. The anger may be expressed overtly and may be directed at the staff for oversights, tardiness, and minor insensitivities. In this phase, the ugliness of reality has made its impact. Displacement of the anger onto others helps soften the impact of reality on the patient. The expression of anger gives the patient a sense of power in a seemingly helpless state. A demanding manner and a whining tone often characterize this stage and represent the patient's primitive attempts to regain the control that appears to have been lost. However, such behavior often alienates the nurse and other personnel. The patient who does not demand or whine has probably withdrawn into depression because of anger directed toward self rather than toward others. This patient will demonstrate verbal and motor retardation, will likely have difficulty sleeping, and may prefer to be left alone.

During this phase, the nurse is likely to hear irrational expressions of guilt. Patients seek to answer the question, "Why me?" They attempt to isolate their human imperfections and attribute the cause of the malady to themselves or their past behavior. Patients and their families may look for a person or object to blame.

Guilt feelings concerning one's own illness are difficult to understand unless one examines the basic dynamic of guilt. Guilt arises when there is a decrease in the feeling of self-worth or when the self-concept has been violated. In this light, the nurse can understand that what is behind an expression of guilt is a negatively altered self-concept. Blame thus becomes nothing more than projection of the unbearable feeling of guilt.

NURSING INTERVENTIONS

During the patient's development of awareness, nursing intervention must be directed toward supporting the patient's basic sense of self-worth and allowing and encouraging the direct expression of anger. Nursing measures that support a patient's sense of self-worth are numerous and include calling the patient by name; introducing strangers, particularly if they are to examine the patient; talking to, rather than about, the patient; and, most important, providing and respecting the patient's need for privacy and modesty. The nurse needs to guard against verbal and nonverbal expressions of pity. It is more constructive and productive to empathize with the patient's specific and temporary feelings of anger, sadness, and guilt rather than with a condition.

The nurse can create outlets for anger by listening and by *refraining from defending* the physician, the hospital, or his or her own actions. A nondefensive, accepting attitude will decrease the patient's sense of guilt, and the expression of anger will avert some of the depression. Later, when the patient apologizes for an irrational outburst, the nurse can interpret the patient's need to make this kind of verbalization as a necessary step toward rehabilitation and health.

Restitution

In this stage, the griever puts aside anger and resistance and begins to cope constructively with the loss. The patient tries new behaviors that are consistent with the new limitations. The emotional level is one of sadness, and time spent crying is useful. As the patient adapts to a new image, considerable time is spent going over significant memories relevant to the loss. Behaviors in this stage include the verbalization of fears regarding the future. Often these go unexpressed and undetected because they are unbearable for the family to hear. Furthermore, after severe trauma, which may have resulted in scarring or removal of a body part or loss of sensation, patients may question their sexual adequacy. They worry about the future response of their mates to their changed bodies. The patient probably also questions a new role in the family. Most likely, the patient has a variety of concerns that are specific to his or her lifestyle. Thus, in the mourning process, such manifestations as reminiscing, crying, questioning, expressing fears, and trying out new behaviors help the patient modify the old self-concept and begin working with and experiencing a revised concept.

NURSING INTERVENTIONS

During restitution, nursing care should again be supportive so that adaptation can occur. Listening to the patient for lengthy periods of time is necessary. If the patient is able to verbalize fears and questions about the future, he or she will be better able to define the anxiety and solve new problems. Furthermore, hearing oneself talk about fears helps put them into a more rational perspective. The patient may require privacy, acceptance, and encouragement to cry so that respite from sadness can be found.

During this stage, the nurse may have the patient consider meeting someone who has successfully adapted to similar trauma. This measure provides the patient with a role model as a new identity is assumed, which often occurs after the crisis period. Many support groups of recovering people with all types of illnesses and injuries will send someone to support and be a role model for patients and families.

The patient, with appropriate support from the nurse, begins to identify and acknowledge changes arising from adaptation to illness. Relationships can and do change. Friends may respond differently to the patient who has suffered a permanent disability, causing the patient to believe that the attitudes and feelings of others have changed as a result of the injury or illness.

During this time, the family has also been going through a similar process. They too have experienced shock, disbelief, anger, and sadness. After they are ready to try to solve their problems, their energies are directed toward wondering how the changes in the patient will affect their mutual relationship and their lifestyle. They too experience the pain of turmoil and uncertainty. Nurses must also help the family. By allowing the family to ventilate their repulsion and fear and by showing acceptance of these feelings, the nurse can help the family be more useful to, and accepting of, the patient. Through intensive listening, the nurse provides a sounding board and then redirects the members of the family back to each other so that they can give and receive each other's support. Asserting the normality of untoward feelings also assists with future acceptance, while decreasing guilt and blame.

Resolution

Resolution is the stage of identity change. At first patients may *over*identify themselves as invalids. They may discriminate against their bodies. Another method patients may use is to detach themselves emotionally from the source of trauma (eg, a stoma, prosthesis, scar, or paralyzed limb) by naming it and referring to it in a simultaneously alienated and affectionate way. Patients are sensitive to the ways in

which health care workers respond to their bodies. A patient may make negative remarks to test the acceptance of the nurse. Chiding or telling the patient that many others share the problem will be less helpful than acknowledging feelings and indicating acceptance by continuing to care for, and talk with, the patient.

As time passes and the patient adapts, the sting of the endured hurt abates, and the patient moves toward an identification as a person who has certain limitations due to illness rather than as a "cripple" or an "invalid." The patient no longer uses a defect as the basis of identity. As the resolution is reached, patients are able to depend on others if necessary and should not need to push beyond their endurance or to overcompensate for an inadequacy or limitation. Often, the patient reflects on the crisis as a time of growth or maturation. Such a patient achieves a sense of pride at accomplishing the difficult adaptation and is able to look back realistically on successes and disappointments without discomfort. At this time, the patient may find it useful and gratifying to help others by serving as a role model for people in the stage of restitution who are experiencing their own identity crises.

Unfortunately, the critical care nurse is rarely in a position to observe the successful outcome of resolution. It is useful to know the process in order to work with and communicate an attitude of hope, especially when the patient is most self-disparaging.

NURSING INTERVENTIONS

The goal of nursing care during the resolution stage is to help the patient attach a sense of self-esteem to a rectified identity. Nursing intervention centers on helping the patient find the degree of dependence that is needed and can be accepted. The nurse must accept and recognize with the patient that periods of vacillation between independence and dependence will occur. The nurse should encourage a positive emotional response to a new state of modified dependence. Certainly, the nurse can support and reinforce the patient's growing sense of pride in rehabilitation. For nurses who have had the experience of successfully working through the process with one person, the problem is to stand back and allow the patient to move away from them.

See the accompanying Nursing Plan of Care for the Patient Experiencing Grief and Loss.

■ SPIRITUALITY AND HEALING

Caring in nursing includes recognition and support of the spiritual nature of human beings. Spirituality refers to the realm of invisible and intangible factors that influences our thoughts and behaviors. This recognition includes not only religious beliefs, but goes beyond. When people sense power and influence outside of time and physical existence, they

NURSING PLAN OF CARE
The Patient Experiencing Grief and Loss

James Saunders, age 41, was admitted to the intensive care unit conscious but unresponsive to verbal questioning. According to the accident report, a large truck had swerved out of control on an icy road, killing Mr. Saunders' fiancée and injuring him. He had been hospitalized for observation and treatment of chest wounds and blood loss. Mr. Saunders' leg was amputated above the left knee as a result of an injury incurred in Vietnam 25 years ago.

While trying to reach Mr. Saunders' family, the nurse learned that his mother had died of cancer about 1 year ago and that 3 months later his father, suffering from depression, had killed himself. He had one sister who was flying to see him.

The primary nursing problems were maintenance of ventilation and vital signs, pain control, and immobility. Mr. Saunders remained uncommunicative, although he was tearful. When he did talk, he expressed hopelessness and said he wanted to die. He asked, "Why me, God? What have I done to deserve this?"

The following plan of care focuses on nursing diagnoses related to Mr. Saunders' psychosocial problems.

Nursing Diagnosis and Outcome Criteria	Nursing Interventions
Grieving: related to the death of his fiancée, loss of parents in past years, and possibly the earlier loss of his leg. Patient will: • Verbally and nonverbally express his grief. • Describe meaning these losses have for him. • Share grief with another person with whom he is close.	1. Ask patient about his feelings. 2. Listen, reflect, and sit quietly with patient. 3. Acknowledge patient's reaction as a normal, expected response to multiple and severe loss. 4. Acknowledge own feelings to self regarding loss and identify separateness from patient in order not to over-identify with patient and lose objectivity. 5. Enlist other staff to act as resources for nurse and patient. 6. Assess stage of grief related to death of parents, loss of leg, and Vietnam experience. 7. Assess patient's stage of grief in relationship to ability to make sound decisions (ie, postdischarge psychiatric follow-up). 8. Support denial, as needed to let patient move at own pace in perceiving degrees of loss. 9. Consult psychosocial liaison nurse and spiritual counselor to assist in coping and facilitating appropriate grieving. 10. Avoid the temptation to reduce pain with false reassurance. 11. Acknowledge depth and breadth of loss. 12. Offer hope by letting patient know that time will ease the degree of pain. 13. Acknowledge that the patient has already demonstrated enormous personal strength by surviving the accident and his other losses. 14. Provide hope that he will recover by talking about the future. 15. Provide positive reinforcement for crying and grieving behaviors. ("Don't apologize for your tears; it's very important that you cry as much as you need to express your grief.") 16. Reframe the catastrophic event from a tragedy to the challenge of a lifetime.
Powerlessness: related to losses, physical injuries, and incapacitation. Patient will: • Demonstrate a sense of control over his own life by making sound decisions.	1. Allow patient as many choices as possible. Acknowledge soundness of choices. 2. Question poor choices in a sensitive way (eg, "You believe that giving up will somehow help you feel better about what has happened?")

NURSING PLAN OF CARE
The Patient Experiencing Grief and Loss (*Continued*)

Nursing Diagnosis and Outcome Criteria	Nursing Interventions
• Experience a decrease in feelings of guilt regarding the collision.	1. Allow expression of irrational thoughts (eg, "I must have done something very very bad to deserve this."). 2. Reflect back statements emphasizing faulty logic (eg, "You believe if you had been a better person, you could have controlled someone else's driving and the weather?"). 3. Teach patient about the stages of grieving and emphasize its necessity for health. 4. Refer patient for mental health follow-up care and support.
Spiritual Distress: related to questions such as "Why me, God?" secondary to death of fiancée and possibly other losses. Patient will: • Share spiritual belief system with nurse. • Reenlist former spiritual sources of empowerment (eg, prayer, rosary, icons, etc.). • Decrease expressions of hopelessness and the wish to die.	1. Ask patient to share religious/spiritual beliefs. 2. Contact appropriate religious or spiritual teacher (eg, priest, chaplain, etc.). 3. Ask patient to share other instances of spiritual distress and their outcomes. 4. Place meaningful spiritual/religious items near patient. 5. Use readings of scripture, verse, or stories with patient as he desires. Perhaps engage a friend or family member in this activity. 6. Assess patient for suicide ideation and impulse control. Observe frequently.

are said to be experiencing the metaphysical aspects of spirituality.

Spirituality includes one's system of beliefs and values. Intuition and knowledge from unknown sources and origins of unconditional love and belonging typically are viewed as spiritual power. A sense of universal connection, personal empowerment, and reverence for life also pertains to the existence of spirituality. These elements also may be viewed as benefits of spirituality.

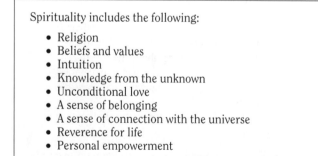

Spirituality includes the following:

- Religion
- Beliefs and values
- Intuition
- Knowledge from the unknown
- Unconditional love
- A sense of belonging
- A sense of connection with the universe
- Reverence for life
- Personal empowerment

Critical care patients and their families frequently pray for miraculous healing. Miracles of healing, when they are experienced by believers, can be viewed as normal healing events occurring in collapsed time. Nursing goals related to spirituality include the recognition and promotion of patients' spiritual sources of strength. By allowing and supporting patients to share their beliefs about the universe

without disagreement, nurses help patients recognize and draw on their own sources of spiritual courage. Recognition of the unique spiritual nature of each patient is thought to assist personal empowerment and healing.

Nurses who find their own spiritual values in religion must acknowledge and respect that nonreligious people may also be spiritual and experience spirituality as a life force. Regardless of personal views, the nurse is obligated to assess patients' spiritual belief systems and assist them to recognize and draw on the values and beliefs already in existence for them.

Furthermore, critical illness may deepen or challenge existing spirituality. During these times, it may be useful for the nurse or family to call on a spiritual or religious leader, hospital chaplain, or a pastoral care representative to help the patient make meaningful use of the critical illness experience.

THE DYING PATIENT

COMPASSION

For the most part, the goals of the critical care nurse are to preserve life and facilitate healing. That is why many nurses experience a sense of disappointment and failure when a patient dies. This is in contrast to nurses who experience sadness when their patients die. Other nurses and colleagues may interpret the signs of compassion and healthy involvement as indications of overinvolvement, but a nurse whose eyes become filled with tears at a sensitive moment conveys a sense of empathy to patients. The major goal for many nurses is to learn to *demonstrate comfortably* the concern and compassion that are already an integral part of their emotional makeup.

COMFORT

The aggressive pursuit of comfort is the primary nursing goal for the dying patient. This is especially important when a decision has been made to discontinue treatments, and the goal changes from curing to supporting and comforting.

Pain relief is an important part of providing comfort for many critical care patients. The nurses must communicate closely with the patient and the physician to create a regimen in which the patient's integrity and peace of mind are not reduced by pain or the need to beg for medication. If a patient is in continuous pain, it is more appropriate to give medication on a predetermined schedule (eg, q3h) rather than as needed (eg, PRN). Furthermore, few patients who are given narcotics for pain develop a serious problem of addiction. In the terminally ill patient, concern for comfort supercedes concern for the problems of addiction. Knowing the patient's concern and desires about the pain experience is of utmost importance. For example, some patients elect not to trade alertness for pain reduction. Many nurses want to medicate these patients because working with people in excruciating pain is trying and frustrating. It also increases the nurse's feelings of helplessness and, therefore, the nurse's anxiety.

In addition, nurses should be made aware that staff attitudes appear to have much to do with the ordering and giving of analgesic medication. In general, young female patients tend to receive more powerful analgesics than others. Age, rather than physical condition, degree of pain, or other variables, may be the determining factor relating to nurses' implementation of PRN medication orders for patients with pain. This phenomenon points out that nurses must be careful to assess the patient's need and capacity for pain medication and separate this assessment from other irrelevant factors. See Chapter 5 for a more detailed discussion on pain and the critically ill patient.

Finally, *every possible comfort measure* that can be used without greatly increasing discomfort should automatically be taken. Mouth care can be easily overlooked in a patient who is not eating. Dryness, drooling, odor, and poor nutrition may cause pain and discomfort. The family can be involved in applying lip balm to the patient's lips and washing saliva from the skin. Positioning, skin care, and massage are all useful measures in promoting comfort. Some family members may choose to participate in this type of care, whereas others may be uncomfortable or fear that they will hurt the patient. Usually, the family's participation means more work for the nurse; however, this participation in care can be a highly significant and useful experience for the grieving family.

Promoting comfort for the dying patient requires constant and judicious decision making. Should a febrile patient be covered when cold? Should someone with depressed respirations be sedated when restless and anxious? Comfort measures that break the usual protocol of the ICU may be required. Honest and direct communication with the patient and family helps guide the actions of nurses and physicians on complicated matters.

COMMUNICATION

Listening well is the cornerstone of effective communication. Some patients do not want to talk about dying; to do so strips them of whatever hope they are holding. Others deal with death in a symbolic way. They speak of autumns and winters and other subjects that symbolize endings. This is an effective way of terminating one's life; no interpretation is necessary, and to do so would be inappropriate.

Communication is also expressed by the nurse's cheerfulness. Empathy and concern do not need to be expressed in a discouraged manner. Even dying people want to be cared for by a pleasant nurse. A good joke can also be appreciated by a dying patient. Sensitivity to the patient's mood and a sense of timing are useful in assessing a patient's receptivity to lightheartedness.

Clinical Applicability Challenges

Self-Challenge: Critical Thinking

1. *You are the nurse caring for a patient who is scheduled for a cardiac catheterization in the morning. In report, you are told the patient has been "acting out all day—crying and very emotional." Explore the possible meaning behind the patient's behavior. Formulate an action plan, including additional data that may be needed.*

2. *You observe an elderly, African-American female patient clutching her Bible to her chest with her eyes tightly shut. She is moving her lips as if in animated prayer. Formulate a nursing plan to provide spiritual support for this patient.*

Study Questions

1. *Anxiety occurs when patients*
   a. *are occupied with internal dialogue.*
   b. *are overly dependent on the nurse.*
   c. *have a long-term recovery ahead.*
   d. *perceive a threat to their well-being.*

2. *The best way to help patients handle anxiety is to*
   a. *reassure them that they will receive the best possible care.*
   b. *assist then to talk about their fears and concerns.*
   c. *be direct and honest with them.*
   d. *limit visitors' time with them.*

3. *The nurse can help provide a sense of control in patients by*
   a. *providing order and predictability.*
   b. *offering as many choices as possible.*
   c. *including them in decision making.*
   d. *All of the above*

4. Cognitive reappraisal is a technique that allows the patient to
   a. identify the stressor and alter the response to it.
   b. ignore a threatening stimulus.
   c. use guided imagery and progressive muscle relaxation.
   d. All of the above

5. A positive effect of laughter is
   a. a psychological sense of well-being.
   b. muscle relaxation.
   c. reduced tension.
   d. All of the above

6. Reassurance will not be valuable for the patient if it
   a. calms excessive fears.
   b. ceases expression of emotions.
   c. decreases respiratory rate.
   d. is combined with presencing.

7. Denial is a response that
   a. is viewed as normal in the early phase of grieving.
   b. helps the patient gather emotional resources to deal with problems ahead.
   c. is a defense that should not be stripped away by the nurse.
   d. All of the above

REFERENCES

1. Henry LL: Music therapy: A nursing intervention for the control of pain and anxiety in the ICU: A review of the research literature. Dimensions of Critical Care Nursing 14(6):295–304, 1995

BIBLIOGRAPHY

Abdullah SN: Towards an individualized client's care: Implication for education. The transcultural approach. J Adv Nurs 22:715–720, 1995

Ackerman MH, Henry MB, Graham KM: Humor won, humor too: A model to incorporate humor into the healthcare setting (revised). Nurs Forum 22(2):15–21, 1994

Astedt-Kurki P, Liukkonen A: Humour in nursing care. J Adv Nurs 20:183–188, 1994

Barnum BS: Spirituality in nursing: Everything old is new again. Nurs Leadersh Forum 1(1):24–30, 1995

Chopra D: Ageless Body, Timeless Mind: The Quantum Alternative to Growing Old. New York, Harmony Books, 1993

Clark C, Heidenreich T: Spiritual care for the critically ill. Am J Crit Care 4(1):77–81, 1995

DeSantis L: Making anthropology clinically relevant to nursing care. J Adv Nurs 20:707–715, 1994

Dossey L: Healing Words: The Power of Prayer and Practice of Medicine. San Francisco, Harper, 1993

Gillman J, Gable-Rodriguez J: Pastoral care in a critical care setting. Crit Care Nurs Q 19(1):10–20, 1996

John SD: Assess carefully before intervening. J Christ Nurs 11(4):6–8, 1994

Lehrer PM, Woolfork RL: Principles and Practice of Stress Management (2nd Ed). New York, Guilford Press, 1993

Mendyka BE: The therapeutic syncretic process: Implications for nursing care delivery. AACN Clin Issues Crit Care Nurs 5(1):86–91, 1994

Mynchenberg TL, Dungan JM: A relaxation protocol to reduce patient anxiety. Dimensions of Critical Care Nursing 14(2):78–85, 1995

Rajan MFJ: Transcultural nursing: A perspective derived from Jean-Paul Sartre. J Adv Nurs 22:450–455, 1995

Shaldham CM, Cunningham G, Hiscock M, Luscombe P: Assessment of anxiety in hospital patients. J Adv Nurs 22:87–93, 1995

Steinbaum E: Acting on faith. Arthritis Today March-April:35–39, 1996

Teasdale K: The nurse's role in anxiety management. Prof Nurse 10(8):509–512, 1995

Teasdale K: Theoretical and practical considerations on the use of reassurance in the nursing management of anxious patients. J Adv Nurs 22:79–86, 1995

3

The Family's Experience With Critical Illness

OBJECTIVES

Based on the content in this chapter, the reader should be able to:

- Discuss cultural factors that may affect the family's critical care experience.
- Describe the characteristics of a crisis event.
- Explore variables that determine the meaning of crisis events for patients and family members.
- Describe nursing behaviors that help families cope with crises.
- Formulate an individualized visitation plan to meet the family's need for proximity to the patient.
- Identify nursing goals and behaviors associated with caring for dying patients and their families.

A holistic approach to critical care nursing includes consideration of and interaction with the patient's family. (For the purposes of this chapter, *family* means any people who share intimate and routine day-to-day living with the critical care patient—in other words, people whose social homeostasis is altered by the patient's entrance into the arena of critical illness or injury.) Anyone who is a significant part of the patient's normal lifestyle is considered a family member. Of significance to the holistic approach is cultural consideration of the family. This chapter addresses families in crisis and nursing care for such families. Death is one of the crises discussed in this chapter.

CULTURAL PERSPECTIVE

Within the biomedical culture of western medicine, a critical illness is often addressed as a disease process with a focus on the physical symptoms, the pathology of organ function, or injury to a body part. The patient and family, having a different cultural perspective, may view the illness in a more psychophysiological manner, focusing on the physical, psychological, personal, and cultural ramifications of the illness. In other cultures, the patient's critical illness may be viewed as a curse or blamed on hot–cold imbalances, the evil eye, or disharmony with the universe.

Cultural characteristics, such as language, values, behavioral norms, diet, and attitudes toward disease prevention, death and dying, and management of illness vary from culture to culture. The beliefs of the highly technological, illness-focused health care system can clash with cultures who believe in folk medicine, rituals, amulets, religious healing, medicine men, or shamans. It is estimated that within the United States, 70% to 90% of illness episodes are self-managed using over-the-counter medications, home remedies, or folk medicine. The patient experiencing chest pain may first try to self-treat symptoms by using an over-the-counter antacid preparation, a home remedy, or a spiritual healer. The patient may be hesitant to share this information with the health care team for fear of being criticized or scolded.

Critical illness may be viewed also from a religious or spiritual perspective. The patient and family may believe that healing will take place only with the assistance of a religious or spiritual specialist who shares their values and beliefs. Referral to clergy, a native healer, or medicine man may be appropriate to provide the patient and family with support.

■ THE FAMILY IN CRISIS

Families typically maintain a steady state of homeostasis. Crises, however, occur in all families and may threaten and alter the family's homeostasis. Often challenges and demands that face one family are similar to demands that present themselves to all families. On the other hand, some families experience many more crises than other families.

The factor of *cognitive appraisal* must be considered. Some people or families assign catastrophic meaning to events that others would not. If family members appraise a situation by giving it the proportions and labels of a crisis event, the emotions, stress, and anxiety associated with a crisis and attempts to cope will follow. This phenomenon implies that crises based on cognitive appraisal are individual and unique; that is, a crisis for one family is not necessarily a crisis for another. The wide range of family behaviors and reactions observed by critical care nurses can in large part be explained by this concept. Cultural and age variables can also be explained in this way.

Threats to Homeostasis

A family member's entrance into a life–death sick role threatens and alters the family's homeostasis. The first stress to the family is fear and anxiety regarding possible death of the family member. Other considerations, which follow, are related to this or a further development as time passes and the patient remains in the intensive care unit (ICU).

Shift of Responsibility

The family loses the contributions of the critically ill member. The patient's responsibilities must now be added to the responsibilities of others. This alters individual and family schedules and activities. When these responsibilities are left undone, family members experience various degrees of discomfort and annoyance. Financial concerns are usually major, and daily activities that previously were of little

---

Insights into Clinical Research

Kleiber C, Halm M, Titler M, Montgomery LA, Johnson S, Nicholson A, Craft M, Buckwalter K, Megivern K: Emotional responses of family members during a critical care hospitalization. American Journal of Critical Care 3(1):70–76, 1994

The purpose of this study was to identify the emotional responses of family members to critical care hospitalization of a relative and to identify interventions perceived as supportive. Fifty-two family members completed a daily log consisting of open-ended questions relating to emotional experiences and perception of support received.

Results indicated the dominant emotion during the first day of the patient's admission was fear of the unexpected or uncontrollable situation. Feelings of anger and hate were directed toward other family members, the life-sustaining equipment, conflicting information received from health care providers, and the situation itself. Family members experienced additional anger at not being able to help the patient and not being able to identify the cause of the illness. Themes of anxiety related to changes in role demands were also identified early in the critical care admission. Fatigue and exhaustion were most evident the first and second day of the patient's critical care stay. Early in the admission, families of infants in the neonatal intensive care unit expressed feelings of guilt and the need to search for answers. Throughout the critical care hospitalization, all families stated that they experienced sadness, despair, and depression.

Positive emotions also were experienced by families during critical care. Happiness and relief were expressed by families on the first and second day of admission as the patient's condition showed signs of improvement or was no worse. The emotions of hopefulness, joy, and appreciation were also reported by families at various times during the critical care hospitalization.

A caring attitude was the most frequently identified supportive intervention. Receiving truthful, understandable information from the health care team was the second most frequently identified support intervention. Other supportive interventions noted by families were presence, open communication, assistance, comfort measures, empathy, spirituality, and distraction.

---

consequence now become important and often difficult to manage. Such activities as packing school lunches for children, keeping the family car filled with gasoline, taking out the garbage, and balancing the checkbook can, when unfulfilled, become critically significant.

Role Performance

In addition to the responsibilities the patient normally carries, the social role that the patient plays in the family is missing. Disciplinarian, provider of affection, lover, humorist, timekeeper, motivator, comforter, and so on, are all important roles in family life. Considerable havoc and even family grief may ensue if these roles are unfulfilled.

Nature of the Event

The nature of the illness event can also influence the family's reaction and increase the likelihood of family crisis. A sudden or unexpected illness or injury, such as a suicide attempt, acute myocardial infarction, stroke, or traumatic injury, can overwhelm the family with massive amounts of unmanageable stress and can throw the family into crisis. The family may receive a phone call from the hospital or police informing them of the patient's condition. They may have little or no time to prepare for the event. The family may not have had experience with the illness or injury and may receive little guidance regarding where to go when arriving at the hospital, what the rules of the ICU are, how to interact with the critically ill patient, or what to expect in terms of prognosis and treatment. Restricted visiting hours and inadequate communication with the health care team may increase feelings of helplessness and loss of control. A prolonged critical illness or a condition in which there are frequent changes in the patient's status will produce an emotional roller coaster for the family and increase the likelihood of crisis.

The family enters into a crisis under several conditions:

- A stressful event occurs and threatens lasting changes for the family.
- Usual problem-solving activities are inadequate or unused and therefore do not lead rapidly to the previous state of balance.
- The present state of family disequilibrium cannot be maintained and will lead either to improved family health and adaptation or to decreased family adaptation and increased susceptibility to crisis events.

Coping Mechanisms

When a family member is in an ICU, other family members may try to maintain their equilibrium at first by either minimizing the significance of the illness or being overprotective. At first, coping mechanisms may seem to work, and the family system may appear to improve despite increasing stress. As stress continues, however, the family system is likely to disintegrate unless intervention occurs based on the reality of the situation. Reactions to crises are difficult to categorize because they depend on individual responses to stress, and within a family, several mechanisms for handling stress and anxiety may be used. In general, the nurse may observe behaviors signifying feelings of helplessness and urgency, such as an inability to make decisions and mobilize resources. A sense of fear and panic may exist. Irrational acts, demanding behavior, withdrawal, perseveration, and fainting all have been observed by critical care nurses. Just as the patient experiences shock and disbelief about the illness, so too does the family. A nurse must be able to perceive the feeling that a person in crisis is experiencing, particularly when that person cannot identify the problem or feeling to self or others. Four generalizations about crises are listed in the accompanying display.

Four important generalizations about crises form a basis for nursing care of families:

- Whether people emerge stronger or weaker as a result of a crisis is not based so much on their character as on the quality of help they receive during a crisis state.
- People are more amenable to suggestions and open to help during actual crises.
- With the onset of a crisis, old memories of past crises may be evoked. If maladaptive behavior was used to deal with previous situations, the same type of behavior may be repeated in the face of a new crisis.
- The only way to survive a crisis is to be aware of it.

Nursing Assessment

Almost all patients and their families experience some degree of discomfort associated with crises. The challenge is first to assess immediate events causing the disruption and then to help the family assign priorities to its needs so that the family can act accordingly.

The nurse identifies current methods of coping and evaluates these in terms of adaptation (see Chapter 2). The nurse should identify, and possibly point out to the family, chronic problems that may result from the threatening crisis. When the situational crisis seems inconsequential or obscure, the nurse should try to understand the meaning the family has attributed to the event. Furthermore, the meaning ascribed to the crisis will help the nurse evaluate current maturational problems with which the family is already coping. Understanding the parameters of the crisis may give direction for action.

Nursing Interventions

The critical care nurse's time with families is often limited because of the nature of the work, so it is important to make every interaction as useful to the family as possible. The

---

CLINICAL APPLICATION:
Examples of Nursing Diagnoses for the Family Associated With Critical Illness and Injury

Risk for Caregiver Role Strain
Decisional Conflict
Ineffective Family Coping (Compromised or Disabling)
Altered Family Processes
Anticipatory Grieving
Impaired Home Maintenance Management
Hopelessness
Ineffective Individual Coping
Altered Parenting
Altered Role Performance
Spiritual Distress
Potential for Enhanced Spiritual Well Being

nurse must take responsibility for directing the conversation and focusing on the *here and now*. He or she must avoid the temptation to give useless advice in favor of emphasizing a problem-solving approach.

Nursing interventions must be designed to help the family accomplish the following:

- Reach a higher level of adaptation by learning from the crisis experience
- Regain a state of equilibrium
- Experience the feelings involved in the crisis to avoid delayed depression and allow for future emotional growth

---

Suggestions for nursing intervention in a family crisis are given in the accompanying display.

USE OF THE NURSE–FAMILY RELATIONSHIP

Establishing an emotionally meaningful relationship with people tends to be easier during crisis than at other times. People in crisis are highly receptive to an interested and empathetic helper. When first meeting the patient's family, the *nurse must demonstrate an ability to help*. Specific help can be given to demonstrate the nurse's interest. Looking up telephone numbers can be extremely difficult for the highly anxious family member. Even deciding who is to be notified of the patient's status can be an overwhelming decision. Assisting the family to determine immediate priorities is essential in the early phase of crisis work.

With this kind of timely intervention, the family will begin to trust and depend on the nurse's judgment. This process then allows family members to believe the nurse when the nurse conveys feelings of hope and confidence in the family's ability to deal with whatever is ahead of them. It is important to avoid giving false reassurance; rather, the reality of the situation can be expressed in statements such as, "This is a complicated problem; we can work on it together."

PROBLEM SOLVING WITH THE FAMILY

As the relationship develops from one interaction to another, the nurse can formulate the dynamics of the problem. Formulations include items such as the following:

- The meaning the family has attached to the event
- Other crises with which the family may be already coping
- The coping behaviors previously used in times of stress, with an idea of why these behaviors are or are not working at this time
- The normal resources of the family, which may include friends, neighbors, relations, colleagues, and so forth

The nurse, having identified these areas, will be able to help the family deal with their predicament.

Defining the Problem

A vital part of the problem-solving process is to help the family clearly state the immediate problem. Often people feel overwhelmed and immobilized by the free-floating anxiety or panic caused by acute stress. Verbalizing the problem helps the patient achieve a degree of *cognitive mastery*. Regardless of the difficulty or threat the problem implies,

---

CLINICAL APPLICATION:
Nursing Intervention Guidelines
Care of the Family in Crisis

- Use the patient's ethnic or cultural background as a clue regarding the family's orientation to illness and death.
- Speak openly to the patient and family about the fact that the illness is a crisis situation in the family.
- Be responsible for directing conversations with the family and for focusing on the present situation.
- Demonstrate a concern about the crisis and an ability to help with the initial relationship.
- Be realistic about the situation, and do not give false reassurance.
- Convey feelings of hope and confidence in the family's ability to deal with the situation.
- Provide opportunities for the patient and family to make choices so they do not feel completely helpless in the situation.
- Try to perceive the feelings that the crisis evokes in the patient or family.
- Help the family identify and focus on feelings.
- Identify and tell the family (when necessary) what chronic problems may result from the threatening crisis.
- Guide the family in defining the current problem.
- Help the family identify its strengths and sources of support.
- Help the family determine their goals and steps to take in facing the crisis.
- Encourage the family members to take respite from the crisis occasionally.
- Recognize the need and help the family find professional help with overwhelming crises.
- Advocate visiting policies that will meet the needs of patient and family.
- Prepare the family for the critical care environment, especially regarding equipment and purposes of the equipment.
- When children are involved, assess whether it is healthy for the child to visit, and prepare the child for such a visit.
- Assist the family in finding ways to communicate with the patient.
- Encourage the family to help with the care of the patient.
- Provide comfort measures for the visiting family.
- Recognize the patient's and family's spirituality, and suggest the assistance of a spiritual advisor if there is a need.

being able to state it as such reduces anxiety by helping the family realize that they have achieved some sort of understanding of what is happening. Defining the problem is a way of delimiting its parameters.

Defining and redefining problems must occur many times before the crisis is resolved. Stating the problem clearly helps the family assign priorities and direct needed actions. For example, in the event of a tragic injury, finding a babysitter may become the number one priority, superseding notification of close relatives. Goal-directed activity will help decrease anxiety and irrational acts that sometimes go with it.

Identification of Support

In high levels of stress, some people expect themselves to react differently. Rather than turning to the resources they use daily, they become reluctant to involve them. Simply asking people to identify the person to whom they usually turn when they are upset and finding out what has gotten in the way of turning to this person now helps direct the family back to the normal mechanisms for handling issues. When the patient or family is reluctant to call on a friend, the nurse can help resolve the indecision by asking, "Wouldn't you want to help her if she were in your place?" Most families are truly not without resources; they only have failed to recognize and call on them.

Defining and redefining the problem may also help put the problem in a different light. It is possible in time to view a tragedy as a challenge and the unknown as an adventure. The process of helping the family view a problem from a different perspective is called reframing.

The nurse can also help the family call on their own strengths. How have they handled stress before? Have they used humor, escape, exercise, or friendship? Do they telephone close friends and relatives who are far away? Even though the family may be threatened financially at this time, some expenditures of this sort may be well worth the money.

Focus on Feelings

A problem-solving technique emphasizing choices and alternatives helps the family achieve a sense of control over part of their lives. It also reminds them, and clarifies for them, that they are ultimately responsible for dealing with the event and that they must live with the consequences of their decisions.

Helping the family focus on feelings is extremely important to avoid delayed grief reactions and protracted depressions later on. The nurse can give direction to the family to help each other cry and to share their fear and sadness. Reflection of feelings or active listening is necessary throughout the crisis. If the nurse can start a statement by saying, "You feel . . . ," he or she is reflecting a feeling. If the nurse says, "You feel *that* . . . ," he or she is reflecting a judgment instead of a feeling. Describing and recognizing one's feel-

ings decreases the need to blame others. Valuing the expression of feelings can help the family avoid the use of tranquilizers, sedatives, and excessive sleep to escape painful feelings. In sad and depressing times, the nurse can authentically promise the family that they will feel better with time. Adaptation takes time.

During the difficult days of critical illness, the family may become dependent on the judgment of professionals. It can be difficult to identify the appropriate areas in which to accept others' judgments. The nurse can best handle inappropriate expectations, such as, "Tell me what I should do" by acknowledging the feelings involved in an accepting manner and stating the reality of the situation; for example, "You wish I could make that difficult decision for you, but I can't, because you are the ones who will have to live with the consequences." This type of statement acknowledges the family's feelings and recognizes the complexity of the problem, while emphasizing each person's responsibility for his or her own feelings, actions, and decisions.

Step Identification

Once the problem has been defined and the family begins goal-directed activity, the nurse may help further by asking them to identify the steps they must take. This anticipatory guidance helps reduce anxiety and make things go more smoothly. The nurse, however, must recognize moments when direction is vital to health and safety. It is often necessary to direct families to return home to rest. This can be explained by stating that family members must maintain their own health so they will be more helpful to the patient at a later time. To make each interaction meaningful, the nurse must focus on the crisis situation and avoid involvement in long-term chronic problems and complaints. For example, when a patient has overdosed, a nurse should help the family deal with the events immediately preceding the suicide attempt rather than with long-standing family problems.

REFERRAL

Some families will benefit most by referral to a mental health nurse clinician, a social worker, a psychologist, or a psychiatrist. A nurse can best encourage the family to accept help from others by emphatically acknowledging the difficulty and complexity of the problem and providing a choice of names and phone numbers. At times it is appropriate for the nurse to set up the first meeting; however, the chances of follow-through are greater if the patient or family makes the arrangements. Many hospitals have skilled mental health nurses and social workers who, with very short notice, can help the nurse intervene.

VISITATION ADVOCACY

A plethora of family-focused research has consistently validated the family's need for emotional and physical contact with the critically ill patient.

The family has the following proximity needs:

- To see the patient frequently and be able to visit at any time
- To have a waiting room near the patient
- To have visiting hours changed for special occasions
- To have visiting hours start on time

Research has indicated that critically ill patients prefer more flexible visiting. Preferences for visiting frequency, number of visitors, and length of visit varied based on patient age, personality type, illness-related factors, and type of unit.

Additional research has indicated that family presence at the bedside may benefit the patient by reducing intracranial pressure, decreasing patient and family anxiety, increasing social support for the patient, and promoting patient control. The findings of these studies support the need for individualized, less restrictive visiting for patients and families. Unfortunately, restrictive visiting policies are still evident in many critical care areas and are based on tradition and nurse preference rather than on the results of sound scientific research.

Critical care nurses must take the responsibility for revising visiting policies to meet the needs of patients and families. When choosing a less restrictive policy, the physical layout and activity level of the unit must be considered. Open visiting with unlimited visitors may not be appropriate for a unit of limited physical size. Inclusive visiting may be most appropriate when visiting is to be limited during change-of-shift report.

Finally, the effectiveness of changes in visiting policies must be evaluated. Interventional research studies must be performed to evaluate the degree to which changes in visiting meet the proximity needs of patients and families.

The patient and family should be prepared for visiting. The family should know the names and roles of various members of the health care team. Family members can easily be overwhelmed by the environment of the ICU. The purpose of monitors and other technological equipment and the meaning of alarms must be explained. Role modeling can be used to increase the family's comfort with touching and communicating with their critically ill member. Placing a chair at the bedside, lowering the side rails (when safe to do so), offering a paper and pencil or a spelling board, or assisting with lip reading are ways to provide proximity for the patient and family. Encouraging the family to provide care for the patient may decrease anxiety and provide control. Direct care activities may include brushing teeth, applying lotion to hands or feet, bathing, or combing hair.

Allowing children to visit an ICU may require special arrangements on the part of the staff. If the patient wishes to see a child or grandchild and if the child wishes to see the patient in an ICU, the child should be offered short, simple explanations concerning the patient's condition. Answering the child's questions in terms that the child can understand helps reduce possible fears. The person who is taking care of the child should be made aware that invasive procedures and equipment, such as nasogastric tubes, are likely to upset the youngster. If a visit from a child is not possible, arrangements for a telephone visit should be made.

■■ DEATH AND DYING

Near-Death Experiences

Advances in medical and nursing technology have increased the number of people who have survived moments of death or a state of near death. Patients who are seriously ill or injured, who move alarmingly close to death and then recover, have provided health care professionals with a growing understanding of near-death experiences (NDEs). Through descriptions of memories of NDEs, remarkable patterns of the experiences have emerged.

There are commonalities in NDEs, even though each experience is unique and individualized. The typical pattern of NDEs nearly always begins with an out-of-body experience. Patients describe floating above their bodies and even moving out of the room. After or concurrent with the out-of-body experience are reports of visitors unseen by staff or family. Usually these visitors are dead family members or other people who have significant meaning to the patient. Patients sometimes talk aloud to these visitors and tell others who the visitors are.

The next phase of the experience includes movement through a long dark enclosure, like a tunnel. Some report a bright, yet comfortable, light at the end of the enclosure. Most report an extraordinary sense of peacefulness. The environment beyond the enclosure is described as inviting and difficult to leave. Feelings of joy, euphoria, and an overwhelming sense of peace pervade the experience.

Some patients recover from NDEs. When the patient "returns" to life and eventually shares the experience with others, the responses of families and staff vary. Whatever the cause or interpretation placed on the experience, the NDE is likely to have a powerful effect on the individual. Attitudes toward life and death can be dramatically altered. Life becomes more meaningful and appreciated, and death becomes less frightening. Although the NDE can end at any point, many who continue with the experience describe being given a choice to return to life, while others are not given a choice but are directed to return to life. Somehow they are told that it is not time for them to enter this new realm. At this point, patients recount returning to their bodies.

There are several compelling explanations for this interesting phenomenon. The biological explanation argues the NDE is nothing more than a hallucination of an anoxic, dying brain, while others interpret the episodes as a close encounter with God and a spiritual domain. In fact, NDEs typically are reported in the context of the culture and faith of the patient.

NURSING INTERVENTIONS

Nurses can assist patients and family members by acknowledging the importance and meaning of the experience to them. Nurses should never attempt to denigrate the reality of the experience by explaining it away as a biochemically induced hallucination that occurs when the brain nears the point of death. Whether the experience is biologically or divinely caused should not detract from its importance for the individual and family. Family members can be told that many have survived years beyond the NDE and that having this experience does not mean that the patient will die. Instead, the nurse genuinely can emphasize the choice to return to life as an important indicator of a positive prognosis. A positive prognosis should not be promised, however. Because reports of NDEs seem to touch emotionally all who hear them, the nurse must be careful to protect the patient's need for time and privacy to process the meaning and significance of the experience.

Dying patients sometimes tell family members that dead relatives are present. Nurses can help teach the family about NDEs, should this happen. If the patient has been suffering and waiting for death, the family is probably ready to let go. The nurse may tell the family that the patient might need their permission to leave this world with those who have come for him or her.

Family members who are unaware of NDEs can become very disturbed when they see the patient talking to someone who is not there. The nurse can support the family through role modeling. The nurse may ask the patient about the visitors and about why he or she believes they are present.

Nursing Implications of Dying

Composure can be described as the ability to be comfortable with the dying patient. For many nurses, being comfortable about death depends on the ability to modify goals that are aimed at preserving life with goals that are designed to preserve personal integrity and family stability when a patient is dying. Rather than considering death as a symbol of failure, nurses can view it as a life-enriching and professionally gratifying experience.

Suggestions for guiding the family through this crisis are given in the accompanying display.

COMMUNICATION

Family members may elect to use the time to go over special memories, reconcile past misunderstandings, and forgive each other for past transgressions. It is hoped that they will have the time and a proper atmosphere to say the things they need to say.

The nurse's responsibility is to establish an atmosphere in which this type of communication can occur. What does the family need to be comfortable on the unit—a cup of coffee, a pillow, a place to sit, permission to leave? Does the family wish to be present at the time of death? How can they

---

CLINICAL APPLICATION:
Nursing Intervention Guidelines
Care of the Family When the Patient is Dying

- Learn to be comfortable with the dying patient and his or her family.
- Acknowledge the meaning and importance of near-death experiences, despite your own interpretation of these events.
- Establish an atmosphere in which the patient and family will feel comfortable sharing memories and correcting misunderstandings.
- Use touch to communicate or convey empathy.
- Keep your sense of humor, and share it with the patient and family as appropriate.
- Reinforce the presence of family members by assuring them they are helping the patient relax or be more comfortable.
- Be tolerant of complaints and criticisms when the family is in crisis.
- Continue to show your interest in the patient and family, even when death is near or you are assigned to other patients on the unit.
- Be an advocate for consistent staff and approaches.
- When death is near, provide comfort measures and a quiet room for the family members.
- Inform the family when death is near, and do not pull any surprises on them.
- Offer to contact a spiritual advisor if the family desires to have someone near.
- Help the health care team identify two team members to inform the family of the patient's death.
- Observe ethnic or cultural customs regarding death and dying.
- Use touch, hugging, or other forms of nonverbal communication to indicate support.
- Prepare the family for viewing of the body, and give them ample time to do so.
- Stay with the family to coordinate paperwork, answer questions, and provide grief education.
- Provide written information or the telephone number of a support group.

---

be reached? All these questions require sensitive timing and a straightforward approach on the part of the nurse. If words escape the nurse, as they often may in difficult moments, or if words seem inadequate, much can be conveyed by touching a shoulder or an arm.

The nurse who keeps a sense of humor and expresses it appropriately offers relief in a difficult situation. Generous smiles and a sense of humor help the family relax and share themselves in their usual ways. Talking to the patient in one's typical fashion helps the family relax and communicate more easily with one another and with the patient. In turn, the patient feels less isolated and alone in this final crisis.

FAMILY INTEGRITY

The family in crisis is vulnerable to all types of stresses. Helping family members provide support for one another is of paramount importance. They may wish to have a family member with the patient at all times. Family members can support one another by providing meal and rest breaks. Being together and being available to one another is sufficient for many families. The nurse may choose to say to some family members that even though it seems they are not doing anything for the patient, their presence seems to relax or comfort the patient or the patient's spouse.

CONSISTENCY OF CARE

Complaints and criticisms are frequently directed toward the nurse during times of crisis. A nondefensive, tolerant attitude and a willingness to continue working with the patient and family are the most effective ways of conveying compassion and understanding. Continued interest in a patient and family demonstrates a sense of worth and respect to those involved.

As patients draw closer to death, nurses are likely to spend less time with them. In some cases, nurses may avoid the client and family because of the nurses' own sadness regarding impending death. Other nurses may feel less physical and emotional care is needed. Regardless of the reason, this decreased contact may evoke feelings of abandonment, sadness, and hopelessness in patients and family. Moreover, changes in staff shifts increase their sense of isolation and cause them to use up energy adjusting to new people. Providing consistent staff who do not withdraw helps the patient and family develop trust and a sense of belonging that can become a rewarding experience for everyone involved.

After the Patient's Death

The patient's death signals the beginning of intense and sometimes overwhelming grief for the family. Research indicates that the manner in which the family is informed of the death has a significant impact on their grief response.

The family is escorted to a quiet, private room. This room should be near the patient's room and accessible to other arriving family members. Emotional support is critical. The family should be met by clergy, a social worker, or another health team member who is trained in bereavement. The family should be provided with a phone, tissues, and offers to call other significant family members or friends. They must be kept informed of the patient's condition on an ongoing basis. Clear, concrete medical information must be provided. If death appears to be the probable outcome, the family must be clearly and compassionately informed of the possibility. Gradually preparing them for the pronouncement will reduce their denial following the death.

The pronouncement of death requires a caring, empathetic approach. Two health team members should be identified to approach the family. This allows one team member to be available should a family member become ill or faint. The term "death" must be used. Abstract phrases will only increase anxiety and confusion. A warm, compassionate, honest tone must be used when communicating with the family. Touching, hugging, or other nonverbal indications of support are appropriate. Repetition of the information may be necessary as the family struggles to overcome their initial denial.

The nurse recognizes the spirituality of death by offering to contact clergy, a spiritual advisor, or other identified family support. Requests by the family for specific people or rituals following the death should be honored to meet cultural needs.

The viewing of the body is the most difficult time for many family members, second only to the pronouncement of death. Viewing of the body has been found to be beneficial to the family by making the loss real, allowing family members to say goodbye, and in cases of sudden death, eliminating any question that the patient is indeed their family member. Health team members must remain neutral in their opinion of whether or not the family should view the body. Family members must be given the option and be allowed to make the decision on an individual basis. It is important to ask more than once, because family members may change their minds after they first decline the offer.

The nurse prepares them for the condition of the body by gently describing the presence of wounds, dressings, tubes, and the coolness of the body temperature. The family is allowed to stay as long as they feel necessary and to come back and forth to spend time at the bedside. Intense emotional reactions, such as screaming, wailing, or fainting, may accompany the family's viewing of the body. Some family members may shake the body or call out loudly for the patient to wake up. Should these behaviors occur, the nurse compassionately confronts the individual and takes him or her to a quiet area until composure is regained.

Children must be assessed for the appropriateness of the viewing. A child should never be coerced into viewing the body and should clearly be given a choice as to whether or not he or she desires a viewing. The child must be well prepared for what will be seen and will require support from an identified staff member. Following the viewing, it is essential that the staff member spend time with the child, discussing what was witnessed and clarifying any misconceptions.

Following the viewing, a health team member should stay with the family to help complete appropriate paperwork; answer questions regarding the death, autopsy, organ donation, or funeral home arrangements; and provide brief grief education. The family must be assured that sleep disturbances, crying, difficulty concentrating, anorexia, and depression are normal symptoms of grief. The family will benefit from written material or the phone number of a grief support group. The family should be escorted to their car when all details are completed. A follow-up phone call should be made by a staff member 24 to 48 hours after the death to answer additional questions, clarify misconceptions, and provide referrals for counseling and support.

CONCLUSION

The nature of the critical care environment is such that the nurse is exposed to repeated losses. If the nurse has experienced loss as a result of death in his or her personal life, dealing with dying patients may reactivate feelings and memories associated with these losses. Therefore, it is essential that the nursing staff support one another, especially by listening in a tolerant way when a colleague is expressing what is generally considered to be unacceptable feelings.

Few nurses come to the ICU with these abilities. Most nurses must request specific educational experiences, consultation, and supervision from appropriate resources. The intensity of emotion and involvement demanded by a nurse in critical care makes these nurses particularly vulnerable to the "burnout" syndrome (see Chapter 9).

Crisis intervention for families undergoing acute stress is an important preventive mental health function for nurses to provide. Their knowledge of and proximity to the problem allow them to be first-line resource professionals. As patient advocates, their role is to realize and point out that dealing with a psychological crisis in the family greatly affects the recovery and well-being of the patient and decreases the chances for further disequilibrium in the family unit.

Clinical Applicability Challenges

Self-Challenge: Critical Thinking

1. Mr. and Mrs. Patel are the parents of a critically ill patient on your unit. They have just arrived in the United States from their home country of India and speak minimal English. Develop criteria you would use to assess their degree of stress and potential for crisis. Compare and contrast how the cultural needs of the Patel family might differ from those of an English-speaking, middle-class American family.

2. Mrs. Jones is a critically ill multiple-trauma patient who has been admitted to your unit. She is not expected to survive her injuries. Mrs. Jones' husband; her two children, ages 6 and 10; and her older parents have just arrived on the unit. Formulate a plan of care to assist the family to deal with the probable death of their loved one.

Study Questions

1. To help the family develop a sense of control, the nurse may
   a. offer reassurance that the patient is receiving the best possible care.
   b. refer family members to a grief counselor or clergy.
   c. offer choices to family members whenever possible.
   d. All of the above

2. Assisting the family members to define or state a problem associated with a crisis is useful because it
   a. increases their sense of understanding of the problem.
   b. implies parameters or limits of the problem.
   c. helps family members achieve a sense of cognitive mastery.
   d. All of the above

3. The family enters a crisis under several conditions. Identify the conditions most likely to increase the probability that a family will enter a crisis:
   a. An event has lasting consequences for a family.
   b. A family's ability to problem-solve is inadequate.
   c. The equilibrium of the family is thrown off.
   d. All of the above

BIBLIOGRAPHY

Borley G, von Hofe K, Blatt L: Holistic care of the critically ill: Meeting both patient and family needs. Dimensions of Critical Care Nursing 13(4):218–223, 1994

Chesla CA: Reconciling technologic and family care in critical-care nursing. IMAGE: Journal of Nursing Scholarship 28(3):199–203, 1996

Davis-Martin S: Perceived needs of families of long-term critical care patients: A brief report. Heart Lung 23(6):515–518, 1994

Furukawa MM: Meeting the needs of the dying patient's family. Critical Care Nurse 16(1):51–57, 1996

Germain CP: Cultural care: A bridge between sickness, illness, and disease. Holistic Nursing Practice 6(3):1–9, 1992

Johnson SK, Craft M, Titler M, Halm M, Kleiber C, Montgomery LA, Megivern K, Nicholson A, Buckwalter K: Perceived changes in adult family members' roles and responsibilities during critical illness. Image 27(3):238–243, 1995

Kirchoff KT, Pugh E, Calame RM, Reynolds N: Nurses' beliefs and attitudes toward visiting in adult critical care settings. American Journal of Critical Care 2(3):238–245, 1993

Krapohl GL: Visiting hours in the adult intensive care unit: Using research to develop a system that works. Dimensions of Critical Care Nursing 14(5):245–258, 1995

LaMontagne L, Hepworth J, Johnson B: Psychophysiological responses of parent to pediatric critical care stress. Clinical Nursing Research 3(2):104–118, 1994

McClelland ML: Our unit has a bereavement program. Am J Nurs 93(1):62–66, 1993

Nicholson AC, Titler M, Montgomery LA, Kleiber C, Craft MJ, Halm M, Buckwalter K, Johnson S: Effects of child visitation in adult critical care units: A pilot study. Heart Lung 22(1):36–45, 1993

Titler MG, Bombei C, Schutte D: Developing family focused care. Critical Care Nursing Clinics of North America 7(2): 375–386, 1995

Tomlinson PS, Kirschbaum M, Harbaugh B, Anderson KH: The influence of illness severity and family resources on maternal uncertainty during critical pediatric hospitalization. American Journal of Critical Care 5(2):140–146, 1996

4

Impact of the Critical Care Environment on the Patient

IMPACT ON COGNITION AND PERCEPTION

Sensory Input
Orientation to Time and Place
Need for Personal Space and Privacy

IMPACT ON CHRONOBIOLOGY

Sleep–Wake Cycles

Periodicity
Variations in Physiological Function

ACUTE CONFUSION (DELIRIUM)

NURSING ASSESSMENT

NURSING INTERVENTIONS

Sensory Stimulation

Sensory Input for the Unresponsive
    Patient
Security Information
Noise Control
Rest and Sleep
Reality Orientation
Personal Space Control

OBJECTIVES

Based on the content in this chapter, the reader should be able to:

- Examine five factors that can adversely affect patients in the intensive care unit.
- Discuss five nursing interventions that can minimize the effects of sensory deprivation and sensory overload.
- Explain how biological rhythms affect the patient in the critical care environment.
- Discuss potential problems caused by sleep deprivation.
- Examine the risk factors and possible nursing interventions related to acute confusion.
- Compare and contrast actions and their effect on the patient's need for personal space and privacy.

*P*atients in today's intensive care units (ICUs) are surrounded by advanced technology that, although essential to save lives, may create an alien and even life-threatening environment for them. Critical care nurses must possess expertise in the use of this technology yet remain aware that a patient's fear of the equipment can create serious stress reactions. While attention to physiological stability is a patient care priority, the nurse also attends to patient re-

sponses produced by interaction with the environment. This chapter discusses ways in which nurses can avoid or minimize the negative effects of the following factors: sensory input, disorientation, lack of privacy, chronobiology, loss of sleep, and acute confusion.

IMPACT ON COGNITION AND PERCEPTION

Sensory Input

The broad concept of sensory input deals with stimulation of all five senses: visual, auditory, olfactory, tactile, and gustatory. Stimuli to all the senses may be perceived in a qualitative manner as pleasant or unpleasant, acceptable or unacceptable, desirable or undesirable, soothing or painful. Individual perceptions vary drastically. Some people may consider the sounds and smells of a metropolitan business district to be pleasant, acceptable, and desirable, whereas others may find them undesirable. Everyday activities, including the choice of food or drink, are based on a person's likes and dislikes. Thus, people tend to choose, whenever possible, the environment or stimuli from the environment most acceptable to them. Patients in the ICU, however, have no control over the choice of their environment or most of its stimuli.

In addition to the *quality* of a stimulus, the nurse must also consider the *quantity*. Too much stimulation is as unacceptable as too little. In the ICU, too many undesirable stimuli, such as excessive and constant noise, bright light, and hyperactivity, can be as distorting and bothersome as too few stimuli, such as gloom, silence, and inactivity.

When trying to control environmental stimuli in an ICU, the nurse must be aware of both the type and the amount of sensory input. If sensory stimuli are diminished too drastically, the patient experiences *sensory deprivation*, which can cause severe disorganization of normal psychological defenses. If sensory stimuli occur in excessive quantity, the phenomenon of *sensory overload* creates an equally undesirable response to the environment, including confusion and withdrawal.

Although all patients are susceptible to sensory deprivation and overload, those who are at highest risk and most likely to be seriously affected include the very young, the very old, those recovering from anesthesia, those with sensory deficits, and those who are unresponsive.

Patients who can communicate are likely to seek out relevant and meaningful information by questioning visitors and those involved in their care. However, the nurse in the ICU serves as the eyes, ears, and voice for those at risk, particularly the unresponsive patient.

SENSORY DEPRIVATION

Sensory deprivation refers to a variety of symptoms that occur after a reduction in the quantity or quality of sensory input. Other terms related to sensory deprivation include *isolation, confinement, informational underload, perceptual deprivation,* and *sensory restriction.* A variety of symptoms have been observed in normal adults after exposure to sensory deprivation for varying periods. These are listed in the display.

Sensory deprivation need not be present for days or weeks for psychopathological reactions to occur. For example, it is well documented that normal young adults undergoing an 8-hour period of sensory deprivation may experience an acute psychotic reaction followed by continuation of delusions for several days and severe depression and anxiety for several weeks.[1]

The degree of sensory deprivation possible in a laboratory setting is greater than that likely to occur in an ICU. However, laboratory subjects are aware of the time involved in the experiment and have the ability to stop whenever they wish. They also possess clinically normal defense mechanisms and total control of the situation. Hospitalized patients do not have these advantages.

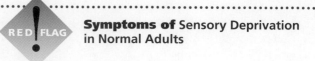

Symptoms of Sensory Deprivation in Normal Adults

- Loss of sense of time
- Boredom
- Presence of delusions, illusions, and hallucinations
- Anxiety and fear
- Restlessness
- Depression
- Any type of behavior or symptom present in psychoses

SENSORY OVERLOAD

The phenomenon of sensory overload has not received as much attention as that of sensory deprivation, but some of its effects on humans are known. Decreased hearing after long-term exposure to high noise levels has been well documented. Also, tension and anxiety increase when people are exposed to continuous noise without quiet periods.

Sounds in ICUs include voices of strangers in large numbers; movement of bed rails; beeping of cardiac monitors, paging systems calling strange names; suctioning of tracheostomies; telephones ringing at all hours; and whispers, laughter, and muffled voices. These are compounded by continuous lighting and strange views of equipment. Such abnormal sounds and sights place additional stress on patients in critical care environments. Therefore, the patient's surroundings must be controlled as much as possible so that environmentally induced stress can be minimized.

Excessive environmental stimuli can cause significant psychological problems for patients in ICUs. In addition, the quantity of noise can be a significant factor in a patient's recovery. For example, high noise levels can increase discomfort and result in an increased need for pain medication, and loud talking and laughing among personnel can cause resentment (see display).

If environmental stimuli exceed the limits to which the human organism can comfortably adapt, the coping system fails. If this occurs, behaviors such as anxiety, panic, confusion, delusions, illusions, or hallucinations may result.

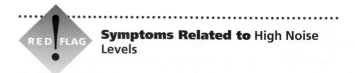

Symptoms Related to High Noise Levels

- Increased need for pain medication
- Inability to sleep
- Feelings of fear, helplessness, forgetfulness, withdrawal
- Reaction to noisy conversation and laughter
- Confusion, delusions, illusions, or hallucinations

Sensory overload also can be related to the amount of directions and information given to the patient. Such information may come from various physicians, nurses, technicians, and the family. A patient with information overload may respond in one of the following ways:

- No processing of information
- Incorrect processing of information
- Selective processing of information
- Escape from the flow of information

THE HOSPITAL PHENOMENON

The hospital environment often deprives patients of normal sensory stimuli while bombarding them with continuous strange sensory stimuli not found in the average home environment. Normal sounds at home include voices of loved ones and friends; barking of neighborhood dogs; automobile, bus, and train traffic and horns; the television or radio on a familiar station; children at play; the washing machine or dishwasher; daytime telephone calls; and many other sounds and sights that diminish when night comes. These are replaced by the unfamiliar and possibly unpleasant sounds of the hospital. This situation, a combination of sensory deprivation and sensory overload, is called *the hospital phenomenon*.

The combination of the loss of familiar stimuli and continuous exposure to strange stimuli elicits different types of defensive responses from patients. Withdrawal is a common coping mechanism and can cause a patient to be mislabeled as confused or disoriented unless a complete assessment is done. Some degree of withdrawal from the frightening reality of the situation is common.

Orientation to Time and Place

For reality testing to occur, there must be continuous input of familiar, meaningful information from the person's outside world. If this information is lacking, the person's internal mental events can be mistaken for external ones. This may explain why some critical care patients appear to have illusions or hallucinations.

As human beings, we take the physical environment for granted. If we suddenly awoke in a world without grass or sunlight or the sounds of traffic or human speech, however, we would not have the necessary stimuli to keep our minds in contact with reality. We would try to interpret unknown stimuli in familiar terms. In reality, however, our interpretations might be wrong. This is especially true of patients who suffer temporary loss of any of the senses, particularly vision or hearing, because people normally use a combination of senses to interpret their environment.

Absence of reality testing may offer at least a partial explanation for the high incidence of psychosis in patients assigned to ICUs for long-term care because of altered levels of consciousness. The following account discusses an unresponsive person's experience.

CLINICAL APPLICATION: Patient Care Study

Carol was a 20-year-old college student with severe basal skull trauma and multiple injuries. She was unresponsive throughout the 8-day period she spent in the intensive care unit.

When Carol began responding verbally, her first words to her mother were, "Am I free now? I was in the hands of the Soviet Union!" An immediate interpretation of such a statement could be that she was totally out of contact with reality because of the injury and had dreamed such an episode. It is just as reasonable to assume that she could have perceived that the actions in the unit and the treatments she received were related to torture and that she was the victim for some unknown reason.

Carol had no noticeable motor control of her facial muscles, so she was "blind." She had a tracheostomy that required frequent suctioning. She was almost immobile because of fractures and spasticity, necessitating plaster casts or soft restraints on all extremities. Because she had no means of interpreting her experience realistically from meaningful cues in the environment, such a situation could have caused her to believe that she was being tortured.

Need for Personal Space and Privacy

All people have an unconsciously marked territory around them that is known as personal space. The actual size of this space is generally thought to be flexible and to provide a margin of safety and security. Factors that influence the size of the space include the social situation, the physical area, the person's cultural background, and the person's relationship to others who are present.

Invasion of one's personal space may cause discomfort, anger, and anxiety. It is normal to defend against such threats to maintain control of the space. In a hospital setting, personal space is severely limited and is often invaded by the nursing staff.

Intrusions also occur in the form of impersonal equipment kept at the bedside (eg, suction machines, monitors, oxygen equipment, and intravenous equipment). This creates a situation in which personal space is limited to the confines of the bed and, possibly, a bedside stand. For this reason, the patient usually clusters all personal possessions on the small stand.

■ IMPACT ON CHRONOBIOLOGY

Chronobiology is the study of biological rhythms. It was once thought that all biological functions were maintained in a steady state, but this is no longer the prevailing view. Chronobiology proposes cyclical variations in biological functions as the norm, rather than a constant state with compensatory return to the steady state. Fluctuations in heart rate, blood pressure, respiratory rate, and urine excretion are just a few biological rhythms that have been shown to vary with time. "Jet lag," which occurs when flying from one time zone to another, is a common example of unsynchronized biorhythms.

By better understanding a patient's typical variation in biological cycles (sleep–wake cycles for example), the critical care nurse can alter the environment to mimic the patient's customary pattern of functioning. The sleep–wake cycle is used here as an exemplar to understand chronobiology; the critical care nurse must remember that similar variations exist with many biological functions.

Sleep–Wake Cycles

Sleep is an essential part of the 24-hour cycle within which human organisms must function. There is a 24-hour periodicity in which the typical major sleep period recurs once a day.[2] People spend about one third of their lives sleeping, and sleep is essential to physical and mental well-being. The purpose of sleep is to prevent physiological and psychological exhaustion or illness; lack of sleep extends the time needed to recover from illness.

There are five stages of sleep, as outlined in the accompanying display. The first four are nonrapid eye movement stages, and the fifth stage is known as rapid eye movement (REM) sleep. The first stage, sleep latency, covers the time between trying to go to sleep and actually falling asleep. The second stage is light sleep from which a person can easily be awakened. Stages three and four are deep slow (delta) wave

---

Stages and Characteristics of Sleep

1. Transitional stage between wakefulness and sleep
   Relaxed state where person is somewhat aware of surroundings
   Involuntary muscle jerking that may waken the person
   Normally lasts only minutes
   Easily aroused
   Constitutes only about 5% of total sleep
2. Beginning of sleep
   Arousal occurs with relative ease
   Constitutes 50% to 55% of sleep
3. Depth of sleep increased and arousal increasingly difficult
   Constitutes about 10% of sleep
4. Greatest depth of sleep (*delta sleep*)
   Arousal from sleep difficult
   Physiological changes in the body—slow brain waves on electroencephalogram; decreased pulse and respiratory rates; decreased blood pressure; relaxed muscles; slow metabolism and low body temperature
   Constitutes about 10% of sleep
5. Sleep with vivid dreaming (REM)
   Rapid eye movement, fluctuating heart and respiratory rates, fluctuating blood pressure
   Skeletal muscle tone lost
   Most difficult to arouse
   Duration of REM sleep increased with each cycle and averages 20 minutes

Adapted from Taylor C, Lillis C, LeMone P: Fundamentals of Nursing 3rd Ed. Philadelphia, Lippincott-Raven, 1997

Insights into Clinical Research

Simpson T, Lee E, Cameron C: Patients' perceptions of environmental factors that disturb sleep after cardiac surgery. American Journal of Critical Care 5(3):173–181, 1996

In this study, 102 patients who had cardiac surgery rated environmental factors that disturbed their sleep both in the intensive care unit (ICU) and after transfer. Researchers adapted the *Factors Influencing Sleep Questionnaire* and administered this tool to patients several days before their hospital discharge. The tool included a wide range of factors, including pain, anxiety, discomfort, procedures, lights, equipment, and different types of sounds.

Eighty-two percent of the patients remembered their experiences during their ICU stay and after transfer. Almost three quarters of the patients rated discomfort as the main cause for their sleep disturbance during their postsurgery hospital stay. The second factor, mentioned by about one half of the patients, was the inability to perform their usual presleep routine while in the ICU. Pain was the second greatest reason for disturbed sleep after transfer from the ICU. These findings indicate a need to control pain and discomfort better throughout hospitalization and to have an overall plan for promoting sleep after cardiac surgery.

---

sleep (SWS). Stage 5 is REM sleep. A person normally experiences four to six cycles of sleep each 24 hours. The average time for a normal sleep cycle is 90 minutes but varies from 70 to 120 minutes. In a normal sleep cycle, people progress from stage one through four, return to stages three and two, and then enter the REM stage.

REM sleep is essential for mental restoration. REM stages become longer and more intense in later sleep cycles, occurring primarily in the last cycles of an uninterrupted night of sleep. Because of REM sleep's importance, it is likely that sleep deprivation is most significant when it occurs during the REM stage. In the ICU, the continuity of sleep cycles is often disrupted, resulting in sleep deprivation in the REM stage.

People who are deprived of SWS and REM sleep for even a few days experience numerous adverse effects, such as irritability and anxiety, physical exhaustion and fatigue, and disruption of metabolic functions, including adrenal hormone production. Even respiratory distress is associated with disrupted sleep, with periods of apnea and hypopnea occurring. Increasing age and certain acute illnesses may further increase sleep apnea or hypopnea.[3]

Periodicity

The broad concept of *periodicity* is another area of knowledge necessary for the nurse in the ICU. Other related terms are *circadian rhythm, biological clock, internal clock,* and *physiological clock*. It has been recognized for many years that all living creatures have not only an identifiable life cycle but also short-term, rhythmic cycles. Disruption of those rhythms can cause deviations from the norm or even cessation of life.

The human organism possesses a 24-hour cycle that is resistant to change, and long-term disruption can be fatal. Many of the biochemical and biophysical processes of the human body have rhythms, with peaks of function or activity that occur in consistent patterns within the daily cycle.

Variations in Physiological Function

Knowing when physiological functions are at their lowest level helps the nurse evaluate the significance of fluctuations. For example, normal variations in the quantity of urine output should be expected, because the kidneys possess their own unique rhythm as demanded by sleep and activity patterns. This accounts for a normal decrease in the quantity of urine produced during the night.

Health care personnel may schedule medication, sleep periods, and stressful procedures on the basis of their knowledge of individual circadian rhythms, thus avoiding further stress on the most vulnerable parts of the cycle and capitalizing on the strongest parts of the cycle.

ACUTE CONFUSION (DELIRIUM)

Patients admitted to an ICU have either a serious trauma or a sudden illness that automatically places them at risk for developing acute confusion. Acute confusion is a common condition seen in all ages but one to which older people are especially prone. It has a rapid onset and is generally reversible, differentiating it from dementias, which develop slowly and are irreversible. An acute confusional state affects cognitive functions, attention, and the sleep–wake cycle. Symptoms of acute confusion are listed in the accompanying display.

NURSING ASSESSMENT

A nursing history taken in the initial phase of planning can provide information to help tailor nursing interventions. Such a history requires that individualized questions be asked of patient and family members. A brief outline of a normal 24-hour period of activity for the patient and his or

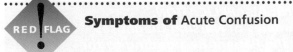

Symptoms of Acute Confusion

General Symptoms
- Fluctuation in the level of awareness
- Visual hallucinations
- Misidentification of people (usually in the form of thinking a nurse is some close relative)
- Severe restlessness
- Memory impairment

Disorders of Cognition
Impairment in perception, memory, and thinking
Behavior includes:
- Disorientation for location and time
- Confusion of unknown person with familiar one
- Memory impairment
- Delusions that food is poisoned

Abnormal Sleep–Wake Cycle
Disorders of attention, vigilance, and sleep dysfunction
Behavior includes:
- Insomnia
- Vivid night dreams
- Agitation as darkness occurs ("sundown syndrome")
- Reduced attention time
- Under-alertness or over-alertness
- Fluctuating awareness from drowsiness to lucidity

Disorders of Psychomotor Behavior
Generally nonspecific
Behavior includes:
- Wandering
- Fluctuation from intense agitation to somnolence
- Combative behavior, usually due to fear

her sleep habits gives the nurse a good starting point in compiling data. A simple rule to use when collecting a nursing history is to determine what is significant or familiar and expose the patient to it, if possible. Additional information included in the nursing history can be anything from food likes and dislikes to favorite types of music or television programs.

Because sensory deprivation and sensory overload can adversely affect patients, the nurse assesses the environment for sensory stimuli (sounds, lights, touches, interruptions) that may occur throughout the day and night. An assessment of this kind includes a record of each type of stimulus and its source, location, duration, and frequency, as well as an evaluation of the quality and quantity of stimuli and how they affect the patient.

When assessing the patient's condition, the nurse considers whether there have been adequate uninterrupted time periods for all stages of sleep to occur. The nursing plan of care must provide such periods as soon as possible after the patient's admission to the unit. The necessity of taking vital signs every 1 or 2 hours during the night must be weighed against the damage caused to the human or-

---

CLINICAL APPLICATION:
Examples of Nursing Diagnoses for the Patient Responding to the Critical Care Environment

Anxiety
Acute Confusion
Fear
Impaired Memory
Sensory/Perceptual Alterations
Sleep Pattern Disturbance
Altered Thought Processes

---

ganism when it is deprived of sleep. Because a cycle of sleep measured from REM stage to REM stage requires 70 to 120 minutes, it is important to provide periods of a minimum of 2 hours of uninterrupted sleep during the night.

Physiological functions reach their lowest levels in the middle of the night; in the later morning hours, functions are beginning to reach a maximum level. Therefore, normal fluctuations in vital signs should be expected, and patients should not be subjected to activity or stressful procedures in the early morning hours. Only life-preserving activities should be allowed to disturb the patient at night.

In addition to assessing the patient's current status, the nurse obtains as much information as possible about recent mental functioning. People who had close contact with the patient before the hospital admission can help with this information. If the patient's functioning was adequate for self-care before admission to the ICU, it should be assumed that any confusion or mental malfunctioning is potentially reversible. Environmental stresses of the unit coupled with the physical and psychosocial impact of illness can precipitate mental impairment that may be labeled as acute confusion. Other causes also need to be considered and are de-

scribed in Table 4–1. Symptoms of acute confusion are listed in a previous display in this chapter.

A sudden change in a person's life, such as a traumatic situation, removal from familiar surroundings, or administration of certain sedative or tranquilizing drugs, can precipitate symptoms of acute confusion. The following situation illustrates these points.

CLINICAL APPLICATION: Patient Care Study

Mrs. Marlow, a 70-year-old retiree, was among several passengers injured when their bus veered off the road and down an embankment. Although apparently not physically injured, Mrs. Marlow had a rapid heart rate, low blood pressure, weakness, and pallor. She was taken to the emergency room, where she described the accident coherently and expressed anxiety and concern about the condition of her injured friend and the loss of her purse and eyeglasses. A physical examination was done, and no injury was evident. Her blood pressure and pulse returned to normal ranges, and her electrocardiogram was normal. During the later part of the examination, however, she displayed increasing confusion and soon became disoriented, not knowing where she was or how she got there. Because of the escalating confusion, she was kept for further observation and evaluation in a four-bed room. Bed rails were raised, and she was instructed to use the call light if she needed to use the bathroom. During the next few evening hours, she was first restless, then agitated; she thought she was home and was frightened by the presence of others in her home. She kept trying to get out of bed and finally climbed over the bed rails. After staff members gently assisted her return to bed, she began screaming and became resistive. She was given 1 mg Haldol intramuscularly and put into a vest restraint in bed.

The shock of these events and the changes they created for this woman were further aggravated by the following:

- Decreased sensory input (due to loss of glasses)
- Misinterpreted sensory input
- Use of restraint
- Use of drugs

TABLE 4-1
Possible Reversible Causes of Acute Confusion

Pharmacological factors:	Narcotics, sedatives, digitalis, tranquilizers, steroids, antihypertensives, antidepressants, diuretics, chemotherapeutic agents, bronchodilators, anticholinergics
Environmental factors:	Abrupt change in environment, sensory deprivation, sensory overload, isolation
Psychosocial factors:	Depression, loss, grief
Nutritional imbalances:	Vitamin deficiencies (B_{12}, folic acid, niacin), starvation
Elimination imbalances:	Fecal impaction, urinary retention
Trauma:	Fractures, surgery, concussion/contusion, subdural hematoma, cerebral hemorrhage
Alcohol abuse:	Alcohol withdrawal when hospitalized
Pain:	Due to trauma of external or internal origin
Fluid or electrolyte imbalances:	Sodium excess of depletion, dehydration, acid–base imbalance
Metabolic factors:	Hypothyroidism or hyperthyroidism, renal impairment, liver malfunction
Cardiovascular factors:	Congestive heart failure, hypotension, myocardial infarction, dysrhythmias
Bacteriological factors:	Infection (eg, pneumonia)
Body temperature:	Hyperthermia, hypothermia

It is easy to see how situations like this can escalate. These events could even lead to placement in an extended care facility if thoughtful assessment, planning, and care do not short-circuit or eventually help reverse the symptoms.

NURSING INTERVENTIONS

Although a comprehensive evaluation is made to determine possible causes that can be corrected, the nurse must use all knowledge available to make the environment a therapeutic tool rather than a stressor for the patient.

Sensory Stimulation

It may be desirable to provide exposure to familiar stimuli by playing a favorite tape from home, finding a favorite radio station, or requesting a taped message from a loved one. Such actions offer meaningful sensory stimulation to the patient in an otherwise unfamiliar environment. Family and friends should be involved in planning and providing such sensory input, especially for unresponsive patients. The potential value of a familiar voice giving information or encouragement is made clear in the following patient situation.

CLINICAL APPLICATION: Patient Care Study

A young woman was admitted to an intensive care unit (ICU) shortly after Christmas. She had a diagnosis of viral encephalopathy and a guarded prognosis. She became unresponsive within a few hours, and her husband was told that she was not expected to live. In spite of this, she held on to life for 2 months, during which the hopeless prognosis remained. Twice more, the husband was told that death was imminent.

After another message from the hospital, the young husband told his 2½-year-old son that his mother was dying, but the child repeatedly told his father not to worry because his mommy would not die. Finally, the father took the boy to the ICU to see his mother for the last time.

While there, the boy said, "I love you, Mommy." To the shock of all except the boy, his mother opened her eyes for the first time. The young woman later told everyone, "I had forgotten everything until I heard his voice say, 'I love you, Mommy.'" She is well on the road to recovery now.

Sensory Input for the Unresponsive Patient

Because unresponsive patients may suffer the greatest psychological trauma related to the effects of the environment, their psychosocial needs require the greatest attention. One barrier to providing this attention may be an attitude of hopelessness about the person's ability to take in sensory input. *Unconscious* denotes a lack of sensory awareness, which cannot currently be measured in the absence of concurrent motor response, whereas *unresponsive* means that

---

CLINICAL APPLICATION:
Nursing Intervention Guidelines
Provision of Familiar, Meaningful Sensory Input

- Collect data from any person who knows the patient. Include such areas as musical tastes, favorite radio stations, hobbies.
- Have as much care given, as much as possible, by the same people.
- Encourage family and friends to visit and communicate.
- Provide instruction and encouragement to family and friends about approaching the unresponsive patient.
- Use simple conversation about everyday activities during your care.
- Provide security information (time and place orientation, explanation of treatment and procedures).

---

motor- and sensory-coordinated responses cannot be elicited. Using the term unresponsive helps remove the connotation of lack of awareness. This paves the way for providing therapeutic sensory input to unresponsive patients.

To provide intentional, meaningful sensory stimulation, the nurse must carefully collect a nursing history. The astute nurse looks for clues and information to make it easier for the patient to keep in contact with the familiar world. Other ways of creating a structured and familiar environment include having care given, as much as possible, by the same person on each shift. Encouraging family and friends to visit and to communicate provides further meaningful sensory stimulation.

Family and friends need instruction and encouragement about approaching the unresponsive patient. The nurse should let them know that they may speak to and then touch the patient. The nurse should communicate to them that it is not only all right but also very desirable for them to touch the patient's hand, arm, or face or to kiss the patient if it is part of their usual relationship (and does not interfere with any equipment attached to the patient). The nurse should not assume that loved ones standing at the bedside know that they may touch the unresponsive person. Most visitors must be given permission and instruction.

One of the most agonizing feelings is that of uselessness on the part of a family member or friend at the bedside of an unresponsive loved one. The scene of a mother, father, husband, wife, or other close relative standing at the bedside and staring with a variety of emotions at the unresponsive patient is an opportunity for intervention. A simple direction or, in some cases, encouragement to touch the patient's hand and talk may bring a look of relief and gratitude to their faces. With further assistance concerning what to say to the patient, visitors can be very effective in diminishing sensory deprivation by discussing familiar people or subjects normally of interest to the patient. The value of conversation about everyday activities is pointed out vividly in the following patient care study.

While caring for a patient in her late 50s who was comatose as a result of metastatic carcinoma of the brain, I carried on a one-sided conversation about many things, including a daily introduction of myself, explanations of care to be given, and discussion of the day and the weather. There was no perceptible response from the patient. Her condition appeared to be slowly deteriorating. I lost contact with her after 4 days because of an assignment change.

While boarding a train about 2 months later, I was approached by a woman on crutches who called me by name and asked if I were a nurse. I answered yes and eventually recognized her as that patient. Our discussion revealed much about our initial relationship. The patient expressed how she had felt during the days she lay in the hospital bed, totally defenseless and at the mercy of those on the nursing team. She said it was very important to her that I had identified myself and talked to her each day.

Of particular interest to the patient was information about when I would leave and when I would return. When I said I would be leaving for another assignment, she cried, she said, because she anticipated receiving no further information about the outside world. The patient recalled much more about the interaction than I did.

Security Information

Security information helps prevent unnecessary anxiety and disorientation, particularly for people with altered levels of consciousness or memory. It includes information about the month, date, year, time of day, and place. It also includes explanation of treatments and procedures. This is particularly important for patients with altered levels of consciousness due to trauma, drugs, or toxicity. The nurse encourages orientation to date and time not only by including the information in conversation, but also by providing large-faced clocks that are readily visible to the patient and calendars that display the day, month, and year in large figures. These simple items increase the patient's comfort by providing information that most people take for granted. It is also necessary to provide this information because an assessment of the patient's state of orientation is often based on answers to questions concerning time and place.

Because many patients cope by withdrawing, the nurse should anticipate a delayed response after calling the patient's name, and provide repetition to orient the patient to time, date, and place. In addition to the voices of the nursing staff, a familiar person's voice can be very helpful in providing such information.

Noise Control

A study of psychosocial parameters in ICUs revealed that noise was a major patient concern. The specific noises patients reported were those from personnel and the sound of chairs squeaking on the floor. Night was reported to be the noisiest time. Suggestions to reduce noise included in-creasing staff awareness of the sources of noise, posting signs, and using drapes and carpeting to muffle sounds.[4]

Hospital personnel can reduce the amount of noise they create, and nursing staff can control the general environmental stimuli, with the exception of some equipment essential to life-support systems. Nurses may be able to control various sounds on monitors that have light alarms instead of sound alarms. Machines that make continuous noise (eg, beeping cardiac monitors, cycling respirators) should not be kept within earshot of patients who are not using them. If individual soundproofed patient units are not provided, at least one unit should be available for use by all patients who are on noisy life-support systems.

Rest and Sleep

For most people, a quiet environment is a prerequisite for falling and staying asleep, progressing from one sleep stage to another, and reaching the later REM sleep stage.[5] Therefore, unnecessary environmental noise should be controlled. Visiting hours should be adjusted to allow for longer periods of rest. For example, allowing visitors a few minutes with the patient every hour makes it impossible to have 70 to 120 uninterrupted minutes to complete a sleep cycle. Instead, longer periods of visiting time can be provided during the nonsleeping hours. Families usually acknowledge the need for their ill member to sleep and can work out an acceptable arrangement for sharing time with the patient.

Rest periods for the patient should be provided with the same emphasis as that given to assessing cardiac status and other aggressive physical measures of care. Some patients are receptive to wearing darkened eye shades (or eye masks) and ear plugs to shut out light and sound and promote rest.

Reality Orientation

Reality orientation requires a rigid, repetitive regimen of giving the security information described earlier at predetermined times around the clock. A concerted effort by the nurses to help the patient achieve reality orientation must be started immediately as a primary treatment, regardless of the cause of symptoms. The monotony of the procedure may make nurses want to give up the regimen when there is no positive response after a few days. However, the regimen should continue until the patient can repeat the information on request. After a few days, the nurse should preface the procedure by acknowledging that the same information has been restated many times, and stressing the necessity of repeating it until the patient is able to repeat it. In addition, the nurse should do the following:

- Answer questions in short simple sentences.
- Demonstrate things concretely and nonverbally.
- Tell the patient if the nurse does not understand him or her.
- Avoid encouraging the disorientation.
- Orient using visual props, such as clocks and calendars.

Considerations for the Older Patient
Possessions

A visit to the home or room of an older person reveals the presence of multiple treasures on walls, tables, and shelves, including pictures, books, and knickknacks. These items, which often depict experiences and relationships, develop increased value for the older person as years pass. When older adults must reduce the size of their living quarters, they take as many treasured possessions as possible. Some personal treasures may even accompany them during an acute care hospital stay. People usually appreciate the health professional's awareness that personal belongings have significance and bring familiarity and comfort.

Other nursing actions that may foster orientation include spending time with the patient, encouraging socialization with family and friends, positioning the bed so the patient can see outside, and possibly turning on the radio or television.

Personal Space Control

Nurses can provide patients with some control over their personal space by practicing common courtesies, such as knocking on the door before entering, asking permission to perform a procedure or inspect a dressing, and using covers and curtains to provide some privacy.

There are also methods to extend the boundaries of a patient's personal space. Radio, television, and telephones are examples that can be used in some ICU settings. The availability of small television sets or radios with earplugs for sound control and of telephones with wall jacks makes it more feasible to use these items in an ICU. A telephone call from a special person may do more than any medication to help a patient relax. Certainly the use of earphones to enjoy a favorite program helps counteract the adverse effects of the strange sounds of the ICU.

Clinical Applicability Challenges

Self-Challenge: Critical Thinking

1. *Evaluate the patient care environment in which you practice for potential environmental stressors.*

2. *Defend the hypothesis that variations in thermoregulatory mechanisms are such that once-a-day temperatures should suffice for fever detection.*

Study Questions

1. Sensory deprivation
   a. will not be a problem for a patient for at least 24 hours.
   b. is a term used to identify symptoms that occur related to a reduction in the quantity or quality of sensory input.
   c. does not occur in a patient with normal defense mechanisms.
   d. is not likely to be a problem in an ICU because there is activity and sound most of the time.

2. The hospital phenomenon is best described as
   a. an ideal environment for anyone who is ill because it is conducive to rest and recuperation.
   b. a situation in which stress is limited for patients because of the structure of the environment.
   c. a combination of sensory deprivation and sensory overload related to the environment.
   d. the desirable control of aspects of patient care by the health care team.

3. Symptoms of acute confusion include
   a. unconsciousness.
   b. disorganized thinking that has worsened over years.
   c. visual hallucinations, restlessness, and fluctuations in the level of awareness.
   d. impaired remote memory.

REFERENCES

1. Curtis GC, Zuckerman M: A psychopathological reaction precipitated by sensory deprivation. Am J Psychiatry 125:255–260, 1968
2. Broughton RJ: Chronobiological aspects and models of sleep and napping. In Dinges D, Broughton R (eds): Sleep and Alertness, pp 72–73. New York, Raven Press, 1989
3. Davis-Sharts J: The elder and critical care: Sleep and mobility issues. Nurs Clin North Am 24:755–767, 1989
4. Williams M, Murphy JD: Noise in critical care units: A quality assurance approach. J Nurs Care Qual 6:53–59, 1991
5. Topf M: Effects of personal control over hospital noise on sleep. Res Nurs Health 15:19–28, 1992

BIBLIOGRAPHY

Davis AE, White JJ: Innovative sensory input for the comatose brain-injured patient. Crit Care Nurs Clin North Am 7(2):351–361, 1885
Evans JC, French DG: Sleep intensive care settings. Dimensions of Critical Care Nursing 14(4):189–199, 1995
Felver L: Patient-environment interactions in critical care. Crit Care Nurs Clin North Am 7(2):327–335, 1995
Foreman MD, Zane D: Nursing strategies for acute confusion in elders. Am J Nurs 96(4):44–52, 1996
Luzure LL, Braum M: Increasing patient control of family visiting in the coronary care unit. American Journal of Critical Care 4(2):157–164, 1995
Parker KP: Promoting sleep and rest in critically ill patients. Crit Care Nurs Clin North Am 7(2):337–349, 1995
Pope DS: Music, noise and the human voice in the nurse-patient environment. Image 27(4):291–296, 1995
Rushton CH: Creating and ethical practice environment: A focus on advocacy. Crit Care Nurs Clin North Am 7(2):389–397, 1995
Southwell MT, Wistow G: Sleep in hospitals at night: Are patients' needs being met? J Adv Nurs 21(6):1101–1109, 1995

Relieving Pain and Providing Comfort

OBJECTIVES

Based on the content in this chapter, the reader should be able to:

- Explain the physiological consequences of undertreated pain.
- Compare and contrast at least five pharmacological options for pain management in the critically ill patient.
- Discuss four nonpharmacological interventions for alleviating pain and anxiety.
- Summarize at least three factors that have contributed to the undertreatment of pain in the critically ill.
- Discuss the AHCPR guidelines for pain management.

*I*ncreased attention has been placed on pain relief needs of critically ill patients. The American Association of Critical Care Nurses (AACN) has identified pain as a research priority for this decade. In 1997, AACN began Thunder Project II, a research project that studies pain perceptions and responses of patients in relation to specific clinical procedures. The study involves a multidimensional pain assessment before and after each procedure and the collection of subjective, objective, and physiological patient data.

Pain is probably the greatest fear of the hospitalized patient and is perhaps the one experience that all patients have in common in the intensive care unit (ICU). Pain becomes a significant issue for ICU nurses because it is often undertreated. Given the life-threatening nature of the ICU patient's illness or injury, pain relief is sometimes relegated to low priority.[1] Efforts to provide pain relief and comfort measures can be complicated by the fact that critical care nurses must sometimes carry out procedures or treatments that cause pain to the patient.

Recent research documents that ICU patients receive significantly less narcotics than are actually ordered.[2-6] In one study,[3] analgesic orders were written nonspecifically, intending to provide flexible dosing guidelines for nursing staff. On average, only 22% to 52% of the mean ordered dose of analgesic was administered. Nurses may be overly concerned about creating problems, such as hemodynamic and respiratory compromise, oversedation, or drug addiction. To minimize these concerns and provide effective pain control, the critical care nurse needs a clear understanding of concepts related to pain assessment and management. This chapter provides an overview of key concepts related to the management of acute pain and discomfort in the critically ill adult patient.

■ AHCPR GUIDELINES FOR ACUTE PAIN MANAGEMENT

In response to the widespread problems in providing adequate pain relief for all patient populations, the Agency for Health Care Policy and Research (AHCPR) was established in 1989. AHCPR's first set of clinical practice guidelines, dealing with acute pain management, was developed in 1992.

The AHCPR guidelines evolved from four main goals[7]:
1. Reduce the incidence and severity of acute postoperative and posttraumatic pain.
2. Educate patients about the need to communicate unrelieved pain so that they can receive prompt evaluation and effective treatment.
3. Enhance patient comfort and satisfaction.
4. Contribute to decreased postoperative complications and in some cases, shorter hospital stays following surgical procedures.

The AHCPR guidelines encourage a proactive, interdisciplinary approach to pain management with patient and family involvement whenever possible. They also incorporate both pharmacological and nonpharmacological interventions with specific recommendations based on research data. Nurses and their health care colleagues now have a research-based, coherent model for pain management. These guidelines are the basis for interventions recommended in this chapter.

■ PAIN IN THE CRITICALLY ILL

Previously it was thought that critically ill patients were unable to remember their pain experiences due to the acute nature of the illness or injury.[8] Recent research, however, demonstrates that ICU patients remember pain experiences and describe their pain as being moderate to severe in intensity.[5,6] Multiple factors inherent in the ICU environment affect the patient's pain experience: anxiety, sleep deprivation, unfamiliar and unpleasant surroundings, loss of control, and separation from family or significant others.[9] The effects of each of these factors increase when they are experienced together.[8] For example, pain and sleep deprivation act in a synergistic fashion to compound each other.

Pain Description

Pain is a complex, subjective phenomenon with several characteristics: intensity, timing, duration, quality, impact, and personal meaning.[9] It is a protective mechanism,

causing one either to withdraw from or avoid the source of pain and seek assistance or treatment. The International Society for the Study of Pain defined pain as *"an unpleasant sensory and emotional experience associated with actual or potential tissue damage or described in terms of such damage."*[10] McCaffery[11] provides an operational definition of pain that considers the subjectiveness and individuality of the pain experience and is based on the premise that the individual experiencing the pain is the true authority:

"Pain is whatever the experiencing person says it is, existing whenever he or she says it does."

The pain most ICU patients experience is caused by an illness, injury, or therapeutic or diagnostic procedure.[12] This type of pain is classified as *acute*, because it has an identified cause and is expected to resolve within a given time frame. For example, the pain experienced during endotracheal suctioning or a dressing change can be expected to end when the treatment is completed. Similarly, pain at an incision or area of injury is expected to cease once healing has occurred.

In contrast, *chronic* pain is caused by physiological mechanisms that are less well understood. Chronic pain differs from acute pain in terms of etiology and expected duration. It may last for an indefinite period and may be difficult, if not impossible, to treat completely.[9]

Physiological Consequences of Pain

In addition to causing stress and suffering, pain produces many harmful physiological effects.[8,13] The autonomic nervous system responds to pain by causing vasoconstriction and increased heart rate and contractility. This increases myocardial workload and oxygen use, both of which can cause or exacerbate myocardial ischemia in the already compromised critically ill person. Respiratory alterations resulting from pain include splinting, decreased respiratory effort, and reduced pulmonary volume and flow. Pulmonary complications, such as atelectasis and pneumonia, can result. Pain also negatively affects the musculoskeletal system by causing muscle contractions, spasms, and rigidity. Because movement increases pain, the patient will be hesitant to move, cough, or breathe deeply. Unrelieved pain impairs the immune system and can delay the healing process after injury.

It has been suggested that patients who are pain free have better outcomes than those stressed by unrelieved pain.[13] The physiological benefits of effective pain relief are summarized in the accompanying display.

Cultural Influences

Many cultures have strong beliefs about pain that influence its assessment and management. A complete discussion of cultural variations and their effect on the pain experience is beyond the scope of this chapter. However, it is important for the critical care nurse to consider the patient's cultural background, because it can significantly influence the patient's pain experience in terms of the following[14]:

- Meaning attached to the pain
- Emotional responses to pain
- Perceived cause of the pain (punishment, lifestyle, fate)
- Reported pain intensity
- How the pain should be treated
- Who should treat the pain

"A key strategy in caring for a patient from a different culture who is in pain is to establish a relationship by listening, showing respect and allowing the patient to help formulate and choose treatment options."[14] The ICU nurse must assess the patient's needs and customs as sensitively as possible. This helps to identify treatment options. Whenever possible, the patient's beliefs and preferences should be respected.[7] For example, a patient's cultural background may be associated with certain spiritual or religious interventions or nontraditional therapies that can be integrated into the plan of care.

If there is a language barrier that affects communication, a word board consisting of translated words, common needs, and phrases can be kept at the bedside.[15] A translator should be located within the hospital or family to develop a simple yet effective plan for pain assessment and management.[7]

Finally, the ICU nurse must recognize that his or her culture, beliefs, past experiences, and attitudes about pain can influence the process of pain assessment and management.[16,17] These personal beliefs can both negatively and positively affect pain management.[16] To overcome these potential barriers to effective pain management, an objective approach to pain management must be used.

◼ PAIN ASSESSMENT STRATEGIES

Assessment of pain is as important as any method used for treatment. The patient's pain should be assessed at regular intervals to determine the effectiveness of therapy, the presence of side effects, the need for dose adjustment, or the need for supplemental doses to offset procedural pain. Pain should be reassessed at an appropriate interval after pain medication has been administered, for example 30 minutes after an intravenous (IV) dose of morphine.[7] A number of conditions may exist, making assessment of the patient's pain and subsequent treatment difficult:

- Acuity of the patient's condition

Benefits of Pain Relief

- Decreases incidence of pulmonary complications
- Promotes ambulation and prevents immobility-related complications, such as deep vein thrombosis
- Minimizes adverse physiological responses to injury
- Promotes positive nitrogen balance
- Enhances metabolic and immune responses to injury

- Inability to communicate pain due to altered level of consciousness (LOC)
- Restricted or limited movement
- Endotracheal intubation

A common misconception among health care professionals is that they are the most qualified to determine the presence and severity of the patient's pain. Absence of physical signs or behaviors is often incorrectly interpreted as the absence of pain. To perform an effective pain assessment, the critical care nurse must elicit a self-report from the patient. Behavioral observation and changes in physiological parameters should be integrated into the pain assessment, if appropriate.[7,9]

Patient Self-Report

Because pain is a subjective experience, the patient's self-report is the most reliable source of information about the presence and intensity of pain.[7,9] The patient's self-report should be obtained not only at rest, but during routine activity, such as coughing, deep breathing, or moving (eg, turning or ambulating).[7] Nurses working with the critically ill frequently are more attuned to objective indicators of pain than to the patient's self-report. The ICU nurse must accept the patient's description of pain as valid. In the conscious and coherent patient, behavioral cues or physiological indicators should never take precedence over the self-report of pain. Behavioral and physiological manifestations of pain are extremely variable and may be minimal or absent, despite the presence of excruciating pain.[7,18]

In assessing pain quality, the nurse should elicit a specific description of the patient's pain, such as "burning," "crushing," "stabbing," "dull," or "sharp." These terms help pinpoint the cause of the pain.

Pain scales and rating instruments based on the patient's self-report can help determine specific characteristics of the pain. Numeric rating and visual analog scales are used to measure pain intensity. With these scales, the patient is asked to choose a number or word that best describes the amount of pain he or she is experiencing. The simplest method is to use a 0-to-10 scale to measure pain intensity. The patient is asked to rate the pain with 0 being no pain and 10 being the worst pain imaginable.[19] Use of these scales may be limited with ICU patients who are unable to speak or move.

Pictures or word boards can also facilitate communication about the patient's pain. The board should include open-ended questions, such as "Do you have pain?" "Where is the pain located?" "How bad is your pain?" and "What helps your pain?" Developing a simple system of eye movements ("blink once for yes and twice for no") or finger movements can also be effective.[1,9]

Pain assessment and subsequent treatment are dilemmas if the patient is unable to use any of the above methods to verbalize or indicate that he or she is in pain. In this situation, it may be appropriate to observe for the behavioral cues or physiological indicators discussed in the next section. However, the absence of physiological indicators or behavioral cues should *never* be interpreted as absence of pain.[7,9,16] AHCPR guidelines recommend that if the procedure, surgery, or condition is believed to be associated with pain, the presence of pain should be assumed and treated appropriately.[7]

Observation

Specific behavioral manifestations may be present in the patient in pain. Protective behaviors, such as guarding, withdrawal, and avoidance of movement, defend against painful stimuli. Attempts by the patient to seek relief, such as rubbing the area, changing positions, or requesting pain medications, are palliative behaviors. Crying, moaning, or screaming are affective behaviors and reflect an emotional response to pain. Changes in facial expressions may also indicate pain.

Patients who are unable to speak may use eye or facial expressions or movement of hands or legs to communicate their pain. Restlessness or agitation may be seen in the unresponsive patient. However, nonverbal cues are difficult to interpret as specific indicators for the presence of pain and its location.[9] In some situations, family input may be helpful in interpreting specific behavioral manifestations of pain that they observed before the patient's hospitalization.

Physiological Parameters

Critical care nurses are skilled in assessing the patient's physical status in terms of changes in blood pressure, heart rate, or respirations. Therefore, it could be reasoned that observation of the physiological effects of pain will assist in pain assessment. With critically ill patients, however, it may be difficult to attribute these physiological changes specifically to pain rather than another cause.[9] For example, an unexpected increase in the severity and intensity of the patient's pain associated with hypotension, tachycardia, or fever must be evaluated immediately. These findings may signal the development of life-threatening complications, such as wound dehiscence, infection, or deep vein thrombosis.

Pain assessment is an ongoing process. In addition to the initial pain assessment, assessment after pain management interventions and prior to procedures is essential. After pharmacological therapy, pain reassessment should correspond to the time of onset or peak effect of the drug administered and the time the analgesic effect is expected to be dissipated. Response to therapy is best measured as a change from the patient's baseline pain level. Occasionally there may be obvious discrepancies among the patient's self-report and behavioral and physiological manifestations. For example, one patient may report pain as a 2 out of 10, while being tachycardic, diaphoretic, and splinting with respirations. Another patient may give a self-report of 8 while smiling. These discrepancies can be due to use of diversionary activities, coping skills, beliefs about pain, cultural background, or fears of becoming addicted or being bothersome to the nursing staff. When these situations occur, they should be discussed with the patient, stressing the importance of a factual self-report.[7] Any misconceptions or knowledge deficits should be addressed and the pain treated according to the patient's self-report.

Documentation

As with any other nursing assessment, pain assessment must be documented. Clear documentation with the nurse's initials and recording of ongoing pain assessment data communicates valuable information to other staff members. Using special flow sheets can promote consistency in the assessment, documentation, and management of pain. An example of a pain assessment and intervention flow sheet appears in Figure 5–1. Computer systems are also available for documentation of pain management.

▩ PAIN MANAGEMENT

The nurse plays an important role in providing pain relief. Nursing management of pain includes physical, cognitive, behavioral, and pharmacological measures. In addition to administering medications or providing alternative therapies, the nurse's role involves measuring the patient's response to those therapies. Because pain may diminish or the pain pattern may change, some therapy adjustments may be needed before improvements are seen. Some guidelines for nursing interventions are listed in the accompanying display.

Pharmacological Interventions

In general, the ideal method of analgesia should allow adequate serum drug levels to be achieved and maintained quickly and easily. Medications should be easily titrated based on the patient's response, and the drug should be quickly eliminated when analgesia is no longer needed. Most clinicians agree that when using a numerical scale for assessment, pain medications should be titrated according to the following goals:

- The patient's reported pain score is less than his or her own predetermined pain management goal (eg, 3 on a scale of 1–10).

A. LOCATION
Chart location of pain on area of figure using letters of the alphabet.

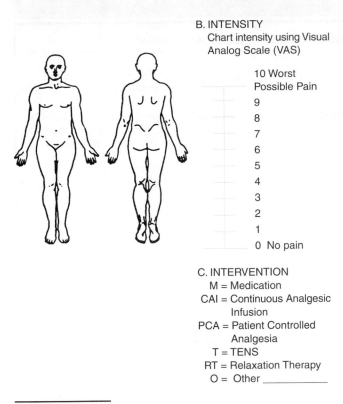

B. INTENSITY
Chart intensity using Visual Analog Scale (VAS)

10 Worst Possible Pain
9
8
7
6
5
4
3
2
1
0 No pain

C. INTERVENTION
M = Medication
CAI = Continuous Analgesic Infusion
PCA = Patient Controlled Analgesia
T = TENS
RT = Relaxation Therapy
O = Other _____

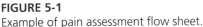

FIGURE 5-1
Example of pain assessment flow sheet.

- Sedation or significant respiratory depression is absent.[7]

The efficacy of analgesia depends on the presence of an adequate and consistent serum drug level. Regardless of the method being used, medications should be administered around the clock for acute pain.[7] The traditional "PRN" analgesic order is a major barrier to effective pain control in all patient populations. The PRN order allows the nurse to administer a dose of analgesic only when the patient requests it and only after a certain time interval has elapsed since the previous dose. Invariably, a delay occurs between the time of the request and the time the medication is actually administered. In some cases, this delay can be up to 1 hour. The PRN order poses another problem when the patient is asleep. As serum drug levels decrease, the patient is suddenly awakened by severe pain, and a greater amount of the drug is needed to achieve adequate serum levels.

NONSTEROIDAL ANTI-INFLAMMATORY DRUGS

Nonsteroidal anti-inflammatory drugs (NSAIDs) decrease pain by inhibiting the synthesis of inflammatory mediators (prostaglandin, histamine, and bradykinin) at the site of injury and effectively relieve pain without causing sedation, respiratory depression, or problems with bowel or bladder function.[7]AHCPR guidelines suggest that NSAIDs be the

initial choice for managing mild to moderate postoperative pain. When NSAIDs are used in combination with opioids, the opioid dose can often be reduced and still produce effective analgesia. This decreases the incidence of opioid-related side effects.[19,20]

Various NSAIDs and their recommended doses are listed in Table 5–1. Most NSAIDs are available only for oral use, which prohibits their use in the patient who is NPO. Presently ketorolac is the only NSAID approved for parenteral use. It is used frequently in the ICU setting as a short-term (less than 5 days) adjuvant to opioids and when opioids are contraindicated, such as head injury or neurosurgery.[7,21] Indomethacin is available in suppository form and can be combined with opioids to provide effective pain relief. Indomethacin should not be used alone for moderate to severe pain.[7]

NSAIDs are associated with risk of gastrointestinal bleeding and platelet dysfunction; these potential complications limit their use in the critically ill patient. For example, ketorolac is contraindicated in patients with recent gastrointestinal bleeding, actual or potential renal impairment, or bleeding disorders.[21]

OPIOIDS

Opioids have been the pharmacological cornerstone of postoperative pain management. They provide pain relief by binding to various receptor sites in the spinal cord, central nervous system, and peripheral nervous system, thus changing the perception of pain.

Morphine sulfate and fentanyl are most commonly used in the ICU setting because, compared with other available opioids, they have a quick onset and short duration of effect (Table 5–2). Other opioids in use include meperidine, hydromorphone, codeine, oxycodone, and methadone. Meperidine is the least potent opioid and is administered in the largest doses. For example, to produce a level of analge-

TABLE 5-1   CLINICAL APPLICATION: Drug Therapy
Dosing Data for NSAIDs

Drug	Usual Adult Dose	Usual Pediatric Dose*	Comments
Oral NSAIDs			
Acetaminophen	650–975 mg q4h	10–15 mg/kg q4h	Lacks the peripheral anti-inflammatory activity of other NSAIDs
Aspirin	650–975 mg q4h	10–15 mg/kg q4h†	The standard against which other NSAIDs are compared. Inhibits platelet aggregation; may cause postoperative bleeding
Choline magnesium trisalicylate (Trilisate)	1,000–1,500 mg bid	25 mg/kg bid	May have minimal antiplatelet activity; also available as oral liquid
Diflunisal (Dolobid)	1,000 mg initial dose followed by 500 mg q12h		
Etodolac (Lodine)	200–400 mg q6–8h		
Fenoprofen calcium (Nalfon)	200 mg q4–6h		
Ibuprofen (Motrin, others)	400 mg q4–6h	10 mg/kg q6–8h	Available as several brand names and as generic; also available as oral suspension
Ketoprofen (Orudis)	25–75 mg q6–8h		
Magnesium salicylate	650 mg q4h		Many brands and generic forms available
Meclofenamate sodium (Meclomen)	50 mg q4–6h		
Mefenamic acid (Ponstel)	250 mg q6h		
Naproxen (Naprosyn)	500 mg initial dose followed by 250 mg q6–8h	5 mg/kg q12h	Also available as oral liquid
Naproxen sodium (Anaprox)	550 mg initial dose followed by 275 mg q6–8h		
Salsalate (Disalcid, others)	500 mg q4h		May have minimal antiplatelet activity
Sodium salicylate	325–650 mg q3–4h		Available in generic form from several distributors
Parenteral NSAID			
Ketorolac tromethamine (Toradol)	• 30 or 60 mg IM initial dose followed by 15 or 30 mg q6h • Oral dose following IM dosage: 10 mg q6–8h • IV dose: 30 mg IV q6h		Intravenous and intramuscular dose not to exceed 5 days

From: Agency for Health Care Policy and Research: Acute Pain Management: Operative and Medical Procedures and Trauma: Clinical Practice Guideline No. 1, US Department of Health and Human Services, pp 18, 19. 1992
Note: Only the above NSAIDs have FDA approval for use as simple analgesics, but clinical experience has been gained with other drugs as well.
*Drug recommendations are limited to NSAIDs for which pediatric dosing experience is available.
†Contraindicated in presence of fever or other evidence of viral illness.

TABLE 5-2 CLINICAL APPLICATION:
Drug Therapy
Comparison of Fentanyl and Morphine

	Fentanyl	Morphine
Dose (mg)		
IV	0.1	11–20
E	0.1	2–5
Time to peak effect (minutes)		
IV	3	30
E	10–20	30–60
Duration (hours)		
IV	1	4
E	2–3	8–24

From: Willens JS: Giving fentanyl for pain outside the OR. Am J Nurs 94:24–29, 1994
IV, intravenous route; E, epidural route

sia comparable to 10 mg of morphine every 4 hours, 100 to 150 mg of meperidine every 3 hours would be needed. Meperidine is commonly underdosed and given at intervals too infrequent to be effective.[7] Meperidine is contraindicated in patients with compromised renal function due to the risk of normeperidine toxicity. Normeperidine, the active metabolite of meperidine, is eliminated by the kidneys. Accumulation of normeperidine can cause central nervous system excitatory effects, such as irritability, delirium, or convulsions.[20] For these reasons, meperidine should be avoided, especially in the critically ill patient.

Dosing Guidelines

Dosing guidelines for opioid analgesics are presented in Table 5–3. Opioid dosage varies depending on the individual patient, the method of administration, and the pharmacokinetics of the drug. Adequate pain relief will occur once a minimum serum level of the opioid has been achieved. Each patient's optimal serum level will be different, and this level can change as pain intensity changes. Therefore, the dosing and titration of opioids must be individualized, and the patient's response and any undesirable effects, such as respiratory depression or oversedation, must be closely assessed. If the patient has previously received an opioid (eg, preoperatively), doses should be adjusted above the previous required dose to achieve an optimal effect.[7] Factors such as age, individual pain tolerance, coexisting disease(s), type of surgical procedure, and the concomitant use of sedatives warrant consideration as well. Older patients may be more sensitive to the effects of opioids; decreasing the initial opioid dose and slow dose titration are recommended for them.[20]

Side Effects

Opioids cause undesirable side effects, such as constipation, urinary retention, sedation, respiratory depression, and nausea. These side effects occur regardless of the route of administration and represent a major drawback to their use. Opioid-related side effects are best managed in the following ways[1,7,20]:

- *Decreasing the opioid dose:* This is the most effective strategy, because it is directed at the *cause* of the side effect. Side effects are usually seen with excessively high serum levels of the drug. Decreasing the opioid dose can alleviate the side effect while still providing effective pain relief. If the patient's pain is adequately managed, the opioid dose can be decreased by 25% to 50%, depending on the severity of the adverse effect.[20]
- *Avoiding PRN dosing:* When opioids are administered on a PRN basis, fluctuating serum drug levels occur, causing a greater tendency toward sedation and respiratory depression. Around-the-clock administration of analgesics, including opioids, is recommended.
- *Adding an NSAID to the pain management plan:* Using an NSAID in addition to an opioid can decrease the amount of opioid needed, still provide effective pain relief, and decrease opioid-related side effects.

Medications can be given to minimize or alleviate some side effects (eg, stool softeners for constipation, antihistamines for pruritus, and antiemetics for nausea). Pasero and McCaffery,[20] however, caution that medications commonly prescribed to treat the opioid-related adverse effects can actually cause other adverse effects. For example, promethazine, a commonly prescribed antiemetic, can cause hypotension, restlessness, tremors, and extrapyramidal effects in the older patient.

Respiratory depression is a life-threatening complication of opioid administration. Significant respiratory depression can be seen as a rate of less than 10 breaths/min, shallow respirations, or an irregular respiratory pattern. Prevention of respiratory depression is preferable to having to treat it. Any variation from the patient's baseline respiratory rate and pattern must be evaluated. When a patient is receiving opioids, it is important to monitor sedation level, because a decrease in LOC can precede the development of respiratory depression.[19,22] Sedation that impairs the patient's ability to cooperate in his or her own care, such as deep breathing or ambulation, should be avoided.[23] An example of a sedation scale used in clinical practice is shown in Table 5–4.

The incidence of significant respiratory depression associated with opioids administered in therapeutic doses is 0.09%.[19] If serious respiratory depression does occur, naloxone (Narcan), a pure opioid antagonist that reverses the effects of opioids, should be administered. The recommended procedure for administering IV naloxone is as follows:

1. Dilute 0.4 mg naloxone in 10 mL of normal saline.
2. Slowly infuse the solution at a rate of 0.5 mL over 2 minutes.

The dose of naloxone is titrated to effect—which means reversing the oversedation and respiratory depression, not reversing analgesia. This usually occurs within 1 to 2 min-

TABLE 5-3   CLINICAL APPLICATION: Drug Therapy
Opioid Analgesics Commonly Used for Severe Pain

Name	Equianalgesic Dose (mg)	Starting Oral Dose — Adults (mg) / Children (mg/kg)	Comments	Precautions and Contraindications
Morphine-like agonists				
Morphine	Oral: 30† Parenteral: 10*	Adult: 15–30 Child: 0.3	Standard of comparison for narcotic analgesics; sustained-release preparations (MS Contin, Roxanol-SR) release drug over 8–12h	For all opioids, caution in patients with impaired ventilation, bronchial asthma, increased intracranial pressure, liver failure
Hydromorphone (Dilaudid)	Oral: 7.5 Parenteral: 1.5*	Adult: 4–8 Child: 0.06	Slightly shorter duration than morphine	
Oxycodone	Oral: 30 Parenteral: —	Adult: 15–30 Child: 0.3		
Methadone (Dolophine)	Oral: 20 Parenteral: 10*	Adult: 5–10 Child: 0.2	Good oral potency; long plasma half-life (24–36 h)	Accumulates with repetitive dosing, causing excessive sedation (on days 2–5)
Levorphanol (Levo-Dromoran)	Oral: 4 Parenteral: 2*	Adult: 2–4 Child: 0.04	Long plasma half-life (12–16h)	Accumulates on days 2–3
Fentanyl	Oral: — Parenteral: 0.1*	— —	Transdermal fentanyl (Duragesic) 25–50 µg/h roughly equivalent to 30 mg sustained-release morphine q8h	Because of skin reservoir of drug, 12-h delay in onset and offset of transdermal patch; fever increases dose rate
Oxymorphone (Numorphan)	Oral: — Parenteral: 1*	— —	5 mg rectal suppository = 5 mg morphine IM	Like IM morphine
Meperidine (Demerol)	Oral: 300 Parenteral: 75*	Not recommended	Slightly shorter acting than morphine	Normeperidine (toxic metabolite) accumulates with repetitive dosing, causing CNS excitation; avoid in patients with impaired renal function or who are receiving monoamine oxidase inhibitors**
Mixed agonist-antagonists				
Nalbuphine (Nubain)	Oral: — Parenteral: 10*	— —	Not available orally; not scheduled under Controlled Substances Act	Incidence of psychotomimetic effects lower than with pentazocine; may precipitate withdrawal in narcotic-dependent patients
Butorphanol (Stadol)	Oral: — Parenteral: 2*	— —	Like nalbuphine	Like nalbuphine
Dezocine (Dalgan)	Oral: — Parenteral: 10*	— —	Like nalbuphine	
Partial agonist				
Buprenorphine (Buprenex)	Oral: 0.4		Not available orally; sublingual preparation not yet in U.S.; less abuse liability than morphine; does not produce psychotomimetic effects	May precipitate withdrawal in narcotic-dependent patients; not readily reversed by naloxone; avoid in labor

*These are standard IM doses for acute pain in adults and also may be used to convert doses for IV infusions and repeated small IV boluses. For single IV boluses, use half the IM dose. IV doses for children > 6 mo = parenteral equianalgesic dose × weight (kg)/100. For babies < 6 mo, see p. 18.
†Some experts argue that 60 mg of oral morphine is the more accurate equivalent dose, and suggest caution in converting patients from high doses of oral morphine to other drugs if the 30-mg equivalent is used (see p. 19 and p. 21).
**Irritating to tissues with repeated IM injection.
Source: American Pain Society: Principles of Analgesic Use in the Treatment of Acute Pain and Cancer Pain (3rd Ed.), Glenview, IL, 1992

TABLE 5-4
Sedation Scale

Score	Patient Response
S	Asleep, easily aroused
1	Awake and alert
2	Occasionally drowsy, easy to arouse
3	Frequently drowsy, arousable, drifts off to sleep during conversation
4	Somnolent, minimal or no response to stimuli

From: Pasero C, McCaffery M: Avoiding opioid-induced respiratory depression. Am J Nurs April: 25–31, 1994

utes. Naloxone can also be given by the intramuscular (IM) or subcutaneous routes; the onset of action by these routes is within 2 to 5 minutes.[19] After giving naloxone, continue to observe the patient closely for oversedation and respiratory depression, because the half-life of naloxone (1½–2 hours) is shorter than most opioids.

Addiction

Some nurses are concerned with the potential for addiction associated with opioid use and fail to differentiate among addiction, pseudoaddiction, tolerance, and physical dependence. According to Salerno, "Patients in pain respond differently to an analgesic than drug-seeking individuals who crave opioids for a euphoric effect (*psychologic dependence or addiction*)."[24] In patients taking opioids for pain relief, addiction rarely occurs regardless of the length of time opioids are taken.[15] *Pseudoaddiction* is often mistaken for addiction. Pseudoaddiction develops in patients inadequately treated for pain and is manifested as a pattern of drug-seeking behaviors to obtain adequate pain control. *Tolerance* requires an increase in opioid dose to achieve the same pain relief that was possible at a previous lesser dose. *Physical dependence* is manifested by withdrawal syndrome when the opioid is suddenly stopped or naloxone is administered. Tapering the opioid dose avoids withdrawal. Although tolerance and physical dependence do not occur in all individuals, these are normal physiological responses that should be expected after seven days of opioid administration.[7,24]

Oral Opioids

Oral opioids are easy to use, inexpensive, and provide effective analgesia. The oral route is used infrequently in the ICU setting, however, because most often, the patient is unable to take anything by mouth. Serum drug levels obtained after oral administration of opioids are variable and difficult to titrate. In addition, the transformation of opioids by the liver causes a significant decrease in serum levels. To achieve adequate serum drug levels, the dose of an oral opioid must be three to six times higher than the dose given intravenously.[7,11]

Intramuscular Injections

IM injections should not be used to provide acute pain relief for the critically ill patient for several reasons:

- IM drug absorption is extremely variable in critically ill patients because of alterations in cardiac output and perfusion.
- IM injections are painful.
- Anticipated discomfort associated with the injection increases the patient's anxiety.[25]
- Repeated IM injections can cause muscle and soft-tissue fibrosis.

Intermittent Intravenous Injections

Intravenous administration is the preferred route for opioid therapy, especially when the patient requires short-term pain relief, for example, during procedures such as chest tube removal, diagnostic tests, suctioning, or wound care. IV opioids have the most rapid onset and are easy to administer. With morphine, the time to peak effect is 15 to 30 minutes; for fentanyl, peak effect is achieved within 1 to 5 minutes.[19] However, the duration of analgesia is shorter with intermittent IV injections, and this can cause serum drug levels to fluctuate.

Continuous Intravenous Infusions

This method has many benefits for critically ill patients, especially those who have difficulty communicating their pain because of an altered LOC or an endotracheal tube. Continuous IV infusions are easily initiated and maintain consistent serum drug levels. For continuous IV opioid infusions, fentanyl and morphine are commonly used because of their short elimination half-life (compared with other available opioids). Before starting a continuous IV infusion, an initial IV loading dose(s) is given to achieve an optimal serum level.[26] Appropriate dosing and titration must be individualized, and this can be difficult because many critically ill patients have hepatic or renal dysfunctions that result in decreased metabolism of the opioid. A disadvantage of continuous IV infusions is that pain occurring during painful procedures is not managed unless additional IV bolus injections are given.[26]

Patient-Controlled Analgesia

Patient-controlled analgesia (PCA) is an effective method of pain relief for the critically ill patient who is conscious and able to participate in the pain management therapy.[12,17,23]

The patient-controlled method of opioid administration produces the most optimal serum drug levels, as shown in Figure 5–2. Effective use of PCA is based on the assumption that the patient is the best person to evaluate and manage his or her pain. PCA individualizes pain control therapy and offers the patient greater feelings of control and well-being.

With PCA, the patient self-administers small, frequent IV analgesic doses using a programmable infusion device. Most often, morphine sulfate or fentanyl will be used. The PCA device only administers the opioid within a specific time period; this helps prevent oversedation and respiratory

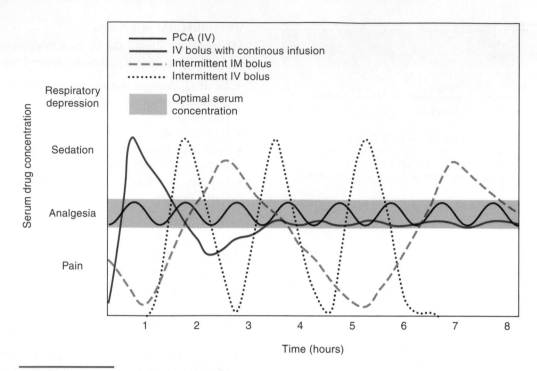

FIGURE 5-2

Comparison of serum drug levels of narcotics according to method of administration. From: Lubenow TR, Ivankovich AD: Patient-controlled analgesia for postoperative pain. Critical Care Nursing Clinics of North America 3(1):35–41, 1990.

depression.[25] The patient should not become oversedated if proper dosing, titration, and assessment tools are used.

Patient-controlled analgesia can also be a valuable pain management option for the chemically dependent patient. Pain management is a complex problem in this patient population. PCA can be used safely with appropriate PCA device programming (lockout interval, dose limits) and when the device is "tamper resistant." For the chemically dependent patient, PCA doses must be titrated to achieve the same analgesic effect as for a nonaddicted patient.[7] Research shows that chemically dependent patients are able to use PCA successfully and that they tend to use the same amount of opioids as nonaddicted patients.[27]

If the patient is physically or cognitively unable to use "conventional" PCA, other adaptations can be made if appropriate. For example, the PCA pump can be activated by a designated family member. This family member will need thorough education in terms of how to assess for the presence of pain, how to administer the medication, and how to assess for oversedation and respiratory depression. In some instances, the PCA pump can be activated by the patient's primary nurse.[27]

If the patient is being started on PCA and has not received any other opioids, a loading dose should be given to achieve adequate serum drug levels. Two methods of PCA delivery are available: intermittent-on-demand (PCA) and continuous IV plus intermittent-on-demand (PCA plus continuous). With the PCA method, the device is programmed to administer the analgesia only when the patient requests it and only after a specific time has elapsed. With PCA plus continuous, the patient receives a continuous background infusion in addition to the PCA doses given on demand. Although both methods provide individualized therapy and consistent analgesia levels, the PCA plus continuous method offers the benefit of maintaining analgesia while

Insights Into Clinical Research

Ashburn MA, et al: Respiratory-related critical events with intravenous patient-controlled analgesia. Clinical Journal of Pain 10:52–56, 1994

This study, which found 14 critical respiratory-related events among 3,785 patients receiving intravenous patient-controlled analgesia (PCA), underscores the necessity for patient and family education in the area of unauthorized PCA use (ie, family members pressing the PCA button when they think the patient is in pain). Adverse outcomes, including ICU stays with intubation, oxygen, or naloxone required, occurred in four of these study patients. Of the 14 critical events, three resulted from a family member activating the PCA pump. There was one instance of tampering, and the majority of the others were a result of prescribing or programming errors.

Educating patients on the correct use of PCA before initiating the therapy will reduce the chance of family members activating the pump. These same principles hold true for staff members or physicians who may be tempted to push the button when they think the patient is in pain. Only the patient knows the degree of his or her pain, and only the patient should control the amount of medication.

the patient is asleep, particularly if shorter-acting opioids are used.[23]

The physician's order for PCA should include instructions for the parameters listed in the display. The patient's PCA prescription should be individualized and followed by close assessment for relief of pain and for undesirable effects, especially respiratory depression or oversedation.

With PCA, physician orders should also include measures to implement when initial settings fail to provide adequate analgesia or when additional doses are needed during painful procedures. Although the incidence of significant respiratory depression with PCA therapy is low, naloxone should be easily accessible and administered if serious respiratory depression occurs.

Subcutaneous and Rectal Routes of Opioid Administration

In some situations, IV access may be limited or impossible to obtain. When this occurs, continuous subcutaneous infusion, subcutaneous PCA, and rectal opioid administration may be used.

Spinal Opioids

Spinal opioids can provide superior pain management for many patients. Spinal opioids selectively block opioid receptors, while leaving sensation, motor, and sympathetic nervous system function intact. This results in fewer opioid-related side effects than oral, IM, or IV routes of administration. Analgesia from spinal opioids has a longer duration than other routes, and less opioid is needed to achieve effective pain relief.[12] Opioids such as fentanyl or morphine can be given as a single injection in the epidural or intra- thecal space or as intermittent injections, continuous infusions through an epidural catheter, or epidural PCA.[7,12,22]

Epidural Analgesia. Epidural analgesia is noted for providing effective pain relief and improved postoperative pulmonary function. This method is especially beneficial for critically ill patients after thoracic, upper abdominal or peripheral vascular surgery, rib fractures, orthopedic trauma, or postoperative patients with a history of obesity or pulmonary disease.[12,17,28] With epidural analgesia, opioids are administered through a catheter inserted in the spinal canal between the dura mater and vertebral arch. Opioids diffuse across the dura and subarachnoid space and bind with opioid receptor sites.[28]

Intermittent injections may be given before, during, or after a surgical procedure. For more sustained pain relief, continuous epidural infusions are recommended. Patient-controlled epidural analgesia (PCEA) provides many benefits for the critically ill patient and should be used whenever the patient is able to participate in the pain management therapy. For PCEA, the same parameters are used as with IV PCA, except that smaller opioid doses are used.[22]

Contraindications to epidural analgesia include systemic infection/sepsis, bleeding disorders, and increased intracranial pressure.[28]

Preservative-free morphine and fentanyl are most commonly used for epidural analgesia (see Table 5–1), because preservatives can be neurotoxic and may cause severe spinal cord injury. Morphine is more water soluble than fentanyl and thus is more likely to accumulate in the cerebrospinal fluid (CSF) and systemic circulation. With increased accumulation, side effects are more likely. Fentanyl diffuses more quickly to the opioid receptors and causes fewer opioid-related side effects.[12,28]

The most serious complication of epidural analgesia is respiratory depression. Early respiratory depression develops within 2 hours of epidural opioid administration and occurs as the drug is absorbed by the epidural veins into the systemic circulation. Late respiratory depression is seen within 6 to 12 hours and occurs as the opioid diffuses into the CSF and combines with opioid receptors in the respiratory centers.[22,28] Although the incidence of serious respiratory depression is less than 1% with epidural analgesia, respiratory assessments should be performed hourly during the first 24 hours of therapy and every 4 hours thereafter.[22,28] Naloxone should be readily available and administered in the event of serious respiratory depression or respiratory arrest.

Because epidural analgesia is more invasive than the other methods discussed, the patient must be closely monitored for signs of local or systemic infection. The insertion site is covered with a sterile dressing, and the catheter is taped securely. To avoid accidental injection of preservative-containing medications, the epidural catheter, infusion tubing, and pump should be clearly marked. The catheter and dressing are usually removed within 72 hours.[28] Other catheter- and opioid-related complications are detailed in Table 5–5.

Patient-Controlled Analgesia (PCA) Physician's Order

Type of drug: Morphine sulfate and fentanyl are most commonly used.

Method: Intermittent-on-demand (PCA) or continuous IV plus intermittent-on-demand (PCA plus continuous) are the methods used.

Loading dose: Typical order for morphine would be 1–2 mg loading dose IV every 15 minutes until adequate relief is obtained.

PCA dose: This is the amount of medication delivered per patient request. For morphine, PCA dose is usually started between 1 and 3 mg.

Lockout interval: The minimum time between PCA doses is usually between 5 to 15 minutes. The lockout interval prevents the patient from administering additional doses until the lockout interval has elapsed.

Continuous dose (if indicated): For IV morphine sulfate, this dose can range from 1–2 mg/h and is meant to be supplemented by intermittent PCA injections.

RED FLAG · **Table 5-5** Complications and Side Effects of Epidural Analgesia

Side Effect/Complication	Treatment/Nursing Intervention
Respiratory Depression Note: Early respiratory depression occurs within 2 h of opioid administration. Late respiratory depression can be seen within 2–16 h.	• Monitor respiratory status and sedation level q1h during first 24 h of therapy, then q4h. • Notify physician for respiratory rate < 8/min. • Administer naloxone as ordered for severe respiratory depression. • Prepare for airway and respiratory support if necessary: oxygen, head tilt-jaw lift, manual ventilation, endotracheal intubation.
Catheter Migration Catheter may be displaced into the subarachnoid space; this causes a larger fraction of opioid to enter the CSF.	• Assess dressing for integrity, wetness. • Observe patient for increased analgesia, seizures, respiratory depression, changes in LOC, circulatory collapse. • Notify physician immediately for any of the above clinical symptoms; prepare to administer naloxone and support respirations and circulation as needed.
Nausea and Vomiting	• Administer antiemetics as needed. • Small amounts of naloxone (0.08–0.12 mg) titrated over 2–3 min may relieve symptoms without affecting analgesia. • Consider nasogastric tube insertion if indicated.
Urinary Retention	• Monitor intake and output. • Assess for bladder distension or urinary catheter patency. • Insert urinary catheter if indicated.
Pruritus	• Observe patient for rash, wheals, or edema, usually over face and neck area. • Administer antihistamines as ordered. • Small amounts of naloxone (0.08–0.12 mg) titrated over 2–3 min may relieve symptoms without affecting analgesia.

Intrathecal Analgesia. With intrathecal analgesia, the opioid is injected into the subarachnoid space, located between the spinal cord and dura mater. Intrathecal opioids are approximately 10 times more potent than those given epidurally; therefore, less medication is needed to provide effective analgesia. The intrathecal method is usually used to deliver a one-time dose of analgesic (such as before or during surgery) and is infrequently used as a continuous infusion due to the serious risk of central nervous system infection.[9]

Intraspinal Opioid–Local Anesthetic Combinations. With epidural or intrathecal analgesia, a local anesthetic, such as bupivicaine, can be added to the continuous opioid infusion. Local anesthetics block pain by preventing nerve cell depolarization. They act synergistically with intraspinal opioid and have a dose-sparing effect.[20] Less opioid is needed to provide effective analgesia, and the incidence of opioid-related side effects is decreased.

This practice is more prevalent with epidural analgesia, because it more commonly uses a continuous infusion. A combination of epidural fentanyl and bupivicaine is usually used. With opioid-local anesthetic combinations, careful dose titration is essential. Local anesthetics are associated with side effects, such as hypotension and motor weakness.[12] Increasing the rate of infusion not only increases the dose of fentanyl, but also increases the dose of bupivicaine, increasing the risk of hypotension and motor weakness. The ratio of concentration of opioid to local anesthetic in the infusion can be changed to deal with this situation.

INTRAPLEURAL ANALGESIA

Intrapleural analgesia is particularly effective for patients who have undergone thoracic surgery or have multiple rib fractures, because these patients are prone to ineffective breathing patterns due to pain at the area of incision or injury.[29] With intrapleural analgesia, a percutaneous catheter is inserted between the parietal and visceral pleura of the lung, or the analgesic is administered through a pleural chest tube. A local anesthetic, such as bupivicaine is administered either as an intermittent injection or a continuous infusion. When given intrapleurally, local anesthetics diffuse across the parietal pleura and relieve pain by blocking intercostal nerve roots, thus providing effective analgesia without the adverse effects of systemic opioids. An intrapleural dose of bupivicaine can last 5 to 6 hours.[29]

Intrapleural analgesia is more invasive than other routes of administration, and catheter insertion is usually performed by an anesthesiologist. Proper catheter placement is crucial for adequate drug absorption. Pneumothorax can occur during catheter insertion, and catheter misplacement into a blood vessel may cause systemic toxicity.

SEDATION AND ANXIOLYSIS

Acute pain is frequently accompanied by anxiety, and anxiety is thought to increase the patient's perception of pain.[7] When treating acute pain, pharmacological anxiolysis can be used to complement analgesia and improve the patient's overall comfort. This is an important consideration, especially prior to and during painful procedures.

Benzodiazepines

Benzodiazepines, such as midazolam, diazepam, and lorazepam, provide sedation and are most often used for anxiolysis in the critically ill patient. In the ICU, benzodiazepines may be given intravenously as an intermittent bolus or continuous infusion and titrated according to the patient's response. Because these medications have no analgesic effect (except for pain caused by muscle spasm), an opioid or NSAID must be administered concomitantly to relieve pain.[7,26] If an opioid and benzodiazepine are used together, the doses of both medications should be reduced, because the risk of respiratory depression is increased.[30] The patient should also be closely monitored for oversedation and respiratory depression.

Midazolam is the benzodiazepine of choice for short-term relief of anxiety because of its rapid onset and short duration. Effects are usually seen 30 to 90 seconds after IV administration.[31] Another advantage is its retrograde amnesia effect, which is particularly beneficial during procedures. The half-life of midazolam ranges from 1.5 to 4.5 hours. However, the half-life may be increased in older or obese patients and those with liver disease, because the drug is eliminated by the liver.[31]

A major advantage of benzodiazepines is that they are reversible agents.[32] If respiratory depression occurs due to benzodiazepine administration, flumazenil can be administered intravenously. Flumazenil is a benzodiazepine-specific reversal agent that reverses the sedative and respiratory depressant effects without reversing opioid analgesics. The dosing of flumazenil should be individualized and titrated so that only the smallest effective amount is used. This will limit the undesirable effects, such as anxiety,

perceptual distortions, and confusion, that can be seen with benzodiazepine reversal. To reverse benzodiazepine-related respiratory depression and sedation, manufacturers' guidelines recommend administering flumazenil slowly IV at a rate of 0.2 to 0.5 mg/min until the desired effects are seen. This usually occurs with a total dose of 3 to 5 mg. If flumazenil is titrated at 0.2 mg/min, effects should be seen within 5 to 10 minutes. (If respiratory arrest is eminent, titrate at the faster rate of 0.5 mg/min.) Oversedation can reoccur because the effects of flumazenil may wear off before the benzodiazepine is cleared from the body. Therefore, the patient should be closely observed for at least 2 hours after reversal, especially when long-acting benzodiazepines (such as lorazepam or diazepam) or large (>10 mg) doses of midazolam are used.

Propofol

Propofol is the newest addition to ICU sedation choices. Classified as a sedative/hypnotic agent, it was previously used exclusively in the operating room for induction of anesthesia. It has no analgesic properties and minimal amnesic effects. Its onset of action is 40 seconds, and half-life is 5 to 8 minutes, depending on the dose and length of infusion. With appropriate airway and ventilatory management, propofol can be an ideal agent for patients requiring sedation during painful procedures. Because of its ultra-short half-life, it is reversible simply by discontinuing the infusion. After the bolus dose, the patient will awaken within a few minutes. Propofol can also be used as a continuous infusion for mechanically ventilated patients who require deep, prolonged sedation. Even after several days of sedation with propofol, the patient awakens quickly after the infusion is discontinued.[33]

Because Propofol is only slightly water soluble, it is formulated in a white, oil-based emulsion containing soybean oil, egg lecithin, and glycerol. It is contraindicated, therefore, in patients allergic to eggs or soy products. Propofol contains no preservatives, and each ampule or vial must be used as a "single-dose" product to minimize the risk of systemic infection. Besides respiratory depression, the most serious adverse effect of propofol is hypotension. This can be seen as a 20% to 30% drop in systolic blood pressure and is more common with bolus administration and in patients who are older or dehydrated.[32]

Figure 5–3 offers a decision-making algorithm to assist in treating the anxious patient. As indicated by the figure, careful and repeated evaluation of the patient's condition is required to provide effective management.

INTERVENTIONS FOR PROCEDURAL PAIN

Procedural pain is a major problem in the critically ill population. In a recent study of patients undergoing endotracheal suctioning and chest tube removal, patients received minimal preprocedural analgesics, although they reported moderate to severe pain during the procedures.[34]

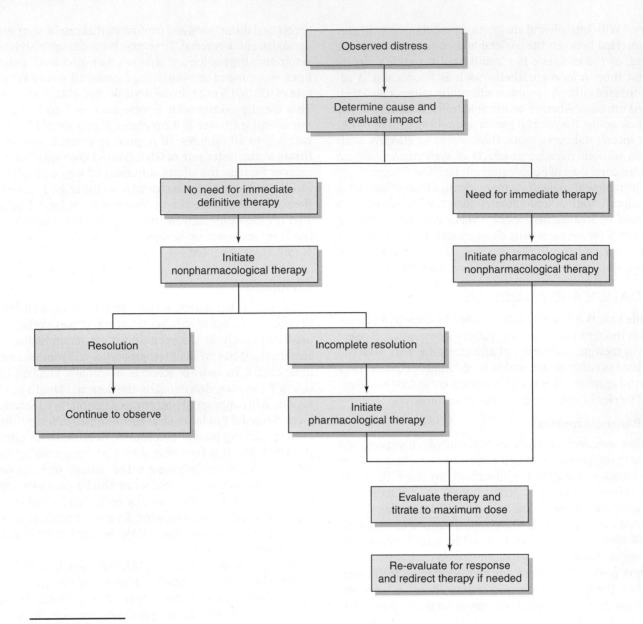

FIGURE 5-3

Flow chart treatment decisions in the management of anxiety. From: Bone, R.C: Recognition, assessment, and treatment of anxiety in the critical care patient. Proceedings of a Consensus Conference. June 13–14, 1993, New York City. Sponsored by Rush-Presbyterian-St. Luke's Medical Center Office of Medical Education.

Most patients received no analgesics in the hour prior to the procedure.

Before performing any procedure known to be associated with pain, patients should be premedicated, and the procedure should be performed only after the medication has taken effect. AHCPR guidelines clearly state that "only when immediate treatment of cardiorespiratory instability is required, or if a competent patient declines treatment, should analgesia be withheld for a painful procedure."[7]

During procedures, IV opioids, such as morphine or fentanyl, are usually used for analgesia. The IV bolus dose of morphine is individualized and depends on the age, weight, pain intensity, and type of procedure being performed. The patient's response must be monitored during the procedure

with additional doses given as needed for breakthrough pain.[7] Anxiolytic medications, such as midazolam or propofol, can be given to relieve anxiety during the procedure; however, these agents should be used as *adjuncts*, because they will not relieve pain associated with the procedure. Using these agents with opioids also increases the risk of respiratory depression.

Nonpharmacological Pain Relief Measures

Nonpharmacological interventions, such as relaxation exercises, touch, distraction music therapy, and guided imagery, are supported by AHCPR guidelines and should be

> ### PATIENT TEACHING
> ### *Instructions Regarding the Quieting Reflex*
>
> 1. Inhale an easy, natural breath.
> 2. Think "alert mind, calm body."
> 3. Smile inwardly (with your internal facial muscles).
> 4. As you exhale, allow your jaw, tongue, and shoulders to go loose.
> 5. Allow a feeling of warmth and looseness to go down through your body and out through your toes.

included in the pain management plan whenever possible to supplement pharmacological interventions. Behavioral therapies promote comfort by placing the patient in control. Working on the cognitive–behavioral level, these interventions reduce pain, anxiety, and the amount of analgesia needed for pain control.[35] Other pain control measures include acupressure, acupuncture, hypnosis, biofeedback, and transcutaneous electrical nerve stimulation.

RELAXATION TECHNIQUES

Relaxation exercises are useful pain relief measures that the patient can learn to perform himself or herself. They promote a sense of detachment but also can give the patient a sense of control over a particular body part. Most relaxation methods require a quiet environment, a comfortable position, a passive attitude, and concentration. The patient may focus on a word, sound, or breathing pattern for concentration.

The quieting reflex as proposed by Stroebel (1982) reduces stress and can easily be taught to the conscious and coherent patient.[36] Instructions regarding the quieting reflex are given in the accompanying display. The nurse encourages the patient to perform the quieting reflex fre-

quently during the day. This relaxation technique requires only 6 seconds to do, calms the sympathetic nervous system, and gives the patient a sense of control over stress and anxiety.

Breathing exercises have been used with much success in childbirth. They can also be used successfully in the critically ill patient. A second display describes one breathing exercise that can be taught to the ICU patient to assist in pain control and anxiety reduction.

Chapter 2 details the interventions of presencing, music therapy, guided imagery, changing internal and external dialogues, and progressive relaxation, which the critical care nurse can use to help the patient control pain and anxiety.

TOUCH

The highly technological ICU environment can contribute to depersonalization of the patient. Before development of all this technology, the greatest contributions a nurse could make were the comfort and caring of his or her presence and touch. These contributions still have an important place in the ICU. Nurses may feel that touching is too simple to be effective. However, few medical advances can replace the benefits of warm and caring touch. The need for

> ### PATIENT TEACHING
> ### *Abdominal Deep Breathing Exercise for Relaxation*
>
> The nurse can instruct the patient in this manner:
> 1. "Lie or sit comfortably."
> 2. "Breathe through your nose whenever possible" (to warm and filter the air).
> 3. "Concentrate on contracting your diaphragm, and breathe from deep within your abdomen." (If clinical situation allows, have patient place hand on abdomen to feel it rise on inhalation to confirm abdominal rather than chest breathing.)
> 4. "Begin to inhale and feel your abdomen begin to rise; inhale a full, deep breath."
> 5. "Slowly exhale as much air as you can, contracting your abdomen towards your spine at the end of the exhalation." (The patient should do this within the limits of condition and at own depth and pace.)
> 6. "Repeat breathing in and out this way several times, concentrating on the rise and fall of your abdomen."
> 7. "Whenever you feel upset, anxious, or uncomfortable, take a few slow, deep breaths in this fashion to help you break the stress cycle and calm yourself down."

touch is thought to intensify during times of high stress and cannot be totally met by other forms of communication. Nurses, when using touch, are usually trying to convey understanding, support, warmth, concern, and closeness to the patient. Touching not only improves the sense of well-being of the patient but also promotes physical recovery from disease. It has a positive effect on perceptual and cognitive abilities and can influence physiological parameters, such as respiration and blood flow. Touch represents a positive therapeutic element of human interaction.

The effects of touch in the clinical environment are far-reaching. Touch has played a major part in promoting and maintaining reality orientation in patients prone to confusion about time, place, and personal identification. Nursing touch may be most helpful in situations in which people are experiencing fear, anxiety, or depression. It may also be beneficial for patients who have a need for encouragement or nurturing, who have difficulty verbalizing needs, or who are disoriented, unresponsive, or terminally ill.

The age of the patient greatly affects the perception of touch. In one study, younger patients felt that touch should be used as an everyday positive component of nursing care, whereas older patients felt it should be used for therapeutic purposes in episodes of pain, loneliness, and depression (see display). Patients also felt the desire for touch increased with the seriousness of the illness and decreased with increased closeness of the family.[37]

In another study, the use of touch by nurses in ICUs did not vary according to the age or sex of the patient.[38] Unfortunately, the high acuity patients—those who probably needed and desired touch the most—were touched the least. A study of touching habits and behaviors of nurses in a geriatric home found that people with little or no evidence of physical impairment were touched the most. Men and those who were physically impaired received little touching.[39]

Patients with hearing or vision loss (or conceivably, distorted sensory input from the ICU environment) demonstrate particularly high needs for effective, creative communication from nurses. The use of deliberate, planned touch seems to give these patients a greater sense of control over the unfamiliar setting of the hospital. Using touch as a planned part of care (eg, in patient teaching) can be an extremely effective nursing intervention. These findings point to the need to include touch as a specific intervention in the plan of nursing care.

If efforts are coordinated by nurses, the use of touch can be more relaxing to a patient than sedatives or tranquilizers. More importantly, there is growing evidence that the nature of nurse–patient interaction influences physical and psychological outcomes of illness.

◼◼◼ PATIENT EDUCATION

To educate the patient about pain and pain relief, the critical care nurse must be familiar with the patient's pain management plan and therapy being used. Communication between the nurse and patient is essential. Any information given should be reinforced periodically during the course of therapy, and the patient should be encouraged to verbalize any questions or concerns. Family members should be included whenever possible.

Plans for pain management should be discussed with patients when they are most able to understand, for example, prior to surgery rather than during the recovery period. Emphasis is on prevention of pain, because it is easier to prevent pain than to treat it once it becomes severe.

Patients need to know that most pain can be relieved and that unrelieved pain may have serious consequences on physical and psychological well-being and may interfere with recovery.[7] The nurse helps patients and families understand that pain management is an important part of their care and that the health care team will respond quickly to reports of pain. It is made clear, however, that total absence of postoperative pain is not a realistic or desirable goal.[7]

Patients should also be given instructions about non-pharmacological interventions and traditional methods to minimize pain. Splinting the incisional area with a pillow while coughing or ambulating is a traditional pain relief measure.

The potential for drug addiction or overdosage is often a major concern for the patient and family. These issues should be addressed and clarified, because they create a barrier to effective pain relief. The patient needs a clear understanding of any specialized pain management technology, such as PCA, to alleviate the fear of overdosage.

◼◼◼ CONCLUSION

Because of its subjective nature, pain management can be a challenge to the critical care nurse. Becoming more aware of the effects of undertreated pain and taking action to make pain control in the critically ill patient a nursing care priority are desirable goals. Misconceptions and knowledge deficits on the part of health professionals and patients must be recognized and corrected. When providing pain management, it is recommended that all available

---

Considerations for the Older Patient
Therapeutic Touch

- Older patients often have an increased need for meaningful touch during episodes of crisis.
- The aging process may make them more prone to sensory deprivation, confusion, and communication difficulties that can sometimes be decreased by the meaningful use of touch in their care.
- Having few visitors and little verbal interaction may intensify their touching needs.

modes of therapy—NSAIDS, opioids, sedatives, and non-pharmacological therapies—be integrated into the plan of care. To manage pain effectively, critical care nurses must continuously familiarize themselves with current research and literature related to practices in pain assessment and management.

Clinical Applicability Challenges

Self-Challenge: Critical Thinking

1. *Mr. J. is 53 years old and 10 hours postoperative from an abdominal aortic resection. His postoperative orders include 2 to 3 mg morphine sulfate every hour IV push as needed for pain. He says his pain is an 8 on a scale of 0 to 10. He appears comfortable, and before you entered his room, he was smiling and in a lively conversation with a family member. You note that his heart rate is 85 and blood pressure is 120/80 mmHg. In view of the discrepancy between Mr. J.'s self-report, behavior, and physical assessment, defend your decision to give or not give the morphine.*

2. *Mrs. S. was admitted for chronic obstructive pulmonary disease and pneumonia. She was intubated and on mechanical ventilation for a week. She is now 24 hours postextubation. She is breathing comfortably on 60% oxygen through a face mask. Her vital signs are stable, but she had been hypotensive during the previous shift. The physician plans to perform a thoracentesis at the bedside shortly. In view of her physical illness, current condition, postextubation status, and recent problem with hypotension, determine whether you should consider holding analgesic or anxiolytic medications during the thoracentesis. Discuss factors that influenced your decision.*

Study Questions

1. *Unrelieved pain may result in all of the following physiological effects* except
   a. *myocardial ischemia.*
   b. *hypotension.*
   c. *atelectasis.*
   d. *musculoskeletal contractions or spasms.*

2. *The critical care nurse should recognize that the most reliable indicator of pain in the conscious patient is*
   a. *observation of patient's behavior.*
   b. *physiological parameters, such as heart rate and blood pressure.*
   c. *the patient's self-report of pain.*
   d. *family input regarding the presence of pain.*

3. *The* best *way to manage an opioid-related side effect is to*
   a. *discontinue the medication.*
   b. *administer medications to treat the side effect, such as antiemetics for nausea.*
   c. *reduce the dose.*
   d. *only give the medication on a PRN basis.*

4. *The patient receiving epidural analgesia must be closely monitored for which of the following complications?*
   a. *Tachycardia*
   b. *Respiratory depression*
   c. *Pneumonia*
   d. *Deep vein thrombosis due to bed rest*

5. *Although respiratory depression is rare with appropriate opioid dosing, which medication should be readily available?*
   a. *Diphenhydramine*
   b. *Nifedipine*
   c. *Naloxone*
   d. *Flumazenil*

REFERENCES

1. Puntillo KA, Wilkie DJ: Assessment of Pain in the Critically Ill. In Puntillo KA (ed): Pain in the Critically Ill: Assessment and Management, pp 45–63. Gaithersburg, MD, Aspen Publications, 1991
2. Gujol MC: A survey of pain assessment and management practices among critical care nurses. American Journal of Critical Care 3:123–128, 1994
3. Sun X, Weissman C: The use of analgesics and sedatives in critically ill patients: Physicians' orders versus medications administered. Heart Lung 23:169–176, 1994
4. Puntillo KA: Dimensions of procedural pain and its analgesic management in critically ill surgical patients. American Journal of Critical Care 3:116–122, 1994
5. Meehan DA et al: Analgesic administration, pain intensity and patient satisfaction in cardiac surgical patients. American Journal of Critical Care 4:435–442, 1995
6. Valdix SW, Puntillo KA: Pain, pain relief and accuracy of their recall after cardiac surgery. Progress in Cardiovascular Nursing 10:3–11, 1995
7. Agency for Health Care Policy and Research: Acute Pain Management: Operative and Medical Procedures and Trauma: Clinical Practice Guidelines No. 1, US Department of Health and Human Services, 1992
8. Dracup K, Bryan-Brown CW: Pain in the ICU: Fact or fiction? American Journal of Critical Care 4:337–339, 1995
9. Puntillo KA: Pain. In Kinney MR, et al (eds): AACN Clinical Reference for Critical Care Nursing, pp 329–347. St. Louis, CV Mosby, 1993
10. International Association for the Study of Pain: Pain terms: A list with definitions and notes on usage. Pain 6:249, 1979
11. McCaffery M: Nursing Practice Theories Related to Cognition, Bodily Pain and Man-Environment Interaction. University of California at Los Angeles, 1968
12. Hess CA: Acute Pain in the Intensive Care Unit. In Ayres SM, et al (eds): Textbook of Critical Care. Philadelphia, WB Saunders, 1995
13. Landow L, Joshi-Ryzewicz W: Anesthesia for Bedside Procedures. In Rippe JM, et al (eds): Critical Care Medicine. Boston, Little, Brown, 1996
14. Bozeman M: Cultural Aspects of Pain Management. In Salerno E, Willens JS (eds): Pain Management Handbook: An Interdisciplinary Approach, pp 67–87. St. Louis, CV Mosby, 1996
15. Ulmer JF: Identifying and Preventing Pain Mismanagement. In Salerno E, Willens JS (eds): Pain Management Handbook: An Interdisciplinary Approach, pp 39–66. St. Louis, CV Mosby, 1996
16. Sullivan LM: Factors influencing pain management: A nursing perspective. Journal of Post Anesthesia Nursing 9:83–90, 1996
17. Alpen MA, Titler MG: Pain Management in the critically ill: What do we know and how can we improve? AACN Clinical Issues 5:159–168, 1995
18. Alspach G: Pain management: Dispelling some myths. Critical Care Nurses 14:13–15, 1994
19. Pasero CL, McCaffrey M: Avoiding opioid-induced respiratory depression. Am J Nurs 94:25–31, 1994
20. Pasero CL, McCaffery M: Managing postoperative pain in the elderly. Am J Nurs 96:38–46, 1996
21. Toradol General Dosing Guidelines, Hoffman-LaRoche, Inc., 1995
22. Willens JS: Giving Fentanyl for pain outside the OR. Am J Nurs 94:24–29, 1994
23. Hauer M, Cram E, Titler M, Alpen M, Harp J: Intravenous patient-controlled analgesia in critically ill postoperative/trauma patients: Research-based practice recommendations. Dimensions in Critical Care Nursing 14:144–153, 1995

24. Salerno E: Pharmacologic Approaches. In Salerno E, Willens JS (eds): Pain Management Handbook: An Interdisciplinary Approach, pp 91–135. St. Louis, Mosby, 1996
25. Lazzara DJ: Patient controlled analgesia in the ICU setting. Critical Care Nursing Quarterly 16:26–36, 1993
26. American Pain Society: Principles of Analgesic Use in the Treatment of Acute Pain and Cancer Pain (3rd Ed). Glenview, IL, 1992
27. Pasero C, McCaffrey M: Unconventional PCA: Making it work for your patient. Am J Nurs 93:38–41, 1993
28. Naber L, Jones G, Halm M: Epidural analgesia for effective pain control. Critical Care Nurse 14:69–85, 1994
29. Martin B, Mehberg D: Intrapleural analgesia: A new technique. Critical Care Nurse 14:31–35, 1994
30. Durbin CG: Sedation in the critically ill patient. New Horizons 2:64–74, 1994
31. Burns SM, Brauer K: Midazolam for conscious sedation and surgery. Critical Care Nurse 13:91–93, 1993
32. Pine LJ: Sedation strategies: Drug selection, costs and treatment protocols. Management of Sedation: A Nursing Perspective. Critical Care Nurse, Suppl:4–9, 1996
33. Huber C, Jain U: Caring for the ICU patient receiving propofol. Dimensions of Critical Care Nursing 15:133–141, 1996
34. Puntillo KA: Effects of intrapleural bupivicaine on pleural chest tube removal pain: A randomized controlled trial. American Journal of Critical Care 5:102–108, 1996
35. Teirnan PJ: Independent nursing interventions: Relaxation and guided imagery in critical care. Critical Care Nurse 14:47–51, 1994
36. Stroebel C: QR: The Quieting Reflex. New York, Berkeley Books, 1982
37. Day F: The Patient's Perception of Touch. In Anderson E, et al (eds): Current Concepts in Clinical Nursing. St. Louis, CV Mosby, 1973
38. Clement JM: A Description. Study of the Use of Touch by Nurses with Patients in Critical Care. Doctoral dissertation. The University of Texas, Austin, Texas, 1983
39. Watson W: The meaning of touch: Geriatric nursing. J Communication 25:104–111, 1995

BIBLIOGRAPHY

Ferrell BR, Ferrell BA: Pain in the Elderly: A Report of the Task Force on Pain in the Elderly of the International Association for the Study of Pain. Seattle, IASP Press, 1996

Guyton-Simmons J, Ehrmin JT: Problem solving in pain management by expert intensive care nurses. Critical Care Nurse 14:37–44, 1994

Henry L: Music therapy: A nursing intervention for the control of pain and anxiety in the ICU: A review of the research literature. Dimensions of Critical Care 14(6):295–304, 1995

Johnson K, Rohaly-Davis S: An introduction to music therapy: Helping the oncology patient in the ICU. Critical Care Nursing Quarterly 18:54–60, 1996

Murray MJ, Plevak DJ: Analgesia in the critically ill patient. New Horizons 2:56–63, 1994

Mynchenberg T, Dungan J: A relaxation protocol to reduce patient anxiety. Dimensions of Critical Care 14(2):78–85, 1995

Titler MA, et al: Research utilization in critical care: An exemplar. AACN Clinical Issues 5:124–132, 1995

Tittle M, McMillan SC: Pain and pain-related side effects in an ICU and on a surgical unit. Nurses' management. American Journal of Critical Care 3:25–30, 1994

Whipple JK, et al: Analysis of pain management in critically ill patients. Pharmacotherapy 15:592–599, 1995

Wong DL: Whaley & Wong's Nursing Care of Infants and Children (5th Ed). St. Louis, CV Mosby, 1995

6

Patient and Family Education in a Changing Health Care Environment

FAMILY PARTICIPATION

THE HEALTH EDUCATION CONTINUUM
Transitioning Education Across Settings
A Concept Map for Education

THE TEACHING–LEARNING PROCESS
Seven-Step Plan
   Motivation
   Knowledge Gap
   Learning Readiness
   Available Resources

Mutual Goal Setting
Psychomotor Change
Feedback
Three Domains of Learning
THE PATIENT TEACHING PLAN

OBJECTIVES

Based on the content in this chapter, the reader should be able to:

- Describe current challenges and strategies to promote patient and family education in a changing health care environment.
- Describe a seven-step process for assessing, planning, and carrying out a patient education plan.
- Discuss specific cognitive, affective, and psychomotor knowledge deficits and related patient goals and outcome criteria.
- Develop and evaluate a patient and family education plan.

*"C*hanges in staffing patterns and personnel, utilization of health care as mandated by federal regulations, increasing patient acuity, and movement of technology-based nursing care into the home have necessitated new approaches to patient education."[1] In today's health care system, the patient leaves the hospital *sicker and quicker*, when neither the patient nor the family is ready for teaching, and the critical care nurse's time for teaching is limited. At the same time, the patient and the family's education is integral to the patient's preparation for leaving the hospital safely.

Another significant health care trend is the initiative to help individuals, families, and communities become more

responsible for managing their own health. Thus, individuals must be better informed about health promotion, health maintenance, and illness prevention and the appropriate use of health care services. In addition, the family is being asked increasingly to provide home care for a family member recovering from serious illness or surgery. As a result of all these changes, nurses face a greater challenge but, at the same time, have a greater opportunity to provide health education to patients and families.

FAMILY PARTICIPATION

Although most of the following discussion focuses on the patient, each of these concepts is applicable to the instruction of family members or support people who are involved with the patient in activities of daily living. The family is often the primary consumer of patient education in the hospital environment because patients are too ill to comprehend adequately and incorporate the information into their self-care. Most of the time, it is necessary and valuable for family members to acquire the same knowledge and skills as the patient. Examples of such involvement include performing a procedure (eg, injection, irrigation, dressing change), shopping or cooking a special diet, offering support, and sometimes even participating with the patient in certain activities (eg, accompanying the patient on a walking regimen).

The nurse assesses the family's ability to care for the ill or recovering family member. Assessing the family's strengths and limitations helps develop an individualized plan that is aimed at achieving desired outcomes. Usually a primary family caregiver is chosen by the family members. This individual may require special education and support from the nurse. In addition, it is important to evaluate the family's cultural norms and beliefs so that what is taught is congruent with their language, health beliefs, and experience. For example, some ethnic groups specify that male relatives care for male patients, and female relatives care for female patients. Other ethnic groups may believe in the healing powers of specific foods that are now restricted on a patient's new diet. Thus, exploring family ethnicity and customs becomes important in helping the patient and family achieve health outcomes.

■ THE HEALTH EDUCATION CONTINUUM

People receive health information from a variety of sources, such as newspapers, magazines, television, radio shows, online computer services, insurance companies, and community events. An emphasis on individual empowerment through knowledge of health and illness has emerged. This emphasis, along with other health care trends, has changed the way people view health education. The hospital is no longer the primary source of health education. Instead, health education has become community based.

Patient and family education has shifted along with aspects of acute care nursing that have shifted from inpatient to outpatient and home settings. Care that was once provided only in hospitals is now provided in home care settings. Many complex pieces of equipment, including home ventilators, dialysis machines, or devices used in parenteral nutrition and tube feeding, are now operated by patients and families at home. As a result, patient education is best viewed as a continuous process. A continuum of health education has emerged.

First, the continuum, illustrated in Figure 6–1, recognizes that patients, families, and health care providers are always moving toward "complete" knowledge of health and

illness care. Complete knowledge is elusive; there is always more to learn. Health care providers, and particularly nurses, play a significant role in assisting the patient and family toward complete knowledge but do not solely control it. Second, the health education continuum reinforces the concept of lifelong learning about health in which hospitalization is but one episode on a person's life trajectory. Third, health education does not begin or end at hospital boundaries.

Transitioning Education Across Settings

An important part of the health education continuum is facilitating the transition of the education plan across settings. Instruction must continue *wherever* the patient receives continuing care. Care may continue at home or in an outpatient, rehabilitation, or long-term care setting. Nurses should send specific information, including what has been taught and the patient and family response, to the agency that will provide continuing care. Areas that were not taught are identified so other nurses do not assume teaching is complete. Documentation is important.

Communicating patient and family education from one setting to another may be the greatest challenge in critical care nursing. The main objective of teaching plans for patients with short hospital stays may focus on essential information and skills the patient and family need between hospital discharge and their next health care visit. Incorporating teaching into daily care provides multiple opportunities for observing and learning. Likewise, preparatory teaching for patients having elective surgery focuses on key messages for properly preparing and getting to surgery and understanding the immediate postsurgical period.

Acute care nurses must communicate the learning achieved by patients and families to nurses who will be providing continued care. This may include nurses in primary care settings, rehabilitation centers, nursing homes, assisted living centers, and home care. Communication with home care and community health nurses will increase as more health education occurs at home. An example is shown in the accompanying display. Nurses who possess knowledge and skills in patient and family education and have a caring relationship with the patient and family are in a crucial position to help them move toward higher levels of learning.

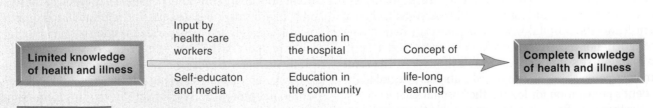

FIGURE 6-1
Continuum of health care education. A person never achieves complete knowledge.

Considerations for Home Care
Communicating Transition of Care Between Critical Care and Home Care Nurses

Knowledge Base

- Expected course of recovery
- Potential risks for client
- Expected outcome(s)
- Essential information and skills needed by patient and family (to experience a complication-free period until next seen by a health care provider); survival skills

Teaching–Learning Process

- Have patient and family as well informed (empowered) as possible.
- Give written instructions (names and numbers of health care providers, especially after hours; what to report; medication and treatment schedules).
- Determine (with multidisciplinary team and patient and family) what additional services and community resources will assist with or maintain recovery.
- Determine what other team members need to be involved (such as a case manager or managed care company), and discuss patient's ongoing health care needs and expected outcomes.
- Initiate referrals, and communicate information that will coordinate and facilitate care.

A Concept Map for Education

Patient and family education is similar to the steps of the nursing process. The concept map presented in Figure 6–2 uses steps in the nursing process and summarizes information used in this chapter.

▉▉ THE TEACHING–LEARNING PROCESS

Despite current health care changes, principles of patient and family education remain unchanged:

- Individualize education.
- Provide necessary information.
- Teach when the patient and family are able to comprehend the information.

Recognizing the patient's response to illness helps predict when teaching will be best absorbed and most useful to the patient. One pattern of adaptation to illness is illustrated in Figure 2–2 and can be applied to learning readiness. Learning is most likely to occur during quiet stages, when the patient's emotional outlook corresponds to physical condition. This means that the patient feels just about as sick or as well as he or she actually is. Providing information during this phase of illness helps the patient move on to the next phase of recovery. When there is less congruence

between the patient's physical condition and emotional acknowledgment of it, motivation for learning is impaired, and teaching is less effective.

Seven-Step Plan

To enhance teaching effectiveness, the nurse can use the following seven-step plan for management of teaching–learning. The seven-step plan is outlined in the display on page 63.

MOTIVATION

Motivation for learning should be assessed in two areas: intrinsic and extrinsic motivation. Intrinsic motivation includes the learner's attitudes, values, personality, and lifestyle. The teaching method and what is taught must be adjusted for these aspects of the patient's life. Extrinsic motivation includes the learning climate, physical environment, time of teaching, possible reinforcers, interpersonal relationship with the teacher, and skill of the instructor. The nurse has far more control over the extrinsic sources of motivation. Does the patient respond best alone or with others? Does he or she prefer the solarium to the bedroom? Do touching, smiling, and encouraging enhance learning? Does the patient like to spend time with the nurse? Has the nurse developed teaching skills and methods for this particular type of learner? Trial-and-error attempts at teaching each patient can be shared with other nurses to increase extrinsic motivation skills.

KNOWLEDGE GAP

Assessing the knowledge gap includes recognizing what needs to be taught and learned to effect behavior change. A knowledge gap can also be assessed in terms of "what is" compared with "what could be." An honest, accurate appraisal leads to realistic, achievable goals rather than unrealistic ones that, if attempted, would result in the patient's experiencing failure. In this phase of the plan, it is important for patients and their families to recognize the advantages inherent in learning the new knowledge, skills, and attitudes. As this phase is completed, patients should become aware that they have a better basis for choice concerning whether they will learn and change. The patient's right to make this choice should be acknowledged and accepted by the nurse. However, the nurse has the responsibility to make certain that the patient is making a knowledgeable choice.

LEARNING READINESS

The step of learning readiness deals with several issues:

- The level of adaptation to illness
- The anxiety level
- The developmental level
- The opportunities for immediate application of new knowledge and skill
- An interpersonally safe learning environment that allows trial and error without recrimination

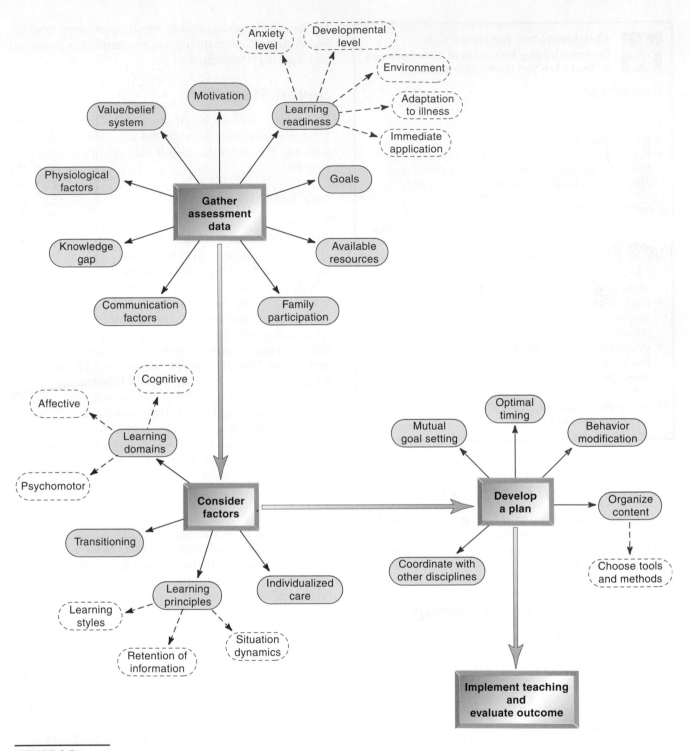

FIGURE 6-2

A concept map for patient and family education in the intensive care unit.

As patients adjust to the sick role, they become more receptive to learning about the illness. Because progress heightens anxiety, teaching is usually more effective during the period of emotional acceptance than during times when the patient is moving either into or out of the sick role. Whenever there is movement forward or backward on the health–illness continuum, there is likely to be an emo-

tional response of anxiety, worry, or depression that can interfere with concentration and learning. Therefore, admission, transfer, readmission to the intensive care unit, and hospital discharge are usually poor times for learning to occur.

Simultaneously, family members progress through levels of adaptation to the critical illness. Each family mem-

---

Seven-Step Management Plan for Teaching in Critical Care

Motivation

ASSESSMENT: INTRINSIC MOTIVATION
- Attitudes, values, personality, lifestyle

ASSESSMENT: EXTRINSIC MOTIVATION
- Learning climate
- Physical environment
- Time of teaching
- Possible reinforcers
- Interpersonal relationship with teacher
- Skill of teacher

Knowledge Gap

ASSESSMENT
- What needs to be taught and learned
- Patient and family recognition of advantages in learning new knowledge, skills, attitudes

Learning Readiness

ASSESSMENT
- Patient's and family's adaptation to illness
- Anxiety level
- Developmental level
- Opportunities for immediate application of knowledge and skills
- Interpersonally safe learning environment

Available Resources

ASSESSMENT
- Equipment
- Finances
- Values and cultural influences
- Family involvement
- Community support
- Learning style preference

Mutual Goal Setting

PLANNING AND ACTIONS
- Contract setting
- Responsibility of nurse
- Responsibility of patient and family
- Establishing achievable goals

Psychomotor Change

NURSING ACTIONS
- Behavior modification
- Reinforcement, support, encouragement
- Community support systems

Feedback

EVALUATION
- Descriptive rather than judgmental feedback
- Specific rather than general feedback
- Positive feedback
- Revision of plan with patient and family

---

ber's learning readiness will depend on his or her response to the critical illness. The nature of the response may increase or decrease learning readiness and the ability to absorb information.

At home, in the patient's own surroundings and with personal routines, nurses can evaluate the patient's and family's knowledge and their ability to apply it. Rehabilitation programs that involve structure and extended periods of time should occur after the crisis, when the patient has reached a fairly stable period of adjustment. Often this stage of readiness does not occur until after hospital discharge. Teaching may also continue in other community-based settings.

Anxiety

Anxiety levels, physiological function, and the patient's own priorities are assessed as part of an evaluation for learning readiness. Worry, pain, and some medications interfere with the patient's ability to learn. The amount and type of information the patient and family need to learn is another consideration. They are likely to experience increased levels of anxiety when they have to learn many facts and change many behaviors.

Because of the high level of anxiety that accompanies critical illness, it is sometimes difficult to reduce anxiety as much as desired. Nevertheless, the best time for learning is when the patient demonstrates only mild anxiety, alertness without fear, motivation to learn, and interest.

Because of anxiety associated with serious illness, patients are likely to have trouble remembering details. It is especially important that they be provided with written material so that they can review what they need to learn. Pamphlets, booklets, and customized lists and directions are useful. These educational items can be personalized by adding handwritten notes and explanations at the bedside. These notes should also address the patient's questions and concerns.

Developmental Level

The patient's developmental level indicates learning readiness. For example, young adolescents do not deal well with philosophical issues regarding their care and life choices as do older adolescents and adults. Their level of abstract thinking is not nearly as well developed as in the older adolescent or adult. Special teaching–learning materials must be developed for both extremes of the age scale. An example of teaching guidelines for the pediatric patient is given in the accompanying display. Considerations for the older adult are summarized in a second display.

The term developmental level pertains not only to the age of the person. Although a patient may be an adult, the person may be mentally challenged or illiterate. Materials

Considerations for the Pediatric Patient
Issues in Teaching the Pediatric Patient

- Children learn from their parents; a parent should be used as often as possible during teaching.
- If parents cannot do the actual teaching, they should be present to answer questions and give the child more confidence.
- Children learn through play (games, role playing) and with toys (dolls).
- Teaching can be more effective if related to home routines so it can be continued at home.
- Teaching should be related to the child's life experiences (developmental level or personal).
- Questions should be answered immediately and in language the child understands.
- Trust is important to teaching. If the nurse says a procedure will not hurt, and it does hurt, the child will not trust the nurse.
- Learning should be evaluated frequently to ensure the child understands.
- The nurse should praise the child often or offer rewards, such as stickers or picture books.
- School-age children usually are eager to learn.
- School-age children can understand cause and effect.
- Children should be included in planning and setting goals.
- Younger children have short attention spans of about 10 minutes; teaching of school-age children should be no longer than 30 minutes; adolescents can have sessions of around 45 to 50 minutes.

Data from Craven RF, Hirnle CJ: Fundamentals of Nursing (2nd Ed). Philadelphia, Lippincott-Raven, 1996

Considerations for Home Care
Features in Planning Learning Experiences for the Older Learner

- Motivation to learn may decrease if the patient feels life is near the end. The nurse can address the quality of life regardless of age.
- Independence is usually valued by the older adult. New knowledge could improve the patient's independence.
- Normal physiological changes of the older adult may hinder learning, especially vision and hearing. Therefore, face the learner; speak in a low, slow voice; and use visual aids with large letters and primary colors.
- Older adults often have short-term memory loss. Nurses should be sensitive to this loss but not assume there is memory loss.
- Sessions should last no more than 20 to 30 minutes.
- Information should be simple. Provide one idea at a time.
- It is helpful to relate new material to the past or past experiences.
- Information should be summarized frequently and positive feedback given.
- Written or recorded summaries of the session are beneficial.

Data from Craven RF, Hirnle CJ: Fundamentals of Nursing (2nd Ed). Philadelphia, Lippincott-Raven, 1996

and methods must be adapted for people with special needs. This also includes hearing and visually impaired patients. Teaching may begin in the hospital, but rarely is it completed by discharge.

Provision of an Interpersonally Safe Environment

Most of the learning required of a patient who is recovering from critical illness involves changes in behavior that will alter his or her lifestyle. Dietary changes that restrict calories, sodium, cholesterol, or carbohydrates are common. A change in activity level may be imposed, exercise may be prescribed, and a decrease in smoking may be imperative. None of these changes is easy to make. Providing information is rarely sufficient to alter behavior. Ongoing support, continued motivation, and reinforcement are also necessary. Group teaching is a technique that is well suited to learning that involves lifestyle changes. Group members can provide needed support, offer encouragement and motivation, and reinforce information and accomplishments. An effective approach to learning includes a combination of informal teaching, group instruction, and specialized learning and evaluation at home.

Providing a safe environment conducive to learning is included in this phase. Learning occurs more easily if security, a sense of belonging, and self-esteem are high. Often, learning about illness means that the patient and family not only must learn facts and techniques but also must apply and adapt what is taught to their own lives. This is difficult if there are high degrees of anxiety, depression, or acute physical dysfunction. It is impossible for patients to respond creatively if they are struggling to maintain basic physiological stability. Therefore, much of the teaching is directed toward the family. A key concept to teach family members is how to support and encourage one another during a change process.

When the teachable moment appears, reminders such as those below will keep communication open:

- Find out about the learner's concerns before teaching.
- Ask for the learner's ideas and perceptions of what is happening.
- Avoid judgmental statements.
- Ask yourself, "Is what the patient or family wants to learn what I want to teach?"

The nursing process helps the nurse answer the last question in the display. The nursing process can be used to determine the teaching plan in the same way that it is used to determine any other nursing action.

AVAILABLE RESOURCES

A careful assessment of the availability of resources has an important effect on the outcome of patient learning. Without a realistic appraisal of family resources, the nurse may spend valuable time teaching the patient activities impossible to implement once he or she is discharged. Equipment, adequate finances, values and cultural influences, family involvements, and community support all are resources that are likely to need careful appraisal to ensure a successfully implemented teaching plan. For example, if the nurse is teaching the patient how to reduce carbohydrate or sodium intake, the nurse should find out the types of foods eaten (a sample meal plan) and the ways they are prepared. This information can then be used to help the patient and family tailor the diet regimen to their meals.

In this phase, learning resources are also assessed. The patient's and family's learning style preferences are evaluated and matched with available resources. For example, many older adults prefer a personal approach rather than videotapes or computer-assisted programs. Written materials may be inappropriate if the person cannot read them because of literacy, language, or visual problems. Reading level, familiarity of terms, and customs and beliefs of the target population are considered when developing written material. Written material for a broad cross-section of people should use short words and sentences and a large print type (12–13 points) and convey key points rather than detailed information. The accompanying display gives guidelines for instructional material used with older adults.

Audio tapes and videotapes on a variety of topics may be purchased. These media are especially valuable because they can be repeated based on patient and family need. They also allow the patient and significant others to view, listen, and discuss the information in privacy. Computer-assisted learning and interactive video programs allow for individualized learning and simulated experiences. Despite the availability of media, nothing can replace a warm, encouraging, supportive relationship between the patient, family, and a skilled and knowledgeable nurse.

MUTUAL GOAL SETTING

The nurse and patient formulate a contract about what is to be learned and how they will know that the specified material has been learned. The nurse and patient agree on what the nurse will do to help the patient learn and what the patient must do to meet the established goal. The actual outcome or objectives to be accomplished provide direction about the content to be taught and prescribe behaviors for teacher and learner. They also measure progress.

Words that define or specify behaviors are more useful and less ambiguous than words that make vague statements about what the patient is to accomplish. For example, "The patient will list 10 common foods that are high in sodium (or salt)" is better than "The patient will develop an understanding regarding high-sodium foods to be avoided." Furthermore, stating the goal in a positive "can do" statement is more likely to lead to success than the negatively stated list of "foods to be avoided." Return demonstrations of how to care for equipment and appliances or how to perform exercises also are specific enough to measure achievements.

> ### Considerations for the Older Patient
> **Guidelines for Printed Materials**
>
> - Type size should be 12 points or greater.
> - Serif type style is preferred over sans-serif type.
> - Avoid script or stylized types.
> - Avoid the use of all upper case letters for body type.
> - Line lengths should be no longer than 5 in.
> - Glossy finish paper should be avoided because glare makes reading difficult.
> - Uncoated or matte finish paper is suggested.
> - Ink color is best when black ink is printed on white or off-white paper.
> - Avoid printing over a designed or customized background.
> - A fourth- to sixth-grade reading level is preferred.

"After 1 week of practice, the patient will be able to make three bed-to-chair or chair-to-bed transfers within 2 hours" is another useful outcome-oriented objective. It tells the nurse and patient how much time is available for learning, the exact behavior expected, and how many times it should be accomplished within a specified time.

Goals can and should be renegotiated as the situation or circumstances change, but more importantly, they should be formulated so that success is achievable. Therefore, goals should be written in increments of complexity and for short periods of time. After one goal is achieved, it can be increased or modified. If it does not appear to be attainable, it should be modified downward so that the patient who makes a reasonable effort does not fail and give up, but rather is reinforced to go on by the feeling of success.

PSYCHOMOTOR CHANGE

The hardest part of adhering to a health or treatment regimen is to change longstanding behavior. Usually this means making long-term lifestyle changes. For example, a person trying to lose 6 lb gained on vacation may feel frustrated, but the situation is in no way comparable to that of a patient who, having experienced the threat of severe illness, must lose and keep off 50 lb. The patient's physical and emotional energies have probably been compromised by the illness and hospitalization. Now, health care providers are demanding extensive lifestyle changes that seem necessary and logical to them for restoring the patient's health. The patient, after the emotional and physical depletion caused by illness, is more likely to experience the demand for change as deprivation.

Giving up smoking, eliminating salt from the diet, and losing weight are difficult objectives, even for the most knowledgeable and motivated health professional. Finding ways to help patients comply with lifestyle changes is a nursing problem that deserves intensive attention and extensive research. Appropriate teaching plans, reinforcement, support, and encouragement, even when there is regression, constitute a beginning. Involving the patient and the family in mutual goal setting and connecting them with community support systems are likely to enhance and sustain the necessary lifestyle changes.

Sometimes, serendipitous changes occur that can be used to encourage behavior modification. For example, a patient who loses 20 of a prescribed 50 lb may be more reinforced by his or her improved self-image than by health improvement. This kind of change in self-image motivates the patient to lose more weight. Nurses can observe changes that improve attitude and use them to reinforce goals and motivate the patient.

FEEDBACK

Feedback is useful for evaluating gains and modifying goals. It must be descriptive rather than judgmental and specific rather than general. Thus, "You've lost 3 lb!" is more constructive than "You're doing well!" Timely feedback is more reinforcing than delayed feedback and is more useful in helping the patient resist temptations to transgress.

Negative feedback can be helpful when it promotes choices rather than guilt. The observation, "You've smoked more cigarettes today than yesterday" provides the patient with more support to modify or control behavior than the statement, "You're ruining your health," a judgment of self-destruction that fills the patient with guilt.

Positive feedback reinforces success and extends motivation. As the teaching plan continues, look for undiscovered knowledge and behavior gaps, and revise the plan with the patient.

Three Domains of Learning

There are three domains of human behavior or learning to consider when developing an education plan: cognitive, affective, and psychomotor. Keeping these domains in mind while assessing for and developing a plan of care can help sharpen teaching interventions. Principal teaching methods for each domain are listed in the accompanying display.

In the cognitive domain of learning, knowledge expands and teaching–learning material is organized from simple to complex. Learning is enhanced when information builds on previous knowledge. Basic ideas should be taught well before teaching hard-to-remember facts.

Affective domain has to do with the patient's values, attitudes, and feelings. When attempting to modify an attitude or emotional response, the nurse must be nonjudgmental and nonthreatening. The nurse who acknowledges the client's power to accept or reject the material thus empowers the client to make more healthy decisions. The nurse listens carefully to what the client values and works with that information.

Psychomotor domains involve the use of muscles and motions in learning a skill. The nurse assembles the equipment prior to the session to save time and prevent interruptions. A written step-by-step guide can be used as a reference during the session and will be a reminder to the

---

> ### Principal Teaching Methods for Use in the Intensive Care Unit Based on Domains
>
> #### Cognitive
> Simple-to-complex organization: clarification of basic concepts and terminology; lecture-type presentation; simulation; models; independent study through pamphlets, written material, and videotapes; tests or quizzes; discussion; question and answer
>
> #### Affective
> Discussion and values clarification, role playing or role modeling, simulation, question and answer, videotapes
>
> #### Psychomotor
> Written material, videotapes, handling equipment, skill demonstration, talking the learner through the skill, return demonstration, repeated practice

---

client when he or she begins to practice the skill independently. The nurse teaches the skill step by step, allowing for questions and comments. Many adults are intimidated by learning a new skill, so encouragement and praise almost always improve performance.

■ THE PATIENT TEACHING PLAN

There are many ways to develop a patient and family teaching plan. Given a homogeneous population, standardized patient teaching plans and records can be developed. Standard plans include information that is essential for most patients but can also be flexible enough to accommodate individual needs. Patient teaching plans include nursing diagnoses, outcome criteria, and interventions (see the Sample Patient Teaching Plan). In addition, clinical pathways that include time-sequenced, interdisciplinary patient education outcomes and interventions may be used.

Defining the knowledge deficit helps the nurse identify the appropriate content to teach. It also helps formulate outcomes that will be used to evaluate the patient's and family's progress and the effectiveness of the teaching plan. Outcomes should be written in measurable terms; for example, *The patient can state the main action of digoxin, or the patient can draw up and administer insulin without contamination.* Teaching should be done in a logical learning sequence that also considers the patient's receptiveness to learning emotionally threatening content.

Nursing interventions include the content, method, and media for teaching. They also include the personal needs that promote learning, such as privacy, reinforcement, a quiet environment, and hearing aids. In the critical care setting, the patient may be too ill or debilitated to cope with essential learning. In these cases, the teaching part of the

SAMPLE PATIENT TEACHING PLAN

Mr. Chang was admitted to the emergency room with a severe myocardial infarction. Within hours after admission, bypass surgery was completed. Mr. Chang is 50 years old, 30 lb overweight, and rarely exercises. As an engineer, he maintains a sedentary lifestyle with his wife. He enjoys high sodium oriental food at least three times a week. Now recovering from surgery, he expresses interest in losing weight and improving his general health.

Nursing Diagnosis and Outcome Criteria	*Nursing Interventions*
Knowledge Deficit related to weight loss strategies, food choices, caloric intake, exercise • Patient will be able to state content presented.	1. Time teaching sessions during minimal interruption for care needs. 2. Include wife in content presentation. 3. Provide written materials to reinforce verbal information. 4. Modify weight reduction program to meet patient needs. 5. Refer patient to full service cardiac rehabilitation program that includes exercise and nutrition. 6. Include dietitian in meal planning. 7. Plan for continued education. 8. Use in-hospital menu selection to validate patient understanding of food choices. 9. If available, give list of cookbooks that prepare foods low in calories, fat, and cholesterol. 10. Gradually increase exercise (ambulation) while assessing physiologic tolerance (eg, heart rate, rhythm, angina).
Health-Seeking Behavior related to desire for weight loss • Patient will participate in goal setting for weight loss. • Patient will carry out exercise plan. • Patient will lose according to personal goal (eg, 1 lb/wk).	1. Plan and set goals with patient for methods of weight loss. 2. Have patient identify favorite moderate exercises. 3. Have patient identify ways to lose weight. 4. Provide chart with caloric values. 5. Refer patient to weight loss group. Provide information about cost and location.
Risk for Anxiety related to fear of failure, lifestyle changes, impact of diet on heart disease • Patient can begin to demonstrate effective coping mechanisms.	1. Have patient discuss feelings about changing diet. 2. Discuss with patient his feeling about his weight loss program. 3. Mobilize patient's resources (family or others) for support. 4. Help patient design chart that will graphically demonstrate weight loss achievement. 5. Acknowledge all questions and responses as meaningful and important (eg, "That's a great idea").

plan should be written and customized for responsible family members or friends. The same points apply, especially in regard to feelings and attitudes, because they affect readiness for learning and motivation to follow through (see Chapter 2). A verbal, or perhaps written, contract among the responsible friend or relative, the patient, and the nurse helps motivate each partner to carry out his or her responsibilities. When designing such a contract, apply the content related to mutual goal setting.

Clinical Applicability Challenges

Self-Challenge: Critical Thinking

1. *Evaluate the teaching materials and documentation system where you practice as to how well they support patient and family education.*

2. *Debate the relative merits of a formal versus informal patient education plan.*

3. Develop strategies for facilitating the transition of patient and family education across health care settings.

Study Questions

1. Learning is most likely to occur under the following conditions:
   a. Anxiety is mild, and acceptance is congruent with the illness.
   b. Anxiety is moderate, and the patient is motivated.
   c. Anxiety is high, and the patient is highly motivated.
   d. Anxiety is low, and the patient denies the severity of the illness.

2. The term "intrinsic learning" deals with the patient's
   a. motivation to learn.
   b. lighting and noise within the environment.
   c. ability to abstract meaning from inner resources.
   d. values, attitudes, personality, and lifestyle.

REFERENCES

1. Rankin SH, Stallings KD: Patient Education: Issues, Principles Practices (3rd Ed), p xi. Philadelphia, JB Lippincott, 1996

BIBLIOGRAPHY

Doak CC, Doak LG, Root JH: Teaching Patients With Low Literacy Skills (2nd Ed). Philadelphia, JB Lippincott, 1996

McGaughey J, Harrison S: Developing and information booklet to meet the needs of intensive care patients and relatives. Intensive Critical Care Nurse 10(4):271–277, 1994

Medaglia M, Shalof T: Meeting families' needs for information. The creation of this booklet, "A critical time: your guide to the intensive care unit." CACCN Summer: 5(2):17–19, 1994

Ott BB, Hardie TL: Readability of written materials: Implications for critical care nurses. Dimensions of Critical Care Nursing 14(6):328–334, 1995

Owens P, Johnson E, Frost C, Porter E, O'Hare E: Reading, readability, and patient education materials. Cardiovascular Nursing 9(2):9–13, 1993

Redman BK: Patient education at 25 years: Where have we been and where are we going. J Adv Nurs 18:725–730, 1993

Professional Practice Issues in Critical Care

Ethical Issues in Critical Care

OBJECTIVES

Based on the content in this chapter, the reader should be able to:

- Explain the way ethics assists clinicians in resolving moral problems.
- Name and describe the ethical principles most frequently appealed to in clinical ethics.
- Describe steps in the process of ethical decision making.
- Identify resources available to nurses to resolve ethical dilemmas.
- Discuss an ethical issue confronted by critical care nurses in practice and how applying ethical principles may assist in its resolution.

*M*echanical replacement of kidney function was once science fiction. Now we can not only mechanically replace the function of the kidneys through dialysis, but also replace the kidney itself through transplantation. The incorporation of sophisticated technology into the clinical arena has made the once simpler questions of life and death increas-

The author's work was done as part of her responsibilities for the U.S. government.

ingly more complex. Progress in health care technology is a double-edged sword. Although there are indisputable benefits from the availability and use of technology, there are also profound ethical, legal, economic, and social challenges and dilemmas.

Questions regarding the appropriate timing and use of technology are fundamental, and nowhere is this more true than in critical care. The intensive care unit (ICU) is dense with complicated technology and is a place where crucial decisions about life and health are made with striking frequency and urgency. Also, patients in the ICU are older and more acutely ill than in the past. Although nurses and other health care providers make moral choices constantly in everyday practice, sometimes the choices are difficult and create feelings of uncertainty, conflict, or distress. The function of ethics is to clarify and illuminate moral issues and obligations and to provide systematic methods for reaching resolutions.

How does ethics illuminate moral conflict? Identifying a problem as a source of moral uncertainty, distress, or dilemma begins the process of reasoning through the complexity. *Moral uncertainty* exists if one is unable to identify clearly a moral conflict within a situation but experiences the troublesome feeling that "something is not quite right." *Moral dilemmas* occur if two or more conflicting principles or alternatives exist, and to choose one would be to violate or compromise another. *Moral distress* is caused if one can clearly identify a moral conflict and the right action to resolve it, but institutional protocol, disagreement between members of the health care team, or rules of professional etiquette prevent morally appropriate action.

Ethics education, interdisciplinary dialogue, collaboration, communication, consultation with institutional ethics committees, and the use of institutional ethics policies can help nurses reason through moral conflicts in the clinical environment. The major purposes of ethical analysis in the clinical area are to clarify the moral issues and principles involved in a situation, to examine one's responsibilities and obligations, and to provide an ethically adequate rationale for the decision. This chapter presents an overview of ethics, some principles and guidelines for nursing ethics, and a process by which to apply them clinically.

ETHICS

The concept of ethics itself is difficult. What exactly is ethics? Are morals and ethics the same? Where do our personal values and feelings fit into such discussions? Does the nursing profession have its own realm of ethics different from that of the medical profession? On what are the tenets of nursing ethics based?

The original meanings of the terms *morals* and *ethics* are similar. The word *moral*, derived from the Latin *mores*, meant customs and habits; the word *ethics*, derived from the Greek *ethos*, meant customs, habitual usage, conduct, and character. In current discussion, the terms are sometimes used interchangeably, although their definitions are somewhat different.

Morals are personal or codified standards of conduct derived from societal expectations of behavior. They are the standards of behavior and values to which we are committed as members of society. *Ethics*, a more formal term, refers to the systematic study of those standards and values. Ethical inquiry, a form of philosophical or theological inquiry, allows us to think reasonably about, to question, to critique, and ultimately to understand the dimensions of moral conduct. The term ethics is used specifically to mean a method of inquiry that helps us answer questions about what is right or good, what ought to be done in specific situations, what kind of people we want to be, and why.

Sometimes the term ethics is used to refer to the formal beliefs or practices of a particular group of people, such as "Jewish ethics" or "business ethics." Most professional groups have formal codes of conduct for their members, and these are usually called codes of ethics. Within the profession of nursing, conduct is guided by the American Nurses Association's (ANA) Code for Nurses with Interpretive Statements[1] (see display). Other professional associa-

---

American Nurses Association Code for Nurses

1. The nurse provides services with respect for human dignity and the uniqueness of the client, unrestricted by considerations of social or economic status, personal attributes, or the nature of the health problems.
2. The nurse safeguards the client's right to privacy by judiciously protecting information of a confidential nature.
3. The nurse acts to safeguard the client and the public when health care and safety are affected by the incompetent, unethical, or illegal practice of any person.
4. The nurse assumes responsibility and accountability for individual nursing judgments and actions.
5. The nurse maintains competence in nursing.
6. The nurse exercises informed judgment and uses individual competence and qualifications as criteria in seeking consultation, accepting responsibilities, and delegating nursing activities to others.
7. The nurse participates in activities that contribute to the ongoing development of the profession's body of knowledge.
8. The nurse participates in the profession's efforts to implement and improve standards of nursing.
9. The nurse participates in the profession's efforts to establish and maintain conditions of employment conducive to high quality nursing care.
10. The nurse participates in the profession's effort to protect the public from misinformation and misrepresentation and to maintain the integrity of nursing.
11. The nurse collaborates with members of the health professions and other citizens in promoting community and national efforts to meet the health needs of the public.

American Nurses Association, 1985

---

tions, such as the American Association of Critical-Care Nurses (AACN), endorse the ANA's code.

Bioethics in Medicine and Nursing

Bioethics, a form of normative applied ethics, is the study of ethical issues and ethical judgments made within the biomedical sciences, including the delivery of health care. Bioethics becomes interesting and relevant when it abandons the ephemeral realm of abstract theory and concentrates on the difficult and practical realities found in the clinical care of people with everyday or unusual health problems and illness. Some have argued that nursing ethics is just a subset of bioethics, that there is little that is morally unique to nursing. According to this schema, nursing ethics is the ethical analysis of judgments made by nurses, and the same moral issues emerge whether one is the nurse, physician, or patient.[2] Others have contended that nursing ethics is a separate and unique field of inquiry built on an understanding of the nature and philosophy of nursing and the nurse–patient relationship.[3] In either case, nursing ethics is best understood as being built on the specific professional roles and responsibilities of the nurse and on the relationships the nurse has with the patient(s), other health care providers, the institutions with which he or she is affiliated, and society. In fact, a nurse never practices in isolation. Decision making, conflict resolution about ethical issues, and many other issues are best accomplished through communication and collaboration with patients, peers, and colleagues on the health care team.

Nursing ethics asks specifically what our obligations are as nurses, what makes a good nurse, and what ends nursing ought to seek. Codes of professional ethics, bioethical principles, and theories all provide nurses with guidance for addressing these questions. They are general guidelines for professional conduct that should be applied to specific clinical situations and when making judgments about individual cases.

Personal Values and Feelings

In addition to the ANA guidelines and general moral principles, personal values, emotions, and judgment help determine the action the nurse takes in a particular situation. In Plato's *Crito*, Socrates states that reason rather than emotion should guide decisions. By definition, ethics involves systematic study, in which reason must play an important part.

How we feel about an issue, however, is a manifestation of our moral convictions that cannot and should not be ignored. To reach an ethical decision allowing reason to temper emotions and emotions to tutor reason would be ideal. Although nursing is a moral endeavor based on the idea of service, the nurse must be allowed to practice in a manner that maintains the practitioner's sense of self-respect while also maintaining the dignity of the patient.

Nursing practice takes place within a team of health care professionals reflecting a multiplicity of values that can be in conflict. Differing personal, professional, and institutional values compound moral conflict; all must be considered. In the end, these competing values must be weighed and assigned priority in light of the ethical norms that guide us.

■ THE TOOLS OF ETHICS

Resolution may seem impossible when we are involved in moral conflict. Systematically applying the tools of ethics, basic moral principles, and nursing's professional guidelines, however, helps us identify our ethical obligations

and decide which "right" actions can help us meet them. A systematic decision-making process is another tool that can help us identify and meet ethical obligations. Multidisciplinary collaboration and dialogue and consultation with ethics committees or experts, when indicated, are also critical to achieving satisfactory resolution of problems.

Ethical decision making does not promise absolute answers, however. Ethical dilemmas are dilemmas precisely because compelling reasons exist for taking each of two or more opposing actions. Decisions about which action to take should be analyzed and justified using guidelines such as the bioethical principles discussed below. Careful ethical reflection and analysis do not preclude the possibility that reasonable people may disagree. However, the value of thoughtful debate and reflection in making ethical judgments cannot be overestimated.

Systems of Ethical Thought

Within normative ethics, there are two major ethical systems used to determine what is right or wrong. The first category, *consequentialist theories,* includes theories that determine an action to be right or wrong on the basis of its consequences. *Utilitarianism* is, today, chief among the consequentialist theories. For utilitarians, the right action is that which offers the greatest good for the greatest number. The second category, *deontologic* or *nonconsequentialist,* includes theories that judge an action right or wrong on the basis of features other than consequences, usually on the basis of the conformity of the action to a moral rule. Both utilitarian and deontologic theories use principles and rules, although for different reasons.

When applying basic moral principles to specific situations, we should remain aware of our own professional values and obligations that color our ethical reasoning. Awareness of differences in professional and personal obligations can provide insight into sources of interprofessional or interpersonal ethical conflict.

Ethical Principles and Care

Four widely accepted bioethical principles apply to ethical problems in health care.[4] These principles are also pertinent to analyzing moral choices and conflicts faced by practicing nurses. These include nonmaleficence, beneficence, respect for autonomy, and justice; they are defined in the display. These principles offer guidance in determining our rights and responsibilities and in judging what is right or wrong for us to do. Two other principles, less frequently discussed in the ethics literature as basic principles but relevant to nursing practice, are fidelity and veracity.[5] *Fidelity* is the duty to be faithful to one's patients, to keep promises, and to fulfill contracts and commitments. It is the moral covenant between individuals in a relationship. *Veracity* is the duty to tell the truth and not to lie or deceive others.

Clinical Terminology: Principles of Bioethics

Nonmaleficence: The obligation never to deliberately harm another

Beneficence: The obligation to promote the welfare of others, to maximize benefits and minimize harms

Respect for autonomy: The obligation to respect, and not to interfere with, the choices and actions of autonomous individuals (ie, those capable of self-determination)

Justice: The obligation to be fair in the distribution of burdens and benefits and in the distribution of social goods, such as health care or nursing care

---

Because the principle-based approach to ethical problem solving has been criticized as too abstract to be helpful in the complex, human dimensions of real cases, a "care ethic" adds an important dimension, especially for nursing. The care ethic is built on the understanding that individuals are unique, that relationships and their value are crucial in moral deliberations, and that emotions and character traits have a role in moral judgment. Caring is considered essential to the nursing role and has been long valued in the nurse–patient relationship. Nurse caring is directed toward the protection of the health and welfare of patients and indicates a commitment to the protection of human dignity and the preservation of human health. Caring has been called a central art and moral virtue of nursing practice.[6]

NONMALEFICENCE AND BENEFICENCE

The principle of nonmaleficence says that we have an ethical duty not to inflict harm or evil. It is a duty foundational to our society. In other words, the duty not to harm others bears more weight than the duty to benefit others. Citing statements from the Hippocratic oath and the words of Nightingale, Jameton argues that "it is more important to avoid doing harm than it is to do good."[7]

Beneficence involves taking deliberate steps to benefit another person. Beauchamp and Childress state that this duty compels us to provide benefits by preventing and removing harm and to balance benefits and harms by performing a risk–benefit analysis, such as weighing the side effects of a drug against its therapeutic actions.[4]

Beneficence and nonmaleficence, like all moral norms, specify what are called prima facie obligations. A prima facie obligation is binding on all occasions unless it is in conflict with another prima facie obligation of equal or stronger claim. Nonmaleficence or the noninfliction of harm usually is given greater weight. The following patient care study illustrates a situation in which appeal to the principles of nonmaleficence and beneficence may facilitate decision making.

CLINICAL APPLICATION: Patient Care Study

George Edwards, a 59-year-old man, came into the emergency room complaining of dizziness and chest pain for the past week. A cardiac monitor showed ventricular tachycardia, and he was successfully cardioverted and placed on Tridil. After admittance to the coronary care unit, Mr. Edwards required multiple cardioversions for recurrent ventricular tachycardia. At one point, he required cardiopulmonary resuscitation (CPR) for sustained symptomatic ventricular tachycardia. Laboratory work indicated a massive myocardial infarction, and an echocardiogram showed an ejection fraction of 25%. Mr. Edwards' cardiologist planned electrophysiology studies, with a possible implantable defibrillator when the patient became stable.

On day 14 of his hospital stay, Mr. Edwards went into congestive heart failure and sustained ventricular tachycardia, requiring CPR and multiple defibrillations. The cardiologist continued to show optimism that the electrophysiology studies and the automatic implantable cardiac defibrillator (AICD) would provide good results. Mr. Edwards was tired, confused at times, and began to seek frequent reassurance from the nurses that he would live long enough for the AICD insertion. He expressed fear about the frequent cardioversions and the discomfort they caused him. The nurses began to question what kind of long-term benefit such treatment would offer this severely compromised patient.

Comfort and Palliative Care

This patient care study shows the dilemma of providing treatment that can offer the benefit of defibrillation for recurrent ventricular tachycardia to a patient already suffering severe cardiac damage. An analysis of the risks and benefits leads to the following questions: Are we helping or harming the patient with recurrent cardioversions? What are the long-term benefits of automatic implantable cardiac defibrillators (AICD)? How do the benefits of recurrent cardioversions in someone with already severe cardiac damage compare with the discomforts and suffering caused by the same procedures? Without the therapy, the patient will die, but do the benefits of avoiding sudden cardiac death outweigh the risks of physical and emotional harm caused by repeated cardioversions and defibrillations while he awaits AICD?

Clinicians who work in the ICU frequently use aggressive treatment to try to stabilize a patient and keep him or her alive. Stepping back to try to ascertain the complex factors that contribute to suffering and comfort for an individual patient is not often easy. Sometimes clinicians forget that relief of suffering is a fundamental goal in health care. In addition to careful pain management, we must be attentive to other components of individual suffering. The desire to prevent harm by postponing death is shaped by beneficence. Perhaps a greater harm than death, however, is the frequent physical and psychological discomfort caused by aggressive treatment. For some people, less aggressive treatment and more comfort may be a more beneficent course. It is crucial to involve the patient or surrogate in discussions about risks and benefits. Another principle that could be very helpful in deciding appropriate action in a case like the previous one is the principle of respect for autonomy.

RESPECT FOR AUTONOMY

Respect for autonomy involves respecting the capacity of an individual to be self-determining, that is, the capacity to deliberate about actions and life choices and to act on those deliberations without interference from others. Informed consent is an application of the principle of respect for autonomy in the health care setting. The nurse's duty regarding informed consent is to see that the patient is adequately informed, has the capacity to understand the options, and can deliberate and make a health care decision. If a patient is incapable of making an informed decision, a surrogate is asked to give consent for the patient. A surrogate is someone who is able to make a "substituted judgment" for the patient; it is usually a spouse, parent, adult child, or someone previously designated by the patient as durable power of attorney for health care. Most importantly, it is someone who knows and can represent the wishes and feelings of the patient regarding the treatment options.

To be fully informed, the patient or surrogate needs all the information a "reasonable person" would need to make a particular decision. If, because of age, physical condition, educational level, position, language, culture, or other factors, the patient or surrogate needs any additional process to understand the information, that must also be supplied. Primary providers are responsible for presenting the information in an understandable manner and for assessing the patient's or surrogate's understanding.

Consistent with respect for autonomy, the consent given as part of informed consent is voluntary. The patient is not to be subject to coercion, fraud, or deceit. A fully informed, freely consenting patient has a right to make an autonomous decision, whether or not it corresponds with what others think he or she should do, as long it does not harm others.

It is not uncommon for patients in the ICU to have compromised autonomy and decision-making capacity due to critical illness and its management. Although important in every health care interaction, assessment of an individual's ability to understand treatment options and make decisions in the ICU should be frequent and careful. Respect for the autonomy of the patient may be manifested through a surrogate decision maker or an advance directive. Respect for people is the overriding principle under which respect for autonomy falls.

Making Treatment and Care Decisions

Historically, most cases in which health professionals and hospitals have sought to override the autonomy of the patient have involved giving the patient treatment or continued treatment deemed necessary for the patient's benefit by the health care team but unwanted by the patient. In most such cases, the patient's or surrogate's wishes have been supported, in both the view of ethics and the law. The right to refuse treatment is a corollary of the right to in-

formed consent and is grounded in the principle of respect for autonomy. The famous words of former Supreme Court Justice Cardozo articulate this respect for a patient's decision to refuse treatment: "Every human being of adult years and sound mind has a right to determine what shall be done with his body . . ."[8] A major concern of the public is being forced to endure an existence supported by machines without hope of a meaningful life and without the ability to have a say in the decision. The Patient Self-Determination Act of 1990 requires all health care facilities that receive federal funds to provide written information to patients about their rights to make decisions about medical care, including the right to accept or refuse care. Included should be information about the right of the patient to formulate an advance directive, such as a living will or a durable power of attorney for health care.

In the United States, most states have statutes regarding advance directives for health care. A living will allows a person to specify in advance wishes regarding treatment and care if he or she loses the capacity to make decisions. A durable power of attorney for health care designates a surrogate, familiar with the patient's treatment preferences, who can make decisions in the event of the patient's incapacity. Advance directives offer the patient an opportunity to express his or her preferences and values for treatment and care in advance of such time when they cannot deliberate and decide for themselves. Encouraging patients to reflect on preferences and to implement a durable power of attorney or living will in case of future need is a demonstration of respect for the autonomy of the patient.

Withholding and Withdrawing Treatment

What does nursing ethics say about withholding or withdrawing treatment, such as medications, mechanical ventilation, intravenous fluids, dialysis, and others? The first provision of the Code for Nurses states that "clients have the moral right to determine what will be done with their own person . . . [and] to accept, refuse, or terminate treatment without coercion." The Code goes on to say that nurses "must protect and preserve human life when there is hope of recovery or reasonable hope of benefit from life-prolonging treatment."

What is meant by the terms "withholding" and "withdrawing"? Withholding refers to never initiating a treatment, whereas withdrawing refers to stopping a treatment once started. Health care professionals often find it emotionally more difficult to withdraw a treatment than to withhold it in the first place. The difference between not starting a treatment and stopping it, however, is not one of moral or legal importance. Ending treatment for sound moral reasons does not violate professional obligations. A presidential commission has acknowledged that "the distinction between failing to initiate and stopping therapy is not itself of moral significance."[9] Because it is not a routine medical order, the presence of both the physician and the nurse at the bedside is encouraged when treatment is to be ended. This offers the opportunity for mutual support to all involved during a time that is often emotionally charged.[10]

The Hastings Center's *Guidelines on the Termination of Life-Sustaining Treatment and Care of the Dying* states that "there is strong reason to prefer stopping treatment over not starting it in some cases . . . . There is often uncertainty about the efficacy of a proposed treatment, or the burdens and benefits it will impose on the patient. It is better to start the treatment and later stop if it is ineffective than not to start treatment for fear that stopping will be impossible."[10]

When the patient or surrogate decides that a proposed treatment will impose undue burdens and refuses such treatment, it is morally correct for the health care professional to respect that decision. If the patient or surrogate decides that a treatment in progress and the life it provides have become too burdensome for the patient, then the treatment may permissibly be stopped. Imposing harmful or futile treatment against the patient's wishes violates the autonomous patient's right to self-determination, and when patients' wishes cannot be known, it violates the nonautonomous patient's best interests. Stopping treatment acknowledges that a patient has an autonomous right to refuse treatment and to determine what constitutes "benefit" for him or her. It also acknowledges the principle of nonmaleficence, or not harming the patient's dignity and quality of life by forcing unwanted, painful, or futile treatment on the patient.

An example of withholding treatment is a "do not resuscitate" (DNR) order, an order not to do cardiopulmonary resuscitation (CPR). The original intent of CPR was to resuscitate or revive patients suffering specific types of sudden cardiac or pulmonary arrest: victims of drowning, electric shock, untoward effects of drugs, anesthetic accidents, heart block, and acute myocardial infarction. In time, CPR became a routine medical intervention extended to almost all patients suffering cardiac or pulmonary arrest, no matter what the underlying disease process. Although CPR has proven dramatically effective for some groups of patients, it is of little, if any, benefit to many others (see display).

The immediate, reflexive intervention to preserve life without the express consent of the patient is supported by the principle of beneficence. Health care personnel assume that a "reasonable person" would wish to be resuscitated and act on the assumption that death is undesirable to the patient. However, some patients can express or have expressed their wishes not to be resuscitated. In such cases, to presume to understand the needs of a patient and act against the patient's expressed wishes (or to avoid ascertaining what those wishes might be) is paternalistic. Paternalism is the act of overriding another's autonomous actions or requests to bring about what is believed to be the most good for that person. Paternalism violates respect for the patient's autonomy.

The perspective of nursing as stated in the Preamble of the *Code for Nurses* acknowledges respect for people as the most fundamental principle in professional practice.[1] Re-

---

Insights Into Clinical Research

Hanson L, Danis M, Mutran E, Keenan N: Impact of patient incompetence on decisions to use or withhold life-sustaining treatment. Am J Med 97(3):235–241, 1994

The purpose of this study was to determine if decisions to withhold treatment were affected by patient competence. Subjects were all patients admitted to a medical service over a 4-month period with congestive heart failure, chronic obstructive pulmonary disease, cancer, or hepatic cirrhosis and with a life expectancy of 6 to 12 months. Competence or incompetence was determined by a daily assessment of cognitive function. The decision to withhold cardiopulmonary resuscitation (CPR) or other forms of treatment or diagnostic testing was based on daily observation and chart review.

The decision to withhold CPR and other life-sustaining treatment occurred significantly more often in the incompetent than in the competent group. Independent predictors of the decision to withhold CPR were incompetence, higher APACHE II scores (sicker patients), and a diagnosis of advanced cancer. Incompetent patients were also more likely to be referred to a hospice on discharge. Of the decisions to withhold CPR for incompetent patients, 79% were made by family members in conjunction with physicians.

These results indicate that family members and physicians place importance on meaningful survival or quality of life, not just on survival.

---

spect for self-determination is essential to respect for people and is undermined whenever intervention takes place without informed consent (if the patient can participate in decision making) or against the patient's wishes. Paternalistic interventions are usually contrary to the spirit and obligations of nursing ethics.

To ensure patient self-determination and the opportunity to refuse treatment, discussion must occur when the patient is alert and has a reasonably clear sensorium. Before making a voluntary and informed decision to accept or to refuse CPR, the patient or surrogate must understand what CPR is and how it will most likely affect the disease process and future quality of life. This process applies to any life-sustaining treatment, hence the need for advance directives.

Decisions should be made jointly by the health care professional and the patient (or patient surrogate). The health care team must supply the necessary information about realistic outcomes and possible interventions. The nurse must ensure that the patient or surrogate understands that information by clarifying technical terms and helping the patient weigh treatment options. By providing the patient an opportunity to discuss personal choices about end-of-life care, the nurse assists the patient. The patient then must consider his or her own values and wishes in the context of prognoses and realistic options. The final decision should reflect the patient's wishes.

It is morally permissible for a nurse to refuse to participate in withholding or withdrawing treatment on the grounds of personal moral conviction or if he or she believes it is against the patient's best interests. In either case, the nurse can remove himself or herself from the situation as long as there is another nurse available to care for the patient.

Questions of Futility and Limits to Autonomy

In contrast to cases in which health care workers wanted to treat patients against their wishes, recently cases have arisen in which the patient or surrogate wanted continued treatment that the physicians or hospital staff felt was inappropriate.

A landmark case of this type involved 86-year-old Helga Wanglie, who had been in a persistent vegetative state and on a ventilator in ICU for more than a year. The health care team treating her felt continued treatment was futile, but her husband disagreed. The court upheld the right of Mr. Wanglie to act as surrogate decision maker for his wife (see Chapter 8 for more details). A more recent case of this type involved a hospital's request to withhold ventilator treatment from Baby K, an anencephalic baby. The court upheld the wishes of the baby's mother for continued ventilation and treatment.[11] These and other cases have stimulated a great deal of discussion among ethicists, health care professionals, and patients' rights groups about futility. Under what conditions, if any, can a patient's request for treatment be denied because of "futility." In addition to lack of consensus on a definition for or criteria for futility, there is concern about whether or not health care providers can be objective enough to make these determinations. In fact, in the most well-publicized court cases involving issues of futility, the courts' decisions focused only on who had the right to make decisions about treatment and have upheld the autonomy rights of family members.

Questions about futility are often raised in relation to the use of CPR. As mentioned previously, current practice is that CPR is used in all situations unless there is a direct DNR order. DNR orders were developed to avoid aggressive efforts to revive a patient when death is imminent and inevitable. Most DNR orders are written with the consent of the patient or surrogate. Debate has focused on the few cases in which the patient or family opts for resuscitation, and the physician or health care team believes CPR is inappropriate. Some have argued that in certain circumstances, a physician should be able to write a DNR order without the consent of the patient or family.[12]

Nurses and other health care professionals promise to act in their patients' best interests, respect their autonomy, and advocate for them. Communicating with patients and their significant others, discussing and respecting their wishes regarding treatment and care, convening patient care conferences for all involved parties, and facilitating the execution of advance directives are all important methods of fulfilling these obligations, as the following patient care study illustrates.

CLINICAL APPLICATION: Patient Care Study

Jack Crawford was a 44-year-old man with severe and persistent pain from metastatic cancer. After a slowly deteriorating stay in the intensive care unit, Mr. Crawford, who was weak, short of breath, anasarcic, and in considerable pain, confided to his primary care nurse, Ms. B, that he was ready to die and did not want any life-sustaining treatments. Ms. B knew that Mrs. Crawford had not accepted her husband's prognosis, was hoping for a miracle, and insisted on aggressive treatment to extend her husband's life. Ms. B dreaded the impending conflict between the unit's aggressive oncologist, the patient with no hope of a life without pain, and the wife who was not ready to let her husband die.

As the primary nurse, Ms. B had worked to develop a trusting relationship with Mr. Crawford and his wife and felt it was her responsibility to act as her patient's advocate. She felt that Mr. Crawford trusted her to communicate his wishes to the physician and the rest of the health care team and to help make sure that they were followed.

Ms. B contacted the physician and set up a family conference to discuss the plan of care with the Crawfords, the physician, the nursing staff, and the social worker. She also spoke to the physician and to Mr. Crawford about the potential usefulness of a written advanced directive and offered some examples. She hoped that the Crawfords and the health care team could discuss Mr. Crawford's prognosis and desires and come to an agreement on what types of treatment would be of benefit to him and consistent with his wishes.

JUSTICE

Justice is a principle of fairness. In the context of health care, the most frequent appeal is to distributive justice, which requires an equitable distribution of burdens and benefits. Is everyone to receive health care, regardless of their ability to pay? If so, is everyone entitled to the same amount (eg, type, quality) of health care? Several substantive criteria have been proposed for answering questions regarding the equitable distribution of social goods, including health care:

- To each person an equal share
- To each person according to need
- To each person according to effort
- To each person according to contribution (including payment)
- To each person according to merit
- To each person according to free market exchanges[4]

Although each of these criteria has strengths and shortcomings, together they provide a basis for deliberation and decision making about how health care is distributed. This applies to the level of how health care resources are distributed in society and how we decide to allocate resources, treatments, and even time and attention between and among patients. Every time a decision is made to offer kidney transplantation to one person and not another, to answer one patient's bell prior to another's, or to put one patient in an ICU bed instead of other(s), criteria such as those listed previously are used. Egalitarians argue that because absolute equality is not possible, fair methods of deciding include only random selection or first-come, first-served, thus avoiding the use of any criteria that make distinctions between people.

Allocation of Resources

Englehardt and Rie[13] identified three major problem situations in the allocation of resources in an ICU:

- When admitting new patients to the ICU endangers the standard of care for all ICU patients; often related to limited personnel, especially nurses
- When potential admissions to the ICU may have greater possible benefit from ICU care than current ICU patients
- When the resources invested in the patient are disproportionate to the anticipated marginal benefits

Incorporated in these problem situations are difficult questions regarding the balance of anticipated benefits and harms for given individuals or groups compared with anticipated benefits and harms for other individuals or groups. They propose the use of an ICU *treatment entitlement index*, which incorporates considerations of likelihood for success, quality of success, length of survival, and costs, to facilitate explicit resource allocation policies.

Zoloth-Dorfman and Carney[14] discuss the case of James Ramsey, a young patient with acquired immunodeficiency syndrome (AIDS) who was admitted through the emergency room (ER) in acute respiratory distress and diagnosed with *Pneumocystis carinii* pneumonia. After the ER physician was unable to obtain a bed in the ICU, Mr. Ramsey was transferred to an AIDS ward. Despite the valiant efforts of the evening shift nurses and the house staff, his condition continued to worsen. The resident was informed that there were "no available beds" in the ICU but later found out that one bed was being reserved for a "code." The patient continued to deteriorate throughout the night, developed acute respiratory distress and hypotensive shock, and a code was called, but the patient died in transit to the ICU.

Hospital staff continued to debate this case, each group feeling their position had been the correct one. ICU staff felt intensive care in this case was futile, and bed space was limited. AIDS unit staff felt their patient had been discriminated against because he had AIDS and worried about the appeal to "futility" as an excuse. This case raises many interesting questions about the way patient selection and resource allocation decisions are made. Perhaps institutional clarification of ICU admitting criteria, including when the bed saved for codes could be used, would have helped in this case.

Distribution of Services

Justice also applies to the distribution of health care services in the country. The "system" (some would say nonsystem) of health care in the United States has been described as fragmented, inefficient, and unjust. The United States spends approximately 14% of its gross national product on health care, and costs have continued to escalate in recent years.[15] Despite these costs, an estimated 35,000,000 or more people have no health insurance. In addition, eligibility, coverage, and reimbursement provided by Medicaid vary dramatically from state to state. During the last few years in the United States, there has been widespread and growing adoption of managed care, in which health insurance companies, industrial health care plans, or groups of patients contract with health care providers to provide a specified level of health care services at a predetermined cost. The goal of managed care is to reduce waste and control costs. Whether managed care plans ultimately save money remains an open question. A recent editorial described managed care as a "work in progress."[16] Recent studies have documented poorer survival and decreased access to treatment for some patients enrolled in managed care plans.[17] Concerns about quality of care have led, among other things, to legislation such as that passed by the U.S. Congress in September 1996, which requires hospitals and payers to provide a minimum of 48 hours of postpartum care for mothers. A major concern expressed by many health care providers is that in striving to "manage" patients efficiently, we may be ignoring significant individualized needs for "care."[18] During the next few years, continued changes in the structure and payment of health care delivery in the United States are likely to occur.

■ ETHICAL DECISION MAKING WITHIN A NURSING PROCESS MODEL

Aspects of a moral conflict include interests of the patient, professional and personal values of health care professionals, institutional values, personal feelings, moral principles, and legal issues. At first glance, it might seem impossible to integrate them into anything other than an incoherent mass of conflicting possible actions.

Ethical decision-making models provide a process for systematically and thoughtfully examining a conflict, ensuring that participants consider all important aspects of a situation before taking action. The steps of ethical analysis and evaluation are much like the steps of the nursing process. Both provide an orderly approach to problems. There are usually five steps to resolution of an ethical problem in the clinical setting.

CLINICAL APPLICATION:
Nursing Intervention Guidelines
Model for Ethical Decision Making

Analysis of an ethical problem in the clinical setting usually involves the following five steps:
1. Gather the relevant facts and identify the decision maker(s).
2. Identify the ethical problem.
3. Analyze the problem using ethical guidance.
4. Analyze action alternatives in light of that guidance, and choose one.
5. Evaluate and reflect.

GATHER THE RELEVANT FACTS

The first step is to identify information needed to understand the situation fully. What are the medical facts (ie, diagnoses, prognoses, treatment alternatives)? Who are the principle agents involved? Who are the decision makers and the stakeholders? Are the values and goals for treatment and care of the patient clear? How do the values, interests, and relationships of others involved affect the problem? Are cultural, religious, or other aspects relevant to this situation? It is important to understand the various contexts of the situation, including the physiological, psychosocial, and legal dimensions. Are there legal ramifications, institutional policies, or economic factors to consider?

IDENTIFY THE PROBLEM

The next step is to identify the ethical problem(s). Is this truly a problem involving conflicting ethical principles or values, or is it primarily a legal issue or a communication problem? Communication problems and legal restrictions are often part of an ethical problem; however, some problems can be resolved simply through better communication or legal counsel without ethical analysis.

ANALYZE THE PROBLEM USING ETHICAL PRINCIPLES AND RULES

It is essential to identify the person who is to make the final decision. Is the patient competent, fully informed, and free to choose (consistent with application of the principle of respect for autonomy)? Is there a family member able to speak to the best interests of a comatose patient (beneficence) or a designated durable power of attorney for health care who knows the patient's wishes (respect for autonomy)? Are there vested interests to consider?

Consider ethical principles. Is harm being avoided or minimized? What are the benefits, and who will benefit? What are the harms, and who will be harmed? Are rights being protected? Have the patient's wishes and interests been articulated? Have promises been made? Has fairness been considered? Which principles are most applicable to the case? There may be competing claims, all of which are reasonable and justifiable, and a conflict of principles. There may also be conflicts between principles and legal or institutional requirements. Consider also whether care and compassion have played a role.

ANALYZE ALTERNATIVES AND ACT

Identify all the possible and reasonable alternatives, and evaluate each of them on their conformity to principles and rules and their compatibility with care and compassion for the patient. Will each of the options respect the autonomy of the patient? Is the patient fully informed and freely consenting? How is the family involved? Is there a designated surrogate? How will each proposed action and its outcome benefit or harm those involved? Will the action strengthen or jeopardize patient–professional bonds and reaffirm society's expectations of health care professionals? After reflec-

tion and careful reasoning, nurses and other health care professionals should choose and act on the option that is most consistent with sound ethical analysis and personal moral convictions.

When considering alternatives, nurses must evaluate their position and involvement in the case. Often the nurse is not the primary decision maker. However, because the nurse is an integral member of the health care team, it is important that she or he contribute to the dialogue, facilitate communication, articulate relevant personal views and values, and cooperate in implementation of the course of action. The nurse's role also includes planning a multidisciplinary conference or arranging for an ethics consultation.

EVALUATE AND REFLECT

After the action has been taken, the ethical problem, the process of resolution, and the outcome must be further analyzed. Compare the outcome with what was hoped for or intended. How can a similar situation be handled with greater sensitivity or wisdom in the future? Evaluation is especially helpful if it is undertaken in a quiet, nonthreatening atmosphere conducive to reflection.

■ BIOETHICS RESOURCES AND SERVICES

Informed clinicians and clear organizational policies and support help in preventing and resolving ethical dilemmas in health care organizations. In addition, most health care organizations have some ethics services, which may consist of an ethics committee or an ethics consultation service or program. Services provided generally include education, policy development, and consultation at the bedside for ethical problems that arise in patient care.

Ethics Committees and Consultant Services

Ethics committees are multidisciplinary and should include representatives of the professions and disciplines involved in patient care (ie, nursing, medicine, social work, spiritual care, and others). In addition, at least one member of the lay community should be a part of the ethics committee. A lawyer, an ethicist, clergy, and others may be members of the committee or serve as *ad hoc* consultants.

Ethics committee members should be involved in self-education as well as education of the professional staff and community on issues related to clinical ethics. Ethics committees may serve as an institutional resource for policy studies and the drafting of institutional policies concerning ethical issues. The Joint Commission on Accreditation of Organizations requires policy statements and guidelines on a number of issues, including the process of addressing ethical issues, informed consent, use of surrogate decision makers, decisions about care and treatment at the end of life, and confidentiality of information.[19] Well thought out and articulated policies about these types of issues offer useful guidance to clinicians in often difficult situations. Ethics consultation is frequently offered in one or both of two modes: an initial bedside consultation or a committee consultation. A bedside consultation by one or more trained consultants may be sufficient to provide the education, clarification, or dialogue necessary to assist decision makers in resolving the problem. In some more complicated cases or when there is conflict among decision makers, consultation by the whole ethics committee may be appropriate. After deliberation, some committees aim to make a single recommendation for the resolution of the ethical problem, while others aim to frame the morally acceptable options and assist key decision makers in choosing an acceptable course of action. In seeking consultation, it is useful to clarify the structure, process, and approach of available bioethics services within each institution.

In addition to services provided by an ethics committee or bioethics consultant service, other valuable resources are available to nurses. Some institutions have nursing ethics committees which, although possibly coordinated with an existing institutional ethics committee, often function independently. These committees are designed to meet the needs of nurses within the institution by providing education and addressing issues unique to nursing, such as refusal of assignment, staffing patterns, and allocation of beds. Some institutions sponsor periodic ethics rounds, which may be general, unit based, or specific to nursing and serve primarily an educational function. Pastoral care, quality assurance, and peer support activities are other examples of institutional resources that may facilitate the resolution of ethical problems.

Professional Nursing Organizations

Professional nursing organizations also address ethical issues of concern to nursing practice. The ANA addresses professional issues and moral dilemmas common to all nurses in the United States. In addition to the aforementioned ANA *Code for Nurses*, the ANA's Center for Ethics and Human Rights publishes position statements and guidelines on many issues for which nurses seek ethical guidance. The AACN also has an active ethics committee, which develops policy statements and position papers that set standards for ethical behavior and decision making for critical care nurses. AACN's ethics committee works closely with other professional nursing organizations and interfaces with other professional organizations, such as the Society for Critical Care Medicine, to examine issues shared by both professions.

Adequate information, multiple perspectives, deliberate thought, ethical principles and guidance, and organizational support are extremely important in enabling clinicians to exercise professional judgment and make sound decisions. Seeking advisory and consultative services from an appropriate resource often assists in this process.

■ CONCLUSION

Sound professional judgment requires clinical excellence, a philosophy of caring, and a determined belief that one of nursing's primary responsibilities is to advocate for the patient, ensuring that the patient's right to self-determination and best interests are both served if possible. Knowledge of basic ethical principles and the ability to apply them systematically are essential to professional nursing practice. Professional responsibility does not end with knowledge, but lies in actively trying to understand patients' values and beliefs and integrating care and compassion into relationships with patients. Nurses have a responsibility to be familiar with the philosophy of nursing and the ethical principles and rules that nursing espouses and to incorporate them into professional practice as habits of thought and action. Maintaining one's professional integrity requires habitual, systematic examination of each patient's plan of care to ensure that the patient receives the information and counseling necessary to make informed decisions, that the patient's informed decisions are respected, that actions are designed to maximize benefits and minimize risks, and that issues of fairness are addressed.

The role of the critical care nurse is to foster an environment in which informed decision making about treatment and care preferences is valued and considered essential to good care. The critical care nurse should help to develop and implement institutional and public policies that reflect a philosophy of care and compassion for patients, balanced with a responsibility to support patient autonomy and protect the free exercise of moral agency by nurses.

Clinical Applicability Challenges

Self-Challenge: Critical Thinking

1. *You believe that CPR is inappropriate for your patient who is terminally ill with metastatic cancer. Construct plans for proceeding. Identify the people with whom you would talk and in what order. Structure arguments you would make to support your position.*

2. *A patient in your unit has severe and intractable pain, which you believe is being inadequately managed. Consider whether or not this is an ethical issue, and state why or why not. Explain what you would do to resolve the problem. Defend your position by using the ANA's Code for Nurses.*

3. *You receive a call from the ER regarding a septic patient who needs to be admitted to your unit. At the time of the call, however, your unit is full. Explain the criteria you would use to determine if there is a patient that could be moved to another unit to accommodate the ER patient. Conclude who would make this decision, and construct how the decision would be made. Choose the ethical principle relevant to this situation.*

Study Questions

1. *Choose the most correct answer to describe the primary purpose of the Patient Self-Determination Act:*
   a. *Requires patients to complete an advance directive*
   b. *Ensures treatment preferences for the terminally ill patient*
   c. *Gives the patient surrogate the power to make decisions for the patient*
   d. *Makes patients aware of their rights to accept or refuse medical treatments so that they can make choices while they are still capable*

2. *Ethics helps people reach answers to moral dilemmas by*
   a. *clarifying the moral issues and principles involved in a situation.*
   b. *helping the person to examine his or her responsibilities and obligations.*
   c. *providing an ethically adequate rationale for a decision.*
   d. *All of the above*

3. *A nurse believes that the medical treatment being given a particular patient is ethically inappropriate and refuses to give the patient care, leaving the workplace that day to avoid being a part of the situation. This is an example of*
   a. *a nurse standing up for his or her right not to participate in morally objectionable care.*
   b. *violation of the principles of beneficence and fidelity through patient abandonment.*
   c. *a nurse's support for the principle of nonmaleficence, noninfliction of harm.*
   d. *the exercise of professional nurse judgment.*

4. *Which of the following is not true?*
   a. *Withholding life-sustaining treatment is ethically acceptable, but withdrawing such treatment is not.*
   b. *To be truly autonomous, a patient must be fully informed and freely consenting.*
   c. *DNR is a medical order to withhold CPR.*
   d. *A nurse's duty always to act in the best interests of his or her patient is based on the principle of beneficence.*

REFERENCES

1. American Nurses Association: Code for Nurses With Interpretive Statements. Kansas City, MO, American Nurses Association, 1985
2. Veatch R, Fry S: Case Studies in Nursing Ethics. Philadelphia, JB Lippincott, 1987
3. Fry S: Toward a theory of nursing ethics. Advances in Nursing Science 11(4):9–22, 1989
4. Beauchamp T, Childress J: Principles of Biomedical Ethics (4th Ed). New York, Oxford University Press, 1994
5. Omery A: Foreword. Journal of Cardiovascular Nursing 9(3):vi–ix, 1995
6. Fry S: Nursing ethics. In Reich W (ed): Encyclopedia of Bioethics, pp 1822–1827. New York, Simon and Schuster Macmillan, 1995
7. Jameton A: Nursing Practice: The Ethical Issues, p 93. Englewood Cliffs, NJ, Prentice-Hall, 1984
8. Schloendorff v. Society of N.Y. Hospital, 211 N.Y. 125, 105 N.E. 92, 93(1914)
9. President's Commission for the Study of Ethical Problems in Medicine and Biomedical and Behavioral Research: Deciding to Forego Life-sustaining Treatment, p 61. Washington, DC, Government Printing Office, 1983
10. The Hastings Center: Guidelines on the Termination of Life-Sustaining Treatment and Care of the Dying. Briarcliff Manor, NY, 1987
11. Fletcher J: Decisions to forego life-sustaining treatment when the patient is incapacitated. In Fletcher J, Hite C, Lombardo P, Marshall M (eds): Introduction to Clinical Ethics, p 155. Frederick, MD, University Publishing, 1995
12. Council on Ethical and Judicial Affairs, American Medical Association: Guidelines for the appropriate use of do-not-resuscitate orders. JAMA 265:1868–1871, 1991
13. Englehardt H, Rie M: Intensive care units, scarce resources, and conflicting principles of justice. JAMA 255(9):1159–1164, 1986
14. Zoloth-Dorfman L, Carney B: The AIDS patient and the last ICU bed: Scarcity, medical futility, and ethics. QRB 17(6):175–181, 1991
15. Spencer E: Economics, case management, and patient advocacy. In Fletcher J, Hite C, Lombardo P, Marshall M (eds): Introduction to Clinical Ethics, p 209. Frederick, MD, University Publishing, 1995
16. Ellwood P, Lundbergh G: Managed care: A work in progress. JAMA 276(13):1083–1086, 1996
17. Ware J, Bayliss M, Rogers W, Kosinki M, Tarlov A: Differences in 4 year health outcomes for elderly and poor, chronically ill patients treated in HMO and fee-for-service systems: Results from the Medical Outcomes Study. JAMA 276(13):1039–1047, 1996
18. Darragh M, McCarrick P: Managed health care; new ethical issues for all. Kennedy Institute of Ethics Journal 6(2):189–297, 1996
19. Fletcher J, Spencer E: Bioethics services in health care organizations. In Fletcher J, Hite C, Lombardo P, Marshall M (eds): Introduction to Clinical Ethics, p 231. Frederick, MD, University Publishing, 1995

BIBLIOGRAPHY

Arras J, Steinbock B: Ethical Issue in Modern Medicine. Mountain View, CA, Mayfield, 1995
Beauchamp, T, Childress J: Principles of Biomedical Ethics (4th Ed). New York, Oxford University Press, 1994
Berrio M, Levesque M, Levesque M: Advance directives; most patients don't have one. Do yours? Am J Nurs 96(8):25–29, 1996
Fletcher J, Hite C, Lombardo P, Marshall M (eds): Introduction to Clinical Ethics. Frederick, MD, University Publishing Group, 1995
Mitchell L: Resources for ethical decision making. J Cardiovasc Nurs 1995; 9(3):78-87.
Omery, A. Care: The basics for a nursing ethic? Journal of Cardiovascular Nursing 9(3):1–10, 1995
Pence T, Cantrall J: Ethics in Nursing, An Anthology. New York, National League for Nursing, 1990

8

Legal Issues in Critical Care

OBJECTIVES

Based on the content in this chapter, the reader should be able to:

- Define the four elements of malpractice (professional negligence).
- Analyze the concept of negligence.
- Delineate allegations commonly made against nurses.
- Explain types of vicarious liability.
- Apply knowledge of advance directives to patient care situations.

*B*ecause society seems to be more litigious than ever, legal issues involving critical care are of increasing concern. The number of malpractice suits that name or in-volve nurses is increasing. Issues such as refusal and termination of treatment have been widely discussed and addressed in the literature. Even legislatures have acted—so-called living will statutes have been enacted in many jurisdictions.

This chapter begins with a discussion of principles of negligence as they apply to the critical care nurse. It then proceeds to identify and address certain current legal issues most applicable to the critical care nurse.

▬▬ NURSING NEGLIGENCE IN CRITICAL CARE

The legal responsibility of the registered nurse in critical care settings does not differ from that of the registered nurse in any work setting. The registered nurse adheres to five principles for the protection of the patient and practitioner. These responsibilities are listed in the accompanying display.

The most common lawsuits against nurses and their employers are based on the legal concept of malpractice, which is negligence by a professional. The following discussion emphasizes the major elements of malpractice and provides some case examples for clarification.

Duty and Breach of Duty

A duty is a legal relationship between two or more parties. Several different kinds of situations can create this type of

---

Five Legal Responsibilities of the Registered Nurse

- Performs only those functions for which he or she has been prepared by education and experience
- Performs those functions competently
- Delegates responsibility only to personnel whose competence has been evaluated and found acceptable
- Takes appropriate measures as indicated by observations of the patient
- Is familiar with policies of the employing agency

---

legal relationship between the nurse and the patient. Most commonly, the duty element in malpractice is established when the patient enters the hospital or health care facility. The admission creates a binding contract on the patient or his insurer to pay for all services rendered. The health care team is obligated to provide reasonable services in exchange for the fees charged.

A nurse who cares for a patient is legally responsible for providing reasonable care under the circumstances present at the time of the incident. The critical care nurse who fails to provide reasonable care under the circumstances has breached (violated) his or her duty toward the patient.

Many different methods are used to determine whether the nurse complied with reasonable standards of care that existed at the time of the incident. Testimony from experts in critical care, agency procedure and protocol manuals, nursing job descriptions, nursing texts, professional journals, medication books, professional organization standards (Advance Cardiac Life Support and Certified Critical Registered Nurse), and equipment manufacturers' instructions can all be used to determine whether or not the care of the critical care nurse was reasonable.

Once the duty is established, a breach of that duty is required; that is, the nurse must have been negligent. Negligence is found or refuted by a comparison of the nurse's conduct with the standard of care. Generally, negligence is either ordinary or gross. Ordinary negligence implies professional carelessness, whereas gross negligence suggests

---

Clinical Terminology: Elements of Malpractice

Duty: A legal relationship between two or more parties
Breach of duty: Failure to comply with reasonable standards of care under the circumstances
Causation: The actions or inaction of the nurse must cause the injury to the patient. Also, the patient's injuries must have been reasonably foreseeable
Injury: The patient must suffer some type of harm as a result of the nurse's actions or inaction

---

that the nurse willfully and consciously ignored a known risk of harm to the patient. Most cases involve ordinary negligence, but gross negligence can be present if a nurse harmed a patient while under the influence of drugs or alcohol.

Causation

Malpractice law also requires that there be a causal relationship between the conduct of the critical care nurse and the injury to the patient, and the injury that the patient suffers must be reasonably anticipated. For example, if a critical care nurse administered digoxin to a cardiac patient who had a pulse of 30, and the patient suffered a cardiac arrest, it is likely that the critical care nurse would be found to have caused the patient's arrest. However, if the patient had a pulse of 70 when the digoxin was administered and the patient suffered a totally unanticipated seizure, it is probable that the nurse would not be found to have caused the seizure because the seizure was not caused by the digoxin and because seizures are not an expected complication of digoxin administration.

Injury

To recover monetary damages in a malpractice suit, the plaintiff has to show that some type of injury or harm occurred as a result of the nurse's actions or inaction. The law allows monetary damages for several different types of harm. For example, injured patients may recover damages for physical injuries, mental harm, pain and suffering, lost income, and emotional distress. In many cases, the spouse of the patient and dependent children can also recover damages for what they suffer as a consequence of the injuries to the patient.

The following case examples may help clarify the legal and professional principles that apply in malpractice cases. Many types of malpractice complaints are lodged against critical care nurses. The following cases illustrate reasons nurses are often named in malpractice suits.

Critical Care Nursing Negligence and Case Law

CASE 1: Failure to Monitor the Patient's Condition Properly

Neonate Loren Dempsey was born with severe breathing difficulties. As a result, shortly after birth, she was intubated and transferred to the neonatal nursery. Fifty minutes after birth, it was discovered that Loren had been improperly intubated. As a consequence of the unrecognized improper esophageal intubation, she experienced oxygen deprivation and was severely impaired.

On her behalf, Loren's parents sued the United States government, because she had been born in a military hospital. Her parents contended that physician and nursing staff had failed to recognize the improper intubation and had inadequately monitored Loren's condition. The magistrate judge hearing the case agreed and awarded $2.8 million to Loren and $1.3 million to her parents for the loss of society and affection of their child.[1]

In this case, Loren was an unstable newborn who required intubation. Reasonable standards of nursing care mandated that her condition be assessed on a regular basis. This included the prompt recognition of complications, such as improper ventilation. Although Loren's initial unstable respiratory status was not due to nursing negligence, the nurse's failure to recognize and treat worsening respiratory status did constitute negligence.

CASE 2: Failure to Comply With Reasonable Standards of Care

On May 11, Mr. Ulmer was admitted to a hospital intensive care unit (ICU) following a boat accident. He sustained rib fractures and internal injuries. On May 17, he was discharged. However, on May 23, he was readmitted with complaints of severe chest pains. Emergency surgery was required at this point to repair a tear in his diaphragm and to remove his spleen.

Postoperatively, Mr. Ulmer was transferred to ICU. His condition deteriorated gradually, and he died on May 26. Death was caused by massive bilateral pulmonary emboli infarction of the right lung.

Testimony at trial revealed Mr. Ulmer had been unable to get out of bed, walk around, or otherwise maintain blood circulation. Experts for Mr. Ulmer's estate testified that with Mr. Ulmer's history, nurses and other hospital personnel should have changed the position of his bed or moved him to maintain adequate blood circulation. However, chart entries demonstrated that they allowed him to remain immobile in bed for unreasonably long periods of time.[2]

CASE 3: Failure to Provide a Safe Patient Environment

Michelle Marie H. was recovering at a medical center from a traumatic brain stem injury. While hospitalized, two members of the hospital staff sexually assaulted her. As a result, she became pregnant, and a therapeutic abortion was performed. Suit was filed against the hospital and various health care providers.[3]

CASE 4: Improper Patient Resuscitation

Pamela Jennings was placed on a respirator in an ICU when she developed respiratory complications from chickenpox. She coughed out her endotracheal tube, and the hospital's respiratory therapist reinserted the tube into her esophagus rather than her trachea. She consequently suffered a respiratory arrest, but none of the hospital staff or her treating physician discovered that the tube was misplaced. Ms. Jennings died from lack of oxygen. The claims against the hospital and hospital personnel were settled. A jury found the treating physician liable for malpractice in this case.[4]

CASE 5: Incorrect Medication Administration

The patient in a North Carolina case testified that the nurse administered an intramuscular injection of meperidine (Demerol) and hydroxyzine (Vistaril) about 3 to 4 inches above her knee. She complained that the injection caused subsequent nerve damage to her leg. Nurse expert witness testimony established that the injection site chosen did not comply with reasonable standards of nursing care. A neurologist testified that the patient's injuries were consistent with the injection. The court ordered a trial on the issue of nursing malpractice.[5]

Vicarious Liability

In some cases, a person or institution can be held liable for the conduct of another. This is called vicarious liability. There are several types of vicarious liability, as follows.

The doctrine of *respondeat superior* is translated as "let the master answer for the sins of the servant." This is the major legal theory under which hospitals are held liable for the negligence of their employees. Respondeat superior is a public policy type of legal doctrine. The philosophy behind respondeat superior is based on the idea that because a hospital typically generates profits from the patients seeking care, if negligence occurs, the hospital should pay for some of the damages caused by hospital personnel. This doctrine applies only when hospital employees act within the scope of their employment.

In some situations, respondeat superior is not applicable. For instance, hospitals are usually not responsible for temporary agency personnel, because they are generally employees of the agency, not the hospital. Physicians, unless they are retained by the hospital, do not typically come within the sphere of this doctrine. Actions by hospital nurses who are not "on the job" rarely fall into the respondeat superior category.

Because the hospital may be held liable for nursing activities conducted by their employees, they carry professional liability insurance for the activities of their employees. Generally, a hospital will defend a nurse named in a malpractice case. However, many nurses also carry their own malpractice insurance for off-the-job nursing activities and so they can retain independent counsel in the event that they are sued.

Another type of vicarious liability is called *corporate liability*. Corporate liability occurs when a hospital is found liable for its own unreasonable conduct. For example, if it is found that a unit is chronically understaffed and a patient suffers an injury as a result of short staffing, the hospital can be held accountable if the short staffing caused the patient's injuries. It is reasonable to expect any hospital that has an ICU or an emergency department to take precautionary measures to ensure that it is adequately staffed. Failure to ensure adequate staffing can lead to payment of monetary damages under the theory of corporate liability.

Corporate liability may also occur with "floating" situations. A nurse working in a critical care setting must be competent to make immediate nursing judgments and to act on those decisions. If the nurse does not possess the theory and skills required of a critical care nurse, he or she should not be rendering critical care. A nurse who is not well versed in critical care should notify the charge nurse or nursing supervisor of this fact. The nurse needs to make it clear which nursing care activities he or she can implement. The display that follows addresses issues about which the floating nurse should inquire. The supervisor and charge nurse must then delegate remaining nursing duties to those with adequate education, training, and experience.

Commonly Asked Questions When Rotating to an Unfamiliar Unit

1. If I am asked to go to another unit, must I go? Generally, you will be required to go to the other unit. If you refuse, you can be disciplined under the theory that you are breaching your employment contract or that you are failing to abide by the policies and procedures of the hospital. Some nursing units negotiate with hospitals to ensure that only specially trained nurses rotate to specialty units.
2. If I rotate to an unfamiliar unit, what types of nursing responsibilities must I assume? You will only be expected to carry out nursing activities that you are competent to perform. In some instances, this will be the performance of basic nursing care activities, such as blood pressures, and uncomplicated treatments.

   If you are unfamiliar with the types of medications used on the unit, you should *not* be administering them until you are thoroughly familiar with them. Remember the medication cards you completed in nursing school? They were assigned because a reasonable, prudent nurse does not give medications without knowledge of their pharmacology,

dosage, method of administration, side effects, and interactions with other medications. The same reasoning applies for any other type of critical care monitoring.

3. What should I do if I feel unprepared when I get on the unit? You need to *immediately* notify the charge nurse or supervisor of your concerns. Suggest that you assist the unit with basic nursing care requirements and that specialized activities (invasive monitoring, cardiac monitoring, administration of unfamiliar drugs) be performed by staff who are adequately prepared. Do not feel incompetent because you are not familiar with all aspects of nursing care. After all, when is the last time you saw the neurologist go to labor and delivery and perform a cesarean section?
4. What if the charge nurse orders me to do something I am not able to do safely? You are obligated to say you are unqualified and request that another nurse carry out the task. The charge nurse also needs to remember that he or she could be held liable for negligent supervision if they order you to do an unsafe activity and a patient injury results.

A third type of vicarious liability is *negligent supervision*. Negligent supervision is claimed when a supervisor fails to supervise people reasonably under his or her direction. For example, if a nurse is rotated to an unfamiliar unit and informs the charge nurse that she has never worked in critical care, it would be unreasonable for the charge nurse to ask her to perform invasive monitoring. If the charge nurse did assign such responsibilities to the floater and a patient injury resulted, the charge nurse could be held accountable to the patient for negligent supervision.

Finally, a fourth type of vicarious liability is known as the *captain of the ship doctrine*. At one time, the physician was viewed as the captain of the ship. Therefore, any order by the doctor was expected to be followed by the nurse. This doctrine has largely been replaced by a legal concept known as *the rule of personal liability*. That is, by virtue of specialized education, training, and experience, nurses are expected to make sound decisions. If they are unsure about the propriety of a physician's order, they need to seek clarification from the physician or, if needed, from their supervisor.

Protocols

If the critical care nurse is required to perform medical acts and is not under the direct and immediate supervision of a delegating physician, the activities must be based on established protocols. These protocols should be created by the medical and nursing departments and should be reviewed for compliance with state nurse practice acts. They must be reviewed frequently so that health care professionals can determine whether they reflect current medical and nursing standards of care. In the event of a malpractice suit, the critical care protocols and procedures can be introduced as evidence to help establish the applicable standard of care.

Although it is important that protocols provide direction, excessive detail restricts the critical care nurse's flexibility when selecting a proper course of action.

The Questionable Medical Order

In addition to protocols, a policy statement should exist (in procedures or by directive) that indicates the manner of resolving the issue of the "questionable" medical order. This is important for all medical orders but particularly for those given for critically ill patients because of the unusual doses of medication that are frequently ordered. The nurse who questions a particular order should express his or her specific reasons for concern to the physician who wrote the order. This initial approach frequently results in an explanation of the order and a medical justification for the order in the patient's medical record. If this approach is unsuccessful, many hospitals require that the attending physician or the nursing supervisor be notified; others have a policy that the chief of service must be consulted about questionable orders. If these options are unavailable or are unsuccessful, a critical care nurse or any other nurse can refuse to give a medication.

An order that is patently wrong can harm the patient if it is followed. A secondary consequence can be liability for the physician and the nurse (and the hospital, as the employer) if the patient suffers harm as a direct result of the order.

Medical Equipment

A medical device, defined as virtually anything used in patient care that is not a drug, includes more complicated pieces of equipment (eg, intra-aortic balloon pumps, endotracheal tubes, pacemakers, defibrillators), along with less obvious ones, such as bedpans, suture materials, patient restraints, and tampons. Before 1976, medical devices were unregulated; since 1976, medical devices have been regulated by the Food and Drug Administration (FDA). Before November 1991, hospitals, their employees, and staffs were permitted but not required to report device malfunctions to the device manufacturer or to the FDA.

On November 28, 1991, the Safe Medical Devices Act of 1990 became effective (Pl 101-629), just after proposed regulations (called the Tentative Final Rule) were published for comment. This act requires user facilities (which include hospitals and ambulatory surgery facilities but not physician offices) to report to the manufacturer medical device malfunctions that result in serious illness or injury to a patient and to report to the FDA those that result in a patient's death. A serious illness or injury includes not only a life-threatening injury or illness, but also an injury that requires "immediate medical or surgical intervention to preclude permanent impairment of a body function or permanent damage to a body structure."[6] Thus, the rupture of an intra-aortic balloon pump that requires that the balloon-dependent patient immediately be transported to the operating room for removal and replacement of the device is a reportable event.

Nursing and other staff now must participate in reporting device malfunctions, even those associated with user error, to a designated hospital department. Personnel in that area are generally responsible for determining which malfunctions engender an obligation to report and to whom.

More recently, the FDA has proposed a new tracking system in which hospitals must participate. As of March 1, 1993, facilities that implant certain devices (eg, pacemakers, heart valves, silicone breast implants) must notify the manufacturer when the devices are implanted and maintain files the hospital can use to determine the identities and certain other information about patients in whom the devices have been implanted.[7]

There is a duty not to use equipment that is patently defective. If the equipment suddenly ceases to do what it was intended to do, makes unusual noises, or has a history of malfunction and has not been repaired, the hospital could be liable for damage caused by it, and nurses could be liable if they know or should know of these problems and use the equipment anyway. The following cases involved liability for defective equipment.

CASE 6: Medical Equipment and Patient Injuries

Mr. Carter was admitted to the hospital for hemorrhaging and underwent a partial gastrectomy. Postoperatively, x-rays were ordered to assess his status. Two nursing students tried to assist transfer of a portable x-ray machine into his room for the x-ray studies. The wheels of the machine became tangled in the cord and the portable x-ray machine fell onto Mr. Carter's abdomen and pinned his left arm and hand. Mr. Carter suffered excruciating pain and had to undergo a second operation for gastric hemorrhaging. Mr. Carter recovered $17,500 actual damages for his injuries.[8]

CASE 7: Defective Equipment and Negligence

An infant suffered a cardiac arrest during surgery and was treated postoperatively with a hypothermia machine. Although the nurse knew that the continuous readout thermometer often malfunctioned, she did not check it with a glass thermometer. After the infant's temperature did not decrease, the nurse did not use other methods to lower body temperature, nor did she call the physician. The infant had a seizure and required mechanical ventilation. The nurse noticed poor air exchange but did not correct a kink in the ventilator tubing. The infant suffered permanent neurological damage. The court held that the injury was proximately caused by the negligence of the hospital's employees and by the defective equipment used in the ICU.[9]

Consent

In most instances, the law requires that the patient be given enough information prior to a treatment to make an informed, intelligent decision. However, in some situations, such consent is not required. An emergency situation does not require informed consent, and a patient can waive informed consent by stating that he or she does not want information about a proposed treatment or procedure. Additionally, some courts allow a physician to avoid full disclosure if the information disclosed might lead to further patient harm. This exception is known as therapeutic privilege.

Generally, obtaining informed consent from the patient or the family is the responsibility of the physician, but many times the nurse will be asked to witness the consent form. In these cases, the nurse is attesting that the signature on the consent form is the patient's or the family member's. When the nurse actually witnesses the physician's explanation concerning the nature of the proposed treatment, treatment risks and benefits, alternative therapies, and potential consequences if the patient decides to do nothing, the nurse may want to place a note on the consent form or in the nurse's notes stating "consent procedure witnessed." This information may be vital in the rare case in which the patient or family sues the physician for lack of informed consent.

▄▄▄ ISSUES THAT INVOLVE LIFE-SUPPORT MEASURES

Several basic issues regarding refusal and termination of treatment can involve the critical care nurse. Do not resuscitate (DNR) orders, refusal of treatment for religious reasons, advance directives, and withdrawal of life support all fall into this category. All of these are complex topics. However, a brief overview of these areas is provided.

Do Not Resuscitate Orders

It has been reported that cardiopulmonary resuscitation (CPR) takes place in 30% of patients who die at a major Boston hospital.[10] However, CPR is not appropriate for all patients who experience a cardiac arrest because it is highly invasive and may constitute a "positive violation of an individual's right to die with dignity."[11] Furthermore, CPR may not be indicated when the illness is terminal and irreversible and when the patient can gain no benefit.

Prestigious authorities (eg, the President's Commission for the Study of Ethical Problems in Medicine and Biomedical and Behavioral Research) have recommended that hospitals have an explicit policy on the practice of writing and implementing DNR orders.[12] Several hospitals and medical societies[13] have published DNR policies.

Whether to resuscitate any patient is a decision that is made by the attending physician, the patient, and the family, although critical care nurses and other nurses often have substantial input into the decision. Generally, however, the consent of a competent patient should be required when a DNR order is written. If the patient is incompetent, the physician and family members make the decision. The situation can be more complex, and the physician and the family or patient can disagree. The President's Commission has published advisory tables regarding the resuscitation of both competent and incompetent patients that take into account the patient's preference and the likelihood that CPR would benefit the patient.[14]

Once the DNR decision has been made, the order should be written, signed, and dated by the responsible physician. It should be reviewed periodically; hospital policies may require review every 24 to 72 hours. More informal methods of designating patients in whom CPR is not to be undertaken can lead to errors if an arrest occurs. For example, the wrong patient can be allowed to die.

If an arrest occurs in an emergency room or in another situation in which a formal DNR decision has not been made and written, the presumption of the medical and nursing staffs should be in favor of life, and a code should be called. A "slow code" (in which the nurse takes excessive time to call or the team takes its time responding) should never be permitted. Either CPR is indicated, or it is not.

Courts may be involved in DNR decisions. In 1978, a Massachusetts appellate court ruled that an attending physician may lawfully write a DNR order for an incompetent patient for whom there is no life-saving or life-prolonging treatment.[15] More recently, a New York grand jury investigated a hospital that indicated DNR decisions by using purple dots stuck to nursing cards that were discarded after the death of the patient. Nurses from the hospital complained that the decals could be stuck to the wrong patient's card; one card had two dots affixed to it. The grand jury found that the dot system "virtually eliminated professional accountability, invited clerical error and discouraged physicians from obtaining informed consent from the patient or his family."[16]

Refusal of Treatment for Religious Reasons

CASE 8: Life-Saving Transfusion for Jehovah's Witness

Gregory Novack, a 16-year-old boy, was seriously injured in an automobile accident. On admission to Kennestone Hospital, he informed the staff not to give him blood because it was against his religious beliefs as a Jehovah's Witness. During orthopedic surgery, Gregory lost a considerable amount of blood. The hospital staff became convinced he would die without a transfusion. The hospital petitioned the court for a guardian ad litem to determine whether a blood transfusion would be in Gregory's best interests. A trial judge conducted an emergency hearing, and a transfusion was ordered against Gregory's and his parents' wishes. Gregory received the transfusion, and subsequently he and his parents claimed his rights of freedom of religion had been violated. The trial and appeals courts found no violation of constitutional rights on the part of the hospital and staff.[17]

The courts are split as to whether or not blood transfusions violate the religious rights of the patient or family. For example, in Vega, the Connecticut Supreme Court found that the hospital cannot "thrust unwanted medical care on a patient who . . . competently and clearly denied that care. . . ." (Stamford Hosp. v. Vega, 646 [1996]). Consequently, ICU nurses need to consult the hospital's risk management department in such situations to ensure proper handling of these types of legal issues.[18]

Advance Directives: Living Wills, Health Care Agents, and Powers of Attorney

A living will is a written directive from a competent patient to family and health care team members concerning the patient's wishes in the event the patient is unable to express these wishes. One difficulty associated with a living will is its limited applicability. In most states, a living will becomes effective only if the patient is terminally ill or permanently comatose. Consequently, when the patient is critically ill or temporarily unable to make health care decisions, the living will is not operative.

To provide broader coverage, many patients opt for a durable power of attorney for health care. A durable power allows the patient to appoint a surrogate decision maker, known as an agent or proxy, who has authority to make treatment and health care decisions in the event that the patient is not able to do so. This type of document allows a trusted friend or relative to "stand in the shoes of the patient" when the patient is not able to make health care decisions.

Many savvy patients elect to combine the living will and the durable power of attorney for health care into one document, commonly called an advance directive. An advance directive allows the patient to communicate his or her wishes in the event of terminal illness or a permanently comatose state. It also names an agent who assists in decision making. Many advance directives give the agent specific instructions concerning health matters. For example, the advance directive may provide instructions concerning artificial nutrition and hydration, or it may outline specific treatments, such as a "no code" status under specified circumstances.

All 50 states have statutes that allow patients to execute living wills, durable powers of attorney for health care, and advance directives.[19] However, each state may place unique requirements on the drafting of these documents. Some states require that the directive be notarized. Other states mandate that the patient be counseled by a state-appointed ombudsman who outlines the pros and cons associated with the advance directive. Witness requirements also vary from state to state. Consequently, it is important to know the laws concerning advance directives that apply in your state. An excellent starting point is an organization called Choice in Dying. This group provides lay people and health care providers with up-to-date information on laws applicable in their state.

In most states, it is likely that a recent living will would be taken as evidence of what the patient would have wanted had he or she been competent when the decision was presented. Although there have not been any cases concerning a written living will, there have been several involving patients who had expressed wishes orally about life-sustaining measures.

CASE 9: Wishes About Life-Sustaining Measures

Brother Fox was an 83-year-old member of a religious order who became permanently comatose during hernia surgery. After hospital officials and physicians refused to cease respirator therapy, Brother Fox's order began court proceedings. New York's highest court, the Court of Appeals, ruled (after the death of the priest) that Brother Fox's oral, solemn statements of his wishes, made to members of his order after the Karen Ann Quinlan case had occurred, was sufficient to authorize termination of treatment.[20]

If a patient or family member reveals the existence of a written living will, a copy should be placed in the medical record, and the attending physician should be notified. If the patient is competent, attempts should be made to clarify the meaning of terminology in the directive; these discussions should be well documented in the medical record. This is necessary to enable nursing and medical personnel to understand exactly what treatment the patient wishes to avoid.

Patient Self-Determination Act

On December 1, 1991, the Patient Self-Determination Act went into effect. This federal statute is applicable to facilities that receive Medicare reimbursement for patient care. As a condition of reimbursement, the law requires that hospitals, nursing facilities, home health care services, hospice programs, and certain health maintenance organizations provide information to adults about their rights concerning decision making in that state. For hospitals, this information must be provided to every adult on admission regardless of diagnosis and regardless of whether the individual is eligible for Medicare coverage. The material distributed must include information about the types of advance directives that are legal in that state. Documentation that the patient has received this information must be placed in the medical record. If the patient is incapacitated on admission, the information must be provided to a family member, if

available. This action, however, does not relieve the hospital of its duty to provide information to the patient once he or she is no longer incapacitated.[21]

Withdrawal of Life-Support Measures

What constitutes life support, when these measures must be used, and when they may be terminated have been issues raised in many court cases. However, the law in these areas is still developing and will continue to do so as each jurisdiction creates its own guidelines.

Given the regularity with which life-support decisions must be made in health care facilities, it is remarkable that it was not until 1976 that the first case, *In re Quinlan*, focused national attention on the "right to die" controversy. The cases have concerned competent minors and adults afflicted with a disease or condition that would eventually be terminal. States have not been consistent in their decisions, even when the situations are arguably similar. For example, the New Jersey court in the case of Karen Ann Quinlan, a 21-year-old woman in a persistent vegetative state, held that the decision about treatment is in the hands of the patient's guardian in consultation with the hospital ethics committee.[22] Massachusetts, however, rejected the New Jersey approach in favor of judicial review of decisions made by physicians and family members.[23] The President's Commission for the Study of Ethical Problems in Medicine and Biomedical and Behavioral Research stated that judicial review of these decisions should be reserved for occasions when "adjudication is clearly required by state law or when concerned parties have disagreements that they cannot resolve over matters of substantial import."[24]

The Florida case of *Satz v. Perlmutter* involved a competent patient and his right to refuse treatment.

CASE 10: Right to Refuse Treatment

Abe Perlmutter was 73 years old, suffered from amyotrophic lateral sclerosis, and was dependent on respirator therapy. He was conscious, competent, and able to speak, although he found speech difficult and painful. He had expressed his suffering and had attempted to disconnect his respirator himself. State officials argued that anyone who helped him disconnect his respirator would be guilty of aiding suicide. The Florida Supreme Court ruled that disconnection of the respirator was not suicide because Mr. Perlmutter's condition was not self-inflicted.[25]

The following three cases concern whether it is necessary to provide patients with fluids and nutrition if they cannot feed themselves.

CASE 11: Food and Fluids

In re Conroy involves an 84-year-old nursing home patient who suffered from severe organic brain syndrome. Her guardian, a nephew, petitioned the court to permit removal of her nasogastric tube, on which she was dependent. The trial court held that the tube could be removed.[26] An appeals court held removal of the tube improper because the bodily invasion suffered by the patient as a result of the treatment was small, and death by dehydration and starvation would be painful.[27] Although the patient had died, the New Jersey Supreme Court held in 1985 that treatment (including artificial feeding and hydration) for nursing home residents may be terminated under certain circumstances and set forth the procedures to be followed. This decision was restricted to nursing home residents who were once competent and who would probably die within approximately 1 year, even with treatment.[28]

Only one case involving the termination of food and fluids has been decided by the U.S. Supreme Court.

CASE 12: Food and Fluids

This case concerned Nancy Cruzan, a young woman who suffered anoxic brain damage in an automobile accident. She remained in a persistent vegetative state in Missouri and was fed by gastrostomy. After rehabilitation was unsuccessful, Ms. Cruzan's parents (as co-guardians) requested withdrawal of the feeding tube. After the employees of the rehabilitation center where she was a patient declined, the Cruzans sought judicial review of their request. After testimony, the trial court approved the parents' request. On appeal, the Missouri Supreme Court reversed the lower court. First, it held that Missouri law does not permit surrogate decision making in decisions of this importance. For a person to exercise the right to terminate artificial feeding in Missouri, that person must have previously expressed his or her wishes, either orally or in writing. Evidence of those wishes had to meet a relatively high evidentiary standard, a standard that the court held had been met in the lower court proceeding.

This case was appealed to the U.S. Supreme Court, and in 1990, it was affirmed on constitutional ground.[29] After the decision was issued, the Cruzans returned to the Missouri lower court and presented further evidence (through additional witnesses) about what their daughter had expressed while competent. The lower court found that they had presented clear and convincing evidence and affirmed the rights of the co-guardians to authorize withdrawal of the feeding tube. After withdrawal of the tube, Nancy Cruzan died on December 26, 1990.

Although this case received much publicity, it did not change the law in any state but Missouri. Most states continue to permit surrogate decision making by relatives and require a lower evidentiary standard than that required in Missouri.

In recent years, as health care providers have become more comfortable recommending termination of treatment in selected cases, they have met resistance from some families who wish to continue treatment no matter what its chance of success. Although no law or legal principle requires that extraordinary, but clearly futile, treatment be provided, it is probably also true that health care providers have no legal recourse against families who refuse to withdraw life support (unless the patient has left written indications of his or her wishes prior to incompetence). There has been one case addressing this complicated problem.

CASE 13: Rights to Terminate Treatment

In December 1989, Helga Wanglie broke her hip. After a complicated course, Mrs. Wanglie, who was 86 years old,

ventilator dependent, and competent, had a cardiopulmonary arrest. After this event, she remained in a persistent vegetative state. Pursuant to the wishes of the family, she was nourished by feeding tube and treated aggressively for recurrent pneumonia. Hospital staff disagreed with the family in this case; intervention by the hospital ethics committee did not resolve the conflict. Therefore, the hospital filed an application for a nonfamily member guardian to decide for the patient. The Minnesota court instead appointed the husband as guardian, finding that he was in the best position to know his wife's wishes. The court found that the hospital had requested the appointment of a nonfamily member not because Mr. Wanglie was incompetent to be guardian, but because he disagreed with hospital staff.[30]

So far there have been no cases in which hospital staff directly challenged a family's decision to continue life support. Most commentators believe that such a challenge to family authority would not prevail, at least in cases where the family is available and interested in making decisions for the patient.

In most states, problems of terminating treatment need not be resolved in court. Decisions regarding treatment or nontreatment that meet accepted medical standards and with which the patient concurs are made virtually every day in health care settings. If the patient is incompetent to decide, generally family members may do so, although they may not refuse therapy that would benefit the patient. Finally, a distinction should be made between termination of treatment and termination of care: Even patients who are not being treated for their terminal condition require competent and sensitive nursing and medical care so that their final days are as comfortable as possible. The families of these patients may also require information along with sensitive emotional support. The need for good nursing care does not end with the decision not to treat.

Brain Death

In 1968, the Harvard criteria established standards for determining brain death. The criteria have been found quite reliable. No case has "yet been found that met these criteria and regained any brain functions despite continuation of respirator support."[31] Some states adopted the Harvard criteria by statute, whereas other states enacted legislation defining brain death in broader, less restrictive terms.

The President's Commission for the Study of Ethical Problems in Medicine and Biomedical and Behavioral Research published *Defining Death* in July 1981. The Commission recommended a uniform statute defining death; it recommended that the statute address "general physiological standards rather than medical criteria and tests, which will change with advances in biomedical knowledge and refinements in technique."[32]

A patient who is brain dead is legally dead, and there is no legal duty to continue to treat him or her. It is not necessary to obtain court approval to discontinue life support on a patient who is brain dead. Furthermore, although it can be desirable to obtain family permission to discontinue treatment of a brain dead patient, there is no legal requirement. However, before terminating life support, physicians and nurses should be sure that organs are not intended for transplant purposes.[33]

Organ Donation

Every state in the United States has a law based on the Uniform Anatomical Gift Act. The statutes establish the legality of organ donation by individuals and their families and set procedures for making and accepting the gift of an organ. Every state also has some provision to enable people to consent to organ donation using a designated place on a driver's license. More recently, many states have enacted "required request" laws. These laws attempt to increase the supply of organs for transplant by requiring hospital personnel to ask patients' families about an organ gift at the time of the patient's death. New York was the second state to enact such a law; it became effective in 1986.[34] A recent Connecticut law goes much further; it requires that hospital personnel ask each patient (aged 18 years or older) whether he or she is an organ donor. The answer must be placed in the medical record.[35] Further proliferation of these statutes is to be expected. It is hoped that new legislation balances the needs of the patient and family and the needs of the organ recipient.

Clinical Applicability Challenges

Self-Challenge: Critical Thinking

1. Mr. C, a critical care patient, is stable after a serious myocardial infarction. Alert and able to make decisions, he tells you if he has another "heart attack," he does not want to be resuscitated.

Explore some of your possible responses to Mr. C. Determine which responses may help you assess his thoughts and feelings about this statement and his current emotional response to his critical illness. Determine which responses indicate your following through on your hospital's policy regarding DNR orders.

Evaluate the Patient Self-Determination Act and advance directives in your state to determine how they can assist Mr. C in further delineating his health care wishes.

Study Questions

1. The doctrine of respondeat superior is the legal theory under which
a. a hospital is directly liable for its corporate hiring decisions.
b. a health care provider is personally liable for acts of negligence.
c. an employer is vicariously liable for the negligent acts of its employees as long as they act within the scope of employment.
d. a hospital is liable for injuries to its employees.

2. The Patient Self-Determination Act went into effect in 1991. This federal law requires that hospitals, nursing homes, and certain other providers
a. provide patients with information about advance directives and require them to execute at least one type of advance directive.
b. provide patients with information about living wills only.
c. provide patients with information about all types of advance directives applicable in that state.
d. provide patients with information about all types of advance directives whether or not applicable in that state.

3. A living will is applicable under which of the following circumstances?
a. If the patient is incapacitated and is terminally ill
b. If the patient is incapacitated and has a life-threatening but curable illness
c. If the patient is competent to express his or her wishes, has a desire to be treated, and has subsequently become incapacitated
d. If the patient is competent but wants his or her grown children to make the health care decisions

---

REFERENCES

1. Dempsey ex. rel. Dempsey v. U.S. No. 92-2042 U.S. Ct. App.(11TH Cir.) April 30, 1993
2. Ulmer v. Baton Rouge General Hospital, 321 So. 2d 1238
3. United Western Medical Centers Incorporated v. Superior Court of Orange County, No. GO18548 (Ct. App., 4th App. Dist.) Feb. 2, 1996
4. Stevens v. Bohlman No. 881548 (Or. Ct. App. Jan. 3, 1996)
5. Holbrooks v. Duke University, Inc. 305 S.E.2d 69 (N.C.App. 1983)
6. Department of Health and Human Services, Food and Drug Administration: Medical devices; Medical device, user facility, distributor, and manufacturer reporting, certification and registration. Federal Register 56:64004–64182 (December 6), 1991
7. Department of Health and Human Services, Food and Drug Administration: Medical devices: Device tracking. Federal Register 57: 22971–22981 (May 29), 1992
8. Carter v. Anderson Memorial Hospital, 325 S.E.2d 78 (S.C.App. 1985)
9. Rose v. Hakim: 335 F. Supp. 1221 (DDC 1971, affirmed in part, reversed in part, 501 F. 2d 806 (DC Cir 1974)
10. Bedell SE, Delbanco TL, Cook EF, Epstein FH: Survival after cardiopulmonary resuscitation in the hospital. N Engl J Med 309:569, 1983
11. Matter of Dinnerstein: 380 NE2d 134, Massachusetts, 1978
12. President's Commission: Deciding to Forego Life-Sustaining Treatment. Washington, DC, Government Printing Office, March 1983
13. Doudera AE, Peters JD (eds): Legal and Ethical Aspects of Treating Critically and Terminally Ill Patients (Appendices B–E). Ann Arbor, MI, Health Administration Press, 1982
14. President's Commission: Deciding to Forego Life-Sustaining Treatment. Washington, DC, Government Printing Office, March 1983
15. Matter of Dinnerstein; 380 NE2d 134, Massachusetts, 1978
16. Panel accuses hospital of hiding denial of care. New York Times, March 21, 1984
17. Novak v. Cobb County Kennestone Hospital Authority, No 94-8403 (11th Cir., Feb. 14, 1996)
18. Stamford Hospital v. Vega 236 Conn. 646 (1996)
19. Sabatino CP: 10 Legal myths about advance medical directives. Journal of Nursing Law 3(1):35–42, 1995
20. In re Eichner (Fox), 420 NE2d 64, New York, 1981
21. Department of Health and Human Services, Health Care Financing Administration: Medicare and Medicaid programs: Advance directives. Federal Register 57:8194–8204, 1992
22. In re Quinlan, 70 NJ 10, 355 A2d 647, New Jersey, 1976
23. Superintendent of Belchertown State School v. Saikewicz: 373 Mass. 728, 370 NE2d 417, Massachusetts, 1977
24. President's Commission: Deciding to Forego Life-Sustaining Treatment, p 6. Washington, DC, Government Printing Office, March 1983

25. Satz v. Perlmutter: 379 So2d 359, Florida, 1980
26. In the matter of Claire C. Conroy: 457 A2d 1232, New Jersey Superior Court, 1983
27. In re Conroy, 464 A2d, 303, New Jersey, 1983
28. In the matter of Claire C Conroy: Slip Opinion 98 NJ:321, A2d, 1985
29. Cruzan v. Director, Missouri Department of Health et al, III L Ed2d 224, 110 STt 2841 (1990)
30. In re the Conservatorship of Wanglie, No. PX-91-283 (Minn Dist Ct. Probate Ct Division, July 1991)
31. President's Commission for the Study of Ethical Problems in Medicine and Biomedical and Behavioral Research: Defining Death, p 25. July, 1981
32. President's Commission for the Study of Ethical Problems in Medicine and Biomedical and Behavioral Research: Defining Death, p 1. July, 1981
33. Robertson J: The Rights of the Critically Ill, p 121. New York, Bantam Books, 1983
34. New York Public Health Law Article 43-A
35. Connecticut Public Act 88-318 (effective 7/1/88)

Rewards and Challenges of Critical Care Nursing

OBJECTIVES

Based on the content in this chapter, the reader should be able to:

- Describe three sources of internal and external work-related stressors for nurses who work in the critical care setting.
- Discuss the condition of burnout in nursing.
- Describe three common coping characteristics of nurses who work in the critical care setting.
- Explore the concepts of hardiness and resiliency as they relate to critical care nursing.
- Evaluate three stress-reducing behaviors that enhance nurses' coping in the critical care environment.
- Compare and contrast the characteristics of assertive, passive, and aggressive behavior and the reaction of others to those characteristics.

*T*he forces of life and death are in endless battle in the critical care environment. Nurses and physicians defend the patient. It is the nurse, however, who attends the patient and family constantly and who is exposed unrelentlessly to illness, suffering, death, and family crisis. The nature of the occupation imposes numerous tensions on the critical care nurse.

CLINICAL APPLICATION: Patient Care Study

Sara delivered a baby 2 weeks before admission to the intensive care unit. She had delivered a healthy girl but had severe headaches after the birth. She returned to the local community hospital several times after the birth, each time complaining of severe headaches. The first visit was resolved when she was sent home with pain relievers. The second visit to the local hospital resulted in Sara's being transferred to the University hospital with a diagnosis of stroke.

On admission, she presented with tachycardia, weakness in her left arm and leg, and lethargy. She was evaluated by the neurosurgery service and then referred to the neurology service. Within the first 24 to 36 hours of admission, Sara developed neurogenic pulmonary edema and respiratory distress; she was intubated and placed on a respirator. Within another 2 days, she developed acute respiratory distress syndrome (ARDS). A Swan-Ganz catheter was inserted, and pressor agents were used.

While the ARDS continued to ravage her lungs, Sara developed bilateral pneumothoraces. Four chest tubes were placed, two into each lung. She was reintubated with a Jet endotracheal tube and placed on a Jet ventilator. Sara was paralyzed with vecuronium bromide (Norcuron) and sedated with midazolam (Versed). She required minute-by-minute assessment by critical care nurses and physicians around the clock, and her course was very rocky during this time. Most of us worried that she would not live to see her new baby.

Exemplar from the excellence in critical care clinical practice award, 1995, American Association of Critical-Care Nurses, Aliso Viejo, California.

Nurses who work in critical care have been the focus of more study and inquiry related to stress than perhaps any other population of nurses. The study of stress is important in understanding the rewards and challenges of providing critical care. By identifying job-related stressors, nurses can construct internal and external responses to combat them and improve the quality of their work experience.

Stress as it relates to the patient's experience is discussed in Chapter 2 and illustrated in Figure 2–1. The critical care nurse can review this material and relate it to the nurse's personal experiences with stress and its management. Figure 9–1, however, schematically diagrams the nurse's personal management of stress in the critical care environment and follows the discussions in this chapter.

This chapter addresses the fact that critical care nursing can be rewarding and challenging at the same time. It examines different types of stressors, reviews the physical and emotional effects of stress on the nurse, and explores helpful stress-reducing behaviors. It also presents the concepts of hardiness and resiliency, two considerations that are important in examining optimism and satisfaction in critical care nursing.

REWARDS OF CRITICAL CARE NURSING

"I feel privileged to be with patients and their families during the critical illness and to be able to help them through the crises."

Some of the other rewards critical care nurses say keep them "excited and still in the business" follow:

- Joy from working hard to save a patient's life
- Participation with the family as agonizing treatment decisions are made
- Presence with someone at the end of his or her life, knowing you helped make it peaceful and dignified.

The rewards of critical care nursing are immeasurable. It is the reason many of us have chosen nursing as a career to provide necessary care when it is needed and to help someone through a life-threatening event (Fig. 9-2). It is rewarding to feel one played a significant role in providing care when a patient recovers from a critical illness or to realize one helped make it possible for the patient to survive. Even when the patient dies, it is rewarding to know that the patient and family were eased through the experience by a caring nurse.

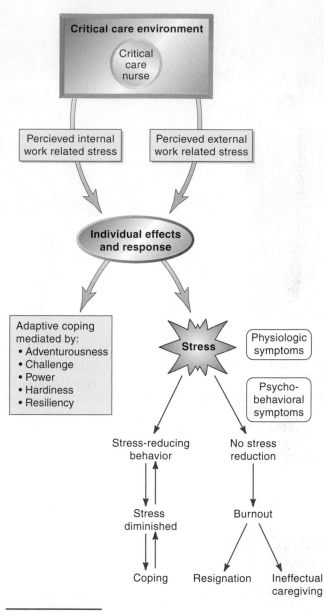

FIGURE 9-1
The pathway for the nurse's personal stress management (or lack of it) associated with the critical care environment.

One nurse, who never gave up hope, describes the reward in the following patient care study.

CLINICAL APPLICATION: Patient Care Study*

A young man nearly died in a motorcycle accident. He had devastating internal injuries and major brain injury and was not expected to survive 12 hours. He was sent to the operating room immediately, and as a result, his mother was not able to see him until his surgery was completed 6 hours later. She said she could not have made it through that time without the help of the nursing staff. During the next few weeks, this young man suffered every major complication possible, including a pulmonary embolism.

I spent hours caring for Patrick and his mother. Without exception, she and I were the only two who believed he would survive, much less recover. He remained in a coma. I remember spending hours talking to him about everything from the weather to the happenings of his favorite television shows. Eventually he had periods when he seemed to be awake but was still unresponsive to most stimuli. Six weeks later, he was transferred to another unit. I heard through the grapevine after several months that he had fully awakened about 1 month after he left us.

That was the last I heard until the next Christmas, 10 months later, when an incredibly handsome young man came on our unit and tapped me on the shoulder. His eyes filled with tears when I asked if I could help him. When his mother rounded the corner, I realized this young man was Patrick. I will never forget what he said: "I don't remember your face, but I will never forget your voice." Patrick had enrolled in college and was doing quite well. His only reminders of the accident were a slight limp and some minor short-term memory problems.

* This personal experience was submitted by a reviewer of this chapter.

These are only a few reasons why nurses continue to care for critically ill patients and their families, despite the stressful challenges of the unit.

STRESSFUL FACTORS IN CRITICAL CARE NURSING

Death and dying are the major stressors in critical care. The unpredictability of the critical care environment is another leading stressor. Other factors include "incessant repetitive routine . . . ; every step must be charted . . . ; floating in nurses from elsewhere . . . ; frequent situations of acute crisis . . . ; physical dangers (inadequate protection from x-rays, needles, isolation patients, and those who are delirious) . . . ; lifting heavy, unresponsive patients . . . ; distraught relatives . . . ; [constant sounds of] moaning, crying, screaming, buzzing, and beeping monitors, gurgling suction pumps, and whooshing respirators . . . ."[1]

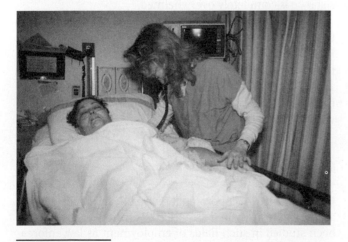

FIGURE 9-2
The nurse helps the patient with physical, mental, and emotional comfort during the critical period of care.

One stress on the nurse that should not be underestimated is that there are bodies everywhere, many of them wasted, mutilated, or discolored. There are exposed genitalia and excretions of feces, blood, chest mucus, vomitus, and urine. Some patients' dressings are soaked with purulent discharge or serous or bloody drainage.[1]

In many cases, all of these stressors add up to a feeling of powerlessness on the part of the nurse. Although he or she can provide responsible care, some factors are outside the realm of the nurse's power of responsibility.

Studies generally classify job-related stress as arising from an internal (within the nurse) or external (stemming from the organizational structure or environment) origin. An understanding of both perspectives is important in comprehending the stress inherent in critical care practice.

Internal Work-Related Stressors

Internal work-related stressors originate from within. Concern regarding patient acuity, apprehension with high technology, and feelings of anxiety or overresponsibility may all contribute to feelings of stress from personal uneasiness. Research has indicated that stressors arising from an internal source occur less frequently than those derived from an external source. Kelly and Cross[2] found that lack of personal knowledge, experience, or skill was an important internally occurring stress variable for critical care staff. Kelly and Cross also described the pressure associated with the need to make rapid decisions relating to patient care as another important variable to personal stress. Norbeck[3] confirmed this finding and specified the top-ranked stressor for critical care nurses as the high number of rapid decisions that must be made in the delivery of care. Interestingly, Norbeck notes that for many critical care nurses, quick decision making is a positive stress; it characterizes the challenge, intrigue, and excitement unique to critical care nursing.

Overresponsibility often manifests itself through the behavior of selflessness. Selflessness is a personality characteristic that is frequently nurtured and praised by nursing administrators and educators. If people are selfless, they deny their own physical or emotional needs in the service of others. Nurses who legitimately refuse to work a double shift, float to another unit, or take on extra assignments because of chronic understaffing usually are not as popular with supervisors as those who deny their own needs and acquiesce immediately. Because in the past selflessness has been a desired trait and one that received praise, many nurses have been socialized into denying their own needs and feelings. Selfless behaviors take their toll on health and well-being unless such behaviors are balanced with behaviors that acknowledge and respect personal feelings and needs.

External Work-Related Stressors

Demands from the organizational structure and the environment are the most commonly cited sources of stress for the critical care nurse. Robinson and Lewis[4] found that shift

---

Stressful Factors in the Critical Care Environment

General Stressors

- Death and dying (frequent acute crises)
- Powerlessness (unpredictability of critical care environment)
- Distraught family
- Personal danger regarding equipment (x-rays, needles, confused or disturbed patients)
- Constant barrage to the senses (noises, smells, sight of exposed bodies and their body fluids)
- Repetitive routines and charting all actions
- Use of float nurses
- Heavy lifting of patients

Internal Work-Related Stressors

- High number of rapid decisions to be made
- Concern regarding the patient's condition
- Apprehension of high technological equipment
- Anxiety or feelings of overresponsibility (selflessness)
- Lack of personal knowledge, experience, or skill

External Work-Related Stressors

- Demands of the critical care environment
- Demands from the organizational structure of the acute care facility
- Higher level politics with nursing administrators and physicians
- Communication problems in unit or with administration
- Low level of experience of medical residents
- Staff utilization and planning (shift rotation and scheduling problems)
- Lack of rewards (including salary, promotion, and educational opportunities)
- Problems in nursing–administration relationships
- Lack of support from non-nursing departments and other health care professionals
- Ethical issues resulting in futility
- Institutional downsizing and changes in staffing mixture, including unlicensed personnel or paraprofessionals

---

rotation and problems with scheduling, lack of rewards, nurse–nursing administration relationships, crowded unit environment, and low experience level of medical residents were common stressors for the critical care nurse. Hart and Moore[5] found that organizational dynamics, such as communication patterns; staff utilization and planning; interdisciplinary politics with division-level nursing administrators and physicians; reward, including salary, promotion, and educational opportunities; and availability of support from non-nursing departments and other health care professionals, were the critical determinants of nurses' job satisfaction and turnover rates.

Ethical issues regarding dying patients and perceptions of futility are also highly stressful to the nursing staff.[6] For instance, futility as a concept in critical care involves medical and nursing interventions delivered at the request of families that the caregivers believe serve no physiological purpose (see Chapter 7). Clinical conditions involving futility are fertile ground for work-related stress because they leave nurses feeling conflicted, frustrated, and unfulfilled.

Current trends of institutional downsizing and changes in staffing mixture to include greater numbers of unlicensed personnel are new stressors for critical care nurses. External demands of delegation, supervision, and evaluation of unlicensed personnel or paraprofessionals place added responsibilities on the nurse.

■ THE EFFECTS OF STRESS

The critical care environment involves a barrage of stressors, events of prolonged duration, and clinical situations in which the course of action is ambiguous and uncertain. The accumulation of stressors from this intense environment can result in an individual's developing physical or psycho-

logical symptoms. Each person's response to stress is unique and individualized. No two nurses will respond in the same fashion to the stressors associated with the critical care setting. Common physiological reactions to stress are listed in the accompanying display. A person reacts to stress not only with biological symptoms but also with behavioral changes. Psychological indicators of stress are highly individualized. Behavioral indicators of stresses are also listed in the display.

When symptoms develop, it is a signal that the body can no longer adapt to the demands being placed on it. These symptoms range on a continuum beginning with occasional, episodic occurrence. These symptoms can progress to moderate intensity and frequency. The most extreme presence of these changes potentially leads to compromise in overall functioning and ultimate death if the person's resistance is completely overwhelmed.

Critical care nurses need to listen to their bodies and thoughtfully consider their sense of individual well-being. Frequent personal assessment for signs of stress is important to longevity and satisfaction in critical care nursing. An awareness of the early warning signs of stress can facilitate rapid identification and swift intervention to enhance individual coping.

■ BURNOUT

People in a variety of professions that deal with behavioral and social aspects may experience burnout. Burnout has been studied in such fields of employment as law enforcement, child day care, and mental health. Burnout in nursing involves physical and emotional exhaustion stemming from the stressors associated with the work of caring for ill people.

Physical and Behavioral Responses to Stress

Common Physiological Reactions to Stress

- Elevation of blood pressure or pulse
- Tightness in chest
- Unexplained shortness of breath
- Dull, aching pain in neck, shoulders, or back
- Increased frequency of headaches
- Insomnia
- Excessive fatigue, insatiable sleep
- Gastrointestinal distress

Behavioral Indicators of Stress

- Anxiety
- Decreased work productivity and contribution
- Irritability
- Forgetfulness
- Disorganization in thinking
- Difficulty concentrating on task
- Decreased interest in relationships
- An increase in consumptive behavior, including alcohol or substance misuse, smoking, and excessive eating or sleeping

Critical care nurses are at risk for burnout. Maslach completed extensive research exploring burnout in nursing and described it as " . . . a syndrome of emotional exhaustion, depersonalization, and reduced personal accomplishment that can occur among individuals who do 'people work' of some kind. It is the response to the chronic emotional strain of dealing extensively with other human beings, particularly when they are troubled, ill, or having personal problems."[7]

Nurses by nature are vulnerable to burnout. Many nurses who enter the profession are highly people oriented and connect easily with patients and their families. Such nurses may describe themselves as selfless or altruistic, a personality trait that has been explored in describing internal work-related stressors. The emotions experienced by these nurses as they work with patients who face illness, crisis, and death may contribute to feelings of burnout.

The condition of burnout renders the individual feeling resigned, ineffective, and hopeless about working in such an environment. The behaviors common in burnout include absenteeism, anger, frustration, anxiety, and loss of commitment. The result of burnout is that the employee either leaves the job or remains in the position functioning ineffectively.

The cost of burnout in health care is significant. Burnout has contributed to many nurses leaving not only critical care settings, but the profession of nursing. Employee turnover is costly to health care institutions; advertisement, recruitment, and orientation of new staff is expensive and time consuming. Burnout is also costly to patients. A nurse who feels ineffective, frustrated, and stressed is unlikely to design and deliver exemplary care.

▬ COPING CHARACTERISTICS AND BEHAVIORS

Reducing stress, enhancing job satisfaction, and preventing burnout are important strategies for nurses working in the critical care environment. Currently there is keen interest in the coping characteristics of critical care nurses. Coping characteristics are used to describe the innate, naturally occurring personal response by an individual confronted with a stressful situation.

Coping is actually a complex process that involves a usually consistent response in each person. For example, a person who copes well in one type of stressful situation usually copes well in all situations. The exceptions are if a person is profoundly fatigued, has had a previous similar experience in which coping failed so that another similar event causes a burst of anxiety, or has experienced several stressful incidents in a brief period of time so that the new stressor is like "the straw that broke the camel's back."

Personality and Coping Characteristics

Because there has been so much emphasis on critical care nursing stress, the question is asked: Are there particular coping abilities or personality styles that help critical care nurses adapt successfully to a stressful environment?

Maloney and Bartz[8] were pioneers in studying the personality and coping characteristics of nurses in intensive care and nonintensive care settings. They examined several factors to determine whether there were differences between the two groups of nurses. Their findings showed that intensive care nurses differed significantly in several ways. Intensive care nurses are more adventurous, feel less powerful, and are more detached than their counterparts.

ADVENTUROUSNESS AND CHALLENGE

These qualities are found more often in critical care nurses than in non–critical care nurses and are believed to contribute to their attraction to the intensive care unit

Personality and Coping Characteristics of Successful Critical Care Nurses

- Adventurous
- Experiences satisfaction in adventure and challenge
- Detached (based on defense mechanisms), which reduces anxiety level
- Strong capacity for coping and adaptation
- Hardiness: control, commitment, challenge, companionship
- Resiliency (bounces back): insight, independence, social support, initiative

(ICU) environment and their capacity to experience satisfaction in it.

POWER

Nurses working in the ICU generally feel less powerful and more controlled by the environment than the non-ICU staff. This is a realistic finding of adaptation in view of the emergency and unpredictable nature of the ICU setting.

DETACHMENT

Nurses who work in the ICU are more detached than their non-ICU counterparts. Maloney and Bartz suggested that this quality helps the nurses cope with the perceptual bombardment present in the ICU setting. The capacity for detachment is based on the use of the defense mechanisms of denial, repression, intellectualization, and similar defenses that reduce the level of anxiety that a person might normally feel in a threatening situation. The generalized conclusion is that ICU nurses have a stronger capacity for coping and adaptation than do nurses attracted to non-ICU settings.

Hardiness and Resiliency

Why do some nurses thrive in a critical care environment while others experience a fairly rapid rate of turnover? Are some people innately more resilient and optimistic, able to cope successfully with work-related stressors? *Hardiness* is a term applied to a particular set of personality characteristics described by Kobassa and Puscetti.[9] Their groundbreaking research revealed that people who are less likely to become ill as the result of stressful life events share the following characteristics:

- They perceive their lives and choices as being under their own control.
- They feel committed to their current goals and lifestyle.
- They experience the strains of life as challenges.

These characteristics were described by the authors as the way a person responds to stress. The concept of hardiness involves the three "C"s and includes the sense of *control* versus powerlessness, *commitment* versus alienation, and *challenge* versus threat.

More recent studies investigating hardiness have identified an additional component to the concept. This component has been termed the fourth C of hardiness: *companionship*.[10] Nurses who have consistent access to social support systems appear more equipped to handle the frustrations and stressors associated with providing critical care. Companionship offered these nurses a verbal outlet for expressing feelings and a sense of connectedness in dealing competently with the clinical situations that may surface.[11]

> **The Four Cs of Hardiness**
> - Control
> - Commitment
> - Challenge
> - Companionship

Based on the extensive study of hardiness, it appears that the use of conscious coping mechanisms, such as reframing one's perspective of a stressful situation, can be important to the critical care nurse. Shifting toward the positive perspectives of control, commitment, challenge, and companionship offers the nurse hope and provides an increased sense of well-being.

Resiliency describes an individual's ability to bounce back or recover in the face of adversity. Resilient nurses are those who are able to deflect, adjust to, or recuperate quickly from tragedy, stress, or change.[12] Strengths inherent in the resilient individual include the qualities of insight, independence, social support, and initiative. Insight refers to a flexibility in thought process and the capacity to understand oneself and others. Independence is the ability to disengage physically and emotionally from situations that are painful or unpleasant. Social support addresses the discovery of strength and nurturance from caring involved people. Initiative involves a sense of control over one's life, coupled with a positive, realistic sense of what can be accomplished in a situation.[13] Continued research in the area of resiliency may further explain variations in nurses' perceptions of work-related stress and the occurrence of burnout.

Stress-Reducing Behaviors

Many nurses who work effectively and productively in the critical care environment would describe themselves as neither hardy nor resilient. For these nurses, active engagement in stress-reducing behavior is an important part of their professional practice. Routine participation in these activities alleviates tension, combats burnout, promotes collegiality, and improves the quality of work life for the critical care nurse. An outline of stress-reducing behaviors is given in the accompanying display. They are discussed further in the following text.

A HEALTHY LIFESTYLE

Many health-promoting activities not only enhance personal wellness, but also combat the negative effects of stress. Routine physical exercise benefits the cardiovascular system and releases the physical and mental tension associated with a challenging work day. A brisk walk every day returns the body's equilibrium to normal. Many people are pleasantly surprised to discover that their emotional state also improves if they begin a regular exercise program. Their depression, anxiety, or fatigue is lessened and may gradually disappear.

> ### *Personal Stress-Reducing Behaviors*
>
> - Develop a healthy lifestyle (physical exercise, balanced diet, balance of daily activity and rest and sleep, self-awareness and self-esteem, personal direction and expectations).
> - Practice relaxation techniques (deep breathing, quieting reflex, yoga, meditation).
> - Develop and use humor (laughing, finding humor in given situations, sharing humor with patients and staff).
> - Acquire and use assertive techniques.
> - Value collegiality, which involves connectiveness, caring, and support.
> - Promote work excitement for self (personal commitment, enthusiasm, creativity, receptivity).
> - Participate in educational opportunities.

A balanced diet rich in fruits, vegetables, and grains is another important consideration to healthful living. Overconsumption is a common American health problem and should be avoided. Limiting the intake of caffeine, saturated fats, alcohol, and raw sugar are believed to enhance the function of the immune system.

A balance of daily activity with rest and sleep is necessary in developing a healthy lifestyle. Sleep is believed to afford the human body a period of recovery from a busy, active day. Time spent in sleep decreases metabolic demands on the body and allows for repair and regeneration. The requirements for sleep are highly individualized, yet most sources recommend between 6 and 8 hours of sleep each night for a healthy adult.

Promoting kindness, patience, and caring toward oneself is another consideration in healthful living. Establishing personal expectations that are realistic is vitally important. Acknowledging strengths, accomplishments, and limitations is critical in developing a realistic self-portrait. Scheduling routine breaks from work (ie, long weekends) and taking vacations demonstrate care and attention toward personal well-being.

RELAXATION TECHNIQUES

Nurses have found relaxation techniques of benefit to themselves and their patients. Such techniques are discussed in Chapters 2 and 5, along with other interventions that promote reduction of stress.

HUMOR

Humor as an activity involves discovering what may be funny in a situation and operationalizing it with laughter. Laughter is a physiological occurrence that provides a release of tension and anxiety. During laughter, muscles relax; the cardiorespiratory system is stimulated, enhancing oxygen exchange; endorphins are released; and a sense of personal well-being is realized. Humor is a useful stress-reducing behavior for nurses who work in the critical care environment.

A number of cautions are necessary when using humor as a stress-reducing behavior. Personal perceptions of humor are widely individualized, and care must be taken not to offend others when using humor. Timing is an important consideration; it should not be used when it could be of detriment to patients, families, or other staff. Conversely, sharing appropriate humor *with* patients can decrease anxiety and stress for the nurse and the recipient. It may also enhance the relationship and the rapport between the patient and care provider. The following patient care study provides an illustration for effective use of humor in the critical care environment.

CLINICAL APPLICATION: Patient Care Study

It all started with the pink flamingo straws! I saw them in a catalog and thought "my patients need these!" I felt that the patients (and nurses) needed diversions, such as the straws, to help them cope with the daily stresses that occur in critical care. I had wanted to develop an intervention that would convey a caring attitude to the patients and families by showing an interest in them. After reading the literature about the benefits and functions of the use of humor, I thought that this would be a good start. Humor, when used appropriately, relieves tension, anxiety, and stress. It also establishes relationships and a comfortable atmosphere. In the "high-tech" environment of the coronary care unit where I have worked as a staff nurse for 5 years and nurse coordinator for the past year, I felt that the use of humor would bring the nurse and patient closer together (high touch). My intent was to use humor as a therapeutic nursing intervention and stress reduction technique. I thought that if the nurse and patient could laugh together, the problems would appear more approachable and manageable (for both of them). With backing from my hospital and a scholarship from the Journal of Nursing Jocularity, I developed and stocked a humor cart that could be pushed from room to room. Additionally, unit funds were used to purchase corkboard strips so patients could hang "get well" cards or pictures of their loved ones on the wall. I thought this might bring a "touch of home" to the hospital.

T.E. was a 43-year-old man admitted to our unit by Medflight from an outlying hospital. An inferior myocardial infarction was suspected, and Streptokinase was given. Early the next morning, T.E. became short of breath and dusky and complained of chest pain. He was taken to the catheterization laboratory where a successful percutaneous transluminal coronary angioplasty (PTCA) was performed on a totally occluded right coronary artery (RCA) and a Swan-Ganz catheter was placed.

Mr. and Mrs. E. were expecting their third child. This is significant because Mrs. E. went into labor on her ride from our hospital and delivered a healthy boy. Unfortunately, she was taken to a different hospital. After providing a phone so that T.E. could receive the good news, the night shift nurses gave him an impromptu baby shower using items from the humor cart. He received a pink flamingo straw, a gold crown, and several plastic duckies. He was thrilled.

Later that morning, T.E. developed chest pain and returned to the laboratory for a second PTCA of the RCA. He returned to the unit pain free. As I was helping his nurse "tuck him in" after the procedure, T.E. joked: "I won't have any visitors today because they all are over with my wife and baby." I was concerned that beneath all of his joking, he was feeling isolated from his family. I wanted to do something to bring this family closer so I called the other hospital and asked if they could take a picture of the baby and fax it to us. This did not produce the best results, but T.E. did not mind; he wanted to save the fax copies. He joked that the dark blob on the paper resembled him.

Because T.E. did not have any visitors that afternoon, we were his only support system. I asked if he were interested in a "dayshift" baby shower. He said he was. After huddling around the humor cart for a minute, we marched into his room singing "Happy Shower to You…" I wore jumbo sunglasses and carried a rubber chicken. His nurse put on a jester hat. A third nurse wore a Goofy hat. When he saw us, T.E. grabbed his gold crown, put it on, and stuck a candy cigar in his mouth. We then presented him with a stuffed animal that was purchased from the gift shop for the baby. This was truly a "Polaroid moment," so pictures were taken to commemorate the event. I recall T.E. stating that he wanted to "save everything" to show his son what happened on the day he was born. While leaving his room, I felt that we had really made a difference in helping him cope with his feelings of isolation, if only for a brief time.

T.E. was discharged home 5 days later. He has returned to visit three times, once with his wife and new baby. I think we left a good impression!

Exemplar from the excellence in caring practice award, 1995, American Association of Critical-Care Nurses, Aliso Viejo, California.

ASSERTIVENESS

Acquiring and using assertiveness techniques may ease the internal work-related stressors of overresponsibility and selflessness. Many people confuse the characteristics of assertiveness with those of aggressiveness. The differences be-tween being aggressive, being assertive, and being passive, or nonassertive, are presented in Table 9–1.

The difference between the passive person and the assertive person is that the passive person is "done unto" by another who has no awareness of the passive person's needs or desires. Passive people seem more like nonpeople. Actually, they often put their faith in others to know what they need, usually with unexpressed expectations (also called *hidden agendas*). If the others fail them in any way, there can be two outcomes:

- They further submerge their "selves" and needs. The implied meaning is "I have no worth."
- They feel resentment. "Why did they do this to me?" Actually, the agency or other person has no idea of the unexpressed needs.

Assertive people, however, are aware of their own needs and the treatment to which they are entitled as human beings. They express these needs when appropriate. If their rights are openly violated, they speak up and express their feelings. Assertive people are not offensive and do not infringe on the rights of other people or institutions. They place value on their own thoughts and beliefs. They place value on themselves.

Aggressive people are offensive people. They impose their beliefs on others, expecting them to agree and becoming angry if the others do not acquiesce. They actually deny others the right to their own thoughts or opinions.

COLLEGIALITY AND CARING

Common to both hardiness and resilience is the concept of social support. Human contact and social relationships are

---

TABLE 9-1
Assertiveness, Passivity, and Aggressiveness

Assertive	Passive	Aggressive
Characteristics		
Open	Weak	Quarrelsome
Honest	Yielding	Bold
Does not impinge on others' beliefs	Self-denying	Degrades others
	Hidden bargaining	Bulldozes over others' opinions, beliefs, and feelings
	Deceptive about real feelings	
Feelings in Self		
At peace inside	Uncertain	Anger
Good self-esteem	Tries to please others	Contempt
Respects others' rights	Resentful	Extreme self-pride
		Anxious when aggressiveness is out of control
Reactions of Others		
Respect	Pity	Indignation
	Uncertainty	Displeasure
	Unconcern	Hurt
	Annoyance	Disgust

an integral aspect of stress reduction and promotion of well-being. Colleagueship in the critical care environment acknowledges the contributions of all caregivers and is respectful of each individual.

Nurses feel a sense of connectedness with their colleagues when they can share common experiences through open and honest communication. Nurses must value exemplary caregiving and recognize the achievements and successes of their peers. It is equally important to be there for one another in clinical situations when there are unfavorable outcomes. This sharing of experience enhances connectedness and gives recognition, support, and strength to one another.

There are a number of positive institutional responses to promoting colleagueship and support among nurses. Identifying needs for continuing education and facilitating access to such programs convey concern and positive regard for the well-being of critical care nurses. If viewed favorably by the nursing unit, formal support groups using a facilitator with a mental health background may prove highly beneficial. The purpose of this type of discussion group is to address any issue of concern to nursing staff. The time is nonstructured with participants raising the issues to be discussed. In the beginning weeks of the group, these issues frequently are centered on the emotional management of problem patients or families. After staff members feel trusting of themselves and their leader, they frequently discuss some of their own psychological reactions to specific incidents, such as the hopelessness of weaning a specific patient from a respirator, grief about the death of a long-term ICU patient, anger about house staff who are not there when needed, frustration with an insensitive nursing administration, or helplessness in dealing with the spouse of a dying 30-year-old patient. Access to such a meeting allows these feelings of grief and loss to be discussed and addressed in a supportive setting.

AN ENVIRONMENT OF WORK EXCITEMENT

Work excitement is an emerging concept in nursing administration. It addresses the conditions of burnout and turnover in nursing. Work excitement, as defined by Simms, is the "personal enthusiasm and commitment for work evidenced by creativity, receptivity to learning, and ability to see opportunity in everyday situations."[14] Work excitement is influenced by individual and work-related factors. Work excitement is believed to be an important component in the delivery of patient care and the development of nurse satisfaction.

Environment-related considerations in promoting work excitement include variety in patient care assignment, opportunity for continuing education, and support by nursing administration.[15] Critical care nurses who are exposed to different and challenging clinical situations report increased enthusiasm, productivity, and commitment to their work. The challenges inherent in new and changing condi-

tions promote interest and excitement. Educational opportunities to enhance personal knowledge and skill development generate a sense of enthusiasm and commitment to critical care nursing. The presence of strong administrative support, which allocates adequate resources for the unit, thereby avoiding understaffing or excessive need for overtime, promotes satisfaction with work. Recognition of staff by nurse administrators for achievements in patient care, knowledge development, or institutional contribution enhances work excitement for critical care nurses.

■ THE NOVICE NURSE IN THE CRITICAL CARE ENVIRONMENT

Development of a Support System

Nurses new to critical care can act on their own behalf by consciously developing a support system. This is a measure that fosters handling of difficult situations and helps novice nurses be in charge of their lives during the adventure of beginning a new job. A support system includes family and friends who give meaning and support to our personal life, regardless of where we work. It also includes colleagues with whom we share common values, interests, and companionship. Strong support systems include people whose words and actions encourage our endeavors.

A support system should also include a mentor. The concept of a mentor as a loyal friend, advisor, teacher, and coach dates from as far back as the Greek Myth of Odysseus. A support system can also include a preceptor, who is often assigned during the orientation period and serves as a clinical resource to help new employees learn the daily aspects of their job.

As with other members of a support system, you will have to seek out a mentor. Because this is a time of increased learning, the mentor should be knowledgeable, should be able to help build confidence and give meaningful feedback, and should be someone with whom the nurse can share concerns. Potential mentors should be willing, and realistically have the time, to develop and maintain the relationship. A mentor is a valuable resource in helping novices grow into new roles, navigate the institution's systems, and maintain values.

Personal Assessment

Periodically reassessing your internal strengths and external supports can help you determine what else you may need to do to manage the challenges of professional growth. Are there family members, friends, and colleagues you can count on for support and companionship? If not, think of ways to expand your support system. A personal inventory can point out coping strengths and vulnerabilities. Recognizing behaviors that do not work in your best interests means you can make a decision to change or abandon them. A work appraisal can help you identify those aspects of the profession that are fulfilling, those you like least, and those that are most stressful. Would more information, practice, confidence, or support improve your satisfaction and performance? Do you need more time to grow into the role? Are resources available to help with these issues?

Strengthening Coping Behaviors

Following are some suggestions that will help you manage personal and professional challenges:

- Develop a broad-based circle of friends and colleagues with whom to share support and have fun.
- Build a relationship with a mentor.
- Adhere to healthy lifestyle practices.
- Recognize internal and external work stresses and the early signs of stress.
- Increase stress-reducing behaviors so they are available when needed.
- Pat yourself on the back periodically, and keep a healthy amount of humor in your life.

Clinical Applicability Challenges

Self-Challenge: Critical Thinking

1. *Nurses need to appreciate humor to use it correctly as a stress-reducing behavior. Thinking back on a stressful situation, analyze how you could have effectively used humor.*

2. *Compare and contrast hardiness and resiliency as human personality characteristics. Personalize the components of these characteristics as they apply to you in day-to-day living.*

3. *Create a personal prescription of stress-reducing strategies in addressing the internal and external sources of tension in your life.*

Study Questions

1. *Effective coping in the critical care environment is assisted by the following personality trait:*
   a. *Boldness*
   b. *Respect*
   c. *Assertiveness*
   d. *Aloofness*

2. *Which one of the following is* not *a normal response to acute anxiety?*
   a. *A change in sleeping patterns*
   b. *An increase in problem-solving ability*
   c. *An increase in blood pressure*
   d. *An increase in pulse rate*

3. *The characteristic believed to be common to both hardiness and resiliency is:*
   a. *Tenacity*
   b. *Self-confidence*
   c. *Ambition*
   d. *Connectedness and support from others*

REFERENCES

1. Hay D, Oken D: The psychological stresses of intensive care nursing. Psychosomatic Medicine 34:109–118, 1972
2. Kelly JG, Cross DG: Stress, coping behaviors, and recommendations for intensive care and medical surgical ward registered nurses. Res Nurs Health 8:321–328, 1985
3. Norbeck JS: Perceived job stress, job satisfaction, and psychological symptoms in critical care nursing. Res Nurs Health 8:253–259, 2985
4. Robinson JA, Lewis DJ: Coping with ICU work-related stressors: A study. Critical Care Nurse 10:80–88, 1990
5. Hart SK, Moore M: The relationship among organizational climate variables and nurse stability in critical care units. Journal of Professional Nursing 3:124–131, 1989
6. Daly B: Futility. AAN Clinical Issues 5:77–84, 1994
7. Maslach C: Burnout: The Cost of Caring. Englewood Cliffs, NJ, Prentice-Hall, 1982
8. Maloney J, Bartz C: Stress-tolerant people: Intensive care nurses compared with non-intensive care nurses. Heart Lung 12:389–394, 1983
9. Kobassa S, Puscetti M: Personality and social resources in stress resistance. J Pers Soc Psychol 45:839–850, 1983
10. Consolvo CA, Brownewell V, Distafano SM: Profile of the hardy NICU nurse. Journal of Perinatology 9:334–337, 1989
11. Chapman M: Assimilating new staff in an intensive care nursery. Nursing Management 24:96B–96H, 1993
12. Kadner KD: Resilience: responding to adversity. J Psychosoc Nurs Ment Health Serv 27:20–25, 1989
13. Chollar S: The miracle of resilience: Why some people keep bouncing back. American Health and Fitness of Body and Mind 13:72–75, 1994
14. Simms L, Erbin-Roesemann M, Darga A, Coeling H: Breaking the burnout barrier: Resurrecting work excitement in nursing. Nursing Economics 8:177–187, 1990
15. Hentemann A, Simms L, Erbin-Roesemann M, Greene JC: Work excitement: An energy source for critical care nurses. Nursing Management 23:96E–96P, 1992

BIBLIOGRAPHY

Bartz C, Maloney J: Burnout among intensive care nurses. Res Nurs Health 9:147–153, 1986
Bohannan-Reed K, Dugan D, Huck B: Staying human under stress: Stress reduction and emotional support in the critical care setting. Critical Care Nurse 8:26–30, 1983
Bolger A, Creamer J, Kitt S: Building a career-resilient workforce: The Northwestern Memorial Hospital career development program. Aspen Advisor for Nurse Executives 10:1–3, 1995
Cooper M: The intersection of technology and care in the ICU. Advances in Nursing Science 15:23–32, 1993
Doran M: Managing the ICU induced stress. Am J Nurs 11:1559–1561, 1988
Topf M: Personality hardiness, occupational stress and burnout in critical care nurses. Res Nurs Health 12:179–186, 1989
Vincent P, Coleman W: Comparison of major stressors perceived by ICU and non-ICU nurses. Critical Care Nurse 6:64–69, 1986

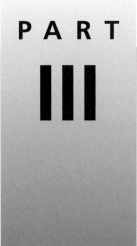

PART

III

Special Populations in Critical Care

The Critically Ill Pediatric Patient

PROMINENT ANATOMICAL AND PHYSIOLOGICAL DIFFERENCES AND IMPLICATIONS
Vital Signs
Neurological System

Cardiovascular System
Respiratory System
Gastrointestinal System
Renal System
Endocrine System

SELECTED PEDIATRIC CHALLENGES
Ventilatory Issues
Pain Management
Interaction With Children and Families
CONCLUSION

OBJECTIVES

Based on the content in this chapter, the reader should be able to:

- Analyze developmental aspects that necessitate the modification of physical assessment parameters and intervention techniques.
- Evaluate pain assessment tools that can be used for the critically ill child.
- Examine important aspects of interaction with the critically ill child and family that will enhance interventions.

*M*ost adult critical care clinicians feel ill-equipped to manage the percentage of children seen in adult intensive care units (ICUs), emergency rooms, procedural suites, and recovery rooms. To facilitate smooth and optimal care of the critically ill child, it is wise to adopt a framework for the modification of the adult critical care practice to include the pediatric patient. A comprehensive framework is beyond the scope of this chapter, but readers are referred to the "PEDS" framework discussed in more detail elsewhere.[1,2] This chapter highlights prominent anatomical and physiological differences and related implications, equipment selection, recognition of the decompensating child, and unique challenges in caring for the pediatric patient in a critical care environment.

▄▄ PROMINENT ANATOMICAL AND PHYSIOLOGICAL DIFFERENCES AND IMPLICATIONS

Vital Signs

The infant and young child have an age appropriate, but higher, heart rate and respiratory rate than the adult. The higher heart and respiratory rate assist in meeting the need for a higher cardiac output, despite a smaller stroke volume and a higher basal metabolic rate. Blood pressure is lower than that of the adult. Vital signs (see Table 10–1 for normal ranges), although important parameters, should not be evaluated in isolation, but rather in a trending fashion. Tachycardia is a nonspecific response to a variety of entities, such as anxiety, fever, shock, and hypoxemia. Although the child is predisposed to bradycardia, tolerance is poor. Bradycardia often produces significant changes in perfusion because cardiac output is heart rate dependent. Bradycardia is most often caused by hypoxemia, but any vagal stimuli, such as suctioning, nasogastric tube insertion, and defecation, may precipitate an event.

As for respiratory rate, the infant or child increases his or her rate to compensate for an increased oxygen demand. Tachypnea is often the first sign of respiratory distress. A

TABLE 10-1
Pediatric Vital Signs

Age	Heart Rate	Respirations	Systolic Blood Pressure
Newborn	100–160	30–60	50–70
1–6 wk	100–160	30–60	70–95
6 mo	90–120	25–40	80–100
1 y	90–120	20–30	80–100
3 y	80–120	20–30	80–110
6 y	70–110	18–25	80–110
10 y	60–90	15–20	90–120
14 y	60–90	15–20	90–130

slow respiratory rate in a sick child often indicates impending respiratory arrest. Associated conditions, such as fever and seizure activity, which further increase the metabolic rate, will also increase oxygen requirements. These conditions can cause rapid deterioration in an already compromised child.

Unlike the adult, the child's blood pressure is the last parameter to fall in the face of shock. Children can compensate for up to a 25% blood loss before the systolic blood pressure falls. A normal blood pressure should never discourage interventions for the child showing signs of circulatory failure. The pulse pressure is often a more reliable indicator for assessing the adequacy of perfusion. Hypertension is uncommon, unless the child has renal disease.

Neurological System

Brain growth occurs at a rapid rate during the first few years of life. Because brain growth is rapid during this time, measurement of head circumference is important in the child until 2 years of age. The circumference of the child's head is related to intracranial volume and estimates the rate of brain growth.

The child's cranial sutures are not completely fused until 18 to 24 months of age. The posterior fontanel closes by 3 months of age, and the anterior fontanel closes by 9 to 18 months of age. The fontanels provide a useful assessment tool in the infant. The characteristics of the fontanels can be used to assess hydration status or the presence of increased intracranial pressure. Bulging fontanels may indicate increased intracranial pressure or fluid overload. Sunken fontanels may be seen with fluid deficit.

Infants, like adults, have intact protective reflexes, such as cough and gag, at birth. There are also several newborn reflexes (the Moro, rooting, grasp, and Babinski), which differ from adult reflexes. For example, the Babinski reflex is present until 9 to 12 months of age or until the child starts walking. A positive Babinski reflex response (fanning of the toes and dorsiflexion of the big toe when the lateral aspect of the sole of the foot is stroked) is expected in the infant yet is considered an abnormal finding in the older child or

adult. In-depth discussion of these reflexes is beyond the scope of this chapter; the reader is referred to a developmental anatomy text for further information.

The infant's and child's mental status is assessed the same way as the adult's, by noting the level of consciousness, interaction with the environment, and appropriateness of behavior for age. Level of consciousness is assessed by noting whether the child is arousable and oriented. This can be done by observing for spontaneous arousability or by providing verbal, tactile, or noxious stimuli. Even though the assessment is the same, the assessment techniques must be age appropriate. Specific techniques are provided in the section in this chapter on interaction. An important difference when interacting with the child is paradoxical irritability. This is present with meningeal irritability, nuchal rigidity, and positive Brudzinski's and Kernig's signs.

Infants and young children are at high risk for ineffective thermoregulation, resulting in physiological instability, due to a variety of maturational and environmental factors.[3] Close monitoring of body temperature and providing a temperature-controlled environment will help manage temperature regulation. The temperature is measured at regular intervals, and external factors affecting body temperature should be controlled.

Cardiovascular System

Decreased perfusion to the skin is an early and reliable sign of shock. Because the skin is thinner than that of the adult, skin characteristics occur easily and rapidly with changes in perfusion. Skin color, texture, and temperature and capillary refill are of great significance during assessment of the child. Prior to assessing the skin, it is important to note the room temperature because some findings may be a normal response to the environment (such as mottling in a drafty operating room). Mottling in a bundled infant or warm environment is reason for further investigation. Assess skin temperature and the line of demarcation between extremity coolness and body warmth. Coolness or the progression of coolness toward the trunk may be a sign of diminishing perfusion.

Peripheral cyanosis is normal in newborns but abnormal in young children and adults. Central cyanosis (circumoral) is always an abnormal finding. Capillary refill is normally recorded in seconds rather than as brisk, normal, or slow and normally is less than or equal to 2 seconds. Estimated blood volume varies with age; despite a higher mL/kg of body weight volume, the overall total circulating volume is small. A small amount of blood loss can be significant in the child.

Respiratory System

The infant's or child's large head (in proportion to body size), weak, underdeveloped neck muscles, and lack of cartilaginous support to the airway lead to an easily compressible or obstructed airway. Avoid overextending or overflexing the neck because the airways are easily collapsible. Head and neck position alone can facilitate a patent airway. Ideal positioning for the decompensating child is in a neutral or sniffing position and can be done by placing a small roll horizontally behind the shoulders. The infant, until 6 months of age, is an obligate nose breather so that any obstruction of nasal passages can produce significant airway compromise and respiratory distress. Secretions, edema, inflammation, poorly taped nasogastric tubes, or occluded nasal cannulas can cause obstructed nasal passages in the infant. The infant's and young child's airways are smaller in diameter and in length, thus requiring smaller artificial airways. Airway compromise can be caused by the slightest amount of inflammation or edema of the natural airway or from a mucous plug in either the natural or artificial airway. The narrowest part of the child's airway (until approximately 8 years of age) is at the level of the cricoid ring as opposed to the glottic opening in the adult.

The young child's thin, compliant chest wall allows for easy assessment of air entry. Air entry is assessed by observing the rise and fall of the child's chest with adequate ventilatory efforts. Unequal chest movement may indicate the development of a pneumothorax or atelectasis but also may indicate endotracheal tube obstruction or displacement into the right mainstem bronchus. The child's flexible rib cage and poorly developed intercostal muscles offer little stability to the chest wall; therefore, suprasternal, sternal, intercostal, and subcostal retractions may be seen during respiratory distress. The presence and location of retractions should be noted. Accessory muscles also are poorly developed, so the infant and the child may use the abdominal muscles to assist with breathing. This gives the appearance of "seesaw" breathing, a paradoxical movement of the chest and abdomen. Seesaw breathing becomes more exaggerated with respiratory distress. Like the adult, the major muscle of respiration is the diaphragm. However, the child is more diaphragm dependent.

Due to the thin chest wall, breath sounds are more audible than in the adult. Additionally, obstructed airways often produce sounds that are easily heard during assessment. Listen for expiratory grunting, inspiratory and expiratory stridor, and wheezing. Expiratory grunting is a sound produced in an attempt to increase physiological positive end-expiratory pressure to prevent small airways and alveoli from collapsing. The infant's and child's thin chest wall may allow breath sounds to be heard over an area of pathology when sounds are actually being referred from another area of the lung. Listen for changes in the breath sounds as well as for their presence or absence.

Gastrointestinal System

The child normally has a protuberant abdomen; however, there are numerous causes of abnormal abdominal distension. A nasogastric or orogastric tube should be inserted early rather than later to minimize the risk of distension. Abdominal distension can interfere with respiratory excur-

sion and may even cause respiratory arrest. Active removal of air with a syringe may be necessary if distension is not relieved by putting the tube to straight drainage. In addition, the abdominal girth is measured every shift or more often if there is a concern about abdominal distension.

Stomach capacity varies with the age of the child. A newborn's stomach capacity is 90 mL, a 1 month old's is 150 mL, a 12 month old's is 360 mL, and an adult's is 2,000 to 3,000 mL. Because stomach capacity is smaller, care is taken when formula and other fluids are instilled into the abdomen. Bolus feedings are of an appropriate amount, consistent with the child's stomach capacity.

The infant and young child have a gastric emptying time of $2\frac{1}{2}$ to 3 hours, which increases to 3 to 6 hours in the older child. An appropriate amount of time to allow for absorption of formula is taken into account when measuring residuals. If the child is receiving chest physiotherapy, the amount of time between therapy and feeding is considered or the gastric contents are checked to avoid problems with reflux and aspiration.

Renal System

The infant has less ability to concentrate urine and therefore has a normal urine output of 2 mL/kg/h. For the child and adolescent, normal urine output is 1 mL/kg/h and 0.5 mL/kg/h, respectively. Because of the infant's limited ability to concentrate urine, a low specific gravity does not necessarily mean that the infant is adequately hydrated. The immaturity of the child's kidney means that the child may not process fluid as efficiently as the adult and will be less able to handle sudden large amounts of fluid, leading to fluid overload.

The infant and young child have a larger body surface area in relation to body weight. Maintenance fluid requirements are determined based on body weight (Table 10–2).

The child has a higher percentage of total body water, most of which is composed of extracellular fluid (ECF), compared with the adult. The ECF comprises 50% of the body weight in the infant but 20% in the adult. In addition, the child has a higher insensible water loss due to a higher basal metabolic rate, higher respiratory rate, and larger body surface area. The child's higher percentage of total body water and higher insensible water loss increase the risk for dehydration. Sudden weight loss or gain may indicate fluid imbalance. The child should be weighed daily at the same time using the same scale.

Signs of dehydration include dry mucous membranes, decreased urine output, increased urine concentration, sunken fontanels and eyes, and poor skin turgor. The severity of dehydration varies with the degree of dehydration and the child's fluid and electrolyte status. Circulatory compromise will accompany severe dehydration. Treating a child's dehydration in an adult ICU requires pediatric consultation. Fluid overload will be manifested by bulging fontanels, taut skin, edema (usually periorbital and sacral), hepatomegaly, and other signs of congestive heart failure.

TABLE 10-2
Calculation of Maintenance Fluid

Body Weight (kg)	Fluid Requirements per Day	Fluid Requirements per Hour
<10	100 mL/kg	4 mL/kg
10–20	1,000 mL/kg + 50 mL/kg for each kg above 10	2 mL/kg for each kg above 10
>20	1,500 mL/kg + 20 mL/kg for each kg above 20	1 mL/kg for each kg above 20

From Samson LF, Ouzts KM: Fluid and electrolyte regulation. In Curley MAQ, Smith JB, Moloney-Harmon PA (eds): Critical Care Nursing of Infants and Children, pp 385–409. Philadelphia: WB Saunders, 1996

Endocrine System

The infant and young child have smaller glycogen stores and increased glucose demand due to their larger brain to body size ratio. The smaller stores and increased demand predispose the infant and young child to the development of hypoglycemia. Blood glucose levels are closely monitored, especially when the infant or child is NPO and numerous adjustments are being made with nutritional support.

◼ SELECTED PEDIATRIC CHALLENGES

Ventilatory Issues

The most common cause of cardiopulmonary arrest in children is respiratory in nature. This mandates that respiratory distress and failure are recognized early and that airway management interventions are immediate (Table 10–3). Signs of respiratory decompensation include diminished level of consciousness, tachypnea, minimal or no chest movement with respiratory effort, evidence of labored respirations with retractions, seesaw breathing, minimal or no air exchange noted on auscultation, and the presence of nasal flaring, grunting, stridor, or wheezing.

The initial intervention for respiratory decompensation is positioning the child to open the airway. If the child does not respond to position alone, manual ventilation with 100% oxygen using a bag-valve mask device is initiated. There are several sizes of pediatric manual resuscitation bags; the correct size is determined by noting the child's tidal volume and deciding if the bag is capable of delivering one and one-half times the child's tidal volume. Even though a pressure manometer may assist in minimizing pressure, the true indicator of delivery of an adequate tidal volume is a clinical one. The adequate amount of tidal volume delivered during a manual resuscitation breath is the amount that causes rise and fall of the child's chest.

If bag-valve-mask ventilation is not successful in restoring the child's ventilatory status, endotracheal intubation is required. Numerous sizes of endotracheal tubes are avail-

able for the infant and child. To estimate the correct size endotracheal tube, the size of the child's little finger or the following formula can be used:

$$\text{internal diameter} = (16 + \text{age in years}) \div 4$$

Because these are both estimations of endotracheal tube size, tubes one-half size smaller and larger should be available for immediate use. Table 10–4 provides information regarding endotracheal tube sizes and other equipment issues. Generally, uncuffed endotracheal tubes are used in the child younger than 8 years of age because the narrow cricoid cartilage provides an anatomical cuff in the presence of anatomically normal lungs. Pediatric endotracheal tubes with cuffs are available for use with stiff lungs that are difficult to ventilate.

Monitoring the patient during intubation is critical to assess for desaturation or bradycardia. Once the child is intubated, observation of chest movement and auscultation of the lungs will help determine correct placement. Confirmation of placement will take place with a chest x-ray. Once placement is confirmed, the tube is securely taped to avoid accidental displacement. In addition, soft restraints should be used to prevent the child from removing the tube. Adequate sedation and analgesia are provided to increase the child's comfort and manage anxiety while intubated.

Medication Administration

Because a child may differ in weight significantly from the average child in the associated age group, medications are prescribed on a microgram, milligram, or milliequivalent per kilogram of body weight basis rather than on a standard dose according to age. Confirming the weight (in kg) that is being used to determine drug dosages is important. This same weight should be used during the child's entire hospitalization unless there is a significant change in the child's weight. Because pediatric dosages may be unfamiliar to the adult clinician, precalculated emergency drug sheets are helpful. The emergency drug sheet should include the recommended resuscitation medication dosages, medication concentration, and the final medication dose

TABLE 10-3
Quick Examination of a Healthy Versus Decompensating Child

Assessment	Healthy Child	Decompensating Child
Airway		
Patency	Child requires no interventions; child verbalizes and is able to swallow, cough, gag.	Child self-positions and requires interventions, such as head positioning, suctioning, adjunct airways. Unmaintainable airway requires intubation.
Breathing		
Respiratory rate	Breathing is within age-appropriate limits.	Breathing is tachypneic or bradypneic compared to age-appropriate limits and conditions.* **Note:** Warning parameter: > 60 breaths/min
Chest movement (presence)	Chest rises and falls equally and simultaneously with abdomen with each breath.	Child has minimal or no chest movement with respiratory effort.
Chest movement (quality)	Child has silent and effortless respirations.	Child shows evidence of labored respirations with retractions. Asynchronous movement (seesaw) is observed between chest and abdomen with respiratory efforts.
Air movement (presence)	Air exchange is heard bilaterally in all lobes.	Despite movement of the chest, minimal or no air exchange is noted on auscultation.
Air movement (quality)	Breath sounds are of normal intensity and duration.	Nasal flaring, grunting, stridor, wheezing are noted.
Circulation		
Heart rate (presence)	Apical beat is present and within age-appropriate limit.*	Heart rate is absent; bradycardia or tachycardia occurs as compared with age-appropriate limits.* **Note:** Warning parameters: Infant: <80 bpm / Child <5 y: >180 bpm / Child >5 y: >150 bpm
Heart rate (quality)	Heart rate is regular with normal sinus rhythm.	Heart rate is irregular, slow, or very rapid; common dysrhythmias include supraventricular tachycardia, bradyarrhythmias, and asystole.
Skin	Extremities are warm, pink with capillary refill $\leq$ 2 s; peripheral pulses are present bilaterally with normal intensity.	Child has pallor, cyanotic, or mottled skin color and cool to cold extremities. Capillary refill time is $\geq$ 2 s; peripheral pulses are weak or absent; central pulses are weak.
Cerebral perfusion	Child is alert to surroundings, recognizes parents or significant others, is responsive to fear and pain, and has normal muscle tone.	Child is irritable, lethargic, obtunded, or comatose; has minimal or no reaction to pain; has loose muscle tone (floppy).
Blood pressure	Blood pressure is within age-appropriate limits.	Blood pressure falls from age-appropriate limits,* a late sign of decompensation. **Note:** A fall of 10 mmHg systolic pressure is significant. Lower systolic blood pressure limit: Infant $\leq$1 mo, 60 mmHg / Infant $\leq$1 y, 70 mmHg / Child, 70 + (2 $\times$ age in years)

* All vital signs are interpreted within the context of age, clinical condition, and other external factors, such as the presence of fever.
Adapted from Moloney-Harmon PA, Rosenthal CH: Nursing care modifications for the child in the adult ICU. In Stillwell S (ed): Mosby's Critical Care Nursing Reference, pp 588–670. St. Louis, Mosby-Year Book, 1992

and volume the individual child is to receive. The recommended dosages should reflect the American Heart Association's Pediatric Advanced Life Support (PALS) standards.

An important recommendation for medication administration in the pediatric patient is the single-dose system. The single-dose system involves preparing one syringe to contain only the prescribed medication dose. The syringe should be properly labeled with the drug name and dose. The nurse administers the entire volume of the syringe to ensure that the prescribed dose has been given. The single dose system prevents overmedication or undermedication of the child.

TABLE 10-4
Recommended Resuscitation Equipment for the Infant and Child

	0–6 mo	6–12 mo	1 y	18 mo	3 y	5 y	6 y	8 y	10 y	12 y	14 y
Weight (kg)	3–5	7	10	12	15	20	20	25	30	40	50
Resuscitation mask	0–1	1	1–2	2	3	3	3	3	3	4	4–5
Laryngoscope (Miller/Mac)	0	1	1	1	2	2	2	2	2	2	3
Endotracheal tube (ETT)	3.0	3.5	3.5	4.0	4.5	5.0	5.5	6.0	6.0	6.5	7.0
Suction (ETT/ tracheostomy)	6	6	8	8	10	10	10	10	10	14	14
Suction (oropharyngeal/ nasopharyngeal)	10	10	10	10	14	14	14	16	16	16	16
Chest tube	10–12	10–12	16–20	16–20	16–20	20–28	20–28	20–28	28–32	28–32	32–42
Nasogastric/ orogastric	8	8	8	8	10	10	10	10	12	12	14
Foley	5	5	8	8	10	10	10	10	12	12	12
Tracheostomy (pediatric)	00	1	1	1–2	2–3	3	3	4	4	5	6

Reprinted from: Moloney-Harmon P, Rosenthal CH: Nursing care modifications for the child in the adult ICU. In Stillwell S (ed): Critical Care Nursing Reference Book, pp 590. St. Louis, Mosby-Year Book, 1992 Adapted form Widner-Kolberg MR: Maryland Institutes for Emergency Medical Services Systems, 1989

Pain Management

Because of the nature of the environment and associated procedures, the critically ill child is at high risk for pain. The first step in assessing pain in children is to understand the child's response to and communication of pain. This is based on a variety of factors, including the child's developmental level, past and present experience with pain, cultural aspects, personality, parental presence, age, and the nature of the illness or injury.[4] For instance, critically ill children may be in severe pain but may be unable to communicate because of sedation, paralytic agents, mechanical ventilation, or coma.

Pain assessment is multidimensional. Pain assessment tools often used include physiological parameters and behavioral response. Physiological parameters include heart rate, respiratory rate, blood pressure, and oxygen saturation. Other parameters described by Anand and Carr[5] include sweating, increased muscle tone, and skin color changes. These parameters will return to normal as physiological adaptation occurs. This adaptation can actually occur within minutes, and the nurse must realize that the child may still be in pain. The physical signs are not necessarily specific for pain but may be the only parameter available to the nurse caring for the critically ill child.

Behavioral responses may be helpful for pain assessment, especially in the child who cannot communicate. The next section on interaction with children and families discusses the continuum of responses related to pain and comfort.

Another dimension of pain assessment is self-report. Many tools are available; however, these often require chil-

dren to interact or use their hands. Because of this, these tools are not usually helpful in the critical care setting. Examples of self-report tools include the visual analog tool, number scale, faces scale, and color scale. If the child is unable or unwilling to give a report, the parent's report of pain is often helpful. Multidimensional scales, such as the COMFORT and Ramsey scales, are helpful because they combine dimensions of behavioral and physiological distress and do not require interaction or use of hands.

Pain management interventions are multidimensional whenever possible, including nonpharmacological and pharmacological approaches. However, pharmacological intervention is never withheld when it is appropriate. Opioids are usually the first-line drugs for pain management in the critically ill child. A variety of pharmacological agents are available, and the choice of drug will depend on the child's response and the practitioner's preference. Nursing responsibilities include assessing the child's need for the drug, administering the appropriate dose, and monitoring the child's response.

Other methods of pain control include intravenous patient-controlled analgesia. This helps the child maintain a steady state of pain relief and also gives the child some control over pain. Epidural analgesia is also helpful for a variety of children. Epidural narcotics provide selective analgesia but do have associated side effects, which include respiratory depression, nausea and vomiting, pruritus, and urinary retention.[6]

Nurses may consider the use of nonpharmacological methods, such as distraction, relaxation, massage, and hypnosis, in conjunction with pharmacological agents. The method must be age appropriate, and parental presence is considered. Whatever methods are used, a critical determinant to their effectiveness is the child's response.

Interaction With Children and Families

Interacting with children demands familiarity with their developmental capabilities and psychosocial needs. Categorization of children into groups according to physical and cognitive age can assist one in predicting the child's expected social, cognitive, and physical capabilities. Developmental and psychosocial assessment is beyond the scope of this chapter; therefore, the reader should consult an appropriate growth and development reference. Although each age group of children has common developmental capabilities, tasks, and fears, it is helpful to recognize the common fears of all children despite their age. These fears include loss of control, threat of separation, painful procedures, and communicated anxiety.[7]

Unlike the adult patient, the young child does not consciously screen most behavior and spoken words. The young child subconsciously communicates behaviorally through verbal, nonverbal (body language, behaviors), and abstract (play, drawing, story telling) cues. Although the child's behavior is more natural in a familiar environment, the cues available to the clinician can suggest how a child is feeling or perceiving an event or the presence of an individual. In general, the child's behavior is more activity oriented and more emotional than that of adults.[8] These qualities of a child's behavior should be expected as the norm of average, healthy children and may be used as parameters with which to contrast the behavior of the critically ill child (Table 10–5).

Behavioral responses are particularly helpful during the assessment of pain or comfort. The infant or child may display body movement that spans the entire activity continuum from minimal movement, such as rigidity and guarding, to high activity, such as thrashing and kicking. Assessing various behavioral responses (eg, gestures, posture, movement, and facial expression) and examining the

---

TABLE 10-5
Contrasting Nonverbal Behavioral Cues of the Healthy and the Critically Ill Child

Healthy	Critically Ill
Posture	
Moves, flexes	May be loose, flaccid
	May prefer fetal position or position of comfort
Gestures	
Turns to familiar voices	Responds slowly to familiar voices
Movement	
Moves purposefully	Exhibits minimal movement, lethargy
Moves toward new, pleasurable items	Shows increased movement, irritability (possibly indicating cardiopulmonary or neurological compromise, pain, or sleep deprivation)
Moves away from threatening items, people	
Reactions/Coping Style	
Responds to parent(s) coming, leaving	Exhibits minimal response to parent presence, absence
Responds to environment and equipment	Exhibits minimal response to presence or absence of transitional objects
Cries and fights invasive procedures	Displays minimal defensive responses
Facial Expressions	
Looks at faces and makes eye contact	May not track faces, objects
Changes facial expressions in response to interactions	Avoids eye contact or has minimal response to interactions
Responds negatively to face wash	Minimally changes facial expression during face wash
Blinks in response to stimuli	Exhibits increased or decreased blinking
Widens eyes with fear	Avoids eye contact
Is fascinated with own mouth	Avoids or dislikes mouth stimulation
Holds mouth "ready for action"	Drools or displays loose mouth musculature
	Sucks intermittently or weakly

Taken from Moloney-Harmon P, Rosenthal CH: Nursing care modifications for the child in the adult ICU. In Stillwell S (ed): Critical Care Nursing Reference Book, pp 590. St. Louis, Mosby-Year Book, 1992

congruency between these responses are particularly help-ful. Interaction with pediatric patients and their families is also facilitated by the appreciation of the child's significant others. The philosophy of family-centered care is essential to the optimal care of the pediatric patient.[9] Gone are the days when parents dropped their children for care at the en-trance of the hospital. Although there are several compo-nents of family-centered care, the salient concept is to value, recognize, and support the family in the care of their child. The family is the constant in the child's life and is ultimately responsible for responding to the child's emotional, social, developmental, physical, and health care needs.[10] Appropri-ate support and incorporation of parents may buffer the threats of the ICU environment on the child.[11] Parents may assist or influence the child's cognitive appraisal of the en-vironment, personnel, and events. The child often uses the reactions of the parent as a barometer in interpreting events in ways ranging from threatening to beneficial.

The tone and manner in which the clinician approaches the bedside of a pediatric patient and his or her family are important. Communicated anxiety relates to the child's un-easy feelings in response not only to the parents' anxiety but also to the anxiety of the health care team members in the child's immediate environment. Interventions to relieve the anxiety of parents and fellow health team members will have a direct impact on the child's well-being. Interventions may include assisting parents and staff in anticipating the child's responses to therapy and illness and guiding parents and staff in therapeutic communication techniques.

CONCLUSION

Caring for the critically ill child in an adult-oriented setting is a challenge. Considering the anatomical and physiologi-cal differences in children and the unique challenges for care will provide tools to help ensure an optimal outcome.

Clinical Applicability Challenges

Self-Challenge: Critical Thinking

1. You are caring for a 1-year-old, 10-kg child. Calculate main-tenance fluids for a 24-hour period, and determine the amount the child should receive per hour.

2. Evaluate aspects of the behavioral assessment in the critically ill child, and formulate a plan of care based on assessment data

that encompasses the child's response to the environment, parents, and pain.

Study Questions

1. An early sign of shock in the child is
   a. increased capillary refill time.
   b. bradycardia.
   c. hypotension.
   d. decreased pulse pressure.

2. You are caring for a 3-year-old, 15-kg child who requires intu-bation. What size endotracheal tube would you select?
   a. 4.0
   b. 4.5
   c. 5.0
   d. 5.5

3. You are caring for a 6-month-old, 5-kg child who is receiving frequent fluid boluses. Appropriate urine output that would in-dicate that the child is responding to fluids is
   a. 50 mL/h.
   b. 40 mL/h.
   c. 20 mL/h.
   d. 10 mL/h.

REFERENCES

1. Rosenthal CH: Pediatric Critical Care Nursing in the Adult ICU: Essentials of Practice. National Conference on Pediatric Critical Care Nursing. New York, Contemporary Forums, 1990
2. Moloney-Harmon P, Rosenthal CH: Nursing care modifications for the child in the adult ICU. In Stillwell S (ed): Critical Care Nursing Refer-ence Book, pp 588–670. St. Louis, Mosby-Year Book, 1992
3. Engler AJ, Rushton CH: Thermal regulation. In Curley MAQ, Smith JB, Moloney-Harmon PA (eds): Critical Care Nursing of Infants and Children, pp 449–467. Philadelphia, WB Saunders, 1996
4. Howe CJ, Mason K, Gordin PC: Pain and aversive stimuli. In Curley MAQ, Smith JB, Moloney-Harmon PA (eds): Critical Care Nursing of Infants and Children, pp 532–554. Philadelphia, WB Saunders, 1996
5. Anand KJS, Carr DB: The neuroanatomy, neurophysiology, and neu-rochemistry of pain, stress, and analgesia in newborns and children. Pediatr Clin North Am 36(4):795–821, 1989
6. Tobias JD, Rasmussen GE: Pain management and sedation in the pe-diatric intensive care unit. Pediatr Clin North Am 41(6):1269–1291, 1994
7. Smith J, Browne AM: Critical illness and intensive care during infancy and childhood. In Curley MAQ, Smith JB, Moloney-Harmon PA (eds): Critical Care Nursing of Infants and Children, pp 15–46. Philadelphia, WB Saunders, 1996
8. Trad PV: Psychosocial Scenarios for Pediatrics. New York, Springer-Verlag, 1988
9. Shelton T, Jeppson E, Johnson B: Family Centered Care for Children With Special Health Care Needs. Washington, DC, Association of the Care of Children's Health, 1987
10. Rushton CH: Family-centered care in the critical care setting: Myth or reality. Children's Health Care 19(2):68–78, 1990
11. Kidder C: Reestablishing health factors influencing the child's re-covery in pediatric intensive care. Journal of Pediatric Nursing 4(2):96–103, 1989

11

The Critically Ill Pregnant Woman

**PHYSIOLOGICAL CHANGES
IN PREGNANCY**
Cardiovascular Changes
Respiratory Changes
Renal Changes
Hematological Changes

**CRITICAL CARE CONDITIONS
IN PREGNANCY**
Severe Preeclampsia
   Physiological Principles
   Medical Management
   Nursing Interventions

Disseminated Intravascular Coagulation
Amniotic Fluid Embolism
Adult Respiratory Distress Syndrome
Trauma
EMOTIONAL SUPPORT
CONCLUSION

OBJECTIVES

Based on the content in this chapter, the reader should be able to:

- Summarize normal physiological changes that occur in the cardiovascular, respiratory, renal, and hematological systems during pregnancy.
- Differentiate the signs and symptoms of preeclampsia and severe preeclampsia.
- Explain the pathophysiology of severe preeclampsia.
- Describe parameters of nursing assessment of a severe preeclamptic patient on intravenous magnesium sulfate.
- Name three obstetrical conditions that predispose a woman to develop disseminating intravascular coagulation.
- Summarize the psychosocial support needed for an obstetrical patient in the intensive care unit.
- Compare and contrast the care of an obstetrical trauma patient to a nonobstetrical trauma patient.

*M*ost women experience a normal pregnancy. A small percentage of women, however, experience life-threatening complications that may result from the pregnancy itself or may be part of a preexisting condition. Such critically ill pregnant women provide a unique challenge to nurses.

The general principles of diagnosis and management are similar to those used for other intensive care unit (ICU) pa-

tients, but physiological changes inherent in pregnancy must be considered in order to decrease morbidity and mortality.[1] Critical care nurses caring for these patients must understand the physiological changes that occur in pregnancy to distinguish normal from abnormal responses. Table 11–1 outlines these changes.

▰ PHYSIOLOGICAL CHANGES IN PREGNANCY

Cardiovascular Changes

Normal cardiovascular changes that occur during pregnancy affect pulse, blood pressure, cardiac output, and blood volume (see Table 11–1). Maternal blood volume increases 40% to 50% above baseline. This increase, which is mostly plasma, begins in the first trimester and continues throughout pregnancy. The increase is necessary to provide adequate blood flow to the uterus, fetus, and changing maternal tissues and to accommodate blood loss at birth. Red blood cell volume increases by 20% and is disproportionate to the plasma increase, resulting in maternal physiological anemia. Heart rate increases 10 to 15 beats/min as early as 7 weeks' gestation and returns to the prepregnancy level by 6 weeks' postpartum.[2] Changes in blood volume and heart

TABLE 11-1
Physiological Changes in Pregnancy

	Change	Pregnancy Levels
Cardiovascular Changes		
Blood volume	>40%–50%	1,450–1,750 mL
Red blood cells	>20%	250–450 mL
Blood pressure		
Systolic	<5–12 mmHg	
Diastolic	<10–20 mmHg	
Cardiac output	>30%–50%	6–7 L/min
Heart rate	>10%–30%	Increased by 15–20 beats/min
Systemic vascular resistance	<20%–30%	$1,210 \pm 266$ dynes/sec/cm^{-5}
Pulmonary vascular resistance	<34%	78 ± 22 dynes/sec/cm^{-5}
Colloid osmotic pressure	<10%–14%	22.4 ± 0.5
Respiratory Changes		
Functional residual capacity	<10%–25%	1,725–2,070 mL
Tidal volume	>30%–35%	700 mL
Renal Changes		
Renal blood flow	>25%–50%	1,500–1,750 mL/min
Glomerular filtration rate	>50%	140–170 mL/min

rate lead to an increase in cardiac output of 30% to 50% (6–7 L/min) during pregnancy.[2] Cardiac output increases slightly more intrapartum as a result of the shunting of blood from the placental–fetal unit. Immediately after birth, a larger increase in cardiac output (65%) occurs when the empty uterus contracts and autotransfuses the systemic circulation with approximately 1,000 mL of blood.[2] A woman loses approximately 500 mL of blood during a vaginal birth and approximately 1,000 mL of blood during a cesarean birth.

Development of the uteroplacental unit provides a low-resistance network for the expanded blood volume, which reduces cardiac afterload.[3] The pulmonary vascular resistance, or right afterload, also decreases in response to increased blood volume and vasodilation. Under hormonal influence, smooth muscles and vascular beds relax, lowering systemic vascular resistance. Blood pressure decreases during the first and second trimesters and returns to prepregnancy levels by the third trimester. Blood pressure is affected by maternal position. Supine hypotension occurs when the mother remains in a flat position. The side lying position is recommended, but if the patient must be supine, the uterus should be tilted away from the inferior vena cava by using a wedge under the hip.

Respiratory Changes

Respiratory changes as shown in Table 11–1 occur to accommodate the enlarged uterus and the increased oxygen demands of the mother and fetus. Mechanical changes include the upward shift of the diaphragm, which decreases functional residual capacity, and rib cage volume displacement, which increases tidal volume by 30% to 35%.[1] Airway mucosal changes include hyperemia, hypersecretion, in-

creased friability, and edema. These changes are significant when inserting nasogastric tubes or nasotracheal tubes because of the risk of epistaxis. Respiratory rate remains unchanged, although some women experience shortness of breath at some time during their pregnancy. The exact cause of dyspnea is unknown, but it may be related to hyperventilation, increased oxygen consumption, or decreased PaCO$_2$.

Oxygen consumption increases 15% to 20% during pregnancy and may increase 300% during labor.[4] This results in an increased PaO$_2$ to 104 to 108 mmHg. PaCO$_2$ decreases to 27 to 32 mmHg and allows for the increased diffusion of CO$_2$ from the fetus to the mother.[1] Renal excretion of bicarbonate causes a slight increase in maternal pH.

Renal Changes

Changes in renal function, outlined in Table 11–1, accommodate the increase in metabolic and circulatory requirements of pregnancy.[2] Renal blood flow increases by 30% and glomerular filtration rate by 50%.[2] These increases allow elevations in the clearance of many substances, such as creatinine and urea, and are reflected in lower serum levels.

Hematological Changes

Hemoglobin (Hgb) and hematocrit (HCT) laboratory values decrease because of the hemodilution effect of increased plasma volume. Normal Hgb levels range between 10 and 12 and HCT 32% to 40% during pregnancy.[5] White blood cell count is elevated to 15,000 to 18,000/mm^3.[6] There is an increase in clotting factors VII through X and a decrease in factors XI and XIII, which inhibit coagulation. Fibrinogen increases to 300 to 600 mg/dL. Bleeding and clotting times and platelet counts remain the same in pregnancy.

CRITICAL CARE CONDITIONS IN PREGNANCY

During pregnancy, normal physiological changes occur to provide for growth of the fetus and to prepare the mother for birth. Medical or obstetrical complications may alter this adaptation and shift an uncomplicated pregnancy into a critical situation. ICU admissions become necessary in 0.5% of pregnancies, with the majority of indications hemodynamic instability and respiratory failure.[1] The most common complications requiring ICU admission are severe preeclampsia, disseminated intravascular coagulation (DIC), amniotic fluid embolus, adult respiratory distress syndrome, and trauma.

Severe Preeclampsia

Hypertensive disorders of pregnancy occur in approximately 7% to 10% of all pregnancies.[7] They are the second leading cause of maternal death in the United States. Terms used to describe the different types of hypertension that may occur in pregnancy are listed in the accompanying display. Preeclampsia is one hypertensive disorder occurring in 6% of pregnancies.[8] The etiology of preeclampsia is unknown; however, predisposing risk factors include nulliparity, multiple gestation, diabetes, age younger than 18 or older than 35 years, and chronic hypertension.

Preeclamptic symptoms include hypertension, edema, and proteinuria. Hypertension is defined as a rise in the systolic blood pressure of greater than 30 mmHg or an increase in the diastolic blood pressure of greater than 15 mmHg over the prepregnancy baseline after the 20th week of pregnancy.[9] If the prepregnancy blood pressure is unknown, a measurement of 140/90 measured twice 6

Clinical Terminology: Hypertensive Disorders of Pregnancy

Pregnancy-induced hypertension: onset of hypertension after the 20th week of pregnancy

Preeclampsia: development of hypertension after the 20th week of pregnancy complicated by renal involvement leading to proteinuria

Eclampsia: preeclampsia complicated by central nervous system involvement leading to seizures

HELLP syndrome: development of hypertension after the 20th week of pregnancy complicated by hepatic and hematological manifestations

Chronic hypertension: hypertension developing prior to the 20th week of pregnancy

American College of Obstetricians and Gynecologists: Technical Bulletin, Hypertension in Pregnancy. American College of Obstetricians and Gynecologists, Washington, DC, 1996

---

hours apart in the same position and using the same arm is used to diagnose this complication. In severe preeclampsia, the systolic blood pressure is >160 mmHg, and the diastolic blood pressure is >110 mmHg.[8] Edema may be generalized but is more pronounced in the hands and face. Proteinuria is diagnosed by protein concentrations of 5 g or greater in a 24-hour urine specimen. Oliguria may occur and is defined as urine output of less than 30 mL/h. Other symptoms of severe preeclampsia include visual and cerebral disturbances, such as blurred vision and headaches, epigastric pain, impaired liver function, thrombocytopenia, and pulmonary edema.

PHYSIOLOGICAL PRINCIPLES

Severe preeclampsia is associated with vascular endothelial damage caused by arteriolar vasospasms and vasoconstriction.[8] Arterial circulation is disrupted by alternating areas of constriction and dilation. Damage to the endothelium results in leakage of plasma into extravascular space and platelet aggregation. Colloidal osmotic pressure (COP) decreases as protein enters the extravascular space, and the woman is at risk for hypovolemia and alteration in tissue perfusion and oxygenation.[8] Pulmonary edema may develop and can be noncardiogenic or cardiogenic. Noncardiogenic pulmonary edema develops because pulmonary capillaries are susceptible to fluid leakage through damaged endothelium and low COP. Cardiogenic pulmonary edema occurs because of left ventricular failure from increased afterload caused by increased hydrostatic pressure in the pulmonary capillaries; this increase occurs because of fluid buildup in the pulmonary bed. Symptoms of pulmonary edema include coughing, dyspnea, chest pain, tachycardia, cyanosis, and pink, frothy sputum.[8]

Arterial vasospasm and endothelial damage also decrease perfusion to the kidneys. The decreased kidney perfusion results in a decreased glomerular filtration rate and leads to oliguria. Oliguria may not be an indication of hypovolemia and should not be treated with diuretics. Glomerular capillary endothelial damage permits protein to leak across the capillary membrane and into the urine, resulting in proteinuria, increased blood urea nitrogen and serum creatinine. If vasospasm and hypercoagulability are long lasting, ischemia will occur in the glomeruli.[8]

The liver is also affected by multisystem vasospasm and endothelial damage. Decreased perfusion to the liver can cause ischemia and necrosis. Liver damage is reflected in elevated liver function studies, such as serum glutamic–oxaloacetic transaminase, lactic dehydrogenase, and serum alanine transaminase.[7] HELLP syndrome (hemolysis, elevated liver enzymes, and low platelets) may accompany severe preeclampsia. Hemolysis occurs when red blood cells pass through vasospastic vessels, producing burr cells or schistocytes.[9] Liver enzymes become elevated as liver damage occurs and platelets are consumed because of the aggregation at endothelial damage sites. Criteria for diagnosis of HELLP also include a platelet count of less than 100,000 mm^3.

Neurological sequelae may include seizures, cerebral edema, and cerebral hemorrhage.[8] Symptoms associated with neurological progression are headaches, blurred vision, hyperreflexia and clonus, and changes in level of consciousness. Increased intracranial pressure and decreased perfusion can lead to hypoxia, coma, and death.[8]

MEDICAL MANAGEMENT

The only cure for severe preeclampsia is delivery of the fetus. The decision to deliver the fetus versus expectant management is individualized.[7]

Usually these patients require invasive hemodynamic monitoring, frequent blood pressure measurements, strict intake and output monitoring, laboratory report monitoring, aggressive anticonvulsant and antihypertensive drug therapy, and if undelivered, fetal surveillance. Management is focused on preventing seizures and respiratory complications, monitoring cardiovascular status, and maintaining fluid status. If the woman does not deliver, fetal monitoring is necessary. Critical care and obstetrical staff must collaborate to provide close fetal observation.[9]

Hemodynamic monitoring permits accurate assessments of cardiac output and fluid volume status. Normal hemodynamic values during pregnancy are listed in Table 11–2.[10] Elevated pulmonary artery wedge pressure (PAWP) and pulmonary artery pressure (PAP) values may indicate hypervolemia, thus placing the woman at risk for cardiogenic pulmonary edema. (See Chapter 16 for a more detailed discussion of hemodynamic monitoring.) Interventions to reduce preload include restricting intravenous fluids, repositioning the patient on her side, and administering diuretics when fluid overload or pulmonary edema is present. Decreased central venous pressure, PAP, and PAWP values indicate hypovolemia, and the patient may need a fluid challenge.

Drug therapy is directed at preventing seizures and hypertensive crises. Intravenous magnesium sulfate is the drug of choice for severe preeclampsia to prevent maternal seizures (see display). Magnesium sulfate blocks the reup-

---

CLINICAL APPLICATION: Drug Therapy
Magnesium Sulfate Administration

Dose concentration: 20 g in 500 mL normal saline or D5W = 2 g/50 mL
Loading dose: 4–6 g IV bolus over 10–20 min
Maintenance dose: 2–3 g/h by intravenous infusion

---

take of acetylcholine at the nerve end synapses and relaxes smooth muscles. Side effects include drowsiness, flushing, diaphoresis, hyporeflexia, hypocalcemia, and respiratory paralysis.[7] A therapeutic serum level of 4 to 6 mEq/L is maintained through a continuous infusion of 1 to 3 g/h. Serum levels higher than 15 mEq/L may result in respiratory arrest.

Hydralazine hydrochloride is the antihypertensive agent most commonly used during pregnancy. It causes arterial vasodilation and decreases mean arterial pressure and systemic vascular resistance. Hydralazine hydrochloride increases cardiac output, heart rate, and renal blood flow. Doses are commonly given in 5- to 10-mg boluses intravenously every 20 minutes until a satisfactory reduction in blood pressure is achieved. Other antihypertensives used include nitroprusside, nifedipine, and labetalol hydrochloride. These drugs may be used when hydralazine therapy fails.

NURSING INTERVENTIONS

The nurse must assess the patient for increased risk of seizures by evaluating neurological symptoms. To reduce the risk of seizures, the nurse can decrease light and sound stimulation to the patient. Treatments and interventions are coordinated to optimize rest periods. If seizures occur, the nurse protects the patient from injury, ensures a patent airway, provides adequate oxygenation, and evaluates possible aspiration.[7] After stabilizing the patient, uterine and fetal activity are quickly assessed. In most instances, immediate delivery of the fetus is indicated.

If the patient is receiving magnesium sulfate therapy, the nurse continuously assesses for symptoms of magnesium toxicity, such as respiratory depression and hyporeflexia. Magnesium is excreted in the urine, and prolonged oliguria allows blood levels to accumulate to toxic levels.[8]

If the patient has delivered, magnesium sulfate therapy should be continued for 24 hours. The nurse must assess uterine bleeding. The uterus should be firm following delivery, and if not, uterine massage and oxytocin therapy are needed.

Disseminated Intravascular Coagulation

Several conditions predispose a pregnant woman to DIC because of changes in the coagulation and fibrinolytic systems. These conditions include preeclampsia, abruptio pla-

---

TABLE 11-2
Hemodynamic Values in Nonpregnant and Pregnant Women

	Nonpregnant	Pregnant
Central venous pressure	5–10 mmHg	1.1–6.1 mmHg
Pulmonary artery pressure		
Systolic	20–30 mmHg	18–30 mmHg
Diastolic	8–15 mmHg	6–10 mmHg
Mean	10–20 mmHg	11–15 mmHg
Pulmonary artery wedge pressure	6–12 mmHg	5.7–9.3 mmHg
Cardiac output	4.3–6.0 L/min	5.2–7.2 L/min

centae, fetal demise, and sepsis.[5] Although the incidence of sepsis has decreased because of antibiotic therapy, it is responsible for 7.6% of the maternal deaths in the United States.[6] Sepsis during pregnancy is a result of bacterial invasion of the uterine cavity. Immunocompetence is a normal consequence of pregnancy and thought to occur so that the fetus is not rejected by the maternal system.[6] This alteration increases the susceptibility to infection and decreases the body's ability to fight infection. Septic shock may develop in a few days or several hours. Manifestations of septic shock include tachycardia, tachypnea, temperature instability, increased cardiac output, and decreased peripheral resistance.

Abruptio placentae is the premature separation of the placenta from the uterine wall and is one of the most common causes of DIC. Blood collects between the uterus and placenta, causing consumption of clotting factors. The placental unit contains high concentrations of thromboplastin. When the placenta prematurely separates, thromboplastin continues to be released systemically, activating the clotting and fibrinolytic systems throughout the body. Parallel to the activation of the fibrinolytic system, the hemostatic system initiates clot formation at the site of the separation.[5] Clinical signs of abruption include acute abdominal pain, uterine tenderness, premature contractions, and vaginal bleeding. Abruptions may be subtle, and blood may not be visible.

Intrauterine fetal death can also lead to DIC. Tissue thromboplastin released from the dead fetus into the maternal circulation causes consumptive coagulopathy. Coagulopathy is gradual and consistent with chronic, low-grade DIC.[5]

MANAGEMENT

Management of patients with DIC includes identifying the underlying condition and initiating appropriate therapy, evaluating and monitoring the coagulation system to restore hemostasis, and preventing further hemorrhage and thrombosis. Management of DIC due to sepsis includes prompt delivery of the fetus and intravenous administration of broad-spectrum antibiotics. For abruptio placentae, prompt delivery of the fetus is necessary to control further bleeding.

Nursing care is aimed at preventing further bleeding, monitoring coagulation studies, and assessing the patient for multisystem involvement, altered tissue perfusion, and fluid volume deficits.[5] Nursing care includes monitoring respiratory status, administering intravenous fluids to prevent hypovolemia, assessing hemodynamic values, and administering and evaluating antibiotics, blood replacement products, and antipyretics.[5] (See Chapter 48 for a more detailed discussion of DIC.)

Amniotic Fluid Embolism

Amniotic fluid embolism (AFE) is responsible for approximately 10% of maternal deaths in the United States.[11] AFE occurs when amniotic fluid gains entry into the maternal circulation. This entry may occur during cesarean section, uterine rupture, or through small tears in the endocervical veins during a vaginal delivery.[11] Once amniotic fluid enters the maternal circulation, it rapidly is transported to the pulmonary vasculature, resulting in pulmonary emboli. The pulmonary response to AFE is vasospasm, which produces transient pulmonary hypertension and profound hypoxia. The maternal system becomes hemodynamically compromised with elevated pulmonary artery pressure and left ventricular failure.[12] Predisposing factors that may lead to AFE include preeclampsia, multiple gestation, hydramnios, low insertion of placenta, post-term pregnancy, hypertonic contractions during labor, abruptio placentae, uterine rupture, and umbilical cord prolapse. Clinical manifestations of AFE include sudden onset of dyspnea, cyanosis, and hypotension, followed by cardiopulmonary arrest.

MANAGEMENT

Management of AFE is directed at maintaining left ventricular output.[11] Interventions include intubation and ventilation with 100% oxygen, intravenous administration of vasopressors and crystalloid fluids, cardiopulmonary resuscitation, administration of blood products, and pulmonary artery catheterization. Potential sequelae include acute pulmonary edema, respiratory distress, DIC, hemorrhage, and multisystem failure.

The nurse must react quickly when AFE is suspected. Following the basic ABCs (airway, breathing, and circulation), the nurse can prioritize interventions needed in this stressful situation. If the patient is not intubated, oxygen must be administered using a face mask and a pulse oximeter to monitor oxygen saturation must be applied. The nurse can anticipate that after intubation, a resuscitation bag or mechanical ventilation will be needed. To maximize venous return, the woman should be positioned on her side or a wedge placed under her hip. A large-bore intravenous line is needed to administer intravenous fluids and blood products and to correct hypotension. Assessment is focused on the cardiovascular, pulmonary, hematological, and neurological systems.

Adult Respiratory Distress Syndrome

Adult respiratory distress syndrome (ARDS) is characterized by progressive respiratory distress, severe hypoxemia, low lung compliance, noncardiogenic pulmonary edema, and diffuse infiltrates on chest radiography.[13] Precipitating factors of ARDS associated with pregnancy include abruptio placentae, severe preeclampsia, pyelonephritis, DIC, sepsis, AFE, aspiration, and fetal death in utero.[14] Maternal hypoxemia can lead to spontaneous labor and fetal hypoxia, acidosis, and death; therefore, it should be aggressively managed. Perfusion to vital organs, including the fetus, must be maintained to reduce morbidity and mortality.

MANAGEMENT

Pregnant women with ARDS require cardiovascular support and mechanical ventilation.[14] Hemodynamic monitoring is essential for evaluating changes associated with ARDS, such as central hypovolemia and noncardiogenic pulmonary edema.[15] Ventilator settings include a rate of 12 breaths per minute, tidal volume of 12 to 15 mL/kg body weight, 100% oxygen, and a positive end-expiratory pressure of 5 cm H_2O.

Nursing care of pregnant women with ARDS is primarily supportive. Interventions are directed at optimizing oxygen transport to tissues and restoring pulmonary capillary integrity.[15] A complete respiratory assessment is made, including evaluation of arterial oxygen saturation using pulse oximetry; observation of respiratory rate, character, and effort; and auscultation of lungs. The nurse should be aware that decreased PAWP and PAP values may indicate the presence of noncardiogenic pulmonary edema. (See Table 11–2 for normal values in pregnancy.) Nursing interventions to improve uteroplacental blood flow include positioning the patient on her side and maintaining adequate fluid volumes.[15]

Nursing care for women who are mechanically ventilated includes psychosocial support to help relieve anxiety, fear, and separation from family. Nurses can facilitate communication between the patient and family and keep them informed about maternal and fetal conditions.

Trauma

Accidental injuries occur in 6% to 7% of all pregnancies and are associated with spontaneous abortion, preterm labor, abruptio placentae, and fetal death.[16] Trauma is the leading cause of nonobstetrical maternal death.[17] Common types of trauma include blunt trauma from motor vehicle accidents, falls, and domestic violence and penetrating trauma from stab wounds or gunshots. Fetal survival is dependent on maternal survival, so immediate care and stabilization of the pregnant woman are essential.

MANAGEMENT

Management consists of immediate stabilization and care. Immediate stabilization of all trauma patients consists of applying the ABCs of resuscitation: establishment of airway, breathing, and circulation. First an airway is established, and oxygen is provided at 10 to 12 L/min to produce a PO_2 level of 60 mmHg or higher. This PO_2 level is necessary for optimal fetal oxygenation. If cardiopulmonary resuscitation is necessary, the anatomical and physiological changes in pregnancy must be considered to maximize efforts.[18] The uterus compresses major abdominal vessels and displaces abdominal contents, which decreases chest compliance. Placing a wedge under the woman's right hip will displace the uterus and decompress the vessels. Standard Advanced Cardiac Life Support procedures are used, including defibrillation and most drugs. The administration of vasopressors should be avoided because the vasoconstrictive action can impair uteroplacental perfusion.[18]

Intravenous access using large-bore catheters is needed, and aggressive intravenous infusions are used to increase stroke volume and maintain cardiac output. If hemorrhage occurs, bleeding must be controlled. A decrease in arterial blood pressure may not be an indication of hypovolemia because of low resistance in the uteroplacental system. A 30% to 35% loss can occur with severe consequence to the fetus before hypotension is noted. Fluid replacement therapy must be administered at a higher rate.[1]

Once the pregnant woman has been stabilized, her neurological status is assessed. After this assessment, a fetal assessment, including determination of life, is made. The fetal heart rate can be auscultated using a fetoscope, stethoscope, fetal Doppler, or ultrasound. Additional assessments can be made on arrival at the hospital or trauma center. These assessments include electrocardiogram, complete physical examination, and laboratory tests, such as arterial blood gases (Table 11–3), complete blood count, platelet count, electrolytes, type and cross-match, and the Kleihauer-Betke test. The Kleihauer-Betke test identifies red blood cells from the fetus that have entered the maternal circulatory system and quantifies fetomaternal hemorrhage.[1]

▰ EMOTIONAL SUPPORT

Emotional support is very important to all critically ill pregnant women and their families. If the woman labors in the ICU, her coach or significant other should be allowed to remain at the bedside. When she gives birth, breast-feeding and bonding should be encouraged when feasible. The mother will need access to her newborn and family during this time. If the newborn is not able to be at the bedside, frequent updates about the newborn are important and can be provided by the staff. Providing a flexible and individualized atmosphere to a new family is a challenge in the ICU.[19] The importance of coordinating obstetrical and critical care cannot be overemphasized.

If the fetus dies as a result of maternal complications, grief support may be needed. The nurse may collaborate with psychiatric liaison nurses, social workers, psychologists, psychiatrists, or clergy to offer emotional support to a grieving mother and family.

TABLE 11-3
Arterial Blood Gas Values in Nonpregnant and Pregnant Women

	Nonpregnant	Pregnant
PaO_2	80–100 mmHg	104–108 mmHg
$PaCO_2$	36–44 mmHg	27–32 mmHg
pH	7.35–7.45	7.40–7.47
Bicarb	24–30 mEq/L	18–21 mEq/L

CONCLUSION

When pregnant women become critically ill and require intensive care, it is essential for ICU nurses to understand the physiological changes that occur during pregnancy. This knowledge can help staff recognize subtle changes to reduce morbidity and mortality. Collaboration between the obstetrical team and the critical care team will facilitate appropriate management for both the mother and her fetus. Childbirth is an emotional experience, and nursing care must address the psychosocial needs of these patients. Providing a supportive, family-centered environment is essential in the care of critically ill pregnant women.

Clinical Applicability Challenges

Self-Challenge: Critical Thinking

1. *Analyze the effect of physiological changes occurring during pregnancy with values found in invasive hemodynamic monitoring.*

2. *Create a plan of care that provides family-centered care in an ICU.*

3. *Compare and contrast the resuscitation of the pregnant trauma patient with the nonpregnant trauma patient.*

Study Questions

1. *Pregnancy produces changes to the cardiovascular system, such as*
   a. *increased blood volume and cardiac output; decreased peripheral vascular resistance and blood pressure.*
   b. *decreased heart rate and cardiac output.*
   c. *passive filling of the placental unit to circulate blood to the fetus.*
   d. *higher cardiac outputs and decreased left ventricular preload.*

2. *The antihypertensive medication of choice for managing severe preeclampsia is*
   a. *magnesium sulfate.*
   b. *labetalol.*
   c. *hydralazine.*
   d. *nifedipine.*

3. *DIC may develop in pregnancy when the following conditions exist:*
   a. *Hemorrhage, sepsis, or preterm labor*
   b. *Hemorrhage, sepsis, mild preeclampsia, or fetal demise*
   c. *Trauma, sepsis, or placenta previa*
   d. *Abruptio placentae, severe preeclampsia, sepsis, or fetal demise*

REFERENCES

1. Lapinsky S, Kruczynski K, Slutsky A: Critical care in the pregnant patient. American Journal of Respiratory and Critical Care Medicine 152(2):427–455, 1995
2. Fallon MK: Physiologic changes of pregnancy. In Simpson KR, Creehan PA (eds): Perinatal Nursing, pp 45–59. Philadelphia, Lippincott-Raven, 1996
3. Ayres SM, Grenvik A, Holbrook PR, Shoemaker WC (eds): Textbook of Critical Care. Philadelphia, WB Saunders, 1995
4. Crapo R: Normal cardiopulmonary physiology during pregnancy. Clin Obstet Gynecol 39(1):3–16, 1996
5. Poole J: HELLP syndrome and coagulopathies of pregnancy. Critical Care Nursing Clinics of North America 5(3):475–487, 1993
6. Simpson K: Sepsis during pregnancy. J Obstet Gynecol Neonatal Nurs 24(6):550–555, 1995
7. Burke M, Poole J: Common perinatal complications. In Simpson KR, Creehan PA (eds): Perinatal Nursing, pp 109–146. Philadelphia, Lippincott-Raven, 1996
8. Surratt N: Severe preeclampsia: Implications for critical care nursing. J Obstet Gynecol Neonatal Nurs 22(6):500–507, 1993
9. Koenigseder LA, Crane P, Lucy P: HELLP: A collaborative challenge for critical care and obstetric nurses. American Journal of Critical Care 2(5):385–392, 1993
10. Kennedy B: Mitral stenosis: Implications for critical care obstetric nursing. J Obstet Gynecol Neonatal Nurs 24(5):406–412, 1995
11. Martin R: Amniotic fluid embolism. Clin Obstet Gynecol 39(1):101–106, 1996
12. Sisson M: Amniotic fluid embolism. NAACOG's Clinical Issues in Perinatal and Women's Health Nursing 3(3):469–474, 1992
13. Papadakos P, Johnson D, Abramowicz J, Sherer D: Adult respiratory distress syndrome: A consideration with rapid respiratory decompensation in association with preeclampsia. American Journal of Critical Care 2(1):65–67, 1993
14. Deblieux P, Summer W: Acute respiratory failure in pregnancy. Clin Obstet Gynecol 39(1):143–152, 1996
15. Surratt N, Troiano N: Adult respiratory distress in pregnancy: Critical care issues. J Obstet Gynecol Neonatal Nurs 23(9):773–780, 1994
16. Harvey C, Troiano N: Trauma during pregnancy. NAACOG's Clinical Issues in Perinatal and Women's Health Nursing 22(6):521–529, 1992
17. Hankins G, Barth W, Satin A: Critical care medicine and the obstetric patient. In Ayres SM, Grenvik A, Holbrook PR, Shoemaker WC (eds): Textbook of Critical Care, pp 50–62. Philadelphia, WB Saunders, 1995
18. Mitchell L: Cardiac arrest during pregnancy: Maternal-fetal physiology and advanced cardiac life support for the obstetric patient. Critical Care Nurse 15(1):56–59, 1995
19. Harvey M: Critical care for the maternity patient. MCN 17(6):296–309, 1992

The Critically Ill Older Patient

OBJECTIVES

Based on the content in this chapter, the reader should be able to:

- Explain physical changes occurring as a result of the normal aging process.
- Describe the developmental tasks of the older person.
- Discuss prevalent conditions that affect the major body systems of the older person.
- Explain cognitive changes that may occur in the older patient.
- Compare and contrast delirium and dementia in the older patient.
- Describe assessment indicators of potential abuse or neglect of the older person.
- Describe why the principle *start low, go slow* is important for the older patient in regard to the absorption, distribution, metabolism, and excretion of medications.

*I*ncreasing numbers of older patients are admitted to intensive care units (ICUs). As a result, critical care nurses need to understand age-related physiological changes that occur normally with aging. All physiological processes alter as a person ages. These alterations are progressive and usually are not apparent or pathological. Because of these age-related changes, however, the older critically ill patient requires more intense observation.

The leading causes of death among older patients are heart disease, malignant neoplasms, cerebrovascular accidents, influenza, and chronic obstructive pulmonary disease. Chronic conditions are prevalent among older people (eg, arthritis, hearing and visual deficits). With advancing age, these conditions become more common and result in increased hospitalizations. A longer life span has been the single most important cause of the increased numbers of older patients with multiple chronic and acute illnesses.

NORMAL PSYCHOBIOLOGICAL CHARACTERISTICS OF AGING

Biological Issues

Changes resulting from the aging process must be distinguished from those resulting from a particular disease process, disuse, or environmental factors, such as ultraviolet radiation. Intrinsic aging refers to characteristics and processes that occur universally with all older adults. The following are examples of intrinsic age changes:

- Reduced resistance to stress
- Poor tolerance to extremes of heat and cold because of hypothalamic and skin changes
- Reduced sensory perceptions
- Greater fluctuation in blood pH

Extrinsic aging is composed of factors that influence aging to varying degrees in different individuals. Extrinsic factors include such things as lifestyle or exposure to environmental influences. Normal aging is defined as the sum of intrinsic aging, extrinsic aging, and idiosyncratic or individual genetic factors specific to each individual.[1]

Aging, in one organ or the entire body, may be premature or delayed in relation to actual chronological age. The effect of aging on cellular tissues is asymmetrical. For example, the changes resulting from aging in relation to the brain, bone, cardiovascular, and lung tissues may be fairly obvious, whereas changes affecting the liver, pancreas, gastrointestinal tract, and muscle tissues are less obvious. Several organic changes that result from aging are listed in the display.

Psychosocial Issues

In addition to physical signs of aging, nurses caring for acutely ill older patients must be aware of the older person's normal *developmental tasks* and the specific dreams or wishes of a particular senior. Developmental tasks of older people are listed in the display.

The need for *support* and *meaningful relationships* continues throughout life. Support can be described as a feeling of belonging or a belief that one is an active participant in the surrounding world. The feeling of mutuality with others in the environment lends strength and helps decrease the sense of isolation. Support by family, friends, and

> **Considerations for the Older Patient**
> **Developmental Tasks of the Older Patient**
>
> - Decision of where and how to live for their remaining years
> - Preservation of supportive, intimate, and satisfying relationships with spouse, family, and friends
> - Maintenance of adequate and satisfying home environment relative to health and economic status
> - Provision of sufficient income
> - Maintenance of maximum level of health
> - Attainment of comprehensive health and dental care
> - Maintenance of personal hygiene
> - Maintenance of communication and adequate contact with family and friends
> - Maintenance of social, civic, and political involvement
> - Initiation of new interests (in addition to former activities) that increase status
> - Recognition and feeling of being needed
> - Discovery of meaning in life after retirement and when confronted with illness of self or spouse and death of spouse and other loved ones; adjustment to death of loved ones
> - Development of a significant philosophy of life and discovery of comfort in a philosophy or religion

the community can provide an older patient with a greater sense of stability and security.

Self-worth and perceived well-being are feelings that usually coincide in older adults. The perception of well-being arises from the satisfaction of meeting an acceptable proportion of one's life goals. It can be described as an inner contentment one has in life as a whole. Related to this, a feeling of self-worth is derived not only from a sense of well-being, but also from satisfaction with one's image or acceptance by others. Self-worth also reflects the quality of interactions with family and friends.

Family environment for the gerontological patient includes, among others, dimensions of interpersonal relationships, personal growth, integrity of the family unit, and adaptation to stress. As family members age, all of these areas of concern intensify because of changes in roles of family members, alterations in the family power structure, and changes in financial and decision-making dynamics. Acute illness increases the urgency for effective cooperation among all family members as the traditional family structure is suddenly challenged.

When older patients are admitted to intensive care, issues of *family cohesion and adaptability* often surface. Frequently, families face immediate changes in roles, with adult children and grandchildren assuming the roles of caretakers and nurturers for the older family members. The family must suddenly adjust to dramatically different demands. Frequent visits to the hospital; dialogues with nurses, physicians, and social workers; and efforts to support and communicate with the patient become primary

> **Considerations for the Older Patient**
> **Organic Changes With Aging**
>
> - Increased amounts of connective and collagen tissue
> - Disappearance of cellular elements in the nervous system, muscles, and other vital organs
> - Reduction in number of normally functioning cells
> - Increased amount of fat
> - Decreased use of oxygen
> - Decreased blood pumped during rest
> - Less air expired by the lungs
> - Decreased excretion of hormones
> - Reduced sensory and perceptual activity
> - Decreased absorption of lipids, proteins, and carbohydrates
> - Presbyesophagus
> - Thickening of arterial lumen

tasks. Amid these activities, families often find themselves being pressed for decisions about immediate and long-term care. At this time, the issue of patient involvement in decision making may arise. Effective communication and a willingness to listen to and respect the wishes of the older patient become foremost. If this is achieved, the stress on families is reduced because of increased acceptance of the plan of care by all family members.

■■ PHYSICAL CHALLENGES .

Changes in one organ system do not predict changes in other systems. For example, decreased renal function does not necessarily mean that the cardiovascular, hepatic, or neurological systems are also impaired. Moreover, there is individual variation in age-related changes. Therefore, each person must be evaluated based on the age-related changes actually present rather than on those that are "normal" for a particular age.

It is equally important to distinguish age-related changes from those associated with a chronic disease or acute illness and to avoid prematurely attributing some findings to age if they are caused by illness. A discussion of the effects of aging on various body systems follows.

Auditory Loss

There is a gradual loss of hearing with age. Common hearing changes, associated physical findings, and appropriate nursing interventions are described in Table 12–1. One source estimates that 7 million people older than 65 years have significant hearing loss, and continuation of current trends indicates that by 2000, more than 11 million people will have this problem.[2] The same source suggests that the aging process affects hearing in two critical ways: reduction in threshold sensitivity and reduction in the ability to understand speech. Threshold elevations that occur between 8,000 and 20,000 Hz are not detectable with a routine hearing test. Therefore, hearing loss because of aging or other factors is not documented clinically until frequencies are at or below 8,000 Hz.

Presbycusis is defined as a hearing loss associated with aging. Presbycusis is characterized by a gradual, progressive, bilateral, symmetrical, high-frequency sensorineural (perceptive) hearing loss with poor speech discrimination. Thirteen percent of people 65 years of age and older, if tested, would show signs of presbycusis.[3] Conductive hearing loss and sensorineural hearing loss are the two other major types of hearing problems in older adults.

Blockage of sound transmission from the external ear through the tympanic membrane and small bones in the middle ear may cause a conductive hearing loss. Sensorineural hearing, the most common type of hearing problem in older people, is due to degeneration or changes in the neural receptors in the cochlea, the eighth nerve, and the central nervous system. Treatment may vary dramatically from simple removal of impacted ear wax to surgical removal of an auditory nerve tumor.

The older patient may retain the ability to hear pure tones, but if these pure tones are grouped to form words, the ability to understand and perceive these sounds as intelligible speech may be lost. This loss is known as impairment of discrimination ability. The patient has increased difficulty hearing high-frequency, stimuli-sibilant sounds (-f-, -s-, -th-, -ch-, and -sh-). Noisy environments further hamper the ability to hear certain sounds.

Impaired Vision

Like all other body systems, the eye is affected by aging. Common visual changes, the physical findings associated with them, and nursing interventions are found in Table 12–2. Structural and functional changes occur slowly and

---

TABLE 12-1
Common Changes in Hearing in the Older Patient With Associated Findings and Nursing Interventions

Characteristics of Hearing Changes	Associated Findings	Nursing Interventions
1. Hearing loss progresses from high- to both high- and low-frequency loss. 2. Consonants are not heard well. 3. Greater sound is needed. 4. Decreased speech discrimination occurs. 5. Cerumen impaction is a reversible and frequently overlooked cause of conductive hearing loss.	1. Increased volume of patient's own speech 2. Turning of head toward the speaker or frequent requests to repeat 3. Inappropriate answers, but otherwise cognitively intact 4. Withdrawal, short attention span, frustrated, angry, and depressed 5. No response to a loud noise	1. Face person directly so he or she can lip read. 2. Touch person to get attention before speaking. 3. Use gestures to help with communication. 4. Speak into the "good ear." 5. Do not shout. 6. Speak slowly and clearly. 7. Allow the person more time to answer your questions.

TABLE 12-2
Common Changes in Vision in the Older Patient With Associated Findings and Nursing Interventions

Characteristics of Vision Changes	Associated Findings	Nursing Interventions
1. Decreased visual acuity 2. Decreased visual fields 3. Decreased dark adaptation 4. Elevated minimal threshold of light adaptation 5. Decreased accommodation 6. Decreased color discrimination 7. Decreased depth perception 8. Increased sensitivity to glare	1. Arcus senilis seen as white circles around the iris 2. Smaller pupil size 3. Decreased ability to read 4. Discomfort from light (glare) 5. Changes in depth perception 6. Tunnel vision 7. Falls or collisions	1. Make sure objects are in patient's visual field. 2. Use large lettering. 3. Allow patient more time to adjust to environment. 4. Avoid glare. 5. Use night lights. 6. Use the colors red and yellow. 7. Mark the edges of stairs and curbs.

---

gradually. Visual perception depends on the integration of various neurosensory systems and structures that age at different rates.

The eyelids lose elasticity and become wrinkled. Ptosis (upper eyelid drooping) may be observed. Changes in tissues beneath the eyelid skin may allow fatty tissue formation and accumulation that result in "pouches."

The conjunctiva may develop a yellowish or discolored membrane or become thickened as a result of environmental hazards, such as dust and exposure to drying and irritating pollutants. Arcus senilis, which is a white or gray ring around the limbus (junction of the cornea and sclera), may be related to a high blood level of fatty substances accumulated with advancing age. Although there is a decrease in the amount of lacrimation with age, overflow of tears may occur due to an impaired drainage of the ductal system.

The iris loses its ability to accommodate rapidly to light and dark and develops an increased need for light. The pupil becomes smaller and fixed. The lens becomes inflexible with less complete accommodation for near and far vision and is the site of cataract formation. The vitreous humor behind the lens may pull on the retina to produce holes or tears, risking detachment. The ciliary muscle becomes stiff, which contributes to the problems of accommodating to distances. By age 60, presbyopia may develop. Presbyopia is the inability to shift focus from far to near. A possible rationale for this loss is that the older, aging lens is less flexible and cannot easily change shape from the action of the focusing muscle to which it is attached. Dark–light adaptation slows as the pupillary response slows and rods degenerate. As the lens yellows with increasing age, color discrimination becomes less acute, especially in the blue-green tones. Peripheral vision may decline because of decreased extraocular muscle strength, and depth perception may decline because of a thickening lens. Therefore, time must be provided for the person to adapt when moving between dark and light environments and when getting out of bed. Selected nursing interventions for vision-impaired patients are listed in the display.

In addition to normal changes in vision, there is an increased incidence of cataracts, glaucoma, senile macular degeneration, and diabetic retinopathy. These pathologies must be studied in relation to normal aging of the eye structure.

CATARACTS

A cataract is a clouding of the normally clear and transparent lens of the eye. When a cataract interferes with the transmission of light to the retina, some loss in visual acuity may result. This loss can progress to complete loss of vision. Cataracts account for one sixth of all cases of visual impairment in the United States and mostly occur in individuals older than 50 years.

GLAUCOMA

Glaucoma is one of the major causes of blindness and is especially prevalent in the older adult. Glaucoma is due to increased intraocular pressure. This pressure may result in compression of the optic disk of the eye and damage the

---

CLINICAL APPLICATION:
Nursing Intervention Guidelines
Visually Impaired Patients

- Identify yourself on approach.
- Approach blind patients from the front.
- Assess impact of failing vision and patient's ability to adapt during hospitalization and after discharge.
- Instill all prescribed medications.
- Assess stress level because increased stress can necessitate higher dosages of eye medication for patients with glaucoma.
- Be alert to side effects that other medications may have on the eyes (ie, medications containing antihistamines, caffeine, and atropine-like substances).
- Provide eye lubrications when eyes are dry.

optic nerve. This results in loss of peripheral vision and visual acuity. Age-related changes in the canal of Schlemm, infection, injury, swollen cataracts, and tumors are etiological factors for glaucoma. Early diagnosis is important because the earlier treatment is begun, the easier it is to control the disease.

RETINAL DEGENERATION

Retinal degeneration, or macular degeneration, is the third major source of visual disability in the older adult. Macular degeneration is a pigmentary change of the macular area of the retina caused by small hemorrhages. Individuals see a gray shadow in the center of the visual area but can see well at the outer border. This condition rarely results in total blindness; however, visual loss can progress to legal blindness. Early symptoms include a slight blurring of vision, followed by a blind spot. Compensation techniques include wearing sunglasses or visors, looking to the side, and use of magnifiers.

DIABETIC RETINOPATHY

Diabetic retinopathy is the leading cause of blindness in the United States. It is caused by the deterioration of the blood vessels nourishing the retina at the back of the eye. Microaneurysms and small hemorrhages in the eye may leak fluid or blood and cause swelling of the retina. If this leaking blood or fluid damages or scars the retina, the image sent to the brain becomes blurred and eventually can progress to blindness.

Other Sensory Changes

Although hearing and vision are the most researched sensory changes occurring in older people, there may be declines in the other three senses also.

The number of taste buds is reported to decrease with age, in conjunction with a decline in the ability to taste substances. Sweet and salty substances are less detectable as one ages; therefore, many older adults complain that food tastes bitter or sour. There is very little information on smell sensation, but it is thought that a decrease in the sense of smell can result from atrophy of the olfactory organ and increased hair in the nostrils. The loss of taste and smell affects the older person's ability to identify food and make odor discriminations. Table 12–3 describes the characteristics of smell and taste changes, associated findings, and appropriate nursing interventions.

The threshold of touch varies with the part of the body stimulated. There is a loss of tactile sensation as one ages, although this varies individually. Older adults may not feel the effects of lying too long in one position. A key nursing intervention is to vary the positions of the immobile older patient. The older adult also has decreased kinesthetic sense, which is the person's awareness of his or her body in space. Decreased kinesthetic sense results in postural instability and difficulty reacting to bodily changes in space.

Sleep Changes

It is estimated that sleep disturbances occur in more than one half of those older than 65 years.[4] An important aspect of the critical care nurse's assessment is to determine whether sleep problems are the result of normal aging, sleep disorders, or sleep disturbances due to the acute care environment.

Although some age-related changes in sleep patterns are the normal consequences of aging, the prevalence and potential for severe sleep disorders call for increased clinical awareness and evaluation. Such complaints as habitual snoring, frequent awakening, nocturnal sweating, and awakening with anxiety may be signs of a genuine sleep disorder.

The daily total number of sleeping hours decreases with age, as does the amount of time in stage IV and rapid eye movement sleep. Sleep changes accompanying normal aging include increased fragmentation of nighttime sleep due to intrusions of wakefulness and less time spent in the deeper stages of sleep (stages III and IV) where slow wave sleep takes place. Common abnormal complaints, such as anxiety, waking up choking, headaches, sweating at night,

---

TABLE 12-3
Common Changes in Smell and Taste in the Older Patient With Associated Findings and Nursing Interventions

Characteristics of Changes	Associated Findings	Nursing Interventions
Smell		
1. Olfactory nerve fibers decrease.	1. Inability to notice unpleasant odors	1. Name food items, and encourage thought about the smell or taste of food.
2. Discrimination of fruity odors persists the longest.	2. Decreased appetite	2. Use strong spices and flavoring.
Taste		
1. Taste buds decrease with age.	1. Complaints that food has no taste	1. Serve food attractively.
2. Sweet and salty tastes are lost first, while bitter and sour remain.	2. Excessive use of sugar and salt	2. Vary food texture.
	3. Decreased appetite	

nocturia, and snoring, are a few of the symptoms the nurse should assess more thoroughly.

The most prevalent and most serious age-related sleep disorder is sleep apnea. There is evidence of an association between sleep apnea and circulatory disorders, including hypertension, stroke, and angina pectoris. There also may be a link between sleep apnea and reduced life expectancy. In addition, there may be an association among habitual snoring, stroke, and angina pectoris in older men.[5]

The prevalence of disordered breathing in the older patient is high. Therefore, care should be taken in dispensing sedative hypnotics for people with risk factors for sleep apnea. Nursing interventions include encouraging older patients with disordered breathing to sleep on their sides and to lose weight if weight affects breathing. Other interventions include giving supplemental oxygen if hypoxemia, caused by chronic lung disease or hypoventilation, is present.

Normal aging, chronic illness, and drug therapy increase the older person's susceptibility to insomnia. Treatment depends on the problem. Before drug therapy is considered, poor sleep hygiene habits should be addressed. Good sleep hygiene includes avoiding daytime naps; maintaining regular bedtimes and rising times; avoiding heavy evening meals, excessive fluids, alcohol, and caffeine; and keeping the sleep environment quiet, sufficiently dark, at a comfortable temperature, and safe. Behavior modification has been used successfully for many sleep problems. The conservative use of medications may be indicated in more problematic sleep disorders, periodic movements of sleep, and dementing illness.[6] Drug treatment is best when accompanied by improved sleep hygiene and patient education about age-related changes in sleep.

Skin Changes

Although a variety of cutaneous changes have been associated with age, some of these changes are due to normal or intrinsic age factors, while others are due to chronic solar exposure.[7] Table 12–4 delineates the changes that occur in the skin associated with normal aging and contrasts those with photoaging. Photoaging is the combined effect of repeated sun exposure and intrinsic aging on the skin, and it is the cause of what is generally associated with the clinical (and histological) changes that are consistent with "aging." With age, there is a thinning of the skin and a decrease in skin flexibility. This puts the older adult at risk of epidermal tearing from shearing forces. Likewise, there is a loss of elasticity resulting in fine wrinkling, looseness, and sagging. Over time, there is a decrease in the number of dermal blood vessels, and these blood vessels become thinner and more fragile. These changes result in the hemorrhaging (known as senile purpura) commonly seen in older adults, and in impaired body temperature management, healing of wounds, and decreased absorption of topical treatments. With age, there is decreased density and activity of the eccrine and apocrine glands and decreased sebum production. Overall, due to a combination of skin changes in older adults, there tends to be a quicker breakdown in the skin barrier and a slower recovery of skin integrity. Common interventions to maintain skin integrity are shown in the display.

Xerosis, or dry skin, is a common problem for the older adult and is the most common cause of pruritus in this group. The treatment for dry skin focuses primarily on the replacement of water, which is the major cause of dryness. Older adults should be encouraged to do the following:

- Maintain a sufficient oral intake of fluid, approximately 2,000 mL of liquids daily.
- Increase bathing time so there is 10 minutes daily of total body water immersion, with water temperature ranging from 32.2° to 40.5°C (90° to 105°F).
- Avoid the use of soaps.
- Use an emollient after bathing.

Cardiovascular Changes

A number of cardiovascular changes occur with aging; they are outlined in Table 12–5. There are increases in heart weight, ventricular septal and left ventricular wall thickness, and valve circumferences. Fat, collagen, elastin, and lipofuscin increase, and arterial compliance decreases. De-

TABLE 12-4
Features of Intrinsic Aging Versus Photoaged Skin

Feature	Intrinsic Aging	Photoaging
Clinical appearance	Smooth/unblemished Decreased elasticity Fine wrinkling	Nodular/leathery/blotchy Deep wrinkling
Epidermis	Thinner than normal	Thicker due to hyperplasia
Keratinocytes	Some cellular irregularity Lower proliferative rate	Marked cellular irregularity Higher proliferative rate
Melanin	Production decreased but uniformly distributed	Production decreased but variability in distribution
Dermis	Decreased fibroblasts; "moth-eaten" fibers	"Microscar"
Microvasculature	Normal architecture	Thickening of vessel walls

spite these changes, in the healthy older adult, cardiac output is normal at least until the age of 80 years. When there is a decrease in cardiac output, it is most likely due to disease or physical deconditioning. There is an impairment in left ventricular compliance, which leads to reduced filling in early diastole. Stroke volume decreases, and the resting heart rate may increase slightly. During exercise, stroke volume increases to compensate for the lower pulse rate, and a rise in cardiac output is maintained. However, in the older adult, the rate increase is less than in younger individuals, and the return to baseline requires more time.

Arteries tend to lose their elasticity with aging and become less compliant with increased output (arteriosclerosis). This may result in a higher systolic pressure, although in the healthy older adult, this remains within the designation of normal (160 mmHg). Diastolic pressure similarly tends to increase, but this levels off by the sixth or seventh decade.

In the absence of vascular disease, these changes should not interfere with normal tissue perfusion. In the older patient, the likelihood of atherosclerosis is increased. The narrowing of vessels, coupled with their decrease in compliance, may produce tissue ischemia. These changes, along with bed rest, contribute to tissue injury and decubitus formation.

The decrease in vessel compliance affects large and small arteries. As a result, even a small increase in intravascular volume can be accompanied by a substantial rise in aortic pressure (and, in turn, systolic blood pressure), which may lead to pressure-produced ventricular hypertrophy.[8]

The older patient may also have a greater amount of pooling in the lower extremities because of decreased muscle mass and poor venous return. If the patient is placed on bed rest, this fluid pool is redistributed and may cause an overload in the cardiovascular system. The nurse must be alert for vascular overload and congestive heart failure.

Another factor to consider is the shifting of fluids when a patient arises after having been on bed rest. The sudden shift in fluid to the lower extremities and the lowered fluid volume that results from bed rest can produce extreme lightheadedness. This is further complicated by a decrease in baroreceptor sensitivity with age. A slow progression of head elevation and dangling before moving the patient to sitting or standing is necessary to prevent syncope and possible injury from falling.

Respiratory Changes

Decreased expansion and flexibility of the pulmonary structure with age results in a decreased volume exchange. In addition, cilia are lost and surfactant diminishes in the alveolar sacs, although mucus production may increase. The number of alveoli is thought to remain constant except in respiratory disease. The older adult with a healthy respiratory system should experience only minimal respiratory difficulty during daily activities. There may be some respiratory compromise with exercise related to decreased exchange.

In many older patients, changes related to disease arise from damage to the lungs from smoking, environmental pollutants, or previous infections. Bony abnormalities, such as kyphosis, may also cause further restriction of respiratory excursion.

The decreased expansion of the thorax, increased secretions, and decreased number of cilia render the older pa-

---

TABLE 12-5
Age-Associated Cardiovascular Changes and Nursing Considerations

Site	Change	Nursing Considerations
Myocardium	Increase in ventricular wall thickness and cardiac mass	Changes relatively mild with no needed interventions.
Cardiac valves	Increase in size Calcification	Change usually does not cause valvular dysfunction.
Aorta	Enlargement and reduction in compliance/thickening	There are increases in pulse wave velocity.
LV* function	Declining LV compliance	Increased blood pressure requires frequent monitoring.
Arteries	Loose elasticity	Increased blood pressure requires frequent monitoring.
Baroreceptors	Decreased sensitivity	Patient at increased risk for orthostatic hypotension.

LV, left ventricular.

tient susceptible to respiratory infections. In addition, a decreased immune response in older adults may contribute to the increased incidence of respiratory infection.

Careful attention to nutrition, especially to sufficient calories, protein, and fluid intake, is needed to reduce the risk of infection. Frequent position changes also assist in the clearance of secretions and aid ventilation and perfusion of the lungs.

Renal Changes

Age-associated kidney changes can be categorized as anatomical or functional. Anatomical changes include the loss of renal glomeruli, decreased kidney size, renal tubular changes, and renal vascular changes. There are also functional kidney changes as described in the accompanying display. The loss of glomeruli, in conjunction with decreased kidney perfusion, results in a decreased glomerular filtration rate (GFR). The decrease in filtration may result in decreased clearance of substances normally excreted. An increase in blood urea nitrogen or creatinine may indicate the extent to which the GFR is diminished. However, creatinine from muscle breakdown may be less than in younger patients and could mask an elevated creatinine. Creatinine clearance is a more accurate measure of renal function for the older patient. Evaluation of renal function is extremely important if the patient is receiving drugs normally excreted by the kidney.

There may also be a lessened response to antidiuretic hormones that can result in a decreased ability to concentrate urine. This decreased ability may lead to problems of fluid and electrolyte balance as excess sodium, potassium, and water are lost. Loss of hydrogen ions may also make the acid–base balance more difficult to maintain.

Older adults tend to have decreased sensations of thirst and consequently drink less fluid. This change leaves them vulnerable to dehydration, especially when medications with diuretic actions are administered. Care must be taken to ensure that the hospitalized older patient has adequate fluid intake by oral, enteral, or parenteral routes. Fluid balance may also be precarious because disease states such as

diabetes can produce diuresis. Further, potassium and sodium levels may already be low when the patient arrives in the unit. Care must be taken to ensure that electrolyte balance remains stable or is restored. Confusion, dysrhythmias, coma, and death can occur quickly in the older patient with altered electrolyte balance.

As bladder muscle tone is lost, incomplete emptying with retention can foster the development of urinary tract infections that can ascend and become renal infections. Hypertrophy of the prostate gland also places older men at risk for urinary tract infection because the enlarged gland interrupts urine flow. Loss of muscle tone, retention with overdistention, and loss of sphincter control lead to incontinence in the older man or woman. For the alert patient, this loss of control is embarrassing and disconcerting. Bladder training, observation for distention, and appropriate medications are nursing measures to assist the patient with maintaining continence. If incontinence does occur, rapid linen changes and proper skin care diminish physical and mental discomfort.

If an older patient develops any type of incontinence or retention during the stay in the ICU, the nurse should evaluate the medication regimen to see if any drugs affect bladder contractility or tone. If an indwelling (Foley) catheter is necessary during acute illness, it should be removed as soon as the primary reason for inserting it (eg, hourly urine measurements) has passed. Early removal may prevent deterioration of bladder function and urinary tract infection.

Gastrointestinal Changes

The gastrointestinal system undergoes many age-related changes. These changes and related nursing implications are summarized in Table 12–6. The mechanical and chemical processes of digestion that begin in the mouth may be impaired because of loss of teeth, poor hygiene, and decrease in salivary secretions. Many older adults experience diminished senses of taste and smell, which may lead to decreased food intake.

Slowing of peristalsis may interfere with swallowing, gastric emptying, and passage through the bowel. The decrease in hydrochloric acid, digestive enzymes, and bile may contribute to incomplete digestion of nutrients. Diminished intrinsic factor in some people and decreased vitamin B_{12} synthesis may produce pernicious anemia.

Data are insufficient to make assumptions regarding changes in absorption in the large and small bowel. Some evidence indicates that absorption is somewhat impaired. Given that the eating patterns of older adults may not include all food groups, deficiencies may arise from lack of intake rather than malabsorption.

The decreased motility of the large bowel is probably not sufficient to produce constipation in the active adult. However, older adults who are on bed rest, have decreased intake of food and fluids, and are exposed to multiple medications may experience constipation and fecal impaction. Dependence on, or misuse of, laxatives must be assessed when the

---

Considerations for the Older Patient
Age-Associated Functional Kidney Changes

- Decreased glomerular filtration rate
- Decreased mean creatinine clearance rate
- Increased mean creatinine concentrations
- Decreased blood flow through the kidneys
- Decreased tubular transport capacity
- Decreased functional nephrons
- Decreased concentrating ability
- Decreased diluting ability
- Decreased plasma renin activity
- Impaired sodium conservation

TABLE 12-6
Age-Associated Gastrointestinal Changes and Nursing Interventions

Site	Change	Nursing Interventions
Esophagus	Decreased motility	Elevate head of bed when patient eats. Monitor for swallowing difficulty.
Stomach	Decreased motility and emptying	Monitor for nausea. Give small, frequent meals.
Small intestine	Possible changes in nutrient absorption	Monitor diet. Watch for malnutrition.
Colon	Possible decrease in motility/constipation common	Monitor bowel activity. Encourage high fiber and fluids. Use natural laxatives (prune juice). Use laxatives as needed to maintain bowel function.

history is taken, because this may further exacerbate the constipation and management of bowel function.

Nursing interventions for gastrointestinal changes begin with a careful history. Eating habits, including time and frequency of food intake, food preferences, usual intake, food intolerances, and intactness of taste and smell, must be assessed. Use of laxatives, enemas, and vitamin supplementation should be explored. Evaluation of the teeth and gums helps to establish how well food can be handled mechanically.

When planning care, the nurse must consider that bed rest slows peristalsis and aggravates any preexisting condition related to motility. Adequate fluid intake, bulk in the diet, use of natural laxatives (eg, prune juice, warm liquids), and as much active or passive exercise as the condition of the patient allows may help maintain a normal pattern of bowel movements. Stool softeners and mild laxatives are often included in the regimen.

Hospitalized patients of any age can become rapidly malnourished secondary to the stress of acute illness, an increased demand for energy, and lack of nourishment. Therefore, it is important to look for indicators of nutritional risk. They include a history of recent weight loss, a diet lacking in protein and calories, an albumin level < 3.5 g/dL, and a lymphocyte count < 1,500 mm^3. The older patient who enters the hospital already mildly to moderately malnourished and who has a poor intake of protein and calories may quickly become severely malnourished. This malnourished state can markedly compromise the immune response and increase the incidence and severity of infection. Therefore, it is crucial to see that critically ill older patients maintain adequate nutritional intake.

Musculoskeletal Changes

Mobility limitations of the older patient may be related to loss of muscle strength. Muscle mass may be lost because of a reduction in the number and size of muscle fibers or an increase in connective tissues. These changes result in less

muscle tension and decreased strength of the contraction. The decrease of lean muscle mass and the loss of elasticity contribute to lost flexibility and increased stiffness.

There may be a loss of bone mass with aging that, in the presence of osteoporosis, increases the risk of fracture. Lack of exercise, poor nutrition, and calcium malabsorption contribute to the loss of bone mass. The patient on bed rest may rapidly lose bone mineral concentration. The calcaneus (heel) and spine are most susceptible, with a loss of approximately 1% per week. This loss is related to lack of weight bearing. Having the patient stand as soon as his or her condition allows will slow the loss of bone mineral concentration.

Forced fasting of the critically ill hospitalized patient may further accelerate muscle loss through catabolism and gluconeogenesis. The added burden of bed rest leads to a rapid loss of mobility, strength, and energy in the older patient. Maintaining nutrition, changing position frequently, active and passive exercise, and getting out of bed as much as permitted by condition are essential to preserving strength, energy, and bone mass. If the patient is comatose or has suffered loss of function, proper positioning and splinting can help prevent permanent deformity.

Endocrine Changes

No significant changes occur in hormone production during the aging process except for the female reproductive hormones. Changes in the circulating hormones, therefore, with the exception of female reproductive hormones, may reflect a disease process or a drug-altered response.

Glucose tolerance decreases with age. An increase in blood glucose to 200 mg/dL occurs in about 50% of people older than 70 years.[9] Interpretation of this glucose intolerance requires the use of age-adjusted parameters to avoid the inappropriate diagnosis and treatment of diabetes mellitus. Evaluating glycosylated hemoglobin (HbA$_{1c}$) or glycosylated albumin may help establish the presence or absence of diabetes mellitus in the older patient with elevated glucose. Because the renal threshold for reabsorption of glucose increases with age, higher degrees of hyperglycemia must be present before glucose spills into the urine. Therefore, monitoring for hyperglycemia with urine testing should be avoided.

Diabetes mellitus is frequently seen in conjunction with acute illness, trauma, or surgery. The end-organ damage of diabetes mellitus is a factor in stroke, myocardial infarction, decreased renal function, and peripheral vascular disease. Longstanding non–insulin-dependent diabetes may only be diagnosed when the patient presents with a stroke or acute myocardial infarction. Therefore, it is important to distinguish among the impaired glucose tolerance of aging, a transient rise in glucose related to acute illness, and the disease process of diabetes.

Recognition of the underlying diabetes and possible end-organ damage may alter the course of the acute illness. For example, knowing that the incidence of congestive heart failure after myocardial infarction is higher in diabetics than in nondiabetics, the nurse can be alert for early signs of fluid retention.

Older diabetics are, for the most part, not insulin dependent. Even if they develop extremely high blood sugars, they are rarely ketoacidotic. In fact, the coma of this age group is usually hyperglycemic, hyperosmolar, and nonketotic (HHNK). Managing this state requires a delicate balance of hydration and rapid reduction of blood sugar without massive brain edema and death. The critical care nurse must be aware that HHNK coma can be triggered by acute illness or surgery. Identification of common problems found in the diabetic older adult and nursing interventions to prevent these problems are shown in Table 12–7.

Although diabetes mellitus is probably the most common endocrine-related disease process encountered in the older critically ill patient, thyroid conditions are also frequently identified. The symptoms of thyroid disease, such as apathy, weakness, and weight loss, may not be as pronounced in the older adult as they are in younger peo-

ple. Moreover, these symptoms are often attributed to old age rather than to hyperthyroidism or hypothyroidism. The older patient with hyperthyroidism is likely to present with atrial tachycardia and is more likely to be anorectic than hyperphagic; this person usually will not suffer from heat intolerance. The hypothyroid older adult may present with increased susceptibility to hypothermia if exposed to cold, a change in cognitive status, fatigue, dizziness and a tendency to fall.

Being aware of the atypical presentation of thyroid disease in older adults leads the critical care nurse to recognize endocrine imbalance. Once identified, the imbalance can easily be corrected by replacing thyroid hormone or changing the dosage of thyroid replacement.

■ PSYCHOLOGICAL CHALLENGES

Cognitive Changes

Cognition refers to the process of obtaining, storing, retrieving, and using information. Some observable and studied changes in cognition occur with aging. They include some decline in perceptual motor skills, concept formation, complex memory tasks, and quick-decision tasks. However, age itself is not the criterion for making decisions about a patient's cognitive functions. Each person's abilities must be judged individually rather than against a norm.

Cognitive function should be assessed and described on admission and monitored routinely over time and whenever the patient's condition changes. While assessing cognitive functions during the patient's stay in intensive care, it is important to remember that physiological deficits, some medications, and internal and external stress, such as environmental stressors, affect cognitive skills. Any acute physical changes in the older adult often initially present as changes in cognitive status. For example, an older adult with an acute urinary tract infection may not have symptoms such as burning with urination or frequency. Rather, this individual may present with changes in cognitive status.

A mental status questionnaire can be used to assess cognitive function systematically. One example is the Folstein Mini-Mental State Examination (MMSE), shown here. The MMSE has 11 questions that provide information about orientation, attention, memory, perception, and thought process. It takes 5 to 10 minutes to complete, and the patient must be able to give oral and written responses.[10] Use of a consistent assessment tool helps the nurse compare responses and monitor results over time. The main drawback to the use of a questionnaire is that some critically ill patients may not be able to hear, see, talk, or write well enough to respond to the questions. Longer, more sensitive tools may also be more fatiguing for the critically ill older patient.

Several common syndromes cause cognitive impairment, including dementia, delirium, and depression (dis-

TABLE 12-7 **Nursing Care of the Older Adult With Diabetes**	
Potential Problem	**Nursing Interventions**
Skin alterations	Monitor for decreased circulation and skin breakdown. Provide foot care to maintain skin integrity. Bathe daily and apply emollient.
Hyperglycemia	Maintain controlled diet. Monitor blood sugars.
Hydration status	Monitor hydration. Encourage 2,000 mL of fluid daily.
End organ disease	Monitor kidney function. Monitor for visual changes (blurred or decreased vision).

Folstein Mini-Mental State Examination

Maximum Score	Factor
	Orientation
5	What is the (year) (season) (date) (day) (month)?
5	Where are we (state) (county) (town) (hospital) (floor)?
	Registration
3	Name three objects; allow one second to say each. Then, ask the patient to repeat the three objects after you have said them. Give one point for each correct answer. Repeat until the patient learns all three. Count trials and record number.
	Attention and Calculation
5	Ask the patient to begin with 100 and count backward by sevens (stop after five answers). Alternatively, spell "world" backward.
	Recall
3	Ask the patient to repeat the three objects that you previously asked him or her to remember.
	Language
2	Show the patient a pencil and a watch and ask him or her to name them.
1	Ask the patient to repeat the following: "No ifs, ands, or buts."
3	Give the patient a three-stage command: "Take a paper in your right hand, fold it in half, and put it on the floor."
1	Show the patient the written item "Close your eyes," and ask the patient to read and obey it.
1	Tell the patient to write a sentence.
1	Tell the patient to copy a design (complex polygon).
30	Total score possible

Scoring: 24 to 30 correct—intact cognitive function
20 to 23 correct—mild cognitive impairment
16 to 19 correct—moderate cognitive impairment
15 or less correct—severe cognitive impairment

Folstein MF, Folstein SE, McHugh PR: "Mini-mental state." A practical method for grading the cognitive state of patients for the clinician. J Psychiatr Res 12(3):189–198, 1975

cussed below). Dementia is based on impairment of memory plus at least one of the following: a personality change or impairment in either abstract thinking, judgment, or higher cortical functions. Delirium is the abrupt onset of clouding of consciousness and is a medical emergency. Table 12–8 identifies factors to differentiate dementia from delirium. Reversible causes of dementia and delirium are listed in the accompanying display.

LEARNING

Older adults may take longer to respond to and assimilate new material. They may also be hesitant to take on new tasks. Motivation continues to be an important aspect of learning new material. If the material is irrelevant or meaningless, motivation is decreased, which is often interpreted as an inability to learn. Sensory abilities and cognition are used to teach older patients. It may be necessary to present information using small segments and varied stimuli, including touching, seeing, hearing, and (if vision permits) writing. If movements are slowed, allow time for the completion of motor tasks, such as manipulating equipment or carrying out exercises.

MEMORY

The older person's memory decline involves short-term memory rather than long-term and remote memory. Recall of memory from the past is least impaired by age. Remote memory recall (items learned many years ago) can be a positive therapeutic strategy for older patients. Reminiscence is an adaptive mechanism that helps the nurse learn about the patient and contributes to feelings of increased self-worth and competence for the patient.

DEPRESSION

Depression disorders are among the most common complaints of older adults and the leading cause of suicide in later life. Symptoms of depression are listed in the display. Based on the diagnostic criteria for major depression, at least five of these symptoms should occur almost daily for at least 2 weeks. These symptoms of depression in the older adult can be masked by normal age changes or disease states. For example, difficulty sleeping, early morning awakening, and lethargy are common physical complaints of the normal aging person. Alternately, depression in the

TABLE 12-8
Distinguishing Delirium From Dementia

Delirium	Dementia
Abrupt onset	Gradual onset
Acute illness (days to weeks)	Chronic illness
Usually reversible	Generally irreversible
Disorientation early	Disorientation late
Variability hour to hour	Generally stable
Clouded consciousness	Consciousness not clouded
Short attention span	Attention not initially decreased
Disturbed sleep–wake cycle (hour by hour)	Day–night sleep reversal (not hour by hour)
Hallucinations common	Hallucinations late
Marked psychomotor changes	Psychomotor changes late

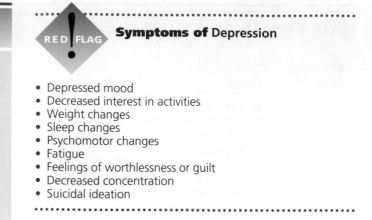

RED FLAG **Symptoms of** Depression

- Depressed mood
- Decreased interest in activities
- Weight changes
- Sleep changes
- Psychomotor changes
- Fatigue
- Feelings of worthlessness or guilt
- Decreased concentration
- Suicidal ideation

older adult may more commonly present with pseudo-hypochondriasis, preoccupation with past life events, and changes in cognitive ability. In some patients, the dominant emotional mood may not be sadness but anger, anxiety, or irritability.

Causes of depression are multifaceted and include multiple losses associated with aging, underlying illness, or drugs.

The accompanying display lists drug groups that may cause depression. Screening tools, such as the Geriatric Depression Scale,[11] shown here, are useful to identify individuals who are depressed. Once identified, appropriate interventions, including drug therapy, behavioral modification, and counseling, can be initiated.

The nurse must also be aware of cardiovascular side effects of tricyclic antidepressive drugs. On the electrocardiograph, ST segment and T wave changes may become evident but are not necessarily indicative of myocardial damage. Ventricular dysrhythmias and disturbances in cardiac conduction are considered serious side effects of some antidepressant drugs, which may result in the drug being reduced or discontinued. The older person may also experience changes related to sleep, appetite, and blood pressure

with antidepressant drugs. Anticholinergic effects, especially in Alzheimer's disease, benign prostatic hypertrophy, or coronary artery disease, may also be seen.

Untreated depression may result in suicide, which is a serious problem among older adults. Of all suicides committed in this country annually, 25% are people older than 65 years. White men older than 85 years are at particular risk.[12] Because of their many losses and changes, suicide may for some older adults fulfill a fantasy of "reunion" with their dead spouse or significant other. The nurse must monitor signs and symptoms of depression, explore the causes of depression, facilitate treatment, and be watchful for suicide attempts or warnings.

Abuse of the Older Person

Mistreatment of older people is a problem that affects more than 4% of the older adults in the United States.[13] Abuse of older adults occurs in homes and institutions and takes many forms. Abuse may be blatant or subtle; it may be physical, psychological, or material (eg, financial). Abuse may involve neglect (by others or by self), exploitation, or abandonment. The abused older person is often physically or mentally frail and unable to report the abusive situation. Abuse can also happen to emotionally and intellectually stable older people who are unable to stop the abuse or report

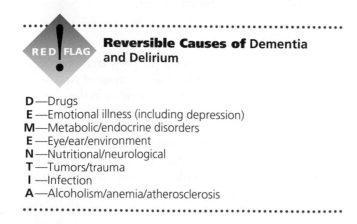

RED FLAG **Reversible Causes of** Dementia and Delirium

D—Drugs
E—Emotional illness (including depression)
M—Metabolic/endocrine disorders
E—Eye/ear/environment
N—Nutritional/neurological
T—Tumors/trauma
I—Infection
A—Alcoholism/anemia/atherosclerosis

CLINICAL APPLICATION: Drug Therapy
Drug Groups That May Cause Depression in the Older Person

Analgesics/anti-inflammatory agents
Anticonvulsants
Antihistamines
Antihypertensives
Antimicrobials
Antiparkinsonian agents
Hormones
Immunosuppressive agents
Tranquilizers

Geriatric Depression Scale (Short Form)

Choose the best answer for how you felt during the past week.

	YES	NO
1. Are you basically satisfied with your life?	☐	☐
2. Have you dropped many of your activities and interests?	☐	☐
3. Do you feel that your life is empty?	☐	☐
4. Do you often get bored?	☐	☐
5. Are you in good spirits most of the time?	☐	☐
6. Are you afraid that something bad is going to happen to you?	☐	☐
7. Do you feel happy most of the time?	☐	☐
8. Do you often feel helpless?	☐	☐
9. Do you prefer to stay at home rather than going out and doing new things?	☐	☐
10. Do you feel you have more problems with memory than most?	☐	☐
11. Do you think it is wonderful to be alive now?	☐	☐
12. Do you feel pretty worthless the way you are now?	☐	☐
13. Do you feel full of energy?	☐	☐
14. Do you feel that your situation is hopeless?	☐	☐
15. Do you think that most people are better off than you are?	☐	☐

TOTAL SCORE _____

The following answers count one point; scores of 5 points or more indicate probable depression.

1. NO	6. YES	11. NO
2. YES	7. NO	12. YES
3. YES	8. YES	13. NO
4. YES	9. YES	14. YES
5. NO	10. YES	15. YES

Yesavage JA, Brink TL: Development and validation of a geriatric depression screening scale: A preliminary report. J Psychiatr Res 17:37–49, 1983

it because of their financial or emotional dependence on the abuser. They may also be afraid of being abandoned.

The abuse can be by people who may or may not live with the older person. Abuse can occur because of lack of knowledge about the older person's basic needs, lack of resources to help, and desire to protect an inheritance. The abuse can be by caretakers who are extremely stressed, or the abused older adult may be the caretaker.

The nurse should be alert to the signs and symptoms of elder abuse as outlined in the display. Any suggestion by the

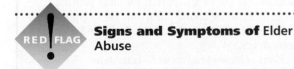

Signs and Symptoms of Elder Abuse

- Lack of compliance with management of health problems
- Unexplained injuries, such as fractures, bruises, lacerations
- Burns
- Poor personal hygiene
- Sexually transmitted disease
- Altered mood
- Depression
- Failure to thrive (underhydration/impaired nutritional status)
- Impaired skin integrity/fungal rashes

patient or family that things are not well at home should be pursued. A statement such as, "My son hasn't been here yet. He sometimes forgets his commitments," should open the door for further conversation. It might uncover a mother who is worried about her son's drinking and perhaps about the way he treats her when he has been drinking. Attempts should be made to compare the history given by the patient with that given by the family. Inconsistencies need to be explored further. Likewise, it is helpful to ask caretakers if they were able to give the care they felt was needed. Indications that the patient was "getting to be a handful" may be a clue to mismanaged care or a caretaker in need of support and assistance. In either situation, the nurse can provide information and support and refer the patient and caregiver to a social worker or mental health nurse for further assistance. In addition, health care workers, including nurses, should know their responsibility under state law for reporting abuse of the older patient.

Alcohol Abuse

Alcohol abuse occurs in the aging population, although there is little documentation about its prevalence. Problem drinking in older adults occurs for similar reasons as during the early to middle adult years. However, smaller amounts of alcohol create larger problems for the older person, and they may be more susceptible to alcohol-induced pathology. Differences in metabolism of alcohol in the older person, the smaller volume of body water, and the decrease in lean body tissue may increase the propensity to alcoholism or alcohol problems. In addition, older adults are high consumers of psychotropic drugs and are at risk for drug–alcohol interactions.

Nursing interventions include screening the older adult for alcohol use. The HEAT screening method,[14] shown here, is useful for screening purposes. A positive response on any item is a reason to obtain a more detailed history of alcohol use. When alcohol abuse is suspected, the immediate goal is to stabilize physiological and psychological responses to alcohol withdrawal and determine its impact on whatever other diagnoses have resulted in the need for critical care. As soon as possible, the nurse should refer the patient to a social worker, psychiatric liaison nurse, or alcohol counselor.

■ CHALLENGES IN MEDICATION USE

The rule for giving therapeutic medications to the older patient is *start low, go slow, and be patient*. Changes related to aging can have a great impact on drug response. Changes in renal function, gastrointestinal secretions and mobility, and cell receptor sites and concurrent disease states can alter the absorption, distribution, and excretion of drugs. These changes are summarized in Table 12–9.

Before admission to the ICU, older patients may have been taking many different medications, including over-the-counter (OTC) medications, such as vitamins, tonics, laxatives, antacids, and pain relievers. They may also have a history of heavy alcohol intake. Any of these drugs can cause problems if combined with medications administered in the hospital.

The nurse needs to elicit a careful history of drug use from the patient and family. The family can be asked to bring in all medications the patient has been using; this includes OTC medications. Although alcohol use may be a sensitive topic, establishing the pattern of use can be essential in preventing untoward drug interactions and anticipating problems with liver damage or withdrawal.

Special considerations concerning administration of drugs to the older patient include knowing the drugs the patient has been taking; assessing renal, hepatic, endocrine, and digestive systems; and evaluating lean body mass. Im-

TABLE 12-9
Age Changes That Impact Pharmacotherapy

Pharmacokinetics	Age Change
Absorption	Increased gastrointestinal (GI) pH
	Decreased GI motility
	Changes in GI villi
Distribution	Decreased total body fluid
	Increased body fat
	Decreased lean muscle mass
	Decreased albumin
Metabolism	Decreased liver and kidney blood flow
	Decreased glomerular filtration
Excretion	Decreased renal blood flow
Altered drug effects	Increased or decreased receptor sensitivity
	Decreased cellular viability
	Decreased homeostatic mechanisms

pairment within body systems may affect the absorption, metabolism, and excretion of drugs. A decrease in lean body mass and an increase in total body fat may alter the distribution of the drug within the body.

Drug Absorption

Drug absorption is affected by the following age-related changes: decreased gastric acid, decreased gastrointestinal motility, decreased gastric blood flow, changes in gastrointestinal villi, and decreased blood flow and body temperature in the rectum. The increased pH of gastric secretions and delayed stomach emptying time can alter the degrada-

---

The HEAT Screening Method for Indications of Alcohol Abuse

How do you use alcohol?
Have you **e**ver thought you used alcohol to **e**xcess?
Has **a**nyone else ever thought you used too much?
Have you ever had any **t**rouble resulting from your use?

❀ *Considerations for the Older Patient*
Medication Use

- Drug dosage guidelines are usually based on studies in younger people, and recommended adult dosage guidelines may not be appropriate for older patients.
- Older people may be taking numerous prescription drugs and may self-medicate with borrowed, old, and over-the-counter drugs.
- The effects of alcohol use must be considered.
- The potential for drug interactions and adverse reactions is increased because of the effects of aging on drug absorption, distribution, metabolism, and excretion.
- Drug toxicities are different than they are in younger people. Fewer symptoms may be identified, and they may develop slower but be more pronounced once they occur.
- Behavioral side effects are more common in older people because the blood–brain barrier becomes less effective. When there is an acute change in mental status, medication should always be considered as the cause.

tion, and thus the absorption, of drugs. Drugs that are not stable in an acid medium can be severely reduced in bioavailability if they remain in the stomach for long periods. Drugs that are designed to be acted on in the small intestine may be affected by the higher pH of the aging stomach. A coated, pH-sensitive medication, such as erythromycin, may lose its coating in the stomach and be degraded before reaching the absorption sites in the small intestine. Coated gastric irritants may lose their coatings and cause bleeding or nausea and vomiting.

Drug Distribution

Distribution of drugs in the body can be affected by a decrease in lean body mass, an increase in total body fat, or a decrease in total body fluid, all of which may accompany aging. Drugs that bind to muscle (eg, digoxin) become more bioavailable as lean body mass diminishes, increasing the risk of toxicity. Fat-soluble drugs (eg, flurazepam [Dalmane], chlorpromazine [Thorazine], phenobarbital) can be deposited in fat and result in cumulative effects of oversedation. In the presence of a volume deficit, drugs that are water soluble (eg, gentamicin [Garamycin]) may have a higher concentration and may reach toxic levels rapidly.

Drug Metabolism

The liver is the major organ for biotransformation and detoxification of medications. In the older patient, there may be some decrease in the metabolism of drugs requiring hepatic enzymes for transformation. This results in an increased plasma level and prolonged half-life of the drug. The benzodiazepines (eg, Valium, Dalmane) may have a half-life increase from 20 to 90 hours in the older patient. Hepatic oxidation of these drugs can further be affected by alcohol-induced changes in the liver. There may be a decrease in drug metabolism with occasional alcohol use. However, in chronic alcohol use, drug metabolism is increased, and excretion is accelerated.

Drug Excretion

The kidney is the primary excretory organ for clearing drugs. Drugs that are excreted unchanged (eg, digoxin, cimetidine, antibiotics) may have a decreased renal clearance. Given the decreased renal function of the older adult, the dosage of these drugs may need to be reduced. Serum creatinine alone is not a good determinant of renal function in older people. A creatinine clearance study reflects a more accurate estimation for drug clearance.

▆▆▆ CONCLUSION

Older adults are being seen more frequently in the ICU. This necessitates critical care nurses' familiarity with normal and abnormal changes in the older patient. Some of these

---

Insights into Clinical Research

Doucet J, Chassagne P, Trivalle C, Landrin I, Kadri PN, Bercoff E: Drug-drug interactions related to hospital admissions in older adults: A prospective study of 1000 patients. Journal of the American Geriatrics Society 44:944–948, 1996

This study investigated the frequency, nature, and side effects of drug–drug interactions (DDI) in a group of older adults in an acute care facility. The focus of the study was on drugs administered at home in the 2 weeks prior to hospitalization. One thousand inpatients older than 70 years (83 ± 7.1 years) were included in the study. All possible two-by-two combinations of drugs administered at home were considered to determine whether drug interactions were actually occurring.

A total of 538 patients were exposed to 1,087 DDIs. The most common interactions were between cardiovascular and psychotropic medications. There were 189 side effects observed in 130 patients. The most frequent side effects were neuropsychological impairment, arterial hypotension, and acute renal failure. The number of side effects did not differ between the 66 contraindicated drug associations and the 1,021 associations that only required precautionary use. DDIs often result in side effects for older adults. The frequency of these side effects can be reduced by limiting the prescription of the most frequent and dangerous DDIs.

---

changes are subtle; therefore, older patients require more intense observation than other patients in the ICU.

Changes in the older adult involve not only body systems, but also psychosocial issues. Psychosocial factors include cognitive changes, abuse, alcoholism, and medication use. Careful assessment and knowledgeable interventions will help in the care of the older patient in the ICU.

Clinical Applicability Challenges

Self-Challenge

1. *Ms. Lopez, an 82-year-old patient, has been admitted to your ICU with an acute myocardial infarction. She has a hearing deficit and wears glasses. Describe nursing actions you would perform to promote optimal use of her senses.*

2. *Investigate the laws in your state regarding the abuse of the older person. Analyze the adequacy of the laws that exist, and suggest laws that should be changed.*

Study Questions

1. *Physical changes that occur as a result of the normal aging process include which of the following?*
   a. *Reduced sensory and perceptual activity*
   b. *Tolerance of extremes of heat and cold*
   c. *Decreased amounts of connective and collagen tissue*
   d. *Increased excretion of hormones*

2. *Major concerns in administration of drugs to older patients include all of the following except*
   a. *status of renal function.*
   b. *assessment of hydration.*
   c. *assessment of muscle strength.*
   d. *medications taken before admission.*

3. *Frequent turning and early ambulation are essential with the older patient for all of the following reasons except*
   a. *to slow bone loss.*
   b. *to maximize loss of strength.*
   c. *to prevent respiratory complications.*
   d. *to prevent skin breakdown.*

4. *Types of abuse of older people are*
   a. *physical, social, biological.*
   b. *social, psychological, biological.*
   c. *material, emotional, social.*
   d. *physical, psychological, material.*

5. *Visual pathologies of aging include*
   a. *glaucoma, diabetic retinopathy, cataracts, retinal degeneration.*
   b. *diabetic retinopathy, cataracts, presbyopia, stria vascularis.*
   c. *cataracts, glaucoma, arcus senilis, retinal degeneration.*
   d. *presbyopia, stria vascularis, diabetic retinopathy, arcus senilis, retinal degenerations.*

6. *Age-related factors that can put older people at greater risk for alcohol-related problems are all of the following except*
   a. *a smaller volume of body water.*
   b. *poor dentition.*
   c. *decreased lean body tissue.*
   d. *alcohol–drug reactions.*

REFERENCES

1. Lamy P: Introduction to the aging process. In Delafuente JC, Stewart RB (eds): Therapeutics in the Elderly, p 8. Cincinnati, Harvey Whitney Books, 1995
2. Weinstein B: Age related hearing loss: How to screen for it and when to intervene. Geriatrics 49(8):40–46, 1994
3. Maguire G: The changing realm of the senses. In Lewis CB (ed): Aging the Health Care Challenge, pp 137–142. Philadelphia, FA Davis, 1996
4. Hays CJ, Blazer DG, Foley DJ: Risk of napping: Excessive daytime sleepiness and mortality in an older community population. J Am Geriatr Soc 44:693–698, 1996
5. Stimmel GL, Guthierrez MA: Psychiatric disorders. In Delafuente JC, Stewart RB (eds): Therapeutics in the Elderly, p 337. Cincinnati, Harvey Whitney Books, 1995
6. Caranasos GJ: Medical approach to the elderly. In Delafuente JC, Stewart RB (eds): Therapeutics in the Elderly, pp 129–130. Cincinnati, Harvey Whitney Books, 1995
7. Lavker R: Cutaneous aging: Chronologic versus photoaging. In Gilchrest B (ed): Photodamage. Boston, Blackwell Sciences, 1995
8. Lipsitz LA, Byrnes N, Hossain M, Douglas P, Waksmonski CA: Restrictive left ventricular filling patterns in very old patients with congestive heart failure: Clinical correlates and prognostic significance. J Am Geriatr Soc 44(6):634–638, 1996
9. Diabetes in American (2nd Ed). National Institutes of Health NIH Publication No. 95-1468, 1995
10. Folstein M, Folstein S, McHugh P: Mini-mental state: A practical method for grading the cognitive state of patients for the clinician. J Psychiatr Res 12:189–198, 1975
11. Yesavage JA, Brink TL, Rose TL, Lum O, Huang V, Adey M, et al: Development and validation of a Geriatric Screening Scale: A preliminary report. J Psychiatr Res 17(1):37–49, 1983
12. Haight BK: Suicide risk in frail elderly people relocated to nursing homes. Geriatr Nurs 16(3):104–107, 1995
13. Rosenblatt DE, Kyung-Hwan C, Durance P: Reporting mistreatment of older adults: The role of physician. J Am Geriatr Soc 44(1):65–70, 1996
14. Rathbone-McCuan E: Promoting help-seeking behavior among elders with chemical dependencies. Generations 12(4):37, 1988

BIBLIOGRAPHY

All AC: A literature review: Assessment and intervention in elder abuse. Journal of Gerontological Nursing 20(7):25–33, 1994

Boykin A, Winland-Brown J: The dark side of caring: Challenges of caregiving. Journal of Gerontological Nursing 21(5):13–19, 1995

Corey-Bloom J, Wiederholt WC, Edlestein S, Salmon DP, Cahn D, Barrett-Connor E: Cognitive and functional status of the oldest old. J Am Geriatr Soc 44(6):671–675, 1996

Delafuente JC, Stewart RB: Therapeutics in the Elderly. Cincinnati, Harvey Whitney Books, 1995

Daniels J: Addiction and aging. Advance for Nurse Practitioners 8:45–49, 1996

Dipiro JT, Talbert RL, Yee GC, Matzke GR, Wells BG, Posey LM: Pharmacotherapy: A Pathophysiologic Approach. Stamford, Appleton & Lange, 1996

Dracup K: Heart failure secondary to left ventricular systolic dysfunction. Therapeutic advances and treatment recommendations. The Nurse Pract 21(9):56–71, 1996

French D: Avoiding adverse drug reactions in the elderly patient: Issues and strategies. Nurse Pract 21(9):90–108, 1996

Frost MH, Willette K: Risk for abuse/neglect: Documentation of assessment data and diagnoses. Journal of Gerontological Nursing 20(8):37–45, 1994

Kavanaugh KM, Tate B: Recognizing and helping older persons with vision impairments. Geriatr Nurs 17(2):68–72, 1996

Lewis CB: Aging the Health Care Challenge. Philadelphia, FA Davis, 1996

Mentes JC: A nursing protocol to assess causes of delirium. Journal of Gerontological Nursing 21(2):26–31, 1995

Mudd SA, Boyd CJ, Brower KJ, Young JP, Blow FC: Alcohol withdrawal: Related nursing care in older adults. Journal of Gerontological Nursing 20(10):17–27, 1994

Planchock NY, Slay LE: Pharmacokinetic and pharmacodynamic monitoring of the elderly in critical care. Critical Care Clinics of North America 8(1):79–90, 1996

Richards KC: Sleep promotion. Critical Care Nursing Clinics of North America 8(1):39–52, 1996

Shannon ML, Lehman CA: Protecting the skin of elderly patient in the intensive care unit. Critical Care Nursing Clinics of North America 8(1):17–28, 1996

St. Pierre J. Delirium in hospitalized elderly patients: Off track. Critical Care Nursing Clinics of North America 8(1):53–60, 1996

13

The Postanesthesia Patient

OBJECTIVES

Based on the content in this chapter, the reader should be able to:

- Compare and contrast anesthetic options used for surgery.
- Differentiate between anesthetic agents appropriate for the conscious patient and those appropriate for the unconscious patient.
- Summarize five potential problems encountered during the immediate postanesthetic period.
- Describe nursing interventions for the patient recovering from anesthesia.

*T*he time immediately after surgery, when the patient is taken to the postanesthesia care unit (PACU) or the intensive care unit (ICU), is the most crucial period in the patient's recovery from anesthesia. Most patients are taken to the PACU for close observation and care by a qualified PACU nurse. Others are taken directly to the ICU, where nurses must be competent in postanesthesia nursing care.

It is important that the anesthesiologist and nurse collaborate in immediate postoperative care. This collabora-

tion is discussed at the beginning of the chapter. Major problems may occur in the immediate postoperative period. Their causes and interventions are the focus of this chapter. The critical care nurse must have a basic understanding of anesthetic options available for use during the intraoperative phase. A Collaborative Care Guide for the patient recovering from anesthesia is included also.

COLLABORATION BETWEEN THE ANESTHESIOLOGIST AND NURSE

The anesthesiologist examines the patient before surgery. From this examination, the anesthesiologist decides which option and technique to use. Decisions are based on the patient's condition, age, previous surgical and anesthetic experiences, ongoing disease processes, operation to be performed, the surgeon's experience, and the position required for the surgical procedure. The anesthesiologist's options range from maintaining a conscious state with the use of minimal, regional, or intravenous agents to induc-

Conscious Sedation

During this state of anesthesia, the patient remains conscious with some alteration of mood, drowsiness, and sometimes analgesia. The patient's protective reflexes remain intact.

Deep Sedation

The patient is asleep with this anesthetic technique but is easily aroused. The patient's protective reflexes are minimally depressed.

General Anesthesia

With this type of anesthesia, the patient has a complete loss of consciousness and is unarousable. It is a reversible state that provides analgesia, muscle relaxation, and sedation. The patient's protective reflexes are partially or more commonly completely lost.

Regional Anesthesia

This state of anesthesia produces analgesia in a specific body part. Regional anesthesia is achieved by placing local anesthetics in close proximity to appropriate nerves to achieve a conduction block.

Spinal Anesthesia

In this type of anesthesia, local anesthetic is injected into lumbar intrathecal space. The anesthetic blocks conduction in spinal nerve roots and dorsal ganglia. Analgesia occurs below the level of injection.

Epidural Anesthesia

With this anesthesia, a local anesthetic is injected into extradural spaces through a lumbar puncture. The effects are similar to spinal analgesia.

Peripheral Nerve Blocks

With this type of anesthesia, a local anesthetic is injected at a specific site to achieve a defined area of anesthesia.

ing an unconscious state with the use of intravenous or inhalation agents. These options are illustrated in Figures 13–1 and 13–2.

What happens in the operating room may affect the patient's immediate postoperative care and the overall recovery. To convey what has occurred in the operating suite, the anesthesiologist gives a detailed and complete report to the nurse who is assuming postoperative care of the anesthetized patient. Information given in the report is listed in the display on page 141.

While receiving report from the anesthesiologist, the nurse simultaneously must assess the patient's condition and individualize the nursing plan of care. Initial assessment parameters reported to the anesthesiologist are the patient's vital signs (blood pressure, pulse, respiration, and temperature), pulse oximetry, and level of consciousness. Cardiac monitoring, pressure readings, and urine output monitoring also may be indicated. Vital signs are monitored

every 5 minutes or more often if the patient's condition warrants. The American Society of PeriAnesthesia Nurses, as endorsed by the American Society of Anesthesiologists, recommends all assessment data be collected and documented on the patient's postoperative record.[1]

CONSCIOUS SEDATION

Conscious sedation is a type of anesthesia that provides analgesia and amnesia during which time the patient remains conscious but relaxed. The patient retains the ability to maintain a patent airway independently and continuously. The advantage of conscious sedation is that it allows the patient to respond to the verbal directives of the physician and to physical stimulation. Conscious sedation is used for certain ambulatory surgical, therapeutic, or diagnostic procedures. The regimen usually consists of an opiate, a phenothiazine, and a local anesthetic.[2] Intravenous (IV) anesthetics may be used also.

A group of 14 nursing societies developed standards for the role of the registered nurse in managing patients receiving IV conscious sedation. These standards are published in Standards of Perianesthesia Nursing Practice (1995)[3] and include management and monitoring before, during, and after the procedure. Among the standards are the following skills required of the registered nurse who is managing the care of patients receiving IV conscious sedation:

- Demonstrate the acquired knowledge of anatomy, physiology, pharmacology, cardiac arrhythmia recognition, and complications related to IV conscious sedation and medications.
- Assess total patient care requirements during conscious sedation and recovery. Physiological measurements should include, but are not limited to, respiratory rate, oxygen saturation, blood pressure, cardiac rate and rhythm, and patient's level of consciousness.
- Understand the principles of oxygen delivery, respiratory physiology, transport, and uptake, and demonstrate the ability to use oxygen delivery devices.
- Anticipate and recognize potential complications of IV conscious sedation in relation to the type of medication being administered.
- Possess the requisite knowledge and skills to assess, diagnose, and intervene in the event of complications or undesired outcomes and to institute nursing interventions in compliance with orders (including standard orders) or institutional protocols or guidelines.
- Demonstrate skills in airway management resuscitation.
- Demonstrate knowledge of the legal ramifications of administering IV conscious sedation or monitoring patients receiving IV conscious sedation, including the registered nurse's responsibility and liability in the event of an untoward reaction or life-threatening complication.

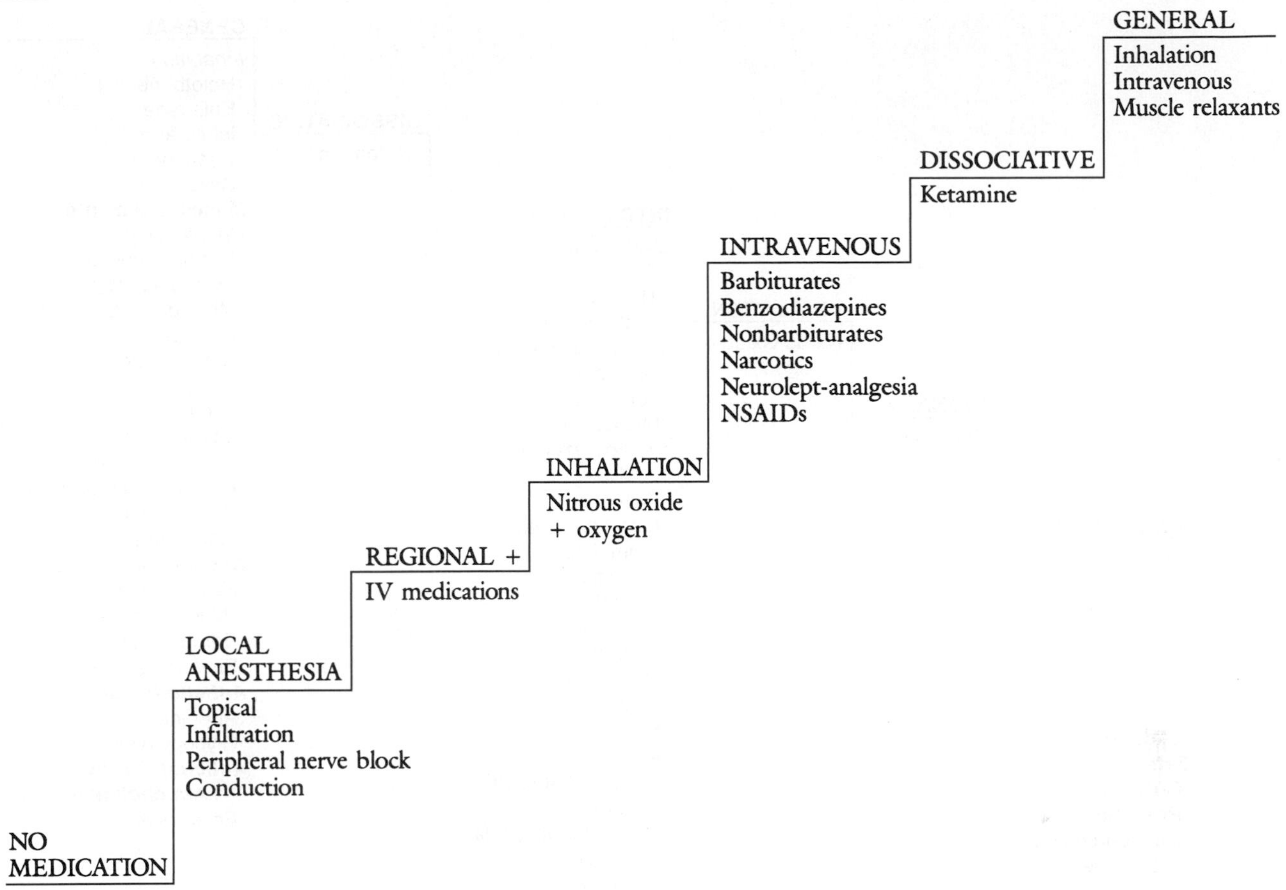

GENERAL
Inhalation
Intravenous
Muscle relaxants

DISSOCIATIVE
Ketamine

INTRAVENOUS
Barbiturates
Benzodiazepines
Nonbarbiturates
Narcotics
Neurolept-analgesia
NSAIDs

INHALATION
Nitrous oxide
+ oxygen

REGIONAL +
IV medications

LOCAL
ANESTHESIA
Topical
Infiltration
Peripheral nerve block
Conduction

NO
MEDICATION

Conscious State	Sedation State	Unconscious State
Protective reflexes are intact	Protective reflexes are minimally depressed	Protective reflexes are diminished or absent
May see alteration of mood, relief of anxiety, and some analgesia	May see patient sleeping but easily aroused	Respiration is automatic and involuntary

NSAIDs, nonsteroidal anti-inflammatory drugs; IV, intravenous.

FIGURE 13-1
Anesthetic options for surgery.

POTENTIAL PROBLEMS IN THE POSTANESTHESIA PATIENT

There are common potential problems in the postanesthesia patient for which the nurse must assess and intervene. They are discussed in the following sections.

Hypoxemia

ETIOLOGY

Hypoxemia is a common occurrence in the immediate postoperative period. Severe hypoxemia is characterized by a PaO_2 less than 50 mmHg and is life threatening. Hypoventilation leads to hypoxia, which is difficult to diagnose because of its multiple presentations. Clinical manifestations of hypoxia can include hypotension or hypertension, tachycardia or bradycardia, cardiac dysrhythmias, dyspnea, tachypnea, hypoventilation, disorientation with agitation, decreased $PaCO_2$, and cyanosis.

When investigating the etiology of hypoxemia related to anesthetic agents, the nurse should consider the effects of a prolonged block that traveled too high; narcotic use; deep sedation; use of inhalation agents, such as enflurane (Ethrane), isoflurane (Forane), halothane, and nitrous oxide; and the use of neuromuscular blockers, particularly if they have not been reversed adequately. Diffusion hypoxia may occur when nitrous oxide is used, but administering 100% oxygen for 3 to 4 minutes after the nitrous oxide is terminated can prevent this complication.

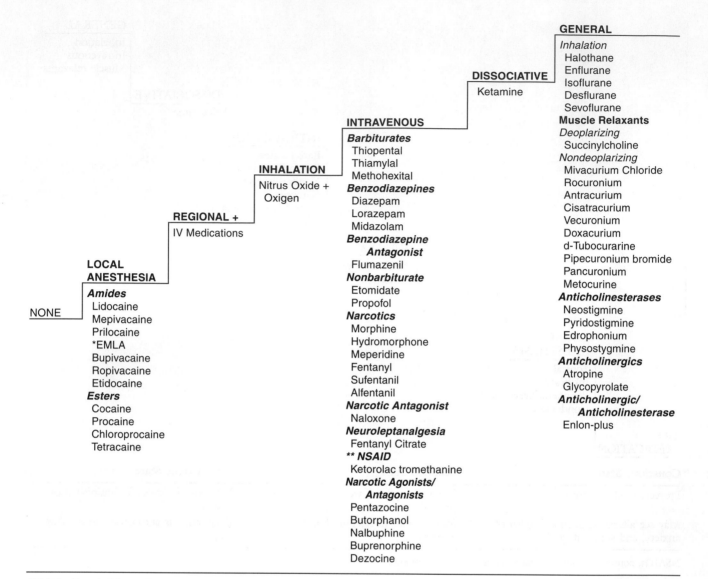

GENERAL

Inhalation
Halothane
Enflurane
Isoflurane
Desflurane
Sevoflurane
Muscle Relaxants
Deoplarizing
Succinylcholine
Nondeoplarizing
Mivacurium Chloride
Rocuronium
Antracurium
Cisatracurium
Vecuronium
Doxacurium
d-Tubocurarine
Pipecuronium bromide
Pancuronium
Metocurine
Anticholinesterases
Neostigmine
Pyridostigmine
Edrophonium
Physostygmine
Anticholinergics
Atropine
Glycopyrolate
**Anticholinergic/
    Anticholinesterase**
Enlon-plus

DISSOCIATIVE
Ketamine

INTRAVENOUS
Barbiturates
Thiopental
Thiamylal
Methohexital
Benzodiazepines
Diazepam
Lorazepam
Midazolam
**Benzodiazepine
    Antagonist**
Flumazenil
Nonbarbiturate
Etomidate
Propofol
Narcotics
Morphine
Hydromorphone
Meperidine
Fentanyl
Sufentanil
Alfentanil
Narcotic Antagonist
Naloxone
Neuroleptanalgesia
Fentanyl Citrate
** NSAID
Ketorolac tromethanine
**Narcotic Agonists/
    Antagonists**
Pentazocine
Butorphanol
Nalbuphine
Buprenorphine
Dezocine

INHALATION
Nitrus Oxide +
Oxigen

REGIONAL +
IV Medications

**LOCAL
ANESTHESIA**
Amides
Lidocaine
Mepivacaine
Prilocaine
*EMLA
Bupivacaine
Ropivacaine
Etidocaine
Esters
Cocaine
Procaine
Chloroprocaine
Tetracaine

NONE

*EMLA - Eutetic Mixture local Anesthetics
** NSAID - Nonsteroidal Anti-inflammatory Drugs

FIGURE 13-2
Medication choices for anesthetic options.

NURSING ASSESSMENT AND INTERVENTIONS

All patients who received a general anesthetic or sedation should be given supplemental oxygen in the immediate postoperative period. The oxygen can be weaned subsequently using pulse oximetry readings. Because pulse oximetry offers a noninvasive method of continuously monitoring oxygen saturation, increasing numbers of patients are receiving supplemental oxygen for 24 hours after surgery.

In addition to being aware of hypoxia, the nurse should use a "stir-up" regimen for every patient in the postoperative period. This regimen involves encouraging the patient to deep breathe, cough, and move in bed. An integral part of recovery from anesthesia, this routine should be included every time vital signs are checked.

Reversal agents may be required while the patient is still under the effects of muscle relaxants, benzodiazepines, and narcotics. Close monitoring always is indicated when reversal agents are administered. The effects of muscle relaxants, benzodiazepines, and narcotics may last longer than the reversal medication, resulting in hypoventilation and hypoxia at some point after the reversal medication is given. Knowledge of the onset and duration of action of reversal agents is important for the nurse.

Hypoventilation

ETIOLOGY

Hypoventilation leading to hypercarbia may result from the following:

- Inadequate respiratory drive secondary to the effects of residual anesthesia (ie, narcotics and inhalation agents)

Anesthesiologist-to-Nurse Report: Information to Convey

Name of patient
Surgical procedure
Anesthetic options (agents and reversal agents used)
Estimated blood loss/fluid loss
Fluid/blood replacement
Vital signs—significant problems
Complications encountered (anesthetic or surgical)
Preoperative condition (eg, diabetes, hypertension, allergies)
Considerations for immediate postoperative period (pain management, reversals, vent settings)
Language barrier

Ideally, the anesthesiologist should not leave the patient until the nurse is satisfied with the patient's airway and immediate condition.

CLINICAL APPLICATION: Drug Therapy
Neuromuscular Blocking Agents

Muscle Relaxants

- Neuromuscular blockers pharmacologically paralyze patients and provide no sedation or analgesia.
- Neuromuscular agents are used to facilitate endotracheal intubation, relax muscles for surgical procedures, terminate laryngospasm, eliminate chest wall rigidity, and provide mechanical ventilation if indicated.
- There are two groups of muscle relaxants: depolarizing and nondepolarizing neuroblockers that work at the myoneural junction, affecting the chemical transmitter, acetylcholine.[4,5]

Depolarizing Agents (Sucostrin, Anectine)

- These drugs combine with acetylcholine receptors at the myoneural junction and mimic the action of acetylcholine.
- Onset of action is 1–2 minutes and duration of action is 4–6 minutes.
- The enzyme pseudocholinesterase removes succinylcholine from plasma, so in conditions involving a decrease in pseudocholinesterase, the length of action of succinylcholine increases, keeping patients paralyzed for longer periods.
- Increased pseudocholinesterase enzyme may be seen in pregnancy, liver disease, malnutrition states, severe anemia, cancer, and with other pharmacological agents, such as quinidine, phospholine eye drops, and propranolol.

Nondepolarizing Agents

- Nondepolarizing agents (atacurium, mivacurium chloride, pipecuronium bromide, vecuronium, *d*-tubocurarine, metocurine, pancuronium, doxacurium, cisatracurium, rocuronium) compete with acetylcholine at the myoneural junction for muscle membrane receptors.
- Onset of action is within 2–3 minutes.
- Duration of action ranges from 20 minutes to 2 hours, depending on the medication and dosage.
- May be reversed pharmacologically with anticholinesterase drugs (neostigmine, pyridostigmine, edrophonium). Duration of action of anticholinesterase is brief, so there is a chance the patient may have continued muscle weakness or respiratory depression. Anticholinesterases may induce muscarinic side effects, including bradycardia, increased salivary and bronchial secretions. These side effects are counteracted with the routine administration of anticholinergic drugs (atropine, glycopyrrolate) in conjunction with the anticholinesterase.

- Inadequate functioning of the respiratory muscles (The lungs may be unable to move an adequate tidal volume because of pain or inadequate reversal of neuromuscular blockade.)
- Intrinsic lung disease, which often requires postoperative ventilatory support of the patient (eg, chronic obstructive pulmonary disease)

NURSING ASSESSMENT AND INTERVENTIONS

The nurse institutes the stir-up regimen in the immediate postoperative phase to stimulate the patient, especially if narcotics and muscle relaxants were used during surgery. Neuromuscular blocking agents are summarized in the accompanying display. Also, the nurse considers the length of time since reversal agents were administered to antagonize neuromuscular blockade. The patient may reparalyze because the effects of the reversal agent were shorter acting than the effects of the original muscle relaxant. Information about various muscle relaxants, their onset and duration, and other comparisons are given in Table 13–1.

Because hypothermia prolongs nondepolarizing blocks, the patient's temperature must be monitored. Other conditions that might potentiate the effect of neuromuscular blocking agents are considered. Such conditions are listed in the display on page 143.

Hypotension

ETIOLOGY

Probably the most common cardiovascular complication seen in the postoperative period is hypotension. It is caused most often by a decreased circulating blood volume.[5] Hypotension refers to a 25% to 30% decrease in systolic blood pressure from resting baseline values. Intervention is indicated if the pressure falls more than 30%. Common causes of hypotension are listed in the display on page 143.

Anesthetic agents can affect the blood pressure in various ways. Regional anesthetics, such as lidocaine and procaine, may decrease blood pressure by sympathetic blockade, vasodilation, and myocardial depression. IV agents, including narcotics, cause vasodilation and histamine release, resulting in lowered blood pressure. Tranquilizers, especially droperidol and chlorpromazine hydrochloride, produce sympathetic blockade and subsequent decreased blood pressure. Barbiturates cause myocardial depression, as do inhalation agents, such as isoflurane, enflurane, halothane,

TABLE 13-1 CLINICAL APPLICATION: Drug Therapy
Muscle Relaxant Comparisons

Drug	Onset	Duration	Dose	Metabolism Elimination	Histamine	Side Effects	Advantages
Depolarizing							
Succinylcholine	1–2 min	4–6 min	1 mg/kg	Plasmacholinesterase Renal, biliary	Possible	↓Pulse Fasciculations Cardiac dysrhythmia Hyperkalemia ↑ICP ↑IOP	Short acting
Nondepolarizing							
Mivacurium chloride (Mivacron)	2–2.5 min	10–15 min	0.1–0.25 mg/kg	Plasmacholinesterase Renal, biliary	Yes	Flushing Hypotension Dysrhythmia Rash, muscle spasm Bronchospasm	Short acting Minimal CV side effects
Atracurium (Tracrium)	Within 2 min	30–45 min	0.4–0.5 mg/kg	Hoffman elimination Ester hydrolysis	Mild		Intermediate acting No CV effect Easily reversed Block not prolonged
Vecuronium (Norcuron)	Within 3 min	30–45 min	0.06–0.1 mg/kg	Hepatic, renal	Very mild to none		Intermediate acting Little or no CV effect Easily reversed
Rocuronium (Zemuron)	1–1.5 min	20–40 min	0.5–1.2 mg/kg	Renal, biliary	Low		Intermediate acting Minimal CV effects
Cisatracurium (Nimbex)	2–3 min	40–60 min	0.15–0.2 mg/kg	Hoffman elimination Renal and hepatic	None	↑PVR	Intermediate acting Hemodynamic stability Excellent for intubating
d-Tubocurarine (Curare)	Within 3 min	45–60 min	Up to 0.6 mg/kg	Renal, hepatic	Yes	Hypotension Histamine-like reaction	Long acting
Metocurine	Within 4 min	>60 min	0.2 mg/kg	Renal and hepatic	Yes	Hypotension Tachycardia	Long acting Useful in CV disease Useful in hypertension
Pancuronium	Within 4 min	1–1½h	0.04–0.1 mg/kg	Renal, hepatic, biliary	Isolated cases	Avoid with: Myasthenia gravis Renal disease Hypersensitivity to bromide Coronary artery disease	Long acting
Doxacurium (Nuromax)	4–6 min	100–160 min	0.05–0.08 mg/kg	Renal	None	Potentiated by inhalation agents, particularly halothane Prolonged recovery in elderly	Long acting
Pipecuronium (Arduan)	3–5 min	60–120 min	0.14 mg/kg	Renal, biliary	None	Hypoglycemia Hyperkalemia CNS depressant Respiratory depressant	Long acting No CV effects

ICP, intracranial pressure; IOP, intraocular pressure; CV, cardiovascular; PVR, peripheral vascular resistance; CNS, central nervous system

sevoflurane, and desflurane. Muscle relaxants can cause hypotension by ganglionic blockade and histamine release.

NURSING ASSESSMENT AND INTERVENTIONS

Because decreased venous return is seen with hypovolemia and myocardial depression, the nurse should consider the adequacy of fluid and blood replacement, bleeding, third spacing, or excessive diuresis. The nurse evaluates the patient for orthostatic hypotension by taking vital signs with the patient supine and after raising the head of the bed 60 degrees (if not contraindicated by the surgical procedure). Cardiac dysrhythmias can produce hypotension, especially when cardiac output is decreased, as it is with supraventricular tachycardia and marked bradycardias. Other causes of early postoperative hypotension include sepsis, pulmonary embolism, transfusion reaction, and pain.

Deliberate, controlled hypotensive techniques are used during specific procedures, such as head, neck, or neurosurgical procedures or shoulder arthroscopy and some cancer operations. The advantage of this technique is that it minimizes blood loss and the need for transfusion, decreases oozing, and requires minimal anesthesia.

Treatment of hypotension is directed to the underlying cause. A complete report from the anesthesiologist, including the techniques used during surgery and any untoward events that occurred will help the nurse identify the underlying cause.

Various interventions may be used to treat hypotension. A priority is to ensure adequate oxygenation and ventilation of the patient. Anesthetic drugs may require reversal, including muscle relaxant reversal with anticholinesterase and anticholinergic agents, narcotic reversal with naloxone, benzodiazepine reversal with flumazenil, or vasopressor drugs to increase blood pressure. IV fluids, including blood, plasma expanders, and crystalloids, should be administered as ordered and dressings and surgical sites inspected frequently for hemorrhage. Elevation of the legs or the Trendelenburg position may be indicated to increase blood pressure.

An important consideration when assessing and treating hypotension is the possibility of technical rather than phys-

Risk Factors for Hypotension
Postanesthesia

Anesthetic Agents
Regional agents
Narcotics
Tranquilizers
Barbiturates
Muscle relaxants
Inhalation agents

Decreased Venous Return
Hypovolemia
   Inadequate replacement
   Continued blood loss
Hypothermia
Myocardial depression
Third spacing
Sepsis
Transfusion reaction
Tight abdominal dressing
Increased intrathoracic pressure

Cardiac
Dysrhythmias
   Supraventricular tachycardia
Myocardial infarction
Congestive heart failure

Pulmonary
Hypoxia
Acidosis
Pulmonary embolism
Pneumothorax

Vasovagal Reactions
Bradycardia
Pain
Bladder/abdominal distention

Technical Problems
Blood pressure cuff size and position
Transducer balance and calibration
Stethoscope position

iological problems. Is the blood pressure cuff the correct size and positioned correctly? Is the stethoscope positioned correctly? Is the patient's position a factor? If an arterial line is present, is the patient peripherally constricted, or does peripheral vascular disease exist? Is the transducer balanced and correctly calibrated?

Hypertension

ETIOLOGY

Hypertension is classified according to its degree of severity, ranging from mild with a diastolic pressure between 90 and 104 mmHg to severe with a diastolic pressure above 115 mmHg to malignant with the diastolic pressure greater than 120 mmHg.

The two most common causes of postoperative hypertension are a history of hypertension, and pain. Hypertension can be associated with peripheral vasoconstriction and shivering. Inhalation and IV anesthetic agents may produce hypoxia and hypercarbia with a resultant increase in catecholamine release and blood pressure elevation. Ketamine (Ketalar), a dissociative drug used for surgery patients, stimulates the sympathetic nervous system and can cause tachycardia and hypertension. Also, if given too rapidly, naloxone may precipitate hypertension, which in turn may precipitate pulmonary edema or cerebral hemorrhage. Other causes of hypertension include hyperthermia, anxiety, urinary bladder distention, fluid overload, pain, a too-narrow blood pressure cuff, and withholding of antihypertensive therapy before surgery.

Transient hypertension may occur during induction, intubation, positioning, making the surgical incision, or on awakening from anesthesia.

NURSING ASSESSMENT AND INTERVENTIONS

The hypertensive patient requires reassurance, close observation, and aggressive postoperative treatment. The treatment is directed first to the cause, if known. Unless contraindicated, patients should be instructed to continue their hypertensive medication up to the time of the surgical procedure. The nurse must administer analgesics if the patient is in pain, starting oxygen if hypoxemia is suspected, and stimulating the patient to deep breathe if hypoventilation occurs. Changing blood pressure cuffs if the wrong size is in use and checking the function of all equipment are integral parts of the nurse's problem solving.

Antihypertensive medications may be ordered if the severity of hypertension indicates. Short-acting peripheral vasodilators, such as hydralazine and nifedipine, may be used. The adrenergic inhibitor, labetalol, also might be prescribed. Continuous vasodilator drips of sodium nitroprusside or nitroglycerin sometimes are needed to bring the blood pressure within safe limits. When hypertension accompanies emergence delirium, narcotics or physostigmine, an anticholinesterase, may be required. If the patient is hypertensive due to anxiety and verbal reassurance is ineffective, tranquilizers, such as diazepam, midazolam, or droperidol, may be indicated. Urinary catheterization and aggressive treatment with diuretics such as furosemide may be used if the hypertension is a result of fluid overloaded during surgery.

Cardiac Dysrhythmias

Discussion of dysrhythmias will be limited to those induced by anesthetic agents and complications frequently seen in the immediate postoperative period (Table 13–2). Refer to Chapter 16 for detailed information on identifying and treating specific cardiac dysrhythmias. There are many causes of cardiac dysrhythmias in the immediate postoperative period. Some of the most common are anesthetic agents, reversal anticholinesterase drugs, hypoxemia, hypoventilation, hypovolemia, fluid overload, hyperthermia, hypothermia, and pain as listed in the display on page 146.

Hypothermia

Hypothermia is present when the body temperature is less than 35°C (95°F). Heat loss during surgery occurs secondary to reduced basal metabolism and the vasodilation caused by inhalation anesthetic agents; vasodilation related to sympathetic blockade with inhibition of motor and sensory nerve fibers when spinal and regional techniques are used; and the inability of the patient to shiver when muscle relaxants are given. Other intraoperative causes include prolonged exposure of body surface, lying under saturated drapes (especially in long procedures), use of antiseptic prepping solutions, use of cold irrigation or IV solutions, and the temperature of the operating suite. As a result, heat is lost through radiation, exposure, convection, and conduction. Older, debilitated patients and newborns are more intolerant of temperature changes and thus more prone to hypothermia. Hats help keep warmth in the body. Warning devices may be used preoperatively, during surgery, and postoperatively.

Hypothermia, with its associated vasoconstriction and initial increase in blood pressure, requires special attention in the postoperative phase. Care must be taken in rewarming because too rapid rewarming of the patient can result in an acute drop in blood pressure and other significant problems. Clinical research regarding rewarming is discussed in the display on page 146.

Hyperthermia

Hyperthermia is a body temperature greater than 39°C (102.2°F). Elevated temperature can occur in the anesthetized patient secondary to thermal insulation from the operating drapes and to the administration of inhalation anesthetics and anticholinergic drugs that can induce a pharmacological loss of thermoregulatory capacity. Most patients with an elevated temperature either arrive in the surgical suite with fever or have a pyrogenic response from septicemia. Other causes of postoperative hyperthermia might include allergic reactions to blood or drugs, central nervous system disorders, or infection.

Malignant Hyperthermia

ETIOLOGY

One of the most catastrophic events that can occur in the immediate postoperative period is malignant hyperthermia. Malignant hyperthermia is a hypermetabolic syndrome that may be triggered by depolarizing neuromuscular blockers, halogenated inhalation agents, and postoperative pain.

This syndrome is a rare, inherited disorder of skeletal muscle and is more prevalent in those with muscular abnormalities, such as ptosis, strabismus, and kyphoscoliosis. Clinical manifestations include an increase in temperature

TABLE 13-2   CLINICAL APPLICATION: Drug Therapy
Cardiac Dysrhythmias Associated With Anesthetic Options

Anesthetic Option	Dysrhythmia
Local anesthesia with epinephrine	Tachycardia
Spinal and epidural	Bradycardia 2° vagal response; PACs, PVCs, supraventricular tachycardia, atrial fibrillation 2° sympathetic stimulation; wandering pacemaker and heart block 2° increased vagal tone
Barbiturates	
Pentothal	Bradycardia, AV dissociation, occasional PVC
Nonbarbiturate etomidate	Sinus tachycardia
Narcotics	
Morphine sulfate	Transient brachycardia
Meperidine hydrochloride	Transient tachycardia
Fentanyl	Bradycardia
Narcotic antagonist	PVCs, ventricular tachycardia, occasional ventricular fibrillation
Neuroleptanalgesia (droperidol component)	Tachycardia
Dissociative agent	Myocardial depression, ventricular ectopy, tachycardia
Inhalation agents	
Halothane	AV dissociation, ventricular dysrhythmias if hypercarbia occurs
Halothane plus aminophylline, cocaine, lidocaine	Bradycardia
Halothane plus pancuronium	PACs and PVCs
Isoflurane	Tachycardia
Enflurane	AV dissociation
Muscle relaxants	
Succinylcholine	Sinus bradycardia, junctional rhythms, PVCs Patients with burns, trauma, paraplegia or quadriplegia prone to ST depression, peaked T waves, widening QRS leading to ventricular tachycardia, ventricular fibrillation, or asystole
Pipecuronium bromide	Atrial fibrillation, ventricular extrasystole
Pancuronium	Tachycardia and nodal rhythms
d-Tubocurarine	Tachycardia
Anticholinesterases	Bradycardia, slowed AV conduction, PVC
Anticholinergics	Tachycardia

PAC, premature atrial contraction; PVC, premature ventricular contraction; AV, atrioventricular.

of 0.5°C or more since the induction of anesthesia, muscle rigidity, unexplained tachycardia, sweating, unstable blood pressure, and very hot skin. Masseter muscle rigidity after the administration of succinylcholine is the earliest warning sign of malignant hyperthermia.[6] If the patient's temperature rises rapidly and the anesthetic is not discontinued, death may occur.

NURSING ASSESSMENT AND INTERVENTIONS

Malignant hyperthermia is treated vigorously with dantrolene sodium, 100% oxygen administration, and correction of acid–base imbalances. Cooling measures, such as icing down the patient and cold fluids, are used. Most institutions that administer anesthesia have a malignant hyperthermia kit that is readily available in the operating suite. The display on page 10 lists the contents of a hyperthermia kit.

Following the acute phase of the malignant hyperthermia crisis, care includes observing in the ICU for at least 24 hours and administering dantrolene 1 mg/kg every 6 hours for 24 to 48 hours. Oral dantrolene may then be used with monitoring of arterial blood gases, creatinine kinase, potassium, calcium, urine, serum myoglobin, and clotting studies every 6 hours. Patients should be referred to the Malignant Hyperthermia Association United States for support and continued education about this entity.

RED FLAG **Risk Factors** That Precipitate Dysrhythmias

Hypoxemia
Sinus bradycardia, sinus tachycardia, PVCs, supraventricular tachycardia

Hypoventilation/Hypercarbia
Sinus tachycardia, PVCs, sinus bradycardia

Hypovolemia
Sinus tachycardia

Fluid overload
PVCs, supraventricular tachycardia, PACs, atrial fibrillation/flutter

Hyperthermia
Sinus tachycardia, PVCs

Hypothermia
Sinus bradycardia, atrial fibrillation, atrioventricular nodal blocks

Pain
Sinus tachycardia, PVCs

PVCs, premature ventricular contractions; PACs, premature atrial contractions.

Nausea and Vomiting

ETIOLOGY

Nausea and vomiting occur frequently in the immediate postoperative period and can be the result of any of the anesthetic options. Other frequent causes include use of preoperative and intraoperative narcotics; increased gastric secretions; anesthesia techniques, particularly spinal anesthesia; and surgical procedures involving manipulation of eye muscles, abdominal muscles, and genitourinary muscles.

NURSING ASSESSMENT AND INTERVENTIONS

The critical care nurse must be cognizant of the potential for regurgitation or aspiration in all patients who have been anesthetized. Vomiting is an active process, whereas regurgitation is a passive one. *Adequate positioning of the unconscious patient is essential*, and the ideal position is on the side with the head and neck extended. If the surgical procedure precludes turning the patient on the side, then the patient must not be left unattended until consciousness is regained.

Antiemetics frequently are ordered in the immediate postoperative period. The critical care nurse should recognize that many antiemetics potentiate the effect of other medications, particularly narcotics. Therefore, decreased doses of narcotic for pain relief may be indicated.

Often, nausea and vomiting can be relieved by identifying the causative factor (gastric distention, hypotension,

---

Insights Into Clinical Research

Krenzischek DA, Frank S, Kelly S: Forced-air warming versus routine thermal care and core temperature measurement sites. Journal of Post Anesthesia Nursing *10(2): 69–78, 1995*

A prospective randomized study was performed at Johns Hopkins Medical Institutions to address whether forced-air warming maintains core temperature better than conventional methods; whether forced-air warming reduces the incidence of postoperative shivering; whether temperature measured in the urinary bladder, oral cavity, and rectum compare with core temperatures measured at the tympanic membrane site; and whether swabbing the oral cavity increases accuracy of temperatures measured orally.

Forced air warming was shown to be more efficacious in maintaining normothermia during the perioperative period as compared with conventional methods, such as warmed cotton blankets. Forced-air warming resulted in a reduced incidence of shivering. The study showed significant differences in temperatures measured at the tympanic, oral, rectal, and urinary bladder sites. Assuming the tympanic temperature is the "gold standard" site for core temperature monitoring because of the proximity of the tympanic membrane to the internal carotid artery, oral temperatures are generally lower, and bladder and rectal temperatures are higher than the tympanic temperature. Swabbing the patient's mouth did not appear to affect oral measurements and therefore was not proven useful in this clinical trial. The concern expressed was that patient discharges from the postanesthesia care unit may be delayed if an adequate temperature is not obtained, which may increase patient or hospital costs.

---

administration of narcotics) and making the appropriate intervention.

POSTOPERATIVE PAIN

Severity of Pain

Patients normally expect to feel pain when their surgical procedure is over. The incidence of pain and its severity depend on the person. All pain assessment in the immediate

---

Contents of Malignant Hyperthermia Kit

Arterial blood gas sets	Methylprednisolone
Blood specimen tubes	Procainamide
Furosemide	Sodium bicarbonate
Dextrose (50%)	Sterile water
Insulin	Nasogastric tubes
Mannitol	Foley catheter tray
	Refrigerated intravenous fluids

postoperative period must be individualized. A number of factors will affect the severity of pain, including the site of the operation, the psychological state of the patient, and the anesthetic technique used.

If the anesthetic option chosen was use of inhalation agents without the use of narcotics or local agents, the patient may have more pain than one who received some form of analgesia during surgery. Patients who have been given analgesic medication during the procedure and who then receive naloxone at the end also may experience severe pain because naloxone will reverse the analgesic effects of any prior medication. Because these patients may renarcotize, the nurse must wait 15 to 45 minutes after the naloxone was given before medicating the patient with an analgesic. The display outlines some factors that can influence the patient's response to pain.

Pain Relief Methods

INTRAVENOUS MEDICATIONS

Intravenous titration of narcotics in the immediate postoperative period offers the quickest and most effective method of pain relief. Because the patient's basal metabolic rate is decreased during surgery, the uptake of intramuscular medication is difficult to predict.

INTRAMUSCULAR MEDICATIONS

One intramuscular medication, ketorolac tromethamine (Toradol), administered during surgery, has proven very effective in the management of postoperative pain. Ketorolac tromethamine is a nonsteroidal anti-inflammatory drug that exhibits analgesic, anti-inflammatory, and antipyretic activity. Peak analgesia occurs in 45 to 60 minutes after intramuscular or IV injection, and the analgesic effect lasts 6 to 8 hours. The medication should not be used for more than 5 days, and no more than a 60-mg loading dose should be used. Ketorolac tromethamine is contraindicated as a prophylactic analgesic prior to surgery and for intraoperative use when hemostasis is critical. The medication is contraindicated for patients with active peptic ulcers, recent gastrointestinal bleeds, or a history of such.[7]

Factors Influencing Pain

Surgical procedure: Site and nature of the operation
Anxiety level: Fear of surgery, disfigurement, death, loss of control
Patient expectations: Effectiveness of preoperative teaching, adequately prepared for outcome
Pain tolerance: Prior use of medications, including analgesics, individual differences
Anesthesia technique: Analgesics used during the intraoperative period, use of naloxone

---

PATIENT-CONTROLLED ANALGESIA AND EPIDURAL MEDICATIONS

Trends in pain control management include use of patient-controlled analgesia (PCA) devices and epidural analgesia. The use of PCA pumps has increased significantly during recent years, and it is believed that patients maintain autonomy when they control administration of narcotics for their pain relief.

Epidural analgesia has proven successful in treating acute pain due to trauma or surgery and for chronic pain as in cancer. Patients receiving epidural narcotics are less sedated and therefore ambulate earlier and have improved respiratory function. Epidural medications may be administered as a bolus injection or by a continuous infusion.

When administering continuous infusions, an infusion pump should be used. Safeguards to be taken include using preservative-free medications in the epidural infusion, using infusion sets that have *no* injection ports, and labeling infusing pump, infusion bag, and infusion tubing with the word *epidural*. The reason for such safeguards is that accidental infusion of vasodilators, chemotherapy medications, antibiotics, and medications with any type of preservative could permanently destroy nerve tissue and paralyze or even kill the patient.

Preservative-free epidural medications frequently used include morphine, hydromorphone, meperidine, and fentanyl. The duration of sensory analgesia varies with the narcotic administered. The more lipid-soluble agents penetrate the dura mater more rapidly, resulting in a more rapid diffusion away from the spinal cord and subarachnoid space and hence a shorter duration of action.[8] The most frequently used narcotics for epidural administration for which average duration times have been identified are morphine, with a duration that varies from 2 to 24 hours; hydromorphone, with an average duration of 10 to 14 hours; meperidine, with an average duration of 6 to 8 hours; and fentanyl, with an average duration of 4 to 6 hours.

Dilute local anesthetic solutions are used either in conjunction with the previously mentioned narcotics or used alone. Local anesthetics used alone and in conjunction with narcotics are lidocaine, mepivacaine, prilocaine, bupivacaine, and etidocaine. The combination of local anesthetics and narcotics has been used to obtain a rapid onset and prolonged duration of analgesia. The local agents work more rapidly, and the narcotics have a more prolonged action. Side effects may occur with the use of narcotics and anesthetic solutions in the epidural space. Nurses have the primary responsibility for recognizing and preventing side effects when caring for patients receiving epidural analgesia, as listed in the display. Adequate pain relief during the postoperative period allows the patient to cough, deep breathe, and ambulate sooner, thus preventing complications.

OTHER MEDICATION METHODS

Other techniques investigated as alternatives in pain management include intrathecal methods, interpleural meth-

---

CLINICAL APPLICATION:
Nursing Intervention Guidelines
Side Effects From Epidural Analgesia

Specific protocols for epidural management are essential for each individual hospital.

Urinary retention
• Catheterize as needed.

Postural hypotension
• Give fluid (volume) replacement.
• Administer ephedrine 5 mg IV as ordered.

Pruritus (itching of face, head, and neck)
• Treat with Benadryl 25 mg PO, IM, IV.
• Treat with naloxone 0.1 mg IV.

Nausea and vomiting
• Administer metoclopramide 10 mg IV.
• Administer droperidol 0.25 mg IV.
• Administer scopolamine patch.
• Administer ondansetron (Zofram) 4 mg IV.

Respiratory depression (risk increases with age)
• Assess for first signs which may include change in level of consciousness.
• Assess for occurrence up to 24-hour after narcotic injection with naloxone 0.1 mg up to a maximum of 0.4 mg IV.
• Observe continuously because naloxone's duration is 30 minutes.
• Make Naloxone and ephedrine available at the bedside of patients who have received epidural narcotics or anesthetics.

---

ods, transdermal patches, and transmucosal–nasal aerosol. Intrathecal analgesia occurs when the anesthesiologist injects, usually as a one-time dose, medication directly into the cerebrospinal fluid of the subarachnoid space.[9] Interpleural techniques involve administration of local anesthetics into the interpleural space. The catheter is placed during the perioperative period but occasionally may be placed in the ICU. Continuous infusions and bolus injections may be given.

Transdermal patches of fentanyl are being studied, as are transmucosal–nasal aerosol delivery systems.[5,9,10] Transdermal fentanyl is an excellent alternative to sustained-release morphine preparations, especially when oral medication is not possible. Patches are constructed as a drug reservoir that are separated from the skin by a microporous rate-limiting membrane and adhesive polymer. The major disadvantage to the transdermal patches is the slow onset and inability to change dosage rapidly in response to changing opioid requirements. Oral transmucosal fentanyl citrate (OTFC) has been evaluated and approved for pediatric premedication and sedation. The onset of sedation is within 5 to 10 minutes, and full recovery is within 60 minutes after administration of the "fentanyl oralet." Plasma levels rise as the patient sucks on the lozenge on a stick. These oralets should be used only in the hospital setting where 1:1 obser-

vation of respiratory function may be measured. Side effects of OTFC include nausea and vomiting and facial pruritus.

■ CONCLUSION

Acute situations arise in the early postoperative period as the patient recovers from anesthesia. An understanding of the anesthetic options and anticipated responses enables the critical care nurse to assist the patient to a safe, uncomplicated, postoperative recovery. The Collaborative Care Guide details the care of the patient recovering from anesthesia.

Clinical Applicability Challenges

Self-Challenge: Critical Thinking

1. *Compare and contrast the actions of the depolarizing muscle relaxants with the nondepolarizing muscle relaxants, and identify medications that can be reversed pharmacologically.*

2. *Develop a plan of care for the patient who has a known family history of malignant hyperthermia.*

3. *Relate any dysrhythmias demonstrated by the anesthetized patient to his or her clinical condition.*

Study Questions

1. *Which of the following medications should be kept at the bedside of the patient who has received epidural narcotics?*
   a. *Naloxone and morphine*
   b. *Naloxone and ephedrine*
   c. *Dopamine and nitroglycerin*
   d. *Benadryl and droperidol*

2. *One of the earliest warning signs for malignant hyperthermia after the administration of succinylcholine is*
   a. *elevated temperature.*
   b. *cyanosis.*
   c. *diaphoresis.*
   d. *masseter muscle rigidity.*

3. *Nondepolarizing muscle relaxants may be reversed with*
   a. *anticholinesterase medications.*
   b. *narcotics.*
   c. *depolarizing muscle relaxants.*
   d. *Acetylcholine.*

4. *An example of a depolarizing muscle relaxant is*
   a. *pancuronium.*
   b. *cisatracurium.*
   c. *succinylcholine.*
   d. *atracurium.*

5. *Which of the following is a specific benzodiazepine antagonist?*
   a. *aminophylline*
   b. *flumazenil*
   c. *naloxone*
   d. *nalbuphine*

COLLABORATIVE CARE GUIDE
for the Postanesthesia Patient

OUTCOMES	INTERVENTIONS

Oxygenation/Ventilation

Depth and rate of respiration after extubation will be normal.
Arterial blood gases are within preoperative normal values.

Airway will be maintained with intact protective reflexes.

- Monitor respiratory rate and breathing pattern q15 min and PRN.
- Assess weaning parameters prior to extubation.
- Monitor end tidal CO_2 and pulse oximeter of mechanically ventilated patients.
- Encourage patient to cough and deep breathe.
- Elevate head of bed if not contraindicated.
- Use jaw thrust, head tilt, or oral or nasal artificial airway to maintain airway.
- Stimulate patient every few minutes (eg, call name, touch).
- Administer antiemetic as indicated.

There will be no evidence of aspiration.

- Position patient on side; suction and maintain airway if patient is vomiting.

Circulation/Perfusion

Heart rate and blood pressure will return to preoperative values within 1–2 h after anesthesia.

- Monitor vital signs q15 min and PRN.
- Assess pulse quality and regularity.
- Monitor for dysrhythmias.
- Monitor for hypotension related to bleeding.
- Monitor for hypotension related to warming and vasodilation.
- Administer IV solution and blood products as ordered.

Body temperature will be within normal limits.

- Anticipate hypothermia; have warming blankets, devices readily available.
- Measure temperature on admission and PRN until normal.
- Warm patient at 1° to 2°C/h.

There will be no evidence of malignant hyperthermia.

- Monitor for malignant hyperthermia, and immediately notify anesthesiologist of temperature increase of 0.5°C.
- Administer dantrolene, and initiate cooling measures.

Fluids/Electrolytes

Patient will have stable blood pressure and heart rate.

- Maintain patient IV.
- Monitor intake and output.
- Assess skin, mucous membranes for signs of hypovolemia.

Urine output will be 30–200 mL/h.
There will be no evidence of hypervolemia.

- Measure specific gravity if indicated.
- Assess for signs of hypervolemia (eg, pulmonary crackles, neck vein distension).
- Measure serum electrolytes if indicated.

Mobility/Safety

Patient will arouse easily and respond appropriately to commands.
Patient will move all extremities purposefully and with normal strength.

- Assess level of consciousness q15 min and PRN.
- Monitor motor and sensory function to assess reversal of neuromuscular blockade.
- Assess level of regional block, epidural, or spinal anesthesia.

Skin Integrity

Skin will remain intact.

- Assess skin immediately postoperatively for pressure areas and burns.

Nutrition

Nutritional intake will be reestablished.

- Resume enteral feeding with return of bowel sounds.
- Begin oral fluids with return of protective airway reflexes.

(continued)

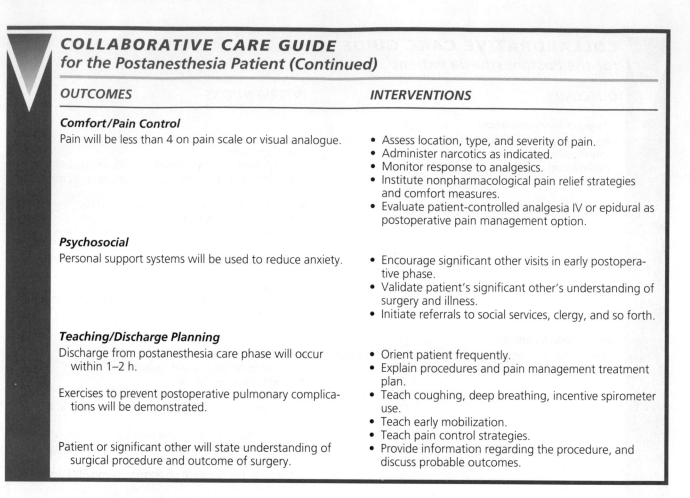

COLLABORATIVE CARE GUIDE
for the Postanesthesia Patient (Continued)

OUTCOMES	INTERVENTIONS
Comfort/Pain Control Pain will be less than 4 on pain scale or visual analogue.	• Assess location, type, and severity of pain. • Administer narcotics as indicated. • Monitor response to analgesics. • Institute nonpharmacological pain relief strategies and comfort measures. • Evaluate patient-controlled analgesia IV or epidural as postoperative pain management option.
Psychosocial Personal support systems will be used to reduce anxiety.	• Encourage significant other visits in early postoperative phase. • Validate patient's significant other's understanding of surgery and illness. • Initiate referrals to social services, clergy, and so forth.
Teaching/Discharge Planning Discharge from postanesthesia care phase will occur within 1–2 h. Exercises to prevent postoperative pulmonary complications will be demonstrated. Patient or significant other will state understanding of surgical procedure and outcome of surgery.	• Orient patient frequently. • Explain procedures and pain management treatment plan. • Teach coughing, deep breathing, incentive spirometer use. • Teach early mobilization. • Teach pain control strategies. • Provide information regarding the procedure, and discuss probable outcomes.

REFERENCES

1. American Society of PeriAnesthesia Nurses. Standards of PeriAnesthesia Nursing Practice. ASPAN, 6900 Grove Road, Thorofare, New Jersey 08086, 1995
2. Eisenhauer LA, Nichols LW, Spencer RT, Bergan FW: Clinical Pharmacology and Nursing Management (5th Ed.). Philadephia, Lippincott-Raven, in press.
3. Standards of Perianesthesia Nursing Practice. American Society of Post-Anesthesia Nurses, Thorofare, NJ, 1995.
4. Drain C: The Post Anesthesia Care Unit (3rd Ed). Philadelphia, WB Saunders, 1994
5. Kirby R, Gravenstein N: Clinical Anesthesia Practice. Philadelphia, WB Saunders, 1994
6. Kaplan R: Malignant hyperthermia. In Barash PG (ed): Refresher Courses in Anesthesia, 22, 1995
7. Morgan G, Mikhail M: Clinical Anesthesiology (2nd Ed). Stamford, CT, Appleton & Lange, 1996
8. Litwack K: Post Anesthesia Care Nursing (2nd Ed). St. Louis, Mosby-Year Book, 1995
9. Rasch D, Webster D: Clinical Manual of Pediatric Anesthesia. New York, McGraw-Hill, 1994
10. Salerno E, Williams J: Pain Management Handbook. St. Louis, CV Mosby, 1996

BIBLIOGRAPHY

Burden N: Ambulatory Surgery Nursing. Philadelphia, WB Saunders, 1993

Carlson K (ed): Certification Review for Perianesthesia Nursing. Philadelphia, WB Saunders, 1996

Drain C: The Post Anesthesia Care Unit (3rd Ed). Philadelphia, WB Saunders, 1994

Kaplan R: Malignant hyperthermia in Refresher Courses in Anesthesia. Paul G. Barash (ed), 22, 1995

Kirby R, Gravenstein N: Clinical Anesthesia Practice. Philadelphia, WB Saunders, 1994

Litwack K (ed): Core Curriculum for Post Anesthesia Nursing Practice (3rd Ed). Philadelphia, WB Saunders, 1995

Litwack K: Post Anesthesia Care Nursing (2nd Ed). St. Louis, CV Mosby, 1995

Ponte J, Green D: Handbooks of Anaesthetics and Perioperative Care. Philadelphia, WB Saunders, 1994

Rasch D, Webster D: Clinical Manual of Pediatric Anesthesia. New York, McGraw-Hill, 1994

Silverman D, Connelly N: Review of Clinical Anesthesia. Philadelphia, JB Lippincott, 1995

Solerno E, Williams J: Pain Management Handbook. St. Louis, CV Mosby, 1996

14

Interfacility Transport of the Critically Ill Patient

MODES OF TRANSPORT
TRANSFER GUIDELINES AND LEGAL
IMPLICATIONS
PHASES OF TRANSPORT
Phase One: Notification and Acceptance
  by the Receiving Facility

Phase Two: Preparation of the Patient
  by the Transport Team
Phase Three: The Transport Process
Phase Four: Turnover of the Patient to
  the Receiving Facility

Phase Five: Post-transport Continuous
  Quality Improvement Monitoring
CONCLUSION

OBJECTIVES

Based on the content in this chapter, the reader should be able to:

- Describe the indications for interfacility transport of the critically ill patient.
- Compare and contrast the advantages and disadvantages of air versus ground transport.
- Explain the physiological effect of stressors associated with air transport and their implications for nursing care.
- Describe key factors necessary for an effective interfacility transfer plan.
- Analyze the role of the registered nurse in the five phases of the interfacility transport of the critically ill.

*C*ritically ill patients are transported between facilities daily. These transfers are linked to a number of factors. Typically, transport is indicated when the patient's need for complex diagnostic procedures or sophisticated medical and nursing expertise exceeds what can be provided at a facility. Family requests may also affect the decision to transport. For example, a family may want their family member transferred to a hospital closer to home.

Outcomes of evolving health care reform also have increased the demands for interfacility transport of critically ill patients. Third party payors may require patients to be transported to a facility that is a member of their network. In addition, many hospitals vie for fewer patients and have developed their own transport teams to provide a flow of patients to their particular facility. The American College of Critical Care Medicine is also investigating the need and benefits of regionalizing critical care, which has the potential to increase tremendously critical care transports.[1]

Whatever the reason for transporting a patient, a risk/benefit analysis of the transport should always be performed. Risks for the patient range from physical safety to physiological compromise to emotional distress.[2,3] Benefits from interfacility transport include access to life-saving assessment techniques and specialized interventions that can improve the patient's outcome. When the benefits for the patient exceed the risks, an interfacility transport is warranted.

MODES OF TRANSPORT

Once the decision has been made to transport, the method of transport must be determined. The two primary methods of interfacility transport are ground and air. Ground transport includes ambulances and mobile intensive care units

(ICUs). Air transport can occur by either a rotary wing vehicle (helicopter) or a fixed-wing vehicle (airplane). When selecting the mode of transport, several factors must be considered, such as distance, the safety of the transport environment, time to and from the receiving facility, the patient's condition and potential for complications, traffic conditions, and weather conditions.[4] In addition, the advantages and disadvantages of ground versus air transport must be considered when selecting the mode of transport. Table 14–1 summarizes the advantages and disadvantages of ground versus air transport.

Whether ground or air transport is selected, potential stressors exist because a moving environment affects the patient, equipment, and crew. Air transport teams must give special attention to additional stressors caused mainly by altitude changes. The effect of these stressors and their implications for nursing care are summarized in Table 14–2.

TRANSFER GUIDELINES AND LEGAL IMPLICATIONS

To facilitate the appropriate transfer of patients, the American College of Emergency Physicians has developed guidelines. These principles of appropriate patient transfer are listed in the display on page 154.

Legislation also exists that provides guidelines, regulations, and penalties for patient transfer. One such law, the Consolidated Omnibus Reconciliation Act (COBRA) of 1985, contains provisions addressing the transfer of patients from hospital to hospital. The purpose of the legislation is to prevent inappropriate transfers of patients who seek emergency department (ED) care and, as a result, has become known as the "antidumping" law.

The following provisions of the COBRA legislation prevent any patient from being denied an initial screening in an ED or from being transferred to another hospital or discharged without receiving care:

1. Hospitals must provide screening examinations for every individual who requests care.
2. If the patient has an emergency medical condition, the hospital must provide stabilizing treatment or transfer the patient to another medical facility. The physician must document that the medical benefits outweigh the risks of the transfer.
3. The receiving medical facility agrees to accept the patient and provide appropriate medical treatment. The receiving medical facility must have adequate space and qualified personnel to care for the patient.
4. The transfer is conducted by qualified personnel and appropriate equipment needed to provide care during the transfer is available.

PHASES OF TRANSPORT

Five phases of transport have been identified: notification and acceptance by the receiving facility, preparation of the patient by the transport team, the actual transport, turnover of the patient to the receiving hospital, and continuous quality improvement monitoring after transport.[5] The keys to the success of transport are a comprehensive assessment, determination of the appropriateness of the transfer, collaboration, communication, evaluation, and education of personnel. Each of these factors is summarized in the display on page 154.

TABLE 14-1
Advantages and Disadvantages of Ground Versus Air Transport

Mode of Tranport	Advantages	Disadvantages
Ground	Adequate work space for personnel and equipment Sensitive monitoring equipment may work better No weight restrictions Adequate lighting Able to travel in most types of weather	Longer transport time Unfavorable road conditions may make transport uncomfortable for patient Interventions difficult to perform in a moving vehicle Ambulance unavailable for other calls in the community
Air	May shorten "out of hospital" time Crew generally composed of advanced level care providers Improved communication capability Ground emergency medical services remain available in the community	Weather conditions restrict availability of the vehicle Potentially more costly Limited space (helicopters) Weight limitations Physiological impact on patient and crew Psychological impact on patient (eg, fear of flying)

Holleran R: Prehospital Nursing: A Collaborative Approach. St. Louis, CV Mosby, 1994

TABLE 14-2
Special Considerations for Air Transport

Stressors	Effect	Nursing Interventions

Altitude change	Hypoxia is due to the following:
	    Decrease in the partial pressure of O_2
	    Decrease in the diffusion gradient for
	        oxygen molecules to cross the alveolar
	        membrane
	    Decrease in oxygen availability
		Provide supplemental O_2.
		Use pulse oximeter and end tidal CO_2 monitor.

Barometric pressure (atmospheric pressure) change	With increasing altitude, the barometric pressure decreases and gases expand. Expansion of gases affects eardrums, sinuses, gastrointestinal tract, pleural spaces, and hollow organs. Expansion of gases affects air splints, pressure bags or cuffs, balloon cuffs on endotracheal tubes, intravenous fluid bags and bottles, pneumatic antishock garments.	Insert a nasogastric tube to decompress the stomach. If possible, fill cuffs with water or saline rather than air. Monitor equipment and decompress with higher altitudes. Vent glass bottles and wrap to protect against breakage. Apply pressure cuffs to IV solution bags.
Thermal change	As altitude increases, temperature decreases. Oxygen demand increases as the body tries to maintain warmth.	Use blankets to keep the patient warm.
Humidity change	As air is cooled, it loses moisture. Mucous membranes dry.	Humidify supplemental O_2. Provide adequate fluid intake.
Gravitational change	Gravitational change affects acceleration and deceleration forces. Transient increase in venous return occurs for patients positioned with head at the back of the aircraft. Potential exists for motion sickness.	Use a head-forward position for patients with fluid overload or increased intracranial pressure. To minimize motion sickness, provide O_2, cool cloth to face, cool air to face. Administer medications, such as transdermal scopolamine patches and promethazine.
Noise	It is difficult to monitor blood pressure, breath sounds, endotracheal tube air leak.	Explain sounds to patient. Monitor blood pressure by Doppler device. Provide continuous airway assessment. Wear head sets or ear plugs.
Vibration	Vibration may distort readings on equipment. Equipment may loosen or move.	Secure all equipment. Check equipment function frequently.

Harrahill M: Interfacility transfer In Kitt S, Selfridge-Thomas J, Proehl J, Kaiser J (Eds): Emergency Nursing:
A Physiologic and Clinical Perspective *(2nd Ed). pp 12–18. Philadelphia, WB Saunders, 1995*

Phase One: Notification and Acceptance by the Receiving Facility

The first phase of transport requires notifying the receiving facility to determine their willingness to accept the patient. Communication is an essential element in this phase of the process. The sending, transporting, and receiving personnel must have the necessary information to make the transport decision. Standards of care and protocols should be in place ahead of time so that the decision to transport and the transport process are carried out in an organized way. A transfer checklist, such as the one shown in the display on page 155, can be used to make sure no steps in the transfer process are missed. In addition, an awareness of the policies and procedures of the transporting agencies used in an area is needed for a smooth transport process.[2,3]

Once a facility is willing to receive a patient, an accepting physician must be identified and an available bed confirmed. The identification of a responsible physician is essential so that a contact person is available for consultation while en route and on arrival. Transport teams should have standard orders and protocols if they are unable to maintain contact with a medical center physician en route.

Current regulations require the patient or a legally authorized representative to give informed consent for the transport. If consent cannot be obtained, documentation of the indications for the transport and the reason consent was not obtained must appear in the medical record.[2,3]

After the transport decision is made, the receiving facility agrees to accept the patient, and the mode of transport is selected, a qualified transport team is notified. Initial information given to the transporting agency includes the patient's name, diagnosis, reason for transfer, vital signs, in-

Principles of Appropriate Patient Transfer

- The health and well-being of the patient must be the over-riding concern when any patient transfer is considered.
- Emergency physicians and hospital personnel should comply with state and federal regulations regarding patient transfer. A medical screening exam should be performed by a physician or by properly trained ancillary personnel according to written policies and procedures.
- The patient should be transferred to another facility only after medical evaluation and, when possible, stabilization.
- The physician should inform the patient or responsible party of the reasons for and the risks and likely benefits of transfer, and document this in the medical record.
- The hospital and medical staff should identify individuals responsible for transfer decisions and clearly delineate their duties regarding the patient transfer process.
- The patient should be transferred to a facility appropriate to the medical needs of the patient, with adequate space and personnel available.

- A physician or other responsible person at the receiving hospital must agree to accept the patient prior to transfer.
- The patient transfer should not be refused by the receiving hospital when the transfer is medically indicated and the receiving hospital has the capability and/or responsibility to provide care for the patient.
- Communication to exchange clinical information between responsible persons at the transferring and receiving hospitals must occur prior to transfer.
- An appropriate medical summary and other pertinent records should accompany the patient to the receiving institution.
- The patient should be transferred in a vehicle that is staffed by qualified personnel and contains appropriate equipment.
- When transfer of patients is part of a regional plan to provide optimal care of patients at specified medical facilities, written transfer protocols and interfacility agreements should be in place.

Adapted from: American College of Emergency Physicians: Principles of Appropriate Patient Transfer. Annals of Emergency Medicine 19(3): 337–338, 1990

travenous (IV) and special monitoring lines, continuous infusion medications, and airway and oxygenation or ventilation status. This information will assist in determining the composition of the transport team and the equipment and medications needed. The American Association of Critical-Care Nurses, the American College of Critical Care Medicine, and the Society of Critical Care Medicine offer guidelines for accompanying personnel for interfacility transport (see display).[2,3]

Individual states define the role of the nurse who may be involved in interfacility transport. Some states require a special certification for nurses involved in an interhospital transport of the critically ill patient.[6] If a nurse is assigned from an inpatient unit to assist with transport, the nurse must be aware of the regulations governing nursing practice in this highly specialized environment and be qualified to meet these expectations. These state regulations should be investigated ahead of time to avoid having a nurse

Key Factors Vital to an Effective Transfer Plan

Assessment and Appropriateness

- Assess and determine available resources (quality and suitability of local technology).
- Appraise level of medical, nursing, and ancillary staff expertise.
- Assess patient benefits versus the risks of transfer.
- Determine appropriateness of transfer and appropriate receiving center.

Collaboration and Communication

- Establish a multidisciplinary team committed to quality patient care and appropriate transfer of critically ill patients.

- Promote interfacility communication that enhances transfer outcomes.

Evaluation and Education

- Approach transfer of critically ill patients as a process requiring specialized knowledge and competencies.
- Monitor and update the essential transfer knowledge and skills of appropriate personnel.
- Develop a comprehensive quality improvement program to evaluate and document problem resolution and patient transfer outcomes.

Guidelines for the Transfer of Critically Ill Patients. Prepared by the American Association of Critical-Care Nurses Transfer Guidelines Task Force and the Guidelines Committee, American College of Critical Care Medicine, Society of Critical Care Medicine, p 6. American Association of Critical-Care Nurses, Aliso Viejo, CA, 1993. Used with permission.

Transfer Checklist

Check the following items as you complete the steps of the transfer process:

____ Risks versus benefits of transfer explained (if possible) and documented

____ Referral center determined

____ Acceptance received from referral center

____ Receiving physician notified

____ Transfer order obtained

____ Transportation arranged

____ Report given to transfer personnel

____ Report called to receiving nurse (if transport nurse is also patient's provider)

____ Medications and treatments given

____ Family/significant other notified of transfer

____ Appropriate consents/forms signed (including orders, protocols for transport)

____ Copies of patient's records obtained (including x-ray and laboratory reports)

____ Patient's valuables secured and documented

____ Needed medications, equipment, and supplies assembled

____ Report called to receiving nurse (if transport nurse is an "additional" provider)

Guidelines for the Transfer of Critically Ill Patients. Prepared by the American Association of Critical-Care Nurses Transfer Guidelines Task Force and the Guidelines Committee, American College of Critical Care Medicine, Society of Critical Care Medicine, 37. American Association of Critical-Care Nurses, Aliso Viejo, CA, 1993. (From Maxwell B, Miller B: Smooth the way for safe emergency transfers. RN 6:36, 1988. Copyright 1988 Medical Economics Publishing, Montvale, NJ. Adapted by permission)

If the sending nurse calls the report, the transporting nurse updates the receiving nurse as needed.

The transport team performs an assessment of the patient and contributes their findings to the previously developed plan of care. If interventions are needed before transport, the transport team and the referral facility personnel determine who will assume responsibility for the interventions. Although resuscitation and stabilization are initiated at the referral hospital, full stabilization may not be achieved until the patient arrives at the receiving hospital.[8]

The psychosocial preparation of the patient and family for transport is an important step before transport begins. The sending nurse ensures that the patient and family understand the reason for transport, the transport mode, the time of transport, and the transport destination. Information about the family is also communicated at this time and includes identification of a family spokesperson and the family's plan for getting to the receiving hospital. If the transport team is unable to meet with the family, the sending nurse supplies information about how to contact the family.

Physical preparation of the patient is the next important step to ensure a safe transport. The ABCs of care (airway, breathing, and circulation) are the top priority. Adequate oxygenation and ventilation are ensured before transport begins. The need for an artificial airway is determined prior to leaving the sending facility so that endotracheal (ET) intubation can be performed in a more predictable environment and the ET tube can be well secured. Most intubated patients are sedated to prevent them from dislodging the ET tube and to decrease fear and discomfort during transport. In addition to the ET tube, a nasogastric tube may be in-

accompanying a patient without knowledge of the role and the responsibilities involved in caring for the patient. The Emergency Nurses Association has published *Guidelines for Pre-Hospital Nursing Curriculum*, which may assist in identification of issues related to the role of the nurse in the field.[7] Additionally, a transfer curriculum and competencies for accompanying staff have been developed.[2]

Phase Two: Preparation of the Patient by the Transport Team

Phase two begins as the transport team arrives at the referral facility. A thorough report about the patient is an essential step in the successful transport of the patient. Not giving an adequate report places the patient at risk. The report should include chief complaint, allergies, medical history, reason for transport, patient's age, vital signs, treatments already performed, and their outcomes. Copies of the chart and of all x-rays also are sent with the patient. To avoid duplication of efforts, the sending and transporting nurses decide who will give the full report to the receiving hospital.

Guidelines for Accompanying Personnel for Interfacility Transfer

- A minimum of two people in addition to the vehicle operator should accompany the patient.
- At least one of the accompanying personnel should be a registered nurse, physician, or advanced emergency medical technician.
- When a physician does not accompany the patient, there should be a mechanism available to communicate with the physician any changes in the patient status and obtain additional orders. If an accompanying physician is not possible, advanced authorization by standing orders to perform acute life-saving interventions must be established.

Guidelines for the Transfer of Critically Ill Patients. Prepared by the American Association of Critical-Care Nurses Transfer Guidelines Task Force and the Guidelines Committee, American College of Critical Care Medicine, Society of Critical Care Medicine, p 11. American Association of Critical-Care Nurses, Aliso Viejo, CA, 1993. Used with permission.

serted to prevent aspiration of stomach contents into the airway. Because auscultation of breath sounds is difficult en route, end tidal CO_2 and oxygen saturation are used to monitor respiratory status. If an endotracheal tube is not indicated, supplemental oxygen may still be used to maintain adequate oxygenation. Usually, any patient traveling by air receives supplemental oxygen, and if the air transport time exceeds 15 minutes, the oxygen should be humidified.[8]

The patient's circulatory and hemodynamic status also are stabilized before transport. Any bleeding is controlled and adequate IV access established and well secured. For a patient with an unstable volume status, several 14-gauge IVs are indicated. If the patient is already on IV drips, the transport team may change over to their own equipment and IV mixtures. The patient's circulatory status is also continuously assessed through cardiac monitoring during the entire transport process. Cardiac arrest medications and a defibrillator should be easily accessible.

Patients with actual or potential spinal injuries should have spinal and neck immobilization devices in place before transport. Patients with any skeletal fractures must have the fracture immobilized before transport to prevent pain and further complications.

Pain control during transport also is addressed. The best agents for a transport patient are those with a rapid onset, short duration, and ease of administration and storage.

Phase Three: The Transport Process

Phase three is the actual transport of the patient. The time spent in careful planning of the transport and stabilization of the patient will ease the transport process. The transport vehicle must contain the essential equipment needed for transporting a critically ill patient. The accompanying display lists the necessary equipment.[2,9]

The ABCs of care continue to be the primary focus of the transport team. Each member of the transport team must have a clear understanding of his or her role in the continuous assessment, planning, and intervention when caring for the patient. Throughout the transport, the team also provides explanations and reassures the patient because transport can be very stressful. The transport team is responsible for documenting the physical and psychosocial care provided during transport and the patient's response to the care.

Prior to arriving at the receiving facility, the transport nurse calls either a full or updated report. This report includes an estimated time of arrival at the receiving facility. The nurse also communicates any special needs, changes in patient status, and unchanged but pertinent findings.

Phase Four: Turnover of the Patient to the Receiving Facility

Phase four of transport involves handing over the patient to the ICU staff at the receiving facility. Back-up plans on how to handle an acutely deteriorating patient in transit be-

---

> ### *Minimally Essential Equipment Necessary for Transport*
>
> - Airway and ventilary management
>   Resuscitation bag and mask of proper size and fit for the patient.
>   Oral airways, laryngoscopes, and endotracheal tubes of proper size for the patient
>   Oxygen source with a quantity sufficient to meet the patient's anticipated consumption with at least 1-hour reserve in addition
>   Suction apparatus and catheters
> - Cardiac monitor/defibrillator
> - Blood pressure cuff and stethoscope
> - Materials for intravenous therapy and devices for regulation of infusion
> - Drugs
>   For advanced cardiac resuscitation
>   For the management of acute physiological derangements
>   For special needs of the patient
> - Spinal immobilization devices
> - Communication equipment
>
> ------
>
> *Guidelines for the Transfer of Critically Ill Patients. Prepared by the American Association of Critical-Care Nurses Transfer Guidelines Task Force and the Guidelines Committee, American College of Critical Care Medicine, Society of Critical Care Medicine, p 13. American Association of Critical-Care Nurses, Aliso Viejo, CA, 1993. Used with permission.*

---

tween the transport vehicle and the ICU should also be identified. This plan may include stopping at the emergency department to stabilize the patient; it is essential for the emergency department staff to be aware of this possibility. Once the patient arrives safely in the ICU, the transport team and the receiving staff determine when the receiving staff will take over the responsibility for the patient's care. A final verbal update and all medical documents are given to the receiving staff. The written report of the transport is also completed.

Phase Five: Post-transport Continuous Quality Improvement Monitoring

The final phase of transport is very important and involves continuous quality improvement monitoring. Ideally, the referring facility, the transport team, and the receiving facility are involved in the review process. The first phase of the quality improvement monitoring involves evaluation of the current transport, including any quality indicators developed by the transporting agency. These indicators may include appropriateness of the transfer, appropriateness of the accompanying personnel, timeliness of the transfer, patient outcome, management of complications, and transfer outcome. The second phase of continuous quality improvement monitoring entails the ongoing review of the transport system. Such reviews focus on system functioning, and indicators may include complications, deaths in transport, and deaths following transport.[2]

The multidisciplinary team responsible for continuous quality improvement monitoring scrutinizes the collected data for patterns and trends, identifies solutions to patient care problems, initiates corrective action, and communicates such action to all involved in the transport process. Through a quality improvement plan, the transport process will be improved and result in optimal care of the critically ill patient during the transport process.[2]

■ CONCLUSION

Interfacility transport provides a vital link between the critically ill patient and expert resources. Whether functioning as the sending, transporting, or receiving nurse, an understanding of the key elements of a successful transfer and the role of each team member is essential (Fig. 14–1).

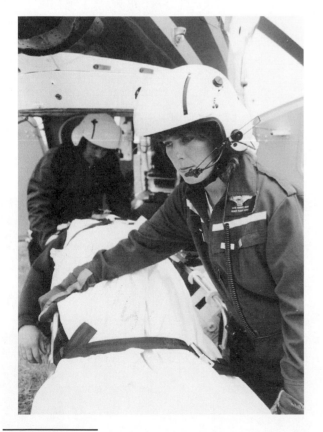

FIGURE 14-1
The nurse involved in interfacility transport has special training and works as a team member to provide a safe and successful transfer. (Photo used with the permission of Bill Rowe, photographer, Rockford Health System, Rockford, IL)

This understanding will ensure that the transport process is safe for the patient and the transport team and that positive outcomes of the transport process are achieved.

Clinical Applicability Challenges

Self-Challenge: Critical Thinking

1. *Analyze the policies and procedures for interfacility transport at an acute care facility. Identify the strengths and weaknesses of the policies and procedures, and develop recommendations for change.*

2. *Compare and contrast the roles and responsibilities of each member of the transport team. Develop a plan to educate staff about the roles and responsibilities of each transport team member.*

Study Questions

1. *Because of altitude changes during air transport, which of the following nursing interventions would be indicated?*
   a. *Run all IV fluids at a KVO (keep vein open) rate.*
   b. *Use blankets to keep the patient warm.*
   c. *Use a cooling blanket to keep the patient cool.*
   d. *Avoid use of humidification with supplemental oxygen.*

2. *The primary physiological concern for a transport patient is*
   a. *maintenance of an airway.*
   b. *placement of at least 2 IV lines.*
   c. *immobilization of a fracture.*
   d. *provision of continuous cardiac monitoring.*

REFERENCES

1. American College of Critical Care Medicine Task Force on Regionalization of Critical Care Medicine: Regionalization of critical care medicine: Task force report of the American College of Critical Care Medicine. Critical Care Medicine 22:1306–1313, 1994
2. American Association of Critical-Care Nurses Transfer Guidelines Task Force and the Guidelines Committee, American College of Critical Care Medicine, Society of Critical Care Medicine: Guidelines for the transfer of critically ill patients. Aliso Viejo, CA: American Association of Critical-Care Nurses, 1993
3. American College of Critical Care Medicine, Society of Critical Care Medicine, and American Association of Critical-Care Nurses Transfer Guidelines Task Force: Guidelines for the transfer of critically ill patients. Critical Care Medicine 21:931–937, 1993
4. Holleran R: Prehospital Nursing: A Collaborative Approach. St. Louis, CV Mosby, 1994
5. Maryland Board of Nursing: Declaratory Ruling 94-4. Re: The Standards of Practice for the Registered Nurse When Managing and Caring for the Critically Ill Patient in Interagency Transport, 1994
6. Maryland Board of Nursing: 10.27.16 Registered Nurse in Inter Agency Transport of the Critically Unstable Patient. Draft, 1995
7. Emergency Nurses Association: National Standard of Guidelines for Prehospital Nursing (2nd Ed). Park Ridge, IL, Emergency Nurses Association, 1995
8. Harrahill M: Interfacility transfer. In Kitt S, Selfridge-Thomas J, Proehl J, Kaiser J (eds): Emergency Nursing: A Physiologic and Clinical Perspective (2nd ed), pp 12–18. Philadelphia, WB Saunders, 1995
9. Barry P, Ralston C: Adverse events occurring during interhospital transfer of the critically ill. Arch Dis Child 71:8–11, 1994

Critical Care Nursing: Alterations in Body Systems

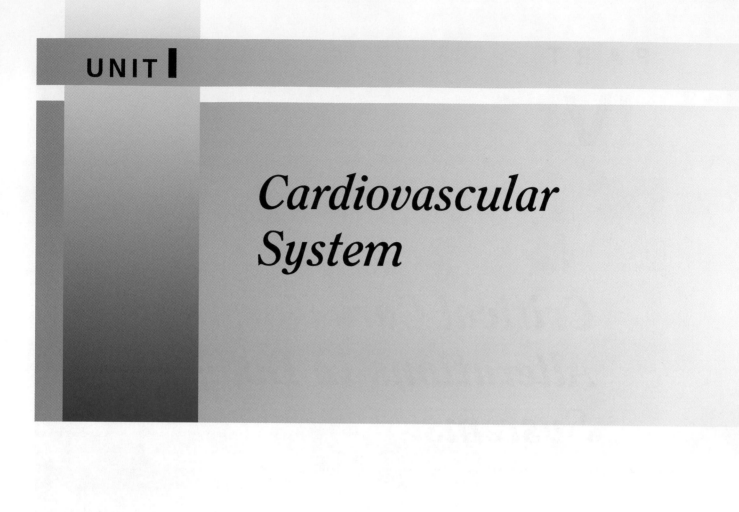

UNIT I

Cardiovascular System

Anatomy and Physiology
of the Cardiovascular System

OBJECTIVES

Based on the content in this chapter, the reader should be able to:

- Briefly describe the characteristics of cardiac muscle cells.
- Differentiate the electrical events from the mechanical events in the heart.
- Explain depolarization.
- Describe the normal conduction system of the heart.
- State the formula for calculating cardiac output.
- Compare and contrast the role of the parasympathetic and sympathetic nervous systems in the regulation of heart rate.
- Explain the three factors involved in the regulation of stroke volume.
- Describe the coronary artery blood source for the cardiac chambers and conduction system.
- Explain the influence of blood volume and blood pressure for peripheral circulation.

*D*uring the 70 years in the life of the average person, the heart will pump approximately 5 quarts of blood a minute, 75 gallons an hour, 57 barrels a day, and 1.5 million barrels in a lifetime. Although the work accomplished by this organ is out of proportion to its size, for most people, the heart functions normally throughout the life span. The pumping action of the heart moves blood, a vital substance, throughout the body, supplying oxygen and nutrients to cells and removing waste. Without this action, cells die. For people in whom cardiac problems develop, the results may be dramatic and the outcome drastic. This chapter reviews the principles of cardiovascular anatomy and physiology.

■ PHYSIOLOGICAL PRINCIPLES

Cardiac Microstructure

Microscopically, cardiac muscle contains visible stripes, or striations, similar to those found in skeletal muscle (Fig. 15–1). The ultrastructural pattern also resembles that of striated muscle. The cells branch and connect freely and form a three-dimensional, complex network. The elongated nuclei, like those of smooth muscle, are found deep in the interior of the cells and not next to the cell membrane as they are in striated muscle.

Cardiac muscle (myocardial) cells are endowed with extraordinary characteristics, most of which belong to the cell

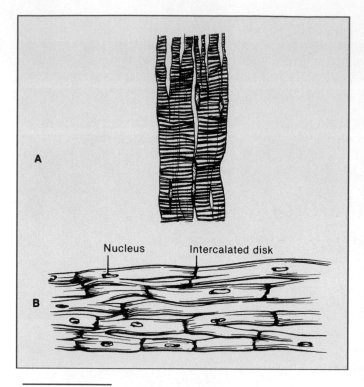

FIGURE 15-1
Histological features of the two types of contractile tissue.
(**A**) Striated muscle. (**B**) Cardiac tissue.

membrane or sarcolemma. To pump effectively, the heart muscle must begin contraction as a single unit. To contract myocardial cells simultaneously, cell membranes must depolarize at the same time. The heart does this, without using much neural tissue, by rapidly conducting impulses from cell to cell through intercalated disks. At each end of every myocardial cell, adjacent cell membranes are folded elaborately and attached strongly. These areas comprise the intercalated disks, where depolarization is conducted extremely rapidly from one cell to the next (see Fig. 15-1B).

Another extraordinary characteristic of myocardial cells, seen mainly in cell membranes, is automaticity. Selected groups of cardiac cells are capable of initiating rhythmic action potentials, and thus waves of contraction, without any outside humoral or nervous intervention.

Within each cardiac cell lie thousands of contractile elements, the overlapping actin and myosin filaments. Figure 15–2 illustrates these elements and the changes seen during diastole and systole. Not shown are the many cross-bridges that extend like rows of oars from the surface of the thicker myosin filaments. During diastole, these bridges are unattached to other filaments. The arrangement of actin and myosin filaments gives cardiac muscle its banded or striated appearance. One grouping of actin and myosin filaments is called a sarcomere.

Mechanical Events of Contraction

Before mechanical contraction, an action potential travels quickly over each cell membrane and down into each cell's sarcoplasmic reticulum (SR). When an action potential causes depolarization of the SR, calcium ions move from the SR into the myocardial cell cytoplasm and bind to troponin molecules on actin filaments. Calcium-bound troponin moves slightly to uncover binding sites on the actin, to which myosin filaments then attach. With a release of energy stored in adenosine triphosphate (ATP), these binding sites move so that actin and myosin slide past each other and new couplings between actin and myosin occur. Rapid, successive uncoupling of cross-bridges and their reattachment to new actin-binding sites lead to rapid and dramatic shortening of the sarcomere (see Fig. 15–2). This shortening is the essence of myocardial contraction (systole). Contraction ceases when the calcium ions return to their storage sites on the SR, thereby causing the binding sites on the actin filaments to be covered again. The separated actin and myosin filaments then slip past each other in the reverse direction, lengthening the sarcomere to its relaxed state.

Contraction requires calcium and energy. The presence of adequate ATP stores and the movement of calcium provide the essential link between the electrical events of depolarization and the mechanical events of contraction in the heart.

Electrical Events of Depolarization

Membranes of all the cells in the human body are charged; that is, they are polarized and therefore have electrical potentials. The charges are separated at the membrane. In humans, all cell membranes, regardless of type, are positively charged at rest, with more positively charged particles at the outer surface of the cell membrane than at the inner surface. Figure 15–3A illustrates this "resting stage."

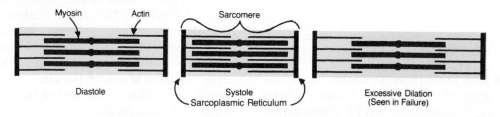

FIGURE 15-2
Contractile elements lying inside a single sarcomere of a myocardial cell.

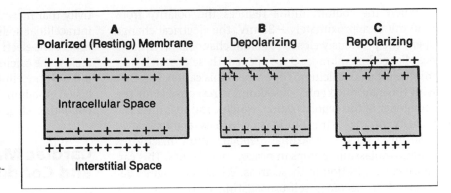

FIGURE 15-3
Electrical events at rest (diastolic) and preceding contraction (systolic).

In the depolarized state, the cell membrane is negatively charged with more negatively charged particles at the outer surface of the cell membrane than at the inner surface. Figure 15–3B illustrates this "depolarized stage."

Cardiac muscle membranes are polarized, and the electrical potential can be measured, as it can in any of the cells in the human body. The potential results from the difference between intracellular and extracellular concentrations of electrolytes. When salt compounds of various elements are dissolved in aqueous solutions, they dissociate into their charged particles, called ions.

In the resting myocardial cell, there are more potassium ions inside than outside the cell and more sodium and unbound calcium ions outside than inside the cell. All three of these positively charged ions (cations) may diffuse through pores, or channels, in the cell membrane. If each ion freely obeyed the law of diffusion, however, potassium would diffuse out of the cell, whereas sodium and calcium would diffuse into it. Very soon there would be equal concentrations of each ion between the intracellular and extracellular fluids, and no resting potential would exist. It is through selective regulation of the concentrations of these ions on either side of the membrane that the resting membrane potential is maintained. Several factors contribute to this regulation. The first factor is the presence of sodium–potassium "pumps" within the cell membrane. These pumps move sodium out of the cell and potassium into the cell, with both movements occurring against the concentration gradients for each of these ions. The second

factor is the active movement of calcium out of the cell against the concentration gradient in response to the passive diffusion of sodium into the cell. The third factor is the regulation of membrane channels, whereby calcium ions can enter the resting myocardial cell. The fourth factor is the presence of intracellular anions (negatively charged particles) that are too large to exit from the cell.

Physiological Basis of the Resting Potential

The cardiac cell contains large anions that cannot exit the cell. These anions attract sodium and potassium cations, which diffuse through membrane channels into the cell. The anions would attract the calcium cation also, except that the membrane channels for the entry of this ion are closed when the cell is at rest. The potassium ions remain within the cell, but the sodium ions are pumped out of the cell almost as fast as they can enter by the sodium–potassium pumps located within the cell membrane. While forcing sodium out of the cell, these pumps actively transport potassium ions into the cell against their concentration gradients. This increase in intracellular potassium still is insufficient to offset all the intracellular anions. Thus, the inside of the myocardial cell remains negative with respect to the outside—as long as the pumps are operative. As a result, the resting potential is approximately -80 mV. For each molecule of an ion pumped from the cell, one molecule of ATP is required to provide the energy necessary to effect the chemical bond between ion and carrier. Maintaining a resting potential thus requires energy.

Physiological Basis of the Action Potential

When a stimulus is applied to the polarized cell membrane, the membrane that ordinarily is only slightly permeable to sodium permits sodium ions to diffuse rapidly into the cell. This rapid diffusion occurs because of inactivation of the sodium active transport enzymes (pumps). The result is a reversal of net charges. The outer surface is now more negative than positive, and the membrane is said to be depolarized (see Fig. 15–3B).

Factors That Maintain Resting Membrane Potential of Myocardial Cell

- Sodium–potassium pumps within the cell membrane
- Active movement of Ca^+ out of cell against its concentration gradient in response to passive diffusion of Na^+ into cell
- Regulation of membrane channels so that Ca^+ ions can enter resting myocardial cell
- Presence of intracellular anions too large to exit from cell

When the sodium influx reduces the polarity from −80 mV to approximately −35 mV, the electrical change opens the previously closed "calcium channels" in the myocardial cell membrane. Once opened, these channels permit the influx of calcium. The entry of this cation, together with the continued entry of sodium, is responsible for the remainder of the depolarization, which continues until the polarity of the extracellular side equals approximately +30 mV. Such a maximal depolarization inactivates sodium–potassium pumps in nearby membranes. This can cause depolarization in these areas. When the original depolarization becomes self-propagating in this way, it is termed an action potential. In a myocardial cell, an action potential triggers the release of intracellular calcium from its storage sites on the SR. This release plus the calcium influx across the sarcolemma elevates intracellular calcium levels, thereby initiating muscular contraction as previously described.

If the depolarization remains below a certain critical (threshold) point, it will die out without having opened any calcium channel or inactivated any adjacent sodium–potassium pumps. Because it does not become self-propagating and remains localized, such a depolarization is termed a local depolarization.

During depolarization, the elevated intracellular sodium concentration frees potassium ions to diffuse out of the cell in accordance with their concentration gradient. Just as this potassium efflux gains some momentum, however, the sodium–potassium pumps automatically reactivate (they can be inactivated only temporarily). Once reactivated, the pumps begin to restore the original resting potential, a process termed repolarization (see Fig. 15–3C). During the initial phase of repolarization, the efflux of potassium and sodium ions exceeds their influx, but as the intracellular sodium ions are removed from the cell, potassium ions remain as the major cation to be electrostatically held within the cell by the intracellular anions. This halts the potassium efflux. The remainder of repolarization consists of pump activity that increases intracellular potassium and decreases intracellular sodium; thus, the resting potential is reestablished. The electrical events at the start of repolarization also reclose the calcium entry channels, thereby halting calcium influx. Intracellular calcium levels are reduced when the diffusion of sodium into the cell causes a movement of calcium out of the cell against the latter's concentration gradient.

Cardiac Macrostructure and Conduction

To pump effectively, large portions of cardiac muscle must receive an action potential nearly simultaneously. Special cells that conduct action potentials extremely rapidly are arranged in pathways through the heart. All these cells have automaticity.

The heart chambers and specialized tissues are diagrammed in Figure 15–4. The sinoatrial (SA) node is located between the opening of the inferior and superior venae cavae in the right atrial wall. The cells of the SA node have the property of automaticity. Because the SA node normally discharges faster than any other heart cell with automaticity (60–100 beats/min), this specialized tissue acts as a normal cardiac pacemaker. Atrial action potentials travel through atrial cells by intercalated disks, although some specialized conductive tissue in the atria has been discovered.

In the lower right portion of the interatrial septum is the atrioventricular (AV) node. This tissue conducts, yet delays, the atrial action potential before it travels to the ventricles. Action potentials reach the AV node at different times. The AV node slows conduction of these action potentials until all potentials have exited the atria and entered the AV node. After this slight delay, the AV node passes the action potential all at once to the ventricular conduction tissue, allowing for nearly simultaneous contraction of all ventricular cells. This AV node delay also allows time for the atria to eject fully their load of blood into the ventricles in preparation for ventricular systole.

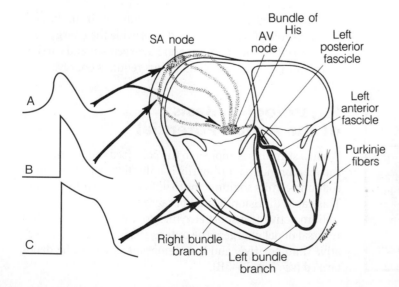

FIGURE 15-4
Conduction system of the heart and action potentials. (**A**) Action potential of sinoatrial (SA) and atrioventricular (AV) nodes. (**B**) Atrial muscle action potential. (**C**) Action potential of ventricular muscle and Purkinje fibers. (From Porth CM: Pathophysiology: Concepts of Altered Health States [4th Ed.]. Philadelphia, JB Lippincott, 1994)

From the AV node, the impulse travels down the bundle of His in the interventricular septum into either a right or left bundle branch and then through one of many Purkinje fibers to the ventricular myocardial tissue itself. An action potential can traverse this conducting tissue three to seven times more rapidly than it can travel through the ventricular myocardium. Thus, the bundle branches, and Purkinje fibers enable a near-simultaneous contraction of all portions of the ventricle, thereby allowing a maximal unified pump action to occur.

ELECTROCARDIOGRAMS

Conduction of an action potential through the heart can be shown by an electrocardiogram (ECG; Fig. 15–5). Because ECGs are extensively covered in a later chapter, discussion here is brief. An ECG does not show mechanical events of the heart, but in the normal heart, coupling of electrical and mechanical events can be assumed (see Chapter 16).

In Figure 15–5, point 1 shows early ventricular diastole, when the atria and ventricles are at rest. Blood is passively filling both atria from the large veins and is spilling over into the ventricles. The AV valves are open.

At point 2, the beginning of late ventricular diastole, both ventricles remain relaxed and are about three-quarters full.

Due to automaticity, the SA node fires spontaneously, and both atria depolarize, generating a P wave. Blood is moved actively from the atria into the ventricles.

At point 3, late in the PR interval, the action potential begun in the SA node is being delayed and "collected" in the AV node and travels to the bundle of His. The atria and ventricles are at rest.

At point 4, the action potential moves to the septum, which depolarizes and leads to the Q wave. Septal depolarization is rapidly followed by action potential movement down the right and left bundles into the Purkinje fibers, to all cardiac muscle cells. These electrical events are seen as the RS waves on the ECG and are followed rapidly by me-

chanical contraction of both ventricles. The AV valves close, and the aortic and pulmonic valves open.

At point 5, the heart returns to early ventricular diastole, and the ventricles repolarize. This repolarization shows as a large, wide T wave. The aortic and pulmonic valves close about midway through repolarization.

RHYTHMICITY AND PACING

Automaticity is an inherent property of myocardial conduction cells and occurs as a result of a spontaneous and rhythmic inactivation of the sodium pumps. Under abnormal conditions, cardiac muscle cells also gain automaticity and can produce their own rhythmic series of action potentials and thus their own stimulus for contraction. Coordination of automaticity is important for rhythmic cardiac contraction and is achieved through the varying rates of automaticity found in different cardiac tissues.

The SA node discharges normally in an adult at a resting rate of 60 to 100 times per minute. The remainder of the conduction system and ventricles have progressively slower rates of firing. The AV node discharges at a rate of 40 to 60 times per minute. The conduction tissues in the ventricles fire about 20 to 40 times per minute. The group of cells with the fastest rate of automaticity paces the heart. Normally, this is the SA node.

If conduction from the SA node to the AV node is disrupted, the fastest pacemaker tissue on both sides of this interruption will govern their respective areas, and the ECG may show independent atrial and ventricular rhythms. Atrial systole is not needed for the ventricle to fill with blood because most ventricular filling is passive and occurs in early diastole. The clinically important rhythm is that of the ventricles; they are the chambers that supply the lungs and the rest of the body with blood. Their systolic rate helps determine true perfusion. The slower the rate, the less able are the ventricles to meet the perfusion needs of the body during exercise or activities of daily living. A very rapid ventricular rhythm also will compromise perfusion needs, because the shorter the diastole, the less time for filling of the chambers. Decreased ventricular filling will reduce cardiac output (CO).

CARDIAC OUTPUT

A traditional measure of cardiac function, CO is the amount of blood, in liters, ejected from the left ventricle each minute. CO is the product of heart rate and stroke volume, which is the volume of blood ejected per ventricular contraction:

$$CO = HR \text{ (beats/min)} \times SV \text{ (liters/beat)}$$

Normal CO for an adult ranges from 4 to 8 L/min. The output can be altered to meet changing bodily demands for tissue perfusion, but the cardiac output equation does not

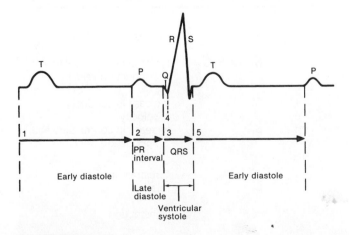

FIGURE 15-5

A comparison of electrical and mechanical events during one cardiac cycle, using a normal electrocardiogram tracing.

account for differences in body size. An output of 5 may be adequate for a 50-kg man but insufficient for a 120-kg man. Because perfusion is a function of body size, a more accurate measure of cardiac function is cardiac index (CI), which represents the amount of blood, in liters, ejected each minute from the left ventricle (or CO) per square meter of body surface area. CI typically averages 3.0 ± 0.2 L/min and ranges from 2.8 to 4.2 L/min/m^2.

$$CI = \frac{CO \ (liters/min)}{body \ surface \ area \ (m^2)}$$

Regulation of Heart Rate

Although the heart has the ability to beat independently of any extrinsic influence, cardiac rate is under autonomic and adrenal catecholamine influence. Parasympathetic and sympathetic fibers innervate the SA and AV nodes. In addition, some sympathetic fibers terminate in myocardial tissues.

Parasympathetic stimulation releases acetylcholine near the nodal cells and decreases the rate of depolarization, thereby slowing cardiac rate. Stimulation of sympathetic fibers causes the release of norepinephrine. This chemical increases the rate of nodal depolarization and has inotropic effects on myocardial fibers, which are discussed later. Thus, sympathetic stimulation increases heart rate (Table 15–1). The adrenal medulla also releases norepinephrine and epinephrine into the bloodstream. These circulating catecholamines act on the heart in the same way as sympathetic stimulation.

Two reflexes adjust heart rate to blood pressure: the aortic reflex and the Bainbridge reflex. In the aortic reflex (Fig. 15–6A), a rise in arterial blood pressure stimulates aortic and carotid sinus baroreceptors to fire sensory impulses to the cardioregulatory center in the medulla. The result is an increase in parasympathetic stimulation or a decrease in sympathetic stimulation to the heart. Thus, a rise in arterial blood pressure reflexively causes a slowing of cardiac rate. The decrease in heart rate results in a decrease in output, which can decrease arterial blood pressure. Conversely, a fall in arterial blood pressure, such as in shock, will reflexively increase heart rate. This aortic reflex is an ongoing regulatory mechanism for homeostasis of arterial blood pressure.

The Bainbridge reflex (see Fig. 15–6B) uses receptors in the venae cavae. An increase in venous return stimulates these receptors, which then fire sensory impulses that travel to the cardioregulatory center. These reflexively cause a decrease in parasympathetic cardiac stimulation and an increase in sympathetic cardiac stimulation, thereby increasing cardiac rate. A fall in venous return causes a decrease in heart rate. Thus, the Bainbridge reflex adjusts cardiac rate to handle venous return.

Regulation of Stroke Volume

Stroke volume is the amount of blood ejected by the left ventricle during systole. Normal values range from 60 to 100 mL/beat. Three factors are involved: preload, afterload (or wall tension), and inherent inotropic myocardial contractility.

TABLE 15-1
α and β Effects of Autonomic Nervous System on the Heart and Vascularity

Effector Organ	Cholinergic Impulses Response	Noradrenergic Impulses	
		Receptor Type	Response
Heart			
Sinoatrial node	Decrease in heart rate; vagal arrest	β_1	Increase in heart rate
Atria	Decrease in contractility and (usually) increase in conduction velocity	β_1	Increase in contractility and conduction velocity
Atrioventricular (AV) node and conduction system	Decrease in conduction velocity; AV block	β_1	Increase in conduction velocity
Ventricles	—	β_1	Increase in contractility and conduction velocity
Arterioles			
Coronary, skeletal muscle, pulmonary, abdominal viscera, renal	Dilation	α β_2	Constriction Dilation
Skin and mucosa, cerebral, salivary glands	—	α	Constriction
Systemic Veins	—	α β_2	Constriction Dilation

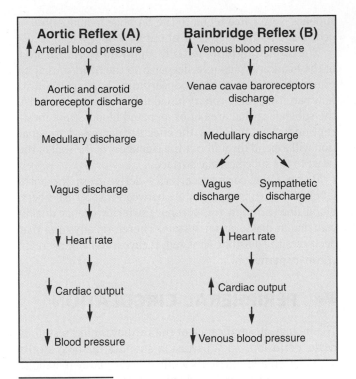

FIGURE 15-6
Effects of (**A**) aortic reflex and (**B**) Bainbridge reflex on heart rate.

PRELOAD

Preload is the amount of stretch placed on a cardiac muscle fiber just before systole. Usually, the amount of stretch in any chamber is proportional to the volume of blood the chamber contains at the end of diastole, before systole.

The concept of preload is related to Starling's law of the heart, which states that the force of myocardial contraction is determined by the length of the muscle cell fibers. Within a certain range (0.05–2.2 μm), increasing myofibril stretch will increase the force of systole. Beyond optimal fibril length (about 2.2 μm), it is hypothesized that too few actin–myosin binding sites overlap to provide an adequate contraction. Below optimal shortening (about 0.05 μm), there is little room for filaments to slide, and cell walls limit further sliding. Also, actin filaments may have begun to overlap, decreasing the number of binding sites available to myosin fibers.

When the force of systole decreases, the chamber pumps poorly and does not empty properly. Excessive blood is left in the chamber at the end of systole. During diastole, when the chamber fills, this extra blood causes overfilling of the chamber and increases stretch. The next systole will be even weaker, as preload increases during every diastole.

Because preload is affected by the volume at the end of diastole, it often is equated with end-diastolic volume or pressure. Thus, left ventricular preload is represented by left ventricular end-diastolic pressure.

An example of rapid and normal adjustments to changes in preload occurs during the Valsalva maneuver. The first part of the Valsalva occurs when one holds one's breath and bears down, such as during defecation or heavy lifting. Bearing down increases intra-abdominal and intrathoracic pressures, decreasing venous return to the right atrium and ventricle. Right heart preload decreases. Bearing down also stimulates the vagus nerve, and the heart rate slows.

On exhalation, during the second part of the Valsalva maneuver, intrathoracic pressures decrease rapidly, allowing a sudden increase in venous return. Right atrial and ventricular preloads increase dramatically, stretch increases, and the right ventricular stroke volume increases. Atrial stretch receptors also signal the medulla and lead to sympathetic nervous discharge. Heart rate increases.

AFTERLOAD

Afterload is the force or pressure against which a cardiac chamber must eject blood during systole. The most critical factor determining afterload is vascular resistance, in the systemic or pulmonic vessels. Afterload often is equated with systemic vascular resistance or pulmonary vascular resistance.

Afterload affects stroke volume by increasing or decreasing the ease of emptying a ventricle during systole. A decrease in systemic vascular resistance, through vasodilation, presents the left ventricle with relatively large, open, relaxed arteries into which it can pump. Because it is easier to pump, the left ventricles will empty easily, which increases stroke volume.

If systemic vascular resistance increases, for example through catecholamine-induced constriction of arteries, it takes a great deal more force for the left ventricle to pump into such a tightened vasculature. Stroke volume will decrease.

CONTRACTILITY

Inotropic capabilities and cardiac workload refer to contractile forces. Cardiac muscle forces change in response to neural stimuli and circulating levels of catecholamines. It is thought that through cyclic adenosine monophosphate mechanisms, cardiac cells change intracellular levels of calcium and ATP. These changes lead to increased inotropic actions, although the mechanisms remain unknown.

However, increased inotropic action increases the oxygen consumption of heart cells. This increased consumption also is called increased workload and increased oxygen demand.

Cardiac output depends on heart rate and stroke volume. Regardless of the initial cause of increased stroke volume (increased preload, increased afterload, or increased inotropic force), an increase in stroke volume increases workload. Similarly, an increased heart rate, no matter what the cause, increases oxygen demand.

CORONARY CIRCULATION

Blood supply to the myocardium is derived from the two main coronary arteries, the left and the right (Fig. 15–7). These arteries originate from the aorta, immediately above the aortic valve. The left main coronary artery has two major branches known as the left anterior descending (LAD) and the left circumflex (LCA). The LAD passes down the anterior wall of the left ventricle toward the apex of the myocardium. The LAD supplies blood flow to the anterior two thirds of the ventricular septum, the anterior left ventricle, the apex, and most of the bundle branches (Table 15–2).

The LCA, the other branch of the left main coronary artery, sits in the groove between the left atrium and the left ventricle and wraps around to the posterior wall of the heart. The LCA supplies blood flow to the left atrium, the lateral wall of the left ventricle, and the posterior wall of the left ventricle. In about 10% of the population, the LCA is the source of blood flow to the posterior descending coronary artery; when this pattern of flow occurs, the patient is referred to as left dominant. Branches of the LCA provide blood flow to the SA node in about 45% of people and to the AV node in about 10% of people.

The right coronary artery (RCA) also comes off the aorta and branches toward the right atrium; the anterior, lateral, and posterior regions of the right ventricle; and the posterior ventricular septum. The RCA provides blood flow to the right atrium, the right ventricle, and the inferior wall of the left ventricle. In about 90% of the population, the RCA is the source of blood flow to the posterior descending coronary artery, a pattern of flow known as right dominant. The RCA

supplies oxygenated blood to the SA node in about 55% of people and to the AV node in about 90% of people.

The coronary arteries initially supply the epicardial layer of the heart and then pass deeper into the heart muscle to provide blood flow to the endocardium. As a result of this flow pattern, poor coronary blood flow will initially deprive the subendocardial area of oxygenated blood. If the interruption to flow continues, the effects of decreased oxygenation will expand throughout the thickness of the wall of the heart to the subepicardial surface.

Because the coronary arteries derive from the aorta (above the aortic valve) and lie between myocardial fibers, blood flow through the coronary arteries occurs during ventricular diastole, not systole. Therefore, anything that decreases the diastolic time (eg, tachycardia) will decrease coronary perfusion.

PERIPHERAL CIRCULATION

The biological significance of the cardiovascular system is tissue perfusion. Such perfusion supplies the body's cells with oxygen and nutrients while carrying away metabolic wastes, including carbon dioxide. Tissue perfusion is directly proportional to the rate of blood flow, which depends on several factors. One factor is the difference between the mean arterial blood pressure and right atrial pressure (usually represented by the central venous pressure [CVP]). The greater this difference, the faster the flow rate (all else being unchanged). Conversely, if arterial pressure falls or venous pressure rises, flow rate, and thus tissue perfusion, will be decreased.

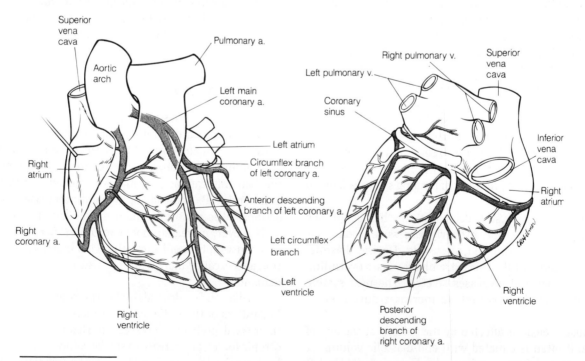

FIGURE 15-7
Coronary circulation through coronary arteries and some of the coronary sinus veins. (From Porth CM: Pathophysiology: Concepts of Altered Health States [4th Ed]. Philadelphia, JB Lippincott, 1994)

TABLE 15-2
Coronary Artery Blood Supply for Cardiac Muscle and Conducting System

Coronary Artery	Cardiac Muscle Supplied	Conducting Tissue Supplied
Left Main Coronary Artery		
Left anterior descending	Anterior ventricular septum Anterior left ventricle The apex	Bundle branches
Left circumflex	Left atrium Left ventricular lateral wall Left ventricular posterior wall	Sinoatrial node in 45% of hearts Atrioventricular node in 10% of hearts
Right Coronary Artery	Right atrium Right ventricle Posterior ventricular septum Inferior wall of left ventricle	Sinoatrial node in 55% of hearts Atrioventricular node in 90% of hearts

Another factor affecting flow rate is vascular resistance. The relationship between vascular resistance and blood flow has two general applications. One is to describe the flow rate through vessels of differing diameters (eg, arteries, capillaries). The other application concerns the ongoing regulation of blood flow by means of adjustments in arteriole diameters (ie, constriction, dilation). Arteriole constriction reduces the radius, thereby increasing resistance and decreasing the flow rate. Conversely, arteriole dilation increases the flow rate.

The other two factors that can affect the flow rate normally are held constant. They are the sum of all vessel lengths and blood viscosity. Because these factors do not normally change significantly, they usually are omitted from flow rate considerations. Their relationships are obvious, however. The greater the length of a vessel, the more resistance and thus the slower the flow rate. Also, the more viscous the blood, the slower the rate of its flow. Blood viscosity is determined by the proportion of solvent (water) to solute and other particles, including blood cells and platelets. The less water and more particles that exist, the more viscous is the blood. The complete equation that describes all four factors is as follows:

$$\text{flow rate} = \frac{\text{mean arterial pressure} - \text{central venous pressure}}{\text{resistance} \times \text{viscosity} \times \text{vessel length}}$$

Because blood volume and pressure have such an important influence on tissue perfusion, the factors that alter and regulate them are examined.

Blood Volume

Urinary output and fluid input are the major normal mechanisms for regulating volume. If output is greater or fluid input is less, the volume is less—if all else is held constant. Factors that alter the volume of urine excreted every 24 hours include those that alter the glomerular filtration rate and the tubular reabsorption of water, with or without electrolytes. (For a more detailed explanation of these factors, see Chapter 41, specifically the discussion of normal endocrine physiology that considers the antidiuretic hormone.) Pathological conditions that promote any type of fluid loss (eg, burns, severe diarrhea, osmotic diuresis) or a shift of water from the vascular to the interstitial compartment have the potential for reducing blood volume.

Blood Pressure

Because the difference between arterial and venous pressures is the driving force for blood circulation and tissue perfusion, factors that influence CVP are examined first and then the factors that regulate arterial blood pressure. CVP is, strictly speaking, the pressure of blood in the venae cavae just before its entry into the right atrium. CVP can be increased by an increase in blood volume (eg, intravenous fluid overload) or a decrease in the pumping ability of the heart (eg, cardiac failure). Because the pulsatile effects of the cardiac cycle are removed by capillary networks, venous pressure is recorded as an average, or mean, and reported in millimeters of mercury (mmHg).

Arterial blood pressure is the pressure of blood in the arteries and arterioles. This is a pulsatile pressure due to the cardiac cycle, and systolic (peak) and diastolic (trough) numbers are reported in millimeters of mercury. Average or mean arterial blood pressure can be clinically useful as an indicator of average perfusion pressures.

Arterial blood pressure is regulated by the vasomotor tone of the arteries and arterioles, the amount of blood entering the arteries per systole (ie, cardiac output), and blood volume itself. The greater the volume or output, the greater would be the blood pressure, and vice versa, if vasomotor tone were held constant. The normal regulation of vasomotor tone involves neural and hormonal mechanisms.

Neural regulation is mediated by the vasomotor center of the medulla oblongata. This center consists of vasopressor and depressor subdivisions. The vasomotor center receives neural input from baroreceptors in the carotid sinuses and aorta, atrial diastolic stretch receptors, the limbic system and hypothalamus, the midbrain, and pulmonary stretch receptors. In addition, the center is directly responsive to local hypoxia or hypercapnia. Neural outputs from the vasopressor center result in increased sympathetic stimulation to arterial smooth muscle cells. This increase in sympathetic stimulation results in arterial constriction and a rise in arterial blood pressure. Stimulation of the depressor area decreases such sympathetic stimulation.

Rapid adjustments in arterial blood pressure are affected primarily by the baroreceptor reflexes. An increase in the pressure on these receptors (directly by elevated blood pressure or manual compression and indirectly by increased blood volume) reflexively stimulates the depressor area. This stimulation of the depressor area results in decreased sympathetic stimulation to major arteries and the aorta, which causes a fall in arterial blood pressure. Decreased baroreceptor stimulation by a fall in arterial blood pressure reflexively stimulates the pressor area and results in increased sympathetic stimulation to arterial muscles, causing a rise in arterial blood pressure. Thus, homeostasis of arterial pressure is maintained.

In orthostatic hypotension, the baroreceptor reflex is sluggish. Arterial pressure is not elevated rapidly enough, so the postural change results in a temporary decrease in brain perfusion that leads, in extreme cases, to syncope.

Various other factors may alter arterial blood pressure reflexively by their influences on the vasomotor center. Nerve fibers from the limbic system and hypothalamus are believed to mediate emotionally produced alterations in blood pressure. An example of this is fainting, caused by neurally mediated vasodilation in response to the sight of blood or very bad (or good) news. Neural inputs from the midbrain and possibly from ascending spinothalamic fibers in the medulla result in the elevation in arterial pressure that initially accompanies severe pain and in the later fall in arterial pressure that occurs when severe pain is prolonged. Lung inflation stimulates pulmonary stretch receptors. Their input to the vasomotor center reflexively decreases arterial pressure. Hypercapnia and to a lesser extent, hypoxia of vasomotor neurons stimulate the pressor area, reflexively causing a rise in arterial pressure. Such stimuli obviously are not part of a normal daily regulatory mechanism but can operate as a normal compensatory mechanism in certain pathological situations. Elevated intracranial pressure can promote medullary hypercapnia and hypoxia. The increase in arterial pressure reflexively produced by these stimuli (Cushing's reflex) increases medullary perfusion, which can ameliorate the medullary hypoxia or hypercapnia or both. Hormonal regulation of arterial blood pressure is affected by adrenal medulla catecholamines and the renin–angiotensin system. In the former, adrenal medullary catecholamines mimic the action of sympathetic fibers innervating the muscle layer or arteries (tunica media),

causing arterial constriction and elevating arterial pressure. The renin–angiotensin system is discussed in Chapter 27. Briefly, a decreased glomerular filtration rate, which can result, for example, from a fall in blood volume or renal perfusion, stimulates the secretion of renin from the juxtaglomerular apparatus. This stimulation of renin leads to the production of angiotensin II, which acts directly on tunica media to promote vasoconstriction. Thus, renin elevates arterial pressure, which increases renal perfusion and glomerular filtration.

Finally, arterial blood pressure can be influenced by alterations in the level of unbound calcium within tunica media cells. Such levels are influenced by factors that open or close calcium channels in the membranes of these muscle cells. Drugs that block calcium channels ("calcium blockers") inhibit the entry of calcium into cells. Such decreased calcium influx can lower intracellular calcium levels sufficiently to decrease muscle contractility, including contractility of the heart, thereby promoting a degree of vasodilation and lowering the arterial pressure.

Clinical Applicability Challenges

Self-Challenge: Critical Thinking

Mr. Smith has been diagnosed with a 90% occlusion of his RCA. Describe which anatomical walls of the heart are affected. Explain which parts of his cardiac conducting system may be affected by the occlusion.

Study Questions

1. Preload refers to
   a. the pressure against which the cardiac chamber must eject blood during systole.
   b. cardiac workload.
   c. the amount of stretch placed on the cardiac muscle fiber just before systole.
   d. the amount of stretch placed on the cardiac muscle fiber just before diastole.

2. Cardiac output is determined by
   a. heart rate times stroke volume.
   b. heart rate times end-diastolic volume.
   c. stroke volume plus end-diastolic volume.
   d. afterload times preload.

3. The LAD coronary artery supplies
   a. the anterior portion of the right ventricle.
   b. the anterior portion of the left ventricle.
   c. the right atrium.
   d. the AV node.

4. In the normal heart, the impulse for cardiac contraction originates in the
   a. AV node.
   b. Purkinje fibers.
   c. bundle of His.
   d. SA node.

BIBLIOGRAPHY

Bullock BL: Pathophysiology: Adaptations and Alterations in Function (4th Ed). Philadelphia, Lippincott-Raven, 1996

Ganong WF: Review of Medical Physiology (16th Ed). Norwalk, CT, Appleton & Lange Medical Publications, 1995

Guyton AC: Textbook of Medical Physiology (9th Ed). Philadelphia, WB Saunders, 1996

Hall-Craggs EC: Anatomy as a Basis for Clinical Medicine (3rd Ed). Baltimore, Williams and Wilkins, 1995

Hole JW Jr: Essentials of Human Anatomy and Physiology (5th Ed). Dubuque, IA, WC Brown, 1994

Lindsay DT: Functional Human Anatomy. St. Louis, Mosby-Year Book, 1996

Memmler RL: Human Body in Health and Disease (8th Ed). Philadelphia, Lippincott-Raven, 1996

Porth CM: Pathophysiology: Concepts of Altered Health States (4th Ed). Philadelphia, JB Lippincott, 1994

Thibodeau GA: Anatomy and Physiology (3rd Ed). St. Louis, Mosby, 1996

16

Patient Assessment: Cardiovascular System

(continued)

OBJECTIVES

Based on the content in this chapter, the reader should be able to:

- Explain the components of the cardiovascular history.
- Describe the steps of the cardiovascular physical examination.
- Discuss the mechanisms responsible for the production of the first and second heart sounds and the phases of the cardiac cycle these sounds represent.
- Discuss the clinical significance of the third and fourth heart sounds and their timing in the cardiac cycle.
- Describe each type of murmur, its timing in the cardiac cycle, and the area on the chest wall where it is most easily auscultated.
- Describe the role of enzyme studies in diagnosing an acute myocardial infarction.
- Compare and contrast the usefulness of creatine kinase (CK) and lactate dehydrogenase (LDH) isoenzyme studies.
- List possible etiologies of serum CK and LDH elevations other than acute myocardial infarction–ischemia.
- Interpret CK and LDH isoenzyme studies when providing patient care.
- Discuss the usefulness of myoglobin and troponin assay determination.
- Describe four current techniques used for diagnostic purposes in cardiology.
- Outline the patient and family teaching appropriate to prepare the patient for exercise electrocardiogram (ECG) studies.
- Explain the preparation necessary before cardiac catheterization.
- Outline the nursing care to be delivered during and after exercise ECG and cardiac catheterization.
- List potential complications of invasive cardiac studies, such as cardiac catheterization.
- Explain the major features of an ECG monitoring system.

- Compare and contrast a hard-wire monitoring system with a telemetry monitoring system.
- Explain correct electrode placement when monitoring the standard leads or the chest leads with a three-electrode system.
- Describe correct electrode placement when monitoring a patient with a four- or five-electrode system.
- Identify approaches for troubleshooting ECG monitor problems.
- List priorities in caring for the patient undergoing ECG monitoring.
- Describe the components of the electrocardiographic tracing and their meaning.
- Explain the steps used to interpret a rhythm strip.
- Describe the etiologies, clinical significance, and treatment for each of the dysrhythmias discussed.
- Discuss the nursing management for patients exhibiting dysrhythmia disturbances.
- Describe the criteria of a normal 12-lead ECG.
- Define electrical axis, and determine the direction of the axis for a 12-lead ECG.
- Explain the etiologies, clinical significance, and treatment for bundle branch blocks, atrial enlargement, and ventricular hypertrophy.
- Describe the ECG changes associated with serum potassium and calcium abnormalities.
- Analyze the characteristics of normal systemic arterial, right atrial, right ventricular, pulmonary artery, and pulmonary artery wedge pressure waveforms.
- Describe the system components required to monitor hemodynamic pressures.
- State nursing interventions that ensure accuracy of pressure readings.
- Discuss the major complications that can occur with an indwelling arterial line and pulmonary artery catheter.
- Describe the thermodilution method of measuring cardiac output.
- Identify the determinants of cardiac output.

- Evaluate the factors influencing oxygen delivery and consumption.
- Use $S\overline{v}O_2$ monitoring to assess oxygen delivery and consumption.

Complex technologies to assess and manage cardiovascular and cardiopulmonary conditions have increased greatly in the last several decades. Technological assessment techniques are discussed in this chapter. Use of these advanced and complex technologies is an integral part of the care of critically ill patients. Nevertheless, the value of a comprehensive cardiovascular history and physical examination should never be underestimated. The chapter begins with a discussion of the cardiac history and physical examination.

Cardiac History and Physical Examination

The cardiovascular history provides physiological and psychosocial information that guides the physical assessment, the selection of diagnostic tests, and the choice of treatment options. During the history, the nurse asks about the presenting symptoms, past health history, current health status, risk factors, and social and personal history. The nurse also inquires about behaviors that promote or jeopardize cardiovascular health and uses this information in guiding health teaching. During the process of taking a thorough history and performing a physical examination, the nurse has an opportunity to establish rapport with the patient and to evaluate the patient's general emotional status.

■ HISTORY

The nurse begins the history by investigating the patient's chief complaint. The patient is asked to describe in his or her own words the problem or reason for seeking care. The nurse then asks for more information about the present illness, including the onset of the problem, its manifestations, and the results of any attempts to resolve the problem. Common cardiovascular symptoms should be investigated in more detail and often include chest pain, dyspnea, edema of feet/ankles, palpitations and syncope, cough and hemoptysis, nocturia, cyanosis, and intermittent claudication.

Presenting Symptoms

CHEST PAIN

Chest pain is one of the most common symptoms of patients with cardiovascular disease. Therefore, it is an essential component of the assessment interview. Chest pain is often a disturbing or even frightening experience for a patient, so the patient may be hesitant to initiate a discussion of chest pain. The accompanying display offers an organized approach to the comprehensive assessment of any symptom and is particularly useful when assessing chest pain.

Because cardiac pain (angina pectoris) is the result of an imbalance between oxygen supply and oxygen demand, it usually builds over time. Typically anginal pain does not start at maximal intensity. Not all chest pain is cardiac in origin. This indicates that careful reporting of the characteristics of the pain and the behaviors (or lack thereof) that precede the onset of pain is required.

Chest pain caused by coronary artery disease is often *precipitated* by physical or emotional exertion, a meal, or being out in the cold. *Palliative* measures to relieve anginal pain may include rest or sublingual nitrates, whereas the pain of a myocardial infarction (MI) usually is not relieved by these measures. The *quality* of cardiac chest pain is often described as a heaviness, tightness, squeezing, or choking sensation. If the pain is reported as superficial, knifelike, or throbbing, it is not likely to be anginal. Cardiac chest pain is usually located in the substernal *region* and often *radiates* to the neck, left arm, or jaw. Although the pain is often referred to other areas, anginal pain is visceral in origin and most complaints will include a reference to a "deep, inside" pain. When asked to point to the painful area, it is unusual for true anginal pain to be localized to an area smaller than a fingertip. Rather, the painful area is around the size of a hand or clenched fist. Using a scale of 1 to 10 with 10 being the worst pain you have ever experienced, the patient is asked to rate the *severity* of the pain. When asked about

---

CLINICAL APPLICATION:
Assessment Parameters
The P, Q, R, S, T Approach to Symptom Assessment for Chest Pain

P	**Precipitating and palliative factors:** Patients are asked to describe what brought on the pain and what measures have helped relieve the pain.
Q	**Quality:** Patients are asked to describe in their own words what the pain feels like.
R	**Region and radiation:** Patients are asked to point to the location of the pain and if the pain goes anywhere.
S	**Severity:** Patients are asked to rate the pain on a scale of 1 to 10 with 10 being the worst pain ever experienced.
T	**Time:** Patients are asked how long the pain lasts and any temporal associations.

time, the patient with cardiac chest pain reports the pain lasting anywhere from 30 seconds to hours.

Pain may be secondary to cardiovascular problems that are unrelated to a primary coronary insufficiency. Therefore, the nurse must consider other causes when obtaining the patient's history. For example, if the patient reports the pain is made worse by lying down, moving, or deep breathing, it may be caused by pericarditis. If the pain is retrosternal and accompanied by sudden shortness of breath and peripheral cyanosis, the patient may be suffering from a pulmonary embolism.

DYSPNEA

Dyspnea is found in patients with both pulmonary and cardiac abnormalities. In cardiac patients it is the result of inefficient pumping of the left ventricle, which causes a congestion of blood flow in the lungs. Dyspnea is differentiated during history taking from the usual breathlessness that follows a sudden burst of physical activity (eg, running up four flights of stairs, sprinting across a parking lot). Dyspnea is a subjective complaint of true *difficulty* in breathing, not just shortness of breath. The nurse determines whether the difficulty in breathing occurs only with exertion or also at rest. If dyspnea is present when the patient lies flat but is relieved by sitting or standing, it is termed *orthopnea*. *Paroxysmal nocturnal dyspnea* is characterized by breathing difficulties starting after approximately 1 to 2 hours of sleep and relieved by sitting upright or getting out of bed.

EDEMA OF THE FEET/ANKLES

Although many other problems can leave a patient with swollen feet or ankles, congestive heart failure (CHF) may also be responsible as the heart is unable to mobilize fluid appropriately. Because gravity promotes the movement of fluids from intravascular to extravascular spaces, the edema becomes worse as the day progresses and usually improves when lying down to sleep at night. Patients or families may report that shoes do not fit anymore, socks that used to be loose are now too tight, and the indentations from sock bands take more time than usual to disappear. The nurse should inquire about the timing of edema development (eg, immediately when lowering the extremities, only at the end of the day, only after a significant salt intake) and duration (eg, relieved with temporary elevation of the legs or requiring constant elevation).

PALPITATIONS AND SYNCOPE

Palpitations refer to the awareness of irregular or rapid heart beats. Patients may report the "skipping" of beats, a rushing of the heart, or a loud "thudding." The nurse asks about onset and duration of the palpitations, associated symptoms, and any precipitating events that the patient or family can remember. Because a cardiac dysrhythmia may compromise blood flow to the brain, the nurse asks about symptoms of dizziness, fainting, or syncope that accompany the palpitations.

COUGH AND HEMOPTYSIS

Abnormalities such as heart failure, pulmonary embolus, or mitral stenosis may cause a cough or hemoptysis. The nurse asks the patient about the presence of a cough or hemoptysis and inquires about the quality (wet or dry) and frequency of the cough (chronic or occasional, only when lying down or after exercise). If there is expectorant with the cough, the color, consistency, and amount as perceived by the patient should be recorded. If the patient reports spitting up blood, the nurse asks if the substance spit up was streaked with blood, frothy bloody sputum, or frank blood (bright or dark).

NOCTURIA

Kidneys that are inadequately perfused by an unhealthy heart during daytime may finally receive enough flow during rest at night to increase their output. The nurse asks about the number of times the patient urinates during the night. If the patient takes a diuretic, the nurse also evaluates frequency of urination in relation to the time of day the diuretic is taken.

CYANOSIS

Cyanosis reflects the oxygenation and circulatory status of the patient. *Central* cyanosis is generally distributed and best found by examining the mucous membranes for discoloration and duskiness; it reflects reduced oxygen concentration. *Peripheral* cyanosis is localized in the extremities and protrusions (hands, feet, nose, ears, lips) and reflects impaired circulation.

INTERMITTENT CLAUDICATION

Claudication results when the blood supply to exercising muscles is inadequate. Usually the cause of claudication is significant atherosclerotic obstruction to the lower extremities. The limb is asymptomatic at rest unless the obstruction is severe. Blood supply to the legs is inadequate to meet metabolic demands during exercise, and ischemic pain results. The patient describes a cramping, charley horse, ache, or weakness in the foot, calf, thigh, or buttocks that improves with rest. The patient should be asked to describe the severity of the pain and how much exertion is required to produce the pain.

Past Health History

When assessing the patient's past health history, the nurse inquires about previous illnesses, such as rheumatic fever, pneumonia, tuberculosis, thrombophlebitis, pulmonary embolism, MI, diabetes mellitus, thyroid disease, or chest injury. The nurse also asks about occupational exposures to cardiotoxic materials. Finally, the nurse seeks information about previous cardiac or vascular surgeries.

Current Health Status and Risk Factors

As part of the health history, the nurse queries the patient about use of prescription and over-the-counter medications, tobacco, drugs, and alcohol and about allergies. The nurse also asks about dietary habits, including usual daily intake, dietary restrictions or supplements, and intake of caffeine-containing foods or beverages. The patient's sleep pattern and exercise and leisure activities also are noted.

Assessment of risk factors for cardiovascular disease is an important component of the history. Risk factors are categorized as major risk factors that cannot be altered, major risk factors that can be altered, and contributing risk factors. The accompanying display summarizes risk factors. For a more detailed discussion of risk factors, see Chapter 20.

Social and Personal History

Although the physical symptoms provide many clues as to the origin and extent of cardiac disease, social and personal history also contribute to the patient's health status. The nurse inquires about the patient's family, spouse or significant other, and children. Information about the patient's living environment, daily life routine, coping patterns, and spiritual beliefs contributes to the nurse's understanding of the patient as a person and will guide the nurse in interacting with the patient and family.

■■■ PHYSICAL EXAMINATION

Cardiac assessment requires examination of all aspects of the individual, using the standard steps of inspection, palpation, percussion, and auscultation. A thorough and careful examination will help the nurse detect not only obvious, but subtle abnormalities as well.

RED FLAG

Risk Factors for Cardiovascular Disease

Major Risk Factors That Cannot Be Altered

Age: There is an increased incidence of all types of atherosclerotic disease with aging. Although 50% of all myocardial infarctions occur in people under the age of 65, 80% of people who die from the myocardial infarction are 65 years or older.[2]

Heredity: The tendency to develop atherosclerosis seems to run in families. The risk is thought to be a combination of environmental and genetic influences. Even when other risk factors are controlled, the chance of developing coronary artery disease increases when there is a familial tendency.[3, 4]

Gender: Men have a greater risk for developing coronary artery disease than women at earlier ages. After menopause, however, women's death rate from coronary disease rises.[2]

Major Risk Factors That Can Be Altered

Cigarette smoking: Smoking increases a patient's risk for peripheral vascular disease. A smoker's risk of sudden death is two to four times greater than the nonsmoker's risk. Smokers have twice the risk of having a myocardial infarction than nonsmokers. Smokers are more likely to die from the infarction. Exposure to environmental smoke also increases the risk of heart disease.[2]

A high blood cholesterol: Middle-aged adults with a blood cholesterol level below 200 mg/dL have a relatively low risk of coronary artery disease. A blood cholesterol level in the range of 200–239 mg/dL represents a moderate but increasing risk. When the level rises above 240 mg/dL, the risk of coronary artery disease is about double.[2]

Hypertension: Known as the "silent killer," hypertension is a risk factor with no specific symptoms and no early warning signs. Men have a greater risk for hypertension than women until the age of 55. The risk of developing hypertension is about the same for men and women between the ages of 55 and 75. After the age of 75, women are more likely to develop hypertension than men.[2] African Americans, Puerto Ricans, Cuban Americans, and Mexican Americans are more likely to have hypertension than white Americans.[5]

Physical inactivity: When lack of regular exercise is combined with overeating and obesity, high cholesterol can result and further increase the risk of heart disease. Even moderate levels of regular low-intensity exercise have been shown to be beneficial in the prevention of heart disease.[2]

Contributing Risk Factors

Diabetes mellitus: Diabetes doubles the likelihood of cardiovascular disease. The associated risk is greater for women than for men.[3] More than 80% of people with diabetes die of some form of heart or blood vessel disease.[2]

Obesity: There is an association between obesity and an increased mortality from coronary artery disease and stroke. Excess weight is also linked with an increased incidence of hypertension, insulin resistance, diabetes, and dyslipidemia.[3]

Psychosocial factors: A relationship has been noted between cardiovascular disease and stress, anxiety, social resources, depression, and cardiovascular reactivity.[3] These psychosocial factors may not be the cause of heart disease but contribute to its development because they affect established risk factors. For example, under stress, a person may be more likely to overeat or to smoke.

Inspection

GENERAL APPEARANCE

Inspection begins as soon as the patient and nurse interact. General appearance and presentation of the patient are key elements of the initial inspection. Critical examination reveals a first impression of age, nutritional status, self-care ability, alertness, and overall physical health.

The ability of the patient to move and speak with or without distress is noted, including posture, gait, and musculoskeletal coordination.

With closer examination, skin is evaluated for moistness or dryness, color, elasticity, edema, thickness, lesions, ulcerations, and vascular changes. Nailbeds are examined for cyanosis and clubbing, which may indicate chronic cardiac abnormalities. General differences in color and temperature between body parts may provide perfusion clues.

CHEST

The chest is inspected for signs of trauma or injury, symmetry, chest contour, and any visible point of maximal impulse (PMI). The PMI is nickel sized and should be located in the left fifth intercostal space in the midclavicular line. Thrusts (abnormally strong precordial pulsations) and thrills (palpable murmurs) are noted. Any depression (sternum excavatum) or bulging of the precordium is recorded.

JUGULAR VENOUS DISTENTION

The height of the level of blood in the right internal jugular vein is an indication of right atrial (RA) pressure because there are no valves or obstructions between the vein and the right atrium. Examination of the patient for the presence of jugular venous distention requires the nurse to position the patient at a 45-degree angle so that the column of blood in the internal jugular vein is visible in the neck. Using a light shining across the distended veins, the internal jugular vein is observed to determine the highest level of visible pulsation.

Next, the angle of Louis is located by palpating where the clavicle joins the sternum (the suprasternal notch). The nurse then slides the examining finger down the sternum until a bony prominence is felt. This prominence is known as the angle of Louis. A vertical ruler is placed on the angle of Louis. Another ruler is placed horizontally at the level of the pulsation. The intersection of the horizontal ruler with the vertical ruler is noted. The intersection point on the vertical ruler is read. Normal jugular venous pulsation should not exceed 3 cm above the angle of Louis.[1] See Figure 19–3 for an illustration of the procedure for assessment of jugular venous pressure. A level more than 3 cm above the angle of Louis indicates an abnormally high volume in the venous system. Possible causes include right sided heart failure, obstruction of the superior vena cava, pericardial effusion, and other cardiac or thoracic diseases. A rise in the jugular venous pressure of more than 1 cm while pressure is applied to the abdomen for 60 seconds (hepatojugular or abdominojugular test) indicates the inability of the heart to accommodate the increased venous return.

EXTREMITIES

A close inspection of the patient's extremities can also provide clues about cardiovascular health. The extremities are examined for lesions, ulcerations, unhealed sores, and varicose veins. Distribution of hair on the extremities also is noted. A lack of normal hair distribution on the extremities may indicate diminished arterial blood flow to the area.

Palpation

PULSES

Cardiovascular assessment continues with palpation and involves the use of the pads of the finger and balls of the hand. Using the pads of the fingers, the carotid, radial, brachial, femoral, popliteal, posterior tibialis, and posterior pedis pulses are palpated. The peripheral pulses are compared bilaterally to determine rate, rhythm, strength, and symmetry. The 0 to 3 scale described in the display is used to rate the strength of the pulse. The carotid pulses should never be assessed simultaneously because this can obstruct flow to the brain.

Pulses can also be described according to their characteristics. For example, pulsus alternans is a pulse that alternates in strength with every other beat; it is often found in patients with left ventricular failure. A pulse that disappears during inspiration but returns during expiration is called pulsus paradoxus. To determine if the condition is pathological, the sphygmomanometer is deflated until the pulse is heard only during expiration and the corresponding pressure noted. As the cuff continues to deflate, the point at which the pressure is heard *throughout* the inspiratory and expiratory cycle is noted. The second systolic pressure reading is subtracted from the first; if the difference is greater than 10 mmHg during normal respirations, it is considered pathological. During the assessment of pulses, compare the warmth and size of the palpated areas to monitor perfusion.

PRECORDIUM

The chest wall is palpated to assess for thrills, abnormal pulsations, and the location of the apical impulse. A systematic

---

Rating Scale Used for Assessing Strength of Pulses

0	Absent
1	Palpable but thready, weak, easily obliterated
2	Normal, not easily obliterated
3	Full, bounding, easily palpable, cannot obliterate

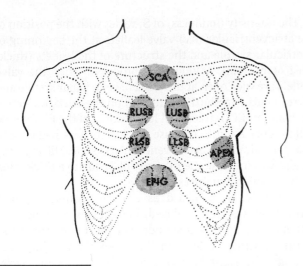

FIGURE 16-1

The seven precordial areas of the precordium. SCA = sterno-clavicular area; RUSB = right upper sternal border; RLSB = right lower sternal border; EPIG = epigastric; LUSB = left upper sternal border; LLSB = left lower sternal border.

palpation sequence is used that includes the seven precordial areas shown in Figure 16–1. Thrills, a fine vibration, are best felt through bone. After placing the patient flat, the seven precordial areas are palpated for thrills by placing the ball of the hand (bone) firmly against the chest. The location of the thrill provides clues as to the cause: If it is in the pulmonic area, the patient should be evaluated for pulmonary artery (PA) stenosis; if it is over the aorta, dilation of the aorta should be suspected. The nurse also palpates for abnormal pulsations in the chest that may be produced by accentuated heart sounds or murmurs. The apical pulse is palpated, noting its location, diameter, amplitude, and duration. Usually, the apical pulse is located in the midclavicular line at about the fourth or fifth intercostal space.

Percussion

With the advent of radiological means of evaluating cardiac size, percussion is not a significant contribution to cardiac assessment. However, a gross determination of heart size can be made by percussing for the dullness that will reflect the cardiac borders.

Auscultation

Data obtained by careful and thorough auscultation of the heart are essential in planning and evaluating care of the critically ill patient. In this section, the basic principles underlying cardiac auscultation, the factors responsible for the production of normal heart sounds, and the pathophysiological conditions responsible for the production of extra sounds, murmurs, and friction rubs are discussed.

To facilitate accurate auscultation, the patient should be relaxed and comfortable in a quiet warm environment with adequate lighting. The patient should be in a recumbent position with the trunk elevated 30 to 45 degrees.

A good-quality stethoscope is essential. The earpieces should fit the ears snugly and comfortably and follow the natural angle of the ear canals. Sound waves that travel a shorter distance are more intense and less distorted; therefore, the tubing of the stethoscope should be approximately 12 inches in length and somewhat rigid. It is best to have two tubes leading from the head of the stethoscope, one to each ear. The head of the stethoscope should be equipped with both a diaphragm and a bell on a valve system that allows the clinician to switch easily between the two components. The diaphragm is used to hear high-frequency sounds, such as the first and second heart sounds (S_1, S_2), friction rubs, systolic murmurs, and diastolic insufficiency murmurs. The diaphragm should be placed firmly on the chest wall to create a tight seal. Low-frequency sounds like the third and fourth heart sounds (S_3, S_4) and the diastolic murmurs of mitral and tricuspid stenosis are best heard with the stethoscope bell, which should be placed lightly on the chest wall only to seal the edges.

The precordium should be auscultated systematically (Fig. 16–2). The nurse should begin the examination by listening with the stethoscope diaphragm at the aortic area where S_2 is loudest, then move to the pulmonic area, and from there, inch the stethoscope down the left sternal border to the tricuspid area and out to the mitral area or apex of the heart, where S_1 is the loudest. This pattern should then be repeated with the stethoscope bell.

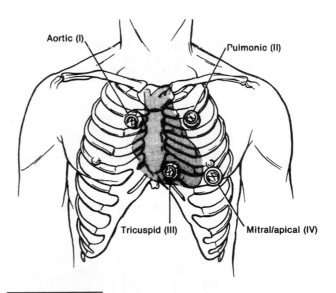

FIGURE 16-2

Areas of auscultation:
  I. Aortic area (second intercostal space to the right of the sternum)
 II. Pulmonic area (second intercostal space to the left of the sternum)
III. Tricuspid area (fifth intercostal space to the left of the sternum)
 IV. Mitral or apical area (fifth intercostal space midclavicular line)

In each area auscultated, the clinician should identify S_1, noting the intensity of the sound, respiratory variation, and splitting. S_2 should then be identified and the same characteristics assessed. After S_1 and S_2 are identified, the presence of extra sounds is noted—first in systole, then in diastole. Finally, each area is auscultated for the presence of murmurs and friction rubs.

FIRST HEART SOUND

S_1 (Fig. 16–3) is timed with the closure of the mitral and tricuspid valves at the beginning of ventricular systole. Because mitral valve closure is responsible for most of the sound produced, S_1 is heard best in the mitral or apical area. The upstroke of the carotid pulse correlates with S_1 and can be used to help distinguish S_1 from S_2.

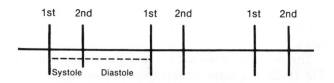

Normal: S_1 is produced by the closure of the AV valves and correlates with the beginning of ventricular systole. It is heard best in the apical or mitral area.

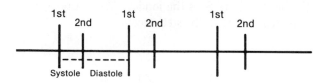

Loud First Sound: The intensity of the first heart sound may be increased when the PR interval is shortened, as in tachycardia, or when the valve leaflets are thickened, as in mitral stenosis.

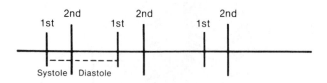

Soft First Sound: A soft S_1 is heard when the PR interval is prolonged.

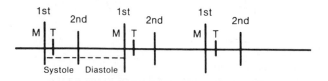

Split First Sound: A split S_1 is heard when right ventricular emptying is delayed. The mitral valve closes before the tricuspid valve and "splits" the sound into its two components.

FIGURE 16-3
Variations in the first heart sound.

The intensity (loudness) of S_1 varies with the position of the atrioventricular (AV) valve leaflets at the beginning of ventricular systole and the structure of the leaflets (thickened or normal). A loud S_1 is produced when the valve leaflets are wide open at the onset of ventricular systole and corresponds to a short PR interval on the surface electrocardiogram (ECG) tracing. A lengthening of the PR interval will produce a soft S_1 because the leaflets have had time to float partially closed before ventricular systole. Mitral stenosis also will increase the intensity of S_1 due to a thickening of the valvular structures.

Generally, S_1 is heard as a single sound. If right ventricular systole is delayed, however, S_1 may be split into its two component sounds. The most common cause of this splitting is delay in the conduction of impulses through the right bundle branch; the splitting correlates with a right bundle branch block (RBBB) pattern on the ECG. Splitting of S_1 is heard best over the tricuspid area.

SECOND HEART SOUND

S_2 (Fig. 16–4) is produced by the vibrations initiated by the closure of the aortic and pulmonic semilunar valves and is heard best at the base of the heart. This sound represents the beginning of ventricular diastole.

Like S_1, S_2 consists of two separate components. The first component of S_2 is aortic valve closure; the second component is pulmonic valve closure.

With inspiration, systole of the right ventricle is slightly prolonged owing to increased filling of the right ventricle. This causes the pulmonic valve to close later than the aortic valve and S_2 to become "split" into its two components. This normal finding is termed *physiological splitting*. Physiological splitting is heard best on inspiration with the stethoscope placed in the second intercostal space to the left of the sternum.

The intensity of S_2 may be increased in the presence of aortic or pulmonic valvular stenosis or with an increase in the diastolic pressure forcing the semilunar valves to close, as occurs in pulmonary or systemic hypertension.

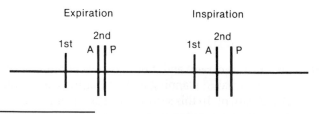

FIGURE 16-4
The second heart sound is produced by the closure of the semilunar valves (aortic and pulmonary). During inspiration, there is an increase in venous return to the right heart, which causes a delay in the emptying of the right ventricle and the closure of the pulmonic valve. This allows the two components of the second heart sound to separate or split during inspiration.

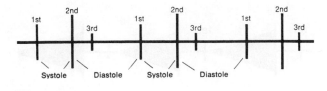

FIGURE 16-5
The third heart sound. An S$_3$ or ventricular gallop is heard in early diastole, shortly after the second heart sound. The presence of a pathological S$_3$ can be indicative of heart failure.

THIRD HEART SOUND

S$_3$ (Fig. 16–5) may be physiological or pathological. A physiological S$_3$ is a normal finding in children and healthy young adults; it usually disappears after 25 to 35 years of age. An S$_3$ heard in an older adult with heart disease signifies ventricular failure. S$_3$ is a low-frequency sound that occurs during the early, rapid-filling phase of ventricular diastole. A noncompliant or failing ventricle cannot distend to accept this rapid inflow of blood. This causes turbulent flow, resulting in the vibration of the AV valvular structures or the ventricles themselves, producing a low-frequency sound. An S$_3$ associated with left ventricular failure is heard best at the apex with the stethoscope bell. The sound may be accentuated by turning the patient slightly to the left side. A right ventricular S$_3$ is heard best at the xiphoid or lower left sternal border and varies in intensity with respiration, becoming louder on inspiration.

FOURTH HEART SOUND

S$_4$ or atrial gallop (Fig. 16–6) is a low-frequency sound heard late in diastole just before S$_1$. It is rarely heard in healthy patients. The sound is produced by atrial contraction forcing blood into a noncompliant ventricle that, by virtue of its noncompliance, has an increased resistance to filling. Systemic hypertension, MI, angina, cardiomyopathy, and aortic stenosis all may produce a decrease in left ventricular compliance and an S$_4$. A left ventricular S$_4$ is auscultated at the apex with the bell of the stethoscope. Conditions affecting right ventricular compliance, such as pulmonary hypertension or pulmonic steno-

sis, may produce a right ventricular S$_4$ heard best at the lower left sternal border; it increases in intensity during inspiration.

SUMMATION GALLOP

With rapid heart rates, as ventricular diastole shortens, an S$_3$ and S$_4$, if both present, may fuse together and become audible as a single diastolic sound. This is called a summation gallop (Fig. 16–7). This sound is loudest at the apex and is heard best with the stethoscope bell while the patient lies turned slightly to the left side.

HEART MURMURS

Murmurs are sounds produced either by the forward flow of blood through a narrowed or constricted valve into a dilated vessel or chamber or by the backward flow of blood through an incompetent valve or septal defect. Murmur classification is based on timing in the cardiac cycle. Systolic murmurs occur between S$_1$ and S$_2$. Diastolic murmurs occur after S$_2$ and before the onset of the following S$_1$. Murmurs are described further according to the anatomical location on the anterior chest where the sound is heard the loudest. Any radiation of the sound also should be noted. The quality of the sound produced is described as blowing, harsh, rumbling, or musical in nature. The intensity or loudness of a murmur is described using a grading system. Grade I is faint and barely audible; grade II is soft; grade III is audible but not palpable; grade IV and V murmurs are associated with a palpable thrill; and a grade VI murmur is audible without a stethoscope.

Systolic Murmurs

As previously described, S$_1$ is produced by mitral and tricuspid valve closure and signifies the onset of ventricular systole. Murmurs occurring after S$_1$ and before S$_2$ are therefore classified as systolic murmurs.

During ventricular systole, the aortic and pulmonic valves are open. If either of these is stenotic or narrowed, a sound classified as a midsystolic ejection murmur is heard. Because the AV valves close before blood is ejected through the aortic and pulmonic valves, there is a delay between S$_1$ and the beginning of the murmur. The murmurs associated with aortic stenosis and pulmonic stenosis are described as

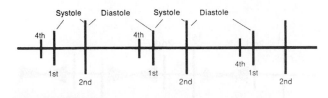

FIGURE 16-6
The fourth heart sound is a late diastolic sound that occurs just prior to S$_1$. It is a low-frequency sound heard best with the bell of the stethoscope.

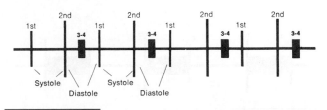

FIGURE 16-7
With rapid heart rates, S$_3$ and S$_4$ may become audible as a single, very loud sound that occurs in mid-diastole. This sound is called a summation gallop.

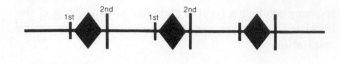

FIGURE 16-8
Blood flow through a stenotic aortic or pulmonic valve will produce a crescendo–decrescendo midsystolic ejection murmur.

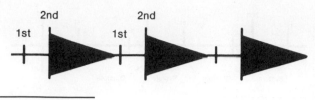

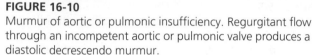

FIGURE 16-10
Murmur of aortic or pulmonic insufficiency. Regurgitant flow through an incompetent aortic or pulmonic valve produces a diastolic decrescendo murmur.

crescendo–decrescendo or diamond shaped (Fig. 16–8), meaning that the sound increases, then decreases in intensity. The quality of these murmurs is harsh, and they are of medium pitch. The murmur caused by aortic stenosis is heard best in the aortic area and may radiate up into the neck. The murmur of pulmonic stenosis is heard best over the pulmonic area.

Systolic regurgitant murmurs are caused by the backward flow of blood from an area of higher pressure to an area of lower pressure. Mitral or tricuspid valvular insufficiency or a defect in the ventricular septum will produce systolic regurgitant murmurs, which are harsh and blowing in quality. The sound is described as holosystolic, meaning that the murmur begins immediately after S_1 and continues throughout systole up to S_2 (Fig. 16–9).

Mitral insufficiency produces this type of murmur, heard most easily in the apical area with radiation to the left axilla. This type of murmur, associated with tricuspid insufficiency, is heard loudest at the left sternal border and increases in intensity during inspiration. This murmur may radiate to the cardiac apex.

A ventricular septal defect also will produce a harsh, blowing holosystolic sound caused by blood flowing from the left to the right ventricle through a defect in the septal wall during systole. The associated murmur is heard best from the fourth to sixth intercostal spaces on both sides of the sternum and is accompanied by a palpable thrill.

Diastolic Murmurs

Diastolic murmurs occur after S_2 and before the next S_1. During diastole, the aortic and pulmonic valves are closed while the mitral and tricuspid valves are open to allow filling of the ventricles.

Aortic or pulmonic valvular insufficiency produces a blowing diastolic murmur that begins immediately after S_2 and decreases in intensity as regurgitant flow decreases through diastole. These murmurs are described as early diastolic decrescendo murmurs (Fig. 16–10).

The aortic insufficiency murmur is heard best in the aortic area and may radiate along the right sternal border to the apex. Pulmonic valve insufficiency produces a murmur that is loudest in the pulmonic area.

Stenosis or narrowing of the mitral or tricuspid valve also will produce a diastolic murmur. The AV valves open in mid-diastole shortly after the aortic and pulmonic valves close, causing a delay between S_2 and the start of the murmur of mitral and tricuspid stenosis. This murmur decreases in intensity from its onset, then increases again as ventricular filling increases because of atrial contraction. This is termed decrescendo–crescendo (Fig. 16–11).

The murmur associated with mitral stenosis is heard best at the apex with the patient turned slightly to the left side. Tricuspid stenosis produces a murmur that increases in intensity with inspiration and is loudest in the fifth intercostal space along the left sternal border.

FRICTION RUBS

A pericardial friction rub can be heard when the pericardial surfaces are inflamed. This high-pitched, scratchy sound is produced by these inflamed layers rubbing together. A rub may be heard anywhere over the pericardium with the diaphragm of the stethoscope. The rub may be accentuated by having the patient lean forward and exhale. A pericardial friction rub, unlike a pleural friction rub, does not vary in intensity with respiration.

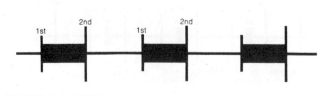

FIGURE 16-9
A holosystolic murmur is caused by the regurgitant flow of blood through an incompetent mitral or tricuspid valve. Flow of blood from the left ventricle to the right ventricle through a ventricular septal defect also will produce this type of murmur.

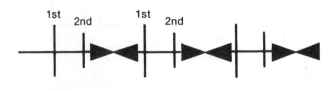

FIGURE 16-11
The murmur of mitral or tricuspid stenosis is a low-frequency murmur heard best with the bell of the stethoscope. It occurs after S_2 and has a decrescendo–crescendo configuration.

Cardiac Laboratory Studies

Knowledge of the purpose and significance of laboratory values in relation to the diagnosis and prognosis of acute MI can enhance the quality of nursing care available to patients. Laboratory studies include routine serum analysis and special studies, such as serum and cardiac enzymes. With a basic understanding of laboratory studies, the nurse can exercise judgment in interpreting results relative to other information about the patient. The ability to use this kind of judgment may well affect the patient's clinical course or prognosis.

■■■ ROUTINE LABORATORY STUDIES

Appropriate assessment of normal and compromised cardiac function is essential to ensure an accurate evaluation and correct diagnosis of the patient experiencing symptoms consistent with a cardiovascular disorder or coronary artery disease. Valuable information can be obtained by assessing hematological, coagulative, electrolyte, and phospholipid levels. Determination of these laboratory studies may vary with institutional techniques and equipment used. Normal and abnormal assay ranges have been universally established. The nurse can more appropriately plan the care of the patient and initiate interventions if an understanding of these laboratory tests and their implications are recognized and understood. A broader explanation of the effects of abnormal laboratory determinations is offered in other sections of this text and is not addressed here. However, a brief listing of frequently ordered laboratory studies with their normal values and their significance can be found in Table 16–1.

■■■ ENZYME STUDIES

Enzymes

Enzymes are found in all living cells and act as catalysts in biochemical reactions. They are present in low amounts in the serum of healthy people. When cells are injured, however, enzymes leak from damaged cells, resulting in serum enzyme concentrations above the usual low levels. No single enzyme is specific to the cells of a single organ. Each organ contains a variety of enzymes, and there is considerable overlap among organs in the enzymes they contain. The distribution of enzymes within the cells of organs is relatively organ specific, however. When organ damage occurs, the presence of abnormally high levels of enzymes in the serum, their distribution, and the time patterns for their serum appearance and disappearance make the clinical use of serum enzyme studies relevant.

CARDIAC ENZYMES

Cardiac enzymes are enzymes found in cardiac tissue. When cardiac injury occurs, as in acute MI, these enzymes are released into the serum, and their concentrations can be measured (Fig. 16–12). Cardiac tissue enzymes are present in other organs also, so elevation of one or more of these enzymes is not a specific indicator of cardiac injury. Because cardiac damage does result in above-normal serum concentrations of these enzymes, however, the quantification of cardiac enzyme levels, along with other diagnostic tests and the clinical presentation of the patient, is routinely used for diagnosing cardiac disease, particularly acute MI.

Only three of the many enzymes present in cardiac tissue have widespread use in the diagnosis of acute MI: creatine kinase (CK), lactate dehydrogenase (LDH), and serum glutamic-oxaloacetic transaminase (SGOT). LDH and SGOT were first used in the 1950s. Since the mid-1960s, CK has become the most important addition to the enzyme diagnosis of acute MI. None of the three is specific to cardiac tissue. CK and LDH, however, can be divided further into components called isoenzymes. In each case, at least one of the isoenzymes is more specific for cardiac disease. The increase in these more specific components of LDH or CK relative to their other isoenzymes has resulted in their common use in diagnosis of acute MI. Because of the nonspecificity of SGOT and the widespread availability of CK and LDH isoenzymes, the routine sampling of serum for SGOT for the diagnosis of acute MI is no longer recommended. The value of drawing blood samples for measuring CK, LDH, and their associated isoenzymes for the diagnosis of acute MI is discussed in the following text.

Creatine Kinase

The level of total CK in plasma usually becomes abnormal 6 to 8 hours after onset of infarction and peaks between 24 and 28 hours. When patients appear at the hospital soon after the onset of symptoms, the initial CK frequently is within normal limits, and at the time of hospital admission, it is not possible to discriminate on the basis of CK those who are having an acute MI from those who are not. For this reason, CK is sampled every 4 to 6 hours for the first 24 hours after the onset of symptoms. Within 2 to 4 days after MI, serum concentration of total CK usually will have returned to normal. Therefore, abnormal total CK levels may be missed in patients who present more than 24 hours after the onset of infarction. The normal level of total CK typically is higher in men than women and in African Americans compared with whites. The upper limit of normal may vary among laboratories, and nurses must be aware of the normal value used in their laboratory. In

TABLE 16-1 CLINICAL APPLICATION: Diagnostic Studies
Common Cardiac Laboratory Studies

Test	Normal Value	Significance
Red blood cell	Men: $4.6–6.2 \times 10^6$ Women: $4.2–5.4 \times 10^6$	May indicate chronic obstructive lung disease, cyanotic congenital heart malformations, diseases of hypoxemia, polycythemia vera
Hematocrit	Men: 40%–50% Women: 38%–47%	May indicate plasma volume deficit/excess, erythrocytosis, polycythemia vera
Hemoglobin	Men: 13.5–18.0 g/100 mL Women: 12.0–16.0 g/100 mL	May indicate anemia producing cardiac symptoms
White blood cell	4,500–11,000/mm³ (total)	May indicate infection or sepsis
Coagulation studies		
Platelet count	250,000–500,000/mm³	May indicate bleeding dyscrasia, abnormal or absent clotting ability, DIC, normal or accelerated response to anticoagulative therapy
Prothrombin time	12–15 s	
Partial thromboplastin time	60–70 s	
Activated partial thromboplastin time	35–45 s	
Activated clotting time	70–105 s	
Fibrinogen level	160–300 mg/dL	
Thrombin time	11.3–18.5 s	
Serum chemistries		
Sodium	135–145 mEq/L	May indicate inability to regulate intracellular functions, cellular and muscular contraction, and fluid balance
Potassium	3.3–4.9 mEq/L	
Chloride	97–110 mEq/L	
Carbon dioxide	22–31 mmol/L	
Glucose (fasting)	65–110 mg/dL	May indicate diabetes mellitus, physiological stress, abnormal endocrine function
Calcium		
Total	8.9–10.3 mg/dL	May indicate neuromuscular deficit, abnormal cellular function and contraction, cellular and capillary permeability
Free (ionized)	4.6–5.1 mg/dL	
Magnesium	1.3–2.2 mEq/L	May indicate abnormal enzyme activity, lipid, carbohydrates, and protein metabolism
Cholesterol		May indicate elevated risk factor for coronary heart disease
Total (desirable)	<200 mg/dL	
LDL (desirable)	<130 mg/dL	
HDL (desirable)	>35 mg/dL	
Serum enzymes		
CK-MM	95%–100%	May indicate myocardial, skeletal muscle, or brain injury
CK-MB	0%–5%	
CK-BB	0%	
LDH-1	Dependent on assay technique ratio	May indicate organ/tissue damage with specific cardiac differentiation
LDH-1:LDH-2 ratio	<1.0%	
SGOT (AST)	<50 U/L	

Adapted from Woods et al: Cardiac Nursing (3rd Ed). Philadelphia, J.B.Lippincott, 1995

general, the amount of total CK correlates with the amount of myocardial damage and is of prognostic importance. With a small infarction, total CK may rise two to three times the initial levels but never reach the upper limit of normal; CK isoenzymes can be valuable in these situations.

Skeletal muscle contains more CK than the heart, whereas the cerebral cortex has slightly less CK. Conditions that result in damage or injury to the brain or skeletal muscle also may result in abnormal levels of CK in plasma. Skeletal muscle diseases, such as polymyositis and muscu-

lar dystrophy, and the effects of alcohol, strenuous exercise, convulsions, trauma, surgery, and intramuscular injections within skeletal muscle may give rise to abnormal CK levels. Cerebrovascular disease also may result in abnormal CK levels. In cerebrovascular disease, the increase occurs later, lasts longer, and is not as high as the abnormal CK levels caused by acute MI. Although the clinical presentation of the patient, the ECG, and the amount and time course of abnormal CK levels are useful in determining whether or not the diagnosis of acute MI is appropriate, it is not always possible to distinguish MI from other clinical conditions. For

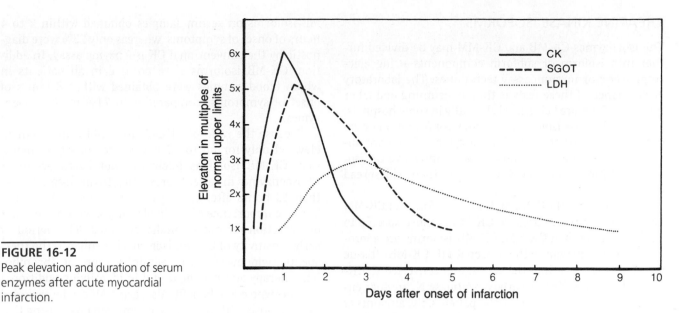

FIGURE 16-12
Peak elevation and duration of serum enzymes after acute myocardial infarction.

this reason, CK isoenzymes, in addition to total CK, generally are obtained serially.

CREATINE KINASE ISOENZYMES

Electrophoresis, glass bead, and radioimmunoassay are techniques used to measure CK isoenzymes. The three CK isoenzymes routinely reported are CK-MM, CK-BB, and CK-MB, found to the greatest extent in skeletal muscle, brain, and heart muscle, respectively. Total CK usually consists entirely of CK-MM, and neither CK-BB nor CK-MB is present. In other words, the normal levels of CK found in healthy people are due entirely to skeletal muscle. Normal skeletal muscle may contain up to 2% CK-MB, and values of CK-MB of up to 5% are not necessarily considered diagnostic. The amount of CK-MB in cardiac muscle is 15% to 22%, with the remainder being CK-MM. When cardiac damage occurs, as in acute MI, total CK rises, and the percentage due to CK-MB is greater than 5%. Although other organs, such as the tongue, small intestine, uterus, and prostate, contain CK-MB, the presence of CK-MB in amounts greater than 5% generally is considered diagnostic for myocardial damage in the presence of chest pain or other symptoms believed to represent myocardial ischemia.

Within 6 to 12 hours after the onset of infarction, CK-MB usually begins to appear in serum, and it peaks at approximately 24 hours. The appearance time and peak, however, may be significantly earlier in patients who have a non–Q-wave infarction or who have undergone successful recannulation of the infarct-related coronary vessel by angioplasty or thrombolytic therapy. Those who present more than 24 hours after the onset of symptoms may not benefit from CK isoenzymes because the levels already may have returned to normal. As with total CK, serial sampling should be performed every 4 to 6 hours for the first 24 hours after the onset of symptoms. Patients who continue to have signs or symptoms of myocardial ischemia after hospital admission should continue to undergo serial CK isoenzyme sampling.

Most laboratories report the absolute amount of each CK isoenzyme present in the serum, although some also report the percentage. Normal values for absolute amounts of each of the CK isoenzymes vary by laboratory and by the measuring technique used. The amount of CK-MB released into the serum after an acute MI offers a better correlation with infarction size than total CK because of its specificity to cardiac muscle.

Because total CK and CK isoenzymes are the cardiac enzymes whose levels become abnormal earliest after the onset of infarction, the routine serial sampling for other cardiac enzymes is unnecessary. Serial analysis of CK isoenzymes is the most specific, sensitive, and cost-effective means of diagnosing acute MI. Perhaps more important, CK isoenzymes also have made possible the ability to "rule out" an acute MI more quickly and reliably. It no longer requires 2 to 3 days of intensive care unit (ICU) hospitalization to determine that SGOT or LDH enzyme levels remain normal; rather, patients can be "ruled out" in less than 24 hours if their CK isoenzyme levels do not become abnormal. Nurses and physicians not only are able to provide earlier reassurance to the patients who are found not to have acute infarction, but patients also can be discharged sooner to a less costly environment than the ICU.

Cardiac disorders other than acute MI also may be associated with abnormal total CK and CK-MB levels. These include pericarditis, myocarditis, and trauma. In addition, CK-MB levels have been reported to be abnormal after cardiac surgery and cardioversion. The clinical presentation of the patient and the ECG usually is helpful in distinguishing patients with acute MI.

CREATINE KINASE ISOFORMS

The isoenzymes CK-MB and CK-MM may be divided further into isoform or subform components using electrophoretic or immunoassay techniques. The laboratory performance of these tests is time consuming and labor intensive. They are being used clinically in some hospitals, however. Because isoforms may offer confirmation or exclusion of MI earlier than CK isoenzymes, efforts are underway to develop faster and less labor-intensive CK isoform measurements that will result in their widespread clinical use.

Two subforms of CK-MB and three subforms of CK-MM have been identified. Because CK-MB is more specific to cardiac muscle than CK-MM, CK-MB isoforms are appropriate for the patient with suspected MI. $CK-MB_2$ (tissue CK-MB) is released into the serum and converted to $CK-MB_1$ (plasma CK-MB) by carboxypeptidase N, another enzyme present in serum. In normal patients, the amounts of $CK-MB_2$ and $CK-MB_1$ present in serum are small, and the ratio of $CK-MB_2$ to $CK-MB_1$ is approximately one. In patients with acute MI, $CK-MB_2$ is released into the serum in larger quantities than normal and the amount of $CK-MB_2$ and the ratio of $CK-MB_2$ to $CK-MB_1$ in the serum of these patients becomes elevated.

Abnormal elevations of $CK-MB_2$ have been reported as early as 2 hours after onset of symptoms of MI.[1] In this study, in patients with acute MI, 59% had diagnostic CK-MB isoforms on serum samples obtained within 2 to 4 hours of onset of symptoms, whereas only 23% were diagnostic by the conventional CK isoenzyme assay. In addition, CK-MB isoforms were positive in all patients in whom blood samples were obtained within 8 hours of onset of symptoms, compared with 71% for CK isoenzymes.

Because the ratio of $CK-MB_2$ to $CK-MB_1$ may remain elevated only for up to 12 hours after onset of infarction, CK-MB isoforms likely will not be as useful as CK isoenzymes in patients presenting to the hospital more than 12 hours after the onset of symptoms. Nevertheless, the importance of a reliable early laboratory marker of infarction cannot be underestimated. The period of early sensitivity of CK-MB isoforms is similar to the therapeutic window for the administration of thrombolytic therapy and may be useful in identifying additional patients who could benefit. Also, acute MI can be excluded as a diagnosis within 8 hours of symptom onset using CK-MB isoform assay, compared with the 18 to 24 hours required for the conventional CK isoenzyme assay (Table 16–2).

Lactate Dehydrogenase

Lactate dehydrogenase may be found in many organs besides the heart, including the liver, skeletal muscle, kidney,

---

TABLE 16-2   CLINICAL APPLICATION: Diagnostic Studies
Biochemical Markers for Diagnosing Acute Myocardial Infarction

Test and Description	Time to Run Test	First Detectable in Serum (After Onset of Symptoms)	Peak Levels	Time Required for Reliable Diagnosis*
CK-MB MB isoenzyme of CK	Electrophoresis: 1–2 h	Electrophoresis: 4–8 h	Electrophoresis: 10–24 h	8–12 h
(more abundant in myocardial tissue)	Monoclonal antibody test: 10–40 min	Monoclonal antibody test: 2–3 h	Monoclonal antibody test: 10–18 h	2–3 h
MB2/MB1 ratio Ratio of subforms of CK-MB isoenzymes: MB2 in the tissue and MB1 in the plasma	25 min	1–6 h; may be detected as early as <1 h	4–8 h	1 h
Myoglobin Heme protein (found in myocardial and skeletal muscle)	10 min	2–3 h; may be detected as early as <1 h	2–4 h (cyclic rise and fall)	2 h
Troponin I, Troponin T Contractile protein (found in myofibrils)	30 min	4–6 h	10–24 h; remains elevated for 5–7 d	2–3 h

* Refers to the minimal time after onset of symptoms.
Source: Apple S: Advanced strategies for diagnosing acute myocardial infarction. Heartbeat 6:1–12, 1995; adapted from a variety of sources.

lung, fat, and red blood cells. Total LDH is less specific than CK for cardiac disease. It usually begins to appear in the serum within 24 hours after the onset of acute MI and does not peak until 2 to 3 days; it may remain elevated for 7 to 10 days before returning to normal levels. The use of LDH in the diagnosis of acute MI is unnecessary if the diagnosis can be confirmed by CK and CK-MB. Patients who present more than 24 hours after the onset of symptoms (CK and CK-MB levels already may have returned to normal) or those who have been having symptoms of myocardial ischemia for several days may be appropriate for sampling for total LDH and LDH isoenzymes. Although LDH rises more slowly and remains elevated longer than CK, the time course of abnormal levels for both enzymes overlaps. A single sample for LDH may be obtained in patients presenting more than 24 hours after symptom onset and if abnormally elevated, may be further analyzed for LDH isoenzymes. Routine serial sampling of LDH or LDH isoenzymes in these patients is not recommended because in the face of nondiagnostic CK isoenzymes, there is no evidence that serial LDH or LDH isoenzyme sampling improves the diagnostic yield.[2]

Because LDH is present in many organs, it may be abnormally elevated in various conditions, including hemolytic anemia; pulmonary infarction; renal infarction; hepatic disorders, such as hepatitis and hepatic congestion; and skeletal muscle disorders. Care must be taken when obtaining blood samples for LDH because hemolysis may result in LDH being released from red blood cells, causing falsely elevated levels.

The upper limit of normal for LDH, like CK, is higher in men than women and varies by laboratory. Nurses must know the normal values for their laboratory.

LACTATE DEHYDROGENASE ISOENZYMES

Electrophoretic techniques are used to measure LDH. The isoenzyme that moves most quickly toward the positive pole of the electrical field, LDH_1, is found most abundantly in heart muscle. Somewhat lesser amounts of LDH_1 are present in kidney, brain, and red blood cells. LDH_5, the LDH isoenzyme that moves most slowly toward the positive electrode, is found most abundantly in liver and skeletal muscle. LDH_2, LDH_3, and LDH_4 are present in intermediate amounts in these organs between the extremes of LDH_1 and LDH_5. In normal healthy people, LDH_1 comprises between 17% and 27% of total LDH, whereas LDH_2 comprises 28% to 38%; LDH_1 is always present in a lesser percentage than is LDH_2. Because the heart contains relatively more LDH_1 than LDH_2, the ratio of the percentage of LDH_1 to LDH_2 usually becomes one or more whenever cardiac injury occurs. This "flip" in the ratio of the percentage of LDH_1 to LDH_2 occurs between 1 and 3 days after the onset of MI. Although LDH isoenzymes are not as specific as CK isoenzymes in the diagnosis of acute MI, they nevertheless are helpful in patients whose CK isoenzyme levels may have returned to normal.

Additional Diagnostic Biochemical Markers

Two newer diagnostic markers are being used in the laboratory for evaluating myocardial damage. Myoglobin and troponin levels have shown high specificity for detecting myocardial damage. Both proteins are evaluated using the same monoclonal antibody technique used for CK-MB subform quantification.

Myoglobin detection can be helpful in the determination of ischemic muscle damage. Found in skeletal and cardiac muscle, it appears in the serum earlier than CK and may be detectable in the serum in less than 1 hour after the onset of symptoms. Myoglobin usually peaks in 2 to 4 hours. It is detected for *any* muscle damage and is not specific for cardiac muscle damage alone. This characteristic facilitates its value in the *exclusion* of an MI. Studies, however, have demonstrated that myoglobin levels may be very sensitive to reperfusion events after thrombolytic therapy and thus may prove to be of significant clinical value in this intervention.[1]

Troponin is highly specific for cardiac muscle damage and is detectable in two subforms, troponin I and troponin T. An advantage of troponin assays is that, unlike myoglobin, troponin is unaffected by skeletal injury.[1,3] Troponin I can be detected within 4 hours after an acute MI and can remain elevated for 1 to 2 weeks. In the healthy individual, this contractile protein is not detectable, and its high sensitivity and specificity can provide rapid diagnostic information in the suspected acute MI patient. Troponin T has been shown to be highly sensitive in detecting minor myocardial injury and may provide valuable prognostic information in patients experiencing angina pectoris. It has been reported that troponin T may detect smaller amounts of myocardial damage than even high-quality serial echocardiograms and may remain elevated in the plasma for up to 1 week after myocardial insult.

Diagnostic Limitations to Enzyme Study

Presently, enzyme determinations can serve only as adjuncts to ECG and clinical diagnosis. To be of most value they should be used with discretion. Consideration must be given to the length of time since the onset of symptoms, because each enzyme rises and returns to normal at different intervals.

Enzyme determinations have been of greatest value to the patient whose ECG and clinical picture are equivocal for diagnosis of MI. Enzyme elevation may well confirm a suspected diagnosis in this case. Sometimes it is difficult or impossible to interpret infarction on ECG because of previous infarction changes; the effects of certain drugs or electrolyte imbalances; conduction defects, such as bundle branch block (BBB) or Wolff-Parkinson-White syndrome; dysrhythmias; or a functioning pacemaker. Enzyme determination may be a distinct advantage here. If a definite diagnosis can be made by ECG, enzyme tests may not be needed, except for academic and prognostic interest.

Because serum enzyme elevations are nonspecific in the diagnosis of MI, they must be considered in view of the total clinical picture. We are in a highly technical age of nursing, and must not forget to look at and listen to the patient before making judgments and decisions.

Cardiovascular Diagnostic Procedures

Cardiovascular diagnostic techniques have expanded dramatically in the past few years, especially in the area of noninvasive testing. This permits a more careful screening of the population for high-risk procedures and low-risk methods for monitoring disease progression and response to treatment. In addition, many technologies are combined for a functional assessment of the patient's cardiac status so the best treatment option can be chosen.

The critical care nurse often cares for patients who undergo one or more of these procedures. Understanding the principles on which the procedures are based enables the nurse to answer questions, incorporate diagnostic findings into the patient's plan of care, and provide high-level nursing care. The critical care nurse also can decrease the anxiety of patients and their families by providing an explanation of the procedure.

■ NONINVASIVE TECHNIQUES

Standard 12-Lead Electrocardiogram

PURPOSE

The standard ECG records electrical impulses as they travel through the heart. In patients with normal conduction, the first electrical impulse for each cardiac cycle originates in the sinus node and is spread to the rest of the heart through the specialized conduction system—the intra-atrial tracts, AV node, bundle of His, and right and left bundles. As the impulse traverses the conduction system, it penetrates the surrounding myocardium and provides the electrical stimuli for atrial and ventricular contraction. The change in electrical potential in cells of the specialized conduction system as the impulse proceeds is very small and cannot be measured from electrodes outside the body. The change in electrical potential of myocardial cells, however, produces an electrical signal that can be recorded from the surface of the body, as is done with an ECG.

Impulses that originate in sites other than the sinus node or impulses that are prevented from traversing the conduction system because of disease or drugs interrupt the normal order of electrical sequences in the myocardium. An ECG may be used to record these abnormal patterns of im-

pulse formation or conduction. The clinician then has a visual record of the abnormal pattern from which to identify the dysrhythmia.

In addition, an abnormal ECG tracing may result from diseased myocardial cells. For example, in patients with left ventricular hypertrophy (LVH), impulses traversing the enlarged muscle mass of the left ventricle produce a bigger electrical signal than normal. In contrast, impulses are unable to traverse myocardial cells that are irreversibly damaged, such as in MI, and no electrical signal is present in the infarcted cells of the left ventricle.

PROCEDURE

The standard 12-lead ECG is so named because the usual electrode placement and recording device permit the electrical signal to be registered from 12 different views. The four limb and six precordial leads are attached to the patient as depicted in Figure 16–13. For the limb leads, the recording device alternates the combination of electrodes that are active during recording of electrical signals from the heart (Fig. 16–14). This results in six standard views or leads (I, II, III, augmented voltage of the right arm [aVR], augmented voltage of the left arm [aVL], and augmented voltage of the left foot [aVF]) that are recorded in the heart's frontal plane. The six precordial leads (V_1, V_2, V_3, V_4, V_5, and V_6) are arranged across the chest to record electrical activity in the heart's horizontal plane, as shown in Figure 16–14. Abnormal localized areas of myocardial conduction, such as occur with ischemia or infarction, may be identified in the leads that are nearest to that part of the heart. For example, an inferior MI produces changes in the leads that view the inferior aspect of the heart, or leads II, III, and aVF.

Used routinely in ICU patients, ECGs assess dysrhythmias and myocardial ischemia or MI. The test is performed easily at the bedside with the patient ideally placed in the supine position and the electrodes arranged as previously described. In some patients, chest bandages may preclude placement of the precordial leads. It is important that the patient remain still during the ECG recording so that skeletal muscle movement does not result in extraneous noise or artifact in the electrical signal. Additional horizontal plane leads may be recorded by placing electrodes on the right side of the chest to view right ventricular (RV) activity (see Fig. 16–13) or the back of the chest to view left ventricular (LV) posterior wall activity.

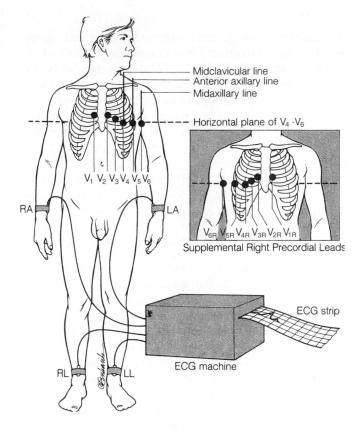

FIGURE 16-13

Electrocardiogram ECG electrode placement. The standard left precordial leads are V_1, 4th intercostal space, R sternal border; V_2, 4th intercostal space, left sternal border; V_3, diagonally between V_2 and V_4; V_4, fifth intercostal space, left midclavicular line, V_5, same line as V_4, anterior axillary line; V_6, same line as V_4 and V_5, midaxillary line. The right precordial leads, placed across the right side of the chest, are the mirror opposite of the left leads.

NURSING ASSESSMENT AND MANAGEMENT

Critical care nurses often record an ECG in the event of a change in patient status. This change in status includes the development of dysrhythmias. Evaluation of a rhythm strip in relationship to dysrhythmias is discussed further later in this chapter. Often, an ECG is obtained during episodes of chest pain before the administration of sublingual nitroglycerin. The ECG provides documentation of ST changes associated with the pain.

Some patients fear being shocked by the ECG recorder. Preparatory instruction for the patient should include an explanation of the manner in which the electrical impulses of the heart are recorded.

Holter Monitoring

PURPOSE

Ambulatory monitoring of coronary care or telemetry patients provides a noninvasive method of assessing for dysrhythmias, response to dysrhythmia treatment, pacemaker failure, and ECG signs of myocardial ischemia. Patients who present to the hospital with syncope, near syncope, or palpitations may not have recurrence of symptoms while at rest. Holter monitoring permits these patients to ambulate while heart rhythm is recorded continuously to ascertain whether the etiology of the symptoms is caused by dysrhythmia. Many patients with unstable angina have tran-

sient episodes of ST segment depression or elevation without associated angina pectoris; Holter monitoring enables the documentation and quantification of these episodes of "silent ischemia."

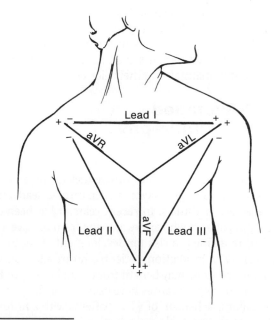

FIGURE 16-14

Frontal plane leads = standard limb leads, I, II, III, plus augmented leads aVR, aVL, and aVF. This allows an examination of electrical conduction across a variety of planes (eg, left arm to leg, right arm to left arm).

PROCEDURE

The Holter monitor is a battery-powered tape recording device that may be worn on a belt around the patient's waist or carried on a shoulder strap. Commonly, two leads are recorded continuously on tape through four or five electrodes placed on the patient's anterior chest; the electrodes are arranged so that one lead reflects the inferior wall of the heart, and the other lead reflects the anterior wall. Continuous recording of ECG leads usually is performed for 24 to 48 hours. The Holter monitor contains a clock so that time also is recorded on the tape. After completion of the test, the tape is removed and played back for identification and quantification of ST segment changes or dysrhythmias.

NURSING ASSESSMENT AND MANAGEMENT

Patients who are scheduled to undergo Holter monitoring should be instructed to bathe before the test because the electrodes cannot be removed during the 24- to 48-hour recording. Skin preparation and electrode placement are crucial to obtaining high-quality ECG recordings. It may be necessary to wrap material or fishnet over the electrodes and cables on the patient's torso to reduce movement artifact. Often, the skin under and around the electrodes becomes irritated, and the patient must be cautioned to avoid pulling at the electrodes because loss of electrical contact can mimic sinus pauses or heart block, making the diagnostic interpretation of the test difficult.

Most Holter monitors have an "event" button that can be pushed whenever symptoms occur; this button sends a signal to mark the tape. Patients are asked to maintain a diary of symptoms and activities and the time they occurred and should be instructed to record the time from the Holter monitor clock. Patients should be encouraged to maintain normal activities while wearing the monitor and told that it is desirable to record an entry in the diary at least every 2 hours. Hospitalized patients may need the assistance of nursing staff in maintaining their diaries.

Signal-Averaged Electrocardiography

PURPOSE

Signal-averaged ECG is a noninvasive method for assessing patients who are at high risk for sudden cardiac death due to ventricular dysrhythmias. In recent years, it has been used primarily in patients who are recovering from or have a history of MI to define the risk for development of ventricular tachycardia (VT). In addition, patients who are admitted with unexplained syncope may benefit from signal-averaged ECG after other noncardiac causes have been excluded.[3]

The major mechanism of VT in patients with a history of MI relates to an area of slow conduction in the left ventricle. This area of slow conduction depolarizes late after most of the ventricle has depolarized, producing small-amplitude and late electrical potentials not visible on the normal 12-lead ECG. The signal-averaged ECG allows these late potentials to be identified by repetitively mapping the patient's QRS complexes onto each other; filtering out noise, such as movement or electrical interference; averaging the repetitively mapped QRS complexes; and amplifying the averaged signal. There is some variation between laboratories in the definition of a positive signal-averaged ECG; however, in general, late potentials are considered to be present if the QRS duration is prolonged, the terminal low-amplitude portion of the QRS complex is prolonged, or the root mean square voltage of the terminal portion of the QRS is less than 20 μV.

PROCEDURE

In addition to a ground electrode, six other electrodes are placed on the patient's chest during the 20 minutes required for performing the signal-averaged ECG. The six electrodes constitute three paired leads that are at right angles to each other; one set of leads is placed horizontally on the mid-right and left anterior chest, a second set is placed vertically at the top and bottom of the sternum, and the third set is placed anteroposteriorly just to the left of the sternum and on the posterior thorax. The patient must rest quietly in a supine position for the duration of the study. Extraneous noise, such as muscle movement, interferes with interpretation of the test, and patients who are restless or agitated or have difficulty lying supine are not good subjects for signal-averaged ECG.

NURSING ASSESSMENT AND MANAGEMENT

The critical care nurse may be responsible for explaining the general format of the test and for emphasizing the need to remain as motionless as possible during the study to achieve accurate data.

Chest Radiography

PURPOSE

Chest radiography is a routine diagnostic test to assess critically ill patients with cardiac disease. The test can be performed easily at the bedside in patients too ill to be transported to the radiology department. The image obtained on a radiograph that allows visualization of vascular and cardiac shapes is based on the premise that thoracic structures vary in density and permit different amounts of radiation to reach the film.

Chest radiography may be used for the evaluation of cardiac size, pulmonary congestion, pleural or pericardial effusions, and position of intracardiac lines, such as transvenous pacemaker electrodes or PA catheters.

PROCEDURE

Cardiac size is evaluated best in the radiology department, where the procedure can be standardized with the patient standing and the radiograph taken from a posterior view at a distance of 6 ft. Portable bedside chest radiographs usually are taken from an anterior view with the patient lying supine or sitting erect and are not standardized.

Patients undergoing radiography of the chest should be instructed not to move while the radiograph is being taken. Proper positioning of the radiographic plate behind the patient is important to ensure that thoracic structures will be aligned on the film. Care should be taken to remove all metal objects, including fasteners on clothing, from the field of view because metal will block the x-ray beam. Patients usually are asked to take a deep breath and hold it when the radiograph is taken to displace the diaphragm downward; this may be uncomfortable for patients who have undergone recent thoracic surgery.

NURSING ASSESSMENT AND MANAGEMENT

The critical care nurse's role in obtaining diagnostic thoracic radiographic films often is limited to the ICU, where portable radiographs are made. With unstable patients, the nurse must decide when the film can be taken. It is important that intravenous (IV) lines not become tangled or loosened while one is trying to place the radiographic plate in the proper position.

Female patients of childbearing potential should have a lead drape placed over the abdomen to protect the ovaries from any radiation scatter. For the same reason, caregivers and family members should leave the patient's room when the radiograph is taken. When caregivers cannot leave the patient's bedside, a lead apron should be worn.

Echocardiography

PURPOSE

The use of echocardiography in diagnosing and monitoring heart disease has increased dramatically since its introduction in the 1960s. It now refers to a group of tests that use ultrasound either alone or in combination with other technologies. For many patients, echocardiography has been an invaluable substitute for more invasive procedures in the management of their heart disease. The growth of echocardiography for clinical application is likely to continue. Because of miniaturization of the equipment, research is being conducted on intravascular ultrasound (IVUS) devices that would permit the identification of intraluminal defects.

Echocardiography is used clinically in many cardiac conditions. The type of echocardiogram that is to be performed depends on the condition being evaluated. In critical care patients, echocardiography is used most often to assess ejection fraction, segmental wall motion, systolic and diastolic ventricular volumes, and mitral valve regurgitation due to papillary muscle dysfunction and to detect the presence of mural thrombi, valve vegetations, or pericardial fluid. Echocardiography is a helpful diagnostic tool in the presence of sudden clinical deterioration in acute MI where significant complications may be observed or suspected. It also may be used in the evaluation of function of all four cardiac valves, including calculation of gradients and orifice size, intracardiac tumors, and aortic dissection. In some centers, echocardiography has made it possible for young

patients unlikely to have coronary artery disease to undergo valve replacement without requiring a preoperative cardiac catheterization. Although M-mode and two-dimensional echocardiography can be performed easily at the bedside, the reduced noise and light levels of the laboratory usually result in better recordings.

PROCEDURE

The first and simplest use of ultrasound in cardiac patients is *M-mode echocardiography*, a technique that provides a rapid assessment of valvular motion and chamber wall thickness. It requires a transducer that acts both as a sound transmitter and a sound receiver. The transducer is placed on the anterior chest in an intercostal space or subcostal position to avoid bony structures. A single ultrasound beam is sent from the transducer and directed toward the heart. As the sound waves reach various structures in the path of the beam, some pass through and around the structures, and some are reflected back to the transducer by the interface between two structures of differing densities. The more distant the interface, the longer it takes for the reflected sound waves to reach the transducer. A recording device is connected to the transducer so that as the reflected sound waves are received, they are converted to an electrical signal. If only one ultrasound wave beam is emitted from the transducer, the recording will contain echoes from structures in the beam's path. For example, based on transducer position #1 in Figure 16–15, the recording would contain

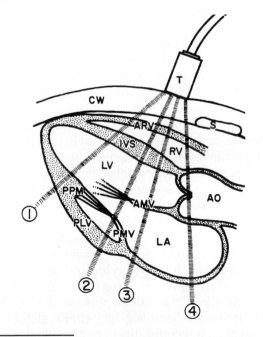

FIGURE 16-15

A cross-section of the heart showing the structures through which the ultrasonic beam passes as it is directed from the apex (1) toward the base (4) of the heart. CW, chest wall; T, transducer; S, sternum; ARV, anterior right ventricular wall; RV, right ventricular cavity; IVS, interventricular septum; LV, left ventricle; PPM, posterior papillary muscle; PLV, posterior left ventricular wall; AMV, anterior mitral valve; PMV, posterior mitral valve; AO, aorta; LA, left atrium.

sound waves reflected from the chest wall, the free RV wall, a space representing the RV cavity, the intraventricular septum, a space representing the LV cavity, and the posterior wall of the left ventricle.

In M-mode echocardiography, ultrasound waves are transmitted intermittently; the remainder of the time, the transducer is receiving the reflected sound waves. Typically, an M-mode recording is made with the reflected sound waves on the vertical axis and time on the horizontal axis. As the heart moves during the cardiac cycle, the recording displays this movement. Because M-mode echocardiography is based on a single beam, the so-called "ice-pick" view, only a small region of the heart can be visualized at any one time. The four positions of the transducer depicted in Figure 16–16 are the typical views used during an M-mode echocardiogram.

Two-dimensional (2D) echocardiography is performed in a similar manner except for two major differences: The ultrasound waves are transmitted in a pie-shaped beam, resulting in a "plane" of reflected echoes, and the recording device is a video camera so that the two dimensions of the plane and movement over time are recorded. In addition to parasternal and subcostal transducer positions, apical and suprasternal positions also may be used in 2D echocardiography.

Recently exercise or pharmacological stress testing has been used in conjunction with 2D echocardiography. A combination of physical exercise and 2D echocardiography has long been recognized as a valuable method to confirm or evaluate the presence of coronary artery disease and the extent of its involvement. An image taken at rest is compared with an image taken immediately after exercise. In patients with significant coronary artery disease, ventricular wall motion abnormalities will develop after exercise in the segments supplied by diseased arteries. In patients who are unwilling or unable to exercise because of physical or psychological constraints, pharmacological agents to physiologically stress the heart have been used appropriately and effectively. Vasodilator agents, such as adenosine and dipyridamole, have been used in the past to induce myocardial ischemia in several imaging modalities (eg, thallium scan testing) and echocardiography. Observation of areas of reduced blood flow can unmask coronary artery disease and quantify myocardium at risk.

In recent years, dobutamine hydrochloride has been proven effective in pharmacological stress testing in combination with echocardiography. Dobutamine is a synthetic catecholamine with beta-1 receptor and alpha-receptor properties, which give the drug both inotropic and chronotropic effects that mimic physical exercise. With dobutamine stress echocardiography (DSE), global or regional wall motion abnormalities in compromised myocardial muscle may be observed before, during, and after titrated dobutamine infusion. Should motion abnormalities be noted, the test is deemed positive and the patient can then be considered for surgical revascularization to improve cardiac performance. Distinct advantages of DSE include the fact that the test is noninvasive, can be safely performed a few weeks after an acute MI, and can illuminate wall motion abnormalities that cannot be assessed with electrographic monitoring.

Doppler echocardiography superimposes Doppler techniques on either M-mode or 2D images. The direction of blood flow can be assessed by measuring echoes reflected from red blood cells as they move away or toward the transducer. This type of study is particularly useful in patients with valvular stenosis or regurgitation; blood flow is quite turbulent through a stenotic valve, and in the opposite direction with regurgitation. When the direction of flow is color encoded, the study is known as a color Doppler echocardiogram. Audio signals usually are recorded during Doppler studies. Contrast material also may be used in conjunction with M-mode or 2D echocardiography. Although many agents have been used as contrast material, almost any liquid injected intravenously contains microbubbles. As the microbubbles travel through the heart, they produce multiple echoes. This technique is especially useful in identifying right-to-left intracardiac shunts because of the early appearance of the microbubble echoes in the left atrium or ventricle.

The most recent type of ultrasound study to be used clinically is *transesophageal echocardiography*. This is made possible by placing a 2D transducer on the end of a flexible endoscope and positioning it at various locations in the esophagus. Doppler and color Doppler also can be added. Because the transducer is closer to cardiac structures, the images are usually superior to those obtained with transthoracic techniques. Transesophageal echocardiography is useful in situations where it is technically impossible to image structures of interest from the usual transthoracic position—in particular, the aorta, atria, and valves. Newer techniques such as transgastric and transthoracic echocardiography are beginning to appear and may demonstrate value in the detection of structural anomalies.

NURSING ASSESSMENT AND MANAGEMENT

There are no specific prestudy restrictions for patients undergoing transthoracic echocardiography. During the study, the patient usually is placed in the supine position or turned slightly to the left side. Noise and light should be kept to a minimum during the test. There is no discomfort associated with transthoracic echocardiographic studies; however, the patient may experience chest wall discomfort after the study due to the positioning of the transducer. Suboptimal imaging may occur in patients who are obese or have obstructive lung disease.

Patients who are scheduled to undergo transesophageal echocardiography should take nothing orally (NPO) for 6 or more hours before the study. Mild to moderate sedation may be administered intravenously both before and during the test. Emergency equipment should be readily available in case of oversedation. A local anesthetic spray usually is applied to the posterior oropharynx to block the gag reflex before the endoscope is inserted orally. After the procedure, the patient should remain NPO until return of the gag reflex.

Phonocardiography

In phonocardiography, heart sounds are recorded by a microphone and converted to electrical activity that is recorded. This procedure may be used to obtain precise measurements of the timing of cardiac cycle events, to determine the characteristics and timing of murmurs and abnormal heart sounds, to measure systolic time intervals, and to teach cardiac auscultation. There are no contraindications or risks associated with this procedure.

PROCEDURE

For a phonocardiogram, the patient is brought to a quiet room and asked to lie on a comfortable table or bed. Microphones are applied to the chest wall over areas where the heart sounds and murmurs are auscultated best. The microphones pick up the sound of the heartbeat and convert it to an electrical impulse that is then amplified, filtered, and recorded. Some of the microphones are allowed to lie free on the chest; others are attached by straps or Ace bandages. A recording of sound waves is obtained, usually in conjunction with an ECG and a carotid pulse wave recording. These accessory recordings provide a reference point for the timing of cardiac events.

Special maneuvers or the use of pharmacological agents may accentuate certain heart sounds and murmurs. These include the inhalation of amyl nitrate, injection of IV isoproterenol or vasopressors, changes in position (sitting or squatting), variations in breathing (deep inspiration and expiration), and the performance of a Valsalva maneuver.

NURSING ASSESSMENT AND MANAGEMENT

Generally, phonocardiography takes 1 to 2 hours. Patients should be told beforehand that they may be asked to perform certain maneuvers or may be given certain agents to facilitate the diagnostic value of the test.

Exercise Electrocardiography

PURPOSE

Exercise ECG is used primarily as an outpatient procedure to assess patients at risk for the presence of coronary artery disease. Its use, however, in coronary care and telemetry units is becoming more widespread. Patients who have presented to the hospital with chest pain but without associated ECG changes, have had the diagnosis of infarction excluded, and have remained symptom free may undergo exercise ECG to evaluate the etiology of their presenting symptoms and whether continued hospitalization is warranted. It also may be used to evaluate patients with dysrhythmias whose symptoms are exacerbated by exercise. Low-level exercise ECG, a modification of the standard exercise test, is commonly performed predischarge in patients hospitalized with acute MI.

Patients with significant coronary artery disease may have normal ECGs at rest when myocardial oxygen supply is sufficient to meet oxygen demands. With increased oxygen demands during exercise, however, coronary blood flow cannot increase adequately owing to coronary artery stenoses, and ECG changes may occur.

Exercise ECG should not be performed in patients who have left bundle branch block (LBBB) or pre-excitation at rest because the baseline QRS abnormalities preclude interpreting the ST segment response to exercise. The test also is less specific in women, especially young or middle-aged, than in men. It is common practice to perform a low-level exercise test before hospital discharge after acute MI to identify patients at risk for ischemic events and to determine exercise prescription. The low-level test exercise target is approximately 70% to 80% of the predicted age-adjusted maximum. In patients with uncomplicated MI, the low-level exercise test has been performed safely as early as 3 days after infarction.[4]

PROCEDURE

Although there are various exercise protocols, most are based on either walking on a treadmill or riding a stationary bicycle. The test usually begins at a low level of exercise and increases every 2 to 3 minutes until the patient reaches a target level of oxygen consumption, manifests signs or symptoms of coronary artery disease, or reaches a predicted heart rate level calculation. Oxygen consumption, the amount of oxygen used in milliliters per minute per kilogram, usually is expressed in metabolic equivalents that take into account the age of the patient. If a treadmill is used to perform exercise, the speed or the uphill slope of the treadmill is increased at the beginning of each 2- to 3-minute stage; in cycling, the resistance of the pedals or braking mechanism is increased at the beginning of each stage.

Patients who have not previously undergone exercise testing should be allowed briefly to practice walking on the treadmill or riding the bicycle. Before starting the test, a resting ECG and blood pressure are obtained with the patient in sitting and standing positions. During the test, an ECG and blood pressure are obtained at the end of each stage of the protocol and immediately before termination. The test usually is terminated when signs or symptoms of myocardial ischemia develop or the patient manifests other symptoms, such as fatigue or dyspnea, and cannot continue. In the absence of myocardial ischemia or serious dysrhythmias, every effort should be made to reach the patient's predicted level of exercise to avoid a nondiagnostic test. During the recovery period, monitoring of the ECG and blood pressure continues until the patient has reached baseline values. It is mandatory that emergency resuscitation equipment and trained personnel be available in areas where exercise testing is performed.

Indications of myocardial ischemia during exercise testing are the development of (1) ST segment depression of 1 mm or more, (2) angina pectoris, or (3) failure to increase systolic blood pressure to 120 mmHg or more or a sustained decrease of 10 mmHg or more with progressive stages of exercise. The ECG leads in which ST segment depression occurs during exercise are not specific to the coronary artery involved. The greater the number of leads with ST segment depression, however, the more likely it is that the patient has multivessel coronary artery disease. The development of ST segment elevation or T wave changes during exercise testing is not specific for myocardial ischemia, and its significance requires further assessment. Often, exercise ECG is performed in conjunction with echocardiography, radionuclide perfusion imaging, or radionuclide ventriculography to assess better the extent of coronary artery disease and its effect on ventricular function.

NURSING ASSESSMENT AND MANAGEMENT

Patients who are scheduled to undergo exercise ECG should abstain from eating or drinking caffeine-containing beverages several hours before testing to prevent abdominal cramps or nausea from developing at maximal exercise and to minimize blood diversion to the gastrointestinal tract, which decreases available coronary blood supply. They also should have available comfortable shoes for walking on a treadmill or riding a bicycle. The ECG lead system is the same as used for the standard 12-lead cardiogram. The limb leads, however, are moved to the torso so that arm or leg movement during exercise will not interfere with ECG recording. Extreme attention is paid to skin preparation and electrode attachment to permit interpretable recordings during maximal exercise. It may be necessary to wrap material or fishnet over the electrodes and cables on the patient's torso to reduce movement artifact.

The critical care nurse may be responsible for explaining the general format of an exercise test to the patient and family. It is important that patients understand why the test is indicated and what will be expected of them. Patients should be reassured that someone will observe them closely throughout the test and encouraged to express any concerns before, during, and after the procedure. Patients also should understand that they may have to continue exercising after the development of angina but will not be expected to do more exercise than is safe.

Radionuclide Imaging

PURPOSE

The noninvasive assessment of cardiac structure and function using radiotracers has increased dramatically in the past few years. In particular, radionuclide perfusion studies are playing a bigger role in the diagnosis and treatment of patients with coronary artery disease. The ability of perfusion studies to separate ischemic, viable myocardium from infarcted, nonviable myocardium is used by clinicians to select noninvasive versus invasive strategies, such as angioplasty or coronary bypass grafting, for treating the underlying coronary artery disease in patients with more severe disease.

Radionuclide perfusion studies provide information not only about the presence of coronary artery disease, but also about the location and quantity of ischemic and infarcted

myocardium. In addition, they offer advantages over exercise ECG when ischemic changes cannot be assessed easily on the ECG, such as in patients with LBBB, with paced rhythm, or those receiving digitalis.

New on the horizon and not discussed in detail here is positron emission tomography (PET). This modality is highly sensitive and is specific for diagnosing coronary artery disease although not superior to single-photon emission computed tomography (SPECT) in diagnostic accuracy. The equipment required for PET is expensive and is available in only a few centers. Because it offers the ability to image and quantify myocardial metabolism and blood flow, however, it is useful in distinguishing viable myocardium and evaluating the response of the myocardium to treatment with pharmacological agents.

PERFUSION IMAGING

Procedure

Cardiac radionuclide perfusion imaging is based on the fact that a radioactive tracer is taken up in abnormal myocardial cells in either increased or decreased amounts compared with normal myocardium. After injection of the tracer, a gamma camera is used to record an image of radioactive counts from the entire myocardium. An abnormal area with decreased uptake is commonly known as "cold spot" imaging and is the type of study used to assess myocardial perfusion. An abnormal area with increased myocardial uptake or "hot spot" imaging is the type of study used to assess myocardial necrosis.

Perfusion studies are performed most commonly in conjunction with exercise testing so that radionuclide scans obtained at rest and with exercise can be compared. Typically, during rest, the radiotracer is spread uniformly throughout the myocardium and the camera reads counts equally from throughout the myocardium. A similar scan is obtained during exercise in patients without significant coronary artery stenosis as blood flow increases uniformly to meet myocardial oxygen demands. In patients with significant coronary artery disease, however, the image during exercise is altered. The amount of coronary blood flow is limited in stenotic arteries, and the quantity of tracer in myocardial segments supplied by stenotic arteries is diminished or absent in comparison to segments supplied by nonstenotic arteries. The presence of an area of decreased tracer uptake during exercise compared to rest is known as a *reversible perfusion defect*.

In patients with previous infarction, decreased uptake may be present on both the rest and exercise scans in the infarcted segments; this pattern is known as a *fixed perfusion defect* and usually signifies nonviable myocardium. It is possible for patients to have fixed perfusion defects in some myocardial segments, reversible defects in others, and normal perfusion in the remaining segments.

Because of the many patients who are physically unable to exercise, pharmacological agents may be used to mimic the heart's response to exercise. Vasodilating agents, such as dipyridamole, adenosine, and dobutamine, administered intravenously mimic exercise conditions in the heart by dilating nonstenotic coronary arteries. Coronary blood flow is increased preferentially through normal, nonstenosed arteries; this results in relative hypoperfusion in myocardial segments supplied by stenosed coronary arteries. A radiotracer injected during the peak action of the pharmacological agent produces images similar to those seen with exercise. As of this writing, only dipyridamole is approved by the Food and Drug Administration for use in perfusion imaging.

Two methods are used to record radioactive images—planar and tomographic. With the planar technique, images of the heart are obtained by the gamma camera from three views—anterior, left anterior oblique (45 degrees to the left of the anterior view), and left lateral, as shown in Figure 16–16. Tomographic or SPECT images are obtained by rotating the head of the camera over a 180-degree arc from the left lateral to the anterior position while stopping to record 32 to 64 times for 20 to 40 seconds each. A computer uses the recorded images to reconstruct multiple slices of the heart along its short axis and both horizontal and vertical long axes.

Three radioactive tracers, thallium-201 (201Tl), technetium (Tc) 99m sestamibi and Tc 99m teboroxime, are approved for perfusion imaging. Because thallium has been available since 1974, most experience in radionuclide perfusion studies has occurred with this agent. Characteristics of the three agents differ and are responsible for the varying imaging protocols used.

Thallium Protocol.   The cardiac half-life of thallium is approximately 7.5 hours, meaning that 50% of the tracer still will be present in myocardial cells 7.5 hours after it is administered. It also redistributes readily, so thallium in normally perfused areas will move to previously underperfused areas after the myocardial blood flow demands in that territory have decreased. The standard protocol for thallium perfusion studies begins first with the exercise portion; thallium is injected at the peak of exercise and imaging starts within 5 minutes of injection. The rest scan is obtained 2 to 4 hours later. Because of redistribution, no additional thallium is required. In some patients with perfusion defects on both the rest and exercise scans, however, significant redistribution may not occur, and it is recommended that an additional dose of thallium be administered.[5]

Sestamibi Protocol.   Perfusion imaging with sestamibi typically begins with the rest scan first. Because significant uptake also occurs in the liver, imaging is delayed for approximately 60 minutes. This time delay allows sestamibi to be cleared from the liver but not the heart. In addition, a glass of milk or small fatty meal is taken shortly after radiotracer injection to enhance hepatic clearance. A second dose of sestamibi is administered during peak exercise, and the exercise scan is obtained 60 minutes after injection, again allowing time for hepatic clearance. Because sestamibi redistributes very slowly, the image obtained 60 minutes after peak exercise reflects the perfusion conditions at the time of injection. Initially, perfusion studies with sestamibi were performed on two different days, but it now is customary to complete both portions of the study in one day. It has been shown that exercise sestamibi myocardial perfusion SPECT can provide incremental prognostic information in patients who have not suffered a previous MI or undergone cardiac catheterization and who are determined to be at low risk.

Teboroxime Protocol.   Because of the very short cardiac half-life of teboroxime, two injections of tracer are required. As with sestamibi, hepatic uptake also occurs. Redistribution is not an issue because of the short half-life. Imaging must begin within 2 to 5 minutes of injection and be completed within 15 minutes. The sequence of imaging, exercise versus rest, is not of concern, and typically the two scans are obtained 60 to 90 minutes apart.

Planar imaging usually is performed with the patient in the supine position, although some laboratories place patients on their right side to obtain the left lateral image.

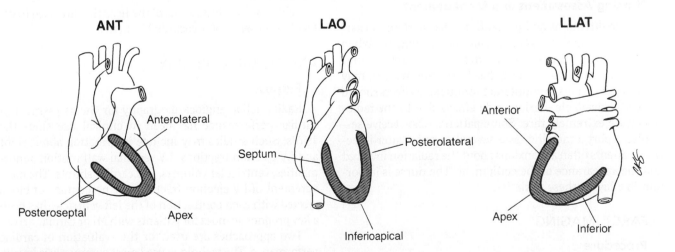

FIGURE 16-16
Ventricular segments as projected on radionuclide planar views. ANT, anterior; LAO, left anterior oblique; LLAT, left lateral.

When teboroxime is used as the radiotracer, scans may be obtained with the patient in a sitting or standing position to avoid hepatic interference. With tomographic studies, it is extremely important that the patient not move during image acquisition because computer reconstruction of the images requires the same reference points. If significant movement occurs, the entire tomographic scan may have to be repeated.

Ultrafast Computed Tomography

Ultrafast computed tomography (CT) is a noninvasive technique that is rapidly showing promise in the assessment of myocardial blood flow. It is similar to conventional CT but differs in the speed at which images can be relayed. A distinct advantage to this modality is the ability to provide high-quality image acquisition that is not contaminated by the artifactual movement that occurs with cardiac contractions. Images are obtained when an electronic beam passes across four tungsten targets creating a fan-shaped x-ray view that is transmitted, digitalized, and reconstructed as with traditional CT scanning. Segmental slices of the heart can then be obtained, which are used to evaluate myocardial perfusion. This is especially useful when clear spatial resolution is required. The technique can be used with or without a contrast media.

Ultrafast CT has demonstrated an increased sensitivity in the detection of coronary calcium, which has been implicated in the development of coronary atherosclerosis. It has been shown that the greater the amount of intimal calcium present, the greater the likelihood of obstructive coronary disease. When used to identify and quantify coronary calcium, no contrast media are required, radiation exposure is minimal, and the physician need not be present. When ultrafast CT is used with contrast media, it has shown a high degree of accuracy in the assessment of myocardial blood flow when flow is normal or reduced. However, it is less accurate when blood flow is increased.

Nursing Assessment and Management

All the directions and precautions that pertain to exercise ECG also apply to exercise radionuclide imaging. When pharmacological agents are used in place of exercise, minor side effects, such as flushing, headache, and nausea, may occur; medications to counteract serious side effects should be readily available. Serious side effects due to the radiotracer are extremely rare. Some patients who receive sestamibi report a metallic taste several minutes after injection. Patients often are anxious about the radiation involved and the appearance of the equipment. The nurse is important in allaying these anxieties.

INFARCT IMAGING

Procedure

Infarct or "hot-spot" imaging may be useful in patients who present to the hospital several days after MI when serum cardiac enzymes have returned to normal. Accumu-

lation of the radiotracer in the area of myocardial necrosis compared to the surrounding normal myocardium is responsible for the hot-spot image obtained.

Tc 99m Sn-pyrophosphate is the only radiotracer currently approved by the Food and Drug Administration for infarct imaging and is sensitive for 1 to 5 days after onset of symptoms. Because aneurysm formation in the area of a previous infarction may result in a false-positive study, a second pyrophosphate scan may be performed 7 to 10 days after symptom onset. In patients with recent infarction, little or no radiotracer uptake will be seen on the repeat scan. The diagnostic sensitivity of pyrophosphate imaging in patients with small or nontransmural infarction is poor.

Indium-111 antimyosin is a monoclonal antibody that binds to damaged myocytes and is under investigation as an imaging agent for myocardial necrosis. Planar or tomographic images are obtained 24 to 48 hours after injection of the indium-labeled antibody. Although the study usually is performed within 1 week of an MI, a positive scan may be obtained for up to 1 year after myocardial necrosis. Initial results suggest that antimyosin is more sensitive than pyrophosphate scans for the detection of infarction. In addition, antimyosin may be useful in other clinical conditions that result in myocardial necrosis, such as myocarditis and rejection after cardiac transplantation. The pattern of radiotracer uptake is more diffuse and global in these conditions, compared with the localized pattern of uptake in infarction.

Nursing Assessment and Management

No special preparation is required for patients undergoing infarct imaging other than an explanation of procedure. Views usually are obtained with the patient in the supine position. If an antimyosin tomographic study is to be performed, the importance of not moving during image acquisition should be reinforced. No serious side effects have been reported with either pyrophosphate or antimyosin administration.

Table 16–3 outlines some of the tests that are used to detect the presence of myocardial ischemia.

ANGIOCARDIOGRAPHY

Purpose

Radionuclide angiocardiography for the assessment of cardiac performance has been in clinical use since the 1970s. Such studies may include information about right and LV ejection fractions, LV regional wall motion abnormalities, ventricular volumes, and cardiac shunts. The measurement of LV ejection fraction, the percentage of blood ejected with each contraction of the left ventricle, has been a key prognostic index for patients with MI or cardiac arrest.

Two approaches are used for the evaluation of cardiac performance. The technique used most commonly is known as equilibrium angiocardiography. It is performed easily at the bedside in patients too critically ill to be transported to the laboratory. The other technique, first-pass angiocardio-

TABLE 16-3   CLINICAL APPLICATION: Diagnostic Studies
Diagnostic Tests Used to Detect Myocardial Ischemia °

Procedure	Adnormal Findings	Special Considerations
Standard 12-lead ECG	Transient ST segment and T wave changes in patients with chest pain at rest or of prolonged duration	
Holter monitoring	Transient ST segment and T wave changes occurring at rest or with activity	Only two ECG leads monitored
Stress echocardiogram	Segmental wall motion abnormality associated with echocardiogram obtained during exercise	May be used in patients with ventricular conduction defects Pharmacological agents may be used in patients who cannot exercise.
Exercise ECG	Transient ST segment and T wave changes occurring with exercise	Cannot be used in patients who are unable to exercise or who have left bundle branch block or paced rhythm Does not provide good information on the location of the cornonary artery disease
Radionuclide perfusion stress study	"Cold spot" image or perfusion defect associated with scan obtained during exercise	May be used in patients with ventricular conduction defects Pharmacologal agents may be used in patients who cannot exercise.
Online ischemia analysis	Myocardial ischemia dynamic analysis (MIDA)* analyzing eight leads to detect ST levels indicating ischemia and QRS changes corresponding to infarct evolution	Noninvasive Hastens clinical decision making Graphic trends monitored online Reocclusion readily identified Helps differentiate chest pain related to ischemia from non-ischemic symptoms

*MIDA CoroNet, Hewlett-Packard, Andover, MA, Product Literature

graphy, likely will enjoy wider use in the future because it can use technetium radiotracers, such as teboroxime or sestamibi, and can be performed at the same time as perfusion imaging.

Procedure

With *equilibrium radionuclide studies*, an aliquot of the patient's blood is drawn, and the erythrocytes are tagged with Tc 99m radiotracer. The blood sample is then returned intravenously to the patient. Imaging can begin within a few minutes after administration and performed serially over a period of 4 to 6 hours because the radiotracer-tagged erythrocytes remain within the vascular system. An ECG signal from the patient is used to separate radioactive counts acquired during systole from those during diastole; imaging continues over several hundred cardiac cycles, and images are averaged for both systole and diastole to obtain a representative cardiac cycle.

At the end of diastole, when the left ventricle is maximally filled with blood containing tagged erythrocytes, the amount of radioactivity will be greatest. As the ventricle contracts during systole, blood is ejected into the aorta. The amount of blood and therefore radioactivity in the left ventricle is lowest at the end of systole. Because radioactive counts are proportional to the blood volume, the difference in counts obtained at the end of systole and the end of dias-

tole permit the calculation of LV ejection fraction. LV impairment due to previous infarction or cardiomyopathy usually results in a reduction in LV ejection fraction from the normal values of 55% to 70%. Comparisons in ejection fractions at rest and with exercise also can be made. An inability to increase LV ejection fraction by at least 5% with exercise is considered abnormal and may represent ischemic myocardium.

Left ventricular volumes and wall motion also can be assessed with equilibrium angiocardiography. By tracing the images obtained during the end of diastole and the end of systole, abnormalities in systolic or diastolic volumes can be ascertained. In addition, global versus regional impairment of ventricular function can be differentiated, including the identification of aneurysm formation after infarction. Baseline data may provide information about the etiology of the ventricular impairment, and serial measurements often are used to assess response to treatment.

First-pass radioangiocardiography also uses Tc 99m tracers; however, they are not tagged to any blood components. An image is obtained immediately after IV injection of the radiotracer as it enters the central circulation. The appearance time of the tracer in the various cardiac chambers and right and LV systolic and diastolic counts provide diagnostic information. Because the time required for the tracer to traverse the central circulation is only a few cardiac cycles, the image acquisition time is very short.

Intracardiac shunts may be diagnosed by first-pass techniques. For example, in a patient with a ventricular septal defect and right-to-left shunt, the tracer appears in the left ventricle at the same time or before its appearance in the left atrium. In addition, this technique allows the amount of shunting to be quantified.

Right ventricular ejection fraction and volumes are measured best by first-pass angiocardiography. Because the tracer is present in the right ventricle before it appears in the left ventricle, there is no contamination of counts from the overlapping left ventricle. The methods for measuring RV volumes and ejection fraction are similar to those used for the left ventricle.

Nursing Assessment and Management

Three planar views similar to those used in perfusion imaging are obtained during equilibrium angiocardiography. If exercise angiocardiography is to be performed, the patient should be instructed to wear comfortable shoes for treadmill walking or bicycle riding. Emergency equipment should be readily available, as is required with other types of exercise testing. Although imaging usually is performed with the patient in the supine position, semierect or erect positioning may be used. It is important that the patient not move during image acquisition for either equilibrium or first-pass studies because of the effect on systolic and diastolic images.

Nurses caring for patients who have undergone radionuclide imaging should be aware of precautions; this information is available through the radiation safety department of their institution. The length of time that any precautions may be necessary is related to the half-life of the radiotracer used. In general, nurses who are pregnant should avoid caring for patients for 24 to 48 hours after the study, and all nurses should wear gloves when handling body fluids during the 24- to 48-hour period.

▬ INVASIVE TECHNIQUES

Cardiac Catheterization

Cardiac catheterization is a generic term that refers to a variety of procedures performed in the catheterization laboratory. Such procedures include selective coronary, saphenous vein bypass graft or internal mammary angiography, ventriculography, and right or left heart catheterization. All of the procedures are performed using invasive techniques and require a sterile environment.

PROCEDURE

Coronary angiography is used to evaluate the presence and location of coronary artery disease. A catheter is introduced via the arterial system under fluoroscopy retrograde to the ascending aorta. The right or left main coronary artery is then selectively cannulated and a radiopaque dye is injected directly into the artery through the catheter. As dye flows down the artery, the lumen of the artery can be visualized and the image recorded on film. Disease in the coronary artery or one of its branches will delay or obstruct the flow of dye and may be visualized on the film as a site of lumen narrowing and slow filling of the artery with dye. In patients who have undergone previous coronary bypass surgery, selective injections of saphenous vein bypass grafts or internal mammary arteries can be performed in a similar manner.

Radionuclide ventriculography is an excellent tool to assess regional decrease in contractility in areas of stenosed vessels and is useful in the evaluation of LV ejection fraction at peak exercise. Ventriculography is accomplished by injecting dye directly into the left ventricle and commonly is performed in conjunction with selective coronary angiography. A catheter is directed retrograde into the left ventricle through the arterial system under fluoroscopy. Dye is injected rapidly, and an image of the LV cavity is recorded on film as the ventricle contracts. LV ejection fraction, the percentage of blood present in the left ventricle during diastole that is ejected during systole, can be calculated from the film images. Outlines of the ventricle during diastole and systole are traced, and the areas inside each outline are proportional to the amount of blood present. In addition, regional ventricular wall motion abnormalities due to MI or severe ischemia can be visualized. The competence of the mitral valve also may be evaluated during ventriculography. In patients with mitral regurgitation, dye is observed being ejected not only into the aorta during systole, but also into the left atrium through an incompetent mitral valve. In patients with suspected aortic regurgitation, dye may be injected into the aorta; if regurgitation is present, the dye will flow retrograde into the left ventricle during diastole.

A *left heart catheterization* is done to measure intracardiac or intravascular pressures in the structures of the left side of the heart. The chambers are accessed with a catheter introduced retrograde through the arterial system under fluoroscopy. If either the mitral or aortic valves are stenosed, the pressures required to eject blood forward will be higher than normal because of the small valve orifice. For example, with normal mitral valve function, the left atrial (LA) pressure and LV pressure are nearly equal during ventricular diastole because blood flows easily from the left atrium through the mitral valve into the left ventricle. In contrast, mitral stenosis will result in a LA pressure that is significantly higher than the pressure in the left ventricle during ventricular diastole because the left atrium has to generate more pressure to force blood forward through the stenosed valve. This difference in pressure is known as a "gradient" and is related to the degree of stenosis present. Similar pressure comparisons are made in the left ventricle and aorta during systole to evaluate aortic stenosis. If a cardiac output measurement is available, the area of either the mitral or aortic valve opening may be calculated.

Mitral or aortic valve regurgitation also may be assessed by pressure measurements and with ventriculography, as previously described. The abnormal retrograde flow of blood into the left atrium during ventricular systole that occurs with mitral regurgitation produces higher-than-normal LA pressures. In patients with severe mitral regurgitation, the pressure in the left atrium may nearly equal the peak systolic pressure in the left ventricle. Similar pressure measurements are made in the left ventricle and aorta to evaluate aortic regurgitation.

A *right heart catheterization* procedure is performed to measure intracardiac and intravascular pressures in structures of the right side of the heart. A catheter is inserted antegrade through the venous system under fluoroscopy; the procedure is similar to the insertion of a PA catheter. Pressures are recorded from the vena cava, right atrium, right ventricle, PA, and pulmonary capillary wedge position. In addition, blood samples may be drawn from each chamber as the catheter is advanced, and the amount of oxygen present in each blood sample is measured. Because the right side of the heart normally contains venous blood, a significant increase in the amount of oxygen present in a blood sample may indicate a left-to-right intracardiac shunt.

Cardiac output, the amount of blood pumped by the heart in a minute, may be measured during a right heart catheterization using the thermodilution technique. Because cardiac output can be expected to vary with body size, the term "cardiac index," which takes height and weight into consideration, is used more often.

Arterial and venous accesses usually are achieved with percutaneous techniques from femoral sites. Typically, a needle is inserted into the artery or vein. A guidewire is then inserted through the needle and advanced to the appropriate position in or near the heart. After removing the needle, a catheter may be placed over the guidewire and advanced to the desired position. Changing catheters over guidewires allows specific preformed catheters to be used during the procedure. In some patients, percutaneous access cannot be accomplished from a femoral site, and a cutdown at a brachial site may be required. A bolus of IV or intra-arterial heparin is administered to patients requiring arterial access to prevent clot formation on the guidewire or catheter.

NURSING ASSESSMENT AND MANAGEMENT

Patients undergoing elective cardiac catheterization are NPO for at least 6 hours before the procedure. Because the dye may be nephrotoxic, hydration with IV fluids may be started before the procedure and continued afterward. Patients with low cardiac output or renal impairment are especially susceptible to dye nephrotoxicity, and their renal function should be monitored closely after the procedure. Patients may be prescribed a mild sedative before the procedure. When percutaneous access is used, pressure usually is applied over the site until bleeding has ceased. A pressure dressing, and in some laboratories, a sandbag, is left in place for several hours after the procedure.

Patients typically are placed on bed rest for 6 hours after the procedure and instructed not to flex the affected extremity. After the procedure, the access site should be checked frequently for signs of bleeding, swelling, or hematoma formation. If a femoral arterial access site was used, peripheral pulses in the affected extremity should be monitored. In addition, bleeding may occur in the retroperitoneal space in patients who have undergone femoral arterial access; close monitoring of blood pressure and heart rate and an awareness that retroperitoneal bleeding frequently presents as low back pain are useful in preventing a significant bleed.

Before catheterization, patients should be informed about the procedures that will be performed and questioned about any possible dye allergies. They should be instructed that they will be placed on a table with rounded sides and that their body will be strapped down so that they will not move as the table rotates from side to side. If they are to undergo ventriculography, they should be instructed that they may experience a temporary hot flash or flushing when dye is injected into the left ventricle. Postcatheterization procedures also should be explained to the patient, including bed rest and monitoring of the access site and vital signs. If the patient is to be discharged after the procedure and a cutdown was used for access, the patient should be instructed to make a follow-up appointment with the physician for suture removal.

Intravascular Ultrasound

A newer approach to the assessment of coronary anatomy is the IVUS technique. Using catheters of various frequencies, miniaturized ultrasound crystals are interfaced to ultrasound imaging consoles. Generally, the higher the frequency, the greater the image resolution. IVUS differs from angiography in that angiography provides a rapid means of assessing the diameter of the vessel lumen in silhouette, whereas IVUS provides a circumferential assessment of the vessel with a 360-degree view. IVUS is capable of providing cross-sectional images of coronary arteries that can illuminate arterial wall layers as well as injured media and adventitia. Vessel diameter and the cross-sectional dimensions can be determined. This evaluation permits identification of plaque composition on the vessel wall and its morphology.

In addition to better assessment of coronary and peripheral arterial atherosclerotic lesions, IVUS has proved useful in the assessment of arterial dissections and clots and aortic and pulmonary arterial disorders and can provide guidance during various catheter-based therapeutic procedures. Studies have shown the IVUS has been useful in the identification of atheromatous disease in vessels that appear normal with angiography and assist in recognition of whether such lesions are soft, fibrous, or calcified. Another common use of IVUS has been for the evaluation of coronary artery stents. Data suggest that IVUS is superior to routine angiography in the determination of expansion and underexpansion of the intracoronary stent postimplantation. IVUS catheters are also used for intracardiac echocardiographic studies. Using 10-MHz ultrasound transducers, atrial and ventricular chambers can be visualized to a greater extent and can provide views of the structures of the left heart through the right atrium and right ventricle. Therefore, IVUS techniques have proven to be superior for intravascular diagnostic assessment over angiographic procedures alone. The ability to characterize plaque composition, arterial wall characteristics, areas at risk, and intracoronary stent expansion has made this a powerful tool in the armamentarium of cardiac diagnostic testing.

Electrophysiology Studies

PURPOSE

Electrophysiology studies are used both for diagnosing and evaluating interventions in the treatment of dysrhythmias. The testing protocol may include the measurement of conduction and recovery times in the specialized conduction system of the heart, identification of abnormal or accessory conduction pathways, and stimulation of atrial or ventricular tissues to induce dysrhythmias. All of the procedures are performed using invasive techniques and require a sterile environment.

Patients presenting with symptoms suggestive of supraventricular tachycardia or VT or syncope frequently are studied with electrophysiological testing. The intracardiac electrodes are used to stimulate atrial or ventricular tissue at various pacing rates and numbers of extra stimuli. The induction and subsequent recording of a supraventricular tachycardia provides information about the mechanism of the dysrhythmia. If an accessory pathway is identified as the mechanism, radiofrequency or surgical ablation of the pathway may be successful in eliminating future episodes of the tachycardia.

The successful induction of VT with electrophysiological testing is of both diagnostic and prognostic value for the risk of sudden cardiac death. Treatment with pharmacological agents can be evaluated with subsequent studies. Antiarrhythmics that prevent induction or slow the rate of a VT in a patient who was inducible in the control state may be used in the long-term management of the dysrhythmia. Ventricular dysrhythmias usually are not treated with ablation methods because the areas of ventricular tissue responsible for the tachycardia are not easily identified and are widespread.

PROCEDURE

To measure electrical activity from the specialized conduction system of the heart, it is necessary to place electrodes at various intracardiac sites. Special catheters with multiple electrodes are inserted through arterial or venous access and advanced to locations within the heart; a separate access site is required for each electrode. In most studies, venous access is adequate for proper positioning of the electrodes; however, arterial access may be required for blood pressure monitoring. The high right atrium, bundle of His, and RV apex sites typically are used for recording and stimulation. In addition, several body surface leads are recorded simultaneously.

Venous and arterial accesses usually are achieved with percutaneous techniques from femoral sites in a manner similar to that used during cardiac catheterization. A sheath may be left in place during the procedure, however, so that electrode catheters may be repositioned as necessary. In some patients, access cannot be accomplished from a femoral site and percutaneous access through the jugular vein or a cutdown at a brachial site may be required. A bolus of IV or intra-arterial heparin is administered to patients requiring arterial access to prevent clot formation on the electrode catheter.

Conduction times from the atria to the bundle of His and bundle of His to ventricles are measured. Sites of block—supra-His or infra-His—can be identified and provide information that is used to direct treatment. In addition, the atrium can be paced over a range of rates to identify the rate at which heart block develops. Sinus node function is evaluated by pacing the atrium at various rates, suddenly stopping pacing, and measuring the amount of time it takes for the sinus node to initiate an impulse. The development of heart block at slow heart rates or prolonged sinus node recovery times may indicate a causal factor in patients presenting with syncope or presyncope.

NURSING ASSESSMENT AND MANAGEMENT

Patients undergoing electrophysiological testing are NPO for at least 6 hours before the procedure, although a sedative administered orally may be prescribed. When percutaneous access is used, pressure is applied over the site until bleeding has ceased. A pressure dressing usually is left in place for several hours after the procedure.

Patients typically are placed on bed rest for 6 hours after the procedure and instructed not to flex the affected extremity. The access site should be checked frequently for signs of bleeding, swelling, or hematoma formation. If a femoral arterial access site was used, peripheral pulses in the affected extremity should be monitored.

Before electrophysiological testing, patients should be instructed that they will be placed on a table with straps over their torso. They should be informed that they may experience palpitations or syncope if rapid tachyarrhythmias are induced. Poststudy procedures also should be explained to the patient, including bed rest and monitoring of the access site and vital signs. If the patient is to be discharged after the procedure and a cutdown was used for access, the patient should be instructed to make a follow-up appointment with the physician for suture removal.

Patients with VT who are being initiated on antiarrhythmic therapy are at risk for sudden cardiac death because some medications may have adverse proarrhythmic effects. These patients often are kept in a monitored setting for most of their hospital stay until appropriate therapies have been identified. Because most of these patients are otherwise healthy and physically active, it becomes a challenge for the nursing staff to care for these patients as well as the more severely ill patient population.

Electrocardiographic Monitoring

Cardiac monitoring is used in a variety of settings. Besides the traditional use in ICU and operating rooms, cardiac monitors are found in other inpatient units where it is necessary to monitor continuously a patient's heart rate and rhythm or the effects of a therapy. Cardiac monitors are used outside the hospital in settings such as paramedic ambulances, surgical centers, outpatient rehabilitation programs, and transtelephonic monitoring clinics.

Although the type of monitor may differ in each of these settings, all monitoring systems use three basic components: an oscilloscope display system, a monitoring cable, and electrodes. Electrodes are placed on the patient's chest to receive the electrical current from the cardiac muscle tissue. The electrical signal is then carried by the monitoring cable to an oscilloscope, where it is magnified over 1,000 times and displayed. The display can be obtained both at the patient's bedside and at a central station, along with displays from other patients' monitors.

■ EQUIPMENT FEATURES

Two types of cardiac monitoring equipment in use are continuous hard-wire monitoring systems and telemetry monitoring systems.

Hard-Wire Monitoring Systems

Hard-wire monitors, which are commonly used in the ICU setting, require the patient to be linked directly to the cardiac monitor through the ECG cable. Information is displayed and recorded at the bedside along with simultaneous display and recording at a central station. Because this type of cardiac monitoring limits patient mobility, patients using this system usually are confined to bed rest or are allowed to be up at the bedside only. Hard-wire monitors operate on electricity but are well isolated so that water, blood, and other fluids do not pose an electrical hazard as long as the machine is maintained adequately.

Telemetry Monitoring Systems

In telemetry monitoring, no direct wire connection is needed between the patient and the ECG display device. Electrodes are connected by a short monitoring cable to a small battery-operated transmitter that the patient carries in a disposable pouch tied to his or her body. The ECG is then sent by radiofrequency signals to a receiver that picks up and displays the signal on an oscilloscope, either at the bedside or at a distant central recording station. Antennas are built into the receiver and may be mounted in the vicinity of the receiver to widen the range of signal pickup. Batteries are the power source for the transmitter, thus mak-ing it possible to avoid electrical hazards by isolating the monitoring system from potential current leakage and accidental shock. Telemetry systems are used primarily for dysrhythmia monitoring in areas where the patient is fairly mobile, such as an dysrhythmia surveillance or "step-down" unit. Because the patient is mobile, stable ECG tracings often are more difficult to obtain. Some hard-wire systems have built-in telemetry capability so that patients may be switched easily from one system to another as monitoring needs change.

Display Systems

Modern electronic technology continues to make sophisticated advances in monitoring equipment, and current display systems incorporate features such as the following:

- Improved freeze/hold modes, which allow the ECG pattern to be held for more detailed examination
- Storage capability, either by tape loops or an electronic memory, which permits retrieval of dysrhythmias
- Automatic chart documentation, in which the ECG recorder is activated by alarms or at preset intervals
- Heart rate indicators, which display the rate either by meter or by digital display (the alarm system is incorporated into the heart rate monitor with adjustments for both the high and low settings)
- Multilead ECG display, which facilitates complex dysrhythmia interpretation
- ST segment analysis for monitoring ischemic events
- Multiparameter displays, which offer display of hemodynamic pressures, temperature, intracranial pressure, and respirations
- Computer systems that store, analyze, and trend monitored data, allowing the information to be retrieved at any time to aid in diagnosis and to note trends in the patient's status

Monitoring Lead Systems

All cardiac monitors use lead systems to record the electrical activity generated by cardiac tissue. Each lead system is composed of a positive or recording electrode, a negative electrode, and a third electrode used as a ground. As the heart depolarizes, the waves of electrical activity move inferiorly, because the normal route of depolarization moves from the sinoatrial (SA) node and atria, downward through the AV node, His–Purkinje system, and ventricles, and to the left as the left heart muscle mass predominates over the right heart. Each lead system looks at these waves of depolarization from a different location on the chest wall and thus produces P waves and QRS complexes of varying configuration.

The terminology used to describe lead systems can be confusing. The wires attached to the patient's chest are called leads, and the pictures produced by these wires are also called leads. A standard ECG uses 10 lead wires with electrodes at the ends (four placed on the limbs and six placed on the chest) and produces 12 electrical views of the heart, known as 12 leads.

Cardiac monitoring systems currently on the market vary from two- and three-electrode telemetry devices to three-, four-, and five-electrode hard-wire systems. The two- or three-electrode systems produce limited selections of leads I, II, or III with only a single lead viewed on the screen at one time (single-channel recording). Five-electrode systems allow the possibility of viewing any of the 12 ECG leads and permit the nurse to view two leads on the monitor screen simultaneously (multichannel recording).

THREE-ELECTRODE SYSTEMS

Monitors that require three electrodes use positive, negative, and ground electrodes that are placed in the right arm (RA), left arm (LA) and left leg (LL) positions on the chest as designated by markings on the monitor cable. When the electrodes are placed appropriately, the standard leads (leads I, II, III) may be obtained by moving the lead selector on the bedside oscilloscope to the lead I, II, or III position (Fig. 16–17). The lead selector automatically adjusts which electrode is positive, which electrode is negative, and which electrode is ground to obtain an appropriate tracing. When lead I is selected, the LA is positive, the RA is negative, and the LL is ground. For a lead II configuration, the LL is positive, the RA is negative, and the LA is ground. To obtain a lead III, the LL is positive, the LA is negative, and the RA is ground. The configuration of leads I, II, and III, as illustrated in Figure 16–18, is known as Einthoven's triangle.

To obtain a chest lead on the monitor that replicates the chest lead from the 12-lead ECG, a five-wire system is needed. When only three wires are available, a modified version of any of the six chest leads may be obtained. To configure a modified chest lead (MCL), the goal is to position the positive elec-

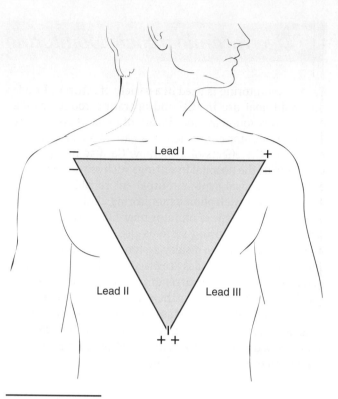

FIGURE 16-18

Leads I, II, and III are known as the standard leads. When placed together over the chest, they form what is known as Einthoven's triangle.

Lead I: Left arm is positive, and right arm is negative
Lead II: Left leg is positive, and right arm is negative.
Lead III: Left leg is positive, and left arm is negative.

trode in the designated chest position. For example, an MCL_1 would require the positive electrode to be placed in a V_1 position (fourth intercostal space, right sternal border). The negative electrode is always positioned under the left clavicle. The ground electrode can be positioned anywhere.

To obtain an MCL_1 lead, the monitor is set to lead I, as shown in the accompanying display. By setting the monitor to lead I, the LA electrode is positive, the RA electrode is negative, and the leg wire is the ground (Einthoven's triangle). The positive electrode (LA) is placed in a V_1 position (fourth intercostal space, right sternal border), and the negative electrode (RA) is positioned under the left clavicle. Although the ground electrode (LL) can be positioned anywhere, if it is placed in a V_6 position, it will be helpful when switching to an MCL_6 lead.

To obtain an MCL_6 lead, the goal is to place a positive electrode in a V_6 position, a negative electrode under the clavicle, and a ground wire anywhere. By setting the monitor to lead II, the LL electrode is positive, the RA electrode is negative, and the LA electrode is ground (Einthoven's triangle). The positive electrode (LL) is placed in the V_6 position, and the negative electrode (RA) is placed under the left clavicle. The ground wire can be placed anywhere. If placed in a V_1 position, it will be helpful when switching to an MCL_1 lead (see Fig. 16–18).

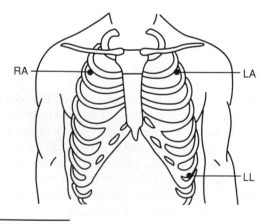

FIGURE 16-17

Three-electrode monitoring system. Leads placed in this position will allow the nurse to monitor leads I, II, or III. The left leg electrode must be placed below the level of the heart.

To monitor MCL_1 using a three-electrode monitor:
1. Select lead I on the monitor.
2. Refer to Einthoven's triangle to remember which electrode is positive, negative, and ground.
3. Place the positive electrode (LA) in a V_1 position (fourth intercostal space, right sternal border).
4. Place the negative electrode (RA) under the left clavicle.
5. Place the ground wire (LL) in the V_6 position (fifth intercostal space, left midaxillary line).

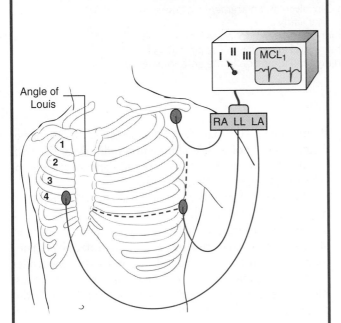

To monitor MCL_6 using a three-electrode monitor:
1. Select lead II on the monitor.
2. Refer to Einthoven's triangle to remember which electrode is positive, negative, and ground.
3. Place the positive electrode (LL) in the V_6 position (fifth intercostal space, left midaxillary line).
4. Place the negative electrode (RA) under the left clavicle.
5. Place the ground wire (LA) in a V_1 position (fourth intercostal space, right sternal border).

Note: The electrodes are in the same position on the chest for the MCL_1 lead and the MCL_6 lead. To view the two leads, the nurse merely switches the monitor from lead I to lead II.

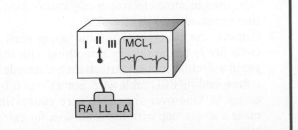

By arranging the electrodes as described previously, the nurse can monitor both MCL_1 and MCL_6 merely by switching the monitor from a lead I to a lead II without changing the electrode placement on the patient's chest. MCL_1 and MCL_6 are ideal leads for detecting BBB rhythms and for differentiating supraventricular wide QRS tachycardias from VT.

FOUR- AND FIVE-ELECTRODE SYSTEMS

Four- and five-electrode systems increase the monitor's capability beyond the three-electrode system. The four-electrode monitor requires a right leg electrode that is the ground for all leads described in the three-electrode system. The five-electrode monitor adds an exploring "chest" electrode that allows one to obtain any one of the six chest leads and the six limb leads. In essence, a five-wire monitor system provides all the capabilities of the 12-lead ECG machine. The only difference is the five-wire monitor has only one chest electrode, whereas the 12-lead ECG machine has six chest electrodes. Newer cardiac monitors now have all six chest electrodes and allow the nurse to view all 12 leads of the ECG simultaneously on the monitor screen.

To monitor a patient with a five-wire system, the four limb electrodes are positioned on the body according to their designations. The fifth chest electrode is placed on the chest in the designated precordial position. For example, if the nurse wants to monitor V_1, the chest electrode is placed in the fourth intercostal space, right sternal border (Fig. 16–19). If the nurse wants to switch to a different chest lead for monitoring, the electrode must be repositioned on the patient's chest. A five-electrode monitor offers the additional advantage of allowing the nurse to view two different leads simultaneously on the monitor screen.

LEAD SELECTION

No single monitoring lead is ideal for every patient. Table 16–4 summarizes the use of various leads with rationale.

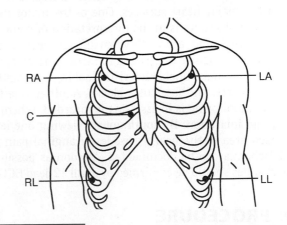

FIGURE 16-19
Using a five-electrode system allows the nurse to monitor any of the 12 leads of the electrocardiogram. The chest electrode must be moved to the appropriate chest location when monitoring the precordial leads.

TABLE 16-4
Suggested Monitoring Lead Selection

Lead	Rationale for Use
II	Produces large, upright visible P waves and QRS complexes for determining underlying rhythm
V_1 or MCL_1	Helpful for detecting right bundle branch block and to differentiate ventricular ectopy from supraventricular rhythm aberrantly conducted in the ventricles
V_6 or MCL_6	Helpful lead for detecting left bundle branch block and to differentiate ventricular ectopy from supraventricular rhythm aberrantly conducted in the ventricles
III, aVF, V_1	Produce visible P waves; useful in detecting atrial dysrhythmias
I	Useful in patients with respiratory distress
	Left arm and right arm electrodes involved and placements less affected by chest motion compared with other leads
II, III, aVF	Helpful in detecting ischemia, injury, and infarction in the inferior wall
I, aVL, V_5, V_6	Helpful in detecting ischemia, injury, and infarction in the lateral wall
V_1 through V_4	Helpful in detecting ischemia, injury, and infarction in the anterior wall

Lead II is used commonly because it records clear upright P waves and QRS complexes that are helpful in determining the underlying rhythm. In addition to lead II, leads III, aVF, and V_1 or MCL_1 show well-formed P waves and therefore are helpful in identifying atrial dysrhythmias. V_1 or MCL_1 is useful in recognizing right bundle branch block (RBBB) and in differentiating ventricular ectopy from supraventricular rhythms with aberrancy; V_6 or MCL_6 is helpful in identifying LBBB and also is useful in differentiating ventricular ectopy from supraventricular rhythms with aberrancy. Lead I may be tried with the respiratory patient who has much artifact on the tracing because there is less movement of the positive electrode in this lead than in a lead II or a V_1.

As mentioned, there is no one ideal monitoring lead for every patient, and in several situations, a multilead recording is desirable. Multilead ECG systems offer multiple views of the heart because they reflect a tracing from each of the major heart surfaces. One of the major uses for this type of system is in the interpretation of complex cardiac dysrhythmias, especially when differentiating aberrancy from ventricular ectopy and in identifying complex atrial dysrhythmias, uncharacteristic-looking ventricular premature beats, and fascicular blocks. Another role for multilead monitoring is in assessing myocardial ischemia, injury, and infarction. By continuously viewing one lead from each area of the heart, episodes of anginal pain or silent ischemia can be documented. As soon as possible, these changes should be confirmed by a full 12-lead ECG.

PROCEDURE

Electrode Application

Proper skin preparation and application of electrodes are imperative for good ECG monitoring. An adequate tracing should reflect (1) a narrow, stable baseline; (2) absence of distortion or "noise"; (3) sufficient amplitude of the QRS complex to activate the rate meters and alarm systems properly; and (4) identification of P waves.

The type of electrode currently used for ECG monitoring is a disposable silver- or nickle-plated electrode centered in a circle of adhesive paper or foam rubber. Most electrodes are pregelled by the manufacturer. They may have disposable wires attached to the electrodes or nondisposable wires that snap onto the electrodes. Electrodes should be comfortable for the patient. If not properly applied, undue artifact and false alarms may result.

When applying electrodes, the following procedure should be followed:

1. Select a stable site. Avoid bony protuberances, joints, and folds in the skin. Areas in which muscle attaches to bone have the least motion artifact.
2. Shave excessive body hair from the site.
3. Rub the site briskly with a dry gauze pad to remove oils and cellular debris. Skin preparation with alcohol may be necessary if the skin is greasy; allow the alcohol to dry completely before applying the electrode. Follow the electrode manufacturer's directions because the chemical reaction between alcohol or other skin-preparation materials and the adhesives used in some electrodes may cause skin irritation or nonadhesion to the skin.
4. Remove the paper backing and apply each electrode firmly to the skin by smoothing with the finger in a circular motion. Attach each electrode to its corresponding ECG cable wire. Sometimes it is necessary to tape over the cable wire connection or make a stress loop with the cable wire for extra stability.

5. Change electrodes every 2 to 3 days, and monitor for skin irritation.

While applying the electrodes, explain the purpose of the procedure to the patient. Reassure the patient that monitor alarm sounds do not necessarily indicate a problem with the patient's heartbeat; alarms often occur when an electrode becomes loose or disconnected.

Monitor Observation

Cardiac monitors are useful only if the information they provide is "observed," either by computers with alarms for programmed parameters or by the human eye, and appropriately acted on by competent, responsible people. Some critical care units use monitor technicians whose main responsibilities are to observe monitors, obtain chart samples, and give appropriate information to the nurse as to each patient's ECG status. Those observing the monitor should know the acceptable dysrhythmia parameters for each patient and should be notified of any interruptions in monitoring, such as those caused by changing electrodes or by changing the patient to a portable monitor. The observer also should be aware of the presence of artifact from chest physical therapy or hiccups so that it may be considered in dysrhythmia diagnosis.

Regardless of the system used for monitor observation, certain practices always should be followed. If the monitor alarm sounds, the nurse should evaluate the clinical status of the patient before *anything else* to see if the problem is an actual dysrhythmia or a malfunction of the monitoring system. Asystole should not be mistaken for an unattached ECG wire, nor should a patient inadvertently tapping on an electrode be misread as VT. In addition, the monitor alarms always should be in the functioning mode. Only when direct physical care is being given to the patient can the alarm system safely be put on "standby." This ensures that no life-threatening dysrhythmia will go unnoticed. If the change on the monitor is not due to artifact or a disconnected wire, a full 12-lead ECG should be recorded to evaluate the rhythm change further.

■ TROUBLESHOOTING ELECTROCARDIOGRAM MONITOR PROBLEMS

Several problems may occur in monitoring the ECG, including baseline but no ECG trace, intermittent traces, wandering or irregular baseline, low-amplitude complexes, 60-cycle interference, excessive triggering of heart rate alarms, and skin irritation. The steps to follow when such problems occur are outlined in Table 16–5.

TABLE 16-5
Troubleshooting: Electrocardiogram (ECG) Monitor Problem Solving

Excessive Triggering of Heart Rate Alarms
- Is high-low alarm set too close to patient's rate?
- Is monitor sensitivity level set too high or too low?
- Is patient cable securely inserted into monitor receptacle?
- Are the lead wires or connections damaged?
- Has the monitoring lead been properly selected?
- Were the electrodes applied properly?
- Are the R and T waves the same height, causing both waveforms to be sensed?
- Is the baseline unstable, or is there excessive cable or lead wire movement?

Baseline But No ECG Trace
- Is the size (gain or sensitivity) control properly adjusted?
- Is appropriate lead selector being used on monitor?
- Is the patient cable fully inserted into ECG receptacle?
- Are electrode wires fully inserted into patient cable?
- Are electrode wires firmly attached to electrodes?
- Are electrode wires damaged?
- Is the patient cable damaged?
- Call for service if trace is still absent.
- Is the battery dead (for telemetry system)?

Intermittent Trace
- Is patient cable fully inserted into monitor receptacle?
- Are electrode wires fully inserted into patient cable?
- Are electrode wires firmly attached to electrodes?
- Are electrode wire connectors loose or worn?
- Have electrodes been applied properly?

- Are electrodes properly located and in firm skin contact?
- Is patient cable damaged?

Wandering or Irregular Baseline
- Is there excessive cable movement? This can be reduced by clipping to patient's clothing.
- Is the power cord on or near the monitor cable?
- Is there excessive movement by the patient? Muscle tremors from anxiety or shivering?
- Is site selection correct?
- Were proper skin preparation and application followed?
- Are the electrodes still moist?

Low-Amplitude Complexes
- Is size control adjusted properly?
- Were the electrodes applied properly?
- Is there dried gel on the electrodes?
- Change electrode sites. Check 12-lead ECG for lead with highest amplitude, and attempt to simulate that lead.
- If none of the above steps remedies the problem, the weak signal may be the patient's normal complex.

Sixty-Cycle Interference
- Is the monitor size control set too high?
- Are there nearby electrical devices in use, especially poorly grounded ones?
- Were the electrodes applied properly?
- Is there dried gel on the electrodes?
- Are lead wires or connections damaged?

Dysrhythmias and the 12-Lead Electrocardiogram

Dysrhythmias and abnormalities of the 12-lead ECG commonly encountered in monitored patients can be recognized with a little practice. The types that occur most frequently are discussed in this chapter. Before presenting the individual dysrhythmias and 12-lead ECG abnormalities, the method for evaluating a rhythm strip is addressed.

To understand the causes, clinical significance, and treatment of dysrhythmias, knowledge of the conduction system is essential. Chapter 15 provides a review of the essential elements of the cardiac conducting system.

◼ EVALUATION OF A RHYTHM STRIP

Electrocardiogram Paper

An ECG tracing is a graphic recording of the heart's electrical activity. The paper consists of horizontal and vertical lines, each 1 mm apart. The horizontal lines denote time measurements. When the paper is run at a sweep speed of 25 mm/s, each small square is equal to 0.04 seconds, and a large square (five small squares) equals 0.20 seconds. Height or voltage is measured by counting the lines vertically. Each small square is 1 mm, and the large square equals 5 mm (Fig. 16–20). Most ECG paper also is marked by vertical slash marks along the top or bottom of the paper. The distance between two vertical markings represents 3 seconds. The distance between 6 seconds is used for rate calculation.

Waveforms and Intervals

During the cardiac cycle, the following waveforms and intervals are produced on the ECG surface tracing (see Fig. 16–20).

P wave: The P wave is a small, usually upright and rounded deflection representing depolarization of the atria. It normally is seen before the QRS complex at a consistent interval.

PR interval: The PR interval represents the time from the onset of atrial depolarization until the onset of ventricular depolarization. Included in the interval is the brief delay of the electrical signal at the AV node that allows time for the blood to move from the atria to the ventricles before the ventricles are depolarized. The interval is measured from the beginning of the P wave to the beginning of the QRS. A normal PR interval is 0.12 to 0.20 second.

QRS complex: The QRS complex is a large waveform representing ventricular depolarization. Each component of the waveform has a specific connotation. The initial negative deflection is a Q wave, the initial positive deflection is an R wave, and the negative deflection after the R wave is an S wave. Not all QRS complexes have all three components, even though the complex is commonly called the QRS complex. A normal QRS complex is 0.06 to 0.11 second in width. Figure 16–21 illustrates different kinds of QRS complexes.

ST segment: The ST segment is the portion of the tracing from the end of the QRS complex to the beginning of the T wave. It represents the time from the end of ventricular depolarization to the beginning of ventricular repolarization. Normally it is isoelectric. An isoelectric ST segment means the ST segment joins the QRS complex at the baseline. ST segments may be elevated or depressed in a variety of conditions. Elevated ST segments could indicate acute myocardial injury. Depressed ST segments may signify acute myocardial injury or myocardial ischemia. For a more detailed discussion of ST segment abnormalities, see Chapter 20.

T wave: The T wave is the deflection representing ventricular repolarization or recovery. The T wave appears after the QRS complex. The atria also have a re-

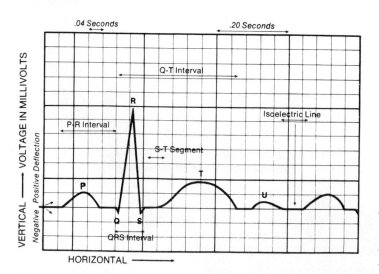

FIGURE 16-20

Schematic representation of the electrical impulse as it traverses the conduction system, resulting in depolarization and repolarization of the myocardium.

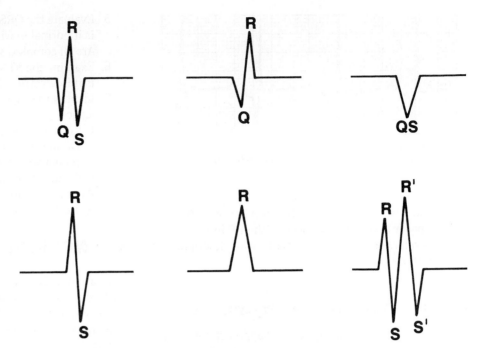

FIGURE 16-21
Different kinds of QRS complexes
An R wave is a positive deflection. A
Q wave is a negative deflection be-
fore an R wave. An S wave is a nega-
tive deflection after an R wave.

polarization phase. However, there is no visible wave on the ECG to represent atrial repolarization because it occurs at the same time as the QRS.

U wave: A U wave is a rarely seen, small, usually positive deflection after the T wave. Its significance is uncertain, but it typically is seen with hypokalemia.

QT interval: The QT interval is the period of time from the beginning of ventricular depolarization to the end of ventricular repolarization. The QT interval is measured from the beginning of the QRS complex to the end of the T wave. Because the QT varies with heart rate, it is necessary to use a table in which QT intervals for various heart rates are listed. Tables such as Table 16–6 are available in most dysrhythmia texts for this purpose. If a table is not available, a corrected QT interval (QT_c) can be calculated for comparison with normal values. A normal QT_c usually does not exceed 0.42 second for men and 0.43 second for women. A quick method for obtaining a QT_c is to use half of the preceding RR interval (described below).

Calculation of Heart Rate

Although cardiac monitors and ECG strips can be used to calculate heart rate, the calculated rate is merely an estimate of the number of times per minute the heart has been electrically excited. In the normal heart, each excitation should be followed by cardiac contraction. However, in some situations, electrical activity can occur without contraction, resulting in a lack of perfusion. Therefore, the heart rate obtained from the cardiac monitor or ECG strip should never be substituted for the determination of heart rate by palpating the pulse.

Both the atrial and the ventricular rates can be estimated by examining the ECG. To determine the ventricular rate, count the number of QRS complexes in a 6-second strip, and

multiply by 10. To estimate the atrial rate, count the number of P waves in a 6-second strip, and multiply by 10. In the normal patient, the atrial and the ventricular rates should be the same. This method of rate calculation provides an estimate of heart rate for regular and irregular rhythms.

Another method of rate calculation can be used if the rhythm is regular. The ventricular heart rate is estimated by dividing 300 by the number of large boxes on the ECG paper between two R waves (the RR interval). The atrial rate

TABLE 16-6
Approximate Normal Limits for QT Intervals in Seconds

Heart Rate per Minute	Men and Children	Women
40	0.45–0.49	0.46–0.50
46	0.43–0.47	0.44–0.48
50	0.41–0.45	0.43–0.46
55	0.40–0.44	0.41–0.45
60	0.39–0.42	0.40–0.43
67	0.37–0.40	0.38–0.41
71	0.36–0.40	0.37–0.41
75	0.35–0.38	0.36–0.39
80	0.34–0.37	0.35–0.38
86	0.33–0.36	0.34–0.37
93	0.32–0.35	0.33–0.36
100	0.31–0.34	0.32–0.35
109	0.30–0.33	0.31–0.33
120	0.28–0.31	0.29–0.32
133	0.27–0.29	0.28–0.30
150	0.25–0.28	0.26–0.28
172	0.23–0.26	0.24–0.26

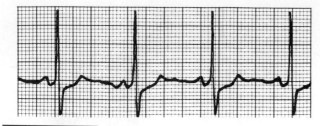

FIGURE 16-22
Normal sinus rhythm. (Rate = 60–100 beats/minute.)

is calculated by dividing 300 by the number of large boxes on ECG paper between two P waves (the PP interval). The reader is referred to a dysrhythmia text for description of other methods.

Steps in Assessing a Rhythm Strip

The following represents a systematic approach for analyzing a cardiac rhythm strip. Whether this method or another method is used, it is important to take the time to go through each step, because many dysrhythmias are not as they first appear.

1. Determine the atrial and ventricular heart rates.
   Are they within normal limits?
   If not, is there a relationship between the two (ie, is one a multiple of the other)?
2. Examine the rhythm to see if it is regular.
   Is there an equal amount of time between each QRS complex (RR interval)?
   Is there an equal amount of time between each P wave (PP interval)?
   Are the PP and RR intervals the same?
3. Look for the P waves.
   Are they present?
   Is there one or more P wave for each QRS complex?
   Do all P waves have the same configuration?
4. Measure the PR interval.
   Is it normal?
   Is it the same throughout the strip, or does it vary?
   If it varies, is there a pattern to the variation?

5. Evaluate the QRS complex.
   Is it normal in width, or is it wide?
   Are all complexes of the same configuration?
6. Examine the ST segment.
   Is it isoelectric, elevated, or depressed?
7. Identify the rhythm and determine its clinical significance.
   Is the patient symptomatic? (Check skin, neurological status, renal function, coronary circulation, hemodynamic status/blood pressure.)
   Is the dysrhythmia life threatening?
   What is the clinical context?
   Is the dysrhythmia new or chronic?

NORMAL SINUS RHYTHM

Normal sinus rhythm (Fig. 16–22) is the normal rhythm of the heart. The impulse is initiated at the sinus node in a regular rhythm at a rate of 60 to 100 beats/min. A P wave appears before each QRS complex. The PR interval is within normal limits (0.12–0.20 second), and the QRS is narrow (< 0.12 second) unless an intraventricular conduction defect is present.

DYSRHYTHMIAS ORIGINATING AT THE SINUS NODE

Table 16–7 summarizes and compares ECG characteristics of sinus rhythm.

Sinus Tachycardia

In sinus tachycardia, the sinus node accelerates and initiates an impulse at a rate of 100 times/minute or more (Fig. 16–23). The upper limits of sinus tachycardia extend to 160 to 180 beats/min. All other ECG characteristics, except for heart rate, are the same as in normal sinus rhythm.

Sinus tachycardia usually is caused by factors relating to an increase in sympathetic tone. Stress, exercise, and stimulants such as caffeine and nicotine can produce this dysrhythmia. Sinus tachycardia also is associated with such clinical problems as fever, anemia, hyperthyroidism, hypo-

TABLE 16-7
A Comparison of the Electrocardiogram Characteristics of Sinus Rhythms

	Normal Sinus Rhythm	Sinus Tachycardia	Sinus Bradycardia	Sinus Arrhythmia
Rate	60–100 beats/min	>100 beats/min	<60 beats/min	60–100 beats/min
Rhythm	Regular	Regular	Regular	Irregular
P waves	Present, one per QRS	Present, one per QRS	Present, one per QRS	Present, one per QRS
PR interval	<0.20 s, equal	<0.20 s, equal	<0.20 s, equal	<0.20 s, equal
QRS complex	<0.12 s	<0.12 s	<0.12 s	<0.12 s

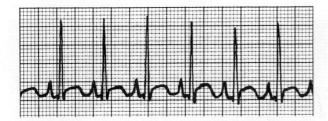

FIGURE 16-23
Sinus tachycardia. (Heart rate = 100–180 beats/min.)

xemia, CHF, and shock. Drugs such as atropine (which blocks vagal tone) and the catecholamines (eg, isoproterenol, epinephrine, dopamine) also can produce this rhythm.

The cause of the sinus tachycardia and the underlying state of the myocardium determine its prognosis. Sinus tachycardia alone is not a lethal dysrhythmia but often signals an underlying problem that should be pursued. In addition, the rapid rate of sinus tachycardia increases oxygen demands on the myocardium and decreases the filling time of the ventricles. In people who already have depleted cardiac reserve, ischemia, or CHF, the persistence of a fast rate may worsen the underlying condition.

Treatment for sinus tachycardia usually is directed toward eliminating the underlying cause. Specific measures may include sedation, oxygen administration, digitalis, and diuretics if heart failure is present, or propranolol if the tachycardia is due to thyrotoxicosis.

Sinus Bradycardia

Sinus bradycardia is defined as a rhythm with impulses originating at the sinus node at a rate of less than 60 beats/min (Fig. 16–24). The rhythm (RR interval) is regular and all other parameters are normal.

Sinus bradycardia is common among all age groups and is present in both normal and diseased hearts. It may occur during sleep, in highly trained athletes, and with severe pain, inferior wall MI, acute spinal cord injury, and certain drugs (eg, digitalis, beta-blockers, verapamil, diltiazem).

Slow rates are tolerated well in people with healthy hearts. With severe heart disease, however, the heart may

not be able to compensate for a slow rate by increasing the volume of blood ejected per beat. In this situation, sinus bradycardia will lead to a low cardiac output.

No treatment is indicated unless symptoms are present. If the pulse is very slow and symptoms are present, appropriate measures include atropine (to block the vagal effect), isoproterenol, or cardiac pacing.

Sinus Arrhythmia

Sinus arrhythmia is a disorder of rhythm (Fig. 16–25). It is said to be present if the RR intervals on the ECG strip vary by more than 0.12 second, from the shortest RR interval to the longest. This dysrhythmia is due to an irregularity in sinus node discharge, often in association with phases of the respiratory cycle. The sinus node gradually speeds up with inspiration and gradually slows with expiration. There also is a nonrespiratory form of this dysrhythmia.

Sinus arrhythmia is a normal phenomenon, seen especially in young people in the setting of lower heart rates. It also occurs after enhancement of vagal tone (eg, digitalis, morphine). Because it is a normal finding, sinus arrhythmia does not imply the presence of underlying disease. Symptoms are uncommon unless there are excessively long pauses, and usually no treatment is required.

Sinus Arrest and Sinoatrial Block

Sinus arrest is a disorder of impulse formation. The sinus node fails to discharge one or more impulses, producing pauses of varying lengths due to the absence of atrial depolarization. The P wave is absent, and the resulting PP interval is not a multiple of the basic PP interval. The pause ends either when an escape pacemaker from the junction or ventricles takes over or sinus node function returns.

An SA block often is difficult to differentiate from sinus arrest on a surface ECG tracing. In SA block, the sinus node fires, but the impulse is delayed or blocked from exiting the sinus node. If the block is complete, the duration of the pause is a multiple of the basic PP interval (Fig. 16–26).

Both dysrhythmias may be due to disruption of the sinus node by infarction, degenerative fibrotic changes, drug effects (digitalis, beta-blockers, calcium-channel blockers), or excessive vagal stimulation. These rhythms usually are tran-

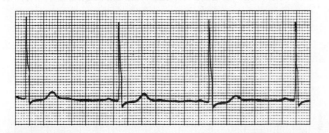

FIGURE 16-24
Sinus bradycardia. (Heart rate less than 60 beats/min.)

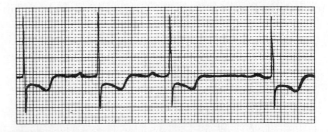

FIGURE 16-25
Sinus arrhythmia. (The difference between the shortest and longest RR interval is greater than 0.12 second.)

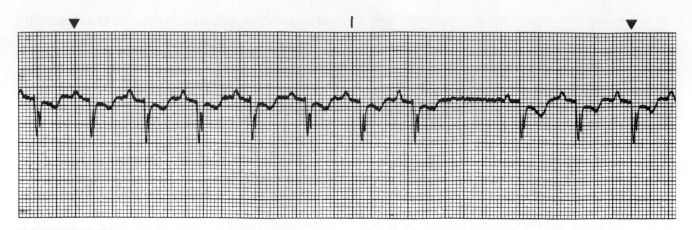

FIGURE 16-26
SA block. The pause is a multiple of the basic PP interval.

sient and insignificant, unless a lower pacemaker fails to take over to pace the ventricles. Treatment is indicated if the patient is symptomatic. The goal is to increase the ventricular rate, which may require the use of atropine or, in the presence of serious hemodynamic compromise, a pacemaker.

Sick Sinus Syndrome

Sick sinus syndrome refers to a chronic form of sinus node disease (Fig. 16–27). Patients exhibit severe degrees of sinus node depression, including marked sinus bradycardia, SA block, or sinus arrest. Often, rapid atrial dysrhythmias, such as atrial flutter or fibrillation (the "tachycardia–bradycardia syndrome") coexist and alternate with periods of sinus node depression.

Management of this condition requires control of the rapid atrial dysrhythmias with drug therapy, and in selected cases, control of very slow heart rates, often requiring implantation of a permanent pacemaker.

◼◼◼ ATRIAL DYSRHYTHMIAS

Premature Atrial Contraction

A premature atrial contraction (PAC) occurs when an ectopic atrial impulse discharges prematurely and, in most cases, is conducted in a normal fashion through the AV conducting system to the ventricles (Fig. 16–28). On the ECG tracing, the P wave is premature and may even be buried in

the preceding T wave; it often differs in configuration from the sinus P wave. The QRS complex usually is of normal configuration but because of timing, may appear wide and bizarre if conducted with some degree of delay (aberrant PAC) or not at all if the atrial impulse is blocked from being conducted to the ventricles (blocked PAC). A short pause, usually less than "compensatory," is present (see later definition of premature ventricular contraction [PVC]).

All age groups experience PACs. PACs may occur in normal people as a result of various stimuli, such as emotions, tobacco, alcohol, and caffeine. PACs also may be associated with rheumatic heart disease, ischemic heart disease, mitral stenosis, heart failure, hypokalemia, hypomagnesemia, medications, or hyperthyroidism.

Alternatively, PACs may be a precursor to an atrial tachycardia, atrial fibrillation, or atrial flutter, indicating an increasing atrial irritability. They also may indicate an underlying condition (eg, CHF). Patients may have the sensation of a "pause" or "skip" in rhythm when PACs are present.

No treatment is necessary in many cases. The patient should be monitored and frequency of premature beats documented. In addition, the patient should be assessed for underlying conditions and treated.

Paroxysmal Supraventricular Tachycardia

Paroxysmal supraventricular tachycardia (PSVT) describes a rapid atrial rhythm occurring at a rate of 150 to 250 beats/min (Fig. 16–29). The tachycardia begins abruptly, in

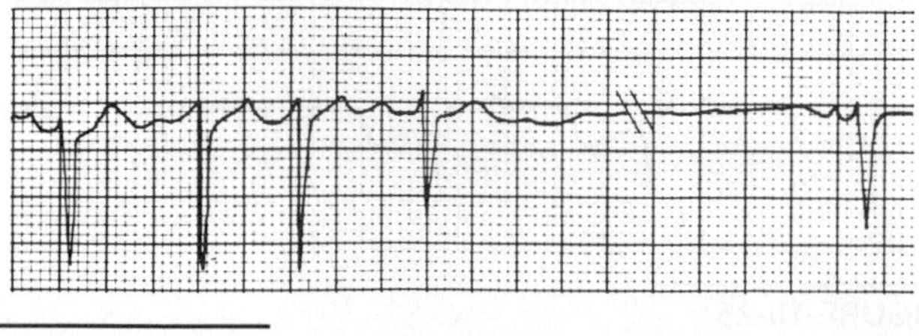

FIGURE 16-27
Sick sinus syndrome. Atrial fibrillation is followed by atrial standstill. A sinus escape beat is seen at the end of the strip.

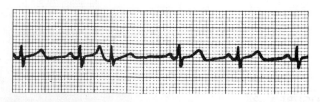

FIGURE 16-28
Premature atrial contraction.

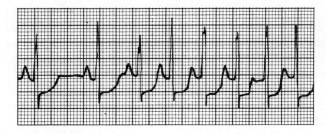

FIGURE 16-29
Paroxysmal supraventricular tachycardia (begins with a premature atrial contraction).

most instances with a PAC, and it ends abruptly. P waves may be seen preceding the QRS but at faster rates, may be hidden in the QRS or preceding T wave. (If some of the P waves are not followed by a QRS, this is referred to as PSVT with block and usually is due to digitalis toxicity.) The P waves may be negative in II, III, and aVF owing to retrograde conduction from the AV node to the atria. The QRS usually is normal unless there is an underlying intraventricular conduction problem. The rhythm is regular and the paroxysms may last from a few seconds to several hours or even days.

The term PSVT is used to identify rhythms previously called paroxysmal atrial tachycardia and paroxysmal nodal or junctional tachycardia, rhythms similar in all respects except in their sites of origin. PSVT also is known as *AV nodal reentrant tachycardia* because the mechanism most commonly responsible for this dysrhythmia is a reentrant circuit or chaotic movement at the level of the AV node.

The PSVT must be differentiated from other narrow QRS (supraventricular) tachycardias. Table 16–8 indicates means of differentiation. The following points favor the diagnosis of PSVT versus a sinus tachycardia:

An atrial premature beat often initiates the rhythm. PSVT begins and terminates abruptly.

The rate often is faster than a sinus tachycardia and tends to be more regular from minute to minute.

In response to a vagal maneuver, such as carotid sinus massage, the ectopic tachycardia either will be unaffected or will revert to a normal sinus rhythm; sinus tachycardia, however, will slow slightly in response to increased vagal tone.

For the same reasons as PACs, PSVT occurs often in adults with normal hearts. When heart disease is present, such abnormalities as rheumatic heart disease, acute MI, and digitalis intoxication may serve as the background for this dysrhythmia.

Often the patient is without underlying heart disease and may experience only palpitations and some light-headedness, depending on the rate and duration of the PSVT. With underlying heart disease, dyspnea, angina pectoris, and CHF may occur as ventricular filling time, and thus cardiac output, is decreased.

Vagal stimulation often will terminate the PSVT, either through carotid massage or the Valsalva maneuver. If vagal stimulation is unsuccessful, IV adenosine is given. If adenosine is not effective in treating the dysrhythmia, IV procainamide is used. Cardioversion or overdrive pacing may be required if drug therapy is unsuccessful. Long-term prophylactic therapy may be indicated for some patients.

Atrial Flutter

Atrial flutter is a rapid atrial ectopic rhythm in which the atria fire at rates of 250 to 350 times per minute (Fig. 16–30). The AV node functions as a "gatekeeper," preventing too many impulses from reaching the ventricle. If the

---

TABLE 16-8
Differential Diagnosis of Narrow QRS Tachycardia

Type of SVT	Onset	Atrial Rate	Ventricular Rate	RR Interval	Response to Carotid Massage
Sinus tachycardia	Gradual	100–180 beats/min	Same as sinus rate	Regular	Gradual slowing
PSVT	Abrupt	150–250 beats/min	Usually same as atrial; block seen with digitalis toxicity and AV node disease	Regular, except at onset and termination	May convert to NSR
Atrial flutter	Abrupt	250–350 beats/min	Occurs with 2:1, 3:1, 4:1, or varied ventricular response	Regular or regularly irregular	Abrupt slowing of ventricular response; flutter waves remain
Atrial fibrillation	Abrupt	400–650 beats/min	Depends on ability of AVN to conduct atrial impulse; decreased with drug therapy	Irregularly irregular	Abrupt slowing of ventricular response; fibrillation waves remain

SVT, supraventricular tachycardia; PSVT, paroxysmal supraventricular tachycardia; AV, atrioventricular; NSR, normal sinus rhythm; AVN, atrioventricular node.

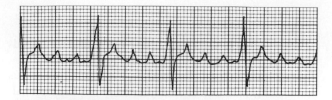

FIGURE 16-30

Atrial flutter. (Atrial rate = 250–350 beats/min. P wave shows characteristic saw-toothed pattern.)

ventricles were stimulated at 250 to 350 times per minute, the ventricles would be unable to respond with effective contractions, and cardiac output would be insufficient to sustain life. The AV node may only allow every second, third, or fourth atrial stimuli to proceed to the ventricles, resulting in what is known as a 2:1, 3:1, or 4:1 flutter block.

The rapid and regular atrial rate produces a "saw-tooth" or "picket fence" P waves on the ECG. It is usual for a flutter wave to be partially concealed within the QRS complex or T wave. The QRS complex exhibits a normal configuration except when aberrant conduction is present.

When the ventricular rate is rapid, the diagnosis of atrial flutter may be difficult. Vagal maneuvers, such as carotid sinus massage or the administration of adenosine, will increase the degree of AV block and allow recognition of flutter waves (see Table 16–8).

Atrial flutter often is seen in the presence of underlying cardiac disease, including coronary artery disease, cor pulmonale, and rheumatic heart disease. If atrial flutter occurs with a rapid ventricular rate, the ventricular chambers cannot fill adequately, resulting in varying degrees of hemodynamic compromise. Likewise, if atrial flutter is accompanied by a very slow ventricular rate, cardiac output will be diminished. A second clinical concern is the loss of "atrial kick" because atrial contraction does not occur with this dysrhythmia. The lack of atrial kick can compromise cardiac output. Finally, without atrial contractions, thrombi can form on the walls of the atria. If these thrombi break loose, the result could be pulmonary embolus, cerebral embolus, or MI.

Treatment goals for atrial flutter are to reestablish sinus rhythm or to achieve ventricular rate control. The use of pharmacological agents to achieve these goals remains controversial and problematic.

When the ventricular rate is rapid, prompt treatment to control the rate or revert the rhythm to a sinus mechanism is indicated. Digoxin alone or in combination with beta-blockers or calcium-channel blockers can be used to control the rate. Quinidine (class IA) has been widely used in the past for the conversion of atrial flutter and for rate control. Because of its side effects and toxicities, quinidine is now used less often. To achieve rate control, drugs such as procainamide and disopyramide may be selected. Flecainide and propafenone have been used in the termination and prevention of recurrence of atrial flutter. Sotalol is effective in the prevention of recurrences of atrial flutter but not in the conversion of the rhythm to sinus. Ibutilide has shown promise in converting the dysrhythmia.[1]

Synchronized cardioversion provides an alternative to drug therapy and is especially useful in the prompt treatment of atrial flutter. The patient should be NPO before the procedure and receives sedation. For a more detailed discussion of cardioversion, see Chapter 17.

A review of the literature indicates that only 50% of patients on antiarrhythmic therapy remain in sinus rhythm after 1 year of treatment.[1] Therefore, other modes of therapy may be indicated for the long-term management of atrial flutter. These modes of therapy include ablation, pacing, and implantable devices.

Atrial Fibrillation

Atrial fibrillation is defined as a rapid atrial ectopic rhythm, occurring with atrial rates of 350 to 500 beats/min (Fig. 16–31). It is characterized by chaotic atrial activity with the absence of definable P waves. Instead, the P waves appear as small quivering fibrillatory waves. Like atrial flutter, the ventricular rate and rhythm depend on the ability of the AV junction to function as a "gatekeeper." If too many atrial stimuli pass through the AV junction, the ventricular response will be rapid. If too few atrial stimuli pass through the AV junction, the ventricular response will be slow. The ventricular rhythm is characteristically irregular.

Although atrial fibrillation may occur as a transient dysrhythmia in healthy young people, the presence of chronic atrial fibrillation is usually associated with underlying heart disease. One or both of the following are present in patients with chronic atrial fibrillation: atrial muscle disease or atrial distention together with disease of the sinus node. This rhythm commonly occurs in the setting of CHF, ischemic or rheumatic heart disease, pulmonary disease, and after open heart surgery. Atrial fibrillation also is seen in congenital heart disease.

The immediate clinical concern in a patient with atrial fibrillation is the rate of the ventricular response. If the ventricular rate is too fast, end-diastolic filling time is decreased and cardiac output is compromised. If the ventricular rate is too slow, cardiac output may again be decreased. Like in atrial flutter, patients with atrial fibrillation have lost AV synchrony and atrial kick, resulting in a compromised cardiac output. Patients also are at risk for the formation of mural thrombi and embolic events, such as stroke, MI, and pulmonary embolus.

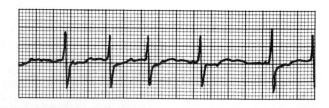

FIGURE 16-31

Atrial fibrillation. (Atrial rate = 400–600 beats/min with a variable ventricular response. Characteristic atrial fibrillatory waves seen.)

The treatment principles for atrial fibrillation are the same as those for atrial flutter. The goal of therapy is to achieve rate control or to convert the rhythm to sinus. Drug therapy as described previously may be used. If the patient has chronic atrial fibrillation, anticoagulant therapy will be added to the drug regimen to prevent an embolic event. Cardioversion is indicated for rhythm control when drug therapy fails or in the setting of hemodynamic compromise. Ablation, pacing, and implantable devices are now part of the therapy options.

Multifocal Atrial Tachycardia

Multifocal atrial tachycardia is a rapid atrial rhythm with varying P wave morphology, resulting from the firing of three or more atrial foci (Fig. 16–32). The atrial rate exceeds 100 beats/min, and the rhythm usually is irregular. The P waves vary in shape because of the multiple foci. The PR intervals may vary also, depending on the proximity of the focus to the AV node. The QRS complexes are normal unless an impulse is conducted with aberrancy.

This rhythm characteristically occurs in patients with severe pulmonary disease. Such patients often exhibit hypoxemia, hypokalemia, alterations in serum pH, or pulmonary hypertension. The patient usually manifests symptoms associated with the underlying disease rather than with the dysrhythmia itself. Treatment is directed toward controlling the underlying pulmonary disease and slowing the ventricular rate if necessary.

■ JUNCTIONAL DYSRHYTHMIAS

Junctional Rhythm

A junctional rhythm, also known as a nodal rhythm, is a rhythm originating in the AV node. When the SA node fails to fire, the AV node usually takes control, but the rate will be slower. The rate of a junctional rhythm ranges between 50 and 70 beats per minute. The P wave in the dysrhythmia can have one of three possible configurations. The first possible configuration is seen when the AV node fires and the wave of depolarization travels backwards (retrograde conduction) into the atria. The impulse from the AV node then moves forward into the ventricle. When this sequence occurs, the P wave appears as an inverted wave before a normal QRS complex. A sec-

ond possible configuration occurs when the retrograde conduction into the atria happens at the same time as the forward conduction into the ventricle. The resulting rhythm strip shows an absent P wave with a normal QRS. In reality, the P wave is not absent. Instead, it is buried inside the QRS complex. The third possible ECG pattern results when forward conduction of the ventricles precedes retrograde conduction of the atria. When this sequence occurs, a normal QRS complex is followed by an inverted P wave (Fig. 16–33).

A junctional rhythm can be the result of hypoxia, hyperkalemia, MI, heart failure, valvular disease, drug effects (digoxin, beta-blockers, calcium-channel blockers) or any cause of SA node dysfunction.

The patient with a junctional rhythm may become symptomatic as a result of the slower rate. Hypotension, decreased cardiac output, and decreased perfusion may result. The benefit of AV synchrony and atrial kick may be lost when the atria are stimulated with or after ventricular depolarization.

Treatment should be directed toward the underlying cause. Symptomatic patients may require immediate treatment. The heart rate can be increased through the use of atropine or cardiac pacing. Interventions are also directed toward improving cardiac output.

Premature Junctional Contractions

A premature junctional contraction (PJC) is an ectopic impulse from a focus in the AV junction, occurring prematurely, before the next sinus impulse (Fig. 16–34). As in all rhythms originating in the AV junction, the QRS will be narrow (< 0.12 second), reflecting normal AV conduction. On rare occasions, the QRS may be wide if the impulse is conducted aberrantly. The atria are depolarized in a retrograde fashion before, during, or after ventricular excitation, producing inverted P waves that may occur before, during, or after the QRS complex. As with PACs, PJCs may occur in normal people or in those with underlying heart disease. Ischemia or infarction may activate an ectopic focus in the AV junction, as may stimulants, such as nicotine or caffeine, or pharmacological agents (eg, digitalis).

Frequent PJCs may indicate increasing irritability and may be a precursor of a junctional rhythm. Although usually asymptomatic, the patient may experience a "skipped beat." Treatment is not necessary for PJCs.

■ VENTRICULAR DYSRHYTHMIAS

Premature Ventricular Contractions

A PVC is an ectopic beat originating prematurely at the level of the ventricles (Fig. 16–35). The beat is ventricular in origin and results in no electrical activity in the atria.

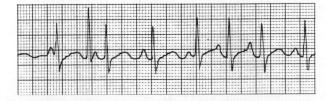

FIGURE 16-32
Multifocal atrial tachycardia. (The atrial rate exceeds 100 beats/min with three or more different P wave morphologies.)

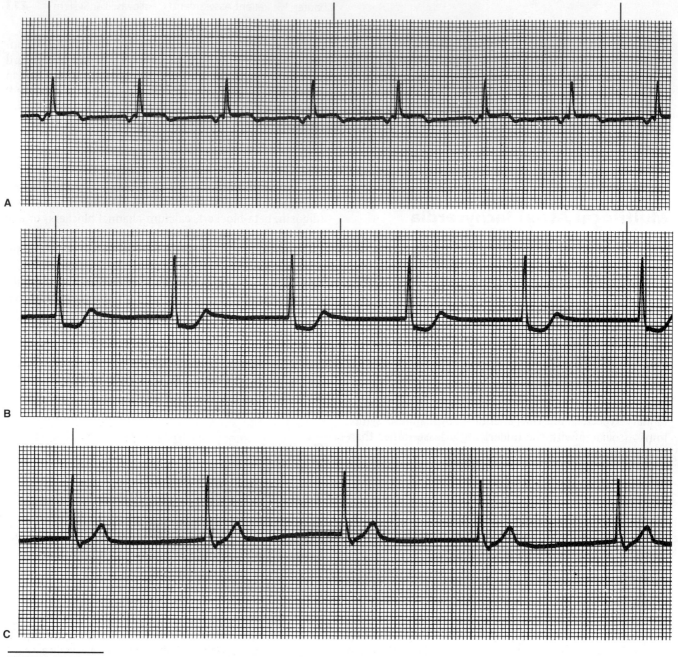

FIGURE 16-33

Junctional Rhythm.

Strip A shows a junctional rhythm in which the inverted P wave appears before a normal QRS complex. Strip B shows a junctional rhythm in which the inverted P wave is buried inside the QRS complex. Strip C shows a junctional rhythm in which the inverted P wave follows the QRS complex.

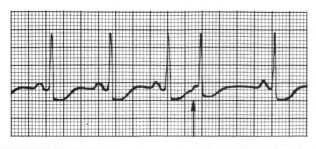

FIGURE 16-34

Premature junctional contraction.

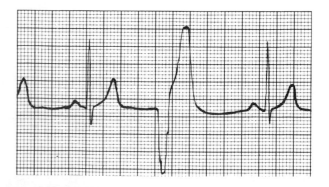

FIGURE 16-35

Premature ventricular contraction.

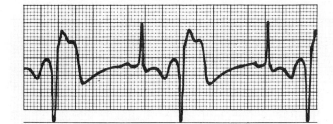

FIGURE 16-36
Ventricular bigeminy. (Every other beat is a PVC.)

As a result, no P waves will appear. The ventricular depolarization does not travel through the normal rapid ventricular conduction system. Instead, ventricular conduction spreads more slowly through the Purkinje system, resulting in a wide QRS complex with a T wave that is opposite in direction to the QRS complex. A compensatory pause often follows the premature beat as the heart awaits the next stimulus from the sinus node. The pause is considered fully compensatory if the cycles of the normal and premature beats equal the time of two normal heart cycles.

Ventricular premature beats can be described by their frequency and pattern. They can be *rare, occasional*, or *frequent*, although it is optimal to describe them in number of PVCs per minute. If PVCs occur after each sinus beat, *ventricular bigeminy* is present (Fig. 16–36). *Ventricular trigeminy* is a PVC occurring after two consecutive sinus beats. When PVCs appear in only one form, they are referred to as *uniformed*, versus *multiformed* when two or more forms of the QRS complex are apparent (Fig. 16–37). Two PVCs in a row are a *couplet* (Fig. 16–38), whereas three in a row are a *triplet* and a short run of VT.

The most common of all ectopic beats, PVCs can occur with or without heart disease in any age group. They are es-

pecially common in a person with myocardial disease (ischemia or infarction) or with myocardial irritability (hypokalemia, increased levels of catecholamines, or mechanical irritation with a wire or catheter).

The presence of PVCs is a sign of ventricular myocardial irritability and in some patients, may lead to VT or ventricular fibrillation (VF). The nature of the patient's underlying heart disease rather than presence of PVCs as such will determine the prognosis. Numerous and multiformed PVCs in the presence of serious heart disease worsens the prognosis. PVCs approaching the apex of the preceding T wave (the R on T phenomenon) are of clinical concern. The T wave represents ventricular repolarization when the heart should not be stimulated. If stimulation occurs during this vulnerable period, VF and sudden death may result.

If infrequent, isolated PVCs require no treatment. Multiple or consecutive PVCs may be managed with antiarrhythmic agents. In the emergency setting, lidocaine followed by procainamide are the drugs of choice. Many antiarrhythmic agents are available for chronic therapy (eg, quinidine, procainamide, amiodarone). If the serum potassium is low, potassium replacement may correct the dysrhythmia. If the dysrhythmia is due to digitalis toxicity, withdrawal of the drug may correct it.

Ventricular Tachycardia

In the previous section, VT was defined as three or more PVCs in a row. VT is recognized by wide, bizarre QRS complexes occurring in a fairly regular rhythm at a rate greater than 100 beats/min (Fig. 16–39). P waves usually are not seen and if seen, are not related to the QRS. VT can present as a short, nonsustained rhythm or be longer and sustained. In the example shown (see Fig 16–40), VT terminates spontaneously, resulting in sinus rhythm.

In adults with normal hearts, VT is rare but is common as a complication of MI. Other causes are the same as de-

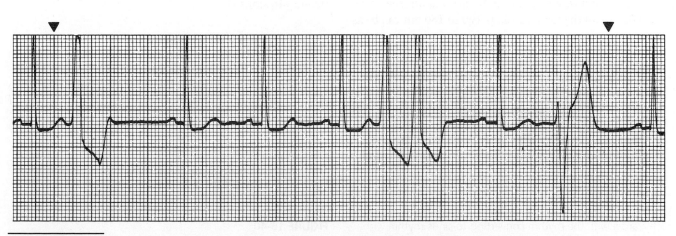

FIGURE 16-37
Multiformed PVCs.

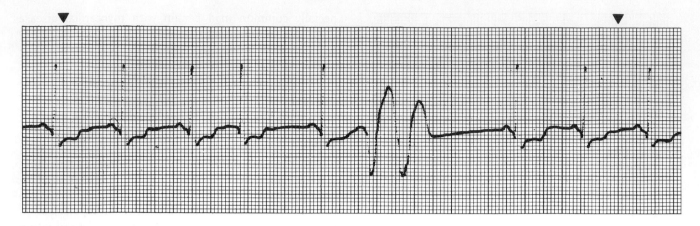

FIGURE 16-38
Couplet (two PVCs in a row).

scribed for PVCs. VT is a precursor of VF; signs and symptoms of hemodynamic compromise (ischemic chest pain, hypotension, pulmonary edema, and unconsciousness) may be seen if the rate is fast and the tachycardia is sustained. Serious dysrhythmia progression depends on the underlying heart disease.

If the patient is hemodynamically stable with the dysrhythmia, lidocaine is the treatment of choice. If the patient becomes unstable, synchronized cardioversion (or in emergency situations, unsynchronized defibrillation) is indicated. Long-term treatment for this dysrhythmia may involve the use of an implantable cardioverter defibrillator (ICD). See Chapter 17 for a more detailed discussion of ICDs.

Torsades de Pointes

Torsades de pointes ("twisting of the points") is a specific type of VT (Fig. 16–40). The term refers to the polarity of the QRS complex, which swings from positive to negative and vice versa. The QRS morphology is characterized by large, bizarre, polymorphous, or multiformed QRS complexes of varying amplitude and direction, frequently varying from beat to beat and resembling torsion around an isoelectric line. The rate of the tachycardia is 100 to 180 but can be as fast as 200 to 300 beats/min. The rhythm is highly unstable; it may terminate in VF or revert to sinus rhythm. This form of VT is most likely to develop with myocardial disease when the underlying QT interval has been prolonged.

Torsades de pointes is favored by conditions that prolong the QT interval. Examples include severe bradycardia; drug therapy, especially with the type IA antiarrhythmic agents (eg, quinidine, procainamide); and electrolyte disturbances, such as hypokalemia and hypocalcemia. Other factors that can precipitate this dysrhythmia include intrinsic cardiac disease, familial QT prolongation, central nervous system disorders, and hypothermia.

Torsades may terminate spontaneously and may repeat itself after several seconds or minutes, or it may transform to VF. Treatment for this dysrhythmia consists of shortening the refractory period (and thus the QT interval) of the underlying rhythm. IV magnesium sulfate, magnesium chloride, or isoproterenol are effective in suppression of the dysrhythmia. Overdrive pacing also can be used in this setting. Treatment is directed at correcting the underlying problem and may necessitate stopping the offending pharmacological agent. Emergency cardioversion or defibrillation is indicated if the torsades does not revert spontaneously to sinus rhythm.

Ventricular Fibrillation

Ventricular fibrillation is defined as rapid, irregular, and ineffectual depolarizations of the ventricle (Fig. 16–41). No distinct complexes are seen. Only irregular oscillations of

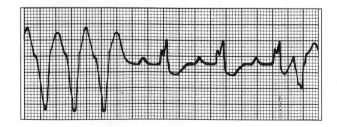

FIGURE 16-39
Ventricular tachycardia. (The first three beats are ventricular tachycardia with the rhythm converting to sinus rhythm with first-degree heart block.)

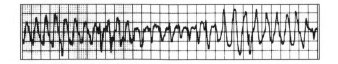

FIGURE 16-40
Torsades de pointes.

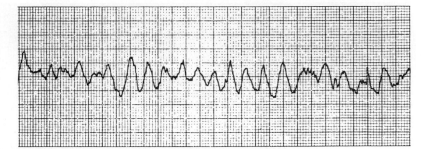

FIGURE 16-41
Ventricular fibrillation.

the baseline are apparent; these may be either coarse or fine in appearance.

Ventricular fibrillation may occur in the following circumstances: myocardial ischemia and infarction, catheter manipulation in the ventricles, electrocution, prolonged QT intervals, or as a terminal rhythm in patients with circulatory failure. As in asystole, loss of consciousness occurs within seconds in the setting of VF. The patient is pulseless and there is no cardiac output. VF is the most common cause of sudden cardiac death and is fatal if resuscitation is not instituted immediately.

If VF occurs, rapid defibrillation is the management of choice (see the discussion of cardiopulmonary resuscitation in Chapter 17). The patient should be supported with cardiopulmonary resuscitation and drugs if there is no response to defibrillation. An ICD may be indicated for long-term management of this problem.

Accelerated Idioventricular Rhythm

Accelerated idioventricular rhythm (AIVR) is produced by a "speeding up" of ventricular pacemaker cells, which normally have an intrinsic rate of 20 to 40 beats/min (Fig. 16–42). When the idioventricular rate accelerates above the sinus rate, the ventricular pacemaker becomes the primary pacemaker for the heart. AIVR is characterized by wide QRS complexes occurring regularly at a rate of 50 to 100 beats/min. AIVR may last for a few beats or may be sustained.

Typically this rhythm is seen with acute MI, often in the setting of coronary artery reperfusion post-thrombolytic therapy. It may occur less commonly as a result of ischemia or digitalis intoxication.

The patient usually is not symptomatic with this dysrhythmia. Adequate cardiac output can be maintained, and degeneration into a rapid VT is rare. In most cases, treatment is not necessary. If the patient is hemodynamically compromised, the sinus rate is increased with atropine or atrial pacing to suppress the AIVR.

◼ ATRIOVENTRICULAR BLOCKS

A disturbance in some portion of the AV conduction system causes an AV block. The sinus-initiated beat is delayed or completely blocked from activating the ventricles. The block may occur at the level of the AV node, bundle of His, or the bundle branches because the AV conduction system contains all of these structures. In first- and second-degree AV block, the block is incomplete—that is, some or all of the impulses eventually are conducted to the ventricles. In third-degree or complete heart block, none of the sinus-initiated impulses are conducted. Table 16–9 summarizes and compares heart block rhythms.

First-Degree Atrioventricular Block

In first-degree block, AV conduction is prolonged, but all impulses eventually are conducted to the ventricles (Fig. 16–43). P waves are present and precede each QRS in a 1:1 relationship. The PR interval is constant but exceeds the upper limit of 0.20 second in duration.

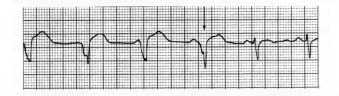

FIGURE 16-42
Accelerated idioventricular rhythm. The first three beats are of ventricular origin. The fourth beat (*arrow*) represents a fusion beat. The subsequent two beats are of sinus origin.

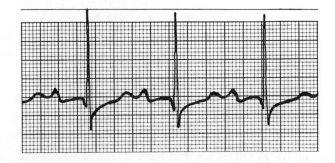

FIGURE 16-43
First-degree AV block (PR interval = 0.36 second.)

TABLE 16-9
A Comparison of the Electrocardiogram Characteristics of Heart Block Rhythms

	First-Degree Heart Block	Second-Degree Heart Block— Mobitz Type I (Wenckebach)	Second-Degree Heart Block— Mobitz Type II	Third-Degree Heart Block
Rate	Usually 60–100 beats/min	Usually 60–100 beats/min	May be slow depending on number of blocked P waves	Rate determined by ventricular focus, usually very slow
Rhythm	Regular	Irregular due to dropped QRS	Often regular but depends on pattern of block	May be regular or irregular ventricular focus
P waves	Present, one per QRS	Present, one per QRS until QRS is missed	Present, more than one P wave per QRS	Present, more than one P wave per QRS; P waves no relationship to QRS complexes
PR interval	> 0.20 s, equal throughout	Progressively gets longer until QRS is missed; pattern repeats	May be normal or prolonged, equal throughout	May be normal or prolonged, unequal throughout
QRS complex	< 0.12 s	< 0.12 s	Usually >0.12 s	>0.12 s

First-degree heart block occurs in all ages and in normal and diseased hearts. PR prolongation may be caused by drugs, such as digitalis, beta-blockers, or calcium-channel blockers; coronary artery disease; a variety of infectious diseases; and congenital lesions. First-degree block is of no hemodynamic consequence to the patient but should be seen as an indicator of a potential AV conduction system disturbance. First-degree block may progress to second- or third-degree AV block.

No treatment is indicated for first-degree heart block. The PR interval should be monitored closely, watching for further block. The possibility of drug effect also should be evaluated.

Second-Degree Atrioventricular Block—Mobitz I (Wenckebach)

In this type of second-degree block, AV conduction is delayed progressively with each sinus impulse until eventually the impulse is completely blocked from reaching the ventricles. The cycle then repeats itself (Fig. 16–44).

On the ECG tracing, P waves are present and related to the QRS in a cyclic pattern. The PR interval progressively

lengthens with each beat until a QRS complex is not conducted. The QRS complex has the same configuration as the underlying rhythm. The interval between successive QRS complexes shortens until a dropped beat occurs.

A Wenckebach or Mobitz type I block usually is associated with block above the bundle of His. Therefore, any drug or disease process that affects the AV node, such as digitalis, myocarditis, or an inferior wall MI, may produce this type of second-degree block.

The patient rarely is symptomatic with this type of second-degree AV block because the ventricular rate usually is adequate. Wenckebach often is temporary, and if it progresses to third-degree block, a junctional pacemaker at a rate of 40 to 60 beats/min usually will take over to pace the ventricles. Of the two types of second-degree block, Mobitz I is the more common. No treatment is required for this rhythm except to discontinue a drug if it is the offending agent. The patient should be monitored for further progression of block.

Second-Degree Atrioventricular Block—Mobitz II

Mobitz type II block is described as an intermittent block in the AV conduction usually within or below the bundle of His. Mobitz type II block is characterized by a fixed PR interval when AV conduction is present and a nonconducted P wave when the block occurs (Fig. 16–45). This block in conduction can occur occasionally or be repetitive with a 2:1, 3:1, or even 4:1 conduction pattern. Because there is no disturbance in the sinus node, the PP interval will be regular. Often there is accompanying BBB, so the QRS will be wide.

A Mobitz II pattern is seen in the setting of an anterior wall MI and various diseases of the conducting tissue, such

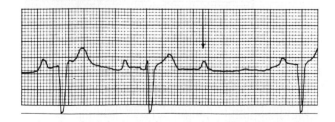

FIGURE 16-44
Second-degree block—Mobitz I (Wenckebach). The arrow indicates the nonconducted P wave in this sequence.

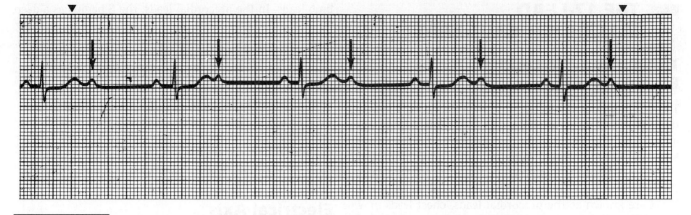

FIGURE 16-45
Second-degree block—Mobitz II. Arrows denote blocked P wave (2:1 block).

as fibrotic disease. Mobitz II block is potentially more dangerous than Mobitz I. Mobitz type II often is permanent, and it may deteriorate rapidly to third-degree heart block with a slow ventricular response of 20 to 40 beats/min. An RBBB often accompanies a Mobitz type II heart block.

Constant monitoring and observation for progression to third-degree heart block are required. Medications, such as atropine or isoproterenol, or cardiac pacing may be required if the patient becomes symptomatic or if this block occurs in the setting of an acute anterior wall MI. Permanent pacing often is indicated for long-term management.

Third-Degree (Complete) Atrioventricular Block

In third-degree or complete heart block, the sinus node continues to fire normally, but the impulses do not reach the ventricles (Fig. 16–46). The ventricles are stimulated from escape pacemaker cells either in the junction (at a rate of 40–60 beats/min) or in the ventricles (at a rate of 20–40 beats/min), depending on the level of the AV block.

On the ECG tracing, P waves and QRS complexes are both present, but there is no relationship between the two. Therefore, complete heart block is considered one form of AV dissociation. The PP and RR intervals will each be regular, but the PR interval will be variable. If a junctional pacemaker paces the ventricles, the QRS will be narrow. A pacemaker site lower in the ventricles will produce a wide QRS complex.

The causes of complete heart block are the same as for lesser degrees of AV block. Complete heart block is often poorly tolerated. The rate and dependability of the ventricular pacemaker depend on its location. If the escape rhythm is ventricular in origin, the rate is slow, and pacemaker site is unreliable. The patient may be symptomatic because of a low cardiac output. A pacemaker site high in the bundle of His may provide an adequate rate and is more dependable. The patient may remain asymptomatic if the escape rhythm supports a normal cardiac output.

A temporary pacing wire is usually inserted immediately, and when the patient is stabilized, a permanent pacemaker is implanted.

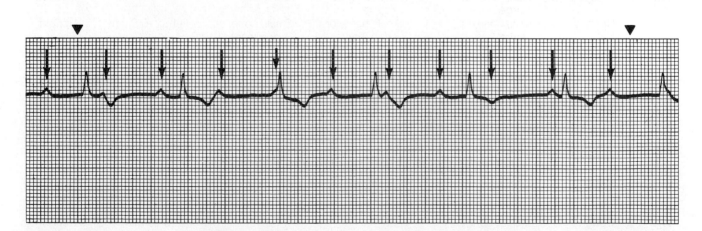

FIGURE 16-46
Third-degree block (complete AV block). Arrows denote P waves. Note the lack of relationship between the atria (P wave) and ventricles (QRS).

■ THE 12-LEAD ELECTROCARDIOGRAM

The Normal 12-Lead Electrocardiogram

The ECG provides 12 electrical views of the heart. The first three electrical views are known as the standard leads and include leads I, II, and III. The next three electrical views are known as the augmented leads and include aVR, aVL, and aVF. The standard and augmented leads are referred to as the limb leads. The remaining six electrical views of the heart are known as the precordial leads, chest leads or V leads. These include V_1, V_2, V_3, V_4, V_5, and V_6.

In the normal 12-lead ECG, the P wave representing atrial depolarization is usually upright and rounded. Each component of the QRS complex (ventricular depolarization) is analyzed separately. The Q wave, the initial downward deflection of the QRS complex, should be absent or small in the 12-lead ECG. The R component is the tallest portion of the QRS complex in the limb leads except aVR. In the precordial leads, the R wave begins as a small wave in V_1 and gradually progresses to a tall wave by V_6. The S wave, the downward stroke following R, is small or absent in the limb leads. In the precordial leads, the S begins as a deep wave in V_1 and gradually disappears by V_6. The ST segment is isoelectric, but may be slightly elevated in V_1 through V_3. The T wave, representing ventricular repolarization, is usually upright, although a variety of configurations can be normal. Table 16–10 summarizes the normal 12-lead ECG.

The 12-lead ECG can be useful in determining the electrical axis of the heart and detecting abnormalities that require more than one electrical view. These abnormalities include BBB, atrial or ventricular enlargement, and patterns of ischemia, injury, or infarction.

Electrical Axis

Electrical axis refers to the general direction of the wave of excitation as it moves through the heart. In the normal heart, the flow of electrical forces originates in the SA node, spreads throughout atrial tissue, passes through the AV node, and moves throughout the ventricles. This flow of forces is normally downward and to the left, a pattern known as normal axis.

The ventricles comprise the largest muscle mass of the heart and therefore make the most significant contribution to the determination of the direction of the flow of forces in

---

TABLE 16-10
The Normal 12-Lead Electrocardiogram

Lead	P	Q	R	S	S-T	T
I	Upright	Small, 0.04, or none	Dominant	<R or none	Isoelectric +1 to −0.5 mm	Upright
II	Upright	Small or none	Dominant	<R or none	+1 to −0.5 mm	Upright
III	Upright Flat Diphasic Inverted	Small or none	None to dominant	None to dominant	+1 to −0.5 mm	Upright Flat Diphasic Inverted
aVR	Inverted	Small, none, or large	Small or none	Dominant	+1 to −0.5 mm	Inverted
aVL	Upright Flat Diphasic Inverted	Small, none, or large	Small, none, or dominant	Small, none, or dominant	+1 to −0.5 mm	Upright Flat Diphasic Inverted
aVF	Upright Flat Diphasic Inverted	Small or none	Small, none, or dominant	None to dominant	+1 to −0.5 mm	Upright
V_1	Upright Flat Diphasic	None May be QS	Small	Deep	0 to +3 mm	Inverted Flat Upright Diphasic
V_2	Upright	None			0 to +3 mm	Upright Diphasic Inverted
V_3	Upright	Small or none			0 to +3 mm	Upright
V_4	Upright	Small or none			+1 to −0.5 mm	Upright
V_5	Upright	Small			+1 to −0.5 mm	Upright
V_6	Upright	Small	Tall	Small or none	+1 to −0.5 mm	Upright

the heart. For this reason, the QRS complex is examined when deciding the electrical axis.

A quick way to estimate the axis of the heart is to examine the direction of the QRS complex in leads I and aVF (Fig. 16–47). If the QRS complex is mainly upright in both leads, the axis is normal. The axis has shifted toward the left when the QRS complex in lead I is upright and in lead aVF is downward. A pattern showing a downward QRS complex in I with an upright QRS in aVF is consistent with right axis deviation. Extreme right axis shift is uncommon and is noted on the ECG by a downward QRS complex in leads I and aVF.

The direction of the flow of forces in the heart can change as a result of an anatomical shift of the heart in the chest wall. An anatomical shift may occur in very obese patients or patients with large abdominal tumors or abdominal ascites. Shifts of the axis to the left can occur with an LBBB, LV enlargement, or inferior wall MI. Right axis deviation can be caused by RBBB, RV enlargement, or an anterior wall MI.

The patient is asymptomatic with an axis shift. The only way an axis shift can be detected is through a 12-lead ECG. The axis shift usually represents some underlying abnormality. Treatment is directed at the underlying cause.

■■■ BUNDLE BRANCH BLOCK

A bundle branch block (BBB) develops when there is either a functional or pathological block in one of the major branches of the intraventricular conduction system. As conduction through one bundle is blocked, the impulse travels along the unaffected bundle and activates one ventricle nor-

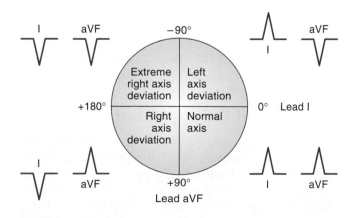

FIGURE 16-47
Determining Electrical Axis
To determine the axis of the heart, examine the direction of the QRS complex in Leads I and aVF.

Lead I	Lead aVF	Axis
negative	negative	Extreme right axis deviation
negative	positive	Right axis deviation
positive	negative	Left axis deviation
positive	positive	Normal axis

mally. The impulse is delayed in reaching the other ventricle, because it travels outside of the normal conducting fibers. The right and left ventricles are thus depolarized sequentially instead of simultaneously. The abnormal activation produces a wide QRS complex, representing the increased time it takes for ventricular depolarization (Fig. 16–48). The broad QRS complex will have two peaks (RSR′) indicating that depolarization of the two ventricles was not simultaneous.

An RBBB and LBBB are diagnosed on the 12-lead ECG but also can be identified on the bedside monitor using a V_1 or MCL_1 tracing and a V_6 or MCL_6 tracing (see section on electrocardiographic monitoring for description of lead selection). To identify the presence of a BBB, the QRS duration must be prolonged to 0.12 second or greater representing the delay in conduction through the ventricles. An RBBB will alter the configuration of the QRS complex in the right sided chest leads, V_1 and V_2. Normally, these leads have a small single-peaked R and deep S wave configuration. With an RBBB, depolarization of the right ventricle is delayed, and the ECG pattern changes. An RBBB is evidenced by an RSR′ configuration in V_1. If the initial peak of the QRS complex is smaller than the second peak, the pattern would be described as rSR′. The "r" is used to describe the first smaller peak and the "R" is used to describe the second taller peak. Likewise, if the initial peak of the QRS complex is taller than the second peak, the pattern would be described as an RSr′. Whenever ventricular depolarization is abnormal, so is ventricular repolarization. As a result, ST segment and T wave abnormalities may be seen in leads V_1 and V_2 for patients with an RBBB.

An LBBB will change the QRS complex pattern in the left sided chest leads, V_5 and V_6. Normally, these leads have a tall single-peaked R wave and a small or absent S wave. Instead, the double-peaked RSR′ pattern is noted. In addition, V_1 will show a small R wave with a widened S wave, indicating delayed conduction through the ventricles. Like RBBB, the ST segments and T waves may be abnormal in the left sided chest leads V_5 and V_6 when the patient has an LBBB (see Fig. 16–48).

The most common causes of BBB are MI, hypertension, heart failure, and cardiomyopathy. RBBB may be found in normal people with no clinical evidence of heart disease. Congenital lesions involving the septum and RV hypertrophy are other causes of RBBB. LBBB is usually associated with some type of underlying heart disease. Long-term cardiovascular disease in the older patient is a common cause of LBBB.

A BBB signifies underlying disease of the intraventricular conduction system. The patient should be monitored for involvement of the other bundles or fascicles or for progression to complete heart block. Progression of block may be very slow or rapid, depending on the clinical setting. A new-onset LBBB in conjunction with an acute MI is associated with a higher mortality rate.[2]

The underlying heart disease determines treatment and prognosis. Patients with an MI and new onset BBB are

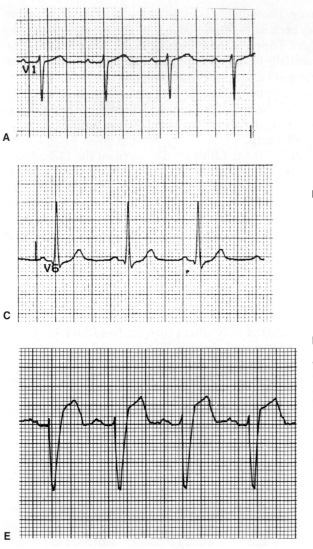

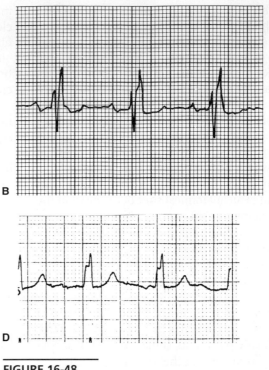

FIGURE 16-48

A Comparison of Right versus Left Bundle Branch Block

Strip A: A normal V_1 tracing. Note the small narrow R and deep narrow S wave.

Strip B: A V_1 tracing showing the wide QRS complex and double peaked R wave indicating a right bundle branch block.

Strip C: A normal V_6 tracing. Note the tall narrow R wave and absent S wave.

Strip D: A V_6 tracing showing the wide QRS complex and double peaked R wave indicating a left bundle branch block.

Strip E: A V_1 tracing. Note the small narrow R and deep wide S wave indicating a left bundle branch block.

closely monitored for the progression to a type of complete heart block. A temporary pacemaker may be inserted.

◼ ENLARGEMENT PATTERNS

Enlargement of a cardiac chamber can be the result of hypertrophy of the muscle or a dilation of the chamber. An ECG is not an ideal diagnostic tool to distinguish the cause of the enlargement. An echocardiogram is more helpful in determining if the enlargement is due to hypertrophy or dilation. The terminology used to describe enlargement patterns on the ECG can be confusing. Because atrial changes on the ECG can result from a variety of causes, including atrial dilation, hypertrophy, or other conditions, the general terms "atrial abnormality" or "atrial enlargement" are often used rather than the specific terms "atrial hypertrophy" or "atrial dilation." In contrast, the term "ventricular hypertrophy" is commonly used because hypertrophy is the

most frequent cause of the enlargement pattern in the ventricles.

Right Atrial Enlargement

When the atria enlarge, changes are seen in the P wave because the P wave represents atrial depolarization. RA enlargement is noted on the ECG by the presence of tall pointed P waves in leads II, III, and aVF. The P wave in V_1 may show a diphasic wave with an initial upstroke that is larger than the downstroke (Fig. 16–49).

The most common causes for any cardiac chamber to enlarge include pumping for a prolonged period against high pressures or pumping for a prolonged period to move blood through narrowed valves. The right atrium is more likely to enlarge as a result of pressures created by pulmonary causes, such as pulmonary hypertension and chronic obstructive pulmonary disease. For this reason, RA enlargement is often referred to as P pulmonale.

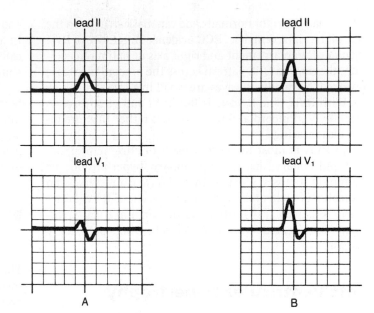

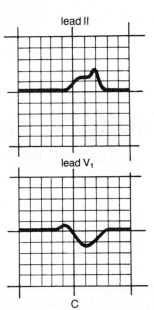

FIGURE 16-49

Right versus left atrial enlargement. (**A**) The normal P wave in leads II and V₁. (**B**) Right atrial enlargement. Note the increased amplitude of the early, right atrial component of the P wave in V₁ and the tall, pointed P wave in lead II. (**C**) Left atrial enlargement. Note the increased amplitude and duration of the P wave in V₁ and the broad, notched P wave in lead II.

The presence of an atrial enlargement pattern may be due to several causes. An echocardiogram will further differentiate the underlying cause. If the right atrium has enlarged, it is often associated with right ventricular hypertrophy.

Treatment is aimed toward the underlying cause. Often, however, the underlying cause may be a chronic condition that cannot be cured.

Left Atrial Enlargement

Left atrial enlargement is noted on the ECG by the presence of broad notched P waves in leads I, II, and aVL. The P wave in V₁ may show a diphasic wave with a terminal downstroke that is larger than the initial upstroke (see Fig. 16–49).

The left atrium is more like to enlarge because of increased pressures created by trying to pump blood through a stenotic mitral valve. For this reason, LA enlargement is often referred to as P mitrale. When a LA enlargement pattern is noted on the ECG, the patient should be evaluated for the presence of mitral stenosis. An echocardiogram is a helpful diagnostic tool in addition to cardiac auscultation. Treatment is aimed toward the underlying cause. The patient may need a valve replacement.

Right Ventricular Hypertrophy

Right ventricular hypertrophy (RVH) may exist without clear evidence on the ECG because the left ventricle is larger than the right normally and can mask changes in the size of the right ventricle. ECG evidence suggestive of RVH includes RA enlargement and right axis deviation. In addition, the normal QRS pattern across the precordial leads is reversed. Normally, R waves are small in V_1 and are tall by V_6. With RVH, The R wave is tall in V_1 and progresses to small by V_6. Precordial S waves persist rather than gradually disappearing.

An RVH is most likely the result of chronic obstructive pulmonary disease, pulmonary hypertension, or pulmonic stenosis. The presence of RVH is most likely an indicator of a chronic pulmonary condition. RA enlargement is usually seen with an accompanying RVH. Treatment is directed toward the underlying pulmonary disease.

Left Ventricular Hypertrophy

Numerous criteria exist for the detection of LVH on the ECG. The simplest criterion involves adding the depth of the S wave in V_1 or V_2 to the height of the R wave in V_5 or V_6. If the sum is greater than or equal to 35 mm and the patient is older than 35 years, LVH is suspected. In addition, the T waves in V_5 and V_6 may be asymmetrically inverted, and the patient is likely to have a left axis shift.

Most likely, LVH is the result of chronic systemic hypertension or aortic stenosis. The presence of RVH is often an indicator of a chronic cardiovascular condition. LA enlargement may result in a displacement of the PMI when palpating the apical pulse. Treatment is directed toward the underlying condition.

◼ ISCHEMIA, INJURY, AND INFARCTION PATTERNS

The 12-lead ECG can be very useful in detecting evidence of myocardial ischemia, injury, or infarction. Ischemia is seen on the ECG by ST segment depressions and T wave inversions. Acute patterns of injury are noted by ST segment elevations. The presence of significant Q waves indicates an MI. For a more detailed discussion of patterns of ischemia, injury, and infarction, see Chapter 20.

Effects of Serum Electrolyte Abnormalities on the Electrocardiogram

Maintenance of adequate fluid and electrolyte balance assumes high priority in the care of patients in any medical, surgical, or coronary ICU. Patients being treated for renal or cardiovascular diseases are especially vulnerable to electrolyte imbalances. The cure may well be worse than the disease if electrolyte abnormalities go undetected or ignored because they frequently are caused by the treatment rather than by the disease itself.

Dialysis can very quickly cause major shifts in electrolytes. Certainly, the often insidious drop of serum potassium levels in the digitalized cardiac patient who received diuretics is well known. Diuretics also are used frequently as part of the medical regimen for the control of hypertension. Any addition, deletion, or change in diuretic therapy warrants close following of serum electrolytes.

A history of any of the aforementioned problems should alert the nurse to check the patient's serum electrolytes on an ongoing basis.

Potassium and calcium are probably the two most important electrolytes involved in the proper function of the heart. Because of their effects on the electrical impulse in the heart, excess or insufficiency of either electrolyte frequently causes changes in the ECG. The nurse who is aware of and is able to recognize these changes may well suspect electrolyte abnormalities before laboratory findings or clinical symptoms appear and hazardous dysrhythmias occur.

◼ POTASSIUM

Potassium is the primary intracellular cation found in the body. Inside the cardiac cell, potassium is important for repolarization and for maintaining a stable, polarized state.

Hyperkalemia

The earliest sign of hyperkalemia on the ECG is a change in the T wave. It usually is described as tall, narrow, and "peaked" or "tenting" in appearance (Fig. 16–50). As the serum potassium level rises, the P wave amplitude decreases

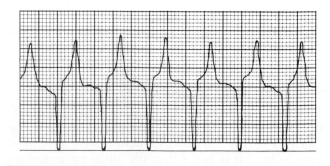

FIGURE 16-50

Hyperkalemia and the presence of peaked T waves.

and the PR interval prolongs. Atrial asystole occurs, along with a widening of the QRS. At high, near-lethal potassium levels, the widened QRS merges with the T wave and starts resembling a sine wave. Various dysrhythmias can occur during this time, with progression to VF and asystole. Clinically, the described changes in T waves begin to appear at serum levels of 6 to 7 mEq/L; QRS widening is seen at serum levels of 8 to 9 mEq/L. Vigorous treatment must be instituted to reverse the condition at this point because sudden death may occur at any time after these levels are reached.

The ECG changes in hyperkalemia also may be associated with other conditions. Tall, peaked T waves may be a normal finding or may occur in the early stages of MI. QRS widening may be seen with quinidine and procainamide toxicity.

Hypokalemia

Hypokalemia is associated with the appearance of U waves. Although the presence of U waves can be normal for many people, they also may be an early sign of hypokalemia (Fig. 16–51). Usually easily recognized (best seen in lead V_3), the U wave may encroach on the preceding T wave and go unnoticed (Fig. 16–52). The T wave may look notched or prolonged when it is hiding the U wave, giving the appearance of a prolonged QT interval. With increased potassium depletion, the U wave may become more prominent as the T wave becomes less so. The T wave becomes flattened and may even invert. The ST segment tends to become depressed, somewhat resembling the effects of digitalis on the ECG. Only at very low serum levels is there reasonable correlation between ECG changes and serum potassium concentrations.

Changes seen in hypokalemia are observed with other conditions also. The U wave may be accentuated in association with digitalis, quinidine, LVH, and bradycardia.

Untreated hypokalemia enhances instability in the myocardial cell. Ventricular premature beats are the most common manifestation of this imbalance, but supraventricular dysrhythmias, conduction problems, and eventually VT and VF can be seen. Hypokalemia also increases the sensitivity of the heart to digitalis and its accompanying dysrhythmias, even at normal serum levels of the drug. The severity of the dysrhythmias associated with hypokalemia requires early recognition of this problem.

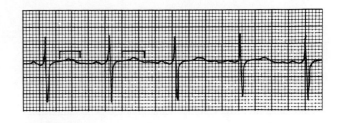

FIGURE 16-52
Fusion of T and U waves (hypokalemia).

CALCIUM

Like potassium, calcium is important in normal cardiac function. It is essential for the initiation and propagation of electrical impulses and for myocardial contractility. Abnormal calcium levels are not commonly seen unless they are associated with an underlying disease, and therefore they are not as common as serum potassium abnormalities.

Hypercalcemia

The major ECG finding associated with this disorder is shortening of the QT interval (Fig. 16–53). Because the QRS and T waves usually are unaffected by changes in serum calcium levels, the shortened QT is a result of shortening of the ST segment. QT shortening also is seen in patients taking digitalis. In addition, the ST segment occasionally becomes depressed and T wave inversion may be seen.

Hypocalcemia

On the ECG, low serum calcium levels prolong the QT interval due to a lengthening of the ST segment (Fig. 16–54). The T wave itself does not prolong but may be inverted in some cases. The prolongation of the QT interval in hypocalcemia should not be mistaken for a prolonged QTU interval seen in hypokalemia. Hypocalcemia may be associated with decreased potassium in the patient with chronic renal failure.

In addition to hypocalcemia, QT prolongation may be seen with cerebral vascular disease and after a cardiac arrest. Several antiarrhythmic agents produce prolonged QT intervals and always should be considered when evaluating the ECG for hypocalcemic changes.

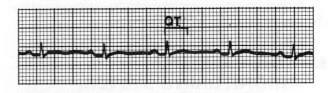

FIGURE 16-53
Shortened QT interval (hypercalcemia). The normal QT interval for the above heart rate of 88 beats/min is 0.28 to 0.36 second. This patient's serum calcium level is 12.1 mg/dL, and the QT interval measures 0.24 second.

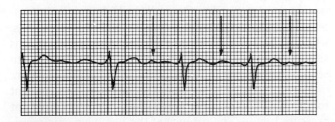

FIGURE 16-51
Presence of U waves (hypokalemia).

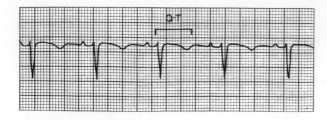

FIGURE 16-54
Prolonged QT interval (hypocalcemia). For this heart rate of 70 beats/min, the QT interval should be between 0.31 and 0.38 seconds. This patient's QT interval measures 0.50 seconds because his serum calcium level is 5.4 mg/dL. (Normal serum calcium is 8.5–10.5 mg/dL.)

SUMMARY

Just as the patient who sustains MI may not have chest pain, the patient who has electrolyte abnormalities may not exhibit any of the ECG changes described (Table 16–11). Conversely, a patient with normal serum electrolytes may show some of these ECG changes for other reasons. Not one of the ECG manifestations described here even approaches being diagnostic. They are valuable primarily in arousing suspicion of electrolyte abnormalities. It is appropriate for the nurse, especially one who cares for the critically ill, to be alert to ECG changes and to interpret observations in the context of known data on the patient.

TABLE 16-11
Electrocardiogram Changes Associated With Electrolyte Imbalances

Hyperkalemia	Tall, narrow, peaked T waves; flat, wide P waves; widening QRS	Sinus bradycardia; sinoatrial block; junctional rhythm; idioventricular rhythm; ventricular tachycardia; ventricular fibrillation
Hypokalemia	Prominent U waves; ST segment depression; T wave flattening or inversion	Premature ventricular beats; supraventricular tachycardia; ventricular tachycardia; ventricular fibrillation
Hypercalcemia	Shortened QT interval	Premature ventricular contractions
Hypocalcemia	Lengthened QT interval; T wave flattening or inversion	Ventricular tachycardia

Hemodynamic Monitoring

The purposes of hemodynamic monitoring are to aid diagnosis of various cardiovascular disorders, guide therapies to minimize cardiovascular dysfunction or treat disorders, and evaluate the patient's response to therapy. To incorporate hemodynamic data into the care of the critically ill, the nurse must understand: (1) cardiopulmonary anatomy and physiology; (2) monitoring system components to measure pressures and cardiac output; (3) rationale for interventions directed toward enhancing cardiac output, oxygen delivery, and oxygen consumption; (4) potential complications; and (5) distinguishing between physiological changes and mechanical or monitoring system problems.

THE PRESSURE MONITORING SYSTEM

Basic equipment necessary to measure hemodynamic pressures includes noncompliant pressure tubing, a transducer, an amplifier, and a means of recording or displaying the information collected (Fig. 16–55).

Hemodynamic pressures are transmitted from the intravascular space or cardiac chamber through the catheter and the fluid in the noncompliant pressure tubing to the pressure transducer. A transducer is a device that converts one form of energy into another. A pressure transducer senses changes in the fluid column generated by the pressures in the cardiac chambers or vessels being monitored. When pressure is applied to the diaphragm of the transducer, sensors are compressed, changing electrical flow to the amplifier or monitor. The monitor then converts the electrical signal generated by the transducer to a pressure tracing and digital value. Generally bedside monitoring systems have the capability to display several digital readings, whereas the oscilloscope displays the pressure waveforms simultaneously. The monitors also include mechanisms to set or adjust alarms and waveform size and zero the system.

Pressure transmission from the catheter in the patient to the transducer occurs through fluid-filled noncompliant pressure tubing. The patency of the hemodynamic monitoring system is maintained by a continuous infusion of flush solution. The flush solution may be normal saline or

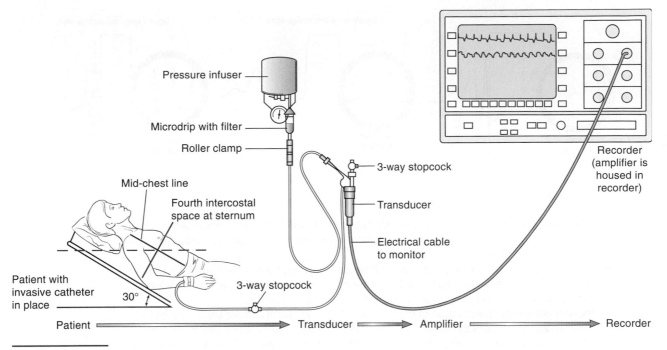

FIGURE 16-55

The indwelling arterial catheter is attached by pressure tubing to a transducer. The transducer is connected to an amplifier/monitor that visually displays a waveform and systolic, diastolic, and mean pressure values. The system is composed of a flush solution under pressure, a continuous flush device, and a series of stopcocks. The stopcock closest to the insertion site is used to draw blood samples from the artery; the stopcock located near the transducer is used for zeroing.

D5W and is usually heparinized. The solution is placed in a pressure bag that is inflated to 300 mmHg to maintain a constant pressure through the transducer and flush device. A continuous flow of approximately 3 mL/h prevents backflow of blood through the catheter and tubing, thereby maintaining system patency and accurate transmission of pressures. The system can be flushed manually by activation of a fast flush device.

Optimal Use of the Monitoring System

Several technical or mechanical factors may cause inaccuracies of the hemodynamic waveforms and values. For instance, air bubbles or blood within the tubing or transducer system will distort pressure readings. Also, as mentioned previously, the system requires continuous pressure of 300 mmHg on the flush solution bag and noncompliant pressure tubing connecting the transducer to the indwelling catheter. The use of soft, distensible tubing will distort and reduce the amplitude of the pressure waveforms. Pressure tubing length is kept to a minimum to decrease the distance in which pressures are transmitted to the transducer. Stopcocks are included in most prepackaged systems for sampling of blood and "zeroing" of the transducer. These stopcocks and any other connections should be as few in number as possible and are Luer-locked to preserve the integrity of the system.

A square wave test helps to identify whether the hemodynamic system is optimized. By activating the fast flush device for 1 or 2 seconds, the pressure waveform on the oscilloscope is replaced by a square wave. The square wave in an optimized system has a straight vertical upstroke from the baseline, a straight horizontal component, and most importantly, a straight vertical downstroke back to the baseline with two of three sharp oscillations. Figure 16–56 depicts a normal square wave and examples of square waves from nonoptimized hemodynamic monitoring systems. The latter may be due to air bubbles, blood, loose connections, cracks, leaks, or soft IV tubing in the system.

ZEROING AND LEVELING

The position of the transducer in relation to the patient's atria and the system calibration will also affect the accuracy of the hemodynamic values. Before obtaining hemodynamic parameters, the transducer is leveled and zeroed. A transducer placed above the reference point will produce erroneously low readings; conversely, a transducer below the reference point will yield falsely elevated readings. Every inch the transducer is above or below the reference point creates a 2-mmHg change in pressure reading.

The zero reference point is established at the intersection of the mid anterior-posterior line and the fourth intercostal space (see Fig. 16–55). This point is known as the phlebostatic axis. Once the zero reference point has been established, the patient's chest must be marked to ensure

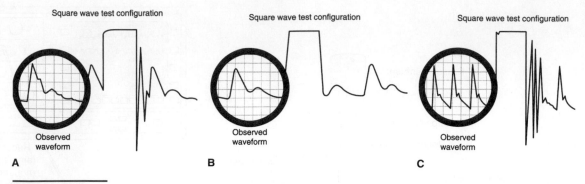

FIGURE 16-56
Square wave test.
(**A**) Optimally damped system; Activation of the fast flush device generates a sharp vertical up-stroke, horizontal line, and straight vertical downstroke ending with one or two oscillations (minimal ringing) and quick return to the baseline.
(**B**) Overdamped system: Activation of the fast flush device generates a slurred upstroke and downstroke with no oscillations above or below the baseline. Causes of an overdamped system include system leaks, blood clots, or air bubbles in the tubing or transducer.
(**C**) Underdamped system: Activation of the fast flush device generates a sharp vertical upstroke and downstroke and ends with numerous oscillations (more than three) above and below the baseline. Usually caused by small air bubbles in the system. From: Darovic GO: Hemodynamic Monitoring: Invasive and Noninvasive Clinical Application, p 161. Philadelphia, W.B. Saunders, 1995.

consistent transducer placement when subsequent pressure readings are obtained by other practitioners.

The patient is placed on his or her back, and the head of the bed may be elevated. With a carpenter type level, the transducer is placed even with the pre-established zero reference point. Further hemodynamic pressure measurements are taken with the patient in the supine position. Measurements should not be obtained in the side lying position because of variability in the readings and inconsistent leveling of the transducer. The head of the bed may be elevated up to 40 degrees, providing the transducer is releveled with any changes in patient position.

Zeroing the system negates any effect of atmospheric pressure on the pressure readings, ensuring measurements reflect only pressure values in the vessel or heart chamber being monitored. After leveling the transducer, the system is zeroed by turning the stopcock on the transducer off to the patient and open to air. Typically, the bedside monitor has a function key that is used to zero the system. When it is activated, the monitor will adjust the digital reading to zero and indicate that the zeroing procedure was successful. The transducer should be zeroed with any change in the bed or patient's position, elevation of the head of the bed, and patient transport; it also should be zeroed every 8 hours.

ARTERIAL PRESSURE MONITORING

Arterial pressure monitoring is achieved through an intra-arterial catheter connected to the pressure monitoring system. This allows continuous monitoring of the systemic arterial blood pressure and provides vascular access for obtaining blood samples by withdrawing blood from a stopcock in the system. Arterial blood pressure monitoring is indicated for patients receiving vasoactive IV infusions or those with fluctuating, unstable blood pressures.

Arterial Line Insertion

The most common sites for arterial catheter insertions are the radial and femoral arteries. Alternate and less frequent sites include the brachial, axillary, or dorsalis pedis arteries in adults or temporal and umbilical arteries in neonates. Artery selection is made after several factors are considered. The size of the artery in relation to the size of the catheter should be considered. The artery should be large enough to accommodate the catheter without occluding or significantly impeding flow. The site chosen should be easily accessible and free from contamination by body secretions. Finally, the limb distal to the insertion site should have adequate collateral flow in the event that the cannulated artery becomes occluded.

The radial artery is the most frequent site for an arterial catheter. It meets the above criteria and is superficially located and therefore easy to palpate. Cannulation of this artery also generally poses the least limitation on the patient's mobility.

Before a catheter is inserted into the radial artery, the presence of adequate collateral circulation to the hand by the ulnar artery is assessed by performing Allen's test (Fig. 16–57). Both the ulnar and radial arteries are occluded. The

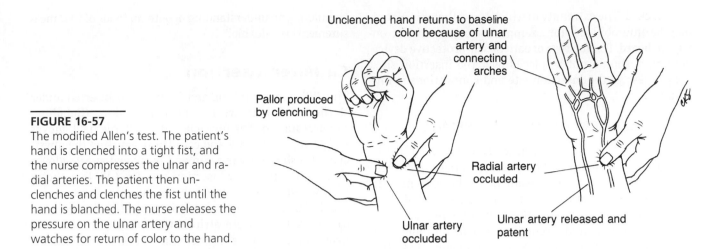

FIGURE 16-57
The modified Allen's test. The patient's hand is clenched into a tight fist, and the nurse compresses the ulnar and radial arteries. The patient then unclenches and clenches the fist until the hand is blanched. The nurse releases the pressure on the ulnar artery and watches for return of color to the hand.

patient then clenches and unclenches the fist until the hand is blanched. Pressure on the ulnar artery is released and observed for color return to the hand. If color returns within 5 to 7 seconds, the ulnar circulation to the hand is adequate. If it takes 7 to 15 seconds for color to return, ulnar filling is impaired. Ulnar circulation is considered inadequate if the hand remains blanched for longer than 15 seconds, in which case the radial artery should not be cannulated.

Regardless of the site chosen for arterial catheter placement, the insertion is performed under sterile technique. The connecting tubing is assembled and flushed, and the transducer is leveled and zeroed and calibrated before the catheter is inserted. Once the catheter is in place, it should be secured and the site dressed according to the policy of the institution.

Arterial Pressure Waveform

The normal arterial waveform should have a rapid upstroke, a clear dicrotic notch, and a definite end-diastole, as shown in Figure 16–58. The initial sharp upstroke of the waveform represents the rapid ejection of blood from the ventricle into the aorta. Note that the QRS complex precedes the rapid rise in arterial pressure. Ventricular depolarization causes ventricular contraction and the sharp rise in pressure. This increase in pressure therefore follows the QRS complex. The dicrotic notch reflects a slight backflow of

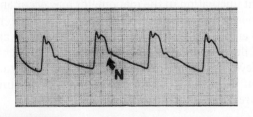

FIGURE 16-58
Normal features of an arterial pressure wave. These include a prominent pulse pressure (50 mmHg in this patient) and a dicrotic notch (N) signifying closure of the aortic valve. The crisp dicrotic notch indicates a properly responsive catheter system.

blood in the aorta, reflecting closure of the aortic valve when the aortic pressure is higher than the LV pressure. The dicrotic notch corresponds with the end of ventricular repolarization and the T wave on the ECG.

The value measured at the peak of the waveform is the systolic pressure. A normal systolic pressure is typically 90 to 140 mmHg. The dicrotic notch then indicates the end of ventricular systole and the beginning of diastole. As blood flows to the periphery, the pressure in the arterial system decreases. The lowest point of the waveform is the diastolic pressure, normally between 60 and 90 mmHg.

Mean arterial pressure (MAP) is used to evaluate perfusion of vital body organs. Normal MAP is 70 to 105 mmHg. Most bedside monitors automatically calculate and continuously display the MAP.

Complications

Primary complications associated with intra-arterial catheters are infection, accidental blood loss, and compromised flow to the extremity.

INFECTION

Proper attention to sterile technique during catheter insertion, care of the insertion site, and blood sampling and maintaining a sterile, closed monitoring system will reduce the risk of infection. The insertion site is assessed frequently for signs of infection. Sterile dressing changes, tubing changes, and flush solution changes are done according to institutional policy, while integrity of the system is maintained. Aspiration removes blood or air in the system through the stopcocks. The stopcocks are flushed and cleaned of any blood residue each time a blood sample is withdrawn. Sterile caps must be used to cover the stopcock ports between use.

ACCIDENTAL BLOOD LOSS

Usually accidental blood loss from an arterial catheter can be prevented. All connections within the system should be

Luer-locked. The extremity in which the catheter is placed may be immobilized, for example placing the wrist on an arm board. If some type of patient self-protective device is used, it should not be placed over the insertion site. Easy access to the insertion site and connections is imperative.

IMPAIRED CIRCULATION TO EXTREMITY

Circulation to the extremity in which the arterial line is placed must be monitored frequently. Initial assessment of color, sensation, and movement of the extremity is made after insertion of the arterial catheter and at least every 8 hours for as long as the catheter is in place. Any indication of impaired circulation may be an indication for catheter removal and is reported immediately to the physician.

Nursing Considerations

Blood pressures obtained from an arterial catheter are compared occasionally with auscultated pressures and whenever the accuracy of the monitored pressure is questioned. Although the two methods of blood pressure measurements reflect different physiological events and are therefore not truly comparable, there is some degree of correlation. The blood pressure from an arterial catheter is usually 5 to 20 mmHg higher than pressures obtained by cuff.

Bedside monitor alarms provide warning that a change has occurred, either within the system or in the patient's physiological status. The high and low alarms are set for systolic, diastolic, and mean pressures within 10 to 20 mmHg of the patient's typical blood pressure. The nurse's assessment of the patient triggered by the alarm sounding includes evaluating the cuff blood pressure, the square wave form test, the monitoring system for disconnections, bleeding at the catheter insertion site, and kinking of the catheter due to extremity involvement.

If catheter patency is questioned, blood and fluid are aspirated from the blood drawing port or stopcock in an attempt to remove a blood clot and then the system is flushed using the fast flush device. The system should not be flushed with a syringe. No IV solution or medication should be administered at any time through the arterial pressure monitoring system.

■ CENTRAL VENOUS PRESSURE MONITORING

Central venous pressure (CVP) reflects the pressure of blood in the right atrium or vena cava. It provides information about intravascular blood volume, right ventricular end-diastolic pressure, and right ventricular function. Although isolated CVP measurements using a water manometer generally have been replaced by hemodynamic monitoring

techniques, an understanding of both methods of CVP measurements is valuable.

Catheter Insertion

The CVP catheter is long and flexible. It is inserted under sterile conditions with a povidone-iodine (Betadine) site preparation. The physician uses a sterile field, gloves and gown, and a mask and cap. Those assisting the physician also should wear a cap and mask and sterile gloves if near the catheter or insertion site. The CVP IV catheter is inserted into an antecubital, jugular, femoral, or subclavian vein and threaded into position in the vena cava close to the right atrium. Occasionally the catheter may advance into the right atrium. If a water manometer is used to measure the CVP, rhythmic fluctuations will appear in the manometer corresponding to the patient's heart rate. If a pressure transducer system is used, the hemodynamic waveform tracing on the bedside monitor will become more pronounced. In this situation, the catheter is withdrawn several centimeters until either the fluctuations cease or the pressure tracing reflects the CVP.

Central Venous Pressure Measurement

WATER MANOMETER

Figure 16–59 illustrates a typical setup for measuring the CVP using a water manometer. A manometer with a three-way stopcock is introduced between the IV solution and the patient's IV catheter. The stopcock is manipulated to open the IV solution flow to the patient, bypassing the manometer, or it is turned off to the IV solution, allowing open communication between the CVP catheter and the manometer. Before the CVP is measured, the manometer is partially filled with solution from the IV bag by turning the stopcock off to the patient and open to the IV solution tubing and the manometer.

To measure the CVP with the water manometer, the stopcock is opened to the manometer and the patient. Pressure in the vena cava equilibrates with the pressure exerted by the column of fluid in the manometer. The point at which the fluid level settles is recorded as the CVP. A slight fluctuation in the manometer may occur and corresponds with the patient's respiratory rate. A patent system is ensured when the fluid column falls freely and the slight fluctuation of the fluid column is apparent. The fluid level in the manometer will fall on inspiration and rise on expiration due to changes in intrapulmonary pressure.

PRESSURE TRANSDUCER

The hemodynamic monitoring system components and preparation for CVP monitoring are identical to that de-

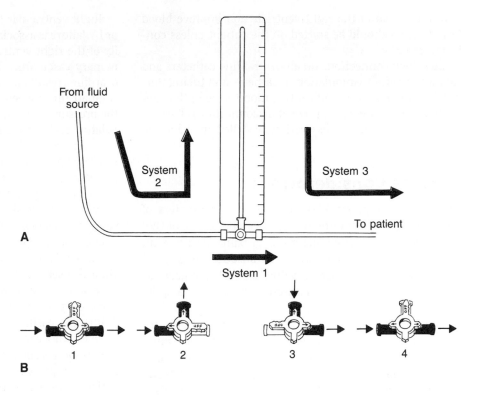

FIGURE 16-59
(**A**) Central venous pressure (CVP) water manometer system. System 1 allows for fluid administration. System 2 fills the manometer with fluid. System 3 allows the flow of fluid from the manometer to the patient and determines the CVP reading. (**B**) Steps in measuring central venous pressure. 1, Stopcock turned so that IV fluid flows to patient. 2, Stopcock in position to fill manometer with fluid. 3, Stopcock turned so that is is open from manometer to patient to obtain reading. 4, Stopcock returned to first position so that IV fluid flows to patient.

scribed for arterial pressure monitoring. Following insertion of the catheter, the pressure tubing is connected to the catheter hub. The CVP waveform and value will appear on the bedside monitor.

Complications

INFECTION

Infection can occur within the catheter or around the insertion site. Systemic infection when the source is the central venous catheter is diagnosed and verified by blood cultures. Signs and symptoms of infection will appear as with any pyrogenic source. Routine catheter and tubing changes, as outlined by the Centers for Disease Control and Prevention and hospital policy, and adherence to sterile technique are primary measures to prevent infection.

THROMBOSIS

Thromboses can vary in size from a thin fibrin sheath over the catheter tip to a large thrombus. The minor thrombosis can be flushed away without sequela, whereas a larger thrombus occluding the catheter and vein should not be flushed into the venous circulation. A large thrombus may be detected by loss of hemodynamic waveform and inability to infuse fluid or withdraw blood from the catheter. The patient may have edema of the arm closest to the catheter site, varying degrees of neck pain (which may ra-

diate), and jugular vein distention. A large thrombus is classified as an emergency because it may impair circulation to a limb. A nurse may attempt to aspirate this clot if hospital policy permits. Frequently hospitals also have protocols to administer small doses of thrombolytic agents to dissolve the clot. At the very least, the nurse is responsible for reporting suspected catheter occlusion to a physician.

AIR EMBOLISM

Air embolism occurs as a result of air entering the system and traveling to the right ventricle through the vena cava. Usually air entry into the catheter is associated with disconnection of the catheter from the IV tubing. Changes in intrathoracic pressure with inspiration and expiration draw air into the catheter and vena cava. Sudden hypotension from decreased cardiac output may be the first indicator of this sometimes lethal problem. Approximately 10 to 20 mL of air must enter the system before the patient becomes symptomatic. Signs of such an emergency may include confusion, light-headedness, anxiety, and unresponsiveness. The physiological event is the creation of foam within the ventricle with each heart contraction and loss of stroke volume due to air instead of blood in the ventricle, causing a sudden decrease in cardiac output. Cardiac arrest may occur.

If this problem is suspected, turning the patient on the left side in the Trendelenburg position may allow the air to rise to the wall of the right ventricle and improve blood flow. Oxygen should be started on the patient unless contraindicated.

Luer lock connections on all central line catheters and tubings, careful manipulation of catheter and tubing during dressing changes, and routine monitoring of the connections are strategies to prevent disconnections. There is no substitute for close observation by skilled and educated nursing staff.

Nursing Considerations

Central venous pressure is measured in centimeters of water or millimeters of mercury. Normal pressure of CVP measured by water manometer is approximately 5 to 8 cm H_2O. A CVP measured by a pressure transducer usually is 0 to 6 mmHg. The trend of the values is most significant as related to the patient's cardiovascular dysfunction and the response to interventions.

The CVP reflects intravascular volume status, right ventricular end-diastolic volume, and right ventricular function. To a very limited degree, the CVP indirectly reflects LV end-diastolic volume and function, because the left and right heart are linked by the pulmonary vascular bed. Usually alterations in volume status or ventricular function are associated with abnormally high or low CVP measurements.

Low CVP values indicate a hypovolemic state often requiring administration of fluids. The anticipated patient response to fluid therapy is an increase in the CVP. Similarly, diuretic therapy reduces intravascular volume and is associated with a reduction in CVP. A low or decreasing CVP also may be related to vasodilation from sepsis or administration of vasodilating drugs. Both create a relative hypovolemia, because blood volume has not changed. Rather, the intravascular space has become greater relative to the patient's blood volume.

Elevated CVP values may be due to a number of complex and interrelated factors, each of which requires scrutiny. Right ventricular failure and mechanical ventilation are two of the more common causes of increased CVP. Rarely is intravascular volume overload and hypervolemia alone a cause of increased CVP.

Mechanical ventilation increases intrathoracic pressure, which is transmitted to the pulmonary vasculature, heart, and great vessels. The CVP value may be directly affected by this pressure. CVP may be elevated as well, because intrathoracic pressure compresses the pulmonary vessels, creating resistance to blood flow from the right to the left side of the heart and causing blood to back up in the right ventricle, right atrium, and vena cava. In extreme cases, the increased intrathoracic pressure associated with mechanical ventilation causes significant right ventricular dysfunction, and the CVP is elevated as a result of reduced forward blood flow and the back up of blood and pressure in the right atrium and vena cava.

Right ventricular failure due to coronary artery disease or LV failure is associated with an elevated CVP. The inability of the right ventricle to pump blood through the pulmonary vasculature because of injured or infarcted myocardium results in increased volume and pressure in the right atrium and vena cava. LV failure may increase CVP as the pressure of blood volume congests the pulmonary vasculature and impairs flow from the right ventricle, causing right ventricular dilation and subsequent failure. Again, the increased pressure is reflected backward to the right atrium and vena cava. In these instances, interventions are directed toward facilitating forward blood flow by improving ventricular contractility and reducing the intravascular blood volume. A decrease in the CVP is an indication of the effectiveness of therapy.

The CVP is always interpreted in conjunction with other clinical observations, such as auscultation of breath sounds, heart and respiratory rate, ECG, neck vein distention, and urine output. For example, elevated CVP associated with pulmonary basilar crackles and decreased urine output is often indicative of LV failure. Distended neck veins but clear breath sounds and a high CVP might be due to increased intrathoracic pressure from the mechanical ventilator effects. Patients who are septic may have a low CVP that is associated with fever, elevated white blood cell count, tachycardia, and tachypnea, whereas a patient receiving vasodilating agents may have low CVP and an increased heart rate, but not the other clinical signs above. A CVP value alone is meaningless, but used with other clinical data, it is a valuable aid in managing and predicting the patient's clinical course.

▬ PULMONARY ARTERY PRESSURE MONITORING

The PA, flow-directed, balloon-tipped catheter has made possible the assessment of right ventricular function, pulmonary vascular status, and indirectly, LV function. Cardiac output, RA, RV, and PA pressures and PA wedge pressure (PAWP) are measured using a PA catheter. The pressures and cardiac output obtained using this catheter allow the clinician to calculate derived parameters and facilitate diagnosis of cardiovascular and cardiopulmonary dysfunction, determine the therapy needed, and evaluate the effectiveness of the interventions.

Pulmonary Artery Catheters

Several types of flow-directed, balloon-tipped PA catheters are available in different sizes. The type of catheter used is determined by the parameters to be monitored and additional requirements governed by the patient's condition. The 7.5-French (Fr. indicates catheter size) thermodilution catheter is the size most commonly used. All PA catheters

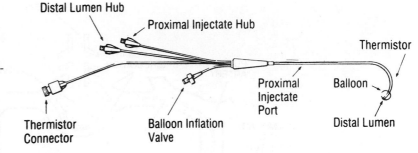

FIGURE 16-60
Pulmonary artery catheter. The distal lumen terminates in the pulmonary artery and the proximal lumen terminates in the right atrium. A syringe is attached to the balloon inflation valve to inflate the balloon at the catheter tip positioned in the pulmonary artery.

have several external ports or lumen hubs corresponding to internal lumens and lumen openings into the right heart and PA (Fig. 16–60).

Four lumens with external hubs or ports are common to all PA catheters: the proximal hub and lumen, distal hub and lumen, balloon inflation valve and lumen, and thermistor connector and lumen. The proximal or RA lumen opens into the right atrium. It may be used for the infusion of fluids or medications and is connected to a transducer allowing RA pressure measurements and display of the RA pressure waveform. The RA lumen port also is used as the injectate port for measuring cardiac outputs.

The distal or PA lumen hub is always attached to a transducer and a continuous flush system. The PA waveform is displayed continuously, as are the PA systolic, diastolic, and mean pressures. Mixed venous blood gases, necessary for oxygen extraction, oxygen consumption, and intrapulmonary shunt measurements, are withdrawn from the PA port. The PA port is not usually used for fluid or medication administration, although some circumstances may require this port to be used for infusions.

The balloon inflation port and lumen enable the clinician to inflate the balloon at the catheter tip with a small volume of air to measure the PA, occlusion, or PAWP. The balloon capacity of most PA catheters is 1.5 mL and should not be inflated with more than this amount of air. Fluid is never infused through the balloon inflation port.

The tip of the PA catheter also contains a thermistor. The external thermistor port is connected to the bedside monitor or to a cardiac output computer. The thermistor permits measurement of the patient's temperature in the PA (core temperature), and it detects the blood temperature change when solution is injected through the RA port to obtain a cardiac output measurement.

Specialty PA catheters include the above components and additional features and lumens. Some of the specialty features include a second proximal lumen that serves as an additional infusion port; a right ventricular lumen that may be used for infusions or insertion of a cardiac pacemaker probe (designated for that particular type of PA catheter) if temporary ventricular pacing is required; a lumen containing fiberoptic filaments allowing continuous measurement of mixed venous oxygen saturation ($S\overline{v}O_2$); continuous measurement and display of cardiac output; and right ventricu-

lar ejection fraction determinations. Several models of PA catheters have combined specialty features, such as the continuous cardiac output and $S\overline{v}O_2$ monitoring catheter or the right ventricular ejection fraction and $S\overline{v}O_2$ monitoring catheter.

Pulmonary Artery Catheter Insertion

Before the catheter is inserted, all necessary equipment should be assembled. The exact setup and equipment used will vary depending on the institution. The flush system is connected to the transducer, which is then placed at the zero reference point, leveled, and zeroed. Each lumen of the PA catheter is flushed with sterile solution from the flush system. (Note: Fiberoptic $S\overline{v}O_2$ monitoring catheters are calibrated prior to flushing lumens of the PA catheter.) The PAWP balloon is inflated with air to ensure proper inflation and evaluate for leaks before the catheter is inserted. The PA port is then connected to the prepared transducer with pressure tubing, and the other lumens are connected to either a pressure monitoring system or to IV solution.

Strict sterile technique is required for the PA catheter insertion procedure. The physician performing the procedure wears a cap, mask, sterile gown, and sterile gloves. The nurse assisting wears a cap and mask and if manipulating the catheter, sterile gloves. A sterile field is also used. The PA catheter is inserted into a large vein through an introducer catheter, which is usually placed by a percutaneous approach. The most common insertion sites are the left or right subclavian veins. Other sites that may be used are the internal or external jugular veins or femoral veins. Occasionally the antecubital vein is used. The antecubital access requires a venous cutdown.

Once the introducer is in place, the PA catheter is inserted by the physician and threaded into place. Determination of the catheter tip location is established by monitoring the waveform and pressures on the bedside monitor as the catheter passes through the vena cava to the right atrium. When the catheter tip is in the right atrium, the PA balloon is inflated with 1.5 mL of air to help "float" the catheter through the tricuspid valve into the right ventricle, across the pulmonic valve into the PA, and eventually into the wedged position (Fig. 16–61). The balloon is allowed to deflate passively after the PA wedge waveform is

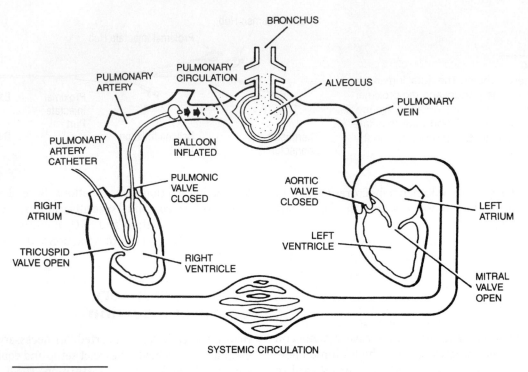

FIGURE 16-61
Position of the pulmonary artery catheter in the right heart and pulmonary artery. When the balloon is inflated and the catheter is in the wedge position, there is an unrestricted vascular channel between the tip of the catheter and the left ventricle in diastole. PAWP thus reflects left ventricular end-diastolic pressure, an important indicator of left ventricular function. (Courtesy of Hewlett Packard.)

noted on the monitor and return of the PA waveform is confirmed. The PA catheter is then secured, and a sterile dressing is placed over the insertion site. Catheter position is also verified with a chest radiograph following the insertion.

Nursing responsibilities during the insertion procedure include monitoring sterile technique, monitoring the changes in hemodynamic waveforms, recording the pressures in each chamber of the heart as the catheter is passed through, and monitoring the patient for complications. Ventricular dysrhythmias are the most common complication during PA catheter insertion (see complications section). Therefore, it is advisable to have a lidocaine bolus and defibrillator available for the insertion procedure.

Waveform Interpretation

All hemodynamic pressures and waveforms are generated by pressure changes in the heart caused by myocardial contraction (systole) and relaxation/filling (diastole) phases of the cardiac cycle. This mechanical activity of the heart is generated in response to the electrical activity, that is, the depolarization and repolarization of myocardial cells. Interpretation of the hemodynamic waveforms is dependent, therefore, on the correlation of mechanical to electrical activities using the ECG. There are three categories of hemodynamic waveforms: atrial, which includes RA, LA, and PA wedge; ventricular, which includes left and right ventricular; and arterial, which includes PA and systemic aortic. The waveforms in each category have similar characteristics because they result from the same cardiac events. The differences are in the pressure measurements because of the different amount of pressure that is generated in the right ventricle and atrium compared with the left side of the heart.

RIGHT ATRIAL PRESSURE

The RA is a low pressure chamber, receiving blood volume passively from the vena cava. The normal pressure is less than 8 mmHg, which reflects the mean RA pressure (RAP).

Atrial waveforms have three positive waves: a, c, and v (Fig. 16–62). The a wave is caused by the increase in atrial pressure during atrial contraction with systole. The c wave reflects the small increase in RAP associated with closure of the tricuspid valve and early atrial diastole. The v wave represents atrial diastole and the increase in pressure caused by filling of the atrium with blood. The v wave of RA diastole is also affected by ventricular contraction and the bulging of the tricuspid valve up into the RA after RA systole.

Accurate identification of the a, c, and v waves requires correlation of the waveform with the ECG. On the ECG, the P wave represents discharge of the SA node and atrial depolarization, which causes LA and RA contraction. Therefore, the a wave occurs after the P wave and usually in the PR in-

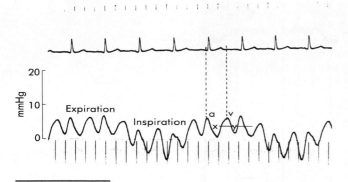

FIGURE 16-62
Normal right atrial (RA) waveform in a spontaneously breathing patient. Vertical lines drawn show the *a* wave following the ECG P wave, and the *v* wave following the ECG T wave. Horizontal line indicates measurement of the mean RAP of approximately 4 mmHg. From: Daily EK, Schroeder JS: Techniques in Bedside Hemodynamic Monitoring. St. Louis, C.V. Mosby, 1994.

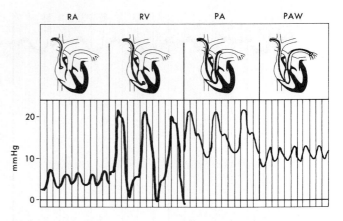

FIGURE 16-63
Waveforms associated with pulmonary artery catheter insertion. Note that the right atrial (RA) pressure is equivalent to the right ventricular (RV) end diastolic pressure, RV systolic is equivalent to the pulmonary artery (PA) systolic pressure, and PA diastolic pressure is equivalent to the PAWP. From: Daily EK, Schroeder JS: Techniques in Bedside Hemodynamic Monitoring. St. Louis, C.V. Mosby, 1994.

terval. The QRS complex represents ventricular depolarization and causes ventricular contraction. Simultaneously the RA relaxes and fills with blood. The v wave generated by these events thus falls after the QRS complex and in the T to P interval. The c wave is not always visible because of the small increase in pressure caused in early diastole and with tricuspid valve closure. If it is visible, the c wave occurs between the a and v waves.

Atrial pressure tracings also have two primary negative waves or descents: x and y. The x descent follows the a wave and represents a decrease in pressure caused by atrial relaxation at the beginning of atrial diastole. The y descent follows the v wave and represents the initial, passive atrial emptying into the ventricle as the tricuspid valve opens.

RIGHT VENTRICULAR PRESSURE

The right ventricle is considered a low-pressure chamber. Right-ventricular end-diastolic pressure is usually 0 to 8 mmHg, equal to the RAP as the tricuspid valve is open (Fig. 16–63). Right-ventricular systolic pressure is normally 20 to 30 mmHg because the right ventricle needs to generate only enough pressure to open the pulmonic valve and move blood through the low-pressure pulmonary vasculature.

As the PA catheter is advanced from the PA into the right ventricle or if the catheter has a right-ventricular lumen that is transduced, the waveform generated has a distinctive square root configuration (Fig. 16–64). Right-ventricular contraction is triggered by ventricular depolarization. The initial rapid rise in pressure represents isovolumetric contraction, which follows the QRS complex of the ECG. The right-ventricular pressure increases as the tricuspid and pulmonary valves are closed until the force

generated exceeds PA pressure. Rapid ejection occurs when the pulmonic valve opens. After ventricular systole, the pulmonic valve closes, and the right-ventricular pressure rapidly decreases, creating a diastolic dip. Next in the cardiac cycle, the tricuspid valve opens and the right ventricle passively fills with blood from the PA. Right-ventricular diastole falls within the period from the T to the next Q wave on the ECG. The point on the waveform just prior to the rapid rise in pressure represents right-ventricular end-diastole.

PULMONARY ARTERY PRESSURE

The pulmonary vasculature is a relatively low-resistance and low-pressure system in normal individuals. Normal PA systolic pressure is 20 to 30 mmHg and is equal to right-ventricular systolic pressure. Normal diastolic PA pressure is 8 to 15 mmHg, and the mean is 10 to 20 mmHg. The PA waveform characteristics are similar to the systemic arterial waveform previously described. PA systolic pressure and the peak of the PA waveform are generated by right-ventricular systolic ejection; therefore, the PA and right-ventricular systolic pressure are the same (see Fig. 16–63). The dicrotic notch in the downward slope of the PA waveform corresponds with pulmonary valve closure at the beginning of right-ventricular diastole and is the beginning of the PA diastolic phase (Fig. 16–65). PA diastolic pressure reflects the resistance of the pulmonary vascular bed and, to a limited degree, LV end-diastolic pressure. PA diastolic pressure theoretically and in absolutely normal conditions is an indirect measure of LV pressure because the pulmonary vasculature, left atrium, and open mitral valve allow equalization of pressure from the left ventricle back to the tip of the PA catheter.

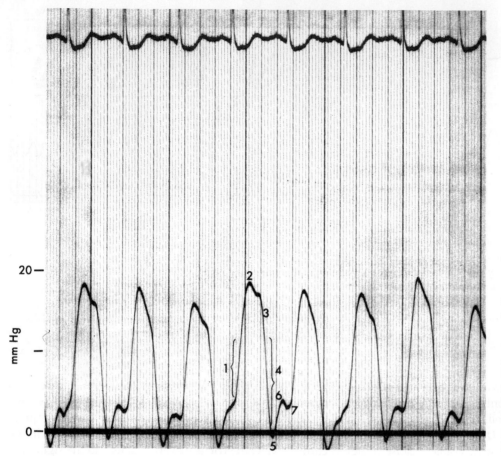

FIGURE 16-64
Normal right ventricle (RV) pressure waveform. (*1*, isovolumetric contraction; *2*, rapid ejection; *3*, reduced ejection; *4*, isovolumetric relaxation; *5*, early diastole; *6*, atrial systole; *7*, end-diastole.) Note rapid upstroke and return to below-zero baseline pressure. From Daily EK, Schroeder JS: Techniques in Bedside Hemodynamic Monitoring, p 128. St. Louis, C.V. Mosby, 1994.

PULMONARY ARTERY WEDGE PRESSURE

When the PA catheter is properly positioned, the PAWP is obtained by inflating the balloon at the catheter tip. The balloon occludes forward flow in the branch of the PA, creating a static column of blood from that portion of the PA through the left atrium, an open mitral valve during diastole, and the left ventricle. In this way, the PAWP reflects LV end-diastolic pressure (see Fig. 16–61). The PAWP more closely measures left atrial and ventricular end-diastolic pressure than the PA diastolic pressure because balloon inflation halts blood flow past the catheter tip and thereby decreases the influence of pulmonary vascular resistance on the pressure reading. Normal PAWP is 8 to 12 mmHg.

Inflation of the PA balloon causes the PA waveform on the monitor to become a PAWP tracing. No more than 1.5 mL of air is used to inflate the balloon. If less than 1 mL of air generates a PAWP tracing, the PA catheter has migrated distally and needs to be withdrawn slightly, usually by a physician, for proper placement.

The PAWP tracing has a, c, and v waves and x and y descents (Fig. 16–66). The electrical and mechanical events of the heart generating these waves are identical to those of the RA waveform, except that the PAWP waveform reflects activity from the left side of the heart. The a wave is

caused by LA contraction, and the v wave corresponds with LV contraction and left atrial filling. The c wave is rarely visible on the PAWP tracing.

The ECG correlation of the PAWP waveform is also the same as the RA waveform. The primary difference from the RA is the slight delay of PAWP a and v waves in relation to the ECG as a result of the distance from the left heart that these pressures are transmitted. The a wave now falls more closely in line with the QRS complex, although it may be within the PR interval. The v wave correlates with the T to P interval.

Complications

PNEUMOTHORAX

Pneumothorax is a complication of PA catheter introducer insertion through the subclavian vein. The anatomy of the patient can make placement of a PA catheter difficult, particularly if the patient is obese or has torturous subclavian veins. The needle or introducer sheath may puncture the lung during insertion and cause an apical pneumothorax. Signs and symptoms of a pneumothorax and routine postinsertion chest radiograph are the diagnostic techniques of this complication.

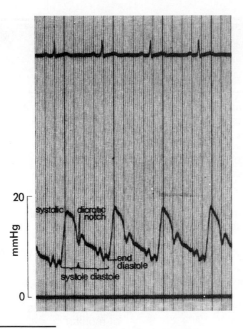

FIGURE 16-65

Pulmonary artery (PA) pressure waveform showing phases of systole, dicrotic notch (pulmonic valve closure), and end-diastole. Normally, PA end-diastole closely represents left ventricular end-diastolic pressure. From Daily EK, Schroeder JS: Techniques in Bedside Hemodynamic Monitoring, p 104. St. Louis, C.V. Mosby, 1994.

INFECTION

Systemic infection and sepsis are caused by contamination of the PA catheter, insertion site, or pressure monitoring system. Careful attention to sterile technique during pressure tubing assembly, insertion, and dressing changes and protocols for changing PA catheter and monitoring sys-

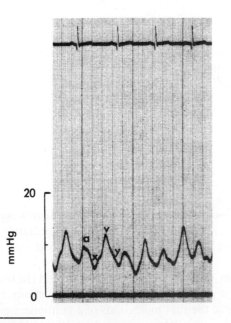

FIGURE 16-66

Normal pulmonary artery wedge pressure (PAWP) waveform showing *a* and *v* waves and *x* and *y* descents. The mean of this PAW pressure is about 8 mmHg.

tem help to prevent infection. Diagnosis of PA catheter-related sepsis is based on blood cultures, white blood cell count, and fever in the absence of other sources of infection.

VENTRICULAR DYSRHYTHMIAS

Ventricular dysrhythmias are common during the insertion of a PA catheter. As the catheter passes through the right ventricle, it may irritate the endocardium and cause PVCs and occasionally VT. The dysrhythmias typically resolve when the catheter is advanced into the PA. After the PA catheter is in proper position in the PA, it may become dislodged if not well secured, and the tip may "fall back" into the right ventricle. The patient may experience dysrhythmias, and the hemodynamic pressures and waveform will reflect those of the right ventricle. Usually in this situation, because of potential contamination at the insertion site, the physician will withdraw the catheter or occasionally inflate the balloon and advance the catheter into the PA. It is essential to have ready access to emergency drugs and equipment should the ventricular dysrhythmias persist.

PULMONARY ARTERY RUPTURE OR PERFORATION

A rare but very serious and potentially fatal complication related to PA catheters is rupture or perforation of the PA. Perforation of the PA may occur during insertion or manipulation of the PA catheter. Patients with friable PA may be at some risk; proper advancement of the catheter with the balloon fully inflated with 1.5 mL of air, however, and avoidance of advancing the catheter too far into a small artery minimize the chance of PA perforation. Rupture of the PA is associated with overinflation of the balloon, particularly if the catheter has migrated distally into a small PA. Close observation of the PA waveform as the balloon is inflated and only filling the balloon with the amount of air to obtain a PAWP tracing prevent overdistending a small PA. As previously stated, the catheter should wedge with 1 to 1.5 mL of air. If less air is required to obtain the PAWP waveform, the catheter has migrated out of proper position.

Nursing Considerations

Nursing care of the patient undergoing PA pressure monitoring is complex. The critical care nurse must be able to interpret waveforms and pressure data and be alert to potential complications. Interventions, outlined previously, that ensure accurate readings and minimize operator error apply to the patient with a PA catheter. Consistency of leveling and measurement techniques are especially important because small variations in the zero reference point will elicit large and erroneous changes in the RAP and PAWP. Table 16–12 outlines problems and trou-

TABLE 16-12
Troubleshooting: Inaccurate Pressure Measurements

Problem	Cause	Prevention	Treatment
Damped waveforms and inaccurate pressures	Partial clotting at catheter tip	Use continuous drip with 1 U heparin/1 mL IV fluid. Hand flush occasionally. Flush with large volume after blood sampling. Use heparin-coated catheters.	Aspirate, then flush catheter with heparinized fluid (*not* in PAW position).
	Tip moving against wall	Obtain more stable catheter position.	Reposition catheter.
	Kinking of catheter	Restrict catheter movement at insertion site.	Reposition to straighten catheter. Replace catheter.
Abnormally low or negative pressures	Incorrect air-reference level (above midchest level)	Maintain transducer air-reference port at midchest level; re-zero after patient position changes.	Remeasure level of transducer air-reference and reposition at midchest level; re-zero.
	Incorrect zeroing and calibration of monitor	Zero and calibrate monitor properly.	Recheck zero and calibration of monitor.
	Loose connection	Use Luer-Lok stopcocks.	Check all connections.
Abnormally high pressure reading	Pressure trapped by improper sequence of stopcock operation	Turn stopcocks in proper sequence when two pressures are measured on one transducer.	Thoroughly flush transducers with IV solution; re-zero and turn stopcocks in proper sequence.
	Incorrect air-reference level (below midchest level)	Maintain transducer air-reference port at midchest level; recheck and re-zero after patient position changes.	Check air-reference level; reset at midchest and re-zero.
Inappropriate pressure waveform	Migration of catheter tip (eg, in RV or PAW instead of in PA)	Establish optimal position carefully when introducing catheter initially. Suture catheter at insertion site and tape catheter to patient's skin.	Review waveform; if RV, inflate balloon; if PAW, deflate balloon and withdraw catheter slightly. Check position under fluoroscope and/or x-ray after reposition.
No pressure available	Transducer not open to catheter	Follow routine, systematic steps for pressure measurement.	Check system, stopcocks.
	Amplifiers still on *cal, zero,* or *off*		
Noise or fling in pressure waveform	Excessive catheter movement, particularly in PA	Avoid excessive catheter length in ventricle.	Try different catheter tip position.
	Excessive tubing length	Use shortest tubing possible (<3–4 ft).	Eliminate excess tubing.
	Excessive stopcocks	Minimize number of stopcocks.	Eliminate excess stopcocks.

PAW, *pulmonary artery wedge;* RV, *right ventricle;* PA, *pulmonary artery.*

bleshooting strategies related to hemodynamic pressure monitoring.

Measurement of all hemodynamic pressures is most accurate when obtained at the end expiration of the respiratory cycle. Because of changes in intrathoracic pressures during inspiration, the least influence of airway pressure transmission to the PA and heart occurs at the point of end expiration. Mechanical ventilation causes increased intrathoracic pressure during inspiration; therefore, end expiration is the lowest point of the hemodynamic waveform

(Fig. 16–67). Spontaneous breathing causes negative intrathoracic pressure; therefore, end expiration is the highest point of the waveform in these patients (see Fig. 16–62).

Alarm parameters are closely set to alert the nurse to potential physiological or technical complications. For example, one of the first indications of a pulmonary embolus is an acute rise in PA pressures. Distal migration of the PA catheter may cause the catheter to wedge spontaneously without balloon inflation, and PA pressures will decrease to

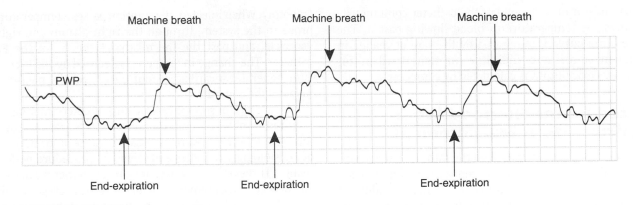

FIGURE 16-67
Pulmonary artery wedge pressure (PAWP) tracing showing respiratory variation from positive pressure mechanical ventilation. PAWP measurement is taken at the mean point of end expiration.

that of a PAWP. Both situations will be detected early if alarms are properly set.

Abnormalities of the RA waveform usually are large, elevated a or v waves. Increased size of the a wave is caused by impaired atrial emptying during atrial contraction and the subsequent increase in atrial pressure. Examples of pathology causing large a waves in the RA waveform are tricuspid stenosis and right ventricular failure. Elevated v waves are related to incompetence of the tricuspid valve, allowing blood to flow from the ventricle back into the atria during ventricular contraction. These abnormalities will also cause the mean RAP to be higher.

Elevation of PA pressures is associated with LV failure, mechanical ventilation, and pulmonary vascular vasoconstriction, for example, because of acute respiratory distress syndrome, primary pulmonary hypertension, or pulmonary embolus.

Abnormal PAWP waveforms are more common than abnormal RA waveforms because LV dysfunction and mitral valve disease tend to occur more frequently than right ventricular or tricuspid valve disorders. Pressure changes caused by left heart disorders are transmitted back through the pulmonary veins to the tip of the catheter in the PA and reflected as changes in the PAWP and waveform. Mitral stenosis creates large a waves as the left atrium contracts against the semiclosed valve, increasing pressure in the left atrium. Mitral regurgitation or insufficiency allows the backflow of blood into the left atrium during ventricular contraction and generates large v waves on the PAWP tracing. In both of these valvular diseases, the PAWP does not accurately reflect LV end-diastolic pressure. LV failure usually causes elevation of both the a and v waves and significantly increases the PAWP because of reduced contractility and forward blood flow. The PAWP waveform configuration is usually normal except for the high pressure reading.

Elevated PAWP frequently is due to LV dysfunction or hypervolemia. In some cases, such as adult respiratory distress syndrome or mechanical ventilator settings that generate extremely high intrathoracic pressure, PAWP will be elevated because of noncardiogenic causes. In these cases, however, the PA diastolic pressure will be greater than the PAWP.

CARDIAC OUTPUT DETERMINATION

Cardiac output is the volume of blood ejected from the heart per minute. It is expressed in liters per minute. Cardiac output is a function of stroke volume, the blood volume ejected with each ventricular contraction, and heart rate. Cardiac output and flow through the aorta are determined by the volume of blood in the ventricle at the end of diastole, impedance to flow from the heart, and the contractile ability of the myocardium. The left ventricle must generate enough pressure in systole to overcome aortic pressure and systemic vascular resistance (SVR) and eject sufficient blood volume to perfuse the organs of the body. The measurement of cardiac output and assessment of its determinants are important adjuncts to the care of the critically ill patient. Routine evaluation of cardiac output is essential when technology such as a PA catheter is used.

Methods

Several methods exist to measure cardiac output. Historically the "gold standard" has been the Fick method, originally developed in the 1800s by Adolf Fick. The Fick method uses the difference between arterial and venous oxygenation, oxygen consumption, and CO_2 production measured by spirometry to determine the cardiac output. Dye dilution is a second method. In this method, a dye indicator is injected into the venous system, and a time–concentration curve is generated from a blood sample obtained from the arterial system. Analysis of the curve allows cardiac output calculation.

The most common method to measure cardiac output is by thermodilution. The indicator is cold or room temperature solution injected into the RA port of the PA catheter.

The thermistor near the end of the catheter continuously measures the temperature of blood flowing past it. The temperature curve is generated by the rate of change in blood temperature after indicator injection. Based on this curve, a cardiac output is calculated by computer.

Procedure for Thermodilution Cardiac Output Measurement

A computation constant, based on the catheter size and volume of injectate, is set on the computer. The injectate solution used for the procedure is sterile normal saline or D5W. Five or 10 mL of solution is drawn into the syringe, which is attached to the RA port. Use of 10 mL enhances accuracy. The syringe is usually part of a closed system that remains intact and attached to the RA port by a stopcock (Fig. 16–68). Iced (0–4°C) or room temperature solution may be used. Room temperature injectate has little effect on accuracy compared with iced injectate. The decision to use iced solution is based on the need to have at least a 10°C difference between the patient's blood temperature and the injectate. Iced solution may be necessary in hypothermic patients and may improve accuracy in very low cardiac output states.

When the injectate syringe is filled, the computer is activated and signals the time for injection. The injectate must be given quickly, in less than 4 seconds, and injected smoothly. When injected, the solution passes a temperature probe in the system, through the right atrium and right ventricle, and past the thermistor at the tip of the PA catheter. The change in temperature sensed by the thermistor generates a cardiac output curve and the measurement by the computer.

The average of several cardiac output determinations is required to obtain a final measurement. Serial measurements and the average are necessary because of the number of physiological variables and technical procedure performance. Three or more consecutive measurements are usually needed. Measurements included in the average should be within 10% to 15% of each other and each associated with a normal cardiac output curve.

Interpretation of Cardiac Output Curves

Many bedside monitors and cardiac output computers are equipped with a strip recorder or modality to visualize the cardiac output curves. A normal cardiac output curve has a smooth upstroke and then a gradual decline (Fig. 16–69). High cardiac outputs generate a smaller curve with a steeper upstroke and decline than curves associated with a low cardiac output. Cardiac output measurements associated with abnormal curves are eliminated from the averaging process.

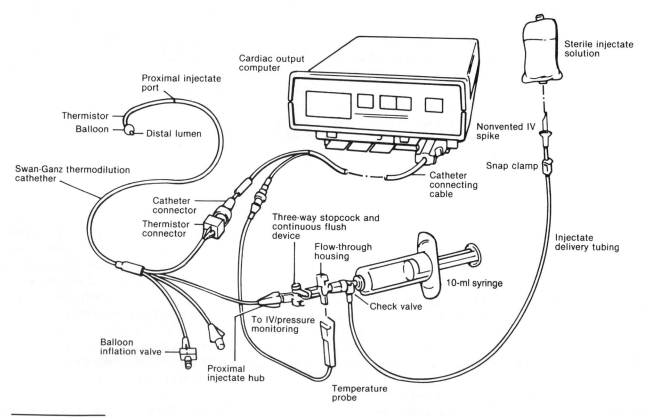

FIGURE 16-68
Sample of a closed injectate delivery system for room-temperature injectate.

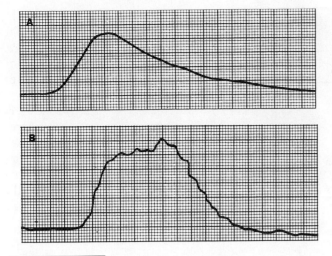

FIGURE 16-69

Examples of accurate and distorted thermodilution curves as produced on strip chart recorder. (**A**) Smooth recording is accurate. (**B**) Irregular recording is distorted, probably from an irregular or uneven emptying of the injectate syringe.

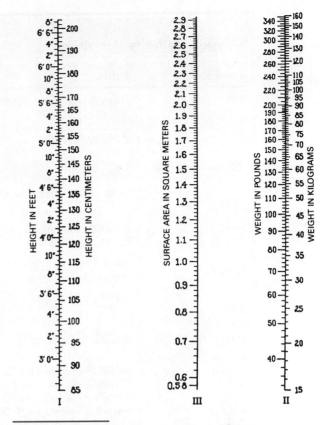

FIGURE 16-70

Dubois body surface chart (as prepared by Boothby and Sandiford of the Mayo Clinic). To find body surface of a patient, locate the height in inches (or centimeters) on scale I and the weight in pounds (or kilograms) on scale II and place a straightedge (ruler) between these two points, which will intersect scale III at the patient's surface area.

DETERMINANTS OF CARDIAC OUTPUT

Normal cardiac output at rest is considered to be 4 to 8 L/min. The measurement may also be calculated to reflect body size and is termed cardiac index. The cardiac index is obtained by dividing cardiac output by the patient's body surface area. Body surface area (BSA) can be determined with the Dubois body surface area chart (Fig. 16–70). Often bedside monitors and computers will automatically calculate cardiac index when the height and weight are entered. Normal cardiac index is 2.5 to 4 L/min/m².

Cardiac output or index is always evaluated by analysis of its determinants, heart rate and stroke volume. Tachycardia may reduce cardiac output as a result of shortened diastole and decreased filling time of the ventricles. Bradycardia is deemed symptomatic when it causes cardiac output and blood pressure to fall.

Stroke volume, the volume of blood ejected by the ventricles with each ventricular contraction, is influenced by preload, afterload, and contractility (see Chapter 15 for detailed discussion). Preload is the volume of blood in the ventricles at the end of diastole. Within physiological limits, increases in end-diastolic volume cause stretch of the myofibrils and increases the force of ventricular contraction (Frank-Starling law of the heart). Preload is primarily influenced by total blood volume. Because the PA catheter measures pressure, not volume, assumptions are made that volume and pressure can be equated. Although many factors alter the pressure–volume relationship, pressures are used to evaluate the adequacy of end-diastolic volume. Right ventricular preload is assessed using the RAP. LV preload is assessed by the PAWP measurement.

Afterload, which is impedance to ejection of blood from the ventricles, is influenced primarily by the status of pulmonary vascular resistance or SVR and the function of the pulmonic and aortic valves. Pulmonary vascular resistance is used to assess right ventricular afterload. LV afterload is evaluated by calculating SVR, as shown in Table 16–13. Indexed values (PVRI and SVRI) are used to account for body surface area.

Contractility is an inherent property of the heart. It is not affected by end-diastolic volume and cannot be directly measured. Sometimes stroke work index for both the left and right ventricles are used to assess contractility. Myocardial contractility is influenced by cardiac oxygen supply and demand balance, electrolytes, and minerals, such as calcium.

Nursing Considerations

Because alterations in cardiac output are caused by changes in heart rate, preload, afterload, and contractility, analysis of these parameters is essential in directing interventions to address the underlying pathophysiology.

Decreased cardiac output may be related to a decrease in preload (RAP and PAWP) caused by hypovolemia or decreased venous return associated with mechanical ventila-

TABLE 16-13
Oxygen Delivery Variables

Parameter	Formula	Normal Values
CO	Heart rate × Stroke volume	4–8 L/min
CI	$\dfrac{CO}{\text{Body surface area}}$	2.5–4 L/min/m²
SVI	$\dfrac{CI}{\text{Heart rate}}$	33–47 mL/beat/m²
MAP	$\dfrac{\text{Systolic BP} + (\text{diastolic BP} \times 2)}{3}$	70–105 mmHg
RAP	Direct measurement	0–8 mmHg
PAWP	Direct measurement	8–12 mmHg
RVEDVI	$\dfrac{\text{Stroke volume index}}{\text{RV ejection fraction}}$	60–100 mL/m²
SVRI	$\dfrac{(\text{MAP} - \text{RAP}) \times 80}{CI}$	1,360–2,200 dyne/s/cm⁻⁵
PVRI	$\dfrac{(\text{MPAP} - \text{PAWP}) \times 80}{CI}$	<425 dyne/s/cm⁻⁵
LVSWI	SVI (MAP-PAWP) × 0.0136	40–70 gm-m/m²/beat
RVSWI	SVI (MPAP − RAP) × 0.0136	5–10 gm-m/m²/beat
CaO₂	(Hb × 1.37 × SaO₂) + (0.003 × PaO₂)	20 mL O₂/dL
CvO₂	(Hb × 1.37 × SvO₂) + (0.003 × PvO₂)	15 mL O₂/dL
DaO₂l	CI × CaO₂ × 10	500–600 mL O₂/min/m²
DvO₂l	CI × CvO₂ × 10	375–450 mL O₂/min/m²

CO, cardiac output; CI, cardiac index; SVI, stroke volume index; RAP, right atrial pressure; PAWP, pulmonary artery wedge pressure; RVEDVI, right ventricular end diastolic volume index; SVRI, systemic vascular resistance index; MAP, mean arterial blood pressure; PVRI, pulmonary vascular resistance index; MPAP, mean pulmonary artery pressure; LVSWI, left ventricular stroke work index; RVSWI, right ventricular stroke work index; CaO₂, arterial oxygen content; Hb, hemoglobin; CvO₂, venous oxygen content; DaO₂l, arterial oxygen delivery index; DvO₂l, venous oxygen delivery index.

tion and elevated intrathoracic pressures. Vasoconstriction causes elevated afterload and has several causes. Increased SVR may be a compensatory response to hypovolemia caused by vasoconstriction to maintain cardiac output in this state. Some medications, hypothermia, and the compensatory vascular response to cardiogenic shock also increase afterload but will reduce cardiac output and increase oxygen demand and the work of the heart. Reduction in contractility decreases cardiac output. Examples include insufficient oxygen delivery to the myocardium, causing myocardial ischemia and infarct; medications, such as beta-blocking agents; or metabolic imbalances, such as low serum calcium, phosphorus, or magnesium levels.

Cardiac output increases with intravascular volume resuscitation, which increases preload. Decreased afterload due to vasodilation reduces resistance to ejection of blood, thus increasing cardiac output. Vasodilating medications, septic states, or allergic and anaphylactic reactions are all causes of vasodilation and will result in elevated cardiac output. Increased cardiac output resulting from enhanced contractility is most often a result of administration of positive inotropic agents or the correction of impaired myocardial oxygenation or metabolic derangements.

EVALUATION OF OXYGEN DELIVERY AND DEMAND BALANCE

One of the primary objectives of hemodynamic monitoring is to apply the data obtained from the PA catheter to the evaluation of oxygen delivery or transport and the consumption of oxygen by the tissues and organs. Adequate oxygen delivery to the body's organs is essential to maintain cellular, tissue, and ultimately organ function. Insufficient oxygen delivery and consumption to meet the cellular requirements for oxygen, oxygen demand, result in hypoxia and the accumulation of an oxygen deficit. Persistent oxygen deficit causes cell and organ dysfunction and eventually leads to cell death and organ failure. Tables 16–13 and 16–14 list the parameters that are used to evaluate oxygen delivery and demand balance, the formulas, and normal values.

TABLE 16-14
Oxygen Use Variables

Parameter	Formula	Normal Values
$S\overline{v}O_2$	Direct measurement	60%–80%
PvO_2	Direct measurement	35–45 mmHg
O_2 extraction	$CaO_2 - CvO_2$	3–5 mL O_2/dL
OER	$\dfrac{CaO_2 - CvO_2}{CaO_2}$	22%–30%
VO_2I	$(CaO_2 - CvO_2) \times CI \times 10$	120–170 mL/min/m²
pHa	Direct measurement	7.35–7.45
BE/BD	Direct measurement	−2–+2
Lactate	Direct measurement	0.5–2.2 mmol/L

OER, oxygen extraction ratio; VO_2I, oxygen consumption index; pHa, arterial pH; BE/BD, base excess/base deficit; all other abbreviations, see Table 16-13.

Determinants of Oxygen Delivery

Oxygen delivery (DaO_2) is the amount of oxygen transported to the tissues. DaO_2 is dependent on arterial oxygen content and cardiac output.

OXYGEN CONTENT

Oxygen content is the total amount of oxygen in the blood that is available to the cells. Most of the available oxygen (fuel) in arterial blood (over 95%) is reversibly bound to hemoglobin (boxcars) in the form of oxyhemoglobin and is measured by arterial oxygen saturation (SaO_2). A very small amount of oxygen, less than 5%, is dissolved in plasma and measured as PaO_2. A sufficient amount of hemoglobin is required to ensure adequate oxygen-carrying capacity. The two primary determinants of oxygen content are hemoglobin and oxygen saturation.

CARDIAC OUTPUT

Cardiac output is required to deliver oxygenated blood to the cells of the body.

Arterial oxygen delivery (DaO_2) is assessed by evaluating the adequacy of cardiac output and arterial oxygen content. In nonstressed states, normal DaO_2 is 1,000 mL O_2/min, or indexed to body surface area, 600 mL O_2/min/m². Increases in the body's oxygen demand associated with injury or illness are initially and primarily met by a compensatory increased cardiac output. Deficiencies of hemoglobin, arterial saturation, or cardiac output decrease DaO_2 to cells and threaten the adequacy of cellular oxygenation.

Determinants of Oxygen Consumption

Oxygen consumption (VO_2) is the amount of oxygen used by the tissues of the body. The primary determinants of VO_2 are the cellular demand for oxygen, the delivery of adequate amounts of oxygen, and the extraction of oxygen from the blood for use by the cells.

OXYGEN DEMAND

Oxygen demand is the requirement of cells for oxygen and is not directly measurable. Oxygen demand increases in any stress state. For example, surgery, infection, mobilization, pain, and anxiety increase the need for oxygen. Reduced oxygen demands are associated with lower metabolic rates, for example, hypothermia, sedation, or pharmacological paralysis. Oxygen demands are met through adequate delivery of oxygen and cellular extraction of oxygen.

OXYGEN DELIVERY

Cellular use of oxygen depends on an adequate supply of oxygen. This is termed delivery-dependent oxygen consumption and is depicted in Figure 16–71. As oxygen delivery increases, oxygen consumption also increases to meet the oxygen demand. When the requirement for oxygen is met, further increases in oxygen delivery will not increase consumption. The level of critical oxygen delivery is the point at which a decrease in oxygen delivery results in decreased VO_2 because of an insufficient oxygen supply.

OXYGEN EXTRACTION

Oxygen extraction ($CaO_2 - CvO_2$) is the amount of oxygen removed from the blood for use by the cells. It is measured by comparing the arterial oxygen content to venous oxygen content. Like arterial oxygen content, venous oxygen content (CvO_2) is primarily determined by the amount of hemoglobin that is saturated with oxygen. Venous saturation is obtained by withdrawing a mixed venous blood gas sample from the distal (PA) port of the PA catheter.

In normal circumstances and provided that oxygen is supplied in adequate amounts, the cells extract the oxygen they need to support tissue and organ function. Increased

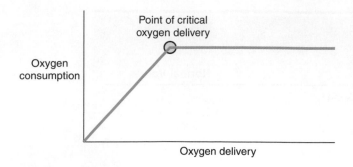

FIGURE 16-71
Delivery dependent oxygen consumption curve reflects the change in oxygen consumption related to oxygen delivery. At the point of critical oxygen delivery, oxygen delivery is sufficient to meet oxygen demand and oxygen consumption does not increase further. However, any decrease in oxygen delivery from this point results in a decrease of oxygen consumption due to an inadequate supply of oxygen.

demand for oxygen results in a compensatory increase in oxygen extraction as more oxygen is "unloaded" from the hemoglobin for cellular use. This is reflected by a reduced amount of oxygen in venous blood and therefore a widened $CaO_2 - CvO_2$ difference. Conversely, as oxygen demands decrease, less oxygen is required and extracted from the blood, and the $CaO_2 - CvO_2$ difference becomes more narrow.

Oxygen Supply and Demand Imbalance

An imbalance of oxygen supply and demand occurs whenever oxygen delivery is inadequate to meet cellular demand or the cells are unable to extract sufficient quantities of oxygen. Specific threats to the balance of oxygen supply and demand are decreased cardiac output, hemoglobin, or arterial saturation; impaired cellular extraction of oxygen; or oxygen demands that are so great that they cannot be met by increased oxygen delivery or extraction.

OXYGEN DEBT ACCUMULATION

Inadequate oxygen consumption causes an anaerobic state and cellular hypoxia. Cells deprived of oxygen begin to acquire an oxygen debt. Over time, oxygen debt accumulation becomes irreversible, cell damage is irreparable, and cell death results. Oxygen debt is a major cause of multisystem organ dysfunction and failure. If oxygen debt accumulation is identified before irreversible cell injury has occurred, the oxygen deficit may be reversed by increasing oxygen availability.

Metabolic Indicators of Oxygen Debt

Several metabolic parameters can be measured to evaluate oxygen debt. When these indicators of oxygen debt are

used in conjunction with hemodynamic monitoring of oxygen delivery and consumption, therapies may be more specifically directed to achieve an oxygen supply and demand balance.

Because hypoxia and oxygen debt are associated with anaerobic metabolism, the byproducts of anaerobic metabolism can be used to assess the presence of an oxygen deficit. Lactic acid accumulation causes a metabolic acidosis in an oxygen debt state. Therefore, laboratory measurement of lactate levels, serum pH, and base deficit/excess are means to evaluate oxygen debt. Serum pH and base deficit/excess are routinely measured and reported with blood gas analysis. Elevated lactate levels (> 2.2 mm/L) or metabolic acidosis (pH < 7.35 with normal $PaCO_2$) correlate with oxygen debt, particularly when the patient has a low or even normal level of DaO_2 and VO_2. As with all assessment parameters, lactate levels, pH, and base deficit should not be viewed in isolation; they should be evaluated in conjunction with other assessment parameters.

CONTINUOUS MIXED VENOUS OXYGEN SATURATION MONITORING

Mixed venous oxygen saturation ($S\overline{v}O_2$) may be used to reflect the balance of oxygen supply, use, and demand. $S\overline{v}O_2$ is the measurement of oxyhemoglobin in desaturated blood returning to the right ventricle and PA. The $S\overline{v}O_2$ is significantly less than arterial saturation due to the extraction of oxygen by the cells and the unloading of oxygen from hemoglobin. $S\overline{v}O_2$ is influenced by the degree of arterial saturation, the quantity of hemoglobin, the cardiac output, the determinants of oxygen delivery, and by the amount of oxygen extracted and consumed by the cells. Under normal conditions of oxygen delivery, oxygen consumption, and demand, approximately 25% of the available oxygen is extracted and used to meet demand. The $S\overline{v}O_2$ is 60% to 80% in this situation. If oxygen delivery is reduced by a decrease in arterial saturation, hemoglobin, or cardiac output, then more oxygen is extracted from the blood to meet cellular demand. The blood returning to the right heart and PA has had a greater quantity of oxygen removed and is more desaturated, which is reflected by a decrease in $S\overline{v}O_2$. Similarly, if oxygen demand rises but oxygen delivery does not increase to meet this requirement, additional oxygen is extracted from the blood and consumed by the cells. Therefore, oxyhemoglobin is reduced in the venous blood, decreasing $S\overline{v}O_2$. Persistently low $S\overline{v}O_2$ is a warning that an oxygen debt may be accruing because of inadequate oxygen delivery or a high oxygen demand not met by the oxygen supply.

Three general conditions result in an increasing $S\overline{v}O_2$:

- When the delivery of oxygen is much greater than the requirement, only a small percent of that oxygen is extracted, causing $S\overline{v}O_2$ to rise.
- In states of low metabolic rate and oxygen demand, the need for oxygen is reduced, and less oxygen is extracted and consumed. $S\overline{v}O_2$ reflects the decrease in

extraction as greater amounts of oxyhemoglobin are returned to the right heart.

- In pathological states where the cells cannot extract oxygen from the blood or where tissue beds are not well perfused with oxygenated blood, oxygen is not extracted from the blood despite the cellular oxygen demand. Oxygen saturation of venous blood, the $S\bar{v}O_2$, returning to the right heart and PA is therefore higher because of the decreased oxygen consumption.

Although the $S\bar{v}O_2$ may be in the normal range, because of the reduced cellular oxygen extraction or the shunting of oxygenated blood past tissue beds, these cells do not use or receive the oxygen they require and begin to accumulate an oxygen debt. In these situations, a normal $S\bar{v}O_2$ may be misleading when viewed in isolation.

$S\bar{v}O_2$ can be continuously measured at the bedside by a PA catheter containing fiberoptic filaments in one of the lumens ending at the tip of the catheter in the PA. The blood in the PA is desaturated, venous blood. An infrared light is emitted that reflects off the red blood cells that are saturated with oxygen. The percent of saturated hemoglobin compared with the total hemoglobin is calculated by the $S\bar{v}O_2$ monitoring computer to yield the venous saturation value. The information is updated every few seconds; thus, a continuous $S\bar{v}O_2$ reading is provided.

Nursing Considerations

When patients are critically ill, careful evaluation of the adequacy of oxygen delivery, oxygen extraction, and consumption with respect to oxygen demand is paramount. Scrutiny of each determinant of cardiac output (heart rate, preload, afterload, and contractility parameters), oxygen content (arterial saturation and hemoglobin), oxygen consumption (DaO_2 and $CaO_2 - CvO_2$), and oxygen debt (lactate, pH, base deficit/excess, $S\bar{v}O_2$) is important to critical care nursing.

Numerous interventions are used to enhance oxygen delivery. Managing these and the patient's response to therapy is necessary. Examples of interventions to increase cardiac output include administration of intravascular volume to increase preload, positive inotropic agents to improve contractility, or vasodilating agents to reduce afterload. Oxygen content may be increased by changes in mechanical ventilator settings, chest physiotherapy, and positioning and mobilization or in nonmechanically ventilated patients by coughing and deep breathing exercises, all of which improve arterial oxygenation. Administration of packed red blood cells increases hemoglobin and oxygen-carrying capacity.

Many of the interventions to reduce oxygen demand and enhance oxygen consumption are important tenants of nursing care. For example, appropriate management of the environment, pain, and anxiety reduce stress and therefore contribute to decreasing the patient's demand for oxygen. Maintaining normothermia by control of the patient's temperature may reduce oxygen requirements associated with fevers and facilitate impaired perfusion and oxygen consumption associated with hypothermia.

$S\bar{v}O_2$ monitoring is helpful to guide nursing interventions. For example, endotracheal suctioning, although a very important intervention, may cause a temporary decrease in arterial oxygenation and increase discomfort and anxiety. Monitoring $S\bar{v}O_2$ allows the nurse to judge the impact this activity has on the patient's oxygen supply and demand. A falling $S\bar{v}O_2$ during suctioning is usually due to the increase in oxygen demand and reduced arterial oxygenation. Hyperoxygenating and hyperventilating before, during, and after auctioning help to lessen the negative effects on oxygen demand and arterial oxygenation. Before proceeding to another activity such as repositioning, the nurse should monitor the $S\bar{v}O_2$ and wait until the value normalizes, thereby avoiding an additional stressor and further increase on oxygen demand.

■ CONCLUSION

Full use of all of the parameters available from a PA catheter supports the use of this invasive and costly technology. Serial monitoring of cardiac output (preload, afterload, and contractility), oxygen delivery, and consumption in conjunction with the indicators of oxygen debt and organ function permits tailoring of interventions to the patient's specific needs. The goal of therapy is to optimize cardiac output and enhance oxygen delivery, maximize oxygen consumption, and normalize indicators of oxygen debt.

Nurses' responsibilities are related to acquiring accurate data, analyzing and interpreting data as an indication for a physician consult, and anticipating the desired response to therapy. Using independent nursing interventions to reduce cardiac work and oxygen demand is imperative. Promoting comfort and pain relief, decreasing anxiety, and treating fever or other causes of increased metabolic oxygen demand are paramount in the care of critically ill patients.

Clinical Applicability Challenges

Self-Challenge: Critical Thinking

1. *Devise strategies to adapt the history and physical examination to a patient who is deaf.*

2. *Determine, in the presence of elevated cardiac enzymes, what other assessment areas the nurse should consider to assist in ruling in or ruling out myocardial damage.*

3. *List and give the rationale for physical and physiological considerations the nurse should address in the planning of invasive and noninvasive cardiac diagnostic procedures.*

4. *You have been newly hired for a position in the coronary care unit. The nurse manager tells you that all patients in the unit are to be monitored using lead II. State your response and explain.*

5. A patient has significant changes in hemodynamic pressure readings following a position change to his right side. Assess the potential causes of the changes and describe appropriate nursing actions.

6. Stressors of any type increase the body's oxygen demand. Develop specific interventions to reduce or minimize oxygen demand and decrease the work of the heart, and outline anticipated interventions to improve oxygen delivery.

Study Questions

Cardiac History and Physical Examination

1. Chest pain associated with a heart problem is usually described as
   a. made worse by taking a deep breath.
   b. superficial and throbbing.
   c. heaviness or tightness that radiates to the left arm.
   d. made worse by movement of the chest and by lying down.

2. S_1 is an important heart sound that is timed with
   a. the beginning of diastole.
   b. the closure of the mitral and tricuspid valves.
   c. the closure of the pulmonic an aortic valves.
   d. the early, rapid-filling phase of ventricular diastole.

3. Which of the following is an important sign of CHF in the adult?
   a. Systolic ejection murmur
   b. Holosystolic murmur
   c. S_3
   d. S_4

Cardiac Laboratory Studies

1. The cardiac enzyme that may be detected as early as 1 hour after the onset of symptoms and usually peaks in 2 to 4 hours is
   a. CK-MB.
   b. SGOT.
   c. myoglobin.
   d. LDH.

2. Which of the following is considered diagnostic for MI?
   a. A latent rise in total CK
   b. CK-MB greater than 5%
   c. An LDH-1 determination greater than LDH-2
   d. An elevated CK-MM

3. All of the following statements are correct except
   a. LDH can be a reliable marker for myocardial damage when the CK determination is inconclusive.
   b. LDH may be abnormally elevated in hemolytic anemia, pulmonary infarction, or hepatic disorders.
   c. cardiac enzyme limits are generally higher for men than for women.
   d. enzymes can be a valuable diagnostic tool for a patient with an inconclusive ECG.

Cardiovascular Diagnostic Procedures

1. For patients who are unable or unwilling to exercise for an ECG study, an alternative approach would be the use of
   a. M-mode echocardiography.
   b. dobutamine stress echocardiography.
   c. a Holter monitor.
   d. transesophageal echocardiography.

2. Radionuclide imaging techniques are playing an increasingly important role in
   a. evaluating and diagnosing MI.
   b. monitoring and diagnosing CHF.
   c. evaluating the etiology of ventricular dysrhythmias.
   d. the diagnosis and treatment of coronary artery disease.

3. A drawback of ultrafast CT in the assessment of myocardial blood flow is that
   a. it is less accurate when blood flow is increased.
   b. it is less accurate when blood flow is normal or reduced.
   c. it cannot detect coronary calcium.
   d. it must always be used with contrast media.

4. Intravascular ultrasound can be very helpful because of its ability to
   a. assess the degree of coronary blood flow.
   b. confirm myocardial ischemia.
   c. assess vessel lumen dimensions with a 360-degree view and illuminate arterial wall layers.
   d. isolate myocardial wall motion abnormalities.

Electrocardiographic Monitoring

1. You have decided to monitor your patient using a modified version of chest lead 1 (MCL_1). To achieve this electrical view of the heart, you would place the lead wires in the following positions:
   a. Negative in the fourth intercostal space right sternal border and positive below the left clavicle
   b. Negative below the right clavicle and positive left midclavicular line below lowest rib
   c. Negative below the right clavicle and positive below the left clavicle
   d. Negative below the left clavicle and positive in the fourth intercostal space right sternal border

2. You have decided to monitor your patient using lead II. To achieve this electrical view of the heart, you would place the lead wires in the following positions:
   a. The positive under the left clavicle and the negative under the right clavicle
   b. The positive on the left side of the body below the heart and the negative below the right clavicle
   c. The positive on the left side of the body below the heart and the negative below the left clavicle
   d. The positive below the right clavicle and the negative on the left side of the body below the heart

3. The best leads to distinguish ventricular ectopy from supraventricular rhythms with aberrancy are
   a. leads II, III, aVF.
   b. leads I, aVL, V_5, V_6.
   c. leads V_1 and V_6.
   d. leads V_1, V_2, V_3.

Dysrhythmias and the 12-Lead Electrocardiogram

1. Mr. Jones, a patient in the coronary care unit, suddenly goes into a sinus bradycardia at a rate of 42, and his BP drops to 88/58. The physician decides to treat Mr. Jones and is likely to order which of the following medications?
   a. IV lidocaine
   b. IV atropine
   c. IV procainamide
   d. IV quinidine

2. Which of the following dysrhythmias results in loss of the atrial component to cardiac output (the "atrial kick")?
   a. Atrial fibrillation
   b. Premature atrial contractions
   c. Sinus tachycardia
   d. Junction rhythm

3. Premature ventricular contractions
   a. have a normal QRS configuration.
   b. are always treated with lidocaine.
   c. are especially dangerous if they fall on the P wave the "vulnerable period."
   d. are caused by an irritable focus in the ventricle.

4. The P wave in junctional rhythm
   a. is absent because the impulse starts at the AV junction.
   b. is normal in configuration and precedes each QRS complex.
   c. may be inverted before, during, or after the QRS.
   d. occurs twice as frequently as the QRS complex because the AV node blocks every other beat.

5. In complete heart block, the
   a. atria and ventricles depolarize at equal rates but very slowly.
   b. atria and ventricles depolarize independently.
   c. atria depolarize slower than the ventricles.
   d. AV node conducts all the stimulus from the sinus node.

Effects of Serum Electrolyte Abnormalities on the Electrocardiogram

1. Which of the following electrolyte abnormalities increases the sensitivity of the heart to digitalis and its accompanying dysrhythmias?
   a. Hyperkalemia
   b. Hypercalcemia
   c. Hypokalemia
   d. Hypocalcemia

2. Hypercalcemia produces which type of change on the ECG?
   a. Prolonged QT interval
   b. Shortened QT interval
   c. Prominent U waves
   d. Tall, peaked T waves

Hemodynamic Monitoring

1. Normal pulmonary artery wedge pressure is
   a. 8 to 12 mmHg.
   b. 12 to 18 mmHg.
   c. 18 to 22 mmHg.
   d. 6 mmHg.

2. PA wedge pressure values reflect
   a. left ventricle preload.
   b. left ventricular afterload.
   c. right ventricular preload.
   d. right ventricular afterload.

3. Which of the following will result in a low central venous pressure?
   a. Hypervolemia
   b. Biventricular failure
   c. Hypovolemia
   d. Left ventricular failure

4. Accurate cardiac output determination is dependent on injection of solution in less than
   a. 2 seconds.
   b. 4 seconds.
   c. 6 seconds.
   d. 8 seconds.

5. Oxygen delivery, extraction, and demand influence
   a. systemic vascular resistance.
   b. preload.
   c. mean arterial pressure.
   d. oxygen consumption.

6. Oxygen debt accumulates when
   a. oxygen delivery is greater than oxygen demand.
   b. oxygen consumption is greater than oxygen demand.
   c. oxygen consumption is less than demand.
   d. oxygen delivery is greater than oxygen consumption.

REFERENCES

Cardiac History and Physical Examination

1. Bates B: A Guide to Physical Examination and History Taking (6th Ed). Philadelphia, J.B. Lippincott, 1995
2. American Heart Association: Heart and Stroke Facts. Dallas, American Heart Association, 1994
3. Roberts R: Acute myocardial infarction. In Kelley WN (eds): Textbook of Internal Medicine (3rd Ed), pp 385–398. Philadelphia, Lippincott-Raven, 1997
4. Bullock B: Coronary artery disease. In Bullock B (ed): Pathophysiology: Adaptations and Alterations in Function (4th Ed), pp 457–472. Philadelphia, Lippincott-Raven, 1996
5. American Heart Association: Heart and Stroke Facts: 1995 Statistical Supplement. Dallas, American Heart Association, 1995

Cardiac Laboratory Studies

1. Adams J, Sicard G, Allen B, et al: Diagnosis of perioperative myocardial infarction with measurement of cardiac troponin I. N Engl J Med 330:670–674, 1994
2. Apple S: Advanced strategies for diagnosing acute myocardial infarction. Heartbeat 6:1–12, 1995
3. Hamm C, Ravkilde J, Gerhardt W, et al: The prognostic value of serum troponin T in unstable angina. N Engl J Med 327:146–150, 1992

Dysrhythmias and the 12-Lead Electrocardiogram

1. Jung F, DiMarco JP: Antiarrhythmic drug therapy in the treatment of atrial fibrillation. Cardiol Clin 14(4):507–517, 1996
2. Catalano JT: Guide to ECG analysis. Philadelphia, J.B. Lippincott, 1993

BIBLIOGRAPHY

Cardiac History and Physical Examination

Marriott HJ: Bedside Cardiac Diagnosis. Philadelphia, J.B. Lippincott, 1993
Myers DG: Review of cardiac auscultation. Part I. Hospital Medicine 29(10):25–52, 1993
Hanson MJ: Modifiable risk factors for coronary heart disease in women. American Journal of Critical Care 3(3):177–186, 1994

Cardiac Laboratory Studies

Puleo P, Meyer D, Wathen C, et al: Use of a rapid assay of subforms of creatine kinase MB to diagnose or rule out acute myocardial infarction. N Engl J Med 331:561–566, 1994
Roberts R, Kleiman N: Earlier diagnosis and treatment of acute myocardial infarction necessitates the need for a "new diagnostic mind-set." Circulation 89:872–881, 1994
Sobel B, Jaffe A: The value and limitations of cardiac enzymes in the recognition of acute myocardial infarction. Heart Disease and Stroke 2:26–32, 1993
Wu A, Abbas S, Green S, et al: Prognostic value of cardiac troponin T in unstable angina pectoris. Am J Cardiol 76:970–972, 1995

Cardiovascular Diagnostic Procedures

Blackwell G, Pohost G: The evolving role of MRI in the assessment of coronary artery disease. Am J Cardiol 75:74D–78D, 1995

Brundage B: Beyond perfusion with ultrafast computed tomography. Am J Cardiol 75:69D–73D, 1995

Budoff M, Georgion D, Brody A, et al: Ultrafast computed tomography as as diagnostic modality in the detection of coronary artery disease. Circulation 93:898–904, 1996

Cerqueira M: Diagnostic testing strategies for coronary artery disease: special issues related to gender. Am J Cardiol 75:52D–60D, 1995

Chirillo F, Cavarzerani A, Ius P, et al: Role of transthoracic, transesophageal, and transgastric two-dimensional and color doppler echocardiography in the evaluation of mechanical complications of acute myocardial infarction. Am J Cardiol 76:833–836, 1995

Coy K, Mauer G, Siegel R: Intravascular ultrasound imaging: A current perspective. J Am Coll Cardiol 18:1811–1823, 1991

Hachamovitch R, Berman D, Kiat H, et al: Exercise myocardial perfusion SPECT in patients without known coronary artery disease. Circulation 93:905–914, 1996

Mancini C, Simon S, McGillem J, et al: Automated quantitative coronary angiography: Morphologic and physiologic validation in vivo of a rapid digital angiographic method. Circulation 75:452–460, 1987

McConnell E: The future of technology in critical care. Critical Care Nurse 16(suppl):3–16, 1996

MIDA CoroNet, Hewlett-Packard, Andover, MA, Product Literature

Nakamura S, Colombo A, Gaglione A, et al: Intravascular ultrasound observations during stent implantation. Circulation 89:2026–2034, 1994

Nissen S, Gurley J, Booth D, DeMaria A: Intravascular ultrasound of the coronary arteries: Current applications and future directions. Am J Cardiol 69:18H–29H, 1992

O'Keefe J, Barnhart C, Bateman T: Comparison of stress echocardiography and stress myocardial perfusion scintigraphy for diagnosing coronary artery disease and assessing its severity. Am J Cardiol 75:25D–34D, 1995

Pandian N, Hsu T: Intravascular ultrasound and intracardiac echocardiography: Concepts for the future. Am J Cardiol 69:6H–17H, 1992

Sherman D, Balady G: What's new in stress testing? Pharmacologic approaches. Hosp Med 31:32–36, 1995

Spears J, Sandor T, Als A, et al: Computerized image analysis for quantitative measurement of vessel diameter from cineangiograms. Circulation 68:453–461, 1983

Thompson E, Detwiler D, Nelson C: Dobutamine stress echocardiography: A new, noninvasive method for detecting ischemic heart disease. Heart Lung 25:87–97, 1996

Tobis J, Mallery J, Mahon D, et al: Intravascular ultrasound imaging of human coronary arteries in vivo. Circulation 83:913–926, 1991

Electrocardiographic Monitoring

Drew BJ: Bedside electrocardiogram monitoring. AACN Clinical Issues in Critical Care 4(1):25–33, 1993

Drew BJ, Adams MGPeter MM, Wung SF: ST segment monitoring with a dreived 12-lead electrocardiogram is superior to routine CCU monitoring. American Journal of Critical Care 5(3):198–206, 1996

Hebra JD: The nurse's role in continuous dysrhythmia monitoring. AACN Clinical Issues in Critical Care 5(2):178–185, 1994

Ide B: Bedside electrocardiographic assessment. Journal of Cardiovascular Nursing 9(4):10–23, 1995

Thomason TR, Riegel B, Carlson B, Gocka I: Monitoring electrocardiographic changes: Results of a national survey. Journal of Cardiovascular Nursing 9(4):1–9, 1995

Dysrhythmias and the 12-Lead Electrocardiogram

Conover M: Understanding electrocardiography (7th Ed). St. Louis, C.V. Mosby, 1996

Futterman L, Lemberg L: Atrial fibrillation: An increasingly common and provacative arrhythmia. American Journal of Critical Care 5(5):379–387, 1996

Huff J: ECG workbook: Exercises in arrhythmia interpretation (3rd Ed). Philadelphia, Lippincott-Raven, 1997

Robinson AW: Common varieties of supraventricular tachycardia: Differentiation and dangers. Heart Lung 25(5):373–383, 1996

Thaler M: The only EKG book you'll ever need (2nd Ed). Philadelphia, J.B. Lippincott, 1995

Effect of Serum Electrolyte Abnormalities on the Electrocardiogram

Nally BR, Dunbar SB, Zellinger M, Davis A: Supraventricular tachycardia after coronary artery bypass grafting surgery and fluid and electrolyte variables. Heart Lung 25(1):31–36, 1996

Thaler M: The only EKG book you'll ever need (2nd Ed). Philadelphia, J.B. Lippincott, 1995

Huff J: ECG workbook: Exercises in arrhythmia interpretation (3rd Ed). Philadelphia, Lippincott-Raven, 1997

Hemodynamic Monitoring

Ahrens T: Changing Perspectives in the assessment of oxygenation. Crit Care Nurse 13:78, 1993

Daily EK, Schroeder JS: Techniques in Bedside Hemodynamic Monitoring (5th Ed). St. Louis, CV Mosby, 1994

Darovic GO (ed): Hemodynamic Monitoring: Invasive and Noninvasive Clinical Application (2nd Ed). Philadelphia, W.B. Saunders, 1995

Doering LV: The effect of positioning on hemodynamics and gas exchange in the critically ill: A review. American Journal of Critical Care 2:208, 1993

Enger EL: Pulmonary artery wedge pressure: When it's valid, when it's not. Crit Care Nurs Clin NA 1:603, 1989

Epstein CD, Henning RJ: Oxygen transport variables in the identification and treatment of hypoxia. Heart Lung 22:328, 1993

Kern L: Hemodynamic monitoring. In Boggs RL, Woolridge-King M (eds): AACN Procedure Manual for Critical Care (3rd Ed). Philadelphia, W.B. Saunders, 1993

Sharkey SW: A Guide to Interpretation of Hemodynamic Data in the Coronary Care Unit. Philadelphia, Lippincott-Raven, 1997

Von Rueden KT, Dunham CM: Evaluation and management of oxygen delivery and consumption in multiple organ dysfunction syndrome. In Secor VH (ed): Multiple Organ Dysfunction and Failure: Pathophysiology and Clinical Implications (2nd Ed). St. Louis, C.V. Mosby, 1996

17

Patient Management: Cardiovascular System

OBJECTIVES

Based on the content in this chapter, the reader should be able to:

- Compare and contrast the most commonly used agents in the treatment of dysrhythmias.
- Describe the indications, normal dose, and side effects of commonly used antiarrhythmic agents.
- Explain the indications, normal dose, and side effects of the commonly used vasoactive agents.
- Discuss the actions and uses of common thrombolytic agents.
- Compare and contrast the indications and contraindications for percutaneous transluminal coronary angioplasty (PTCA),

coronary stenting, atherectomy, laser, and percutaneous balloon valvuloplasty (PBV).
- Summarize interventions for complications associated with PTCA, stenting, atherectomy, laser, and PBV.
- List potential nursing diagnoses and the interventions for each diagnosis in the patient undergoing an interventional cardiology procedure.
- Describe the physiological effect of intra-aortic balloon pump (IABP) counterpulsation therapy.
- Explain indications and contraindications for IABP therapy.
- Describe a ventricular assist device and its indications and mechanism of action.
- Discuss nursing interventions for the patient receiving IABP therapy or ventricular circulatory assistance.

- Define autologous blood transfusion and its indications for use.
- Explain three methods of autologous blood reinfusion.
- Describe the nursing assessments and interventions necessary for the patient undergoing autotransfusion.
- Describe indications and contraindications of cardiopulmonary resuscitation.
- Explain the role of each member of the hospital resuscitation team.
- Explain the steps of cardiopulmonary resuscitation according to advanced cardiac life support guidelines.
- Analyze the first-line pharmacological therapy for cardiac arrest, including indications, dose, route, and side effects.

- Describe the indications, procedure, and nursing management for cardioversion and radiofrequency catheter ablation.
- Describe the components of the pacing system and pacemaker functioning.
- Use the pacemaker code to describe modes of pacing.
- Explain complications of pacing and appropriate interventions.
- Discuss the nursing management of the patient with a pacemaker.
- Describe the indications for an implantable cardioverter defibrillator (ICD).
- Describe the ICD system and its functioning.
- Explain the nursing management of a patient with an ICD.

Pharmacological Therapy: Antiarrhythmic, Vasoactive, and Thrombolytic Agents

Critically ill patients often experience altered cardiac output. The variables affecting cardiac output are stroke volume (preload, afterload, contractility) and heart rate. The cardiac rhythm and the synchronization between atrial and ventricular activity also influence cardiac output.

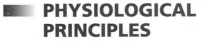

PHYSIOLOGICAL PRINCIPLES

Multiple medications are used to manipulate cardiac output variables in an attempt to ensure adequate oxygen delivery to the body's cells. The critical care nurse must have an understanding of these agents and adverse reactions that can occur. The following section addresses major pharmacological agents used to manipulate stroke volume and heart rate.

ANTIARRHYTHMIC AGENTS

Altered heart rate or rhythm can affect cardiac output, thus necessitating the need for antiarrhythmic agents. The goal is to restore a normal rhythm and prevent life-threatening dysrhythmias. In 1969, Vaughan Williams proposed a way of classifying antiarrhythmic agents based on their effect on action potential and conduction. Table 17–1 lists the agents commonly used. The reader might find it helpful to review the section on action potential discussed in Chapter 15 to understand better how cardiac drugs work. Features of those agents most commonly used for management of dysrhythmias are listed in Tables 17–2.

Digitalis Preparations

Digoxin

Digoxin may be selected for patients with supraventricular dysrhythmias, such as paroxysmal atrial tachycardia, atrial fibrillation, and atrial flutter. Digoxin has little effect on

multifocal atrial tachycardia. Digitalization often produces reversion to a normal sinus rhythm or in the case of atrial fibrillation or flutter, slowing of the ventricular rate to a more satisfactory level. Digoxin should not be used to treat sinus tachycardia except when the tachycardia is secondary to congestive heart failure (CHF). The reduction in heart rate in such instances results from improved cardiac output.

Table 17–3 lists the chief characteristics of three digitalis preparations. Because digoxin is used most often, it merits further discussion.

Approximately 70% to 80% of an oral dose of digoxin is absorbed. Digoxin also is absorbed when given intramuscularly, but this route is painful and has few advantages. When given by the intravenous (IV) route (preferable for many seriously ill patients), the usual starting dose is 0.5 mg, followed by 0.25 mg every 2 to 4 hours. Total dosage requirements vary widely, although most patients will respond to a total dose of 1.0 to 1.5 mg IV. Some patients will not respond to customary doses of digoxin.

To minimize the risks of *digitalis toxicity*, a serious and sometimes lethal complication, the following options should be considered for the patient with a supraventricular tachycardia:

- Stop treatment if the heart rate has reached a satisfactory, although not ideal, level and further doses of digoxin produce no further slowing (an example is atrial fibrillation with a ventricular rate of 100–120 beats/min).
- Choose a second drug for control of heart rate, such as propranolol or verapamil.
- Attempt electrical cardioversion.
- Use an agent such as quinidine, procainamide, or amiodarone, which may reestablish normal sinus rhythm.

Alternate forms of digitalis are useful in specific circumstances.

TABLE 17-1   CLINICAL APPLICATION: Drug Therapy
Commonly Used Antiarrhythmic Agents

Class	Action	Drug
I	All class I antiarrhythmic agents block sodium movement into the tissue, resulting in a reduced maximal velocity of phase 0 depolarization.	
IA	Slows depolarization at all heart rates and increases the duration of action potential	Quinidine Procainamide Disopyramide
IB	Slows phase 0 depolarization at fast heart rates	Lidocaine Tocainamide Phenytoin Mexilitene
IC	Slows phase 0 depolarization at normal rates, does not affect the action potential duration	Flecainide Propafenone Moricizine
II	Blocks sympathetic stimulation of the conduction system	Beta-blockers (propranolol) Acebutolol Esmolol
III	Prolongs the action potential duration	Amiodarone Bretylium Sotalol Ibutilide
IV	Blocks influx of calcium into the cell and decreases conduction velocity	Calcium channel blockers (verapamil, diltiazem)

TABLE 17-2   CLINICAL APPLICATION: Drug Therapy
Pharmacokinetics of Antiarrhythmic Drugs

Drug	Effect on ECG	Dose and Interval	Route	Adverse Effects
Digoxin	Prolongs PR (±) ST depression	0.5 mg initially; 0.25 mg q2–4h total 1.0–1.5 mg first 24 h	IV or PO	Nausea, vomiting, abdominal pain, blurred or colored vision, weakness, psychosis, PVCs, heart block
Quinidine	Prolongs QRS, QT, and PR (±)	100–600 mg q4–6h	PO	GI symptoms, cinchonism, thrombocytopenia, hypotension, heart block, ventricular tachycardia
Procainamide	Prolongs QRS, QT, and PR (±)	500 mg–1 g; then 2–5 g/d 250–500 mg q3–6h 100 mg q5min to 1 g total Maintenance: 2–4 mg/min	PO IM IV	GI symptoms, psychosis, hypotension, rash, lupus-like syndrome
Disopyramide	Prolongs QRS, QT, and PR	Loading: 200–300 mg Maintenance: 100–200 mg q6h	PO	Anticholinergic effects, hypotension, heart failure, heart block, tachydysrhythmias
Lidocaine	None	1 mg/kg; may repeat at 0.5 mg/kg	IV	Drowsiness, seizures
Propranolol	Prolongs PR, no change QRS, shortens QT	10–80 mg q6h 0.3–5 mg total (not >1 mg/min)	PO IV	Hypotension, heart failure, heart block, asthma
Verapamil	Prolongs PR	5–10 mg 80–120 mg tid–qid	IV PO	Hypotension, bradycardia, dizziness, GI disturbance
Tocainide	No effect on PR, QRS, QT	400–600 mg q8h	Oral	Nausea, vomiting, abdominal pain, dizziness, tremor

(continued)

TABLE 17-2   CLINICAL APPLICATION: Drug Therapy (Continued)
Pharmacokinetics of Antiarrhythmic Drugs

Drug	Effect on ECG	Dose and Interval	Route	Adverse Effects
Mexilitene	No effect on PR, QRS, QT	150–400 mg 3–4 times/d	Oral	Nausea, vomiting, dizziness, tremor
Flecainide	Prolongs PR, QRS; may slightly prolong QT	100–200 mg twice daily	Oral	Dizziness, blurred vision
Amiodarone	Prolongs QRS, QT; may slightly prolong PR	Loading dose—800–1200 mg/d for 10–14 d; then 200–400 mg/d	Oral	Corneal microdeposits, hyper/hypothyroidism, pulmonary fibrosis, skin sensitivity (blue skin), nausea, tremor, headache, ataxia
Bretylium	None	5–10 mg/kg	IV	Hypotension, nausea, vomiting
Sotalol	Prolongs PR and QT	80 mg bid	Oral	Hypotension, bradycardia, fatigue
Ibutilide	Prolongs QT	1 mg IV over 10 min May repeat 1 mg 10 min after end of previous dose	IV	Nausea and vomiting; ventricular dysrhythmias
Propafenone	Prolongs PR and QRS	150–300 mg every 8 h	Oral	Nausea, bitter taste, hypotension, exacerbation of ventricular ectopy
Moricizine	Prolongs PR and QRS	200–300 mg every 8 h	Oral	Dizziness, headache, nausea, exacerbation of ventricular ectopy
Adenosine	Prolongs PR	6–12 mg	IV	Hypotension, facial flushing, dyspnea

Ouabain

Given only IV, ouabain exerts an effect on atrial dysrhythmias within minutes. Its chief benefits are for the two following types of patients: those in whom speed of rhythm control is important and those in whom the status of digitalization is uncertain. In each group, small increments of ouabain (0.1 mg IV every 30 minutes) may produce either a favorable response or evidence of toxicity, such as the development of ventricular premature beats. The latter indicates that safe levels of digitalization have been exceeded. The small, stepwise doses and the shorter half-life make this approach somewhat safer than the use of digoxin for this purpose.

Digitoxin

By virtue of its relatively slow excretion, digitoxin is especially useful in some patients with chronic atrial fibrillation or atrial flutter who continue to exhibit rapid ventric-ular rates. The vagotonic action of digitoxin on the atrioventricular (AV) node is more consistent than that of digoxin, leading to more dependable rate control.

DIGITALIS TOXICITY

All digitalis glycosides should be used with great caution in patients with Wolff-Parkinson-White (WPW) syndrome in whom atrial fibrillation or flutter develops. Digitalis reduces the refractory period of the accessory pathway. This action leads to transmission of potentially rapid atrial rates to the ventricle; ventricular fibrillation may result.

Excessive doses of digitalis can be avoided if consideration is given to some principles of its metabolism. When renal function is normal, one third of the digoxin stored in the body is excreted daily. The renal clearance of digoxin directly relates to the creatinine clearance. When serum cre-

TABLE 17-3   CLINICAL APPLICATION: Drug Therapy
Digitalis Preparations

Agent	Onset of Action (min)	Peak Effect (h)	Average Half-life	Principal Excretory Path	Average Digitalizing Dose		Usual Daily Oral Maintenance Dose
					Oral	IV	
Ouabain	5–10	½–2	21 h	Renal; some GI	—	0.3–0.5 mg	—
Digoxin	15–30	1–2	33 h	Renal	1.25–1.5	0.75–1.0 mg	0.25–0.5 mg
Digitoxin	25–120	4–12	4–6 d	Hepatic	0.7–1.2 mg	1.0 mg	0.1 mg

atinine is elevated to 2 to 5 mg/dL, the maintenance dose of digoxin should be reduced by at least one half. More severe levels of renal failure require an even further reduction of dosage. Because creatinine levels rise only after considerable loss of renal function, a normal serum creatinine does not ensure a normal clearance of digoxin.

It is prudent to reduce the maintenance dose of digoxin in the older patient. Creatinine clearance declines with age. A second factor that favors accumulation of digoxin in this age group is the age-related decrease in muscle mass. Skeletal muscle is the major body depository for digoxin; a decrease in muscle mass is reflected in increased glycoside concentration in the serum and in the heart. Features of digitalis toxicity are listed in the accompanying display.

Other conditions that may lead to digitalis toxicity include hypokalemia, hypomagnesemia, hypothyroidism, pulmonary hypertension, and severe heart disease of any etiology. Concomitant therapy with quinidine or verapamil also is known to increase the serum digoxin level. Some of these states, such as severe heart failure, are themselves associated with atrial dysrhythmias. The utmost care is required when choosing the dose of digitalis for these patients.

Cases of life-threatening digoxin or digitoxin intoxication or overdose may be treated with Digibind Digoxin Immune Fab, an antibody that binds with digoxin, rendering it unable to react at receptor sites on the myocardium and allowing for its elimination through the kidneys.[1] Digibind Digoxin Immune Fab has been demonstrated to be effective in reversing the cardiac effects of toxicity. Dosing is based on how much drug was ingested, serum levels, and body weight. Digibind should be administered over 30 minutes through a 0.22-µm filter; however, in the case of cardiac ar-

rest, it may be administered as an IV bolus. An initial response to treatment can be expected to occur within 1 hour. Serum potassium levels should be monitored because as the digoxin level is lowered, hypokalemia may result.

Measurements of serum digoxin levels have assisted in many cases in dysrhythmia management. The normal serum digoxin range is 0.8 to 1.8 ng/mL. The serum level is only a guide and not an absolute indicator of the adequacy of digitalization. The clinical status of the patient, in particular the adequacy of rate control, often provides more useful information about the status of digitalization than absolute serum levels. As a common clinical example, a patient with chronic atrial fibrillation may require larger than customary doses of digoxin for maintenance of a satisfactory ventricular rate. A serum level above the "therapeutic range" in this instance may be misleading as an indicator of toxicity.

Class IA Antiarrhythmic Agents

QUINIDINE

Quinidine is effective in the management of atrial and ventricular ectopic rhythms. These include supraventricular tachycardia, atrial fibrillation, atrial flutter, multifocal atrial tachycardia, ventricular premature contractions, and ventricular tachycardia. Because of drug intolerance mainly from gastrointestinal side effects, quinidine is often discontinued. Additionally, the proarrhythmic effects resulting in torsades de pointes and sudden death have limited the use of quinidine.

Quinidine has two modes of action. First, it is vagolytic and thus enhances conduction through the AV node. This action tends to speed the ventricular rate in atrial fibrillation or flutter; prior digitalization prevents this undesirable effect. Second, quinidine exerts a direct myocardial effect that prolongs AV conduction, His–Purkinje conduction times, and the duration of repolarization (the QT interval on the electrocardiogram [ECG]).

Quinidine sulfate is well absorbed orally and reaches a peak serum level at about 1.5 hours. In contrast, quinidine gluconate is absorbed more slowly, with a peak level occurring at about 4 hours. Quinidine gluconate can be given less frequently (every 8–12 hours) than the sulfate compound (every 6–8 hours) because of the more prolonged absorption of the gluconate salt, which also results in lower peak levels. The effective dose in any patient will vary widely as a result of patient variation, the disease state, the presence of other drugs, and differences in composition of other products. An initial total dose of 600 to 900 mg daily usually is given. The dose should be increased gradually as needed with attention directed to ECG signs of toxicity (prolonged QRS and QT intervals).

Blood levels offer a guideline for management and should be obtained after the first six to eight doses. With current techniques, the therapeutic levels range from 2.3 to 5.0 µg/mL. An occasional patient may show signs of toxic-

---

CLINICAL APPLICATION: Drug Therapy
Manifestations of Digitalis Toxicity

Gastrointestinal
Anorexia
Vomiting
Abdominal pain
Diarrhea
Unexplained weight loss

Neurological
Weakness
Blurred or colored vision
Psychosis

Cardiac (Entirely Manifest as Dysrhythmias)
Atrial tachycardia, commonly with AV block
Junctional tachycardia
Ventricular ectopic rhythm
SA node depression
AV block
Bidirectional tachycardia

ity with "therapeutic" serum levels. In some of these patients, the QT interval may show considerable prolongation over the pretreatment ECG and warn of impending toxicity. Excessive serum levels are associated with a high frequency of toxicity. Conversely, some patients may be controlled at "subtherapeutic" blood levels. The dosage of the drug should not be raised further in this situation. Concomitant administration of quinidine with digoxin can raise digoxin levels.

Quinidine should not be given intramuscularly because of erratic absorption and the tendency to produce pain at the injection site. The IV route is hazardous because quinidine produces vasodilation and sometimes circulatory collapse.

Quinidine Toxicity

About 30% of the patients on quinidine cannot tolerate the drug because of troublesome side effects. Diarrhea is the most common and often is associated with nausea and vomiting. The gastrointestinal side effects do not seem to be related to plasma concentrations. Cinchonism (headache and visual, auditory, and vestibular symptoms) occurs with increased plasma concentrations. Dysrhythmias, especially ventricular ectopic rhythms, occur more frequently in patients with advanced cardiac failure. A very slow ventricular rate in patients with atrial fibrillation or flutter also predisposes to ventricular dysrhythmias. Transient ventricular flutter or fibrillation may produce the entity known as "quinidine syncope." This proarrhythmic effect—a worsening of ventricular dysrhythmias—has been seen in the class IA and IC agents.

Sudden death occurs in a small percentage of patients on maintenance quinidine. A retrospective look at patients with quinidine syncope reveals a prolonged QT interval in many cases. Other patients may show AV block. Finally, idiosyncratic reactions occur in some patients; these include fever, rash, thrombocytopenia, hemolytic anemia, and hepatic dysfunction.

As a rule, the maintenance dose of quinidine should be reduced to 70% in the presence of congestive failure and to 50% with renal failure. The blood level should be checked at the peak serum concentration (1.5 hours after oral use) and at the trough (1 hour before the next dose).

PROCAINAMIDE

Procainamide is highly effective for atrial and ventricular ectopic rhythms, whether given orally, intramuscularly, or IV. Like quinidine, procainamide has a mild vagolytic effect on the AV node, which in some patients will prove deleterious by increasing the ventricular rate. Procainamide has the potential for myocardial depression. It decreases conduction throughout the heart and can prolong the QRS and QT intervals. A reduced cardiac output and hypotension may occur after rapid IV use or when the oral dose accumulates as a result of renal failure.

A metabolite of procainamide, *N*-acetylprocainamide (NAPA), also has antiarrhythmic activity. NAPA has a longer serum half-life than procainamide. Renal failure produces a toxic level of NAPA that is not detected by the usual serum measurements. Patients with renal failure therefore should be treated with lower doses of procainamide and followed closely to detect QRS prolongation.

Procainamide is well absorbed orally, reaching a peak level at 1 hour. The usual dose ranges from 250 to 500 mg every 3 to 6 hours. Therapeutic plasma levels range between 4 to 10 μg/mL. Earlier investigations indicated that the serum level fell to subtherapeutic levels after 3 to 4 hours. Many patients, however, exhibit a continued response for longer periods. This effect probably results from the more prolonged antiarrhythmic action of NAPA.

Procainamide is given IV in initial doses of 100 mg by slow infusion and repeated every 5 minutes until either a therapeutic effect is obtained or toxicity (hypotension or widening of the QRS complex) is noted. The total IV dose should not exceed 1 g. The loading dose is followed by a maintenance infusion of 2 to 3 mg/min. The dose should be reduced in patients with heart failure or hepatic or renal insufficiency.

Procainamide Toxicity

Commonly encountered side effects of procainamide include nausea, vomiting, and diarrhea with the oral route. Rash, fever, agranulocytosis, and frank psychosis are seen occasionally. Long-term use leads to a very high incidence (80%) of antinuclear antibodies. Thirty percent of patients manifest a lupus-like syndrome characterized by high antinuclear antibody titer, fever, pleuropericarditis, and arthritis. Cessation of the drug usually reverses these findings.

DISOPYRAMIDE

Disopyramide is effective for both atrial and ventricular dysrhythmias. By prolonging the refractory period of the accessory pathway, disopyramide may be especially effective in patients with WPW syndrome in whom supraventricular tachydysrhythmias develop. Although disopyramide is used less than quinidine and procainamide, it has been useful in treating the dysrhythmias associated with hypertropic cardiomyopathy and neurally mediated syncope.[2]

Disopyramide is well absorbed by the oral route. Peak plasma levels occur in 2 hours; plasma half-life approximates 6 hours. Excretion occurs mainly by the renal route. Oral doses range from 100 to 300 mg every 6 hours. Effective plasma levels occur at about 2 to 8 μg/mL. The IV route has not been approved for general use.

Disopyramide Toxicity

Disopyramide causes a slight to moderate decrease in cardiac output. It may precipitate overt cardiac failure in patients with limited myocardial reserve. The drug should be avoided in patients with advanced heart block. The most frequent side effects of this drug are anticholinergic, namely, dry mouth, blurred vision, and, especially in men with prostatic enlargement, urinary retention.

Disopyramide, like quinidine and procainamide, can prolong the QT interval. Patients with marked prolongation of this interval appear especially susceptible to malignant ventricular rhythms and sudden death.

Class IB Antiarrhythmic Agents

LIDOCAINE

Lidocaine is of great value in the management of ventricular ectopic rhythms in the critically ill. Lidocaine has the advantages of rapid effectiveness and minimal effect on cardiac contractility.

An initial IV bolus of 50 to 100 mg or 1 mg/kg usually will suppress ectopic activity for approximately 20 minutes. Recurrence of ventricular premature contractions calls for a repeat IV bolus followed by a sustained IV infusion of 1 to 4 mg/min. The dosage is adjusted to control ventricular ectopic beats. Care is taken to avoid excessive doses, which produce agitation or seizures. As a rule, lidocaine is not helpful in the management of supraventricular dysrhythmias.

Because lidocaine is metabolized by the liver, the dose should be reduced when hepatic blood flow is decreased, as in CHF. AV block with a slow junctional or ventricular focus also is a contraindication to the use of lidocaine. Therapeutic levels range from 1.5 to 6 µg/mL.

PHENYTOIN

Phenytoin usually is ineffective for atrial dysrhythmias. Phenytoin is reserved largely for digitalis toxicity rhythms, in which it has moderate success. Such rhythms include atrial tachycardia, with or without block, and atrial fibrillation or flutter with a very slow ventricular rate and multiple ventricular premature contractions. In this setting, phenytoin may increase the ventricular rate to a more normal range and abolish the ventricular ectopic activity.

Phenytoin should be given IV, slowly and undiluted from the vial because it can cause severe bradycardia or asystole. The rate of administration should not exceed 50 mg/min. The drug should be given until the dysrhythmia is controlled or a maximal dose of 1 g is given. Phenytoin seldom is used in maintenance by the oral route.

TOCAINIDE

This drug is an analogue of lidocaine, but unlike lidocaine, tocainide is effective orally. Tocainide is useful primarily in the therapy of ventricular dysrhythmias. The dose ranges from 400 to 600 mg every 8 hours. Adverse effects involve the gastrointestinal tract (nausea, vomiting, abdominal pain, or constipation) and the central nervous system (dizziness, tremor, or paresthesias). Half-life of this drug is 9 to 20 hours. Because tocainide is excreted through the kidneys, the dose should be reduced in patients with renal impairment.

MEXILETINE

Mexiletine also is structurally similar to lidocaine. It may be given IV or orally. The oral dose is 150 to 400 mg given three to four times daily. Half-life of mexiletine is 12 to 13 hours.

Effectiveness has been established for ventricular dysrhythmias, whether given IV in the setting of acute myocardial infarction or administered orally for chronic symptomatic ventricular dysrhythmias. Dose-related neurological and gastrointestinal adverse effects are common, but hemodynamic reactions are minor. Periodic blood counts should be obtained because mexiletine has been shown to cause agranulocytosis. This side effect decreases its use in the treatment of dysrhythmias.

Class IC Antiarrhythmic Agents

FLECAINIDE

Flecainide has been shown to be effective in the treatment of ventricular dysrhythmias but currently is used only in the treatment of life-threatening dsyrhythmias. During the Cardiac Arrhythmia Suppression Trial, flecainide was removed due to an increase in mortality in the patients treated with this agents. It was shown to exhibit a proarrhythmic effect, a worsening of ventricular dysrhythmias.[3] Flecainide has been shown to be effective in the treatment of supraventricular dysrhythmias. Flecainide has a long half-life of 12 to 27 hours. Doses of 100 to 200 mg/d can be given with slow increases every 4 to 7 days up to 400 mg/d. The drug exerts a negative effect on cardiac performance, probably of importance only in patients with markedly compromised ventricular function. Other major side effects include dizziness and blurred vision.

PROPAFENONE

This drug is approved for the treatment of life-threatening ventricular dysrhythmias. In addition to its class IC properties, it also exhibits a beta-blocking and calcium channel blocking effect.[4] Dosing ranges from 150 to 300 mg every 8 hours. Propafenone's half-life is from 2 to 10 hours. The chief adverse effects include nausea, bitter taste, hypotension, and, in susceptible patients with AV nodal disease, heart block. Due to its beta-blocking and calcium channel blocking effects, propafenone can lower heart rate and depress cardiac function. There is a risk of proarrhythmic activity, as with the other class IC agents.

MORICIZINE

Moricizine is classified mainly as a IC agent because it slows atrial, AV nodal, and intraventricular conduction.[5] It is used in the treatment of severe, life-threatening ventricular dysrhythmias. Moricizine is metabolized in the liver and excreted in the feces and kidney. Dosing ranges from 200 to 300 mg every 8 hours but should be decreased in the presence of hepatic and kidney dysfunction. Moricizine's half-life is 10 hours. The most common side effects are central nervous system (dizziness and headache) and gastrointestinal (nausea). Moricizine also has been shown to be proarrhythmic, thus causing new or worsened ventricular dysrhythmias.

Class II Beta-Blocking Agents

Beta-blocking adrenergic agents interfere with stimulation of the sympathetic nervous system, thus slowing heart rate and conduction through the AV node and decreasing automaticity. Beta-blockers have been effective in the treatment of both ventricular and supraventricular dysrhythmias. They are categorized as cardioselective (inhibition of beta 1 receptors) or nonselective (inhibition of beta 1 and beta 2 receptors).[5] Inhibition of beta 1 receptors causes a slowing of heart rate, decreases conduction through the AV node, and depresses cardiac function. Inhibition of beta 2 receptors causes bronchoconstriction, vasoconstriction, and a decrease in glycogenolysis. Table 17–4 indicates the beta activity of the various beta-blocking agents. Although these agents can be used in the treatment of angina and hypertension, only three of them are used in the treatment of dysrhythmias: propranolol, acebutolol, and esmolol.

PROPRANOLOL

Propranolol is the most commonly used beta-blocker for treatment of dysrhythmias in the United States. It is useful for a variety of atrial and ventricular tachydysrhythmias. Propranolol increases the degree of block at the AV node and reduces the heart rate in patients with atrial fibrillation or flutter. In some, these rhythms may revert to a sinus rhythm. Propranolol may be useful alone or as an adjunct to digitalis or quinidine. Beta blockade is especially helpful in some patients with chronic atrial fibrillation or flutter in whom digitalization is insufficient to control the ventricular rate. Propranolol is the agent of choice for rapid atrial dysrhythmias due to hyperthyroidism.

The oral dose of propranolol varies over a wide range owing to differences in the rate of removal by the liver. The usual dose is between 80 and 320 mg/d given in three or four divided doses. On occasion, however, even low doses of propranolol (10–20 mg/d) increase the degree of block at the AV node and provide satisfactory control of the heart rate. The dose in each situation must be "titrated," beginning with small amounts of the drug and adjusting further

doses according to the degree of response. Therapeutic serum level measurements have not been established. Beta blockade usually is present at 50 to 100 ng/mL.

The IV use of propranolol requires great caution. Hypotension, acute pulmonary edema, and cardiovascular collapse may occur with IV doses as low as 1 mg. Doses of 0.3 to 0.5 mg IV should be used initially with close ECG and blood pressure monitoring. The dose should be repeated every 1 to 2 minutes and increased slowly as needed. The total IV dose should not exceed 7 to 10 mg in the first 2 to 3 hours.

Propranolol Toxicity

Side effects are common. Sinus bradycardia, usually well tolerated, need *not* be regarded as a complication. Fatigue, depression, nausea, diarrhea, alopecia, impotence, increased peripheral vascular insufficiency, and hypoglycemia have been noted.

Propranolol depresses cardiac output in patients with preexisting CHF and therefore may be contraindicated in such patients. An exception may be the patient with heart failure due to atrial fibrillation or flutter with a very rapid ventricular response. Reduction of the ventricular rate in this instance may improve cardiac output and offset the depressant action of propranolol on the heart.

The drug should be used with great caution in patients with asthma, in whom it may induce irreversible and fatal bronchospasm. Finally, in the insulin-dependent diabetic patient, propranolol may mask the symptoms of hypoglycemia and therefore should be given with great care.

ACEBUTOLOL

Acebutolol is a cardioselective beta-blocker used in the treatment of ventricular dysrhythmias.[5] Its effectiveness in the treatment of supraventricular dysrhythmias still is under investigation. Acebutolol exhibits some intrinsic sympathomimetic activity properties, which allow it to have a lesser effect on slowing of heart rate and depression of cardiac function than propranolol. Dosing ranges from 600 to 1,200 mg orally per day. Acebutolol's half-life ranges from 9 to 20 hours. Major adverse effects include bradycardia, hypotension, heart failure, anxiety, dizziness, nausea, and abdominal pain.

ESMOLOL

Esmolol is an ultra–short-acting, cardioselective beta-blocker effective in slowing the ventricular rate in supraventricular dysrhythmias and to a lesser extent, conversion to sinus rhythm. Because of its short half-life of 9 minutes, adverse effects resolve quickly. Adverse effects include hypotension, bradycardia, and pulmonary edema. Esmolol is administered by the IV route and titrated to the desired effect. A loading dose of 500 µg/kg/min is administered over 1 minute, followed by 50 µg/kg/min over 4 minutes. After 30 minutes, if the desired effect is not achieved, the dose may be doubled. An infusion of 25 to 50 µg/kg/min may

TABLE 17-4 CLINICAL APPLICATION: Drug Therapy
Beta-Blocking Agents

Drug	Cardioselective	Nonselective
Propranolol		X
Acebutolol	X	
Esmolol	X	
Atenolol	X	
Labetalol		X
Metoprolol	X	
Nadolol		X
Timolol		X

be used to maintain the desired effect for 24 to 48 hours. Esmolol has been shown to be effective in treating the cardiovascular hyperactivity exhibited during surgery and anesthesia.[6]

Class III Antiarrhythmic Agents

AMIODARONE

Initially introduced in the 1960s as an antianginal agent, amiodarone has shown great promise as an antiarrhythmic drug. A unique feature of amiodarone is that it has an extraordinarily long duration of action, with a half-life of 14 to 52 days. This characteristic makes less frequent dosing possible but increases the duration of toxic effects when they occur.

Amiodarone is useful for recurrent supraventricular and ventricular tachydysrhythmias not responsive to conventional agents. The oral dose ranges from 200 mg 5 days a week to 600 mg once a day. Adverse effects are seen commonly and sometimes are life threatening. Corneal microdeposits can be found in nearly all cases; impaired vision occasionally is present. Hyperthyroidism and hypothyroidism both have been reported. Cutaneous problems include photosensitivity and skin pigmentation. Other problems include neurological toxicity and an increase in hepatic enzyme levels. The most dreaded complication is pulmonary fibrosis, which may reverse when the drug is discontinued but progresses in some instances to respiratory impairment and death. Due to its ability to prolong the QT interval, amiodarone may be proarrhythmic.

BRETYLIUM

Bretylium tosylate IV has been approved for life-threatening ventricular dysrhythmias (recurrent ventricular tachycardia or fibrillation) occurring during myocardial infarction that fail to respond to lidocaine or procainamide. The recommended dose, 5 to 10 mg/kg, is delivered IV over 10 to 12 minutes and is followed by an IV infusion of 1 to 2 mg/min. Hypotension, which may occur even when the patient is supine, and nausea and vomiting are the most common adverse effects.

SOTALOL

Sotalol is an agent that exhibits properties of class III agents (prolonged repolarization) and beta-blockade (noncardioselective).[7] It is useful to treat ventricular dysrhythmias. Sotalol is excreted in the urine, therefore the dose should be carefully titrated in those with renal failure. Side effects are related to the effect of beta-blockade and include bradycardia, hypotension, and fatigue. Studies have shown that sotalol is less of a myocardial depressant than other beta blockers. Of concern is its ability to prolong the QT interval and therefor cause serious ventricular dysrhythmias.

IBUTILIDE

Ibutilide is a class III agent that has been recently released for the conversion of atrial fibrillation/flutter. It prolongs the action potential by enhancing the slow inward sodium current.[8] Like other class III agents, ibutilide prolongs the QT interval and thus may be proarrhythmic. Ibutilide is excreted in the kidneys and has a half life of 2 to 12 hours. The recommended dose is 1 mg IV over 10 minutes. The drug may be repeated 10 minutes after the end of the previous dose.

Class IV Calcium Channel Blockers

VERAPAMIL

Given IV, verapamil is used in the treatment of paroxysmal supraventricular tachycardia (PSVT). The drug also has antianginal and antihypertensive properties. Verapamil has a potent depressant action on the AV node, thereby slowing conduction and prolonging the effective refractory period in the AV node. Verapamil interrupts the pathways used by reentrant atrial rhythms, such as PSVT, and when given IV, causes reversion to normal sinus rhythm in most cases. The agent also is useful in retarding the ventricular response in patients with atrial fibrillation or atrial flutter and often is used alone or in conjunction with digoxin for this purpose. Verapamil is less successful in restoring sinus rhythm in patients with atrial fibrillation or flutter.

The usual dose of verapamil is 5 to 10 mg IV given over 1 to 3 minutes. The dose may be repeated in 20 minutes if necessary. When administered orally, the dose ranges from 80 to 120 mg given three to four times daily.

Verapamil Toxicity

Adverse effects include hypotension (especially with IV use), bradycardia, gastrointestinal intolerance, headache, anxiety, and edema. In susceptible patients with sinoatrial or AV nodal disease, verapamil should be avoided. The drug also should not be given to patients on beta-blocking agents if such patients exhibit left ventricular dysfunction or significant bradydysrhythmias. Verapamil may be used safely in combination with digoxin, but because verapamil increases the serum level of digoxin by 50% to 70%, the maintenance dose of digoxin should be adjusted downward.

DILTIAZEM

Diltiazem is a calcium-channel blocker that has actions similar to those of verapamil. It has been approved for treatment of supraventricular dysrhythmias. Diltiazem has been shown to decrease the ventricular rate in atrial flutter and atrial fibrillation, and in some cases, convert PSVT to sinus rhythm by slowing conduction through the AV node. Plasma half-life ranges from 3.5 to 6 hours. Adverse effects include hypotension, flushing, and junctional dysrhythmias. Diltiazem is metabolized by the liver and excreted through the kidneys. The initial dose is 0.25 mg/kg administered over 2 minutes. If the response is not sufficient, then it may be repeated at 0.35 mg/kg. An infusion of 5 to 15 mg/h may be infused for a period of 24 hours to maintain the desired effect.

Other Antiarrhythmic Agents

ADENOSINE

Adenosine is an antiarrhythmic agent that is effective in converting PSVT to normal sinus rhythm by slowing conduction through the AV node. It has not been shown to be effective in converting atrial flutter or fibrillation to sinus rhythm but may slow the ventricular rate.[9] Adenosine has a half-life of 10 seconds; thus, side effects are short lived. A dose of 6 mg is administered rapidly IV, followed by a saline flush. The dose can be repeated at 12 mg in a few minutes if the desired effect is not obtained. Adverse effects include a brief period of hypotension, facial flushing, and dyspnea. As the rhythm is converted, various degrees of AV block, sinus bradycardia, or ectopic beats may be seen before sinus rhythm is established.

ATROPINE

Atropine is a parasympatholytic agent used for treatment of symptomatic bradycardias and slowed conduction at the AV node. It reduces the effects of vagal stimulation, thus increasing the heart rate and improving cardiac function. Doses of 0.5 to 1 mg given IV are recommended. The dose can be repeated in a few minutes but not to more than a total of 2 mg. It is important not to increase the heart rate to an excessive degree in patients with ischemic heart disease because myocardial oxygen consumption can be increased and the ischemia worsened.

MAGNESIUM

Magnesium sulfate is the drug of choice in the treatment of torsades de pointes. It is also effective in the treatment of some supraventricular dysrhythmias. Its mechanism of action is unclear but has calcium-channel blocking properties. The dose is 1 to 2 g over 1 to 2 minutes. Side effects include hypotension, nausea, and flushing.

◼ VASOACTIVE AGENTS

Like heart rate, stroke volume is an important variable that alters cardiac output. Stoke volume is affected by preload, afterload, and contractility. Agents used to manipulate these variables are called inotropes, vasopressors, and vasodilators. This section discusses these major agents.

Inotropic and Sympathomimetic Agents

Several classes of agents are used to increase the force of myocardial contraction. They are listed in Table 17–5. Cardiac

TABLE 17-5 CLINICAL APPLICATION: Drug Therapy
Action and Dosage of Common Vasoactive Agents

Name	Cardiac Glycoside	Action — Adrenergic Agent: Alpha	Beta 1	Beta 2	Dopaminergic	Phosphodiesterase Inhibitor	Dosage
Digoxin	X						0.25 mg
Dopamine		High dose	Middle dose		Low dose		1–20 µg/kg/min
Dobutamine			X	X			2.5–20 µg/kg/min
Epinephrine		X	X				0.01–0.2 µg/kg/min
Norepinephrine		X	X				0.05–0.17 µg/kg/min
Phenylephrine		X					0.5 titrate down to 0.25 µg/kg/min
Amrinone						X	Loading dose—0.75 mg/min then 5–10 µg/kg/min
Milrinone						X	Loading dose—50 µg/kg over 10 min, then 0.375–0.75 µg/kg/min

glycosides (ie, digoxin) enhance myocardial performance by inhibiting the sodium–potassium pump, thus allowing for an increase in intracellular calcium and increased contraction. Adrenergic agents act by stimulating receptor sites on the cells in the heart and blood vessels. Some of these agents stimulate more than one receptor. Those that stimulate alpha 1 receptors cause vasoconstriction and elevation in blood pressure. Stimulation of beta 1 receptors results in an increase in myocardial contractility (inotropic effect), an increase in heart rate (chronotropic effect), and an increase in speed of conduction (dromotropic effect). Stimulation of beta 2 receptors causes brochodilation and vasodilation. Action on dopaminergic receptors causes an increase in blood flow to the renal and mesenteric arteries. Phosphodiesterase inhibitors increase contractility by inhibiting the enzyme phosphodiesterase, thus allowing increased levels of cAMP in the cell. This class of agents also has a vasodilating effect, thus allowing the heart to pump against a lesser force.

Inotropic agents are used in low output states (ie, shock, heart failure) in an effort to make the heart pump more effectively and deliver oxygen to the tissues. Enhanced contraction increases stroke volume and blood pressure, cardiac output, and perfusion to the coronary arteries. As the ventricles empty more completely, ventricular filling pressures, preload, and pulmonary congestion are decreased. This allows for a decrease in myocardial oxygen needs. However as contractility and heart rate are increased, myocardial oxygen needs can go up. If this need is not met, ischemia can occur. The nurse must closely monitor the patient for evidence of angina, myocardial infarction, and dysrhythmias.

Vasopressors

Vasopressor agents act by stimulating alpha receptors on the blood vessels, thus causing vasoconstriction and an elevation in blood pressure and systemic vascular resistance. These agents are used in patients with low blood pressures and shock states when inotropic agents and fluids are inadequate to maintain an adequate blood pressure. Some vasopressors have both alpha- and beta-stimulating properties. An increase in blood pressure increases perfusion to the heart, brain, kidneys, and other vital organs. Adversely, vasopressors can cause a strain on a diseased heart muscle, causing it to work harder, thus stroke volume, cardiac output, and blood pressure may decrease.

Vasodilators

Vasodilating agents are used to decrease preload and afterload. Preload is affected by the amount of volume in the ventricles at the end of filling. The greater the stretch of the myocardial cells, the better the contraction. However, if the cells are overstretched (increased preload) contractile force goes down. Afterload is the force against which the heart has to work to eject its contents. If afterload is too low, blood pressure and tissue perfusion may be low. If afterload is too high, the heart has to work harder.

CLINICAL APPLICATION: Drug Therapy
Vasodilators

Direct acting
  Nitroglycerin
  Sodium nitroprusside
  Hydralazine
Calcium channel blockers
  Nifedipine
  Diltiazem
  Verapamil
ACE inhibitors
  Captopril
  Enalapril
Alpha/beta adrenergic blocker
  Labetolol

Patients with ischemic states (ie, myocardial infarction for heart failure) have an increase in preload and afterload, placing a further strain on the heart. Nitroglycerin decreases preload, therefore lowering filling pressures and myocardial oxygen needs. Decreasing afterload lowers the force against which the heart has to work, thus allowing it to pump better. Vasodilating agents act by relaxing the smooth muscle in the arteries or veins or both. Major agents are listed in the accompanying display. Potential disadvantages in decreasing preload and afterload are hypotension, tachycardia, and decreased perfusion to the coronary arteries and other tissues.

Calcium channel blocking agents block the influx of calcium into the cell, thus causing arterial vasodilation and a lowering of blood pressure. These agents also exert a negative inotropic effect on the heart, thus decreasing contractility.

Angiotensin-converting enzyme (ACE) inhibitors are another group of agents that decrease afterload. They are not true vasodilators. Vasoconstriction is a compensatory mechanism seen in low output states. It occurs when the renin–angiotensin system is activated and angiotensin II, a powerful vasoconstrictor, is produced. ACE inhibitors block the conversion of angiotensin II, thus lowering the force against which the heart has to work. Side effects include hypotension, rash, and cough.

Alpha-adrenergic blockers directly block the alpha receptors, thus causing vasodilation. Labetalol is an agent in this group. It also has beta-blocking activities that prevent an increase in heart rate as blood pressure goes down.

◼ THROMBOLYTIC AGENTS

An acute thrombus superimposed on an atherosclerotic plaque is a major cause of an acute myocardial infarction. Thrombolytic agents are administered to dissolve the clot, thus restoring blood flow and perfusion to the myocardium, decreasing infarct size, and improving

TABLE 17-6   CLINICAL APPLICATION: Drug Therapy
Thrombolytic Agents

Name	Action	Use	Note
Streptokinase	Binds to plasminogen Complex breaks down fibrin clot	Acute MI Pulmonary embolus Deep vein thrombosis	Half-life—18–20 min Allergenic properties
Eminase/APSAC	Combines with plasminogen Complex breaks down fibrin	Acute MI	Half-life—90 min Allergenic properties
Tissue plasminogen activator (rTPA)	Converts plasminogen to plasmin at the site of the clot	Acute MI Pulmonary embolus	Short half-life—5 min
Urokinase	Directly converts plasminogen to plasmin	Pulmonary embolus	Half-life—10–20 min

APSAC, Anisoylated plasminogen streptokinase activator

myocardial function. Thrombolytic agents act directly or indirectly on converting the inactive protein plasminogen to its active form, plasmin. Plasmin is an enzyme that lyses the clot. As the clot dissolves, fibrin split products are formed. Because an anticoagulant state is produced, bleeding is a major adverse effect. Major agents are listed in Table 17–6. Thrombolytic agents are also used to dissolve pulmonary thrombi and arterial thrombi in the extremities. More recently, thrombolytics have been used in the treatment of nonhemorrhagic stroke. For a more detailed discussion of the use of thrombolytic therapy in patients with an acute myocardial infarction, see Chapter 20.

Percutaneous Transluminal Coronary Angioplasty and Percutaneous Balloon Valvuloplasty

■ PERCUTANEOUS TRANSLUMINAL CORONARY ANGIOPLASTY

In percutaneous transluminal coronary angioplasty (PTCA), a coaxial catheter system is introduced into the coronary arterial tree and advanced into an area of coronary artery stenosis. A balloon attached to the catheter is then inflated, increasing the luminal diameter and improving blood flow through the dilated segment. PTCA is a nonsurgical technique applied as an alternative to coronary artery bypass surgery in the treatment of obstructive coronary artery disease (CAD). When indicated and if successful, PTCA can alleviate myocardial ischemia, relieve angina pectoris, and prevent myocardial necrosis.

Historical Background

Cardiovascular disease is the number one cause of death in the United States. The American Heart Association estimates that 1,500,000 Americans will have a heart attack and about 500,000 of them will die each year.[1]

The first major advance in the palliative treatment of CAD was the implantation of an aortocoronary saphenous vein bypass graft in 1967. Since that time, coronary artery bypass graft surgery (CABG) has been refined continually and has been the treatment of choice for many patients with CAD. The first PTCA, however, performed by Gruentzig in 1977, marked another major innovation in the treatment of CAD.

The path to PTCA began in 1964, when Dotter and Judkins introduced the concept of mechanically dilating a stenosis in a blood vessel with a technique of inserting a series of progressively larger catheters to treat peripheral vascular disease. After experimenting with this technique, Gruentzig modified the procedure by placing on the tip of a catheter a polyvinyl balloon, which was passed into a narrowed vessel and then inflated. Because it produced a smoother luminal surface with less trauma than the Dotter–Judkins approach, this new method reduced the risk of complications such as vessel rupture, subintimal tearing, and embolism. At first, Gruentzig continued to apply his technique only to peripheral vascular lesions. Then, after successful dilation of more than 500 peripheral lesions, he designed a smaller version of the dilation catheter for use within the coronary arterial tree. This new design was tested initially on dogs with experimentally induced coronary artery stenoses. After extensive canine experimentation, Gruentzig performed the first human PTCA in 1977. Since then, considerable improvements in technique and equipment have made PTCA the treatment of choice for appropriate cases of CAD.[2]

Physiological Principles

The process that leads to successful dilation is complex and not clearly defined. Angiographic evaluation and animal and human histological studies indicate that PTCA stretches the vessel wall, often leading to fracture of the in-elastic atheromatous plaque and to tearing or cracking within the intima and media. This cracking or slight dis-section of the inner lumen of the vessel may be necessary for successful dilation.[3]

Comparisons Between PTCA and CABG

As an alternative treatment in appropriate cases of CAD, an-gioplasty compares favorably to bypass surgery in terms of risk, success rate, the patient's physical capacity after the procedure, length of hospital stay, and cost.

Mortality rates associated with first-time angioplasty and CABG are similar. The in-hospital death rate for patients undergoing angioplasty ranges from 0% to 2%; the CABG mortality rate ranges from 1.5% to 4%.[3] If a second surgi-cal operation becomes necessary to alleviate the symptoms of progressive disease, the mortality and complication rates for the bypass procedure are significantly greater than for second angioplasty.

Successful PTCA, which often is defined as a significant reduction of the luminal diameter stenosis without in-hospital death, myocardial infarction, or CABG surgery, ranges from 80% to 95%, depending on the severity of the patient's angiographic and clinical presentation. Long-term survival also is excellent. In a study by Bentivoglio and coworkers, cumulative 2-year survival was 96% and 95% among patients with stable and unstable angina, re-spectively, with event-free survival (ie, no death, myocar-dial infarction, or CABG) in 79% and 76%, respectively.[4] Among patients with multivessel PTCA, actuarial survival was 97% at 1 year and 88% at 5 years in a study by O'Keefe and colleagues.[5] At 7 years after PTCA, Dorros and associ-ates reported a survival rate of 90% in patients with sim-ple single-vessel angioplasty and 95% in patients with sim-ple multivessel angioplasty.[6]

In the Coronary Artery Surgery Study, graft patency after CABG was 90% at 2 months, 82% at 18 months, and 82% at 5 years. Ten-year survival was 82%.[7]

Restenosis or patency data differ greatly between CABG and PTCA. Within 6 months after angioplasty, 20% to 30% of lesions recur or restenose. The mean occlusion rate for bypass grafts is approximately 18% during the first 5 years and 4% to 5% between 5 and 10 years.[7]

Psychological advantages of PTCA over surgery may argue favorably for the procedure. The emotional stress of awaiting dilation is less than that of awaiting surgery. This reduction in anxiety, however, is partly offset by the risk of psychological crisis if the angioplasty fails and surgery—especially immediate surgery—is needed. The psychological impact of this discouraging situation is sig-nificant, but it occurs in a relatively low percentage of cases (1%–5%).

If there are no complications with either procedure, PTCA requires a hospital stay of 1 to 2 days, whereas CABG requires a stay of 5 to 7 days. Because the average hospital stay is shorter with PTCA and because PTCA is performed in the cardiac catheterization laboratory under local anesthe-sia, the average cost of PTCA may be substantially lower than that of CABG. The following factors, however, can in-crease the cost of PTCA:

- Complications occurring during the procedure, re-quiring emergency surgery
- Lesions that recur, requiring repeat dilation or bypass surgery
- Surgical standby, which is provided in different levels to correspond to the risk associated with each PTCA

A factor in favor of PTCA is the lower morbidity after the procedure compared with CABG. Percutaneous translumi-nal coronary angioplasty patients often return to work within 7 to 10 days after angioplasty, whereas bypass pa-tients return to work within 6 weeks.

In short, the major advantages of angioplasty over bypass surgery may include reduced mortality and morbidity, shorter convalescence, and lower cost to the patient.

Diagnostic Tests for PTCA and CABG Patient Selection

Before deciding between PTCA and CABG, all objective ev-idence of coronary insufficiency must be documented. Noninvasive methods of evaluation that may be used be-fore and after PTCA include standard *treadmill stress test-ing* and *thallium stress and redistribution myocardial imaging*. These tests allow the physician to discover the areas of ischemia in the myocardium when the patient is subjected to stress (ie, exercise; see Chapter 16 for a dis-cussion of these tests). The nurse should be familiar with the results of the thallium stress test indicated on the ex-amination report because an understanding of the pa-tient's diagnosis and related symptoms, and thus of the reasons for interventional angioplasty therapy, promotes more informed patient care.

Coronary arteriography with cardiac catheterization, another method of documenting coronary insufficiency, is done if the previous tests indicate coronary disease. Al-though this procedure is more invasive than treadmill test-ing and thallium imaging, it is required to pinpoint the lo-cation of any stenoses and the degree of involvement of the artery or arteries (see Chapter 16 for a discussion of this test). This procedure yields a 35-mm or VHS tape cinean-giogram of the coronary artery anatomy. The physician can then analyze closely areas of narrowing, gaining precise in-formation with which to decide the mode of treatment (Figs. 17–1 and 17–2).

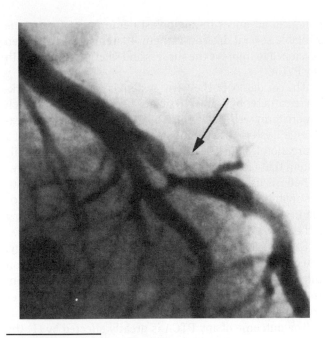

FIGURE 17-1

An eccentric stenosis in the left anterior descending artery. The term "eccentric" defines a plaque involving only one side of the intraluminal wall. (Courtesy of John B Simpson, MD, Palo Alto, CA)

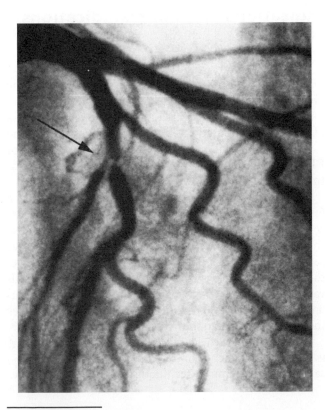

FIGURE 17-2

A coronary arteriogram of the circumflex artery illustrating a concentric stenosis. The term "concentric" defines a plaque involving the intraluminal wall circumferentially, giving a dumbbell appearance. (Courtesy of John B Simpson, MD, Palo Alto, CA)

Equipment Features

Since the introduction of PTCA, the equipment has been continually refined, resulting in fewer contraindications and lower rates of mortality and emergency bypass surgery.

The guiding catheters used to direct and support the advancement of the dilation catheter into the appropriate coronary artery ostium have an outer diameter of 6 to 10 Fr. Like the Judkins and Amplatz coronary angiography catheters, the tips of the guiding catheters have curves that are preshaped for selective access to either the right or left coronary artery (Fig. 17–3).

Balloon dilation systems have evolved since Gruentzig's original design, in which the guidewire tip and catheter shaft were integral. In the early days of angioplasty, physicians were limited by catheter performance and could address lesions only in the proximal anatomy. In 1982, Simpson introduced a coaxial "over-the-wire" system, an improvement that has become predominant in current catheter designs. The main innovation is an independently movable guidewire within the balloon dilation catheter. This guidewire can be manipulated to select the correct vessel despite side branches and permits safe advancement of the dilation catheter across the lesion. Currently, the available guidewires measure between 0.010 and 0.018 inches in diameter and thus usually pose little threat of interference with the blood flow through a stenosis.

Coronary dilation catheter shafts range in size from 1.9 to 4.2 Fr, small enough for easy passage through the guiding catheter and for visualization around the catheter during contrast injection (Fig. 17–4). The dilation catheter has

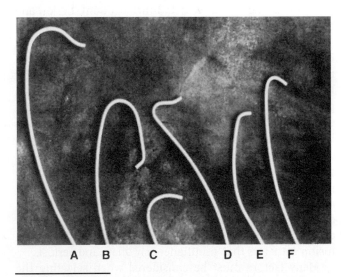

FIGURE 17-3

A variety of guiding catheters with preshaped tips suitable for selectively engaging the appropriate coronary osita, from left to right: (**A**) left Amplatz guiding catheter; (**B**) left Judkins guiding catheter; (**C**) hockey stick guiding catheter; (**D**) right Amplatz guiding catheter; (**E**) right Judkins guiding catheter; (**F**) left internal mammary guiding catheter. (Reprinted with permission of Advanced Cardiovascular Systems [ACS] Inc., Santa Clara, CA)

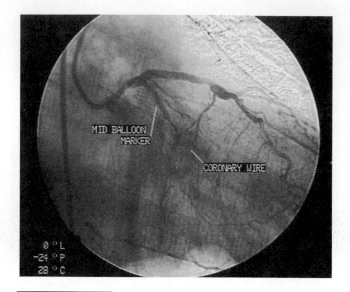

FIGURE 17-4

Contrast injection through the guiding catheter to verify position. The coronary guidewire tip is located at the occlusion of the circumflex artery, and the coronary balloon is positioned in the proximal vessel. (Reprinted with permission of Advanced Cardiovascular Systems [ACS] Inc., Santa Clara, CA)

a radiopaque marker that can be imaged by fluoroscopy (Fig. 17–5). Thus, the physician can position the balloon accurately across the lesion. The inflated balloon size ranges from 1.5 to 5.0 mm in diameter and from 10 to 40 mm in length. The size (inflated diameter) of the balloon to be used for a particular PTCA is usually the same as the smallest-diameter segment of the coronary artery proximal or distal to the stenosis (eg, 3-mm vessel, 3-mm balloon). Lesion and balloon length also are approximated.

The physician manually inflates the balloon with a contrast-filled, disposable inflation–deflation device that connects to the side arm or balloon lumen of the coronary dilation catheter (see Fig. 17–5). The device incorporates a pressure gauge that indicates the amount of pressure exerted against the balloon wall during balloon inflation. Balloon pressure is measured in pounds per square inch (psi) or atmospheres (atm). The average initial inflation is between 60 and 150 psi or 4 to 10 atm and lasts from 1 to 3 minutes. Longer inflations may promote a smoother, more regular vessel wall as assessed by angiography and are used primarily for the treatment of major dissections and abrupt closure. Extended inflations are performed safely with perfusion catheters that simultaneously dilate and perfuse.

Many factors must be considered when selecting the most appropriate equipment for performing PTCA. Tech-

nological advances in angioplasty equipment have made available several dilation catheter systems that have been developed to improve the success and safety associated with any PTCA.

The coaxial "over-the-wire" system is considered a workhorse catheter by many physicians because it can approach any anatomy well. A physician also might select a "rapid-exchange" system to accomplish more easily the dilation of a bifurcation lesion. This type of device incorporates a "rail" system that facilitates the exchange process. A "fixed-wire" catheter is used to reach and dilate lesions in distal, tortuous anatomy, and its small shaft also makes it an option for the use of two coronary dilation catheters in one guiding catheter when the strategy calls for side-by-side balloons.

Each strategy also encompasses an inflation strategy. The main elements of an inflation strategy are the duration and pressure of balloon inflation required to open a lesion. Today, balloons are available that can withstand greater pressure for the treatment of calcific lesions.

The outcome of any PTCA is greatly affected by (1) the selection of a guiding catheter that provides a platform for the advancement of the dilation system while preserving flow to the coronary artery and (2) the selection of a dilation system that best addresses the vessel's anatomy and the lesion's location.

Indications and Contraindications for PTCA

INDICATIONS

When choosing to treat with PTCA (as with CABG), the physician's purpose is to alleviate angina pectoris unrelieved by maximal medical treatment and to reduce the risk of myocardial infarction in symptomatic patients and asymptomatic patients with severe stenosis. Indications for PTCA have expanded as equipment, technique, and operator experience have improved.

In patients with coronary arteries that have at least a 50% narrowing, PTCA is indicated. Lesions with less narrowing are not considered appropriate for PTCA because they are equally at risk for abrupt closure, which can have serious consequences. Patients with severe surgical risk factors, such as severe underlying noncardiac diseases, advanced age, and poor left ventricular function, are particularly suited for PTCA because successful dilation obviates the need for an operation that would be poorly tolerated.

An example of the wide spectrum of candidacy for PTCA is the accepted practice of treating patients with multivessel disease. The common technique for dilating multiple le-

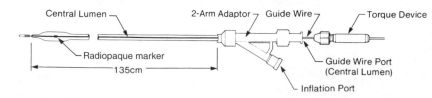

FIGURE 17-5

PTCA balloon dilation catheter illustrating the key components of the system. (Reprinted with permission of Advanced Cardiovascular Systems [ACS] Inc., Santa Clara, CA)

sions is to dilate the most critical stenosis first. With successful dilation of this "culprit" lesion, remaining lesions are dilated in stages (ie, at different intervals during the procedure or over several days). Dilation of multiple vessels, however, is technically more demanding and carries a higher risk of complications.

Another expanded indication is the approach to treating the patient with a totally occluded vessel. Early in PTCA practice, total occlusion disqualified a patient for the procedure because the stenosis could not be crossed with the guidewire and dilation catheter without causing severe trauma to the artery. Currently, due to refinement of equipment, technical advances, and greater physician experience, dilation of total occlusions may be attempted in appropriate candidates. Total occlusions of a short duration (eg, 3 months or less) are easier to cross and dilate successfully than total occlusions of a longer duration. Therefore, dilation of chronic total occlusions should be attempted only in selected patients.

Other candidates for PTCA are those who have undergone CABG in whom symptoms have recurred due to stenosis and graft closure or progression of coronary disease in the native vessels. For these candidates, successful angioplasty makes second surgery, with its increased potential for complications, unnecessary. It is thought that the proliferative disease in the graft wall generates fibrous stenosis that is much less dense than most fibrotic tissue in the native vessels, so certain vein graft stenoses respond favorably to dilation.

In the past, if a patient had an acute myocardial infarction documented by significant ST segment elevation, increased cardiac enzyme levels, and pain unrelieved by medication, surgery or pharmacological treatment with complete bed rest in a coronary care unit were the only treatment alternatives. Now, if thrombosis and underlying stenosis are causing the infarction, thrombolytic therapy, PTCA, or both offer alternatives. When a blood clot has impeded flow to the distal myocardium and thus caused an ischemic episode, a thrombolytic agent (eg, streptokinase, urokinase, tissue-type plasminogen activator) can be administered IV. On successful lysis of the thrombus, delayed dilation of the underlying stenosis often further enhances blood flow to the reperfused myocardium, reducing the risk of rethrombosis or critical narrowing caused by normal or spastic vasomotion superimposed on an organic stenosis.

Primary coronary angioplasty is a dilation of an infarct-related coronary artery during the acute phase of a myocardial infarction *without* prior administration of a thrombolytic agent. Meyer and associates first used PTCA in the acute myocardial infarction setting in 1982.[8] They reported an 81% success rate in PTCA of the infarct-related artery after intracoronary thrombolytic therapy. In 1982, Hartzler and associates reported a stand-alone PTCA success rate of 93% with a patency rate of 89% 7 days after PTCA.[9] Parameters routinely assessed in patients selected to receive primary angioplasty are depicted in the accompanying display.

In the setting of acute myocardial infarction, PTCA may benefit patients deemed ineligible for traditional medical

---

CLINICAL APPLICATION:
Assessment Parameters
Parameters Evaluated in Patients Selected to Receive Primary Angioplasty

- Age
- Hemodynamic status
- Angiographic anatomy:
  - Single-, double-, or triple-vessel disease
  - Vessel involvement: LAD, RCA, LCX
  - Lesion location: proximal, mid, or distal disease
  - Percent grade stenosis
  - Thrombolytics in myocardial infarction (TIMI) flow: 0, I, II, III
  - Left ventricular ejection fraction
- Presence of chest pain consistent with acute myocardial infarction
- ECG evidence of acute myocardial infarction:
  - 1 mm ST elevation in two contiguous leads
  - or
  - 1 mm ST depression believed to represent reciprocal changes to an area of infarction

LAD, left anterior descending artery; RCA, right coronary artery; LCX, left circumflex artery

---

therapy. Such patients include those in cardiogenic shock, those believed to be at high risk for bleeding complications (cerebrovascular accidents, prolonged cardiopulmonary resuscitation (CPR), bleeding diathesis, severe hypertension, or recent surgery), and those of advanced age (older than 75 years). Primary angioplasty does not preclude the use of thrombolytics if residual thrombus is observed. Primary angioplasty may offer distinct advantages in reducing the length of hospital stay and eliminating the need for additional interventional procedures in many cases.[10,11] Indications for PTCA are summarized in the display.

Complications of primary angioplasty include retroperitoneal or vascular hemorrhage, other bleeding requiring transfusion, late restenosis, and early acute reclusion.[12] These complications occur at the same rate as those experienced in routine elective coronary angioplasty.

CONTRAINDICATIONS

There are very few contraindications for PTCA. Patients with left main CAD generally are not considered candidates for angioplasty. The obvious drawback of PTCA in left main artery disease is the possibility of acute occlusion or spasm of the left main artery during the procedure, which would result in severe left ventricular dysfunction. The only exception to this rule is the patient who has a "protected" left main (ie, has had previous bypass surgery to the left anterior descending or circumflex arteries with patent grafts present). Only then might a physician consider dilating a left main artery stenosis. At present, however, most of these patients still are considered surgical candidates.

Indications	Contraindications
Clinical	
Symptomatic (angina unrelieved by medical therapy)	
Asymptomatic but with severe underlying stenosis	
Stable/unstable angina	
Acute myocardial infarction	
High-risk surgical candidates	
Anatomical	
Severe stenosis (≥50%)	Mild stenosis (<50%)
Proximal and distal lesions	"Unprotected" left main coronary artery
Single and multivessel disease	
Bifurcation lesions	
Ostial lesions	
Totally occluded vessels	
Bypass graft lesions	
"Protected" left main coronary artery (previous LAD or LCX CABG)	

LAD, left anterior descending artery; LCX, left circumflex artery; CABG, coronary artery bypass graft.

and replaced by a valved introducer sheath. The sheath provides support at the puncture site in the groin and hemostasis and reduces potential arterial trauma if multiple catheter exchanges are necessary. The guiding catheter is preloaded with a 0.038-inch J wire and introduced into the sheath. The 0.038-inch J wire is advanced over the arch and the guiding catheter is advanced over the wire. The 0.038-inch J wire is removed, and the guiding catheter is rotated precisely to the appropriate coronary ostium. The procedure also may be accomplished by the Sones approach, in which a brachial cutdown is used to isolate the brachial vein and artery. A small arteriotomy is made, and the catheter is passed to the level of the aortic arch.

Regardless of the mode of access, repeat coronary arteriography is then carried out in both the left anterior oblique (30 degrees) and right anterior oblique (60 degrees) views. These views allow for visualization of the heart along its transverse and longitudinal planes. Opposing views provide a thorough assessment of both the lesion and the anatomical approach. A "freeze frame" of each view is obtained as a "road map" or guide throughout the procedure. A final lesion assessment is made, confirming lesion severity and vessel diameter for appropriate balloon sizing.

If PTCA is indicated, surgical standby is confirmed, and the patient is anticoagulated with 10,000 U heparin to prevent clots from forming on or in the catheter system during the procedure. Intracoronary nitroglycerin is kept on

For high-risk patients (eg, patients with left main vessel disease, severe left ventricular dysfunction, or dilation of the last remaining patent artery), percutaneous support devices may improve the safety of PTCA. Among the devices and techniques being investigated are perfusion balloons, intra-aortic balloon counterpulsation, coronary sinus retroperfusion, cardiopulmonary support, and partial left heart bypass.

The display, in addition to summarizing indications for PTCA, also lists factors that usually contraindicate the procedure.

Procedure

The PTCA procedure is carried out in a sterile fashion, with the use of local anesthesia and either the Judkins (percutaneous femoral) approach or, less often, the Sones (brachial cutdown) approach (Fig. 17–6).

With the Judkins approach, the physician cannulates the femoral vein and artery percutaneously by inserting a needle (usually 18-gauge) containing a removable obturator. The obturator then can be removed to confirm by the presence of blood flow that the outer needle is within the lumen of the vessel. Once proper placement is established, a guidewire is introduced through the needle into the artery to the level of the diaphragm. The needle then is removed

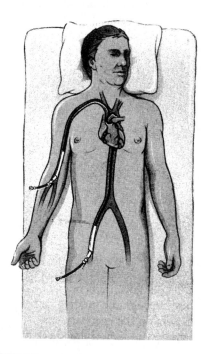

FIGURE 17-6

Two approaches to left heart catheterization. The Sones technique uses the brachial artery, and the Judkins technique uses the femoral artery. With either method, the catheter is passed retrograde through the ascending aorta to the left ventricle. (Reprinted with permission of Advanced Cardiovascular Systems [ACS] Inc., Santa Clara, CA)

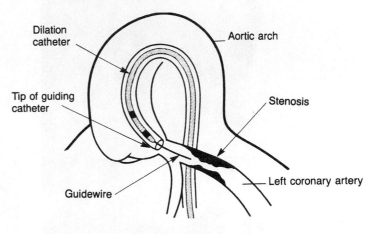

FIGURE 17-7

The advancement of the coronary dilation catheter to the tip of the guiding catheter, which is positioned in the left coronary artery, is facilitated by fluoroscopy. (Reprinted with permission of Advanced Cardiovascular Systems [ACS] Inc., Santa Clara, CA)

the sterile field throughout the procedure and given intermittently as needed for vasospasm and for dilation to facilitate visualization of the coronary artery.

The dilation catheter is introduced into the guiding catheter through a bifurcated adapter that provides access and is a port for contrast injections and aortic pressure measurement. The dilation catheter and guidewire are advanced to the tip of the guiding catheter while their position is checked by fluoroscopy (Fig. 17–7). The guidewire then is advanced and manipulated to negotiate branch vessels. Proper advancement can be confirmed by injecting contrast through the guiding catheter and fluoroscopically visualizing the coronary tree.

Once the guidewire is positioned safely beyond the stenosis, the dilation catheter can be advanced slowly over the guidewire into the narrowing without risk of injury to the intima (Fig. 17–8).

Exact placement of the dilation balloon within the stenosis is facilitated under fluoroscopy by the radiopaque marker on the balloon and by contrast injections for visualization. Initially, the balloon is inflated at 1 to 2 atm to confirm its position. Many PTCA balloon catheters expand at both ends and not in the center, where they are pinched by the stenosis (Figs. 17–9 and 17–10). The central indentation usually disappears as the stenosis is dilated. After each inflation, the physician injects a small bolus of contrast medium to assess any changes in coronary blood flow through the stenosis and to assess any increase in luminal diameter. At this time, the need for additional inflations is determined and a waiting period of 10 to 15 minutes is observed. Complications such as vessel recoil and abrupt closure occur most often during this early phase; however, their incidence is low, and redilation can be done readily at this time. After dilation is complete, the guiding catheter and the dilation catheter are removed. Postdilation arteriography is performed to define more clearly the results of the PTCA.

Reasons for failure to complete a PTCA procedure include inability to cross the target lesion with a guidewire or dilation catheter due primarily to chronic total occlusions; inability to dilate the lesion due to rigid lesions or severe dissection; and embolization of friable vein graft material or embolization of thrombus.

Successful dilation of a lesion commonly is defined as a reduction of the luminal diameter stenosis by about 40% or 50%. Clinical success commonly is defined as angiographic success with clinical improvement and without significant in-hospital complications, such as death, myocardial infarction, or CABG.

Angiography after successful angioplasty demonstrates an immediate increase in the intraluminal diameter of the involved vessel (Fig. 17–11). Clinical improvement of the patient is demonstrated by improved or normalized myocardial perfusion deficits, as shown by comparison of a post-PTCA thallium stress image to the pre-PTCA stress image. Postangioplasty treadmill test results compared to the preprocedure test results reveal increased exercise endurance and a decrease in exercise-induced chest pain.

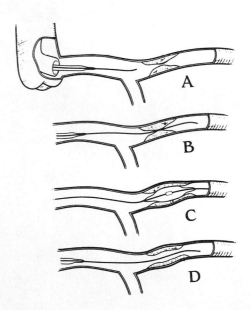

FIGURE 17-8

(**A**) PTCA dilation catheter and guidewire exiting the guiding catheter. (**B**) Guidwire advanced across the stenosis. (**C**) Dilation catheter advanced across the stenosis and inflated. (**D**) Dilation catheter pulled back to assess luminal diameter. (Reprinted with permission of Advanced Cardiovascular Systems [ACS], Inc., Santa Clara, CA)

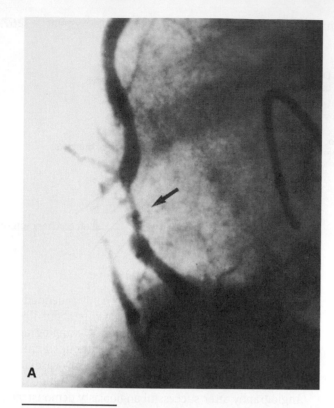
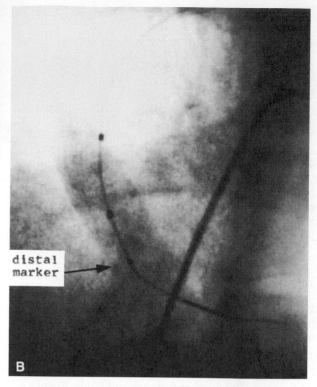

FIGURE 17-9

Thirty-five-spot frames showing (**A**) stenosis involving the midright coronary artery and (**B**) the first and second radiopaque markers revealing the position of the dilation balloon across the stenosis, with the distal marker referring to the tip of the catheter beyond the narrowing. (Courtesy of John B Simpson, MD, Palo Alto, CA)

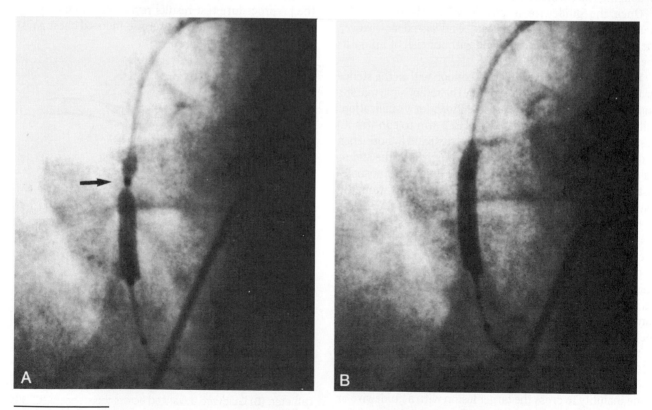

FIGURE 17-10

Thirty-five-spot frames showing (**A**) inflation of the balloon, revealing the position of the stenosis by the "dumbbell" effect, and (**B**) absence of stenosis after dilation. (Courtesy of John B Simpson, MD, Palo Alto, CA)

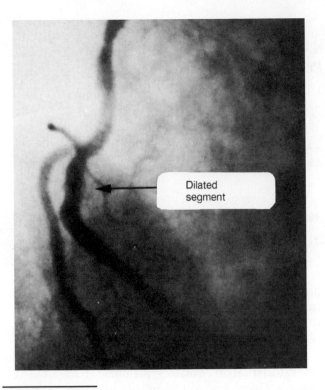

FIGURE 17-11
Repeat angiography after PTCA of a right coronary artery stenosis showing increased flow and increased diameter of the dilated segment. (Courtesy of John B Simpson, MD, Palo Alto, CA)

Results

Excellent short- and long-term results have been achieved in patients undergoing coronary angioplasty. The results vary depending on the patient's clinical presentation (eg, stable or unstable angina) and angiographic characteristics (eg, subtotal or total occlusion). Among patients undergoing either single-vessel dilation or multivessel dilation, in-hospital clinical success ranges from 85% to 95%.[13] In-hospital complications are low, with a reported mortality rate of 1% to 2% in both these patient groups.[13] Long-term survival is high, although repeat PTCA may be necessary for recurrent or progressive disease.

Among patients with higher risk clinical or angiographic presentations, success rates may be lower; however, PTCA often is preferable to surgical revascularization because of the latter's increased risk in patients such as older adults or those with depressed left ventricular function.

Assessment and Management

PATIENT PREPARATION

Laboratory Tests

When the decision has been made to proceed with coronary angioplasty, the patient usually is admitted to the hospital the day of the procedure. The nurse should monitor all preliminary laboratory tests, such as evaluations of cardiac enzymes, serum electrolytes, and prothrombin time (assessing coagulability), and should notify the physician of any abnormalities. The serum levels of potassium, creatinine, and blood urea nitrogen (BUN) are particularly important.

Potassium levels must be within normal limits because low levels result in increased sensitivity and excitability of the myocardium. The cardiac muscle also is sensitive and becomes irritable when the flow of oxygen-rich blood decreases, as happens for a controlled period of time during placement and inflation of the dilation balloon across the lesion. The irritability arising from hypokalemia or ischemia or both can give rise to ventricular dysrhythmias that pose a threat to the patient.

Elevation in the levels of serum creatinine, BUN, or both may indicate problems in kidney function. Good kidney function is important because during angioplasty, radiopaque contrast material (which allows fluoroscopic visualization of the coronary anatomy and of catheter placement) is introduced into the bloodstream. This contrast material is a hyperosmotic solution that the kidneys must filter from the blood and excrete. High levels of creatinine and BUN may reflect decreased renal filtration capability and vulnerability of the kidney in processing the extra load of radiopaque solution. Instances of acute renal failure have resulted from high doses of radiopaque contrast. Because false high serum levels may result from hypovolemia, however, the nurse should take care to keep the patient adequately hydrated, either by mouth with clear liquids or by means of IV solutions. If the efficacy of kidney function is in question, it can be monitored best by trends in creatinine and BUN levels, in conjunction with measurement and documentation of urine output.

Informed Consent

After it is determined that the physical condition permits angioplasty, the physician must obtain from the patient an informed consent to the procedure. The physician will explain how the angioplasty is done, the reasons for the treatment, and the risks and potential benefits of PTCA and of the available alternative, surgery. The nurse should answer any questions that the patient may have and should explain the course of post-PTCA care.

Preoperative Medications

Twenty-four hours before the procedure, the patient's medications should include aspirin, 325 mg once a day for its antiplatelet effect. Medications may be prescribed to reduce vasospastic events, including nitroglycerin and calcium-blocking agents, such as nifedipine 10 mg three times a day, and diltiazem 30 mg three times a day.

Surgical Standby

Surgical standby for PTCA is arranged before the procedure. Surgical availability is required, but the degree to

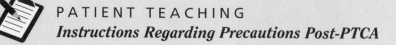

PATIENT TEACHING
Instructions Regarding Precautions Post-PTCA

- Remain on bed rest for 6 to 8 hours.
- Maintain the involved leg in a straight position (for Judkins technique).
- Avoid an upright position.
- Avoid vigorous use of the abdominal muscles, as in coughing, sneezing, or moving the bowels.

which the operating room is held for availability varies according to patient's risk factors, hospital policies, or both.

NURSING MANAGEMENT DURING PTCA

During the preparation for angioplasty and throughout the procedure, nurses in the cardiac catheterization laboratory are responsible for understanding all aspects of equipment use and patient care. They should be experienced in advanced life support and knowledgeable about the proper administration of emergency medications and the correct application of emergency equipment, including the defibrillator, the ventilator, and the pacemaker. They should observe and communicate with the patient intermittently and report any changes in patient status to the physician. The nurse monitors the ECG and arterial pressure scopes constantly and is aware of changes in tracing that may accompany the administration of drugs, symptoms of ischemia, or chest pain. The nurse must recognize signs and symptoms of contrast sensitivity, such as urticaria, blushing, anxiety, nausea, and laryngospasm. The nurse should understand the proper assembly and use of all angioplasty equipment and should be able to "troubleshoot" any malfunction that might arise.

The patient's anticoagulation status during the PTCA procedure is of utmost importance. Subtherapeutic levels may result in serious complications, including acute closure or thrombotic events. An activated clotting time (ACT) should be measured in the catheterization laboratory at baseline (prior to the PTCA), 5 minutes after the heparin bolus (usually 10,000 U), and every 30 minutes thereafter for the duration of the procedure. ACT levels of 250 to 300 seconds are desirable following the initial heparin bolus. Subsequent boluses of 2,000 to 5,000 U of heparin may be required to achieve and maintain these ACT levels during the PTCA procedure.

After the PTCA is complete, the nurse instructs the patient in the precautions necessary *to prevent bleeding from the puncture site*. The accompanying display reflects patient teaching.

Following the procedure, the patient is transferred to a telemetry unit for observation. Common nursing diagnoses and collaborative problems for PTCA patients are listed in a display.

NURSING MANAGEMENT POST-PTCA

The nurse in the coronary care or telemetry unit plays an important role in observing and assessing the patient's recovery. Postangioplasty care is designed to monitor the patient closely for signs and symptoms of myocardial ischemia. The most overt symptom of a possible complication—early recurrence of angina pectoris after PTCA—requires prompt nursing action.

As soon as possible on receiving the patient from the cardiac catheterization laboratory, the nurse attaches the ECG monitor, which allows a quick initial cardiac assessment and establishes a baseline if the patient's condition should change suddenly. The nurse assesses the patient's status from head to toe, noting the overall skin color and temperature and

---

CLINICAL APPLICATION:
Examples of Nursing Diagnoses and Collaborative Problems for the Patient Having PTCA or PBV

Risk for Decreased Cardiac Output related to mechanical factors that affect preload, afterload, and left ventricular function

Risk for Decreased Cardiac Output related to electrical factors affecting rate, rhythm, or conduction

Risk for Decreased Cardiac Output related to structural changes (dissection, thrombus, or arterial spasm at PTCA site), resulting in myocardial ischemia or infarction

Risk for Decreased Cardiac Output related to increased preload and pulmonary congestion related to temporary mechanical factors (eg, balloon inflation during PBV)

Risk for Decreased Cardiac Output related to left-to-right shunt with mitral PBV or late cardiac tamponade

Risk for Altered Peripheral Perfusion related to hematoma, thrombus formation, or infection associated with cannulation site

Risk for Altered Cerebral Perfusion related to embolism from procedure site, left ventricle, or left atrium

Risk for Pain related to angina or stretching of the valve during dilation

Risk for Fluid Volume Deficit related to renal sensitivity to contrast material or diuretic therapy

Knowledge Deficit related to illness and impact on patient's future

Anxiety/Fear related to lack of knowledge of PTCA/PBV, acute care environment, and potential for surgery

carefully observing the level of consciousness. After the patient is transferred to the bed and attached to the monitor, the nurse listens closely to heart and breath sounds. The nurse evaluates the peripheral circulation by noting peripheral skin color and temperature and the presence and quality of dorsalis pedis and posterior tibialis pulses in the limbs.

Because the Judkins technique is used most often in PTCA to access the vasculature, most patients will have an entry port in either the right or the left groin through which sheaths will have been placed percutaneously in a vein and artery to allow catheterization. (If the Sones technique was used, there will be an arterial catheter in the brachial area— see Fig. 17–6.) The sheaths are not removed immediately after PTCA because the patient was anticoagulated at the start of the procedure to avoid complications of clot formation; consequently, the effects of the heparin are not reversed but allowed to dissipate naturally, over 3 to 4 hours. Indwelling arterial and venous sheaths should not be removed until ACT levels fall below the 160-second level. A variety of mechanical devices and clamps may be used to facilitate hemostasis after sheath removal. Following sheath removal, the nurse pays careful attention to the area distal to the puncture site, checking pulses frequently and reporting immediately to the physician any changes that may indicate bleeding. Bleeding at the sheath site may result in a major hematoma that can require surgical evacuation or compromise distal blood flow to the lower extremity. To prevent excessive bleeding and to aid hemostasis, the physician may order a 5-lb to be sandbag placed over the puncture site.

The nurse instructs the patient on the importance of keeping the involved leg straight and the head of the bed angled up no more than 45 degrees. To prevent clotting within the lumens of the introducing sheaths, an IV infusion is attached to the venous sheath, and a pressurized arterial flush is attached to the arterial line. This arrangement also ensures patency should an immediate return to the cardiac catheterization laboratory be necessary because of a complication. The physician chooses both the type of solution infused (through the venous sheath) and the rate of infusion, which depends on the patient's fluid volume state.

Initial post-PTCA laboratory blood tests should include prothrombin time to assess the patient's coagulability; cardiac enzymes, with particular attention to creatine kinase (CK) and CK isoenzymes; and serum electrolytes. Elevation of the cardiac enzymes can indicate that a silent myocardial infarction has occurred (ie, infarction unannounced by prolonged chest pain). If an abnormal cardiac enzyme laboratory value appears, the nurse notifies the physician immediately because the patient's postoperative care might need to be modified to prevent further injury.

The nurse plays a significant role in observing and assessing angina that recurs soon after PTCA. Any chest pain demands immediate and careful attention because it may indicate either the start of vasospasm or impending occlusion. The patient may describe angina as a burning, squeezing heaviness or as sharp midsternal pain. Other signs and symptoms of myocardial ischemia include ischemic ECG changes (elevation of the ST segments or T wave inversion), dysrhythmias, hypotension, and nausea. The nurse notifies the physician immediately of any such change in the patient's condition because it is impossible to tell merely by observation whether the change indicates a transient vasospastic episode, which can be resolved with vasodilation therapy, or an acute occlusion requiring emergency surgery.

If vasodilation therapy is indicated, it may be administered as described subsequently unless the patient is severely hypotensive; in that case, vasodilation is contraindicated. At the first sign of vasospasm, the nurse gives oxygen by mask or nasal cannula. For fast, temporary (and possibly permanent) relief, 0.4 mg of nitroglycerin, 5 mg of isosorbide, or 10 mg of nifedipine is administered sublingually. In addition, the IV drip of nitroglycerin should be titrated to maintain a blood pressure adequate to ensure coronary artery perfusion and to alleviate chest pain.

In conjunction with the onset of the chest pain, a 12-lead ECG reading is recorded to document any acute changes. If the angina resolves and any acute ECG changes caused by medical therapy disappear, it is safe to assume that a transient vasospastic episode occurred; however, if the angina continues and the ECG changes persist, redilation or emergency bypass surgery should be considered.

If the postangioplasty course is uncomplicated, the sheaths are removed after 3 to 4 hours, and a pressure dressing is applied to the site. A variety of mechanical clamps or hemostasis devices may be used to facilitate hemostasis following sheath removal. The patient must continue complete bed rest for 6 to 8 hours after the sheaths are removed. A normal, low-sodium, or low-cholesterol diet may be resumed, depending on the preference of the physician and the needs of the patient.

During the recovery period, the nurse can introduce the patient to the rehabilitation process, emphasizing ways to combat the advance of CAD. Efforts should be made during this instruction to reinforce the importance of aerobic conditioning with regular, moderate exercise and reasonably paced increases. Also, the nurse explains that such abuses as frequent stress, excessive weight, and smoking promote CAD and that the patient has the power and responsibility to avoid these abuses by behavior modification.

As preventive therapy for 6 months after angioplasty, the patient will take medications that help prevent thrombus formation and maintain maximal dilation at the angioplasty site. All patients should be routinely sent home on aspirin for the antiplatelet effect. Often, long-acting nitrates or calcium channel blockers are added to the medical regimen. The nurse may be responsible for explaining to the patient the indications for the specific medications ordered by the physician, including side effects and signs of overdose, and should answer any questions the patient may have on the follow-up care, making sure that all aspects are clearly understood. The display on page 272 summarizes medications currently associated with PTCA.

Four to six weeks after the patient's discharge, an exercise treadmill stress test and a thallium rest–stress imaging study may be performed to test the efficacy of the PTCA. In com-

CLINICAL APPLICATION: Drug Therapy
Summary of Medications Most Often Associated With PTCA

Anticoagulants/Antiplatelets

Aspirin
Indications: Prophylaxis of coronary and cerebral arterial thrombus formation
Actions: Blocks platelet aggregation
Dosage: 80–325 mg qd, PO
Adverse effects: Well tolerated; nausea, vomiting, diarrhea, headache, and vertigo occasionally

Heparin
Indications: Prophylaxis of impending coronary occlusion and prophylaxis of peripheral arterial embolism
Actions: Inhibits clotting of blood and formation of fibrin clots; inactivates thrombin, preventing conversion of fibrinogen to fibrin; prevents formation of a stable fibrin clot by inhibiting the activation of fibrin stabilizing factor; inhibits reactions that lead to clotting but does not alter normal components of blood; prolongs clotting time but does not affect bleeding time; does not lyse clots
Dosage: Varies with indications; IV or IA: 10,000 U at start of PTCA
Adverse effects: Uncontrollable bleeding, hypersensitivity

Coronary Vasodilators

Isosorbide dinitrate (Isordil, Sorbitrate)
Indications: Prophylaxis of angina
Actions: A nitrate that acts as a smooth muscle relaxant; causes coronary vasodilation without increasing myocardial oxygen consumption; secondary to general vasodilation, blood pressure decrease
Dosage:
1. Sublingual: 2.5–10 mg q2–3h prn angina
2. Oral: 5–40 mg qid
3. Sustained action oral: 40 mg q6–12h
Adverse effects:
1. Cutaneous vasodilation that can cause flushing
2. Headache, transient dizziness, and weakness
3. Excessive hypotension

Nitroglycerin
Indications: Control of blood pressure and angina pectoris
Actions: Potent vasodilator that affects primarily the venous system; selectively dilates large coronary arteries increasing blood flow to ischemic subendocardium
Dosage:
1. Sublingual: 0.3–0.4 mg prn chest pain
2. Topical (patch): 2.5–10 mg/d; indicated for primary, secondary, or nocturnal angina due to more sustained effect
3. IV: 5 μg/min to start—titrate to patient response (no fixed dose due to variable response in different patients)
Adverse effects:
1. Excessive and prolonged hypotension

2. Headache
3. Tachycardia, palpitations
4. Nausea, vomiting, apprehension
5. Retrosternal discomfort

Calcium Channel Blockers

Nifedipine, Diltiazem
Indications:
1. Angina pectoris due to coronary artery spasm and fixed vessel disease
2. Hypertension
3. Dysrhythmias
Actions: Inhibits calcium ion flux across the cell membrane of the cardiac muscle and vascular smooth muscle without changing serum calcium concentration; decreases afterload through peripheral arterial dilation and
1. Reduces systemic and pulmonary vascular resistance
2. Vasodilates coronary circulation
3. Decreases myocardial oxygen demands and increases myocardial oxygen supply
Dosage:
1. Nifedipine (Procardia): 10–30 mg tid-qid, PO
2. Diltiazem (Cardizem): 30–90 mg tid-qid, PO
Adverse effects:
1. Contraindicated in patients with sick sinus syndrome
2. Hypertension after IV use
3. GI distress
4. Headache, vertigo, flushing
5. Peripheral edema, occasional increase in angina, tachycardia

Vasopressors

Norepinephrine (Levophed)
Indications: Restoration of a normal systemic blood pressure in acute hypotensive states
Actions: Alpha-adrenergic action causing an increase in systolic and diastolic pressures; peripheral vascular resistance increasing in most vascular beds and blood flow reduced through the liver, kidney, and usually skeletal muscle
Dosage: IV concentration: 2 mg/250 mL solution; initial IV infusion of 2–3 mL (8–12 μg/min), rate of infusion adjusted to reestablish and maintain a normal blood pressure (80–100 mmHg) sufficient to maintain blood flow to vital organs
Note: Before administering, hypovolemia corrected
Adverse effects:
1. Anxiety, bradycardia, severe hypertension, marked increase in peripheral vascular resistance, headache, decreased cardiac input
2. Necrosis and sloughing can occur with extravasation at infusion site.
3. Reduced blood flow to vital organs (kidney, liver)

See text for full discussion of antiarrhythmics.

parison to the pre-PTCA tests, an increase in exercise capacity and a decrease in or disappearance of exercise-induced chest pain (without ST segment changes) suggest improved blood flow and normalization of cardiac function in the previously hypoperfused muscle. Treadmill stress testing should be repeated at 6 months and 1 year after angioplasty.

Complications

Although indications for PTCA have expanded to include patients with more severe CAD (eg, total occlusions, multivessel disease, recent or ongoing myocardial infarction, poor left ventricular function), the rate of complications associated with dilation has not increased. Complications from angioplasty can occur during the procedure or after it is completed. Thus, close observation and monitoring of the patient are imperative after successful PTCA. Major complications that can result in ischemia and possible severe left ventricular dysfunction necessitating emergency surgery include angina unrelieved by maximal administration of nitrates and calcium channel blockers (see the previous display), myocardial infarction, coronary artery spasm, abrupt reclosure of a dilated segment, coronary artery dissection leading to occlusion, and restenosis.

ANGINA, INFARCTION, AND VASOSPASM

Normally angina is an anticipated complication during coronary angioplasty due to the temporary occlusion of the involved vessel during dilation. Such incidence of angina is handled with intracoronary nitroglycerin or removal of the dilation catheter while the guidewire is left across the lesion. Evidence of persistent chest pain after PTCA, reflected in changes in heart rate and blood pressure and elevated ST segments, indicates ischemia predisposing to an insult to the myocardium and requiring immediate intervention. Coronary artery spasm sometimes requires surgical intervention when the vasoconstriction, occlusion, and ischemia cannot be reversed through the administration of nitrates.

ABRUPT RECLOSURE OF DILATED SEGMENT

Abrupt reclosure is a serious complication of coronary artery dilation that occurs in approximately 3% of those undergoing angioplasty.[14] An estimated 70% to 80% of abrupt reclosures occur while the patient is still in the cardiac catheterization laboratory. Approximately one third to one half of those patients whose vessel recloses undergo a successful repeat dilation. Abrupt reclosure can be caused by coronary artery dissection, coronary artery spasm, and thrombus formation. Treatment options include immediate repeat dilation, emergency surgery, or pharmacological therapy. To maintain blood flow through the occlusion while the patient is being prepared for emergency surgery, the physician can use a perfusion balloon catheter, which has side holes along its shaft to allow blood to flow through the catheter at the site of occlusion and perfuse the distal myocardium.

CORONARY ARTERY DISSECTION

Coronary artery dissection or an intimal tear in the inner lining of the artery can be visualized in the form of intraluminal filling defects or extraluminal extravasation of contrast material. Mild interruptions in the intraluminal wall are an expected result of the splitting and stretching of the intima on inflation of the dilation balloon at the lesion site. Therefore, in the absence of adverse effects early after PTCA, angiographically apparent dissection usually does not represent a major complication. A dissection sometimes may cause a major luminal obstruction associated with coronary artery occlusion, however, leading to a deterioration in blood flow with resultant severe ischemia or myocardial infarction that requires emergency bypass surgery.

RESTENOSIS

Restenosis of a dilated lesion occurs in about 20% to 30% of PTCA cases within the first 6 months after angioplasty. Various pharmacological agents that reduce restenosis are being investigated. These include fish oil, prostacyclins, anticoagulants, platelet antibodies, and corticosteroids. None of these agents have shown promising results to date.

The development of new devices to remove atherosclerotic plaque (atherectomy catheters) and implantable devices to maintain the opening mechanically (stents) may provide effective adjuncts or alternatives to angioplasty for the problem of recurring lesions. Restenosis of previously nondilated stenoses after atherectomy is similar in character and prevalence to that in PTCA; however, intracoronary stenting may result in a lower restenosis rate in native and vein graft lesions.

The cause of restenosis still is unclear. It appears to be the result of an excessive healing response to balloon dilation that exposes the subintimal structures of the vessel to circulating blood. These exposed areas are then potential sites for platelet adhesion and aggregation and for thrombus formation. The degree of this "healing" response varies from lesion to lesion and may be influenced by the clinical and angiographic factors associated with restenosis that were discussed previously. The restenosis rate remains at a discouraging 20% to 30% despite a clearer understanding of its mechanism. Factors associated with increased incidence of restenosis are listed in the display.

OTHER COMPLICATIONS

Other major complications of PTCA requiring medical intervention are bradycardia, which requires temporary pacing; ventricular tachycardia or ventricular fibrillation, which requires immediate defibrillation; and a central nervous system event causing transient or persistent neurological deficit.

Peripheral vascular complications occurring primarily at the catheter site include arterial thrombosis, excessive bleeding that causes a significant hematoma, pseudoaneurysm, femoral arteriovenous fistula, and arterial laceration. If any of these complications persists or compromises

---

CLINICAL APPLICATION:
Assessment Parameters
Factors Associated With Increased Incidence of Restenosis

Clinical Factors
Severe angina
Absence of prior myocardial infarction
Diabetes
Smoking cigarettes

Angiographic Factors
Lesion location
Lesion length
Lesion severity before and after PTCA
Adjacent arterial diameter

distal blood flow to the involved extremity, surgical intervention may be required.

Table 17–7 is a summary of complications that may result from PTCA, including general signs of the complications and possible interventional actions.

See the Collaborative Care Guide on the next page for a complete outline of care for the patient undergoing PTCA.

Other Interventional Cardiology Techniques

The immediate and long-term efficacy of coronary angioplasty in treating symptomatic patients with single-vessel disease has been well established. In many centers, PTCA also is routinely and successfully applied to patients with multivessel disease. The safety and efficacy with which angioplasty has been applied have fostered research into treating patients with unstable angina, acute myocardial infarction, and cardiogenic shock.

New technologies are being developed to address the challenges associated with complex angioplasty. These include laser angioplasty, atherectomy, and intracoronary stents. Percutaneous removal of plaque using directional or rotational atherectomy catheters has been used in coronary arteries with good results. Laser technology has progressed and is being used to ablate plaque or as an adjunct to PTCA to make a pathway in total occlusions. Implantations of intravascular stents to reinforce arterial walls have been successful and are well suited for repairing acute occlusive dissection.

RED FLAG   **Table 17-7**   Complications of PTCA

Complications	General Signs/Symptoms	Possible Interventions
Prolonged angina	Angina pectoris	CABG
Myocardial infarction	Dysrhythmias: tachycardia, bradycardia, ventricular tachycardia/fibrillation	Redo PTCA
		Oxygen
Abrupt reclosure	Marked hypotension	Medications:
Dissection/intimal tear	Acute ECG changes (ST segment change)	vasodilators (nitrates), calcium channel
Hypotension	Nausea/vomiting	blockers, analgesics, anticoagulants, vasopressors
Coronary branch occlusion	Pallor	Complete bed rest
Coronary thrombosis	Restlessness	Increase IV fluid volume within patient tolerance
	Cardiac/respiratory arrest	
Restenosis	Angina pectoris	Redo PTCA
	Positive exercise test	CABG
Marked change in heart rate: bradycardia, ventricular tachycardia, ventricular fibrillation	Rate below 60 beats/min	Temporary pacemaker
	Rate above 250 beats/min	Defibrillation
	No discernible cardiac rhythm	Medications:
	Pallor	antiarrhythmics,
	Loss of consciousness	vasopressors
	Hypotension	
Vascular: excessive blood loss	Hypotension	Possible surgical repair
	Decreased urine output (from hypovolemia)	Fluids
	Decreased hemoglobin/hematocrit	Transfusion
	Pallor	Oxygen
	Hematoma at puncture site	Flat in bed or in Trendelenburg position
Allergic	Hypotension, urticaria, nausea/vomiting, hives, laryngospasm, erythema, shortness of breath	Medications: antihistamines, steroids, antiemetics
		Clear liquids/NPO
		Oxygen
		With anaphylaxis: fluids for volume expansion, epinephrine, vasopressors for hypotension
Central nervous system events	Changes in level of consciousness	Oxygen
	Hemiparesis	Discontinue/hold sedatives
	Hypoventilation/respiratory depression	Medication: narcotic antagonist as a respiratory stimulant

Miscellaneous complications: conduction defects, pulmonary embolism, pulmonary edema, coronary air embolism, respiratory arrest, febrile episode, nausea, minor bleeding.
PTCA, percutaneous transluminal coronary angioplasty; CABG, coronary artery bypass graft; ECG, electrocardiogram.

COLLABORATIVE CARE GUIDE
for the Patient Undergoing PTCA

OUTCOMES	INTERVENTIONS
Oxygenation/Ventilation Patient will maintain normal arterial blood gases, or pulse oximeter reading.	• Provide supplemental oxygen per face mask or nasal cannula per hospital post-PTCA protocol. • Monitor blood gases/pulse oximeter per protocol. • Auscultate breath sounds when taking vital signs. • Monitor for signs of pulmonary edema or respiratory distress.

Circulation/Perfusion The patient will have stable vital signs following PTCA.
 	
There is no evidence of post-PTCA myocardial ischemia or infarction due to coronary reocclusion (eg, no ECG changes or angina).
 	
There is no evidence of cardiac dysrhythmias post-PTCA.
 	
There is no evidence of bleeding at the puncture site.
 	
There is no evidence of arterial occlusion at puncture site.
	• Monitor BP, HR, RR, arterial puncture site, distal pulses, and distal motor function and sensation:
	    q15min × 4, q30min × 4
	    q1h × 4, then q4h
	• Monitor cardiac rhythm in leads specific to myocardium most affected by PTCA location.
	• Administer medications to treat coronary artery spasms (eg, niphedipine and nitroglycerin).
	• Administer heparin per protocol.
	• Report type and frequency of dysrhythmias.
	• Administer antiarrhythmic medication as indicated and ordered.
	• Temporary transvenous or external pacemaker and defibrillator are readily available.
	• Monitor site for hematoma as above with vital signs.
	• Assess for tenderness, ecchymosis, warmth over puncture site.
	• Apply direct pressure to puncture site for 15 to 30 minutes after sheath is removed.
	• Apply sandbag to puncture site if oozing continues, per hospital protocol.
	• Apply a pressure dressing to puncture site when oozing has stopped.
	• Monitor ACT, PT, PTT, and platelets, reporting coagulopathies per protocol.
	• Monitor involved extremity with vital signs for mottling, coolness, pallor, diminished pulses, numbness, tingling, pain, and so forth.

Fluids/Electrolytes Patient is euvolemic. Renal function is maintained following administration of radiographic IV contrast.	• Monitor intake and output. • Obtain type and cross-match, CBC, electrolytes prior to PTCA. • Maintain IV patency. • Obtain pre-PTCA and post-PTCA BUN, creatinine, and electrolytes. • Closely monitor urine output; report if less than 30 mL/h. • Monitor urine specific gravity or osmolarity for clearance of IV contrast. • Administer diuretic agents as ordered.
Mobility/Safety	• The patient is on bed rest for 6 to 8 hours post-PTCA per hospital protocol. • While sheath is in place and while on bed rest, keep head of bed less than 45 degrees.
Skin Integrity Patient's skin will remain intact.	• Assess skin immediately post-PTCA for pressure areas.

(continued)

COLLABORATIVE CARE GUIDE
for the Patient Undergoing PTCA (Continued)

OUTCOMES	INTERVENTIONS
	• Reposition to relieve pressure from bony prominences, maintaining alignment of extremity involved in procedure. • Consider pressure relief/reduction mattress.
Nutrition Nutritional intake is reestablished.	• Resume PO fluids and diet per protocol. • Monitor swallowing and protective airway reflexes while patient is receiving sedatives or narcotics.
Patient does not experience nausea or vomiting post-PTCA.	• Monitor nausea and vomiting. • Administer antiemetic medication as appropriate.
Comfort/Pain Control Patient will not experience anginal pain.	• Instruct patient to verbalize discomfort and pain. • Evaluate severity and location of pain, distinguishing angina from other causes of discomfort. • Administer nitrates or narcotics per order or protocol for angina. • Evaluate patient response to medication.
Patient will not experience pain from mobility restrictions.	• Reposition patient frequently, keeping involved extremity straight. • Use mattress overlay or egg crate for comfort. • Administer analgesics as appropriate, after distinguishing joint or muscular pain from angina.
Psychosocial Patient and family state risks associated with PTCA.	• Provide information for informed procedural consent. • Encourage verbalization of questions, concerns, and fears.
Patient uses personal support systems to reduce anxiety.	• Encourage significant other to visit in early postprocedural recovery phase. • Validate patient/significant others' understanding of surgery and illness. • Initiate referrals to social services, clergy, and so forth as necessary.
Teaching/Discharge Planning Patient and family are prepared for possibility of emergent repeat PTCA or cardiac surgery.	• Preprocedure teaching includes discussion regarding causes for coronary reocclusion or perforation and rationale for surgery or repeat PTCA.
Patient cooperates with post-PTCA mobility restrictions.	• Provide preprocedure and postprocedure instruction and rationale for bed rest and limited movement of involved extremity.
Patient states lifestyle changes required to reduce risk of worsening coronary artery disease.	• Provide verbal and written instruction/information regarding risk factors and pathophysiology, activity, diet, stress reduction, medication administration, and appropriate times/indications to seek medical attention.

LASER ANGIOPLASTY

Laser angioplasty has become an exciting addition to the interventional cardiology arsenal. A laser is a device that generates a directional beam of monochromatic light. The acronym LASER means *l*ight *a*mplification through *s*imulated *e*mission of *r*adiation. Through a series of mirrors and lenses, the laser beam is directed into a catheter containing numerous glass fibers. These fibers transmit the light energy through the catheter to the plaque that is to be ablated.[1,5]

Laser angioplasty is performed much like a standard balloon angioplasty procedure. The guide catheter is advanced to the ostium of the coronary artery targeted by fluoroscopy. Once the lesion location is ascertained through contrast injection, a guidewire is advanced up and through the lesion. Before the laser is activated, everyone in the room (including the patient) must don protective eyewear. The laser catheter is then advanced through the guidewire and brought into contact with the lesion. Depending on anticipated lesion morphology, energy settings are chosen that will presumably suffice to ablate the plaque. The laser settings include the fluency (mJ/mm²) to be delivered and the repetition rate (pulses per second). The plaque is then vaporized by the laser energy. Several passes down the length of the lesion may be performed. Laser success is determined by fluoroscopy and coronary injections with contrast dye. If there is residual stenosis after use of the laser, adjunctive angioplasty balloon inflations can be performed to achieve an optimal final result.

Stenotic lesions best suited for laser angioplasty include those that are long and diffuse (longer than 15–20 mm), ostial in location, highly calcified, in vein grafts, and totally occluded. Risks associated with laser angioplasty include perforation of the coronary artery, dissections, aneurysm, and blood vessel damage.

ATHERECTOMY

Atherectomy is the process of removing atherosclerotic plaque from the coronary artery by cutting or ablating and thus "debulking" the lesion. Atherectomy devices include directional coronary atherectomy (DCA), transluminal extraction catheter (TEC), or rotational ablation (Rotoblator).

Potential complications of all atherectomy devices include perforation of the coronary artery, abrupt closure, embolization distal to the lesion site, and myocardial infarction.[11] The rate of restenosis and other complications is comparable to that of PTCA.

Directional Coronary Atherectomy

The DCA device is a cutting catheter that is inserted over a guidewire into the coronary artery across the stenotic lesion. It is positioned so that the opening for the blade faces the lesion. A low pressure balloon on the opposite side of the catheter is inflated, thus forcing the atherosclerotic plaque into the opening near the cutting blade. The cutting blade turns at approximately 1,200 revolutions per minute (RPM) and is then slowly advanced along the length of the lesion, cutting the plaque and collecting it in the catheter nosecone. The DCA catheter is turned a complete 360 degrees in the artery to shave all sides of the atherosclerotic plaque with repeated passings. The procedure is repeated until the atherosclerotic plaque is sufficiently removed. The catheter, laden with plaque, is then withdrawn from the patient.

Transluminal Extraction Catheter

The TEC device is a percutaneous over-the-wire, motor-driven cutting and aspiration system.[16] The TEC device is unique in that it has a detachable vacuum bottle. The TEC device simultaneously cuts the atherosclerotic plaque and then sucks the plaque and thrombus into the vacuum bottle. The cutting device is advanced over the guidewire and positioned 1 to 2 mm proximal to the stenotic lesion. The cutting blade and the vacuum suction are then activated. The cutting blade rotates at 750 RPMs and is manually advanced along the length of the stenotic lesion, pulling excised plaque and thrombus through the TEC catheter and into the vacuum bottle. Several passes across the lesion are performed. Adjunctive balloon angioplasty may be performed following use of the TEC device.

Rotational Ablation Device

The Rotoblator device is a high-speed rotating abrasive burr-tipped catheter that ablates the atherosclerotic plaque within the coronary artery. The Rotoblator has proved to be especially effective in complex stenotic lesions that are calcified, tortuous, small in diameter, ostial, or diffuse in character. The device consists of a football shaped, diamond-studded burr attached to a drive shaft. The Rotoblator is advanced over a guidewire to the lesion site. The burr rotates at 160,000 to 190,000 RPMs and pulverizes the atherosclerotic plaque into small microparticles that are absorbed into the patient's circulatory system. The spinning burr is advanced across the lesion several times to debulk the stenotic lesion. Adjunctive balloon angioplasty may be performed following the Rotoblator device.

STENTS

Intracoronary stents are hollow stainless steel tubes that act as "scaffolding" in the coronary artery. The Palmaz Schatz stent and the Gianturco Roubin stents are currently approved by the Food and Drug Administration with many more designs on the horizon. Following predilation with a PTCA balloon catheter, most stents are premounted on a balloon catheter and inserted through the guide catheter along a guidewire to the lesion site. Once placed across the stenotic lesion, the balloon is inflated, and the stent is expanded and left in the coronary artery.

Many stent designs are stainless steel and thus a potent thrombogenic prosthetic material. Stent thrombus is a major short- and long-term complication. Success of the stenting procedure depends on endothelialization of the stent to provide a smooth flow of blood within the coronary artery and through the stent yet controlled as to prevent stent thrombosis. Anticoagulation and antiplatelet medication regimens are crucial to successful stenting and long-term prognosis. Preliminary results with stenting are promising in reducing restenosis rates and improving long term prognosis. Complications may include bleeding at the access site, stent migration, coronary artery dissection, and abrupt closure.

OTHER TECHNOLOGY

Devices for viewing the vasculature directly, such as angioscopy and intravascular ultrasound, are used to assess lesion severity and type before inflation and to determine change in lesion diameter and arterial structure after deflation. Angioscopy and ultrasound also may provide information to help determine which interventional technology (eg, PTCA, atherectomy, stent implantation) is best suited to the lesion.

A major factor limiting the expansion and long-term efficacy of PTCA is the problem of restenosis. Pharmacological treatment before and after dilation, procedure techniques, and patient identification continue to be investigated as ways to reduce the recurrence rate.

With the various tools and technologies available to the interventional cardiologist and improved pharmacological adjunctive therapy, the future should bring further improvement in the efficacy and predictability of PTCA and in the long-term patency of involved atherosclerotic vessels.

PERCUTANEOUS BALLOON VALVULOPLASTY

Percutaneous balloon valvuloplasty (PBV) is a nonsurgical technique for increasing blood flow through stenotic cardiac valves using dilation catheters. This relatively new procedure is similar to PTCA in that a catheter system is inserted percutaneously and advanced to the region of narrowing using fluoroscopic guidance. A dilation catheter then is inflated to increase the valvular opening and improve blood flow.

Historical Background

The first cases of balloon dilation of stenotic cardiac valves were reported in 1979 and 1982, when physicians successfully dilated pulmonary valve stenoses. This technique was considered an effective alternative to open heart surgery, although long-term results could not yet be evaluated. Because surgical commissurotomy was successful in treating mitral valve stenoses and because of the initial success with pulmonary valve dilation, physicians began percutaneous dilation of mitral valves in 1984 to avoid the need for thoracotomy. In 1984 and 1985, physicians successfully dilated congenital aortic valve stenoses (AVS). A calcific AVS was first dilated in 1985. These procedures improved cardiac function with no serious procedural complications.

The number of PBVs does not approach the volume of coronary angioplasty. This is due partly to the lesser incidence of valve disease compared with CAD.

Assuming patients have long-term clinical improvement associated with PBV, the advantages compared with surgery are similar to PTCA versus CABG surgery. PBV is less traumatic, requires no anesthesia, is associated with lower morbidity and a shorter hospital stay, causes no scarring, and is less expensive.

Pathophysiology of Stenotic Valves

Stenotic valves are caused by calcific degeneration, congenital abnormalities, or rheumatic heart disease. Calcific aortic and mitral valve degeneration now appears to be the most frequent causes of valve disease requiring surgical treatment. Refer to Chapter 21 for a discussion of the pathophysiology and clinical manifestations of specific stenotic valves.

Diagnostic Tests for PBV and Valve Replacement

Before deciding the appropriate intervention, the physician evaluates the patient for evidence and severity of valvular stenosis. A variety of noninvasive tests allows the physician to determine the degree of left atrial or left ventricular hypertrophy, pulmonary venous congestion or hypertension, valvular rigidity, and transvalvular gradient. In a 12-lead ECG, the magnitude of the R wave in the precordial leads reflects the presence of left ventricular hypertrophy associated with AVS. The presence of broad notched P waves reflects left atrial hypertrophy associated with mitral valve stenosis. A chest radiograph illustrates the presence of calcium within or around the valve, left ventricular or atrial hypertrophy, and pulmonary venous congestion or CHF. A two-dimensional echocardiogram is used to scan the cardiac valves and chambers. A Doppler ultrasound study allows measurement of the transvalvular gradient, indirect calculation of valve area, and assessment of valvular regurgitation. With this information, the physician is able to estimate the size of the valve orifice, (2) visualize the degree of valve leaflet movement, and (3) determine the extent of left ventricular or atrial hypertrophy.

Right and left heart catheterization is done if the previous tests indicate valvular disease. Although this procedure is invasive, it is required to determine the pressures within each of the cardiac chambers and to confirm transvalvular gradients. Once the pressures and gradients are obtained, a series of radiographs may be taken by injecting radiopaque contrast medium, either in the aorta to visualize aortic regurgitation or in the left ventricle to visualize mitral regurgitation. This procedure yields a cineangiogram illustrating the function of the cardiac valves and chamber sizes.

After this series of tests, the physician can analyze the valves closely, gaining precise information with which to decide the mode of treatment. The nurse should be familiar with the results of these tests because a better understanding of the patient's diagnosis and related symptoms, and thus of the reasons for intervention, promotes better care.

Equipment Features

Although PBV and PTCA catheters are based on similar designs, there are important differences, primarily because of the larger diameters of heart valves compared with coronary arteries. One major difference is the outer diameter of the catheters. PBV catheter shafts range from 7 to 9 Fr. PBV balloons range from 15 to 25 mm in diameter when inflated. A 10- to 14-Fr introducing sheath may be used at the arterial or venous puncture site to allow for introduction of the valve dilation catheter. A large guidewire, 0.035 to 0.038 in, also is used to provide the added stiffness and support required to introduce the dilatation catheter. PBV dilation catheters have radiopaque markers similar to PTCA dilation catheters for fluoroscopic imaging.

Indications and Contraindications for PBV

The use of PBV initially was limited by the fear of embolization of calcific debris, disruption of the valve ring, acute valvular regurgitation, and valvular restenosis. The incidence of these complications continues to be a concern. Both major and minor complications have been reported in numerous early studies; however, these complications must be assessed in terms of the patient population in which the procedure is performed.

Although surgical valve replacement is an effective treatment for those with AVS and operative mortality is low, operative mortality significantly increases in patients with multisystem disease (who often are older). PBV initially has proven to be a safe and efficacious alternative for these patients. It also is an effective therapy for children who are high surgical risks, because it delays the need for surgery until the child is older and can better tolerate an operation. In addition, the longevity of both mechanical and bioprosthetic valves is approximately 10 years, so PBV delays or prevents the need for a second operation. Also, the long-term anticoagulation therapy required with mechanical valve prostheses is undesirable in younger patients and pregnant women. PBV also is effective for stabilizing those with poor left ventricular function before surgery; it is contraindicated in patients with moderate to severe valvular regurgitation due to a small but significant risk of increasing valvular insufficiency with the procedure (see the display).

A complication associated with PBV is excessive bleeding at the puncture site due to the large catheters required to perform dilation. The development of smaller catheters may reduce the incidence of bleeding. As with PTCA, PBV catheters are being refined continually to increase procedural safety, time, and efficacy.

CLINICAL APPLICATION:
Assessment Parameters
Indications and Contraindications for PBV

Clinical Indications
High-risk surgical patients (advanced age, severe pulmonary hypertension, renal failure, pulmonary dysfunction, left ventricular dysfunction)
Unstable presurgical patients
Patients not candidates for chronic anticoagulation

Anatomical Indications
Moderate to severe valvular narrowing
Moderate to severe valvular calcification
Mild valvular regurgitation

Anatomical Contraindications
Inability to access vasculature
Thrombus
Severe valvular regurgitation
History of embolic events

Procedure

The PBV procedure is performed in the cardiac catheterization laboratory and involves many of the same steps as PTCA (see earlier section on PTCA procedure). Right and left heart catheterization is repeated to evaluate hemodynamic status and to obtain baseline transvalvular gradients. Coronary angiography, when indicated, is repeated to determine whether the patient still meets the criteria for valvuloplasty. Thorough repeat evaluation is necessary because a patient's status can change, precluding treatment with this intervention.

The angiographic catheter is replaced either by an introducing sheath or a dilation catheter. In mitral PBV, a venous puncture is made in the right femoral vein. During both aortic and mitral PBV, maintaining patent IV and radial or femoral arterial lines is important to administer medications and draw blood samples.

In aortic PBV, once the sheaths are in place, the patient is anticoagulated with 5,000 to 10,000 U heparin to prevent clot formation within the catheter system. The dilation catheter and guidewire then are advanced to the root of the ascending aorta. The guidewire is advanced across the stenotic aortic valve, and the dilation catheter is advanced over the guidewire (Fig. 17–12). Exact placement of the dilation catheter is facilitated by fluoroscopy and radiopaque markers on the balloon.

In mitral PBV, a pacing catheter may be positioned through a separate venous sheath at the level of the inferior vena cava or right atrium and placed on standby. The mitral valve then is approached either by way of the femoral artery and aortic valve or in most cases, through the right heart by perforating the atrial septum to enter the left atrium. Once the mitral valve has been accessed, the patient is anticoagulated with 5,000 to 10,000 U heparin. The dilation catheter is then advanced over the guidewire through the atrial septal puncture and across the mitral valve (Fig. 17–13). Again, exact placement of the dilation catheter within the valve is facilitated by fluoroscopy and radiopaque markers on the balloon.

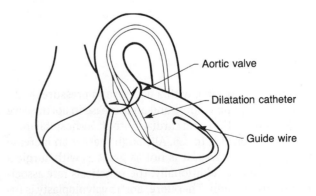

FIGURE 17-12
Cross-sectional view of heart illustrating guidewire and dilation catheter positions across the aortic valve. The guidewire is curved to prevent ventricular dysrhythmias or puncture.

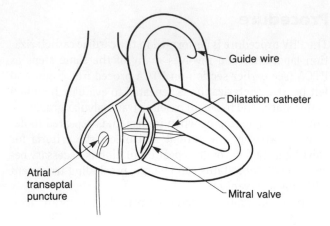

FIGURE 17-13
Cross-sectional view of heart illustrating guidewire and dilation catheter placed through an atrial transseptal puncture and across the mitral valve. The guidewire is extended out the aortic valve into the aorta for catheter support.

Average inflation time of the dilation catheter is 15 to 60 seconds in aortic valvuloplasty and 10 to 30 seconds in mitral valvuloplasty. During dilation of either valve, the nurse monitors blood pressure closely because of the imposed decrease in cardiac output. Once the dilation catheter has been deflated, blood pressure should return to normal. During dilation of the mitral valve, there is a temporary increase in the pulmonary artery wedge pressure (PAWP). Once the dilation catheter has been deflated, the PAWP should return to baseline. Dysrhythmias such as ventricular tachycardia, ventricular fibrillation, or sinus bradycardia also may occur during dilation.

Once maximum dilation has been obtained, the catheter is removed. Hemodynamic measurements, including transvalvular gradients, are repeated to determine efficacy of the procedure. Repeat angiography is done to assess for valvular regurgitation. When the procedure is complete, to prevent bleeding complications associated with the large puncture site, the anticoagulant effects of heparin are reversed.

Results

Aortic PBV is associated with a decrease in pressure gradient and end-systolic volume and an increase in aortic valve area, ejection fraction, and cardiac output. In-hospital mortality ranges from 1% to 3%. Although there is an increase in the aortic valve area, it is not as great as with surgical valve replacement. Additionally, the restenosis rate associated with PBV is high. Therefore, aortic valvuloplasty is indicated primarily for older and high-risk surgical patients and generally is considered a palliative, not a curative, procedure.

Results of mitral valvuloplasty are more dramatic. There is a more significant increase in valve area and cardiac output and a decrease in valve gradient, PAWP, and mean pulmonary arterial pressure. Operative mortality has been reported as 1.5%, and sustained clinical improvement has been reported in 63% to 90% of cases. Late deaths occur in approximately 5% to 10%.

Three mechanisms have been postulated for the improvement of valvular function due to PBV: (1) fracture of calcific nodules adherent to leaflets (most frequent); (2) separation of fused commissures; and (3) stretching of the anulus and leaflet structure.

Assessment and Management

PATIENT PREPARATION

The patient is admitted to the hospital the day of the PBV procedure. The goal of nursing care is to reduce the cardiac workload, monitor fluid and electrolyte balance, and reduce psychological stress so the patient remains hemodynamically stable.

In most cases, the patient will not have invasive pressure monitoring lines in place before the procedure. The nurse, therefore, carefully monitors signs and symptoms of CHF: narrowing in the arterial pulse pressure, more frequent increases in heart rate during activity, peripheral edema, presence of a cough, complaints of dyspnea, or rales in lung fields. The nurse also must note any changes in sensorium, color, skin temperature, pulse volume, and any decrease in urinary output. To monitor fluid and electrolyte balance, the nurse obtains a baseline serum electrolyte level and baseline body weight. In addition, daily fluid intake and output are recorded.

The patient's medications before admission may have included diuretics, digoxin, and anticoagulants. Before the procedure, any anticoagulant medication will be discontinued because of the possibility of emergency surgery. Therefore, patients with chronic atrial fibrillation who have the potential for systemic embolization due to thrombus should be monitored closely. The nurse also monitors preliminary laboratory tests and notifies the physician of any abnormalities. (See the section on PTCA patient preparation for further information on these tests.)

After the patient fully understands the procedure, the physician must obtain an informed consent for PBV, anesthesia, and surgery. Surgical standby usually is provided during PBV due to possible complications requiring emergency valve replacement.

NURSING ASSESSMENT AND MANAGEMENT

During Percutaneous Balloon Valvuloplasty

The nurse continuously monitors pulmonary artery pressure and PAWP and is aware of changes in tracings that may suggest symptoms of CHF or pulmonary edema. In the presence of severe hypotension, the nurse should be prepared to start an IV infusion of dopamine or norepinephrine (Levophed). In the case of ventricular dysrhythmias, a lidocaine drip should be available for infusion.

Post-PBV

The nurse is important in the patient's recovery. The goal of postvalvuloplasty nursing care is to maintain adequate cardiac output, maintain fluid and electrolyte balance, and verify hemostasis at the puncture site. Alterations in cardiac output can be caused by dysrhythmias secondary to valve manipulation, resulting in edema near the bundle of His; left-to-right atrial shunt through the transseptal puncture created during mitral valvuloplasty; cardiac tamponade; alteration in circulating fluid volume; or blood loss. Alteration in fluid and electrolyte balance results from diuretic therapy and contrast medium used during catheterization. Bleeding at the puncture site is secondary to the combined effect of systemic anticoagulation and the large diameter of catheters used.

Because fluids are important in the hemodynamic balance of the patient with valvular disease, the volume of IV fluids is recorded to establish an accurate intake and output. The decreased circulating volume from diuretic medications given before PBV combined with improved stroke volume after successful PBV can be reflected as a decrease in cardiac output. Therefore, careful monitoring of central venous pressure, pulmonary artery pressure, PAWP, and blood pressure, in addition to heart rate, urinary output, and electrolyte balance, are essential in the evaluation and assessment of circulating fluid volume and cardiac pumping status.

Additionally, the nurse assesses the patient's status from head to toe, noting overall skin color and temperature and carefully observing the level of consciousness and neurological signs. The nurse also listens closely to heart and breath sounds. Circulation distal to the puncture site is evaluated by noting peripheral skin color and temperature in addition to the presence and quality of the dorsalis pedis and posterior tibial pulses.

Finally, the presence of any drainage on the puncture site dressing or tenderness during palpation should be noted to establish a baseline for the possibility of increased pericatheter bleeding. The nurse reports immediately any changes that may indicate excessive bleeding. Bleeding at the sheath site may result in a hematoma requiring surgical evacuation. To prevent excessive bleeding and to aid hemostasis, the physician may order a sandbag or clamp placed over the puncture site.

If the patient has documented CAD, the physician also may request a serum cardiac enzyme panel. Particular attention should be paid to CK and CK isoenzymes (see section on nursing assessment and management post-PTCA). The nurse should be aware of the signs and symptoms of myocardial ischemia in addition to the appropriate interventions.

The nurse instructs the patient about the importance of keeping the involved leg straight and the head of the bed flat for the first 6 hours after valvuloplasty.

Post-PBV laboratory evaluation may include prothrombin time, hemoglobin and hematocrit, coagulation studies, serum electrolytes, CK, ECG, and chest x-ray. In the section Nursing Management During Percutaneous Transluminal Coronary Angioplasty, a display on nursing diagnoses and collaborative problems lists problems for PBV patients.

Complications

A common in-hospital complication associated with PBV is bleeding at the arterial puncture site due to the large diameter of the catheters needed to dilate the valve anulus. Additionally, in mitral PBV, a common complication is left-to-right shunting secondary to septal dilation, again due to the large diameter of the dilation catheters. Systemic embolization in both mitral and aortic PBV is a potential and significant complication, although its incidence is low. There have been few reports of significant increase in valvular regurgitation. Complications associated with PBV are listed in the accompanying display.

▬ CONCLUSION

The PTCA and PBV procedures can be performed successfully in catheterization laboratories. Long-term clinical outcome and restenosis rates continue to be assessed to determine the efficacy of these treatments as compared to surgery. Both procedures provide a cost-effective means to treat cardiac disorders and are usually associated with shorter length of stays, faster recovery times, and fewer complications than surgical interventions.

Complications Associated With PBV

- Embolization of calcific debris
- Valve ring disruption
- Valvular regurgitation
- Valvular restenosis
- Bleeding at arterial puncture site
- Left ventricular perforation
- Severe hypotension
- Transient ischemia
- Vascular trauma
- Atrial septal defect (with mitral PBV)
- Aortic dissection
- Aortic rupture
- Cardiac tamponade
- Chordae tendineae rupture

Intra-aortic Balloon Pump Counterpulsation and Ventricular Assist Devices

■ INTRA-AORTIC BALLOON PUMP COUNTERPULSATION

Intra-aortic balloon pump (IABP) counterpulsation was first introduced clinically by Kantrowitz and associates in 1967. This therapeutic approach was instituted for treatment of two patients with left ventricular failure following acute myocardial infarction. Since that time, IABP has become a standard treatment for medical and surgical patients with acute left ventricular failure that is unresponsive to pharmacological and volume therapy.

Therapeutic goals are directed toward increasing oxygen supply to the myocardium, decreasing left ventricular work, and improving cardiac output. Before IABP, no single therapeutic agent was capable of meeting these three goals.

The IABP counterpulsation is designed to increase coronary artery perfusion pressure and blood flow during the diastolic phase of the cardiac cycle by inflation of a balloon in the thoracic aorta. Deflation of the balloon, just before systolic ejection, decreases the impedance to ejection and thus left ventricular work. Inflation and deflation counterpulse each heart beat. With improved blood flow and effective reduction in left ventricular work, the desired results are improved myocardial pump function and increased cardiac output.

Physiological Principles

Greater work is required to maintain cardiac output in the failing heart. With this added work requirement, oxygen demand increases. These circumstances may occur at a time when the myocardium already is ischemic and coronary artery perfusion is unable to meet the oxygen demands. As a result, left ventricular performance diminishes even further, resulting in decreased cardiac output. A vicious cycle ensues that is difficult to interrupt (Fig. 17–14). Without interruption of the cycle, cardiogenic shock may be imminent. This cycle can be broken with IABP therapy by increasing aortic root pressure during diastole through inflation of the balloon. With increased aortic root pressure, the perfusion pressure of the coronary arteries will be increased.

Effective therapy for the patient in left ventricular failure also involves decreasing myocardial oxygen demand. Four major determinants of myocardial oxygen demand are afterload, preload, contractility, and heart rate. Intra-aortic balloon pump counterpulsation therapy can have an effect on all these factors. It will decrease afterload directly and will affect the other three determinants indirectly as cardiac function improves. Because IABP therapy assists the left heart, only the left ventricle is discussed here.

AFTERLOAD AND PRELOAD

The greatest amount of oxygen required during the cardiac cycle is for the development of afterload (see Chapter 15). With greater impedance to ejection, afterload increases, thus resulting in increased myocardial oxygen demand. Impedance to ejection is caused by the aortic valve, aortic end-diastolic pressure, and vascular resistance. Greater aortic end-diastolic pressures require higher afterload to overcome impedance and ejection. Vascular resistance will increase impedance when vessels become vasoconstricted. Vasodilation or lower vascular resistance will decrease afterload by decreasing impedance to ejection. Deflation of the balloon in the aorta just prior to ventricular systole will lower aortic end-diastolic pressure. This will decrease impedance to ejection and decrease left ventricular workload. In this way, IABP can effectively decrease the oxygen demand of the heart.

A person in acute left ventricular failure has increased volume in the ventricle at end-diastole (preload; see Chapter 15) as a result of the heart's inability to pump effectively. This excessive increase in preload increases the workload of the heart. IABP therapy helps to decrease excessive preload by decreasing impedance to ejection. With decreased impedance, there is more effective forward flow of blood and more efficient emptying of the left ventricle.

CONTRACTILITY

Contractility refers to the velocity and vigor of contraction during systole. Although vigorous contractility requires more oxygen, it is a benefit to cardiac function because it ensures good, efficient pumping, which increases cardiac output. In failure, contractility is depressed. The biochemical status of the myocardium directly affects contractility. Contractility is depressed when calcium levels are low, catecholamine levels are low, and ischemia is present with resultant acidosis.

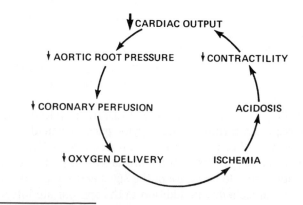

FIGURE 17-14
Cycle leading to cardiogenic shock.

Intra-aortic balloon pump counterpulsation can increase oxygen supply, thereby decreasing ischemia and acidosis. In this way, IABP therapy contributes to improved contractility and better cardiac function (see Fig. 17–14).

HEART RATE

Heart rate is a major determinant of oxygen demand because the rate determines the number of times per minute the high pressures must be generated during systole. Normally, myocardial perfusion takes place during diastole. Coronary artery perfusion pressure is determined by the gradient between aortic diastolic pressure and myocardial wall tension. It can be expressed by the following equation:

Coronary perfusion pressure =
Aortic diastolic pressure − Myocardial wall tension

Tension in the muscle retards blood flow, which is why approximately 80% of coronary artery perfusion occurs during diastole. With faster heart rates, diastolic time becomes shortened, with very little change occurring in systolic time. A rapid heart rate not only increases oxygen demand but also decreases the time available for oxygen delivery. In acute ventricular failure, a person may not be able to maintain cardiac output by increasing the volume of blood pumped with each beat (stroke volume) because contractility is depressed. Cardiac output is a function of both stroke volume and heart rate:

Cardiac output = Stroke volume × Heart rate

If stroke volume cannot be increased, heart rate must increase to maintain cardiac output. This is very costly in terms of oxygen demand.

By improving contractility, IABP therapy helps improve myocardial pumping and the ability to increase stroke volume. Decreasing afterload also increases pumping efficiency. With improved myocardial function and cardiac output, the need for compensatory tachycardia diminishes. Intra-aortic balloon pump counterpulsation will increase coronary artery perfusion pressure by increasing aortic diastolic pressure during inflation of the balloon, resulting in improved blood flow and oxygen delivery to the myocardium.

Physiological effects of IABP therapy are summarized in the display. Proper inflation of the balloon will increase oxygen supply, and proper deflation of the balloon will decrease oxygen demand. Timing of inflation and deflation is crucial and must coincide with the cardiac cycle.

Equipment Features

The intra-aortic balloon catheter and the balloon mounted on the end are constructed of a bicompatible polyurethane material. Filling of the balloon is achieved with a pressurized gas that enters through the catheter. Because of its low molecular weight, helium is the pressurized gas of choice. With inflation, the addition of 40 mL of volume into the aorta acutely increases aortic pressure and retrograde blood flow back to-

---

> ### *Direct Physiological Effects of IABP Therapy*
>
> #### *Inflation*
> ↑ Aortic diastolic pressure
> ↑ Aortic root pressure
> ↑ Coronary perfusion pressure
> ↑ Oxygen supply
>
> #### *Deflation*
> ↓ Aortic end-diastolic pressure
> ↓ Impedance to ejection
> ↓ Afterload
> ↓ Oxygen demand

ward the aortic valve. With deflation, the sudden evacuation of 40 mL of volume out of the balloon acutely decreases aortic pressure. Catheters have a central lumen with which aortic pressure can be measured from the tip of the balloon.

Indications for IABP Counterpulsation

Two major applications of IABP therapy are for treatment of cardiogenic shock after myocardial infarction and for acute left ventricular failure after cardiac surgery. Other applications of IABP therapy for patients with cardiac pathophysiological conditions are noted in the display.

CARDIOGENIC SHOCK

Treatment of cardiogenic shock is complicated, and the mortality remains high. Cardiogenic shock will develop in approximately 15% of patients with myocardial infarction.

Patients initially are treated with various inotropic drugs, vasopressors, and volume. A lack of or minimal response in cardiac output, arterial pressure, urine output, and mental status after this therapy will indicate a need for assisted circulation with IABP therapy. Once hypotension is present, the self-perpetuating process of injury will be in effect. Control of further injury and improvement in survival require early reversal of the shock state.

> ### *CLINICAL APPLICATION:*
> ### *Assessment Parameters*
> ### *Indications for IABP Therapy*
>
> - Cardiogenic shock after acute infarction
> - Left ventricular failure in the postoperative cardiac surgery patient
> - Severe unstable angina
> - Postinfarction ventricular septal defect or mitral regurgitation
> - Short-term bridge to cardiac transplantation

Response Patterns

Once IABP therapy is instituted, improvement should be observed within 1 to 2 hours. At this time, steady improvement should be seen in cardiac output, peripheral perfusion, urine output, mental status, and pulmonary congestion. With improved cardiac function, a decrease in central venous pressure and PAWP also should be seen. Average peak effect should be achieved within 24 to 48 hours.

POSTOPERATIVE LEFT VENTRICULAR FAILURE

Successful reduction in mortality has been achieved by using IABP therapy for patients with acute left ventricular failure after cardiac surgery. Two major conditions might lead to postoperative pump failure: severe preoperative left ventricular dysfunction and intraoperative myocardial injury.

Intra-aortic balloon pump counterpulsation therapy can be used to wean patients from cardiopulmonary bypass and to provide postoperative circulatory assistance until left ventricular recovery occurs. In these situations, early recognition of failure is evidenced by the heart's inability to support circulation after cardiopulmonary bypass. Early recognition and treatment are crucial if left ventricular failure is to be reversed.

UNSTABLE ANGINA

Intra-aortic balloon pump counterpulsation therapy may be used during cardiac catheterization for patients with unstable angina or mechanical problems. In this situation, cardiac catheterization studies generally are followed by emergency cardiac surgery. Patients in this category include those with unstable angina, postinfarction angina and postinfarction ventricular septal defects, or mitral regurgitation from papillary muscle injury with resultant cardiac failure. IABP counterpulsation therapy has been used successfully to control the severity of angina in patients in whom previous medical therapy has failed. The use of IABP therapy for patients with cardiac failure after ventricular septal rupture or mitral valve incompetence will aid in the promotion of forward blood flow, which will decrease shunting through the septal defect and decrease the amount of mitral regurgitation.

Contraindications to IABP Counterpulsation

There are few contraindications associated with the use of IABP therapy.

A competent aortic valve is necessary if the patient is to benefit from IABP therapy. With *aortic insufficiency*, balloon inflation would only increase aortic regurgitation and offer little, if any, augmentation of coronary artery perfusion pressure. In fact, the patient's heart failure could be expected to become worse.

Severe peripheral vascular occlusive disease also is a relative contraindication to the use of IABP therapy. Occlusive disease would make insertion of the catheter difficult and possibly interrupt blood flow to the distal extremity or cause dislodgement of plaque formation along the vessel wall, resulting in potential emboli. In patients who absolutely require IABP therapy, insertion can be achieved through the thoracic aorta, thus bypassing diseased peripheral vessels. Any previous aortofemoral or aortoiliac *bypass graft* would contraindicate femoral artery insertion.

The presence of an *aortic aneurysm* also is a contraindication to the use of IABP therapy. A pulsating balloon against an aneurysm may predispose the patient to dislodgement of aneurysmal debris with resultant emboli. A more serious complication would be rupture of the aneurysm. It is possible that the catheter could perforate the wall of the aneurysm during insertion.

Procedure

INSERTION

Proper positioning of the balloon is in the thoracic aorta just distal to the left subclavian artery and proximal to the renal arteries (Fig. 17–15). The most commonly used method of catheter placement is percutaneous insertion using a Seldinger technique, although other approaches have been described. The most common alternative is direct insertion into the thoracic aorta. Because this requires a median sternotomy incision, it is restricted to cardiac surgery patients whose chests have been opened for the surgery.

Once in place, the catheter is attached to a machine console that has three basic components: a monitoring system, an electronic trigger mechanism, and a drive system that moves gas in and out of the balloon. Monitoring systems have the capability of displaying the patient's ECG and an arterial waveform showing the effect of balloon inflation–deflation. Consoles also are capable of displaying a balloon waveform that illustrates the inflation and deflation of the balloon itself. The standard trigger mechanism for the balloon pump is the R wave that is sensed from the patient's ECG. This trigger will signal the beginning of each cardiac cycle for the drive system. Other possible triggers include systolic arterial pressure or pacemaker spikes on the ECG. Adjustment of exact timing is controlled on the machine console. The drive system is the actual mechanism that drives gas into and out of the balloon by alternating pressure and vacuum.

TIMING

Two methods of timing can be used with IABP therapy: conventional timing and real timing. Conventional timing uses the arterial waveform as the triggering mechanism to determine both inflation and deflation of the balloon. Real timing uses the same point of reference (the dicrotic notch on the arterial waveform) for balloon inflation but uses the ECG signal as the trigger for balloon deflation. Real timing is discussed briefly after conventional timing.

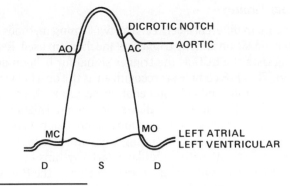

FIGURE 17-16

Cardiac cycle of the left heart with aortic, left ventricular, and left atrial pressure waveforms. AO, aortic valve opening; AC, aortic valve closure; D, diastole; MO, mitral valve opening; MC, mitral valve closure; S, systole.

Closing of the aortic valve creates an artifact on the arterial waveform that is called the dicrotic notch. The dicrotic notch is used as a timing reference to determine when balloon inflation should occur. Inflation should not occur before the notch because systole has not been completed.

After aortic valve closure, two phases of diastole begin: isovolumic relaxation and ventricular filling. After aortic valve closure, there is a period in which neither the aortic nor mitral valve is open. The mitral valve remains closed because left ventricular pressure still is higher than left atrial pressure. This phase is isovolumic relaxation. When left ventricular pressure falls below left atrial pressure, the mitral valve is forced open by the higher pressure in the left atrium. This begins the filling phase of diastole. Balloon inflation should continue throughout diastole. Deflation should be timed to occur at end-diastole, just before the next sharp systolic upstroke on the arterial waveform.

Figure 17–16 illustrates the cardiac cycle with left atrial, left ventricular, and aortic pressures superimposed on one another. Figure 17–17 illustrates a radial artery waveform with the beginning of systole and diastole marked.

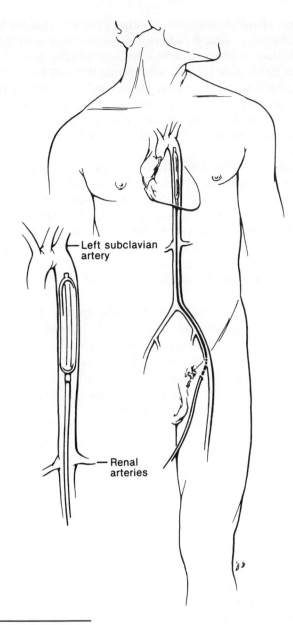

FIGURE 17-15

Proper position of the balloon catheter; illustrating percutaneous insertion.

Conventional Timing

The first step to proper timing of the balloon pump using conventional timing is the identification of the beginning of systole and diastole on the arterial waveform. Systole begins when left ventricular pressure exceeds left atrial pressure, forcing the mitral valve closed.

There are two phases to systole: isovolumic contraction and ejection. Once the mitral valve is closed, isovolumic contraction begins and continues until enough pressure is generated to overcome impedance to ejection. When ventricular pressure exceeds aortic pressure, the aortic valve is forced open, initiating ejection, or phase two. Ejection continues until pressure in the left ventricle falls below pressure in the aorta. At this point, the aortic valve closes, and diastole begins.

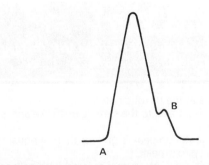

FIGURE 17-17

Arterial waveform, with *A* representing the point of balloon deflation before the systolic upstroke, and *B* representing balloon inflation at the dicrotic notch, at diastole.

Real Timing

The main difference between the two timing methods is balloon deflation and the triggering mechanism used. Real timing uses the ECG as the trigger signal for balloon deflation. The QRS complex is recognized as the onset of ventricular systole, and balloon deflation occurs at this time. Triggering off of the R wave allows for balloon deflation to occur at the time of systolic ejection and not before (as with conventional timing). This timing mechanism is more effective in patients with irregular heart rhythms because balloon deflation will occur on recognition of the R wave (systolic ejection). It does not need to be approximated by the operator or an algorithm, as in conventional timing. Both a rapid deflation mechanism and a reliable ECG signal are necessary for the IABP using real timing to augment blood pressure effectively. Balloon inflation, using real timing, occurs at the onset of diastole as triggered by the dicrotic notch on an arterial waveform just as in conventional timing.

Interpretation of Results

WAVEFORM ASSESSMENT

Analysis of the arterial pressure waveform and the effectiveness of IABP therapy is an important nursing function. Nurses must be able to recognize and correct problems in balloon pump timing.

Step 1. The first step in timing assessment is the ability to recognize the beginnings of systole and diastole on the arterial waveform, as shown in Figure 17–17. Systole begins at point A, where the sharp upstroke begins. Point B marks the dicrotic notch, which represents aortic valve closure. At this point, diastole begins and the balloon should be inflated. Balloon deflation occurs just before point A, at end-diastole.

The accompanying display lists five criteria that can be used to measure the effectiveness of IABP therapy on the arterial pressure waveform. To evaluate the waveform effectively, the patient's unassisted pressure tracing must be viewed alongside the assisted pressure tracing. This can be accomplished through adjustment of the console so that the balloon inflates and deflates on every other beat (ie, a 1:2 assist ratio). Most patients will tolerate this well for a brief period of time. Machine consoles are capable of freezing the waveform on the console monitor so that it would be necessary to assist 1:2 only for one screen. Another alternative would be to obtain a strip recording of the 1:2 assistance for analysis.

Step 2. After identification of the patient's dicrotic notch, a comparison is made with the assisted tracing to see that inflation occurs at the point of the dicrotic notch. Inflation before the dicrotic notch will shorten systole abruptly and increase ventricular volume as ejection is interrupted. Late inflation, past the dicrotic notch, will not raise coronary artery perfusion pressure. The peak-diastolic pressure may not be as high as it would be with proper timing.

Step 3. Next, the slopes of systolic upstroke and diastolic augmentation should be compared. The diastolic slope should be sharp and parallel the systolic upstroke. The slope always should be a straight line. The greater the peak in diastolic pressure, the greater the increase in aortic root pressure. For this reason, balloon assistance is adjusted until the highest peak possible is achieved.

Step 4. Deflation should occur just before systole, causing an acute drop in aortic end-diastolic pressure. This quick deflation displaces approximately 40 mL of volume. The result is an end-diastolic dip in pressure that reduces the impedance to the next systolic ejection. The end-diastolic pressure without the balloon assistance should be compared to the end-diastolic pressure with the dip created by balloon deflation. Optimally, a pressure difference of at least 10 mmHg should be obtained. Better afterload reduction is achieved with the lowest possible end-diastolic dip.

The point of deflation also is crucial. Deflation that is too early will allow pressure to rise to normal end-diastolic levels preceding systole. In this situation, there will be no decrease in afterload. Late deflation will encroach on the next systole and actually increase afterload owing to greater impedance to ejection from the presence of the still inflated balloon during systolic ejection.

Step 5. Finally, if afterload has been reduced, the next systolic pressure peak will be lower than the unassisted systolic pressure peak. This implies that the ventricle did not have to generate as great a pressure to overcome impedance to ejection. This may not always be seen because the systolic pressure peak also represents the compliance of the vasculature. If the vasculature is noncompliant due to atherosclerotic disease, the systolic peak may not change very much. Figure 17–18 illustrates the five points that are assessed on the waveform, while Figure 17–19 demonstrates possible errors in timing.

Balloon Fit. The fit of the balloon to any particular patient's aorta will determine how well these criteria are met. Ideally, approximately 80% of the aorta is occluded with balloon inflation. In a dilated aorta, in which less than 80%

CLINICAL APPLICATION:
Assessment Parameters
Criteria for Assessment of Effective IABP Therapy on the Arterial Pressure Waveform

- Inflation occurs at the dicrotic notch.
- Inflation slope is parallel to the systolic upstroke and is a straight line.
- Diastolic augmentation peak is greater than or equal to the preceding systolic peak.
- An end-diastolic dip in pressure is created with balloon deflation.
- The following systolic peak (assisted systole) is lower than the preceding systole (unassisted systole).

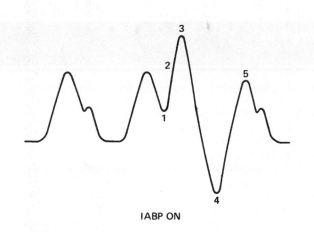

FIGURE 17-18

Inspection of the arterial waveform with intra-aortic balloon assistance should include observation of (1) inflation point; (2) inflation slope; (3) diastolic peak pressure; (4) end-diastolic dip; (5) next systolic peak.

occlusion occurs, the effect of inflation and deflation will not be as dramatic on the waveform. When a patient is hypotensive or hypovolemic, the balloon will not have as pronounced an effect on the waveform because there is less volume displacement as the balloon inflates or deflates.

Assessment and Management

Patients requiring IABP are managed much like any other critically ill patient in cardiogenic shock or acute left ventricular failure. Nursing assessment and management of these conditions are discussed in Chapters 19 and 49. Additional nursing skills and assessment considerations specific to IABP therapy must be included in the care of these patients. These are summarized in the Nursing Intervention Guidelines on the next page.

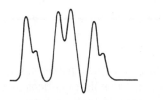

Early inflation   Late inflation

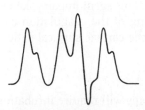
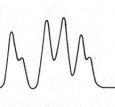

Early deflation   Late deflation

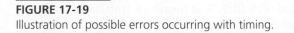

FIGURE 17-19

Illustration of possible errors occurring with timing.

SYSTEM MONITORING

Cardiovascular System

Monitoring the cardiovascular system is extremely important in determining the effectiveness of balloon pump therapy. The basis for this assessment includes vital signs, cardiac output, heart rhythm and regularity, urine output, color, perfusion, and mentation.

Vital Signs.   Three important vital signs with respect to IABP therapy are heart rate, mean arterial pressure (MAP), and PAWP. Effective IABP therapy will cause a decrease in all three parameters. Acute changes in the MAP may indicate volume depletion. Critically ill patients tolerate little change in their volume status. The PAWP is an important parameter for monitoring volume and will provide the clinician with an early indication of volume depletion or overload.

Blood pressure readings require special consideration. Because the balloon inflates during diastole, peak-diastolic pressure may be higher than peak-systolic pressure. Most IABP consoles have monitoring systems capable of distinguishing systole from peak diastole; however, some monitoring equipment can only distinguish peak pressures from low-point pressures. For this reason, a monitor's digital display of systolic pressure actually may represent peak-diastolic pressure. It is advisable to record blood pressure as systolic, peak-diastolic, and end-diastolic—that is, 100/110/60. These pressures can be read from a strip recording of the arterial waveform.

Heart Rhythm and Regularity.   Heart rhythm and regularity are important considerations. Early recognition and treatment of *dysrhythmias* are crucial for effective IABP support. Irregular dysrhythmias may inhibit efficient IABP therapy with some types of consoles because timing is set by the regular RR interval on the ECG. A safety feature of all balloon pump consoles is automatic deflation of the balloon for premature QRS complexes. One particular IABP model tracks real time versus any average of beats so it more effectively tracks dysrhythmias. If the dysrhythmia persists and timing is ineffective, another alternative might be use of the systolic peak on the arterial waveform as the trigger mechanism for balloon inflation. The primary goal in dysrhythmias is to treat the dysrhythmia.

Other Observations.   *Urine output, color, perfusion,* and *mentation* all are important assessment parameters for determining the adequacy of cardiac output. All should improve in patients responsive to IABP therapy. Any deterioration in these signs also might indicate a fall in cardiac output. Cardiac output measurement is indicated when deterioration is evident, when a major change in volume or pharmacological therapy has been instituted, and during weaning from IABP support.

The left radial pulse and the cannulated extremity should be frequently assessed. A decrease, absence, or change in character of the left radial pulse may indicate that the balloon has advanced up the aorta and may be partially obstructing or has advanced into the left subclavian artery.

CLINICAL APPLICATION: Nursing Intervention Guidelines
IABP Counterpulsation

IABP Timing

- Verify correct timing using assist ratio of 1:2, and document settings, hourly.
- Reevaluate timing for any change in heart rate greater than 10 beats/min.
- Maintain proper balloon volume and refill as needed every 2 to 4 hours. Use automatic filling mode if available. Avoid hip flexion, which may impair gas movement in and out of IABP catheter.
- Maintain good arterial waveform and adequate ECG signal for evaluation of timing.
- Reduce or eliminate situations that will interfere with the IABP's ability to maintain proper assist ratio. Notify physician of the development of tachycardias or irregular rhythms, and treat dysrhythmias with drug therapy or pacing as ordered.
- Notify physician immediately if IABP starts to fail.

VAD Pump Flow

- Assess and maintain adequate filling pressures during immediate postoperative phase.
- Monitor and assess HR, BP, MAP, pump flow, urine output, and mental status hourly. Treat changes as ordered.
- Assess and change equipment level for devices that require specific placement of equipment for adequate pump flow.
- Evaluate pump flow and rate of VAD in relation to native heart rate and activity level of patient.
- Manage VAD function and volume status as ordered to maintain adequate device output.

General

- Monitor and record temperature every 4 hours and prn.
- Observe all insertion sites and incisions for signs of infection. Maintain sterile technique with dressing changes.
- Change any dressing that is wet or not intact.
- Change all infusion lines and infusion bags per unit protocol.
- Culture any site with suspicious drainage, redness, or swelling.
- Notify physician of an elevation in WBCs.
- Treat patient with antibiotics as ordered.

- Auscultate and document breath sounds every 2 to 4 hours.
- Assist patient with pulmonary toilet activities (ie, coughing, deep breathing, frequent turning). Suction intubated patients as needed.
- Use pulse oximetry to monitor more closely those patients with abnormal blood gases, excessive secretions, or respiratory difficulty.
- Extubate patients and increase their activity level as tolerated, particularly those with the implantable VADs.
- Document quality of peripheral pulses and neurological status prior to IABP or VAD insertion. Assess and document quality of pulses, skin perfusion, and neurological status per protocol. Evaluate peripheral perfusion with any complaints of leg/foot pain by patient.
- Notify physician of any changes in pulses or neurological status.
- Maintain anticoagulation as ordered.
- Avoid hip flexion, which might obstruct flow to the affected extremity, by keeping the cannulated leg straight and the bed at an angle less than 15 degrees.
- Always maintain balloon motion to avoid thrombus formation on the balloon.
- Assess skin integrity, and document any redness and ulcerations over bony prominences.
- Use sheepskin, foam pads, and specialty beds as needed. Turn patient every 2 hours.
- Ensure that skin remains clean and dry.
- Maintain adequate nutrition by encouraging oral intake or implementing use of parenteral or enteral nutrition when necessary.
- Maintain alarm volumes, monitor noise at lowest level possible, and minimize unnecessary noise in room.
- Talk with patient and reorient to date and time frequently.
- Encourage family visits.
- Explain all procedures and activities to the patient.
- Organize care to allow for periods of uninterrupted sleep. Turn the lights off in room at night if possible.
- Sedate patient if necessary and as tolerated per physician orders.

The presence of the balloon catheter in the femoral or iliac artery predisposes the patient to impaired circulation of the involved extremity. The affected extremity will need to be kept relatively immobile. Because flexion of the hip may kink the catheter and impair balloon pumping, it may be helpful to use a knee immobilizer to remind the patient to avoid hip flexion. The head of the bed should also not be elevated more than 30 degrees. Hip flexion also contributes to decreased perfusion to the distal extremity. Extremities should be checked hourly for pulses, color, and sensation. Any deterioration in the affected extremity should be reported to the physician. Severe arterial insufficiency will necessitate removal of the catheter.

Physicians advocate the use of heparin therapy to prevent possible thrombus formation around the catheter and

vascular insufficiency, especially in medical patients. Each physician will determine whether the risks of anticoagulation outweigh the benefits for the specific patient. Low-molecular weight dextran is another possible choice of therapy to prevent thrombus formation. This agent impairs platelet function and prevents triggering of the coagulation cascade. It is usually preferred in the cardiac surgical patient for the first 24 hours.

Pulmonary System

Many patients on IABP therapy will require intubation and ventilatory assistance. Some of these patients may have respiratory insufficiency secondary to fluid overload associated with CHF. The immobile, intubated patient is always at risk for respiratory infections and the development of atelectasis. Turning the patient is appropriate provided modifications are implemented to keep the extremity cannulated by the balloon catheter straight. Daily chest roentgenograms are needed to follow pulmonary status and to inspect IV catheter placement. The position of the balloon catheter also can be determined in this manner.

Renal System

Patients in cardiogenic shock or severe left ventricular failure are at risk for the development of acute renal failure. In the shock state, the kidneys suffer the consequences of hypoperfusion; therefore, urine output and quality should be monitored closely. Serum BUN, creatinine, and creatinine clearance should be monitored daily to assess renal function. Creatinine clearance will indicate renal dysfunction and possible failure much earlier than elevated serum creatinine. Any acute, dramatic drop in urine output might be an indication that the catheter has slipped down the aorta and is obstructing the renal arteries.

WEANING

Indications for Weaning

Weaning patients from balloon assistance generally can begin 24 to 72 hours after insertion. Some patients will require longer periods of support. Weaning can begin when there is evidence of *hemodynamic stability* that does not require excessive vasopressor support. Ideally, vasopressor support is minimal when weaning begins. After the balloon is removed, it is much easier to increase vasopressor support than to reinsert a balloon catheter for hemodynamic support.

The patient should exhibit signs of *adequate cardiac function*, demonstrated by good peripheral pulses, adequate urine output, absence of pulmonary edema, and improved mentation. *Good coronary artery perfusion* will be evidenced by an absence of ventricular ectopy and no evidence of ischemia or injury on the ECG.

Complications may require abrupt cessation of IABP. This may or may not result in reinsertion of another balloon catheter. Severe arterial insufficiency evidenced by a loss of pulses in the distal extremity, pain, and pallor is definitely an indication to remove the balloon catheter from that particular insertion site. Any balloon that develops a leak also requires removal. The physician may choose to reinsert the balloon catheter in another extremity or to replace the faulty balloon if the patient is hemodynamically unstable. Depending on the philosophy of the institution and physician, a deteriorating, irreversible situation also might be an indication for weaning or discontinuing balloon pump support. The accompanying display lists major indications for weaning from IABP therapy.

Approaches to Weaning

Weaning is commonly achieved by decreasing the assist ratio from 1:1 to 1:2 and so on until the minimum assist ratio is achieved on any particular console. A patient might

---

CLINICAL APPLICATION:
Assessment Parameters
Indications for Weaning From IABP

- Hemodynamic stability
    Cardiac index >2 L/min
    PAWP <20 mmHg
    Systolic blood pressure >100 mmHg
- Minimal requirements for vasopressor support
- Evidence of adequate cardiac function
    Good peripheral pulses
    Adequate urine output
    Absence of pulmonary edema
    Improved mentation
- Evidence of good coronary perfusion
    Absence of ventricular ectopy
    Absence of ischemia on the ECG
- Severe vascular insufficiency
- Balloon leakage
- Deteriorating, irreversible condition

---

be assisted at the first decrease for up to 4 to 6 hours. The minimum amount of time should be 30 minutes. During this time, the patient must be assessed for any change in hemodynamic status. An increase in heart rate, a decrease in blood pressure, and a decrease in cardiac output indicate a deterioration in hemodynamic status. Weaning should be discontinued temporarily and therapy should be adjusted before another weaning attempt. If the first decrease in assist ratio is tolerated, the assist ratio is decreased to minimum, with 1 to 4 hours allowed for each new assist ratio. The patient must be assessed continually for any indications of intolerance to the process.

Complications Specific to IABP Therapy

Patients with IABP counterpulsation need to be monitored for development of poor blood flow to the cannulated extremity, which could lead to compartment syndrome. It may occur within the first 24 hours of support or not until several days after catheter insertion. Compartment syndrome is caused by a rise in the tissue pressure in one of the compartments of the affected lower extremity. Bone, muscle, nerve tissue, and blood vessels all are enclosed by a fibrous membrane called the fascia, and this enclosed space is called a compartment. It is nonyielding, so a rise in volume in the compartment will increase the pressure in the compartment. The IABP patient in whom limb ischemia develops from decreased capillary flow can suffer cellular and capillary damage that leads to increased capillary permeability. The resultant transudation of fluid into the closed compartment space increases tissue pressure to a level that can interfere with capillary blood flow. When this degree of tissue pressure is reached, tissue viability may be threatened. Treatment is directed at improving blood flow. Pressure release by fasciotomy may be needed to prevent tissue death.

Decreased circulating platelets in the first 24 hours of IABP therapy and a minimal decrease in red blood cell count have been reported; however, they are not thought to be significant problems. There is a low incidence of balloon leakage and rupture. These complications might result from balloon inflation against a calcific, atherosclerotic plaque in the aorta. This disruption in the balloon surface may be as small as a pinhole or may be a large tear. The associated danger is gas embolism.

Insertion of the catheter in the face of severe atherosclerotic vascular disease might result in arterial perforation or occlusion. Any leak is an indication for immediate balloon removal. Iatrogenic dissection of the aorta is rare but has been reported. Arterial insufficiency is the most common complication of IABP therapy. Arterial insufficiency may be permanent, or it may be relieved by aortofemoral or ileofemoral bypass grafting. Neuropathy in the catheterized extremity is another reported complication.

■ MECHANICAL CIRCULATORY SUPPORT

When there is profound myocardial injury, the augmentation of systemic blood pressure by the IABP may not be adequate for patient survival. Use of the IABP for circulatory support requires that a patient have a functioning left ventricle because the IABP only augments cardiac output by 8% to 10%. Patients with severe, acute left ventricular failure after a myocardial infarction, after a surgical procedure, or from end-stage CHF may need a mechanism for replacing left ventricular function. Circulatory support with a ventricular assist device (VAD) has become a successful treatment for patients with cardiac failure refractory to pharmacological therapies, revascularization procedures, and IABP counterpulsation. These devices are capable of supporting circulation until the heart recovers or a donor heart is obtained for transplantation.

Interest in the research and development of artificial circulatory support devices has existed since the 1930s. Cardiopulmonary bypass, an early example of these efforts, was successfully implemented in the 1950s. In 1964, a National Institutes of Health initiative helped to organize and support these efforts on a national level. Michael Debakey became the first clinician to support successfully a postcardiotomy patient with a left ventricular bypass pump in 1966. An impetus for continued research during the 1960s and 1970s was the limited early success with heart transplantation. The focus of research at that time was to develop a device that could support the failing heart until sufficient cardiac function had returned. Current research focuses on the use of these devices as a bridge to heart transplantation and as a method of permanent cardiac support for patients with end-stage cardiac disease.

Physiological Principles

Patients who are candidates for ventricular assistance suffer from heart failure resulting from ischemic or myopathic heart disease. Both disease processes lead to a reduction in cardiac output and oxygen delivery. The physiological response of the body to this low output state is vasoconstriction and increased systemic vascular resistance. While these compensatory mechanisms are meant to protect and preserve cardiovascular function in the short term, a vicious cycle develops that is characterized by compromised cardiac contractility and a low ventricular ejection fraction. Hypotension will ensue, leading to hemodynamic instability requiring the use of pharmacological agents and possibly the IABP for cardiovascular support. Should the patient continue to deteriorate despite drug therapy and the IABP, a VAD may be necessary for survival. Hemodynamically, these patients usually demonstrate a cardiac index of < 2.0 L/min/m^2, a PAWP of > 20 mmHg, and a systolic blood pressure of < 80 mmHg despite pharmacological therapies and the use of IABP counterpulsation.

Restoration of adequate blood flow and preservation of end-organ function are the fundamental goals of short- or long-term VAD use. Hemodynamics and perfusion improve as the VAD(s) assumes the workload of the failing ventricle(s). Ventricular assistance may involve supporting one or both ventricles depending on the extent of myocardial damage and ventricular failure.

Left ventricular support usually requires cannulation of the left ventricle with a conduit that leads to the device. The ascending aorta, which receives the output from the device, is also cannulated with a conduit. In certain situations, the left atrium may be cannulated instead of the left ventricle. Circulation in the patient supported by a left ventricular assist device (LVAD) is similar to the normal circulatory process. Venous blood returns to the right heart, passes through the lungs to be oxygenated, and then returns to the left atrium through the pulmonary veins. Blood then passes from the left atrium through the left ventricle and into the LVAD. The LVAD will then eject blood into the ascending aorta during pump systole.

In situations that necessitate biventricular support, two pump units function in synchrony to assume the roles of the native right and left ventricles. One pump supports right heart circulation while the other supports left heart circulation. The addition of right ventricular assistance requires cannulation of the right atrium for inflow to the pump and the pulmonary artery for outflow from the right ventricular assist device (RVAD). During biventricular assistance, blood is diverted from the right atrium to the lungs through the RVAD, bypassing the right ventricle. Circulation continues to the left heart where the LVAD undertakes support of systemic circulation. Univentricular or biventricular assistance relieves the ventricle(s) of its workload by acting as the primary pump supporting pulmonary circulation or systemic blood pressure. Reducing ventricular workload decreases cardiac oxygen demand.

Devices

Several VADs are available for use. Certain devices are commercially available, while others require special exemption for investigational purposes. Although no universal classification system exists, the devices can be categorized according to four general functional characteristics: the intended duration of support (short term versus long term), the type of support provided (univentricular versus biventricular), the actual physical placement of the device (internal versus external), and the type of blood flow produced (pulsatile versus nonpulsatile). Short-term support usually refers to assistance for patients expected to recover from episodes of acute left ventricular failure secondary to myocardial infarction or surgical procedures. Long-term ventricular assistance may be an option for individuals awaiting heart transplantation, or it may provide an alternative method of permanent cardiac support.

NONPULSATILE PUMPS

Centrifugal and roller pumps are examples of nonpulsatile VADs capable of providing univentricular (to either ventricle) or biventricular support. They are primarily used for short-term ventricular assistance when myocardial recovery is expected. These devices have been used, infrequently, as bridges to transplantation. Both types are approved by the Food and Drug Administration (FDA) and commercially available. Centrifugal and roller pumps are extracorporeal devices designed to support circulation of the patient's blood. Because these devices do not generate pulsatile blood flow, the IABP is often used in conjunction with them to create a pulse. Blood is transported from the cannulated chamber to an external pump console that circulates the blood back to the corresponding great vessel by a separate cannula. Should right ventricular failure be identified after placement of an LVAD, an RVAD can be added for additional support with these devices.

These devices can be inserted relatively quickly and are adequate methods of deploying short-term circulatory assistance. Methods of cannulation and physical placement of the equipment limit the mobility and activity level of the patient. Patients supported by these VADs are often sedated and paralyzed. A commonly used centrifugal pump is the Biomedicus.

Extracorporeal membrane oxygenation (ECMO) or cardiopulmonary bypass (CPB) systems are alternative methods of temporary CPR involving circulatory support and oxygenation of the patient's blood. CPB is primarily used for operative situations but has demonstrated effectiveness as a mechanism of support for patients unable to wean from the pump perioperatively or for those requiring cardiopulmonary support refractory to conventional efforts. Circulation of blood between the patient and an external pump is supported by cannulation of the femoral vessels. Venous blood is diverted from central venous circulation; pumped through a membrane oxygenator, where oxygen and carbon dioxide are exchanged; and returned to the arterial circulation through the femoral artery cannula. A heating mechanism within the pump console helps to maintain body temperature during circulatory support.

Rapid deployment without the need for surgical intervention and the ability to provide hemodynamic stabilization for a brief period are the major advantages of these resuscitative devices. CPB and ECMO allow time for further assessment and intervention during episodes of acute hemodynamic decompensation. Disadvantages include the need for continuous anticoagulation and the inability to provide extended circulatory support. The presence of occlusive peripheral vascular disease could be a contraindication to use of these devices.

PULSATILE PUMPS

Implantable Pumps

Implantable pumps were designed with the intention of providing long-term, left ventricular support while allowing the patient a certain amount of physical independence. A few devices have successfully supported a patient for greater than 1 year while awaiting heart transplantation. Many patients with the implantable devices have been physically rehabilitated by participating in regular physical therapy programs and normal activities of daily living while being supported with a VAD. This might better prepare them physically to endure the transplantation process. One day these devices may provide an alternative to heart transplantation as the number of potential transplant recipients far exceeds available donors. Examples of the implantable devices are the TCI Heartmate and the Novacor LVAS. The Novacor device operates on electrical energy. Thermo Cardiosystems has two devices: one that operates by electrical energy and one that operates by pneumatic energy.

Surgical implantation of the VAD necessitates a sternotomy and the use of CPB. Device placement is in an abdominal pocket just below the left diaphragm. Typically the inflow conduit is tunneled through the diaphragm and anastomosed to the apex of the left ventricle. The outflow conduit is brought around the diaphragm and is anastomosed to the ascending aorta. Drive lines extending from the implanted device are tunneled through the patient's skin and connected to a portable, external power source. This power source may be a portable console or battery pack that is worn by the patient (Fig. 17–20). Either situation allows the patient mobility and independence during the recovery period.

Pump units of the implantable VADs are encapsulated in rigid housing and consist of a blood pump sac and single or dual pusher plates (depending on the particular device). Inflow and outflow conduits have valves that support unidirectional blood flow. These devices work on the principle of converting electrical or pneumatic energy to mechanical energy. This mechanical energy activates the pusher plates causing them to compress the blood sac at the appropriate time. Blood sac compression causes ejection of the blood out of the pump sac and into the ascending aorta through

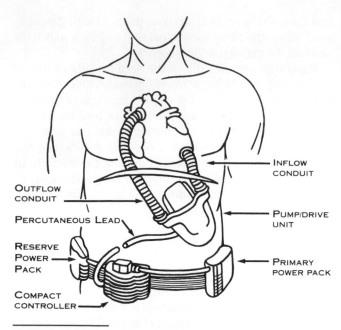

FIGURE 17-20
Portable, implantable left ventricular assist device. (Artwork courtesy of the Novacor Division, Baxter Healthcare Corporation)

the outflow conduit. These devices have stroke volumes of 70 to 83 mL and can support pump outputs of greater than 10 L/min. Depending on the device implanted, long-term anticoagulation may be necessary to prevent thromboembolic events.

External Pumps

Two commonly used external pulsatile devices are the Thoratec VAD and the Abiomed pump. Both devices have successfully supported postcardiotomy patients and patients bridged to heart transplantation.

The Thoratec VAD is a pneumatically driven device that is positioned externally on the recipient's upper abdomen. Placement of this device requires a sternotomy incision and use of CPB. The structure of the pump drive, the inflow and outflow conduits, and the cannulation techniques of the chambers and great vessels are all similar to that of the implantable devices. A major difference is that the cannulas supporting the blood flow pass through the patient's chest wall to the externally positioned pump. One advantage of this device is the ability to provide univentricular or biventricular support, depending on the extent of heart failure. Figure 17–21 is an example of biventricular support. Another advantage is that due to its external placement, small patient body size is less of a contraindication when considering the need for ventricular assistance.

Another external VAD, the Abiomed pump, is designed for short-term univentricular or biventricular support. It has been used in patients when myocardial recovery is expected and as a bridge to transplantation. Components consist of cannulas for venous and arterial access, blood pumps to support unidirectional blood flow and systemic circula-

tion, and a pneumatically driven console that provides the power source. Cannulation sites for this device are either atria, the pulmonary artery, and the ascending aorta. Filling of the blood pumps occurs passively by gravity; therefore, the blood pumps must be positioned securely below the level of the heart to promote adequate blood flow into their chambers (Fig. 17–22). The internal bladders operate in a fill-to-empty mode. Pumps positioned too high will insufficiently fill and pumps that are too low will prolong filling time, each adversely affecting patient hemodynamics. Nursing interventions specific to the Abiomed include monitoring and adjusting the level of the blood pumps and monitoring filling pressures to ensure adequate volumes necessary to support optimal flow through the system. Use of this device significantly impairs patient mobility.

Modes of Operation

With the exception of the Abiomed device, the pulsatile pumps have several modes of operation. Two primary modes depend on the patient's ECG or the rate of blood flow through the pump during each cardiac cycle. In the ECG trigger mode, the pump initiates blood ejection in conjunction with the patient's QRS complex; the R wave acts as

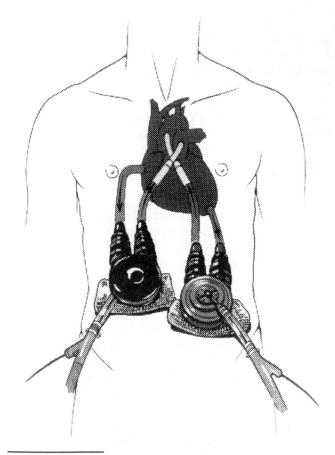

FIGURE 17-21
Thoratec pneumatic ventricular assist device. External placement with biventricular assist capabilities. (Courtesy of Kathy J. Vaca, RN; Department of Surgery, St. Louis Health Sciences Center, St. Louis, MO)

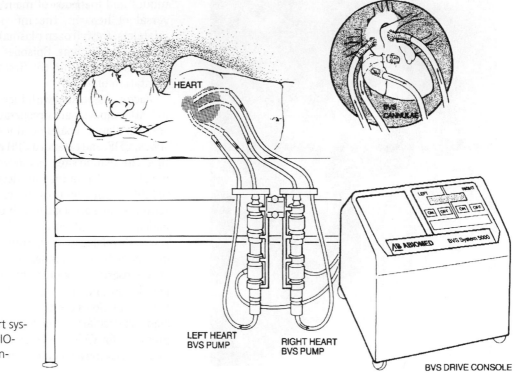

FIGURE 17-22
Abiomed biventricular support system. (Artwork courtesy of ABIO-MED Cardiovascular, Inc., Danvers, MA)

LEFT HEART BVS PUMP

RIGHT HEART BVS PUMP

BVS DRIVE CONSOLE

the trigger for pump systole. The second mode is a dynamic mode that allows the pump to respond to the changing heart rate, depending on patient activity level. Pump systole and cardiac output will depend on the blood flow sensed by the device, which is programmed to respond to changes in pump filling rate as blood passes from the left ventricle into the blood sac of the pump drive. This ability is particularly important as a patient's level of activity increases during the recovery phase after implantation. A third mode of operation, rarely used clinically, is a fixed rate mode that functions independently of the native heart.

Nursing Implications

Historically, VAD recipients have received care in the intensive care unit (ICU), usually intubated and sedated. Evolution of the technology and the use of portable devices as bridges to transplantation have changed the mode of care. Now, patients are encouraged to be independent, pursue physical rehabilitation, and engage in normal activities of daily living when possible (Fig. 17–23). Certain patients may even be discharged from the hospital. Nursing has an opportunity to be instrumental in the coordination of patient care and outcomes management with this new patient population.

During the immediate postoperative phase, the critical care nurse must be cognizant of the physiological responses expected and the common postoperative complications associated with device implantation. The nurse determines whether the equipment is functioning appropriately by monitoring parameters associated with adequate tissue perfusion and improved end-organ function because these are the primary goals of VAD implantation. Hemodynamic instability and the maintenance of adequate filling pressures are critical issues in the immediate postoperative period. Other issues the critical care nurse encounters include, but are not limited to, dysrhythmias, bleeding complications, infections, thromboembolic events, and possible mechanical problems associated with the devices.

Psychosocial issues and patient education dominate the nursing focus during periods of extended support with a VAD; the majority of these patients require minimal direct nursing care once stabilized and discharged from the ICU. Increased independence in activities of daily living, continued physical rehabilitation, and patient education are emphasized. All aspects of the rehabilitation phase should include the recipient's family members or identified support person. As patients are discharged, they and their primary caregivers will need to be educated on the operation of the equipment and how to troubleshoot malfunctions. An individual capable of operating the VAD will need to accompany the patient at all times. Nursing must facilitate the integration of the patient's lifestyle with the boundaries created by having a VAD implanted for extended support. Feelings of isolation may unfold as investigational device protocols governed by the FDA may restrict the patients' social activity and geographical mobility.

An advanced practice nurse is in a pivotal position to assume the role of case manager facilitating the implementation of clinical paths, protocols, and procedures related to

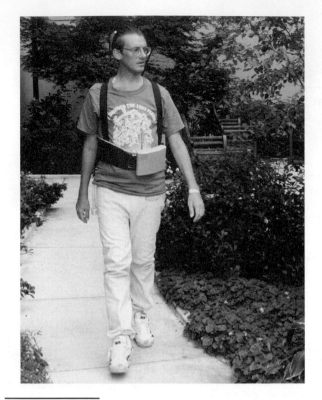

FIGURE 17-23
Wearing the portable left ventricular assist system, a patient is able to enjoy the independence of outdoor activites. Some patients may take day trips or be discharged form the hospital. (Photograph courtesy of Stanford Health Services, Stanford, CA)

patient progress from the acute to chronic phases of rehabilitation. Nursing education facilitated by a clinical nurse specialist will be vital to patient care as increasing numbers of nurses on the general floors, and possibly the outpatient setting, are exposed to this patient population. As more patients receive the portable devices and approach the possibility of hospital discharge, case management will be a principal facet of patient care.

COMPLICATIONS ASSOCIATED WITH IABP THERAPY AND CIRCULATORY SUPPORT

BLEEDING

Prolongation of bleeding times is a side effect of exposure to CPB, which is normally reversed in the early postoperative period. With the use of mechanical circulatory support, the continued exposure of blood to an artificial surface causes trauma to platelets. A cascade of events involving the platelets, white blood cells, fibrinolytic system, and complement system will occur. The frequency and severity of bleeding associated with artificial circulatory devices have been reduced by improved surgical tech-

niques and methods of maintaining hemostasis, the reversal of heparin, the infusion of coagulation factors (platelets, fresh frozen plasma), and continued experience with the equipment. Episodes of severe bleeding are usually corrected within the first 24 hours after surgical implantation of a VAD.

Factors associated with increased postoperative bleeding in VAD recipients are preoperative and postoperative use of anticoagulants; coagulopathies secondary to cardiogenic shock, CHF, and extended CPB exposure; and the use of multiple cannulation sites. Hemodynamic instability, a reduction in native cardiac output and device output, a risk of ischemia to target organs, and possible cardiac tamponade are all deleterious events associated with uncontrolled bleeding in the patient supported with a VAD. In the IABP patient, bleeding is usually related to use of continuous anticoagulation or the development of coagulopathies. Bleeding commonly occurs at the insertion site of the balloon catheter. In both patient populations, nursing interventions include observing external cannulation sites for oozing, monitoring changes in vital signs (particularly hemodynamic parameters, such as filling pressures for VAD recipients) and laboratory values, and regularly assessing adequate tissue perfusion.

THROMBOEMBOLIC EVENTS

Placement of the IABP puts a patient at risk for thromboembolic events. At the time of insertion, plaque may become dislodged from the vessel wall or emboli may break off a thrombus that has formed on the indwelling catheter or balloon. Both situations can impair circulation to distal extremities and other vital organs or cause a cerebrovascular accident. Continuous anticoagulation with a heparin infusion is required during IABP therapy; dextran infusions may also be used.

The development of a thrombus and the migration of emboli have been reported with the use of mechanical circulatory support. Anticoagulation regimens and the prevention of embolic events are unresolved issues in the clinical management of VAD recipients. Currently, anticoagulation therapy is managed differently depending on the device that is inserted. Devices used for short-term support require prophylactic use of low-dose heparin infusions. Similar to the IABP, dextran infusions may be used in conjunction with heparin. Patients supported with the Novacor, Heartmate, and Thoratec devices requiring long-term support are at greater risk secondary to extended periods of exposure to the device. These patients are usually managed with heparin infusions in the immediate postoperative phase. During the extended support period, the heparin is weaned and coumadin therapy is initiated to maintain the prothrombin time at an International Normal Ratio (INR) of 3.0 to 4.0.[1] Antiplatelet agents, such as dipyridamole, may be used in conjunction with coumadin therapy. Obtaining baseline and postimplant neurological assessments; monitoring peripheral pulses, especially those distal to cannulation sites; and assessing tissue perfusion are critical to the early recognition and intervention of any embolic event.

RIGHT VENTRICULAR FAILURE

Right ventricular failure continues to be a significant problem associated with LVAD implantation. Twenty to twenty-five percent of LVAD recipients develop right ventricular failure after device implantation secondary to the physiological effects the LVAD has on systemic circulation.[2,3] Because the pumping capabilities of the device exceed those of the impaired left ventricle, systemic circulation and right ventricular preload will increase, subsequently increasing right ventricular workload. Right ventricular output will be increased in a patient with a healthy right ventricle. A patient with underlying right ventricular failure, however, may not be able to handle this augmentation in circulatory volume. Evidence of primary right ventricular dysfunction may not become apparent until the right heart is challenged by the cardiac output of the LVAD.[3,4] When right ventricular failure develops after LVAD implantation, vasodilators and IV inotropes, such as PGE$_1$, isoproterenol, and epinephrine, are used to reduce pulmonary pressures and improve right ventricular contractility. It may be possible to add an RVAD for additional support if pharmacological intervention is unsuccessful. Clinical practice has shown that the addition of an RVAD after LVAD placement has been a poor prognostic indicator.[2]

INFECTION

Individuals requiring mechanical circulatory assistance and IABP therapy are at increased risk for infection secondary to the surgical procedures and the presence of external cannulas, pumps, drivelines, and so forth. Many of these patients suffer from chronic illness rendering them more immunocompromised. Infection may be related to surgical wounds after device insertion, invasive monitoring lines, drain placement, pulmonary status, or nutritional status. Early recognition of signs and symptoms of infection and early intervention can prevent the development of sepsis. Early detection is particularly important as some of these patients await heart transplantation, and an infection could preclude transplantation. Diligent handwashing, changing or removing invasive lines or drainage tubes when appropriate, adherence to sterile dressing techniques and schedules, and the use of appropriate prophylactic antibiotics are effective barriers to the development of infection. Early extubation and mobilization are goals for patients with the implanted devices. Primary nursing interventions include monitoring invasive sites for signs of infection, encouraging good pulmonary toilet, increasing activity level as tolerated, and promoting adequate nutrition.

DYSRHYTHMIAS

Most patients with cardiomyopathy who require some form of circulatory assistance experience dysrhythmias prior to insertion of a device. These dysrhythmias often continue after device implantation and may hinder device function depending on the rhythm. Dysrhythmias should be treated when they occur, and attempts should be made to restore sinus rhythm.

Circulatory assistance with the IABP is affected by dysrhythmias. Diastolic augmentation and systolic assistance decrease in the presence of irregular rhythms, such as atrial fibrillation or sinus rhythm with frequent ectopy. These rhythm changes make it difficult to manage the timing of balloon inflation and deflation. Lethal ventricular dysrhythmias need to be treated conventionally as the IABP is designed only to augment existing cardiac output.

Right ventricular function and the maintenance of adequate pump output are of primary concern in LVAD recipients with lethal ventricular rhythms. These patients may lack sufficient right ventricular function to support cardiac output during ventricular dysrhythmias even though left ventricular function has been assumed by the LVAD. Although LVAD flow and mean blood pressure have been known to decrease by approximately 20%, it has been demonstrated that patients with LVADs do tolerate sustained lethal ventricular rhythms without the need for RVAD support. Symptoms associated with these rhythms and low flow states are usually weakness and palpitations.[5] Patients receiving biventricular support should be able to maintain adequate device outputs despite the dysrhythmia because left and right ventricular function has been taken over by the VAD. Atrial fibrillation is usually tolerated by these patients even though it may have some effect on right heart function. Severe bradycardia and tachydysrhythmia need to be addressed because they will change pump flow and output. Cardiac rhythms require close monitoring for any acute changes.

NUTRITIONAL DEFICITS

Nutritional status is an important element of any recovery process. Many patients have had end-stage CHF and are nutritionally depleted prior to any surgical intervention, placing them at a higher risk for nutritional deficits during the postoperative phase. Adequate nutrition is necessary for wound healing. Obtaining dietary consultation, encouraging increased oral intake, and providing flexibility with meals will assist these patients in meeting their nutritional goals. Patients supported by the IABP and VADs that require intubation and sedation will require parenteral or enteral feedings. Those with implanted devices will eventually progress to a regular diet but may need smaller, more frequent meals. Experiencing feelings of fullness or early satiety is not uncommon for these patients due to the abdominal placement of the device.

PSYCHOSOCIAL FACTORS

Balloon and VAD insertion are usually unplanned, emergent interventions for a deteriorating condition. Abundant monitoring is frightening for both patient and family;

therefore, explanations of procedures and surroundings are very important. Family members need to be prepared prior to visiting their loved one immediately after device insertion. The goal is to alleviate anxiety and to help the patient and family feel more secure in a foreign environment. Honest communication is important. This will help the family members recognize changes in their loved one's condition and make informed, realistic decisions regarding the patient's care. Putting the family in contact with nonmedical personnel who can objectively provide emotional support is often beneficial. Issues that families and patients struggle with are fear, hopelessness, and death.

Critically ill patients often suffer from disorientation and sleep deprivation. Immobility and unfamiliar noises of the ICU tend to increase stress and anxiety. Mechanisms to help alleviate this stress and anxiety include frequent reorientation by the nursing staff and contact with family members. Better organization of time and procedures will also reduce stress because this will allow the patient longer periods of uninterrupted rest.

Autologous Blood Transfusion

Autologous blood transfusion (autotransfusion, ATS) is the collection, filtration, and reinfusion of the patient's own (autologous) blood. The purpose of autotransfusion is to avoid or decrease the requirements for allogeneic (homologous, bank, donor) blood and its potential risks and complications, including disease transmission and transfusion reaction. Autologous blood is the safest type of blood for transfusion when guidelines established by the American Association of Blood Banks are followed. Although reported by Blundell in 1818, performed successfully in 1914, and used as a means to meet the increased demand for blood caused by advances in open heart surgery in the 1970s, the major shift toward the use of autologous blood transfusion has occurred during the last decade. This has been due in large part to the acquired immunodeficiency syndrome (AIDS) epidemic and recognition of the risk of transfusion transmission of the human immunodeficiency virus (HIV).[1,2]

Because postoperative bleeding in surgical patients can be significant, postoperative and intraoperative autotransfusion systems have been developed. Although associated primarily with perioperative cardiovascular management, autotransfusion is used widely in other areas with requirements for large volumes of blood replacement, such as trauma, and orthopedic procedures, such as hip fractures, spinal fusion, and hip, knee, and shoulder arthroplasty procedures that require an average transfusion volume exceeding 1 U.

The addition of autologous perioperative plasmapheresis facilitates complete autotransfusion of both washed red blood cells and platelet-rich plasma, significantly reducing the need for supplemental use of allogeneic components. Both whole blood and component autotransfusion are now well accepted procedures that in many instances are life saving.

This section of the chapter includes a review of physiological principles of allogeneic and autologous blood, the equipment and methods available for collection and reinfusion of shed postoperative blood, indications and contraindications for the use of autologous blood transfusion, and principles of assessment and management. Although it is beyond the scope of this chapter to provide a comprehensive discussion of all aspects of autologous blood transfusion, a comprehensive list of references and supplemental bibliography has been provided.

Physiological Principles

The primary function of red blood cells is oxygen delivery. Oxygen delivery is maximal when hemoglobin is within the normal range. When hematocrit is below 21% to 24% and the hemoglobin level below 7 to 8 g/dL, adequate tissue oxygen delivery cannot be ensured.[3] The most common indication for blood transfusion is a low hemoglobin, with increased oxygen delivery as the therapeutic goal. When this physiological need exists, transfusion should provide a significant benefit. To determine the need for transfusion, the physician assesses the patient's disease status, estimated or anticipated blood loss, and ability to compensate for anemia. Once the decision to transfuse is made, the method of transfusion is determined by the timing of the transfusion (preoperative, intraoperative, postoperative), the status of the patient (extent and location of the blood loss), and availability of the best blood component, either allogeneic or autologous.

ALLOGENEIC BLOOD

Allogeneic blood transfusion is the transfer or transplantation of living tissue from one person to another. In 1995, the risk of disease transmission and transfusion reaction with allogeneic blood was approximately 1/450,000 to 1/660,000. Serological tests for transfusion-transmitted diseases, such as hepatitis and HIV, now include specific assays for antibodies to HIV, human T-lymphotropic virus type I (HTLV-I), and hepatitis C virus (HCV) and surrogate tests to supplement HCV detection.[1] The accompanying display gives statistics regarding infectious and noninfectious risks in allogeneic blood transfusions. The time between infection with HIV and the formation of enough antibodies to be detected by laboratory tests (the window period) has now been reduced to approximately 25 days. The newer, more sensitive tests have reduced the risk of disease transmission by reducing the window period.

Infectious and Noninfectious Risks of Allogeneic Transfusion

Infectious Risks of Allogeneic Transfusion Per Unit Transfused

- Hepatitis B: ?
- Hepatitis C: 1/300 to 1/3,300
- HIV: 1/40,000 to 1/225,000
- HTLV I or II: 1/50,000

Other infectious vectors or diseases:
- Cytomegalovirus, Epstein-Barr virus, delta virus, *Treponema pallidum,* malaria, babesiasis, toxoplasmosis filariasis

Incidence of post-transfusion hepatitis:
- 1986 to 1989: 10.97% decreased to 4.29% Prior to hepatitis C screening (no data after 1989–1990)

No hepatitis in autologous recipients

Noninfectious Risks of Allogeneic Transfusion

- ABO-Rh incompatibility: 1/2,000 to 1/6,000
- Fatal hemolytic transfusion reaction: 1/100,000
- Septic unit: ? perhaps 1/100,000
- Alloimmunization: Cross-match more difficult; transplant match more difficult
- Immunosuppression
- Volume overload, hyperviscosity overtransfusion
- Graft-versus-host disease reaction (potentially fatal 1/4,000 in Japanese population)

Source of data: Speiss, BD: Autologous blood should be availbale for elective cardiac surgery. J Cardiothorac Vasc Anesth, 8(2):231–237, 1994

Although the risks associated with the use of today's allogeneic blood supply have been decreased by advances in donor screening, they still remain significant. These are summarized in the previous display. For example, it is estimated that approximately 12% to 15% of all allogeneic blood products are being transfused into CPB patients, causing approximately 8,000 patients per year to receive viral transmission.[4] In addition, it has been documented that patients receiving allogeneic transfusion are at increased risk of postoperative infection resulting from the immunosuppression associated with the transfusion of allogeneic blood products. One study documented postoperative infection in 32% of hip replacement patients receiving allogeneic blood compared with only 3% of patients receiving only autologous blood transfusions.[5] Other studies have demonstrated significantly fewer postoperative infections in the patient group (cardiac surgery, abdominal trauma, Crohn's disease, colon cancer, open fractures) receiving only autologous blood.[4] It is believed that the increased risk of perioperative infection may be due to allogeneic blood transfusion depressing lymphocyte activity, increasing suppressor cell activity, and causing a reduction in interleuken-2 production.[4]

Patients continue to have a high level of anxiety related to disease transmission by exposure to allogeneic blood.

Reactions to allogeneic transfusion, which can occur with as little as 10 to 15 mL of incompatible blood, include hemolytic reactions, transfusion-induced graft-versus-host disease, hemoglobinuria, purpura, fever, circulatory overload, thrombophlebitis, urticaria, hyperkalemia, asymptomatic hemoglobinuria, pulmonary edema, and allergic and anaphylactic reactions.[6–13] The most dangerous reaction to a blood transfusion, an acute hemolytic transfusion reaction, occurs in one out of every 3,000 to 10,000 allogeneic transfusions.[14,15] It is caused by incorrect cross-matching; improper handling or administration, which causes hemolysis; and the number of previous allogeneic transfusion.

Characteristics of allogeneic blood include decreased red blood cell wall integrity, causing an increase in serum potassium; nonviable platelets within 24 hours of storage; anticoagulants; no 2,3-diphosphoglycerate (DPG) after 10 days of storage, causing left shift of oxyhemoglobin dissociation curve with impairment of oxygen transfer at tissue level; reduced clotting factors V (labile), VIII (antihemophilic), and IX (Christmas); and immunological differences between donor and recipient, which may increase the risk of perioperative infections. Because increased oxygen delivery is the therapeutic goal of transfusion, the low level or absence of 2,3-DPG (essential to adequate tissue oxygenation) may be a factor in transfusion decisions. A summary of autologous versus autogeneic blood appears in the accompanying display.

Autologous Versus Allogeneic Blood

Autologous Blood

- Morphologically, physiologically, and biochemically superior to allogeneic blood
- Normal levels of 2,3-DPG
- Higher platelet count
- Higher hematocrit
- Normal PTT, potassium, ammonia levels
- Near normal RBC clotting factors V, VIII, and IX
- Near body temperature
- Eliminates transmission of donor-related diseases
- Eliminates allogeneic transfusion reactions
- Lower incidence of postoperative infections

Allogeneic Blood

- Decreased RBC wall integrity causing increase in serum potassium
- Platelets nonviable within 24 hours of storage
- Anticoagulants
- No 2,3-DPG after 10 days storage, causing left shift of oxyhemoglobin dissociation curve with impairment of oxygen transfer at tissue level
- Reduced clotting factors V (labile), VIII (anti-hemophilic), and IX (Christmas)
- Immunosuppression causing increased risk of postoperative infection

AUTOLOGOUS BLOOD

Autologous blood is considered the safest type of blood for transfusion in most patients for a variety of reasons, including elimination of disease transmission and elimination of transfusion reaction. In addition, the quality of autologous blood is morphologically, physiologically, and biochemically superior to that of allogeneic blood. A study involving patients having CABG demonstrated that the autotransfusion of shed mediastinal blood reduced the amount of allogeneic blood used postoperatively with no significant difference in hematological data during a 3-month follow-up period.[16]

Platelets in autologous blood remain viable with nearly normal platelet count and function. 2,3-DPG, which is essential to adequate tissue oxygenation, is within normal levels in fresh autologous blood. Fresh autotransfused erythrocytes have a near-normal survival time. Also, levels of clotting factors V (labile factor), VIII (antihemophilic factor), and IX (Christmas factor) remain near normal in autologous blood but not in allogeneic blood. In addition, autologous blood has normal partial thromboplastin time and potassium and ammonia levels, and is near body temperature.

Mediastinal blood is defibrinated by its contact with serosal surfaces and the beating action of the heart. Defibrinated blood is devoid of fibrinogen with prolonged prothrombin activity (30%–50% of normal) and partial thromboplastin time and increased levels of fibrin split products. This eliminates the need for use of regional anticoagulants in most shed blood. Values usually return to normal by the second postoperative day (Table 17–8).

Hemolysis, the primary effect of autotransfusion systems on blood, causes a reduction in hematocrit, an increase in serum and urine hemoglobin, and accumulation of erythrocyte debris. Correct collection techniques, filtration, and washing procedures reduce the risk of associated pathophysiology.

Equipment Features

A variety of autologous blood transfusion systems (ATS) are available for whole blood autotransfusion and component (washed or processed) autotransfusion. Whole blood autotransfusion is used most frequently with emergency/trauma patients and during the postoperative management of cardiovascular patients. Whole blood systems are easier to set up and use, provide faster access to blood for reinfusion, and return all blood components to the patient.

An inexpensive, disposable, sterile autotransfusion chest drainage unit is most often used to collect whole blood from the mediastinal or pleural cavity after surgery and after emergency hemothorax evacuation. The water seal, usually set to provide a constant negative pressure of 20 cm H_2O to the thoracic cavity, provides a visual confirmation of any air leak. The blood from the chest tubes passes through a gross filter within the chest drainage unit to remove clots and gross debris.[17] Because postoperatively shed mediastinal blood usually is defibrinated, regional anticoagulant seldom is added to the collection chamber. Regional anticoagulant is added routinely to mediastinal–pleural blood that is not defibrinated, such as with emergency hemothorax or postoperative thoracic hemorrhage, where the blood has not remained in the chest cavity long enough to become defibrinated. Unit dose vials of regional anticoagulants are available for syringe transfer into the blood collection chamber or bag. The blood may be reinfused as whole blood using an intermittent or continuous reinfusion technique or transferred to a cell washer system for processing before reinfusion.

The cell washer–processor is used most commonly in operating rooms, blood banks, and for postoperative orthopedic drainage. A cell washer–processor is a centrifuge device that separates the plasma from the red blood cells. The red blood cells are washed and resuspended in normal saline by

---

TABLE 17-8
Comparison of Autologous and Allogeneic Blood

Blood Elements	Autologous Blood	Allogeneic Blood
• Hematocrit (% of RBCs)	22%–30%	41%–45%
• RBC life span	Normal	Decreased
• Platelets	15,000–67,000	0
	Varies with patient status; become viable after infusion	Depleted of viable platelets within 24 h
• 2,3-DPG (oxygen-releasing enzyme in blood)	100%	0%–6%
	Ensures normal delivery of oxygen to the tissues	
• Fibrinogen	Will not clot with normal slow bleeding due to defibrination in chest cavity	More normal clotting as defibrination does not occur; however, anticoagulant prevents clotting
• Clotting factors	Near normal levels	Lower than normal levels
• pH	7.4 (normal)	6.3 (acidotic)
• Anticoagulants	Seldom; ACD or CPD for rapid bleeding PRN	CPD (1:7 ratio)
• Typing and cross-matching	No	Yes

(Adapted with permission by Atrium Medical Corporation, Hudson, NH)

continuous centrifugation. Systems specifically designed for use on orthopedic patients during surgery and for postoperative wound drainage now are available. Devices that wash red blood cells remove approximately 90% of the debris, irrigating solutions, activated clotting and complement factors, anticoagulants, free hemoglobin, platelet aggregates, and hemolyzed red cells. In addition to reducing the risk of microemboli, washed–processed blood provides increased hemoglobin and hematocrit secondary to volume reduction. Enteric contamination is reduced, but not eliminated, by cell washing.

Blood parameters that remain relatively unchanged by cell washing include mean corpuscular volume and 2,3-DPG levels. There may be a slight drop in white blood cells.

Disadvantages of washed–processed blood include cost, complexity, time delay, and loss of clotting factors, white blood cells, plasma proteins, and platelets. Systems now are available for perioperative recovery of platelet-rich plasma, used in conjunction with washed erythrocytes.

Specially trained operators are required for cell washer–processor autologous blood systems. Smaller portable systems with disposable cassettes that are easier and faster to set up are being used more extensively in postanesthesia care units (PACUs) and ICUs.

Indications for and Advantages of Autologous Blood Transfusion

Because of concerns about the risks associated with allogeneic blood, blood quality, and blood shortages, candidates for transfusion should be evaluated for autotransfusion. Autotransfusion offers many advantages to the patient, the staff, and the hospital (see display). Cost savings with ATS are based not only on the cost of a unit of blood, but on the cost of reinfusion equipment, nursing time, the risk of infectious diseases to patient and staff, and avoiding other complications of allogeneic blood transfusion.

Contraindications to Autologous Blood Transfusion

The use of postoperative shed blood my be contraindicated in some clinical situations. Contraindications are listed in the accompanying display. Excessive hemolysis, such as

---

RED FLAG ! Contraindications to Autotransfusion

- Malignancy
- Sepsis
- Enteric contamination
- Coagulopathy or DIC
- Pulmonary/respiratory infection or infestation
- Impaired renal function
- Intraoperative thoracic/mediastinal cavity use of topical agents or antibiotics

---

found in injuries more than 6 hours old, is also a contraindication to autotransfusion.

Contamination of the blood with abdominal contents, such as feces, urine, or bile, is a relative contraindication. If allogeneic blood is available, its use is recommended. Cell washing reduces but does not eliminate enteric contamination. When contamination of the blood is suspected, autologous blood is used only if failure to transfuse would be life threatening.

Procedure

Many different autotransfusion systems and methods are used before and during surgical procedures, including predeposit phlebotomy (autodonation or predonation),[18] perioperative phlebotomy with hemodilution,[19] and intraoperative autotransfusion.[20]

PREDEPOSIT PHLEBOTOMY (AUTODONATION OR PREDONATION)

Predeposit phlebotomy involves the collection of one or more units of whole blood, red blood cells, plasma, or platelets before an elective surgical procedure for retransfusion into the same person during or after the surgical procedure. Standards for autologous blood donors have been established by the American Association of Blood Banks.

Autologous blood donors often take iron supplements before donation and may continue the supplements if indicated. Autologous blood donors are encouraged to drink fluids immediately before and after phlebotomy. In some instances, IV fluids, usually normal saline, are administered to prevent hypovolemia in older or underweight patients.

PERIOPERATIVE PHLEBOTOMY WITH HEMODILUTION

Perioperative phlebotomy with hemodilution is used primarily with open heart surgery. One or two units of blood is withdrawn immediately after induction of anesthesia and before heparinization. The blood is replaced with equivalent amounts of crystalloids or colloids, such as Ringer's lactate, 5% serum albumin, or 5% dextran, to produce normovolemic anemia. This replacement decreases the blood viscosity, decreasing the workload on the heart and increasing

---

Advantages of Autotransfusion

Elimination of disease transmission
Elimination of transfusion reaction
Absence of anticoagulants
Availability
Superior blood quality
Reduction of religious objections
Conservation of bank blood
Cost effectiveness

microcirculation. All blood removed is reinfused into the patient during surgery, usually after reversal of heparin. Because this blood has not been exposed to air, damaged tissue, or CPB equipment, it contains labile plasma coagulation factors, platelets, and fresh red blood cells. The patient may be given a diuretic after surgery to lower plasma volume before reinfusion of the autologous blood.

INTRAOPERATIVE AUTOTRANSFUSION

Intraoperative autotransfusion usually consists of collecting anticoagulated blood during surgery, processing the cells, and reinfusing whole blood or washed, packed red blood cells in the operating room. Pooled blood is aspirated from a body cavity during surgery and reinfused during or after the procedure. Regional anticoagulation of the aspirated blood with citrate phosphate dextrose (CPD), acid citrate dextrose (ACD), or heparin is routine. This regional anticoagulation is used most often during thoracic and cardiovascular surgery. Its use also has been reported with gastric liver resection, orthopedic surgery (hip resection), gynecological surgery (for ruptured ectopic pregnancy), and neurosurgical (spinal fusion) procedures.

The use of intraoperative ATS is increasing as a means of preventing the transmission of viral diseases, such as hepatitis C, decreasing perioperative infections secondary to the immunosuppressive effects of allogeneic blood and decreasing costs.[21]

POSTOPERATIVE AUTOTRANSFUSION

Collection (Blood Recovery)

Autotransfusion with shed mediastinal blood was initially reported in 1978.[16] Postoperative autotransfusion chest drainage systems are used to collect shed mediastinal blood through chest tubes after cardiac surgery. Multipurpose systems combine standard water-seal chest drainage with a system for collecting, filtering, and reinfusing autologous blood. These systems can be set up in approximately 5 to 10 minutes.[22] Aseptic technique is used with all autotransfusion procedures. Anticoagulation usually is not required because shed mediastinal blood is normally defibrinated. The autologous blood may be reinfused as whole blood or washed (component) blood. The use of regional anticoagulants may be indicated in patients with rapid blood loss (> 100 mL/h) through chest tubes, as with postoperative hemorrhage or hemothorax. With rapid blood loss, the blood may not be in contact with the serosal surfaces of the lung long enough to defibrinate. The aggressive stripping (milking) of chest tubes may cause the blood to be removed from the mediastinum before it has become defibrinated, causing clotting of shed blood.

Depending on the system used, the blood is collected in a single-use blood bag that is attached to a chest-drainage unit or in a chamber specifically designed for the collection of blood for reinfusion (Fig. 17–24). If a regional anticoagulant is ordered, it may be placed into the blood bag through the infusion port either before or during blood collection. The patient's shed blood will pass through a gross

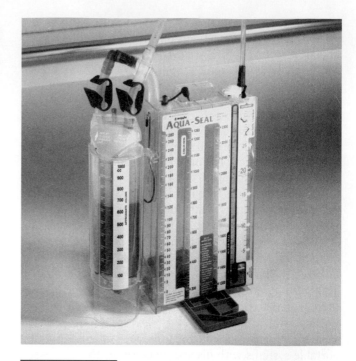

FIGURE 17-24
Autotransfusion chest drainage unit with water-seal chest drainage system for collection and reinfusion of shed mediastinal/pleural cavity blood. (Argyle Aqua-Seal Autotransfusion Chest Drainage Unit. Courtesy of Sherwood-Davis & Geck, St. Louis, MO)

filter located within the blood bag, which removes large blood clots and other debris. Most units have safety overflow designs that divert blood into the chest-drainage unit if the filter clogs, facilitating replacement of the blood bag, and continuous chest drainage. Reinfusion of the blood is based on volume, time, and method, using a gravity, pressure, or continuous reinfusion technique.

REGIONAL ANTICOAGULANTS

Regional (local) anticoagulants (CPD, citrate phosphate dextrose adenine, ACD, ADSOL, Nutricel, and Optisol), may be added directly to the ATS collection system for mixture with the harvested blood to prevent or minimize clotting after heparin reversal with protamine postoperatively, during thoracic hemorrhage and evacuation of traumatic hemothorax. CPD, the same anticoagulant used in allogeneic blood, and ACD-A are the most commonly used regional anticoagulants. The usual ratio and maximum recommended dosage is one part anticoagulant to seven parts blood, the same ratio used in allogeneic blood. The citrate chelates calcium, preventing the blood from coagulating, with the dextrose and phosphate providing metabolic support of the blood. Because rapid infusion of anticoagulated blood may cause citrate toxicity and myocardial depression, blood pH and serum calcium levels are analyzed during rapid infusions, and the patient is monitored for hypotension, narrowed pulse pressure, elevated pulmonary artery pressure, dysrhythmias, stomach cramps, and tingling around the mouth.[23] Cardiovascular patients receiving intraoperative autotransfusion are usually systemically anticoagulated with heparin during surgery. Heparin prevents clotting by interfering with the formation of thromboplastin and thrombin. When the heparin is reversed during surgery, a regional anticoagulant is added to the autologous blood collection system.

REINFUSION

The three methods for reinfusing autologous blood are continuous, by gravity, or pressure cuff. It is recommended that autologous blood be reinfused within 4 to 6 hours of initiating blood collection. A 20- to 40-µm depth or screen microaggregate filter is used for reinfusion so that microaggregate debris (consisting of degenerating platelets, white cells, red cells, fibrin, and fat particles) can be eliminated. Adult respiratory distress syndrome has been reported less frequently with filtered autologous blood than with allogeneic blood.

Before initiation of reinfusion by gravity or pressure cuff, all air is removed from the blood collection system (Fig. 17–25). Although mediastinal blood usually is defibrinated, some clotting may occur. The presence of clots in the gross filter is not a contraindication to reinfusion of the shed mediastinal blood. Reinfusion may be expedited by placement of the blood in a pressure administration cuff inflated to a maximum of 150 mmHg.

Continuous Reinfusion Method

This method facilitates continuous collection and continuous reinfusion of blood adjusted to the amount of blood loss and need for volume replacement. Advantages of this method include providing continuous infusion of fresh blood; reducing the amount of nursing time required, resulting in cost savings; eliminating the need for new blood bags and microaggregate blood filter and IV sets for each infusion; and using a closed system, which reduces the risks of system contamination and exposure of personnel to blood.

For continuous autotransfusion, a blood-compatible bedside infusion pump with a bubble-detector (air-in-line pump alarm) is added to the postoperative autotransfusion system. The pump should be located below the level of the patient's chest. Defibrinated blood may be reinfused directly from the postoperative autotransfusion chest drainage unit chamber or bag being used for collection. A microemboli blood filter and nonvented, blood-compatible IV administration set primed with saline connects the spike port of the collection chamber to the infusion pump. The pump is set with "volume to be infused" and "ml per hour rate." Continuous autotransfusion systems are used most commonly during short periods (< 24 hours) of blood loss. A typical reinfusion cycle lasts 1 hour, during which the previous hour's blood collection is reinfused.

If a regional anticoagulant has been added, it is recommended that the collection unit be separated from the chest drainage unit before reinfusion; this facilitates maintaining the 1:7 ratio between anticoagulant and collected blood. The pump is programmed to reinfuse continuously the

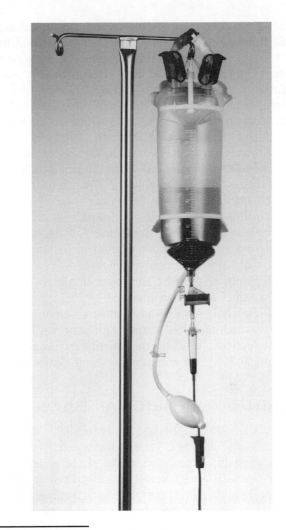

FIGURE 17-25
Reinfusing autologous blood with pressure infusion cuff inflated to a maximum of 150 mmHg for rapid reinfusion of blood.

amount collected in one collection device, whereas a second device is used to continue collection.

EMERGENCY AUTOTRANSFUSION

Emergency autotransfusion is categorized as postoperative autotransfusion. Although most commonly used for hemothorax, emergency autotransfusion also can be used in primary injuries of the lungs, liver, chest wall, heart, pulmonary vessels, spleen, kidneys, inferior vena cava, and iliac, portal, and subclavian veins.

Because the source of bleeding is not always apparent in an emergency situation, a regional anticoagulant, most commonly CPD or ACD, is added to the collection device before or during blood collection. Although a 1:7 ratio of CPD to blood usually is used, ranges between 1:7 and 1:20 are acceptable. If the blood is known to be mediastinal in origin and defibrinated, regional anticoagulants sometimes are omitted.

Blood usually is collected through chest tubes into a sterile, disposable liner with a gross particulate filter (170 µm) that has been primed with CPD or ACD. A vacuum of 10 to 30 mmHg is maintained so that hemolysis can be reduced. Should there be a loss of vacuum during blood collection, the chest tube must be clamped immediately. Failure to do so may result in pneumothorax. Before discontinuing autotransfusion vacuum, an underwater seal must be established.

During aspiration of blood, the quantity of added anticoagulant is controlled to provide approximately 100 mL of anticoagulant for every 700 mL of blood.

Reinfusion is initiated when all blood is evacuated from the site, when immediate transfusion is clinically indicated, or when the autotransfusion collection liner is full.

A microaggregate (microemboli) filter and recipient set are attached to the disposable autotransfusion collection container, usually a flexible, sterile liner. All air should be removed from the blood container before initiation of reinfusion so that risk of air emboli is reduced.

Blood pumps or pressure administration cuffs may be used to expedite rapid blood infusion.

Although whole blood is used most commonly in an emergency situation, a cell washer–processor may be used in selected patients to salvage the patient's erythrocytes for reinfusion and discard contaminants and debris in the plasma.

WOUND DRAINAGE AUTOTRANSFUSION

Orthopedic autotransfusion systems are available for postoperative wound drainage. Various-size wound drains are placed during hip, knee, and spinal surgery. The sanguineous wound drainage usually is washed before reinfusion to prevent platelet or complement activation. Activation of the complement cascade and complement-induced granulocyte aggregation may be a mechanism of noncardiogenic pulmonary edema.

Assessment and Management
GENERAL MEASURES

Before using autotransfusion, hospital protocols for infection control, blood anticoagulation, collection, reinfusion, and disposal of blood and ATS devices should be reviewed. In some hospitals, unused autologous blood is sent to the blood bank for use as allogeneic blood. The practice of crossing over of autologous blood is controversial at this time.[24] The changing health care environment includes an increased awareness of issues of blood safety, blood conservation, blood costs, and medicolegal aspects of blood transfusion. A malpractice jury award of $12 million was based on a physician ordering a unit of allogeneic blood when autologous units may have been sufficient.[25] The decision of when and how to transfuse is made on clinical assessment and evaluation of the adequacy of oxygen delivery against risks associated with transfusion.

RECORD KEEPING

Patient records should include laboratory values, such as platelet count and hemoglobin; the amount of whole blood or washed components reinfused; the length of time between initial collection of autologous blood and completion of reinfusion; and disposition of unused blood. The type and amount of anticoagulant used in whole blood reinfusion are noted. The amount of vacuum used and any complications encountered, such as clots, are recorded. When the continuous method of reinfusion is used, the reinfusion rate per hour, which is usually the amount collected during the previous hour, is recorded hourly.

Complications Associated With Autologous Blood Transfusion

Although autologous blood transfusion has proven to be safe and effective, some adverse reactions have been reported with the procedures. These include hemolysis, air and particulate emboli, coagulation, and thrombocytopenia. Knowledgeable selection of equipment used according to the manufacturer's instructions makes risks negligible. Nursing diagnoses and collaborative problems for patients undergoing autologous blood transfusion are listed in the display.

COAGULOPATHY

Although the incidence is small, coagulopathy associated with autologous blood collection and reinfusion techniques, multiple transfusions, hypothermia, and shock has been reported. When a preexisting blood dyscrasia or clotting anomaly is present, the risk of hemorrhage and prolonged clotting times is increased by reinfusing autologous blood that lacks the necessary clotting factors.

The incidence of coagulopathy has been reduced by the use of autologous perioperative plasmapheresis. To obtain 600 to 1,000 mL of platelet-rich plasma, approximately 20% of the total blood volume is used. For patients with normal weight, body build, hematocrit, and cardiovascular compliance, this volume usually is well tolerated. Because heparin may activate platelets and cause a hypercoagulable state, ACD is the recommended anticoagulant. The temperature of the platelet-rich plasma should be maintained at 36° to 37°C before reinfusion.

Troubleshooting

Table 17–9 outlines some guidelines for troubleshooting problems with autotransfusion.

CLINICAL APPLICATION:
Examples of Nursing Diagnoses and Collaborative Problems for Patients Undergoing Autologous Blood Transfusion

Fluid Volume Excess related to autologous blood transfusion

Risk for Infection related to vascular access line

Risk for Altered Body Temperature related to reinfusion of autologous blood or infection

Knowledge Deficit related to risks of transfusion

TABLE 17-9
Autotransfusion Troubleshooting Guidelines

Complication	Cause	Intervention
Coagulation	Insufficient anticoagulant added	Add regional anticoagulant such as CPD or ACD at a ratio of 1:7 CPD to blood. Shake collection device periodically to mix blood and regional anticoagulant.
	Mediastinal blood not defibrinogenated	Check reversal of heparin. Strip chest tubes PRN only.
Hemolysis	Blood trauma secondary to turbulence or roller pumps	Avoid using equipment containing roller pumps. Maintain vacuum below 30 mmHg when collecting blood from chest tubes.
Coagulopathies	Hypothermia, shock, multiple transfusions	Patients autotransfused with more than 4,000 mL of blood may require transfusion of fresh frozen plasma or platelet concentrate.
	Decreased levels of platelets and fibrinogen	
	Platelets trapped in filters	
	Increased levels of fibrin split products	
Particulate and air emboli	Microaggregate debris	Wash blood as indicated. Use 20 to 40 µm microaggregate filter during reinfusion.
	Air emboli	Use only infusion pumps with a bubble detector system. Remove air from blood bags and IV circuit prior to reinfusion. Use nonvented, blood-compatible IV set.
Sepsis	Breakdown of aseptic technique	Use broad-spectrum antibiotics as indicated. Maintain good aseptic technique. Reinfuse within 4 to 6 h of initial collection.
	Contaminated blood	Avoid use of blood from infected areas and/or with known contaminants, such as stool and urine.
Citrate toxicity (rare and unpredictable)	Chelating effect of citrate in the CPD/ACD on calcium	Monitor for hypotension, dysrhythmias, and myocardial contractility; when more than 2,000 mL of CPD anticoagulated blood is given over a 20-min period, calcium chloride may be given prophylactically.
	Hyperkalemia, hypocalcemia, acidosis, hypothermia, myocardial dysfunction, and liver or renal dysfunction disposing factors	Slow down or stop CPD infusion; correct acidosis. Monitor toxicity with frequent blood gases and serum calcium levels.
Gradual rise of blue water in water seal chamber during continuous ATS	Negative pressure caused by volume of blood being reinfused greater than volume of blood being drained from chest tube	Depress negative pressure relief valve periodically (manual vent).

CPD, citrate-phosphate-dextrose; ACD, acid-citrate-dextrose.

◼◼ CONCLUSION

Autotransfusion is a safe, cost-effective method for conserving blood and reducing the risks associated with allogeneic (homologous, bank, donor) blood transfusion in selected patients. Although prevention of the transmission of transfusion-related HIV was a catalyst to the development and growth of autologous blood transfusion, concern about AIDS is not the major indication for autotransfusion. Substituting autologous blood transfusion for allogeneic blood transfusion potentially eliminates risk of disease transmission, post-transfusion immunosuppression, and transfusion reaction associated with allogeneic blood transfusion.

Autologous blood is life saving for patients who are bleeding rapidly and for those who have rare blood types. The blood is compatible and often immediately available, saving allogeneic blood for use when no other alternative is available. A comprehensive blood recovery program uses both perioperative and intraoperative autologous blood transfusion systems to minimize the use of allogeneic blood and reduce transfusion-related costs.

Cardiopulmonary Resuscitation

For nearly 40 years, CPR has been in use. Success rates, defined as return of adequate vital signs with long-term survival without disabling complications, remain distressingly low. The procedure is based on external cardiac massage, begun in 1960, and IV drug use, which has been updated continuously over the decades. Many other interventions have been introduced from time to time, but only a few have proven useful.

Out-of-hospital cardiac arrests have gained more attention recently, especially those without acute myocardial infarction. These patients usually are candidates for more intense investigation of their dysrhythmia potential and frequently undergo electrophysiological studies. Ongoing clinical studies will clarify the best approach to these patients.

Some of the common terms associated with CPR are defined in the following paragraphs.

Cardiac arrest is the abrupt cessation of effective cardiac pumping activity, resulting in cessation of circulation. There are only two types of cardiac arrest: cardiac standstill (asystole) and ventricular fibrillation (plus other forms of ineffective ventricular contraction, such as ventricular flutter and ventricular tachycardia). The condition called profound cardiovascular collapse is not specifically included because its recognition and definition are nebulous, and management is less specific. One form, called *cardiogenic shock*, is discussed in Chapters 20 and 49.

Resuscitation, liberally interpreted, is the restoration of vital signs by mechanical, physiological, and pharmacological means. The application of CPR is made possible by the concept of clinical versus biological death.

Clinical death is defined as the absence of vital signs, and *biological death* refers to irreversible cellular changes. As determined experimentally and clinically, the interval between clinical and biological death is approximately 4 minutes. The following section addresses major features of CPR.

Indications and Contraindications

It is easier to determine who should *not* be resuscitated than who should be resuscitated. People who should not be resuscitated include those with known terminal illness and those who have been clinically dead for longer than 5 minutes. Both represent situations in which resuscitation likely would prove impossible, and survival would be brief and meaningless.

All others should be regarded as candidates for resuscitation. Resuscitation always can be abandoned, but it cannot be instituted after undue delay.

The term *the very elderly* often is used to differentiate likely degrees of vitality and therefore of survival probability. On the surface, this is perhaps reasonable, but age alone should rarely, if ever, determine treatment. Regardless of chronological age, an older person is a candidate for resuscitation unless that person has clearly stated otherwise in the presence of witnesses.

The Hospital Resuscitation Team

An organized approach to resuscitation is essential. Resuscitation should be conducted by a team made up of trained personnel, including nurses, physicians, ECG technicians, respiratory therapists, and unlicensed personnel to transport special instruments (eg, defibrillators, pacemakers, and special tray sets). Unlicensed personnel also are helpful in making phone calls and performing other miscellaneous duties that are a necessary part of every resuscitation attempt. In some hospitals, a patient representative is a member of the team. The patient representative provides support to the family and keeps the family informed of what is occurring.

A common method of organizing a resuscitation team is to designate specific people who will respond to all cardiac emergencies; this works well, but it is not the only method, nor is it always feasible. The following is an illustration of a successful method of resuscitation geared to an institution with trained resuscitative personnel. The team includes a nurse who serves as the primary member. The first nurse present becomes the initial captain of the team, who also institutes the resuscitation attempt as outlined.

A single call by anyone should immediately summon the entire team and those who will immediately transport the necessary equipment (defibrillator, monitor, and pacemaker instrument) to the site of the emergency.

An important member of the team is the hospital operator, who must immediately alert the entire team in preference to all other duties. A single digit on the telephone dial should be used to alert the operator. The hospital operator often will know where to find key physician members of the team and can summon them individually.

Hospitals with house officers who carry emergency electronic communication equipment can be alerted directly.

Many smaller institutions, however, may have only nursing personnel and well-trained technicians available in the institution who initiate resuscitation efforts until a physician arrives.

Two additional factors are crucial to the team's success. The team must have a definite routine that is kept up to date by all members. Furthermore, nursing personnel and other key nonphysician members must be sanctioned to act spontaneously.

Assessment of Cardiac Arrest

The recognition of cardiac arrest depends on the finding of signs of absence of circulation:

- Unconscious state preceded by less profound states of mental obtundation
- Pulselessness
- Dilated pupils
- Minimal or absent respirations

Pulselessness is best determined by palpation of either the carotid or femoral arteries. Palpation of the carotid almost always is immediately available, whereas palpation of the femoral is not. Brachial or radial pulse palpation is of lesser value. Pulselessness should not be determined by attempting to obtain a blood pressure nor by merely viewing a monitor.

The pupils require a certain amount of time to dilate, which has been estimated at approximately 45 seconds but may be longer than 1 minute. It therefore occasionally may be a valuable sign for pinpointing the time of cardiac arrest.

Inadequate respiratory excursions may be noted in the early seconds of cardiac arrest, and these should not cause delay in recognition of the other signs. Respiratory distress may quickly progress to apnea.

Procedure for Cardiopulmonary Resuscitation

The Advanced Cardiac Life Support (ACLS) guidelines developed by the American Heart Association for adult emergency cardiac care (the Universal Algorithm and the Asystole Treatment Algorithm) are outlined in Figure 1 of Appendix 1. Related ACLS guidelines can also be found in Appendix 1.

There are two hospital settings in which health care personnel may encounter a person in need of CPR: that of a patient whose ECG is being monitored continuously, as in the ICU, and that in an area where the patient is not under continuous monitoring, such as a regular hospital room or unit.

For the continuously monitored patient, the dysrhythmia sets off the alarm, and if ventricular fibrillation is confirmed, CPR is initiated until the defibrillator is readied for use. The patient is immediately defibrillated, after which a physician and the team are summoned.

The following steps are those used for CPR in the unmonitored patient.

DETERMINE RESPONSIVENESS

The rescuer who encounters an adult victim of collapse should first determine the patient's level of responsiveness. A "shake and shout" maneuver is used. If the patient is responsive, the patient is closely monitored, and appropriate treatment as indicated is initiated promptly. If the patient is unresponsive, actions to obtain help are begun.

CALL FOR HELP

To call for help, the rescuer simply relays the cardiac arrest message to a member of the hospital personnel using the appropriate terminology for the institution, such as "code zero" or "red alert." The second individual then places the emergency call to bring the team together, being certain to relate the exact location of the patient.

POSITION THE VICTIM

The patient should be placed in a supine position on a firm, flat surface. This position enables the rescuer to open the airway and assess for the presence and effectiveness of any spontaneous breathing. If the patient is in a standard hospital bed, a resuscitation board should be placed under the torso of the victim when help arrives. If the patient is in a specialty bed, the CPR setting on the bed is selected.

If the patient is found to be breathing effectively and there is no evidence of trauma, the patient is placed in the recovery position. The recovery position is used to reduce the possibility of airway obstruction by the tongue or by secretions or emesis. To place the patient in the recovery position, the rescuer kneels next to the shoulder of the patient. The rescuer lifts the arm of the patient nearest the rescuer and bends it at the elbow. The arm is then positioned so that the patient's palm of the hand is turned upward and moved toward the patient's face. The rescuer then lifts the leg of the patient furthest from the rescuer and crosses it over the patient's body, moving it toward the rescuer. One hand of the rescuer will support the patient's head during turning and the second hand will be used to turn the patient's hips toward the rescuer.

ESTABLISH AN ADEQUATE AIRWAY

Artificial ventilation (by mask or ambu bag) is instituted immediately. The head is tilted back and the chin raised to stretch the airway and advance the tongue in preparation for ventilation (Fig. 17–26). Two complete ventilations are provided. Newer techniques advise a 1.5- to 2-second ventilatory pause and less force and pressure on exhalation so that the esophagus is not opened (which would allow air under pressure into the stomach). Breaths are delivered once every 5 to 6 seconds. Slow full breaths should be delivered to the patient with a duration of 1.5 to 2 seconds per breath.

PERFORM EXTERNAL CARDIAC COMPRESSION

External cardiac compression is a simple technique performed by standing at either side of the patient, placing the

If one person must apply both ventilation and massage, it is best to give two complete ventilations mouth-to-mouth or by other readily available means, followed by 15 external cardiac compressions. This routine may be maintained until additional members of the team arrive. The patient's pulse is checked at regular intervals.

Mechanical compression devices for CPR were developed in the 1960s to decrease the number of people needed to perform CPR and to regulate the rate and depth of compressions. Additional advantages to mechanical compression devices include avoidance of rescuer fatigue, effective delivery of compressions in the obese person, and ability to provide compressions in a moving vehicle. Disadvantages of using mechanical compression devices include the cost of the device, the time required to position the device, the training required to use the device, and the potential for mechanical failure.[1]

The mechanism that results in blood flow during chest compressions is not fully understood.[2] One perspective, the cardiac pump theory, asserts that blood moves as a result of the heart being compressed between the sternum and the vertebral column. A second hypothesis, the thoracic pump theory, contends that blood flow is a result of changes in intrathoracic pressure. This change in pressure is transmitted to vascular structures in the chest, resulting in forward flow of blood.[3] It is likely that both mechanisms play a role in the movement of blood and that the patient's chest size and shape are important determining factors.

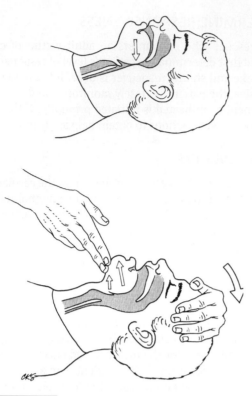

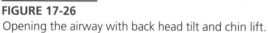

FIGURE 17-26
Opening the airway with back head tilt and chin lift.

heel of one hand two to three finger breadths above the xiphoid process, and placing the heel of the other hand over the first. Firm compressions are applied directly downward, and the sternum is depressed between 1.5 and 2 in and released abruptly. This rhythm is maintained at the rate of 80 to 100 times per minute. A 5:1 compression–ventilation ratio is used with a pause to provide the ventilation. To be effective, this technique must be learned correctly and applied skillfully (Fig. 17–27).

DELIVER AN EXTERNAL COUNTERSHOCK

If indicated, an external countershock should be applied as soon as the instrument is available. The defibrillator paddles are positioned so that the heart is in the current pathway. The anterior apex, also known as the anterolateral or sternum-apex position, is used most often. The anterior paddle is placed firmly on the patient's upper right chest below the clavicle and to the right of the sternum. The apex paddle is

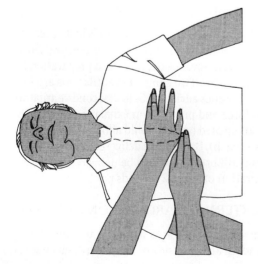

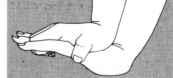

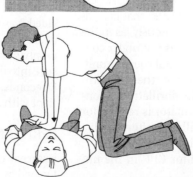

FIGURE 17-27
External chest compression. *Left,* proper hand position over lower portion of sternum; *Right,* correct rescuer position.

positioned firmly on the patient's lower left chest in a mid-axillary line (Fig. 17–28). The initial shock is delivered at 200 J. If subsequent shocks are needed, a second shock is administered at 200 to 300 J, and a third shock is administered at 360 J. All personnel are advised to avoid touching the patient or bed when the shock is delivered. Immediate resumption of artificial circulation and ventilation should occur after each countershock if no pulse returns.

This procedure should be done on a pulseless unresponsive patient, even if the specific rhythm diagnosis is unknown (eg, if there has been a delay in determining this). After the initial countershocks are administered, a specific rhythm diagnosis is used to guide the determination of continued therapy.

Appropriate personnel should demonstrate competence in defibrillation techniques and be expected to execute defibrillation without need of supervision. Regularly scheduled training sessions may be necessary to help staff maintain competency.

In more recent years, automated external defibrillators (AED) have been used rather than manual defibrillators. The AED is a type of defibrillator that is capable of analyzing the patient's rhythm and automatically defibrillating the patient based on specific ECG criteria. In essence, the device, rather than the user, determines the need for defibrillation. The 1993 standards developed by the Association for the Advancement of Medical Instrumentation recommends that the sensitivity (correct identification of ventricular fibrillation) be 90% or more for AEDs and the specificity (correct identification that the rhythm is not ventricular fibrillation) be 95% or more.[4]

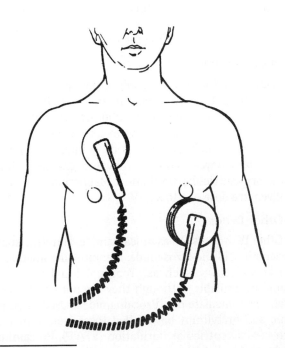

FIGURE 17-28
Standard positioning of defibrillator paddles.

ASSIST WITH ENDOTRACHEAL INTUBATION

Endotracheal intubation is required for the patient in whom spontaneous cardiac rhythm and respiration have not resulted from the measures already outlined. The lung fields should be auscultated immediately following intubation to determine proper placement of the tube. If IV access has not been established, epinephrine, lidocaine, and atropine may be administered through the endotracheal tube. Approximately two and a half times the usual dose is given, and the medication is diluted in 10 mL of normal saline.

ADMINISTER MEDICATIONS

Establishing and maintaining IV access is the responsibility of a very important member of the team—the first nurse who is available after two members are applying ventilation and compression. This person will be in charge of the emergency cart and therefore responsible for preparing the drugs and the IV infusion sets. The importance of this function cannot be minimized because most drug therapy will require IV access and infusion by the most feasible route. To avoid drug interactions due to incompatibilities, it may be necessary to stop the patient's current medications while the emergency medications are delivered. The nurse also is responsible for careful documentation of the time each medication is administered.

The simplest method of all to establish IV access is the insertion of a needle or cannula into an arm vein. Internal jugular or subclavian venipuncture sites are excellent, readily available, and accessible. The internal jugular is used most commonly because it is a simpler approach and recently trained physicians feel more comfortable with it. Both the internal jugular and subclavian sites may be used for rapid infusion, blood withdrawal for laboratory studies, or monitoring of central venous pressure and oxygen saturation.

The intracardiac route or endotracheal route of drug administration should be reserved for situations in which urgency takes precedence over availability of the IV route. This should be a rare occurrence.

Guidelines for the administration of pharmacological therapy are now classified as being "definitely helpful" to "not indicated, may be harmful." (See Fig. 4, Asystole Treatment Algorithm, Appendix 17–1.)

Pharmacological agents and appropriate preparations to be made available immediately include the following:

Epinephrine

Epinephrine in a 1:10,000 aqueous solution is given if ventricular fibrillation persists after defibrillation. This drug has been used in cardiac arrest due to its beta-adrenergic effect. More recent evidence suggests that its alpha-adrenergic effect is the basis for its effectiveness. The dose of epinephrine is 1 mg, which can be repeated every 3 to 5 minutes. Experience with high-dose epinephrine has yielded results that support further study. The use of up to 5 mg IV epinephrine every 3 to 5 minutes is considered "acceptable, possibly helpful." Defibrillation is repeated at 360 J 30 to 60 seconds after the drug is administered.

If cardiac standstill is present, epinephrine (1:10,000) should be given routinely, usually 1 mg IV, and artificial ventilation and circulation should be continued; if unsuccessful, epinephrine should be repeated every 3 to 5 minutes. Possible causes should be determined and treated (see Fig. 1 in Appendix 17–1).

Lidocaine

Lidocaine should be given next at doses of 1 to 1.5 mg/kg IV push and repeated in 3 to 5 minutes up to a dose of 3 mg/kg. A single dose of 1.5 mg/kg in cardiac arrest is acceptable. The agent should be allowed to circulate for 1 minute before defibrillation is again attempted. If a normal rhythm is restored, a lidocaine drip should be started at 2 to 4 mg/min.

Bretylium Tosylate

Bretylium tosylate is a second-line antiarrhythmic used in ventricular fibrillation when lidocaine has failed to convert the life-threatening dysrhythmia. Bretylium often causes hypotension and has a delayed onset (often 20 minutes), requiring resuscitative efforts to continue until the drug's action is apparent.

Bretylium's actions are complex and include adrenergic influences that give it a modest inotropic effect (unlike other antiarrhythmics). Its major action is a striking antifibrillatory effect produced by prolongation of both the action potential duration and the effective refractory period. Occasionally, it causes defibrillation without use of countershock. This sharp rise in threshold for ventricular fibrillation and ventricular tachycardia makes bretylium extremely effective when these rhythm disturbances are recurrent, and it is becoming the drug of choice in this circumstance. Bretylium is given by IV bolus, in a usual dose of 5 mg/kg IV push. It can be repeated in 5 minutes at 10 mg/kg up to a total dose of 35 mg/kg.

Sodium Bicarbonate

Sodium bicarbonate in a 5% solution may be given in 50-mL prefilled syringes in a dose of 1 mEq/kg and may be repeated every 10 minutes based on individualized patient assessment. Sodium bicarbonate administration is classified as "acceptable, probably helpful" in the following situations: if there is a known preexisting bicarbonate-responsive acidosis, if the patient overdosed with tricyclic antidepressants, or if there is a need to alkalinize the urine in a drug-overdose patient. The administration of sodium bicarbonate is considered "acceptable, possibly helpful" if the patient is intubated and there has been a continued long arrest interval or on return of spontaneous circulation after a long arrest interval. In the situation of hypoxic lactic acidosis, sodium bicarbonate administration is classified as "not indicated, may be harmful."

It has been argued that giving sodium bicarbonate IV results in a rise in $PaCO_2$ (by the reaction $HCO_3 + H \rightarrow H_2CO_3 \rightarrow H_2O + CO_2$) and an increase in osmolality. For this reason, this alkalizing agent has been reexamined and is used less frequently for cardiac arrest. Usually, pH, PaO_2, and $PaCO_2$ are followed with arterial blood sampling and often show normal or only moderately abnormal values. Due to the invariably poor perfusion during CPR, venous blood reflects rising $PaCO_2$ from reduced pulmonary perfusion, where CO_2 is normally lost. Thus, adding sodium bicarbonate may worsen this gap, causing deterioration in metabolic status. Sodium bicarbonate is used primarily in patients with hyperkalemia, drug overdose, or in those who were in metabolic acidosis at the time of arrest.

Vigorous correction of metabolic acidosis during a cardiac arrest should be attempted by overventilation with a hand-held ventilation bag. This technique will reduce $PaCO_2$ and hyperinflate the alveoli, while delivering higher levels of PaO_2. If sodium bicarbonate is overused, alkalosis may result. Metabolic alkalosis will shift the oxygen dissociation curve and cause less oxygen to be released from hemoglobin at the tissue level (see Chapter 15). The PaO_2 blood levels may remain high, and the tissue level suffers from hypoxemia.

Calcium Chloride

Calcium chloride is no longer used routinely in CPR. Due to lack of efficacy in clinical studies in cardiac arrest, calcium has fallen into disfavor. Calcium chloride is thought detrimental owing to its raising of plasma levels, and it may even intensify the increased intracellular concentration already present in cardiac arrest victims. Use of calcium chloride is limited largely to instances of hypocalcemia, excessive calcium-channel blockage, and hyperkalemia, although it still is used by some in the presence of electromechanical dissociation.

Isoproterenol

Isoproterenol is not useful as a routine drug in cardiac arrest and is reserved for "medical pacing" in bradycardia for temporarily maintaining the heart rate.

Magnesium Ion

Magnesium ion is second only to potassium in intracellular concentration and is vital in energy metabolism (including membrane transport function). Studies have shown its administration to be effective in certain life-threatening dysrhythmias, such as torsades de pointes (polymorphic ventricular tachycardia) or in a hypomagnesemic state of refractory ventricular fibrillation. Magnesium sulfate may be given in a dose of 1 to 2 g IV.

Other Drugs

Other IV drugs, such as procainamide; diuretics, such as ethacrynic acid and furosemide; mannitol; dexamethasone; and beta-blockers, such as propranolol and metoprolol, should be available, although they are not prepared routinely for immediate use. Procainamide is used when lidocaine and bretyllium have failed to convert ventricular tachycardia/ventricular fibrillation (VT/VF). Procainimide is administered at 20 to 30 mg/min with a maximal dose of 17 mg/kg.

The catecholamine *dopamine* has emerged as perhaps the inotropic agent of choice. Its central inotropic effect is comparable to that of isoproterenol, but it has the advantage of augmenting renal blood flow. Dopamine largely has replaced isoproterenol and norepinephrine for enhancing perfusion pressure (although isoproterenol still is more effective as a temporary medical "pacemaker").

Other drugs that have become useful in cardiopulmonary emergencies include dobutamine and the class called *calcium antagonists* (eg, verapamil). These drugs have not been fully evaluated but are unlikely to be important except in very special situations (eg, recurrent dysrhythmias associated with variant angina). Calcium antagonists may prevent microvascular spasm, a potential factor in ischemia and necrosis. Their use in CPR for this purpose is uncertain, although it appears promising.

Dobutamine, a derivative of isoproterenol, has the advantage of possessing minimal chronotropic effect. When dopamine produces tachycardia, dobutamine may provide potent inotropy without the harmful effects of excess heart rate.

An additional advantage of dobutamine is its effects in reducing PAWP (left sided preload), which may be important in some patients. Thus, dobutamine may be combined with dopamine in certain patients to take advantage of the augmented renal blood flow and reduced PAWP.

Transcutaneous Pacemakers

Transcutaneous pacemakers should be part of the standard equipment available for a patient in cardiac arrest. Large pacing electrodes are positioned externally on the patient's chest and connected to an external pacing device. Many models of defibrillators have the capability to provide transcutaneous pacing. The pacing stimulus is passed through the patient's chest to the heart. The patient may experience chest discomfort with each pacing stimulus. Transcutaneous pacing can be an effective means to pace the heart in an emergency situation until a transvenous pacing wire can be inserted.

Other Possible Procedures

If CPR measures fail, a pericardial tap may be performed, preferably by the subxyphoid route, to treat a possible cardiac tamponade. Although an uncommon factor in cardiac arrest, pericardial tap may result in dramatic recovery. Tamponade is hallmarked by electrical–mechanical dissociation, distended jugular veins, absence of central pulses despite adequate CPR, and inadequate physiological responses to all other therapies.

Other underlying causes requiring immediate treatment also need to be considered in a cardiac arrest situation. A pneumothorax necessitates insertion of chest tubes; pulmonary embolism may require assisted circulation, surgery, thrombolysis, or heparin; and ventricular aneurysm or rupture of papillary muscle or interventricular septum may be treated with assisted circulation or surgery. The nurse also may need to prepare for the insertion of a pulmonary artery catheter or IABP.

Nursing Management

DURING RESUSCITATION

The nurse plays a vital role in the efforts to resuscitate a patient. As mentioned, the nurse often is the one who first assesses the patient and initiates CPR and calling of the team. The patient's primary nurse should be present to answer questions about the arrest. Roles of the nurses who respond to the arrest situation include continuing CPR, monitoring heart rhythm and other vital signs, defibrillating, administering drugs, recording of events, controlling any crowds, and notifying the attending physician and family members. Support to the patient's family and friends is important at this time and should be provided by other nurses and health care professionals until the primary nurse and physician are available to speak with them.

If resuscitation efforts fail, the decision to terminate resuscitative attempts is imminent, based on central nervous system changes or the assumption of a nonviable myocardium. Once the physician pronounces death, the patient's primary nurse and physician should spend time with the patient's family and friends while other nurses and personnel prepare the body. Often family members want to view their lost loved one before they leave the hospital. It is essential that the body be cleaned, all resuscitation equipment removed, and the room straightened.

POSTRESUSCITATION

After a successful resuscitation, the nurse and physician need to monitor closely the vital signs and hemodynamics of the patient and any signs of complications. Prompt recognition and treatment of abnormalities are important in the care and outcome of the patient. The specific approach in the postresuscitative period will depend not only on the patient's condition at the time, but also on the underlying disease process, the previous condition of the patient, and the events in the immediate postresuscitative period.

If there is resumption of spontaneous cardiac activity, the situation should be evaluated thoroughly as to the clinical state, underlying causes, and complicating factors to determine proper management. A portable chest x-ray and arterial blood gases are done. Oxygen therapy is maintained; appropriate IV infusions are continued. Routine measurements in addition to continuous ECG monitoring include frequent blood pressures (ideally done by intra-arterial cannula), hourly urine volumes, frequent beside estimates of tissue perfusion, and central venous pressure and O_2 saturation measurements.

If central nervous system damage is evident, consideration should be given to the administration of mannitol and dexamethasone. If oliguria or anuria is present, large doses of furosemide should be given. If there is no response, management like that used in acute renal failure should be instituted (see Chapter 30).

Complications of Resuscitation

The art of resuscitation has come a very long way; it has changed drastically with time and undoubtedly will continue to do so. Resuscitation has proved its worth beyond doubt. Potential complications include injuries to sternum, costal cartilages, ribs, esophagus, stomach, liver, pleura, and lung, any of which can be serious; permanent central nervous system damage, which renders the patient dependent; and medicolegal considerations. When resuscitation is performed by an organized competent team, these complications can be minimized or avoided.

■ CONCLUSION

Many modifications of the mechanical, pharmacological, and physiological approach to CPR have been instituted in the last several decades. When correct CPR technique is used by competent personnel, the patient's chance of survival is improved. The national initiative to have widespread availability of automated external defibrillators may be the next step in helping cardiac arrest victims have a positive outcome.

Management of Dysrhythmias

Other techniques have been developed for management of dysrhythmias. Those discussed here are cardioversion, radiofrequency ablation, cardiac pacemakers, and implantable defibrillators.

■ CARDIOVERSION

Electrical countershock therapy is useful in converting supraventricular and ventricular dysrhythmias to sinus rhythm, especially when the patient becomes hemodynamically unstable or does not convert to a normal rhythm with pharmacological agents. As opposed to defibrillation, which delivers an unsynchronized current to the heart through the chest wall in an attempt to convert pulseless ventricular tachycardia/fibrillation to sinus rhythm (see section on CPR), cardioversion delivers a shock that is synchronized with the heart's activity. By setting the defibrillator to the synchronized mode, the device detects the patient's R wave and delivers the shock during ventricular depolarization. As a result, there is no danger of the shock being delivered during ventricular repolarization (T wave) which could result in spontaneous ventricular fibrillation. Indications for cardioversion and recommendations for initial joules used are listed in Table 17–10.[1]

The energy needed to convert unstable ventricular tachycardia with a pulse may be as low as 10 J, but often the use of 100 J initially, followed by 200, 300, or 360 J, is necessary for conversion. The energy required for conversion of PSVT and atrial flutter ranges from 50 to 100 J initially. Further increases in energy may be needed for conversion. The energy required to convert atrial fibrillation is greater, starting at 100 J with increases to 360 J if necessary. After conversion to sinus rhythm, further antiarrhythmic therapy should be initiated. Although recommendations are made for the amount of joules needed to convert various rhythms, the actual energy needed varies with the duration of the dysrhythmia, rate, morphology, and underlying cause of the dysrhythmia.

Procedure

The steps for cardioversion are as follows:

1. Restrict the patient's food and water for 6 to 8 hours before cardioversion, unless emergency cardioversion is required.
2. Ideally, withhold digitalis for 24 hours before cardioversion, although cardioversion may be attempted in an emergency situation without this precaution.
3. Explain the procedure to the patient, and obtain informed consent.
4. Record a 12-lead ECG and vital signs, establish an IV line, and ready all necessary resuscitation equipment.
5. Turn on the defibrillator and monitor, and attach the electrodes to the patient's chest to monitor the rhythm. Avoid placing the electrodes in the

TABLE 17-10	
Energy Requirements for Cardioversion	
Indications	**Energy in Joules (J)**
Unstable ventricular tachycardia with a pulse	50–360
Supraventricular tachycardia	75–100
Atrial flutter	25 initially
Atrial fibrillation	100 initially

area where the defibrillation paddles will be positioned. Some devices permit both monitoring and defibrillation through disposable defibrillation patches.

6. Select a monitoring lead that provides a good ECG pattern with a tall R wave. If monitoring by way of the disposable defibrillator patches, select "paddles" lead.

7. Turn on the synchronizer mode button. The size of the R wave may need to be adjusted until the synchronization marker appears on each R wave.

8. Sedate the patient, and maintain an adequate airway.

9. Remove paddles and apply a generous amount of electrode jelly to them, or apply gel pads to the chest wall. This is done to prevent skin burns and decrease electric resistance. Disposable defibrillator patches may be selected rather than using gelled standard paddles.

10. Apply paddles, one just below the right clavicle and the other over the apex of the heart. If anterior–posterior paddles are used, place the anterior paddle over the precordium and the posterior one on the back opposite the anterior one. Make sure the paddles are away from electrode wires and any pacemaker battery.

11. Set the desired energy level.

12. Press the charge button. A light will flash until paddles are fully charged.

13. Reconfirm the synchronization markers on the R waves on the monitor.

14. Call out "clear" to make sure no one is touching the patient or the bed.

15. Discharge the paddles while applying 25 to 30 lb of pressure. Push and hold both paddle discharge buttons until the defibrillator discharges. Maintain contact on the chest wall until the machine has delivered the shock. There will be a momentary delay from the pressing of the discharge button to delivery of the shock because of the synchronization with the R wave. Failure to keep the paddles on the chest can result in failure to cardiovert and burns to the chest.

16. Remove the paddles, and assess the patient's rhythm and vital signs.

17. Subsequent shocks may need to be delivered. If so, be certain to select the synchronized mode.

18. After cardioversion, observe the patient for changes in rhythm, blood pressure, and respirations. Further antiarrhythmic agents may need to be administered to maintain sinus rhythm. Monitor the patient's respiratory status and level of consciousness because sedation was delivered before the procedure. Inspect the chest wall for any signs of burns and treat appropriately.

19. If the patient's rhythm deteriorates to ventricular fibrillation, turn off the synchronizer and immediately defibrillate the patient, starting with 200 J and increasing to 360 J as needed.

20. Clean the paddles thoroughly before storing them in the device.

21. Document the procedure, the outcomes of the procedure, and the patient's status in the medical record.

■ RADIOFREQUENCY CATHETER ABLATION

Radiofrequency catheter ablation is an invasive procedure used for the treatment of dysrhythmias. The technique involves the localized destruction, isolation, or excision of cardiac tissue that is responsible for the initiation or conduction of the dysrhythmia.

Attempts to ablate portions of cardiac tissue were begun in 1964. Direct current countershocks were delivered to the cardiac tissue through a catheter attached to a defibrillator. Because this technique was associated with high mortality and morbidity rates, safer means to ablate tissue were investigated.

Radiofrequency energy is now used as the means to ablate cardiac tissue. A form of electrical energy, radiofrequency energy is produced by high-frequency alternating current that is passed through tissue. Heat is created as the energy dissipates, which results in a small localized lesion in cardiac tissue. If properly targeted, this localized area of damage can prevent the initiation of the dysrhythmia or interrupt the conduction of the dysrhythmia. The amount of heat produced and the size of the resulting lesion depend on the frequency, amount, and duration of the alternating current used. The size and shape of the ablating electrode also influence the resulting lesion.

Indications for Ablation

A PSVT can be treated with radiofrequency ablation. Most PSVT dysrhythmias are caused by either AV *nodal* reentrant tachycardia (AVNRT) or by AV reentrant tachycardia (AVRT). PSVT also can be caused by intra-atrial reentrant tachycardia. Recurrent symptomatic or life-threatening ventricular dysrhythmias also may be indications for ablation.

Reentry occurs in myocardial tissue when conduction of an impulse is slowed or blocked in one direction. Tissue near the slowed area has time to repolarize and may conduct the previously delayed signal in a retrograde (backward) direction. As a result, a circular reentrant pattern of conduction occurs, which is the most common mechanism associated with PSVTs.

ATRIOVENTRICULAR NODAL REENTRANT TACHYCARDIA

Two pathways for conduction exist in the AV node: slow pathways and fast pathways. AVNRT, the most common type of PSVT, occurs when the AV node is stimulated by a premature atrial contraction. The fast pathways of the AV node are still in their repolarization phase and do not conduct the premature atrial impulse. Instead, the impulse travels down the slow pathways of the AV node and activates the ventricles. The impulse then returns to the atria through the fast pathways, which have now completed their repolarization phase. Selective ablation of either the slow or the fast pathways may be used to treat AVNRT.

ATRIOVENTRICULAR REENTRANT TACHYCARDIA

In the normal heart, the AV node and the bundle of His serve as the connection between the atria and the ventricles for the conducting system. AVRT rhythms are characterized by the presence of additional accessory pathways that link conduction between the atria and the ventricles. Conduction through accessory pathways may be from the atria to the ventricles (antegrade conduction), from the ventricles to the atria (retrograde conduction), or in both directions. AVRT rhythms result when circular movement of the impulse occurs because of the ability of the accessory pathways to conduct signals in either direction.

In WPW syndrome, a cardiac congenital abnormality, the person has accessory pathways linking the atria and the ventricles. Because of the presence of these accessory pathways, the person with WPW syndrome is prone to AVRT. Ablation therapy may be used to interrupt the flow of the impulse in the accessory pathway.

ATRIAL FIBRILLATION OR FLUTTER

Ablation therapy may be indicated for patients with atrial fibrillation or flutter with a rapid ventricular response that has not been controlled by pharmacological therapy. Portions of the AV node may be ablated to control the ventricular response. Successful ablation usually results in a nodal rhythm at a rate of 40 to 70 beats/min. A permanent pacemaker also is often inserted to ensure the presence of a reliable rhythm and adequate rate.

VENTRICULAR DYSRHYTHMIAS

The success of ablation for the treatment of ventricular tachycardia depends on the cause of the dysrhythmia. Radiofrequency ablation has been shown to be effective in patients with structurally normal hearts and in patients with ventricular tachycardia due to bundle branch reentry.[1] The technique also has been successful in patients with hemodynamically stable sustained ventricular tachycardia associated with CAD or cardiomyopathy.[1]

Procedure

Several days or just prior to an ablation, the patient will undergo an electrophysiological study (EPS) to evaluate the electrical activity of the heart. The EPS is an invasive test in which catheters are placed in the heart to record intracardiac ECGs. The test provides information about the sequence of activation of the heart during sinus rhythm and any abnormal sequence of activation during a dysrhythmia. (For a more detailed discussion of EPSs, see Chapter 16).

Once a diagnosis of the dysrhythmia is made by EPS, an ablating catheter is positioned in the targeted area of the heart. Four additional catheters are positioned in the right heart to stimulate atrial and ventricular tissue and to help localize the target area. The ablation catheter contains multiple electrodes designed to localize the site of the dysrhythmia and to deliver the ablation current. The shaft of the catheter can be extended or flexed at the tip to provide access to the abnormal tissue and to ensure direct contact with the tissue. Fluoroscopy and the electrogram pattern from the catheter help the physician determine the appropriate target area.

Once all catheters are positioned, a loading dose of heparin is administered, and a continuous heparin infusion is initiated. Baseline ECG recordings are made from the surface electrodes on the patient's chest and from the intracardiac electrodes. A programmed electrical stimulation (PES) is then performed to induce the dysrhythmia so that its mechanism and pathway can be evaluated. Next, the radiofrequency current is applied for about 30 seconds. Enough lesions are created until the abnormal conducting tissue is eliminated. Successful elimination of the target site is determined by examining the surface and intracardiac tracings. When the procedure is finished, the intracardiac catheters and arterial sheath are removed, and efforts to attain hemostasis at the insertion site are implemented.

Nursing Management

The nurse plays a vital role in the care of the patient undergoing radiofrequency ablation. In collaboration with the physician, the nurse will provide information for the patient and family about what to expect before, during, and after the procedure. The psychosocial support provided by the nurse may be key in helping the patient and family cope with the uncertainties of dysrhythmia management.

PREABLATION

The nurse participates in educating the patient and family about radiofrequency ablation. The accompanying display provides a guide for patient and family education. During the preablation period, the nurse records a 12-lead ECG, continuously monitors the patient's cardiac rhythm, and treats any dysrhythmias per the physician's orders. Other baseline data obtained include vital signs, breath sounds, fluid status, serum chemistries, prothrombin time, and complete blood counts. Antiarrhythmic drugs are usually stopped 2 to 3 days before the procedure. The patient receives nothing by mouth for about 8 hours before the procedure. Because of x-ray exposure during the test, it is important to verify that a female patient is not pregnant. No activity restrictions are imposed before the procedure.

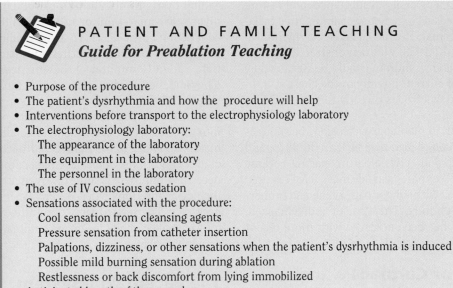

PATIENT AND FAMILY TEACHING
Guide for Preablation Teaching

- Purpose of the procedure
- The patient's dysrhythmia and how the procedure will help
- Interventions before transport to the electrophysiology laboratory
- The electrophysiology laboratory:
    The appearance of the laboratory
    The equipment in the laboratory
    The personnel in the laboratory
- The use of IV conscious sedation
- Sensations associated with the procedure:
    Cool sensation from cleansing agents
    Pressure sensation from catheter insertion
    Palpations, dizziness, or other sensations when the patient's dysrhythmia is induced
    Possible mild burning sensation during ablation
    Restlessness or back discomfort from lying immobilized
- Anticipated length of the procedure
- Potential for placement of a permanent pacemaker

DURING ABLATION

The nurse in the electrophysiology laboratory is responsible for monitoring of the patient throughout the procedure and assisting the physician with necessary interventions. The nurse must be competent in advanced cardiac life support so that an emergency situation can be handled appropriately.

Once the patient arrives in the laboratory, the nurse explains all procedures to the patient and helps to put the patient at ease. The nurse connects the patient to an automatic external defibrillator, physiological recorder, cardiac monitor, automatic blood pressure device, and pulse oximeter. Oxygen is provided by a nasal cannula. If not already in place, an IV line is inserted. IV conscious sedation is administered to ensure patient comfort. A urinary catheter is inserted if the procedure is anticipated to be lengthy. Both groins and the right subclavian sites are shaved and the skin prepared. A sterile field is established and maintained throughout the procedure. A lead apron is placed over the patient's abdomen.

Throughout the procedure, the nurse monitors hemodynamic status, ACT, sedation level, and other parameters. Communication with the patient is essential so that the patient is kept informed about the progress of the procedure, and anxiety and fear are minimized. The nurse also warns the patient that a burning sensation may be felt for a very brief time during the actual ablation.

POSTABLATION

Thorough assessment and monitoring of the patient are continued after the ablation procedure. Essential components of the assessment include vital signs, cardiac rhythm, catheter insertion sites, peripheral pulses, and level of consciousness. The patient may remain drowsy for several hours and experience nausea and vomiting as a result of the

Table 17-11 Potential Complications of Radiofrequency Ablation and Associated Signs and Symptoms

Complications	Signs and Symptoms
Cardiac perforation	Tachycardia, hypotension, dyspnea, pleuritic chest pain
Cardiac tamponade	Hypotension, distended neck veins, muffled heart sounds, pulsus paradoxus, change in level of consciousness
Pneumothorax	Dyspnea, decreased oxygen saturation
Cerebral embolus	Slurred speech, blurred vision, headache, seizures
Pulmonary embolus	Chest pain, dyspnea, tachycardia

medications. When an arterial site has been used, leg immobilization and bed rest are maintained for about 6 hours. If only venous sites were used, the patient may begin ambulation in about 3 to 4 hours. The nurse assesses the patient for any pain or discomfort and provides comfort measures if indicated. Fluid volume status is checked, and when stable, the urinary catheter is removed.

During the postablation period, the nurse carefully assesses the patient for any evidence of complications. Table 17–11 lists potential complications of radiofrequency ablation and associated signs and symptoms.

■ CARDIAC PACEMAKERS

Electrical stimulation of the heart was tried experimentally as early as 1819. In 1930, Hyman noted that he could inject the right atrium with a diversity of substances and restore a heartbeat. He devised an "ingenious apparatus" that he labeled an artificial pacemaker, which delivered a rhythmical charge to the heart. In 1952, Zoll demonstrated that patients with Stokes-Adams syndrome could be sustained by the administration of current directly to the chest wall. In 1957, Lillehei affixed electrodes directly to the ventricles during open heart surgery.

From 1958 to 1961, implantable pacemakers became accepted treatment for complete heart block. In the 1970s and 1980s, AV synchrony and "physiological" pacing became available. Currently, technological advances have resulted in smaller pacemakers with longer battery life and numerous programmable options. The goal of individualized, physiological pacing has been achieved with more recent types of pacemakers.

Indications for Cardiac Pacing

Cardiac pacing is indicated for conditions that result in failure of the heart to initiate or conduct an intrinsic electrical impulse at a rate adequate to maintain perfusion. Pacemakers are necessary when dysrhythmias or conduction defects compromise the electrical system and the hemodynamic response of the heart. The original pacemakers were designed to treat bradydysrhythmia, whereas today's pacemakers are intended to treat bradydysrhythmias and tachydysrhythmias.

Critical care nurses work with members of the health care team to assess potential pacemaker patients who may exhibit dysrhythmias, atherosclerotic heart disease, acute myocardial infarction, or other conditions that alter the conduction of the heart. To assist medical professionals in determining the clinical criteria for pacemaker implantation, a Joint Committee of the American College of Cardiology and the American Heart Association was formed to establish uniform criteria for pacemaker implantation.[1] The committee divided its recommendations for implantation into three classes. Class I includes conditions when a pacemaker implantation is considered necessary. Class II includes conditions when pacemaker implantation may be necessary, but there is some divergence of opinion. Class III includes conditions when pacemaker implantation is not necessary. The revised 1991 Committee recommendations for pacemaker implantation are summarized in the accompanying display.

The Pacemaker System

Consisting of a pulse generator and a lead with electrodes, a pacemaker system performs two main functions: diagnosis and treatment. The diagnostic function is to sense cardiac intrinsic activity; the treatment function is to emit an electrical impulse that excites endocardial cells and produces a wave of depolarization in the myocardium.

THE PULSE GENERATOR

The pulse generator for a permanent pacemaker is composed of a lithium iodide battery source and electronic cir-

---

Indications for Permanent Cardiac Pacing

Disorder

Atrioventricular block

Class I: Symptomatic second-degree AV block; symptomatic complete heart block; asymptomatic complete heart block with a heart rate ≤ 40 beats/min

Class II: Asymptomatic second-degree type II heart block; complete heart block with a heart rate >40 beats/min

Class III: First-degree AV block; asymptomatic type I second-degree AV block

Bifascicular or trifascicular block

Class I: Bifascicular block with intermittent complete heart block associated with symptoms; bifascicular or trifascicular block with intermittent type II second-degree AV block without symptoms

Class II: Bifascicular or trifascicular block associated with syncope; other causes of syncope not identifiable; prolonged His–ventricular (HV) interval on electrophysiological study

Class III: Asymptomatic fascicular block or asymptomatic fascicular block with first-degree AV block

Sinus node dysfunction

Class I: Sinus node dysfunction with documented symptomatic bradycardia

Class II: Sinus node dysfunction with heart rate <40 beats/min with no clear association between symptoms and bradycardia

Class III: Sinus node dysfunction in asymptomatic patients; sinus node dysfunction in patients in whom symptoms are clearly documented not to be associated with bradycardia

Neurogenic syncope

Class I: Recurrent syncope associated with clear, spontaneous events provoked by carotid sinus stimulation, asystole of >3 seconds induced by minimal carotid sinus pressure

Class II: Recurrent syncope without clear, provocative events and a hypersensitive cardioinhibitory response; syncope associated with bradycardia reproduced by a head-up tilt

Class III: Recurrent syncope in the absence of a cardioinhibitory response; a hyperactive cardioinhibitory response in the absence of symptoms

Tachydysrhythmias

Class I: Symptomatic recurrent supraventricular tachycardia when drugs fail to control the dysrhythmia or produce intolerable side effects

Class II: An alternative to drug therapy in patients with recurrent supraventricular tachycardia

Class III: Tachycardias that are accelerated or converted to fibrillation by pacing

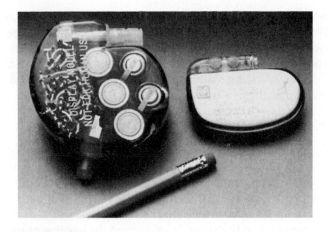

FIGURE 17-29
Permanent pulse generators, old and new. Note the decrease in size and weight that has been achieved over the years. The smaller unit is an example of an activity-responsive pulse generator and is four times smaller than the larger 1968 unit.

cuits enclosed in a hermetically sealed metal container. The generator weighs 20 to 30 g and is 5 to 7 mm thick (Fig. 17–29). The longevity of most permanent pacemakers is about 10 years, depending on the percentage of pacing the heart requires over time. Most permanent pulse generators

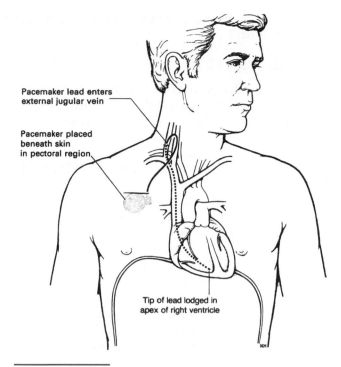

Pacemaker lead enters external jugular vein

Pacemaker placed beneath skin in pectoral region

Tip of lead lodged in apex of right ventricle

FIGURE 17-30
Implanted transvenous pacing electrode and permanent pacemaker generator.

Clinical Terminology Regarding Pacemakers

Active fixation lead
A pacing lead with some design at the lead tip (corkscrew, barbed) that allows the tip to be embedded in heart tissue, thus decreasing the likelihood of dislodgement

Asynchronous pacing
A pacemaker that fires at a fixed rate regardless of the intrinsic activity of the heart

Bipolar lead
A pacing lead containing two electrodes. One electrode is at the tip of the lead and provides stimulation to the heart. A second electrode is several millimeters proximal to the tip and completes the electrical circuit. Both electrodes provide sensing of the intrinsic cardiac activity.

Capture
The depolarization of a cardiac chamber in response to a pacing stimulus

Demand pacing (inhibited pacing)
A pacemaker that withholds its pacing stimulus when sensing an adequate intrinsic heart rate

Dual-chamber pacing (physiological pacing)
Pacing in both the atria and the ventricles to restore artificially atrioventricular synchrony

Electromagnetic interference
Electrical or magnetic energy that can interfere with or disrupt the function of the pulse generator

Milliamperage (mA)
The unit of measure used for the electrical stimulus (output) generated by the pacemaker

Overdrive pacing
A method to suppress a tachycardia by pacing the heart at a rate faster than the patient's intrinsic rate

Oversensing
Inhibition of the pacemaker by events other than those that the pacemaker was designed to sense. These may include tall T waves and electromagnetic interference.

Pacing threshold
The minimum electrical stimulation required to initiate atrial or ventricular depolarization consistently

Passive fixation lead
A pacing lead that lodges in the trabeculae of the heart without actually penetrating the cardiac wall

Rate responsive pacing (rate adaptive, rate modulated)
A pacemaker that alters pacing rate in response to detected changes in the body's metabolic demand

Sensing
The ability of the pacemaker to detect intrinsic cardiac activity and respond appropriately. How the pacemaker responds depends on the programmed mode of pacing.

Sensing threshold
The minimum atrial or ventricular intracardiac signal amplitude required to inhibit or trigger a demand pacemaker

Triggered
A response to sensing in which the pacemaker fires a stimulus in response to intrinsic cardiac activity. In pacemaker terms, triggered is the opposite of inhibited.

Undersensing
Failure of the pacemaker to sense the heart's intrinsic activity. As a result, the pacemaker fires inappropriately.

are inserted into subcutaneous tissue below the clavicle (Fig. 17–30, p. 315).

THE LEAD SYSTEM

The lead is a wire that provides the communication network between the pulse generator and the heart muscle. One or more electrodes are at the distal end of the lead and provide sensing and pacing of the heart muscle. In a bipolar lead, the negative pacing electrode is at the tip and the positive sensing electrode is approximately 1 cm proximal to the tip (Fig. 17–31).

The connecting lead is placed either through a subclavian vein or a cephalic vein through the chest wall. The lead is then threaded through the right atrium into the apex of the right ventricle where the electrode is lodged. The lead must provide adequate electrical conduction, sufficient insulation, and the endurance to withstand pulsatile turbulence.

The lead can be affixed to the myocardium with a lead fixation device. Called active fixation, these devices include screws, barbed tips, tines, or coils (Fig. 17–32). Another alternative is to use passive (smooth tipped) and steroid-eluding electrodes (tips designed to reduce cardiac inflammation) placed in the trabeculae of the heart. Over time, fibrous tissue forms around the tip to secure placement and ensure proper function of the electrode.

Temporary Pacing Systems

Temporary pacemaker systems are used in emergency and elective situations. In life-threatening situations, temporary pacemakers can be used for asystole, complete heart block, severe bradydysrhythmias, or during cardiac arrest. Electively, temporary pacemakers are used while evaluating the need for permanent pacing, after cardiac surgery, or for pace-terminating rapid supraventricular tachydysrhythmias. Temporary pacing systems can be transvenous, epicardial, transcutaneous, or transthoracic.

METHODS OF TEMPORARY PACING

A *transvenous* pacemaker system consists of an external pulse generator and a temporary transvenous pacing wire. The temporary transvenous lead system usually includes the use of a bipolar catheter. A bipolar catheter contains a negative (distal) electrode attached to the negative generator terminal on the pulse generator and the positive proximal electrode attached to the positive generator terminal on the pulse generator.

For temporary transvenous pacing, the catheter is introduced into a superficial vein, using local anesthesia. The brachial, internal jugular, or subclavian veins are the preferred sites. The subclavian and internal jugular sites afford catheter stability and allow for patient mobility. The pacing catheter is threaded through the vein, the vena cava, the right atrium, and into the right ventricle. The catheter tip is placed in contact with the endocardial surface of the right ventricle (Fig. 17–33). The insertion procedure may be done with or without fluoroscopy.

The pulse generator for a transvenous pacing system is an external device powered by a 9-volt replaceable battery (Fig. 17–34). Often called a temporary pacemaker, the device contains several controls that regulate the current output, rate, sensitivity, and the mode of pacing.

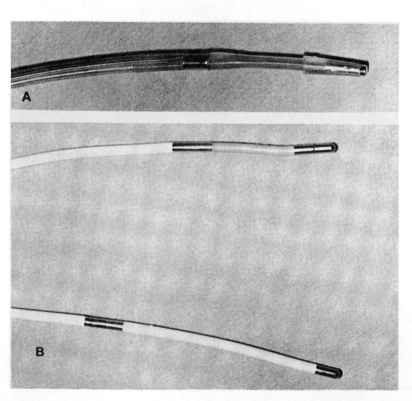

FIGURE 17-31
(**A**) Permanent bipolar pacing catheter. (**B**) Temporary bipolar pacing catheters.

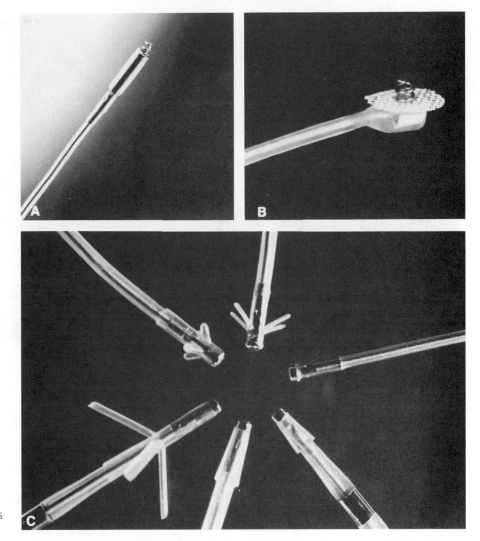

FIGURE 17-32
Lead wires with screws, barbs, or tines ensure fixation to the myocardium.

Placement of *epicardial* wires provides another method for temporary pacing. This method can be accomplished by thoracotomy or through a subxyphoid incision with the placement of pacing electrodes directly on the surface of the heart. Epicardial wires often are used as a temporary adjunct during and after open heart surgery. The pacing wires are sutured or screwed to the epicardial surface of the heart, brought outside through the chest incision, and either connected to a temporary pacemaker generator or capped and then connected if the need arises. An example of a screw-in type electrode is shown in Figure 17–35. The wires are extracted without reopening the incision, even after scar tissue has formed over the tips.

Another method of temporary pacing is known as external *transcutaneous* pacing. This method involves placing large gelled electrode patches directly on the chest wall anteriorly and posteriorly. The electrodes are connected to an external transcutaneous pacemaker (Fig. 17–36). When first developed, transcutaneous pacing required higher amounts of electricity for pacing, resulting in pain, burns, and skeletal muscle twitching. Because of these problems,

the method was abandoned. Today's technology has permitted the use of lower amounts of electrical current, eliminating many of these earlier problems. Transcutaneous pacing is used in an emergency situation until a temporary transvenous wire or a permanent pacemaker can be placed.

Transthoracic pacing is a temporary pacing method used as a last resort in an emergency situation. This method involves introduction of a pacing lead into the heart through a needle in the anterior wall. Transthoracic pacing has limited success rates and a high potential for complications.

Pacemaker Functioning

When the pacemaker system functions appropriately, it will diagnose and treat the heart rhythm dysfunction. To diagnose appropriately, the pacemaker wire must sense the inability of the heart to initiate or conduct an impulse. This ability of the pacemaker to detect the heart's intrinsic activity is known as the *sensing* function of the pacemaker

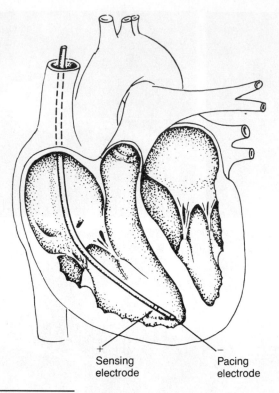

FIGURE 17-33
Transvenous bipolar pacing catheter in place.

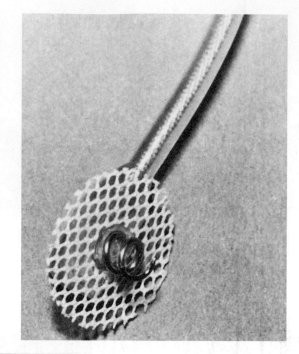

FIGURE 17-35
Screw-in type electrode for permanent epicardial pacing.

system. Once proper sensing occurs, the pacemaker usually will respond by inhibiting a pacing stimulus if the intrinsic activity of the heart is adequate. If the intrinsic rate is not adequate, the pacemaker will function. When the pacemaker fires, a pacemaker artifact known as a pacing spike appears on the ECG, as shown in Figure 17–37. As a result of the firing, the cardiac chamber containing the pacemaker lead will be depolarized. *Capture* is the term used to indicate depolarization of the atria or ventricle in response to a pacing stimulus. The minimal amount of voltage required from the pacemaker to initiate consistent capture is known

as the *pacing threshold*. This threshold level is determined by establishing successful pacing at higher energy and then gradually decreasing the energy output of the generator until capture ceases. The threshold is expressed as milliamperage (mA) at this level. The generator output is then set at several milliamperes above the threshold to allow for the usual increase in threshold level that occurs over a period of time after pacing has been initiated.

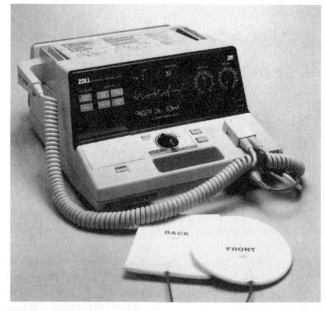

FIGURE 17-36
Commercially available transcutaneous cardiac pacing generator and surface patch electrodes.

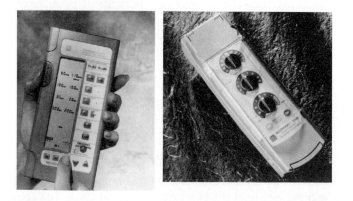

FIGURE 17-34
Two types of temporary pacemakers. (**A**) Microprocessor-based single chamber pacemaker. (**B**) description of this pacemaker photo. Courtesy of Medtronic, Minneapolis, MN.

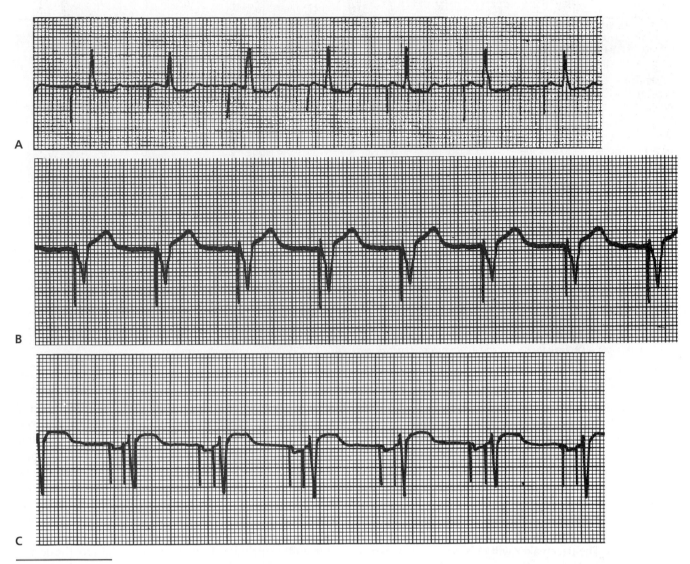

FIGURE 17-37
Strip **A** shows an atrial pacemaker. Note that each pacing stimulus is followed by a P wave. Strip **B** shows a ventricular pacemaker. Note that each pacing stimulus is followed by a wide QRS complex. Strip **C** shows a dual-chamber pacemaker. Note that the first spike is followed by a P wave and the second spike is followed by a QRS complex. All strips show 1:1 capture.

Many factors affect the pacing threshold. The pacing threshold usually is increased during hours of sleep, possibly due to lowered catecholamine levels. Other factors that may increase pacing thresholds include hypoxia, hyperkalemia, beta-blocking drugs, and type I antiarrhythmic drugs. In contrast, thresholds may be decreased with increased catecholamines, digoxin toxicity, and corticosteroids.

The *sensing threshold* is the minimal atrial or ventricular intrinsic signal that is consistently sensed by the pacemaker. The smallest number on the sensor control represents the most sensitive setting. The amplitude of the intrinsic depolarization wave at the site of the sensing electrode is measured. The sensitivity setting should allow for adequate sensing without oversensing artifact.

The Pacemaker Code

Since the initial use of cardiac pacemakers, the technology has become so complex and diverse that a coding system has been formed to identify the various modes of pacemaker operation. Initially developed in 1974, the pacemaker coding system has undergone several revisions. The most recent version of the code was developed in 1987 through the joint efforts of the North American Society of Pacing and Electrophysiology (NASPE) and the British Pacing and Electrophysiology Group (BPEG).[2] The NASPE/BPEG Generic Pacemaker Code is shown in Table 17–12 and is simply called the NBG pacemaker code.

The first three letters of the code are intended exclusively for describing antibradycardia pacing functions. The first letter describes the chamber or chambers of the heart in

TABLE 17-12
The NASPE/BPEG Generic Pacemaker Code

Position/ Category	I	II	III	IV	V
	Chamber(s) paced	Chamber(s) sensed	Response to sensing	Programmability rate modulation	Antitachyarrhythmia function(s)

Letter Codes	0 = None
	A = Atrium
	V = Ventricle
	D = Dual
	(A + V)
		0 = None
		A = Atrium
		V = Ventricle
		D = Dual
		(A + V)
			0 = None
			T = Triggered
			I = Inhibited
			D = Dual
			(T + I)
				0 = None
				P = Simple
				    Programmable
				M = Multiprogrammable
				C = Communicating
				
				R = Rate modulation
					0 = None
					P = Pacing
					    (antitachyarrhythmia)
					S = Shock
					D = Dual
					    (P + S)

Manufacturer's designation only	S = Single (A or V)	S = Single (A or V)			

Note: *Positions I through III are used exclusively for antibradyarrhythmia function.*
NASPE, North American Society of Pacing and Electrophysiology: BPEG, British Pacing and Electrophysiology Groups.
From Bernstein AD, Camm AJ, Fletcher RD, et al: The NASPE/BPEG generic pacemaker code for antibrady-arrhythmia and adaptive-rate pacing and antitachyarrhythmia devices. PACE 10:795, 1987; used with permission

which pacing occurs: A, atrium; V, ventricle; and D dual chamber. The second position of the code indicates the chamber or chambers in which intrinsic cardiac activity is sensed: A, atrium; V, ventricle; and D dual chamber.

The third position denotes the pacemaker's response to sensed intrinsic cardiac activity. The letter I means the pacemaker is inhibited from firing in response to a sensed intrinsic beat. For example, if the pacemaker is set to a rate of 70, the pacemaker will not fire if the patient's rate exceeds 70 beats/min. The pacemaker will only fire if the patient's intrinsic rate drops below the paced rate. Thus, the pacemaker functions on demand and is known as a *demand pacemaker*. Because the pacemaker is inhibited by intrinsic heart activity, there is no danger of the pacemaker firing at a time that could initiate a dangerous cardiac dysrhythmia, such as ventricular tachycardia. The letter T in the third position of the code indicates a pacemaker that triggers pacing stimuli in response to a sensed intrinsic beat. This function is not frequently used in cardiac pacing. However, in selected situations, it may be helpful to have a pacemaker capable of sensing intrinsic atrial activity that results in a triggered ventricular pacing stimulus for each sensed atrial stimulus. The letter O in the third position designates a mode in which the pacemaker does not respond to sensed intrinsic activity. The inability of the pacemaker to respond to sensed intrinsic activity is known as *asynchronous pacing*. Permanent pacemakers may be switched to an asynchronous mode temporarily by placing a specialized magnet over the pulse generator. This maneuver will cause the pacemaker to fire in an asynchronous mode, allowing the physician to assess for appropriate firing and capture.

The fourth position of the pacemaker code describes the externally programmable features of the pacemaker and the presence or absence of rate modulation. The letter P is used to denote simple programmability, indicating a device with one or two programmable features. When more than two features can be programmed, the letter M is used to represent multiprogrammability. The letter C in the fourth position refers to communicating and is used to describe telemetry capability. This capability involves the noninvasive transmission of data from the implanted pulse generator to an external receiver. Examples of data that can be transmitted include information on the status of the device, such as the internal resistance of the pacemaker battery, or physiological data, such as an intracardiac electrogram signal. The letter R in the fourth position means rate modulation. This is a feature in which the pacing rate varies in response to a physiological variable rather than being set at a fixed pacing rate. The physiological variable used most often is muscle motion. When patients increase their activity, the pacer detects vibrations from muscle and increases the pacing rate to meet increased metabolic demands. The letter R is considered hierarchical, meaning a pacemaker with R function also is multiprogrammable with communicating ability. The letter O in the fourth position indicates the absence of externally programmable or rate-modulated features.

The fifth position of the code designates the presence of one or more antitachydysrhythmia functions that can be initiated manually or automatically. The letter P in the fifth position means that a pacing stimulus is used to convert the tachydysrhythmia. This is known as *overdrive pacing*. An S indicates a shock intervention for cardioversion at low energy or defibrillation at high energy. The letter D denotes a device capable of pacing and shocking either simultaneously or sequentially. If there is an absence of any antitachydysrhythmia features, the letter O is used in the fifth position of the code.

Pacing Modes

Knowledge of the five-letter pacemaker code will help the critical care nurse determine the type of implanted device, the intended mode of operation, and the actual mode of operation. Modes of operation can be classified as single- and dual-chamber modes.

SINGLE-CHAMBER MODES OF OPERATION

A VVIRO mode is a commonly used mode of operation for permanent ventricular pacemakers. Devices with this mode of operation are characterized by ventricular demand pacing, ventricular sensing with inhibited ventricular response to sensing, rate modulation, multiprogrammability, communicating, and no antitachydysrhythmia functions. The rate modulation feature offers the benefit of adjusting the paced rate in response to metabolic demand. This rate modulation feature is not used in temporary pacing, so the mode would be designated as VVIOO. A disadvantage of the VVIRO and the VVIOO modes is the lack of hemodynamic benefits from atrioventricular synchrony.

An AAIMO is a mode of operation for permanent atrial pacemakers. With this mode of operation, there is atrial demand pacing, atrial sensing with inhibited atrial response to sensing, multiprogrammability, and no rate modulation or antitachydysrhythmia functions. Temporary atrial pacemakers most often are set to an AAIOO mode. These modes of pacing can only be used for patients with normal functioning of the AV node and intraventricular conduction system. If needed, the pacemaker will provide atrial depolarization, but the patient's AV node must conduct the signal to the ventricles. An advantage of these modes is the presence of AV synchrony.

DUAL-CHAMBER MODES OF OPERATION

Temporary and permanent dual-chamber pacemakers can operate in a variety of modes. The most common mode is DDDOO for temporary pacemakers and DDDRO for permanent pacemakers. A DDDOO mode provides dual-chamber pacing, dual-chamber sensing with both inhibited and triggered responses to sensing, and no programmability, rate modulation, or antitachydysrhythmia functions. The DDDRO mode has the additional features of rate modulation, multiprogrammability, and communicating. Other modes of single- and dual-chamber operation are listed in Table 17–13.

Complications of Pacing

Numerous possible complications are associated with cardiac pacemakers. The critical care nurse plays a vital role in the early detection and management of these complications. Table 17–14 describes troubleshooting strategies for complications resulting from pacemaker malfunction.

TABLE 17-13

Examples of Modes of Pacing According to the NASPE/BPEG Pacemaker Code

Code	Explanation
VVIMD	Ventricular demand pacing; ventricular sensing with inhibited ventricular response to sensing; multiprogrammable; defibrillation, cardioversion, or cardioversion/defibrillation and antitachyarrhythmia pacing functions
DDDMO	Dual-chamber "physiological" pacing, dual-chamber sensing with both inhibited and triggered response to sensing; multiprogrammable; no rate modulation or antitachyarrhythmia functions
VVIPP	Ventricular demand pacing; ventricular sensing with inhibited ventricular response to sensing; simple-programmable, with antitachyarrhythmia-pacing function
VVIRP	Ventricular demand pacing; ventricular sensing with inhibited ventricular response to sensing; rate modulation, with antitachyarrhythmia-pacing function
DDDRD	Dual-chamber "physiological" pacing, dual-chamber sensing with both inhibited and triggered responses to sensing; rate modulation with defibrillation, cardioversion, or cardioversion/defibrillation and antitachyarrhythmia pacing functions

NASPE, North American Society for Pacing and Electrophysiology; BPEG, British Pacing and Electrophysiology Group.

FAILURE TO DISCHARGE

Because stimulus discharge from the pacemaker causes an artifact, or "spike," to appear on the ECG, failure to discharge results in absence of the artifact (Fig. 17–38). The cause of this failure may be within the generator itself (either mechanism or battery failure), at the site of lead attachment to the generator, or within the lead due to wire fracture. When failure occurs in the temporary pacemaker, the nurse checks the connections at the generator terminals, replaces the batteries in the generator, or replaces the generator. If these efforts do not solve the problem, it must be assumed that wire fracture is the culprit. If only one wire is fractured, conversion to a unipolar system, with a chest electrode to replace the fractured wire, may provide successful pacing. When the permanent pacemaker fails to discharge a stimulus, the problem must be solved operatively. If the situation is emergent, the physician may insert a temporary transvenous pacemaker to support the patient hemodynamically until the permanent pacemaker problem can be corrected.

FAILURE TO CAPTURE

Failure of the pacing stimulus to capture the ventricles or atria will be noted by the absence of the QRS or P wave im-

---

TABLE 17-14
Troubleshooting a Temporary Pacemaker

Problem	Cause	Intervention
Failure to discharge: No evidence of pacing stimulus	Pacemaker too sensitive Battery depletion or pulse generator failure Output or timing circuit failure Loose, broken, or disconnected wire Short circuit of wire Lead fracture without insulation break	Check connection of lead to pacer. Reduce sensitivity. (Turn sensitivity dial toward asynchronous or higher mV value.) Change battery. Change pulse generator. Repair or replace pacing lead.
Failure to capture: Pacing stimulus not followed by ECG evidence of depolarization	Lead malpositioned or disconnected Battery depletion Lead insulation break or lead fracture Output setting (mA) too low Perforation Increase in pacing threshold due to medication or metabolic changes	Check connection of lead to pacer. Increase output (mA). Reposition patient. Reposition lead. Change battery. Change pulse generator. Change lead. Alter medication regimen. Correct metabolic changes.
Oversensing: Device detects noncardiac electrical events and interprets them as depolarization Device detects tall T waves and interprets them as R waves Pacer inappropriately inhibited from pacing	Electrical interference Improperly grounded electrical devices Tall T waves on ECG Sensitivity set too high	Check connection of lead to pacer. Reposition or replace the pacing lead. Identify the source of electrical interference, and eliminate it. Make certain all equipment is properly grounded. Decrease sensitivity. (Turn sensitivity dial toward asynchronous or higher mV value.)
Undersensing: Device fails to detect intrinsic cardiac activity and fires inappropriately	Lead disconnected from pacer Lead malpositioned or dislodged Lead fracture Battery depletion	Check connection of lead to pacer. Reposition or change lead. Change battery. Increase sensitivity. (Turn sensitivity dial to a lower mV value.)

---

mediately after the pacemaker artifact on the ECG (Fig. 17–39). If the pacing threshold has increased, the milliamperage may need to be increased until capture occurs. Displacement of the pacing electrode also may cause failure to capture. It sometimes is possible to regain capture by repositioning the patient, often in the left lateral decubitus position, until the electrode can be repositioned.

Battery failure also can cause failure to capture. If the patient is pacemaker dependent and becomes symptomatic, drug therapy (atropine, isoproterenol), transcutaneous pacing, or CPR may be required until the cause of the problem is found and corrected.

FAILURE TO SENSE

Failure of the pacemaker to sense intrinsic beats is known as *undersensing* and results in inappropriately placed pacemaker artifacts on the ECG (Fig. 17–40). Undersensing may be caused by improper electrode placement, battery or component failure, or lead wire fracture. Ventricular dysrhythmias caused by the pacemaker firing during the vulnerable phase of the T wave is of concern with undersensing. The most likely cause for sensing failure in the temporary pacemaker is electrode displacement.

To correct undersensing problems, the nurse makes sure the lead is properly connected to the temporary pacer. The

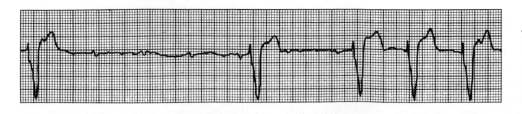

FIGURE 17-38
VVI pacemaker. Failure to discharge is indicated by lack of pacemaker spikes at appropriate intervals.

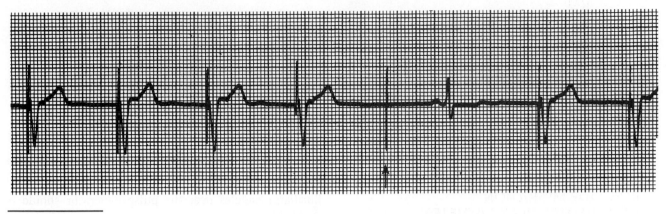

FIGURE 17-39
ECG strip showing evidence of failure to capture. Note pacing stimulus is not followed by a QRS complex.

battery for the pulse generator may need to be changed. The problem may also be corrected by increasing the sensitivity of the device, which is done by turning the dial to a lower millivolt (mV) value. If problems persist, the physician may need to reposition or replace the lead.

Oversensing is the term used to describe a sensing malfunction when the pacemaker detects events other than those that the pacemaker was designed to sense. For example, if tall T waves are present on the ECG, they may be mistaken for QRS complexes, causing the pacemaker to be inhibited. Similarly, electromagnetic interference may result in inappropriate sensing and as a result, incorrectly activate the inhibited or triggered mode of the pacemaker.

To correct oversensing problems, the nurse checks the connection between the temporary pacemaker and the lead. A thorough assessment of potential sources of electromagnetic interference is made. The grounding wires of all electrical equipment should be checked. The sensitivity may be decreased by turning the dial toward asynchronous, which is toward a higher millivolt value. If these efforts fail, the physician may need to reposition or replace the lead.

If sensing malfunctions render the pacemaker totally ineffective, it may be advantageous to turn the pacemaker off until the cause can be identified and corrected. This strategy requires knowledge of the patient's underlying rhythm.

Again, it may be necessary to institute emergency measures in the interim.

VENTRICULAR IRRITABILITY

Ventricular irritability at the site of the endocardial catheter tip is a frequent occurrence after initial catheter insertion. The premature ventricular complexes usually appear similar in configuration to the pacemaker complexes. Irritability from the catheter as a foreign body usually disappears after 2 or 3 days (Fig. 17–41).

PERFORATION OF VENTRICULAR WALL OR SEPTUM

Perforation of the ventricular wall or septum by the transvenous catheter occurs in a small number of patients. This may or may not result in noncapture. Perforation can be suspected on cardiac monitoring if the patient is monitored in a V_1 or modified V_1 lead. Right ventricular pacing should provide a negative QRS in this lead. Often, ventricular perforation results in pacing from the left ventricle, and the QRS becomes positive in polarity. Pericardial tamponade, causing a decrease in blood pressure and an increase in sinus node discharge rate, must be evaluated after ventricular wall perforation.

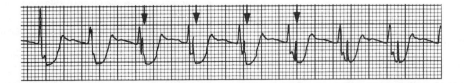

FIGURE 17-40
ECG strip showing evidence of undersensing. Failure of the ventricular demand pacemaker to detect the intrinsic rhythm is shown by pacemaker spikes at inappropriate intervals after spontaneous QRS complexes.

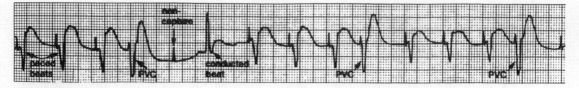

FIGURE 17-41
Ventricular demand pacemaker with PVCs. This strip also shows one noncaptured pacemaker spike followed by a spontaneous conducted beat.

RETROGRADE MIGRATION OF RIGHT VENTRICULAR CATHETER

Retrograde migration of the right ventricular pacing catheter into the right atrium may result in atrial pacing (pacing artifact followed by P wave) or inhibition of the pacemaker by atrial depolarizations. The effects on the patient depend on the ability of the AV node to conduct atrial impulses and on the ability of a lower escape focus to emerge at an adequate rate.

ABDOMINAL TWITCHING OR HICCUPS

Abdominal twitching or hiccups occur occasionally as a result of electrode placement against a thin right ventricular wall and resultant electrical stimulation of the abdominal muscles or diaphragm. This complication usually is very uncomfortable for the patient, and the electrode should be repositioned as soon as possible.

INFECTION AND PHLEBITIS

Infection and phlebitis can occur at the temporary pacemaker insertion site, and infection or hematoma may occur at the site of permanent generator implantation. These sites must be inspected for swelling and inflammation and kept dry. Sterile technique must be used when dressings are changed.

PERMANENT GENERATOR MIGRATION

Migration of the permanent generator from its initial site of implantation may occur in patients who have very loose connective tissue. This may or may not require reimplantation. Erosion at the implantation site occurs rarely.

MALFUNCTION DUE TO DEFIBRILLATION

Defibrillation of the patient while the temporary pacemaker system is intact may affect various components of the generator and cause it to malfunction. The temporary generator should be turned off and the catheter wires disconnected from the generator, if at all possible, before defibrillating. When defibrillating a patient with a permanent pacemaker, placement of the de-

fibrillator paddles over the pulse generator should be avoided.

Nursing Management

Critical care nurses play a key role in caring for patients with a pacemaker. The nurse is responsible for comprehensively assessing the patient, educating the patient and family, monitoring the ECG, and maintaining patient safety. The accompanying display lists nursing diagnoses and collaborative problems for patients with a cardiac pacemaker.

PATIENT ASSESSMENT

The critical care nurse may be the first to detect the patient's dysrhythmia that will necessitate pacing. Knowing the indications for pacing and how to initiate emergent transcutaneous pacing is essential for the critical care nurse. After a comprehensive assessment and stabilization of the patient, the critical care nurse may need to assist the physician in the insertion of a transvenous or permanent pacing system.

An important aspect of preimplantation of a pacemaker includes an assessment of patient activity. The

---

CLINICAL APPLICATION:
Examples of Nursing Diagnoses and Collaborative Problems for the Patient With a Pacemaker

Decreased Cardiac Output related to abnormal cardiac rate, rhythm, or conduction
Anxiety related to life-threatening cardiac disease requiring pacemaker
Knowledge Deficit related to impending pacemaker insertion
Decreased Cardiac Output related to pacemaker system failure
Risk for Infection related to invasive procedure and presence of foreign body
Ineffective Individual Coping related to change in body image and dependence on pacemaker

patient's activities of daily living and recreational activities should be discussed before permanent pacing to ascertain an appropriate site for implantation. For example, the right pectoralis muscle should not be used in the right-handed rifle hunter. Abdominal implantation may be preferable for the avid swimmer because of strenuous arm activity.

To assess patients with pacemakers accurately, the nurse must understand the pacemaker code to know the type of pacer used and the intended mode of the device.[3] The nurse must be aware of the patient's underlying rhythm so that if the pacemaker fails, the nurse will be prepared to treat any life-threatening dysrhythmias.

A thorough assessment also will help the nurse determine the patient's physiological response to pacing therapy. Important parameters to assess include pulse rate, underlying cardiac rhythm, blood pressure, activity tolerance, and evidence of dizziness, syncope, dyspnea, palpitations, or edema. The nurse should be attentive to results of chest radiographs, blood tests, and other relevant laboratory tests. If a permanent pacemaker has been implanted, the incision should be examined for swelling, redness, drainage, hematoma, and tenderness.

A psychosocial assessment is another essential component of comprehensive care of the patient with a cardiac pacemaker. Patients' psychosocial responses to the need for cardiac pacing may differ. Some may be relieved to have a device that will support the functioning of their heart, whereas others may be anxious about the technology and express fears of dying. If a permanent pacemaker is implanted, patients and families should be encouraged to join support groups where they can share their fears and concerns with others who are dependent on pacing technology.

PATIENT AND FAMILY EDUCATION

A planned and systematic approach to teaching the patient and family about cardiac pacing is a vital part of nursing care. Patient teaching relative to pacemakers begins at the time the decision for pacemaker insertion is made. The nurse can begin by eliciting the patient's previous knowledge of pacemakers and clarifying any misconceptions. Nothing is assumed about the patient's understanding. If appropriate, the difference between heart block and heart attack is clarified. The patient may confuse cardiac monitoring with pacing and become anxious when the monitoring electrodes are removed.

The patient and family should be told why the pacemaker is necessary. The anatomy of the heart should be discussed in general terms when explaining the need for pacing and how the pacemaker takes the place of or complements spontaneous rhythm. The insertion procedure and the immediate postinsertion care that can be expected should be explained.

Many booklets and media presentations are available to aid the nurse in teaching the pacemaker patient. Visual and written guidelines are helpful for the patient and family to review after discharge from the hospital.

The depth of teaching that is appropriate and the teaching tools used depend on such variables as the patient's age, intellect, attention span, vision, and interest in learning. Initial teaching should be confined to the positive aspects of life with a pacemaker. Knowledge of the function and care of the pacemaker are of no interest until this patient is able to accept it as part of life. The display provides a guide for teaching patients and families about pacemakers.

ELECTROCARDIOGRAM MONITORING

Careful monitoring of the ECG of the patient with a cardiac pacemaker is an essential component of comprehensive patient assessment. The first step in the analysis involves examining the strip for evidence of discharge. This evidence is noted by the presence of pacing spikes on the strip. Each pacing spike should result in capture. If the pacing lead is in the atria, a pacing spike is followed by a P wave. If the pacing wire is in the ventricle, the spike is followed by a wide QRS complex. When both the atrial and ventricles are paced, appropriate capture would be seen as a pacing spike followed by a P wave and another pacing spike followed by a wide QRS complex.

The sensing function of the pacemaker is evaluated next. If the pacemaker does not sense intrinsic cardiac activity (undersensing), inappropriate pacemaker spikes may appear throughout the underlying rhythm. An oversensing problem can be detected when the pacemaker senses events other than the intrinsic rhythm and is activated inappropriately in the inhibited or triggered mode.

The third step in evaluating the ECG is to measure various intervals in milliseconds. Each small box on the ECG paper represents 40 ms, and one large box represents 200 ms. The duration of each interval is compared with the programmed setting for that interval.

The first interval, the pacing interval, is the amount of time between two consecutive atrial pacing spikes or two consecutive ventricular pacing spikes. This interval is used to determine the pacing rate. To calculate the pacing rate, the nurse counts the number of milliseconds between two consecutive atrial spikes or two consecutive ventricular spikes (Fig. 17–42). To convert from milliseconds to beats per minute, the following formula is used: 60,000 ms/min divided by the number of milliseconds between pacing spikes equals the pacing rate.

The next interval to measure is the AV interval, also known as the AV delay. This interval is analogous to the PR interval on the ECG. The AV interval is measured from the beginning of an intrinsic P wave or an atrial pacing spike to the beginning of the intrinsic QRS complex or the ventricular pacing spike (see Fig. 17–42).

The third interval to measure is the ventriculoatrial (VA) interval, also called the atrial escape interval. The VA

PATIENT TEACHING
Living With a Pacemaker

Patient Activity

- Start passive and active range-of-motion exercises on the affected arm 48 hours after pacemaker implantation in the pectoralis major muscle to avoid "frozen shoulder."
- Repeat these exercises several times daily until the implantation site is completely free of discomfort through all ranges of arm motion.
- Touch or bathe the implantation site without hesitation. The pacemaker is sturdy, and touching and bathing will not damage it.
- Avoid activities that may result in high impact or stress at the implantation site. This includes all contact sports.
- Report any activity that may have damaged your pacemaker.
- Return to work at the discretion of your physician after discussing the type of work you do and what your job entails.
- Return to whatever degree of sexual activity you prefer.
- Be prepared for your pacemaker to set off the alarm on metal-detector devices in airports.

Signs of Pacemaker Malfunction

- Be alert for symptoms of pacemaker malfunction: those associated with decreased perfusion of the brain, heart, or skeletal muscles.
- Report any dizziness, fainting, chest pain, shortness of breath, undue fatigue, or fluid retention. Fluid retention includes sudden weight gain, "puffy ankles," "tightness of rings," and so forth.
- Take pulse once daily upon awakening. Report a pulse rate of more than 5 beats/min slower than that at which pacemaker is set.
- Be aware that pulse may be somewhat irregular if it is a demand pacemaker and has some spontaneous beats and paced beats. This does not signify pacemaker malfunction.

Signs of Infection

- Report any redness, swelling, drainage, or increase in soreness at the implantation site.

Pulse Generator Replacement

- Follow instructions regarding the expected life of pacemaker battery.
- Be aware that generator replacement requires hospitalization for about 1 day and that usually only the generator will need to be replaced.

Medications

- Follow instructions regarding medications.
- Know the name of the medication and the dose, frequency of administration, side effects, and use of each medication.

Safety Measures

- Inform any physician or dentist of the pacemaker and of the medications being taken.
- Carry a pacemaker identification card at all times. This card shows the brand and model of pacemaker, the date of insertion, and the programmed settings.
- Wear a medical alert bracelet or necklace stating a pacemaker is worn.

Follow-up Care

- Adhere to schedule of follow-up visits with your physician or clinic. The follow-up visit will include an interval history and physical examination and a 12-lead ECG. Many pacemaker clinics have specialized equipment available to measure the rate, amplitude, duration, and contours of the pacemaker artifact. This information is very helpful in predicting battery depletion. Some clinics have the capability for obtaining this information by telephone, reducing the necessity for travel to the clinic.

---

interval is the amount of time from a ventricular paced or sensed event to the next atrial paced stimulus (see Fig. 17–42). The sum of the AV and the VA interval equals the pacing interval.

PATIENT SAFETY

Electrical safety precautions must be observed when the patient has a temporary pacemaker. Electrical equipment in the room is kept at a minimum and must be properly grounded. Use of a nonelectric bed is preferable. If an electric bed is used, it must be properly grounded or remain disconnected from AC current. Only battery-operated electric shavers, toothbrushes, or radios are recommended. An AC-powered television may be used if it is operated by someone who is not in contact with the patient. The nurse should avoid simultaneous contact with the patient and any electrical equipment. The patient's bed must be kept dry at all times. Diathermy and electrocautery equipment should not be used because their waves may be sensed by and inhibit the demand pacemaker.

To date, there is no research to guide the practice of ensuring electrical safety when handling the pacing wires or pulse generator. The use of rubber gloves to handle pacing leads and electrodes is often recommended. Some institu-

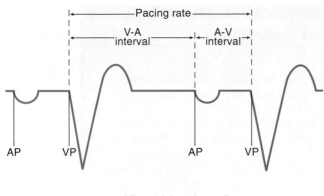

AP = atrial pacing spike
VP = ventricular pacing spike

FIGURE 17-42
The intervals measured on a ECG strip for a patient with a pacemaker. The pacing interval is the amount of time between two consecutive atrial pacing spikes or two consecutive ventricular pacing spikes. The atrioventricular (AV) interval is measured from the beginning of a P wave or an atrial pacing spike to the beginning of an intrinsic QRS complex or the ventricular pacing spike. The ventriculoatrial (VA) interval is measured from a ventricular pacing or sensed beat to the next atrial pacing spike. The sum of the AV and VA interval equals the pacing interval.

tions wrap pieces of rubber gloves around leads or connections to provide insulation.[4]

The plastic cover supplied with the temporary generator must be kept in place over the dials to prevent inadvertent change in settings. The generator should be attached securely to the patient's arm or abdomen. The catheter should be taped securely to the patient's skin without direct tension on the catheter. Motion of the extremity nearest the catheter entry site should be minimized, especially if the femoral site has been used.

According to manufacturers of permanent pacemaker generators, there are very few electrical hazards associated with the permanent generators currently in use. These generators are shielded from external electrical sources and usually are not affected by microwave ovens or small appliances. There have been rare reports of unipolar pacemakers being affected by large electromagnetic fields, such as radio transmitters.

Conclusion

Nurses who care for patients with a pacemaker must have thorough knowledge of the heart, the pacemaker, and the patient as a person. This knowledge is applied continuously from the time the decision for device insertion is made until the patient is discharged from the hospital and sometimes beyond, to follow-up care. The nurse plays a vital role in en-

suring success after implantation and in reassuring the patient, whose well-being depends on the device.

◼ IMPLANTABLE CARDIOVERTER DEFIBRILLATORS

Approximately half of all deaths resulting from cardiovascular disease are sudden and unexpected. Each year in the United States, about 250,000 adults die from sudden death.[6] This sudden rapid loss of heart function is the result of an unresuscitated cardiac arrest that may be caused by any type of heart disease. Most cardiac arrests, however, are caused by ventricular tachycardia or ventricular fibrillation.

In the late 1960s, Dr. Michel Mirowski and Dr. Morton Mower developed a device called an implantable cardioverter defibrillator (ICD) to treat patients at risk for sudden death due to ventricular dysrhythmia. In 1980, the first device was implanted successfully in a person. The device was found to be safe and effective and, as a result, received FDA approval in 1985. Since its initial use in 1980, the ICD has undergone many improvements in design and function. Currently, the ICD is used frequently for long-term therapy for patients at risk for sudden death.

Indications for Implantable Cardioverter Defibrillators

A joint committee of the American College of Cardiology and the American Heart Association developed guidelines for the use of ICDs.[7] Class I includes indications for which there is general agreement that the device should be implanted. Class II consists of conditions for which ICDs are frequently used, but there are differences of opinion regarding the necessity of insertion. Conditions for which there is general agreement that ICDs are unnecessary are considered class III. Further research is underway comparing the ICD with drug therapy, and results of these studies may influence acceptable indications for ICD therapy. The display lists the indications for use of ICD therapy.

The Implantable Cardioverter Defibrillator System

The purpose of an ICD is to monitor continuously the patient's rhythm, diagnose rhythm changes, and treat life-threatening ventricular dysrhythmias. Similar to a pacemaker, the ICD consists of a lead system and a pulse generator containing the battery, capacitors, and circuits. The lead system and the pulse generator have undergone significant changes in design and function since their initial use in 1980.

Indications for Implantable Cardioverter Defibrillators

Class I

One or more documented episodes of hemodynamically significant ventricular tachycardia or ventricular fibrillation in a patient in whom electrophysiological testing and ambulatory monitoring cannot be used to predict efficacy of therapy accurately.

One or more documented episodes of hemodynamically significant ventricular tachycardia or ventricular fibrillation in a patient in whom no drug was found to be effective or no drug currently available and appropriate was tolerated

Continued inducibility at electrophysiological study of hemodynamically significant ventricular tachycardia or ventricular fibrillation despite the best available drug therapy or despite surgery or catheter ablation if drug therapy has failed

Class II

One or more documented episodes of hemodynamically significant ventricular tachycardia or ventricular fibrillation in a patient in whom drug efficacy testing is possible

Recurrent syncope of undetermined origin in a patient with hemodynamically significant ventricular tachycardia or ventricular fibrillation induced at electrophysiological study in whom no effective or no tolerated drug is available or appropriate

Class III

Recurrent syncope of undetermined cause in a patient without inducible tachydysrhythmias

Arrhythmias not due to hemodynamically significant ventricular tachycardia or ventricular fibrillation

Incessant ventricular tachycardia or fibrillation

THE PULSE GENERATOR

Early ICD pulse generators were large and heavy in comparison to the pacemaker pulse generator. Because of their size and weight, these ICD pulse generators required implantation in the patient's abdomen. Currently used ICD pulse generators are not much larger than pacemakers and can be implanted in the pectoral area. The size of the device is shown in Figure 17–43. Lithium batteries provide the power source for ICDs and generally last 3 to 5 years. Improved circuit design has expanded the capabilities and functions of the ICD.

THE LEAD SYSTEM

Lead systems sense the life-threatening ventricular rhythm and deliver a shock to convert the rhythm. Previously, one of two lead systems was used for the ICD. The first lead system consisted of a patch sewn on the epicardial surface of the heart and a transvenous superior vena cava spring coil electrode. The second lead system was entirely epicardial and consisted of epicardial leads and epicardial patches. These types of lead systems required a median sternotomy or thoracotomy for placement. As a result, lead placement was often associated with expensive hospitalization, potential complications of thoracic surgery, and lengthy recovery time.

Dramatic improvements have been achieved in lead system design. Current systems consist of a single tripolar transvenous lead capable of sensing and delivering the shock. One electrode of the tripolar lead is in the superior vena cava, the second is high in the right atrium, and the third is in the apex of the right ventricle. An alternative is to use a two- or three-electrode lead system. In some situations, a submuscular or subcutaneous patch may be placed in the left anterior axillary area if defibrillation thresholds are not adequate through the transvenous lead. The newer lead systems are inserted through a transvenous approach and have eliminated the need for a median sternotomy or thoracotomy. As a result, patient discomfort is decreased, and recovery time is shortened. In addition, hospital costs are greatly reduced, length of stay is shorter, and complications are minimized.

Implantable Cardioverter Defibrillator Functioning

Based on their functioning, ICDs have been categorized into "generations." The first-generation ICDs were nonprogrammable devices that used a preset rate criterion to detect ventricular dysrhythmias and deliver a shock at a preset energy level. In the mid-1980s, the second generation of the device became available and included more programmable features.

Today's ICDs are known as third-generation devices and have many programmable features that allow the physician to tailor the device to the patient's needs. To improve identification of the dysrhythmia, the rate detection criteria can be programmed rather than being preset. A first-shock

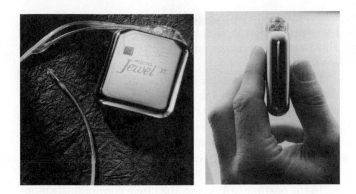

FIGURE 17-43
Two views of an implantable cardioverter defibrillator device. The lead carries the electrical impulse to the heart. Impulses pass through the heart and return to the device, which serves as the second electrode. The device weighs about 3½ ounces. Courtesy of Medtronic, Minneapolis, MN.

delay feature also is used in current devices. This feature involves a programmed amount of time the rhythm must be sustained before the shock is delivered. A first-shock delay prevents shocking of nonsustained ventricular dysrhythmias.

In current devices, tiered therapy is the term used to describe different levels of therapy the device can provide to terminate the dysrhythmia. The first tier of therapy is usually antitachycardia pacing, which involves the carefully timed delivery of low-energy pacing stimuli. If antitachycardia pacing is not successful, the second tier of therapy will be initiated by the device. With the second tier, a low-energy synchronized cardioversion is delivered. The joules for cardioversion can be programmed anywhere from 0.1 to 37 J, depending on the specific device. Some devices allow multiple attempts at cardioversion. If cardioversion is not successful, the third tier of therapy, defibrillation, is used. The energy delivered for defibrillation can be programmed

to a maximum of 37 J. The number of defibrillation attempts varies with different devices, but six attempts is usually the maximum. If the patient is successfully converted to a life-compatible rhythm, but the rate is slow, ventricular demand pacemaker will be initiated. This fourth tier of therapy is usually intended for brief periods of pacing. Those patients requiring sustained or frequent pacing support would need a separate pacer implanted.

Third-generation defibrillators have additional features, including memory and event retrieval. Event retrieval may involve R wave to R wave analysis or the recording of an electrogram. These methods document the dysrhythmia before and after the therapy, allowing the physician to analyze the problematic rhythm. Ideally these data can be related to any patient symptoms to help further evaluate the patient's condition.

Some devices also have the ability to deliver a PES. The PES will induce the patient's dysrhythmia so that the physician can test the device's ability to detect the rhythm and treat it appropriately. This feature of the device minimizes the need to test the device in a laboratory situation where catheters are placed in the patient's heart to induce the rhythm disturbance. Instead, testing is done within the device itself, thus minimizing patient discomfort and potential complications.

The Implantable Cardioverter Defibrillator Code

The cardiac pacemaker code previously discussed has limited ability to describe modes of ICD function. As a result, in 1993, NASPE and BPEG developed the NASPE/BPEG Defibrillator Code[8] (Table 17–15). Known as the NBD defibrillator code, it describes ICD capabilities and operation.

Although the pacemaker and defibrillator codes are similar, they have some important differences. The pacemaker code offers detail about antibradycardia pacing and little specific information about shock capability. The defibrilla-

	TABLE 17-15		
	The NASPE/BPEG Defibrillator Code		
I	II	III	IV
Shock Chamber	Antitachycardia Pacing Chamber	Tachycardia Detection	Antibradycardia Pacing Chamber
0 = None	0 = None	E = Electrogram	0 = None
A = Atrium	A = Atrium	H = Hemodynamic	A = Atrium
V = Ventricle	V = Ventricle		V = Ventricle
D = Dual (A + V)	D = Dual (A + V)		D = Dual (A + V)

NASPE, North American Society of Pacing and Electrophysiology; BPEG, British Pacing and Electrophysiology Group.
From Bernstein AD, Camm AJ, Fisher JD et al: The NASPE/BPEG defibrillator code. PACE 16:1777, 1993; used with permission.

tor code provides more specific information about shock functions with few details about antibradycardia function. Positions I, II, and IV of the defibrillator code describe the location of shock, antitachycardia pacing, and antibradycardia pacing through use of the letters A (atrium), V (ventricle), D (dual), and O (none). The third position of the defibrillator code designates the means used to detect the tachycardia by using H (hemodynamic) or E (electrogram). The letter H is hierarchical, meaning that a device that monitors hemodynamic variables also monitors the intracardiac electrogram.

In medical documentation and device labeling, often the first three letters of the defibrillator code are used, followed by a hyphen and the first four letters of the pacemaker code. For example, a device labeled VOE-VVIR would designate a ventricular defibrillator with no antitachycardia pacing function that detects the tachycardia by means of an electrogram. The device is able to function as a rate-modulated ventricular demand pacemaker.

Nursing Management

The critical care nurse plays a key role in the preimplant and postimplant management of patients with an ICD. Patient teaching is one of the most important roles for the critical care nurse. Topics for discussion are included in the accompanying display. Patients and families need to understand why an ICD is indicated, the purpose of an ICD, the basic parts of the ICD system, and how the ICD functions. Once the physician has determined the type of system to be used, the nurse reinforces the physician's explanation of how the device will be implanted and where the leads and pulse generator will be placed. The patient and family should be informed of the expected length of hospitalization and plans for follow-up care. Many resources for patient education are available from manufacturers of ICDs, including printed materials and videotapes.

In addition, the patient and family may find it helpful to meet with a person who has an ICD. This person may be able to allay any fears or clarify misconceptions about living with an ICD.

During the immediate postimplant phase, it is essential for the nurse to know the type of ICD system that was implanted. If a transvenous system was used, the postimplant care is similar to postpacemaker implant patient care. If the ICD implant necessitated a thoracotomy or median sternotomy, the postimplant care is similar to any patient postthoracic surgery.

In the postimplant period, the nurse continuously monitors the patient for the development of any ventricular dysrhythmias and intervenes immediately if necessary. The nurse should not wait for the ICD to fire in the presence of ventricular tachycardia or ventricular fibrillation. Instead, CPR is initiated immediately, and if needed, defibrillation with external paddles is performed.

The nurse must be aware of the programmed settings and features of the patient's ICD to provide safe and competent care. Device information should be readily available at the bedside and clearly documented in the patient's chart. If the device fires, the status of the patient and the patient's rhythm is assessed and documented.

In collaboration with the physician, the nurse provides discharge instructions about resuming daily activities. Patients are usually instructed to avoid swimming or boating alone, climbing ladders, operating heavy equipment, or playing contact sports. Emergency plans listed in the display should be reviewed with the patient and family.

Discussion of psychosocial issues regarding living with an ICD also should be part of the discharge preparation. Although the emotional adjustment varies with each patient, many have fears about receiving their first shock. Other potential patient concerns the nurse should discuss include loss of independence, uncertainty about the future, alterations in body image, return to work,

---

PATIENT TEACHING

Topics for Patient and Family Using an Implantable Cardioverter Defibrillator (ICD)

- Why an ICD is indicated
- Purpose of an ICD
- Components of an ICD
- How the ICD works
- How the ICD will be implanted
- Expected length of hospitalization
- Postimplant activities of daily living
- Plans for follow-up care
- When to call the doctor
- Importance of an ICD identification card and medical alert bracelet or necklace
- What the patient and family should do if a shock occurs
- Safety precautions
- Support groups

> ### PATIENT TEACHING
> ### *Instructions for an ICD Emergency*
>
> - Carry an ICD identification card.
> - Wear a medical alert necklace or bracelet.
> - Carry a list of your medications and dosages.
> - Keep emergency phone numbers readily available.
> - Call your physician within 24 hours of receiving a shock.
> - Call your physician immediately if you receive a second shock the same day.
> - Inform family, significant others, coworkers, traveling companions about your ICD.
> - When traveling by air, inform airline security personnel of your ICD.
> - Encourage your family members to take a CPR course.

participation in recreational activities, and reaction of family and friends to the device. If support groups are available, the patient and family should be encouraged to join.

CONCLUSION

The ICD has revolutionized the care of patients at risk for sudden cardiac death. The device design and function have improved significantly since its initial use, and refinements are likely to continue. The critical care nurse can help patients and families understand the device and adjust to its presence in their life.

Clinical Applicability Challenges

Self-Challenge: Critical Thinking

1. *Mr. B. Has been experiencing recurrent ventricular dysrhythmias and is placed on sotalol for treatment. Determine what specific side effects you would monitor as you begin to administer this agent. Formulate a teaching plan for Mr. B. as he prepares to go home.*

2. *Compare and contrast the postprocedure care of patients undergoing a PTCA and a PBV.*

3. *Many different interventional devices are available for the treatment of CAD. Categorize these devices by the specific lesion types that are best suited for that device.*

4. *Develop an educational tool that experienced critical care nurses might use to teach new graduates the basic similarities and differences between IABP support and VAD support. Discuss issues such as hemodynamic support capabilities, target patient populations, contraindications and limitations, patient outcomes, and patient teaching.*

5. *Examine the ethical issues surrounding the implementation of long-term cardiac support with a VAD as an alternative to cardiac transplantation.*

6. *Multiple complications can result from the use of IABP therapy. From a systems approach, describe an assessment of end-organ function as it applies to nursing assessment and intervention when caring for this patient population in the ICU.*

7. *Compare risks associated with allogeneic blood to risks associated with autologous blood.*

8. *Develop a cost analysis for your unit comparing the cost of intermittent reinfusion of autologous blood to continuous reinfusion, including reduced cost of administration systems, nursing time, and reduced risks to patients and staff.*

9. *Mrs. M. has been admitted to your unit with an acute myocardial infarction. As you observe her, she goes into ventricular fibrillation. Relate the steps you and your team would go through to resuscitate her.*

10. *While you are providing preprocedure instruction for your patient, she tells you she does not know what conscious sedation means. Describe how you would instruct the patient.*

11. *Critique a clinical pathway for a patient with a cardiac pacemaker.*

12. *Develop a plan of care for the patient who is going home with a new permanent pacemaker.*

13. *Generate a list of nursing diagnoses for the patient with an ICD.*

Study Questions

Pharmacological Therapy: Antiarrhythmic, Vasoactive, and Thrombolytic Agents

1. *Which of the following class III antiarrhythmic agents prolongs repolarization and possesses beta-blocking properties?*
   a. *Sotalol*
   b. *Amiodarone*
   c. *Ibutilide*
   d. *Bretyllium*

2. *Which of the following is the drug of choice for the treatment of torsades de pointes?*
   a. *Amiodarone*
   b. *Quinidine*
   c. *Magnesium*
   d. *Procainamide*

3. Stimulation of beta 1 receptors causes
   a. bronchoconstriction.
   b. decreased contractility.
   c. decreased heart rate.
   d. increased contractility.

4. A major side effect of thrombolytic agents is
   a. elevated blood pressure.
   b. depressed left ventricular function.
   c. bleeding.
   d. renal failure.

Percutaneous Transluminal Coronary Angioplasty and Percutaneous Balloon Valvuloplasty

1. Percutaneous transluminal angioplasty compares favorably to coronary artery bypass surgery in terms of
   a. risk, success rate, length of hospital stay, and restenosis.
   b. risk, success rate, cost, and restenosis.
   c. risk, success rate, length of hospital stay, and cost.
   d. risk, success rate, cost, and acute closure.

2. Primary angioplasty may be performed
   a. 1 hour after administration of a thrombolytic.
   b. 4 to 6 hours after administration of a thrombolytic.
   c. without prior administration of a thrombolytic.
   d. after a thrombolytic has failed.

3. Restenosis is defined as
   a. a reoccurrence of the blockage in a coronary artery.
   b. platelet adhesion on the coronary valves.
   c. excision of plaque from the coronary artery.
   d. dissolving the thrombus within the coronary artery.

4. The signs and symptoms of an access site infection following an interventional cardiology procedure are
   a. fever, oozing from the catheter insertion site, and chest pain.
   b. fever, headache, and chest pain.
   c. fever, chest pain, and back pain.
   d. fever, pain, and drainage from the catheter insertion site.

5. Complications associated with an interventional cardiology procedure include all except which of the following?
   a. Bleeding at the catheter insertion site
   b. Myocardial infarction
   c. Hyperlipidemia
   d. Restenosis

6. Which of the following are treatments for CAD?
   a. PTCA, laser, ECG, and directional coronary atherectomy
   b. PTCA, stents, laser, and directional coronary atherectomy
   c. Medication, PTCA, and ECG
   d. Medication, smoking cessation, and ECG

Intra-Aortic Balloon Pump Counterpulsation and Mechnical Circulatory Support

1. The primary purpose of an intra-aortic balloon pump is to
   a. provide rest for the left ventricle.
   b. improve coronary artery perfusion and decrease afterload.
   c. improve the contractility of the left ventricle.
   d. reduce the fluid load on the lungs.

2. All of the following are contraindications to IABP therapy except
   a. aortic aneurysm.
   b. previous aortofemoral bypass graft.
   c. terminal cancer.
   d. aortic valve incompetence.

3. The primary goal of univentricular and biventricular assistance is
   a. to support the patient until heart transplantation.
   b. the restoration of adequate blood flow and preservation of end-organ function.
   c. to keep the patient flat in bed until the device is removed.
   d. to increase ventricular workload.

4. An important psychosocial intervention by the nurse caring for a patient on IABP or ventricular assistance is
   a. to limit conversation with the patient so he or she is able to rest.
   b. to intervene at the bedside as much as possible.
   c. to explain procedures and nursing activities to the patient.
   d. to limit family visitation.

Autologous Blood Transfusion

1. Major hematological differences between allogeneic and autologous blood include the following:
   a. Autologous blood has normal levels of 2,3-DPG, a higher platelet count, and a higher hematocrit than allogeneic blood.
   b. Allogeneic blood has normal levels of 2,3-DPG, a higher platelet count, and a higher hematocrit than autologous blood.
   c. Autologous blood has normal levels of 2,3-DPG, a lower platelet count, and a higher hematocrit than allogeneic blood.
   d. Bank blood has normal levels of 2,3-DPG, a higher platelet count, and a lower hematocrit than autologous blood.

2. A complication associated with autotransfusion is
   a. transfusion reaction.
   b. coagulopathy.
   c. HIV.
   d. hepatitis.

Cardiopulmonary Resuscitation

1. The following drug can be put down the ET tube when there is no IV access:
   a. Epinephrine
   b. Bretyllium
   c. Magnesium
   d. Adenosine

2. Following three consecutive shocks in a ventricular fibrillation arrest, which drug should be administered next?
   a. Atropine
   b. Lidocaine
   c. Bretyllium
   d. Epinephrine

3. Which of the following is correct regarding defibrillation for ventricular fibrillation?
   a. Initiate at 200 J.
   b. Initiate at 360 J.
   c. Delay until the physician arrives.
   d. Initiate at 50 J with the "sync" button is on.

Management of Dysrhythmias

1. When a patient is cardioverted, the shock is synchronized with
   a. the P wave (atrial depolarization).
   b. the R wave (ventricular depolarization).
   c. the ST segment (the time between ventricular depolarization and ventricular repolarization).
   d. the T wave (ventricular repolarization).

2. Mr. Taylor has just returned to the unit after having a radiofrequency ablation. During your assessment, you note that his blood pressure has dropped from 130/82 to 90/60. His pulse has increased from 86 to 104 beats/min. He tells you he is having difficulty breathing. You decide to
   a. recheck his vital signs in 30 minutes.
   b. check for evidence of cerebral embolus.
   c. notify the physician of a suspected cardiac perforation.
   d. Record a 12-lead ECG.

3. The ability of the pacemaker to detect the heart's intrinsic cardiac activity and respond appropriately is known as
   a. the telemetry function.
   b. the sensing function.
   c. the capture function.
   d. the output function.

4. Mr. Cooper has received a transcutaneous pacemaker. Which of the following best describes a transcutaneous pacemaker?
   a. The pacing wires are implanted transvenously, and the power box is outside the body.
   b. The pacing wires and the power box are implanted in the body.
   c. The pacing wires and the power box are outside the body.
   d. The pacing wires are implanted epicardially, and the power box is outside the body.

5. You are caring for Mrs. Carlson who has just come back from the operating room with a DDDRO pacemaker. Which of the following best describes a DDDRO pacemaker?
   a. The ventricles are paced at a rate based on metabolic demand.
   b. Both the atria and the ventricles are paced at a rate based on metabolic demand.
   c. Both the atria and the ventricles are paced to control tachydysrhythmia.
   d. The atria are paced at a fixed rate, and the ventricles are paced at a rate based on metabolic demand.

6. You are assessing for evidence of electrical capture for your patient's temporary ventricular pacemaker. The best evidence would be
   a. a pacer spike followed by a QRS complex.
   b. a pacer spike preceding each T wave.
   c. a change in the monitor rate from 58 to 64.
   d. a change in blood pressure from 98/60 to 104/64.

7. The ICD is designed to terminate which of the following dysrhythmias?
   a. Supraventricular tachyarrhythmias
   b. Ventricular tachyarrhythmias
   c. Both supraventricular and ventricular tachyarrhythmias
   d. Only ventricular fibrillation

8. Mr. Smith suffers with episodes of ventricular tachycardia and now has an ICD. His ventricular tachycardia is usually at a rate of 200 beats/min. As a result, his rate sensitivity parameter on the ICD is most likely to be set at
   a. 260 beats/min.
   b. 220 beats/min.
   c. 190 beats/min.
   d. 125 beats/min.

9. Some models of the ICD have tiered therapy. Tiered therapy means

   a. the device is capable of shocking both atrial and ventricular tachyarrhythmias.
   b. a wide range of electrical shocks (joules) can be programmed to meeet individual patient needs.
   c. the device can convert the rhythm by either a pacing stimulus, a low-voltage cardioversion, or a higher voltage shock followed by antibradycardia pacing if needed.
   d. the device can be externally programmed, and printouts of the features of the device can be obtained.

REFERENCES

Pharmacological Therapy: Antiarrhythmic, Vasoactive, and Thrombolytic Agents

1. Deglin JH, Vallerand AH: Davis's Drug Guide for Nurses (4th Ed). Philadelphia, F.A. Davis, 1995
2. Ewald GA, McKensie C (eds): Manual of Medical Therapeutics: The Washington Manual (28th Ed). St. Louis, Little Brown, 1995
3. Tomuselle G: Clinical implications of antiarrhythmic drug classification. Journal of Critical Illness S15–S21, 1996
4. Brzozowski L: Antiarrhythmic propafenone: Improving patient outcomes. DCCN 12(3):116–122, 1993
5. Vukmir R: Cardiac arrhythmia therapy. Am J Emerg Med 13(4): 459–470, 19
6. Pifarre R, Blakeman B, Darovic G: In Darovic G (ed): Hemodynamic Monitoring: Invasive and Non-invasive Clinical Applications (2nd Ed), pp 807–835. Philadelphia, W.B. Saunders, 1995
7. Hohnloser S, Woosley R: Sotalol. N Engl J Med 331(1):31–37, 1994
8. Cummins R: Textbook of Advanced Cardiac Life Support. Dallas, American Heart Association, 1994
9. Young G, Hoffman J: Thrombolytic therapy: Advances and updates. Emerg Med Clin North Am 13(4):735–753, 1995

Percutaneous Transluminal Coronary Angioplasty and Percutaneous Balloon Valvuloplasty

1. American Heart Association: 1996 Heart and Stroke Facts. Dallas, American Heart Association, 1996
2. Faxon DP: "Introduction and Historical Background" In Faxon DP (ed): Practical Angioplasty. New York, Raven Press, 1994
3. Faxon DP: "Mechanisms of Angioplasty and Pathophysiology of Restenosis" In Faxon DP (ed): Practical Angioplasty. New York, Raven Press, 1994
4. Bentivoglio LG, Holubkov R, Kelsey SF et al: Short and long term outcome of percutaneous transluminal coronary angioplasty in unstable versus stable angina pectoris: A report of the 1985/1986 NHLBI PTCA registry. Cathet Cardiovasc Diagn 23:227–238, 1991
5. O'Keefe JH Jr, Rutherford BD, McConahay DR et al: Multi-vessel coronary angioplasty from 1980 to 1989: Procedural results and long-term outcome. J Am Coll Cardiol 16:1097–1102, 1990
6. Dorros G, Iyer SS, Hall P, Mathiak LM: Percutaneous coronary angioplasty in 1001 multivessel coronary disease patients: An analysis of different patient subsets. Journal of Interventional Cardiology 4:71–80, 1991
7. Alderman EL, Bourassa MG, Cohen LS et al for the CASS investigators: Ten year follow-up of survival and myocardial infarction in the randomized coronary artery surgery study. Circulation 82:1629–1646, 1990
8. Meyer J, Merx W, Schmitz H et al: Percutaneous transluminal coronary angioplasty immediately after intracoronary streptolysis of transmural myocardial infarction. Circulation 66:905–913, 1982
9. Hartzler GO, Rutherford BD, McConahay DR et al: Percutaneous transluminal coronary angioplasty with and without thrombolytic therapy for treatment of acute myocardial infarction. Am Heart J 106:965–973, 1983
10. Coombs VJ, Brinker JA: Primary angioplasty in the acute myocardial infarction setting. AACN Clin Issues 6(3):387–397, 1995
11. Coombs VJ: Keeping up with interventional cardiology. Office Nurse Nov/Dec:12–16, 1993

12. Simari RD et al: Coronary angioplasty in acute myocardial infarction: Primary, immediate, adjunctive, rescue or deferred adjunctive approach? Mayo Clin Proc 69:346–358, 1994
13. Ryan TJ: "Patient Selection: Current Status" In Faxon DP (ed): Practical Angioplasty. New York, Raven Press, 1994
14. Waller BF, Pinkerton CA: "The Pathology of Interventional Coronary Artery Techniques and Devices" In Topol EJ (ed): Textbook of Interventional Cardiology (2nd Ed). Philadelphia, W.B. Saunders, 1994
15. Goodkind J, Coombs VJ, Golobic RA: Excimer laser angioplasty. Heart Lung 22(1):26–35, 1993
16. Krause KR, Sketch MH, Stack RS: Extraction Atherectomy, pp 27–40. Baltimore, Williams and Wilkins, 1996

Intra-aortic Balloon Pump Counterpulsation and Ventricular Assist Devices

1. Holman WL, Bourge RC, McGriffin DC, Kirklin JK: Ventricular assist: Experience with a pulsatile heterotopic device. Seminars in Thoracic and Cardiovascular Surgery 6(3):147–153, 1994
2. McCarthy PM, Sabik JF: Implantable circulatory support devices as a bridge to heart transplantation. Seminars in Thoracic and Cardiovascular Surgery 6(3):174–180, 1994
3. Farrar DJ: Ventricular interactions during mechanical circulatory support. Seminars in Thoracic and Cardiovascular Surgery 6(3): 163–168, 1994
4. Dasse KA, Frazier OH, Graham TR: "The Physiology of Left Ventricular Assistance" In Lewis T, Graham TR (eds): Mechanical Circulatory Support, pp 13–25. London, Edward Arnold, 1995
5. Oz MC, Rose EA, Slater J et al: Malignant ventricular rhythms are well tolerated in patients receiving long-term left ventricular assist devices. J Am Coll Cardiol 24:1688–1691, 1994

Autologous Blood Transfusion

1. Kruskall MS et al: On improving the cost-effectiveness of autologous blood transfusion practices. Transfusion 34(3):259–264, 1994
2. Busch MP: "Transfusion-Associated AIDS" In Rossi EC et al (eds): Principles of Transfusion Medicine, pp 699–707. Williams & Wilkins, 1996
3. Menitove JE: "Transfusion in the Hypoproliferative Anemias" In Rossi EC et al (eds): Principles of Transfusion Medicine, pp 161–165. Williams & Wilkins, 1996
4. Spiess BD: Autologous blood should be available for elective cardiac surgery. Journal of Cardiothoracic and Vascular Anesthesia 8(2):231–237, 1994
5. Murphy P, Heal JM, Blumberg N: Infection or suspected infection after hip replacement surgery with autologous or homologous blood transfusions. Transfusion 31:212–217, 1991
6. Greenberger PA: "Plasma Anaphylaxis and Immediate Type Reactions" In Rossi EC et al (eds): Principles of Transfusion Medicine, pp 765–770. Williams & Wilkins, 1996
7. Stack G et al: "Febrile and Nonimmune Transfusion Reactions" In Rossi EC et al (eds): Principles of Transfusion Medicine, pp 773–782. Williams & Wilkins, 1996
8. Koff RS et al: "Transfusion-Transmitted Hepatitis A, B, and D" In Rossi EC et al (eds): Principles of Transfusion Medicine, pp 675–683. Williams & Wilkins, 1996
9. Alter HJ: "Transfusion-Transmitted non-A, non-B and Hepatitis C Virus Infections" In Rossi EC et al (eds): Principles of Transfusion Medicine, pp 687–698. Williams & Wilkins, 1996
10. Hjelle B: "Transfusion-Transmitted HTLV-I and HTLV-II" In Rossi EC et al (eds): Principles of Transfusion Medicine, pp 709–714. Williams & Wilkins, 1996
11. Gunter KC, Luban NLC: "Transfusion-Transmitted Cytomegalovirus and Epstein-Barr Virus Disease" In Rossi EC et al (eds): Principles of Transfusion Medicine, pp 712–728. Williams & Wilkins, 1996
12. Shulman IA: "Transmission of Parasitic Infections by Blood Transfusion" In Rossi EC et al (eds): Principles of Transfusion Medicine, pp 733–736. Williams & Wilkins, 1996
13. Ness PM: "Bacterial Transmission by Transfusion" In Rossi EC et al (eds): Principles of Transfusion Medicine, pp 739–744. Williams & Wilkins, 1996
14. Huston CJ: Hemolytic transfusion reaction. Am J Nurs 96(3):47, 1996
15. Brecher ME: "Hemolytic Transfusion Reactions" In Rossi EC et al (eds): Principles of Transfusion Medicine, pp 747–761. Williams & Wilkins, 1996
16. Schmidt H et al: Autotransfusion after coronary artery bypass grafting halves the number of patients needing blood transfusion. The Society of Thoracic Surgeons 61:1177–181, 1996
17. Smith RN: Underwater chest drainage. Nursing95 (2) 60–63 February, 1995
18. Sassetti RJ: "Preoperative Autologous Blood Donation" In Rossi EC et al (eds): Principles of Transfusion Medicine, pp 593–598. Williams & Wilkins, 1996
19. Stehling L, Zauder HL: "Preoperative Hemodilution" In Rossi EC et al: Principles of Transfusion Medicine, pp 601–604. Williams & Wilkins, 1996
20. Kruskall MS: "Intraoperative Autotransfusion" In Rossi EC et al (eds): Principles of Transfusion Medicine, pp 607–612. Williams & Wilkins, 1996
21. Valbonesi M et al: Intraoperative blood salvage (IOBS) in cardiac and vascular surgery. The International Journal of Artificial Organs 18(3):130–135, 1995
22. Smith RN et al: Instilling the facts about autotransfusion. Nursing95 25(3):52–55, 1995
23. Fakhry SM et al: "Metabolic Effects of Massive Transfusion" In Rossi EC et al (eds): Principles of Transfusion Medicine, pp 615–624. Williams & Wilkins, 1996
24. Myhre BA: Crossing over of autologous and directed donor blood. Ann Clin Lab Sci 22(5):343–352, 1992
25. Robberson F, Simon TL: "Medicolegal Aspects of Blood Transfusion" In Rossi EC et al (eds): Principles of Transfusion Medicine, pp 925–934. Williams & Wilkins, 1996

Cardiopulmonary Resuscitation

1. Wong M, Linehorn K: Advances in cardiopulmonary resuscitation. Critical Care Nursing Clinics of North America 7(2):227–230, 1995
2. Chandra NC: Mechanisms of blood flow during CPR. Ann Emerg Med 22(part 2):281–288, 1993
3. Hazinski MF: Basic life support: Controversial and unresolved issues. Journal of Cardiovascular Nursing 10(4):1–14, 1996
4. Association for the Advancement of Medical Instrumentation: Automatic external defibrillators and remote-control defibrillators (DF-39). Arlington, VA, AAMI, 1993

Management of Dysrhythmias

1. Cummins R: Textbook of Advanced Cardiac Life Support. Dallas, American Heart Association, 1994
2. Dreifus LS, Fisch C, Griffin JC, Gillette PC, Mason JW, Parsonnet V: Guidelines for implantation of cardiac pacemakers and antiarrhythmia devices. A report of the American College of Cardiology/American Heart Association Task Force on assessment of diagnostic and therapeutic cardiovascular procedures. (Committee on Pacemaker Implantation). J Am Coll Cardiol 18(1):1–13, 1991
3. Bernstein AD, Camm AJ, Fletcher RD et al: The NASPE/BPEG generic pacemaker code for antibradyarrhythmia and adaptive-rate pacing and antitachyarrhythmia devices. PACE 10:794–799, 1987
4. Morton PG: The pacemaker and defibrillator codes: Implications for critical care nursing. Critical Care Nurse 17(1):50–59, 1997
5. Baas LS, Beery TA, Hickey CS: Care and safety of pacemakers electrodes in intensive care and telemetry nursing units. Am J Crit Care 6(4):302–311, 1997
6. American Heart Association: Heart and Stroke Facts. Dallas, Texas, American Heart Association, 1995
7. Dreifus LS, Fisch C, Griffin JC, Gillette PC, Mason JW, Parsonnet V: Guidelines for implantation of cardiac pacemakers and antiarrhythmia devices. A report of the American College of Cardiology/American Heart Association Task Force on assessment of diagnostic and therapeutic cardiovascular procedures. (Committee on Pacemaker Implantation). J Am Coll Cardiol 18(1):1–13, 1991
8. Bernstein AD, Camm AJ, Fisher JD et al: The NASPE/BPEG Defibrillator Code. PACE 16:1776–1780, 1993

BIBLIOGRAPHY

Pharmacological Therapy: Antiarrhythmic, Vasoactive, and Thrombolytic Agents

Antz M, Cappato R, Kuch K: Metropolol versus sotalol in the treatment of sustained VT. J Cardiovasc Pharmacol 26(4):627–635, 1995

Burns D: Review of thrombolytic agents use in acute myocardial infarction, pulmonary embolus, and cerebral infarction. Critical Care Nursing Quarterly 15(4):1–12, 1993

Ching K, Williamson B, Niebaaur N et al: Physiologic effects of sotalol and amiodarone in patients with monomorphic VT. Am J Cardiol 74:1119–1123, 1994

Collier W, Holt S, Wellford L: Narrow Complex tachycardias. Emerg Med Clin North Am 13(4):925–954, 1995

Dorian P, Naccarelli G et al: A randomized comparison of flecanide versus verapamil in paroxysmal supraventricular tachycardia. Am J Cardiol 77:89A–95A, 1996

Ellenbogen K, Dias V et al: Safety and efficacy of intravenous diltiazem in atrial fibrillation or atrial flutter. Am J Cardiol 75:45–49, 1995

Kerin N, Faibel K, Nuini M: The efficacy of intravenous amiodarone for the conversion of chronic atrial fibrillation. Arch Intern Med 156:49–53, 1996

Kochs M, Eggeling T, Hombach V: Pharmacologic therapy in coronary artery disease: Prevention of life threatening ventricular tachdysrhythmis and sudden cardiac death. Eur Heart J 14(Supp. E):107–119, 1993

Lipka L, Dizon J, Reiffel J: Desired mechanisms of drugs for ventricular arrhythmias: class III antiarrhythmic agents. Am Heart J 130:632–640, 1995

Morton PG: Update on new antiarrhythmic drugs. Critical Care Nursing Clinics of North America 6(1):69–83, 1994

Olson J: Clinical pharmacology made ridiculously simple. Miami, Medical Master, 1994

Pill MW: Ibutilide: A new antiarrhythmic agent for the critical care environment. Critical Care Nurse 17(3):19–22, 1997

Reiffel JA, Estes N et al: A consensus report on antiarrhythmic drug use. Clinical Cardiology 17:103–116, 1994

Roden D: Risks and benefits of antiarrhythmic therapy. N Engl J Med 331(12):785–791, 1994

Scherer J, Roach S: Introductory Clinical Pharmacology (5th Ed). Philadelphia, J.B. Lippincott, 1996

Symanski J, Gettes L: Drug effects on the electrocardiogram. A review of their significance. Drugs 46(2):219–248, 1993

Wyze D, George D: Pharmacologic therapy in patients with ventricular tachyarrhythmias. Cardiol Clin 11(1):65–82, 1993

Percutaneous Transluminal Coronary Angioplasty and Percutaneous Balloon Valvuloplasty

Albert NM: Laser angioplasty and intracoronary stents: Going beyond the balloon. AACN Clinical Issues 5(1):15–20, 1994

Baim D, Kent K, King SI et al. Evaluating new devices, acute results from the new approaches to coronary intervention registry. Circulation 89:471–481, 1994

Barbiere CC: A new device for control of bleeding after transfemoral catheterization. Critical Care Nurse 15(1):51–53, 1995

Davis C, Van Riper S, Longstreet J, Moscucci M: Vascular complications of coronary interventions. Heart Lung 26(2):118–127, 1997

DeJong MJ, Morton PG: Control of vascular complications after cardiac catheterization: A research-based protocol. Dimensions of Critical Care Nursing 16(4):170–180, 1997

Ellis SG, Holmes DR: Strategic approaches in coronary intervention. Baltimore, Williams and Wilkins, 1996

Fischman D, Leon M, Baim D et al: A randomized comparison of coronary stent placement and balloon angioplasty in the treatment of coronary artery disease. N Engl J Med 331(8):496–501, 1994

Gardner E, Joyce S, Iyer M, Mowery MA, Olson K, Piontek S: Intracoronary stent update: Focus on patient education. Critical Care Nurse 16(2):65–75, 1996

Holloway S, Feldman T: An alternative to valvular surgery in the treatment of mitral stenosis: Balloon mitral valvotomy. Critical Care Nurse 17(3):27–36, 1997

Meany TB, Leon MB, Kramer BL et al: Transluminal extraction catheter for the treatment of diseased saphenous vein grafts: A multicenter experience. Cathet Cardiovasc Diagn 34(2):112–120, 1995

Meluch F, Mitchell SB: Decreasing intracoronary stent complications. Dimensions of Critical Care Nursing 16(3):114–121, 1997

O'Neill WW, Brodie BR, Ivanhoe R et al: Primary angioplasty for acute myocardial infarction. Am J Cardiol 73:627–634, 1994

Perra BM: Managing coronary atherectomy patients in a special procedure unit. Critical Care Nurse 15(3):57–68, 1995

Ryan TJ, Bauman WB, Kennedy W et al: Guidelines for percutaneous transluminal coronary angioplasty. A report of the American Heart Association/American College of Cardiology Task Force on Assessment of Diagnostic and Therapeutic Cardiovascular Procedures (Committee on Percutaneous Transluminal Coronary Angioplasty). Circulation 88(6):2987–3007, 1993

Schickel S, Cronin SN, Mize A, Voelker C: Removal of femoral sheaths by registered nurses: Issues and outcomes. Critical Care Nurse 16(2):32–36, 1996

Vaska PL: Ischemic heart disease. AACN Clin Issues. 6(3):369–495, 1995

Intra-Aortic Balloon Pump Counterpulsation and Ventricular Assist Devices

Bruzeese J, Jobin CI, Quaal SJ: Intra-aortic balloon pumping in the community hospital setting. Critical Care Nursing Clinics of North America 8(4):465–470, 1996

Cadwell CA, Quaal SJ: Intra-aortic balloon counterpulsation timing. American Journal of Critical Care 5(4):254–261, 1996

Hobson KS: Physiologic aspects of the TCI Heartmate mechanical left ventricular assist device. Journal of Cardiovascular Nursing 8(2):16–35, 1994

Lewandowski AV: The bridge to cardiac transplantation: Venticular assist devices. Dimensions in Critical Care Nursing 14(1):17–26, 1995

Lewis T, Graham TR (eds): Mechanical Circulatory Support. London, Edward Arnold, 1995

Nastala CJ: Bridge to cardiac transplantation: Current practice. Critical Care Nurse Quarterly 18(1):65–76, 1995

Oz MC, Levin HR, Rose EA: Long term, implantable ventricular assist devices: What are they and who needs them? Comprehensive Therapy 21(7):351–354, 1995

Quaal SJ (ed): Cardiac Mechanical Assistance beyond Balloon Pumping. St. Louis, Mosby, 1993

Quaal SJ: Caring for the intra-aortic balloon pump patient: Most frequently asked nursing questions. Critical Care Nursing Clinics of North America 8(4):471–176, 1996

Quaal SJ (ed): Comprehensive Intra-aortic Balloon Counterpulsation (2nd Ed). St. Louis, Mosby-Year Book, 1993

Quaal SJ: Maintaining competence and competency in the care of the intra-aortic balloon pump patient. Critical Care Nursing Clinics of North America 8(4):441–450, 1996

Sitzer VA, Atkins PJ: Developing and implementing a standard of care for intra-aortic balloon counterpulsation. Critical Care Nursing Clinics of North America 8(4):451–458, 1996

Stavarski DH: Complications of intra-aortic balloon pumping: Preventable or not preventable. Critical Care Nursing Clinics of North America 8(4):409–422, 1996

Vaca KJ, Lohmann DP, Moroney DA: Current status and future trends of mechanical circulatory support. Critical Care Nursing Clinics of North America 7:249–258, 1995

Vargo RL: Bridging to transplantation: Mechanical support for heart failure. Critical Care Nursing Clinics of North America 5:649–659, 1995

Wojner AW: Assessing the five points of the intra-aortic balloon pump waveform. Critical Care Nurse 14(3):48–52, 1994

Autologous Blood Transfusion

Guidelines for Quality Assurance Programmes for Blood Transfusion Services, pp 21–30. World Health Organization, 1993

Rossi EC et al: "Transfusion Into the Next Millennium" In Rossi EC et al (eds): Principles of Transfusion Medicine, pp 1–11. Williams & Wilkins, 1996

Sobel M: "Diagnosis and Management of Intraoperative and Postoperative Hemostatic Defects" In Rossi EC et al (eds): Principles of Transfusion Medicine, pp 649–659. Williams & Wilkins, 1996

Cardiopulmonary Resuscitation

American Heart Association: 1996 Handbook of Emergency Cardiac Care for Healthcare Providers. Dallas, American Heart Association, 1996

Chandra NC, Hanzinski M (eds): Basic Life Support for Healthcare Providers. Dallas, American Heart Association, 1996

Crockett PJ, Droppert BM, Higgins SE, Richards RK: Defibrillation: What you should know. Redmond, WA, Physiocontrol, 1996

Cummins R (ed): Advanced Cardiac Life Support. Dallas, American Heart Association, 1994

Ivy SS: Ethical considerations in resuscitation decisions: A nursing ethics approach. Journal of Cardiovascular Nursing 10(4):47–58, 1996

Kirby AK, Sanders A: Developing and revising the American heart Association guidelines for advanced cardiac life support. Journal of Cardiovascular Nursing 10(4):15–23, 1996

O'Hearn P: Early defibrillation: Lessons learned. Journal of Cardiovascular Nursing 10(4):24–36, 1996

Stewart J: A more effective approach to in-hospital defibrillation. Journal of Cardiovascular Nursing 10(4):37–46, 1996

Tucker K, larsen J et al: Advanced cardiac life support: Update on recent guidelines and a look at the future. Clin Cardiol 18:497–504, 1995

Management of Dysrhythmias

Akhtar M, Jazayeri M, Sra J, Dhala A, Deshpande S, Blank Z, Axtell K: Implantable cardioverter-defibrillator therapy for prevention of sudden cardiac death. Cardiol Clin 11(1):97–108, 1993

Axtell K: Implantable cardioverter-defibrillator therapy for prevention of sudden cardiac death. Cardiol Clin 11(1):97–108, 1993

Barbiere C: From emergent transvenous pacemaker to permanent implant and follow up. Critical Care Nurse 13(2):39–45, 1993

Beery TA, Baas LS, Hickey CS: Infection precautions with temporary pacing leads: A descriptive study. Heart Lung 25(3):182–189, 1996

Bernstein AD, Parsonnet V: "Pacemaker and Defibrillator Codes" In Ellenbogen KA, Kay GN, Wilkoff BL (eds): Clinical Cardiac Pacing, pp 279–283. Philadelphia, W.B. Saunders, 1995

Brenner S, McCauley K, Axtell K: A follow-up study of patients with implantable cardioverter defibrillators. Journal of Cardiovascular Nursing 7(3):40–51, 1993

Burke L: Securing life through technology acceptance: The first six months after transvenous internal cardioverter defibrillator implantation. Heart Lung 25(5):352–366, 1996

Collins M: When your patient has an implantable cardioverter defibrillator. Am J Nurs 94(3):34–39, 1994

Craney J, Powers M: Factors related to driving in persons with an implantable cardioverter defibrillator. Progress in Cardiovascular Nursing 10(3):12–17, 1995

Davidson T, VanRiper S, Harper P, Wenk A: Implantable cardioverter defibrillators: A guide for clinicians. Heart Lung 23(3):205–217, 1994

Dunbar S, Warner C, Purcell J: Internal cardiovascular defibrillator device discharge: Experiences of patients and family members. Heart Lung 22(6):454–501, 1993

Finch N, Leman R, Kratz J Gillette P: Driving safety among patients with implantable cardioverter defibrillators. JAMA 270(13):1587–1588, 1993

Gallagher R, McKinley S, Mangan B, Pelletier D, Squire J, Mitten-Lewis S: The impact of implantable cardioverter defibrillator on quality of life. American Journal of Critical Care 6(1):16–24, 1997

Futterman LG, Lemberg L: New indications for dual chamber pacing: Hypertrophic and dilated cardiomyopathy. American Journal of Critical Care 4(1):82–87, 1995

Hauser R, Kurschinski D, McVeigh K, Thomas A, Mower M: Clinical results with nonthoracotomy ICD systems. PACE 16(1):Part II:141–148, 1993

Hayes DL, Wang PJ, Reynolds DW, Estes NA, Griffith JL, Steffens RA, Carlo GL, Findlay GK, Johnson CM: Interference with cardiac pacemakers by cellular telephones. N Engl J Med 336(21):1473–1479, 1997

Horwood L, Van Riper S, Davidson T: Antitachycardia pacing: An overview. American Journal of Critical Care 4(5):397–404, 1995

Jordaens L, Vertongen P, Provenier F, Trowerbach J, Poelaert J, Herregods L: A new transvenous internal cardioverter-defibrillator: Implantation technique, complications and short-term follow-up. Am Heart J 129(2):251–258, 1995

Kleman J, Castle G, Kidwell G, Maloney J, Morant V, Trohman R, Wilhoff B, McCarthy P, Pinski S: Nonthoracotomy- versus thoracotomy-implantable defibrillators: Intention to treat comparison of clinical outcomes. Circulation 9(6):2833–2841, 1994

Luceri RM, Zilo P, Weiss DN: Management of patients with tiered-therapy defibrillators. Primary Cardiology 21(3):24–33, 1995

Manion P: Temporary epicardial pacing in the postoperative cardiac surgical patient. Critical Care Nurse 13(2):30–38, 1993

Morton P: The pacemaker and defibrillator codes: Implications for critical care nursing. Critical Care Nurse 17(1):50–59, 1997

Moser S, Crawford D, Thomas A: Updated care guidelines for patients with automatic implantable cardioverter defibrillators. Critical Care Nurse 13(2):62–73, 1993

Nichols K, Collines J: Update on implantable cardioverter defibrillators: Knowing the differences in devices and their impact on patient care. AACN Clinical Issues 6(1):31–43, 1995

Porterfield L, Porterfield J: Third generation pacemaker–cardioverter–defibrillator: A case study. Critical Care Nurse 15(1):43–45, 1995

Rasmussen M, Mangan D: Third generation antitachycardia pacing implantable cardioverter-defibrillators. Dimensions of Critical Care Nursing 13(6):284–291, 1994

Schurig L: Educational guidelines: Pacing and Electrophysiology. Armonk, NY, North American Society of Pacing and Electrophysiology Council of Associated Professionals, Futura Publishing Company, 1994

Sirovatka B: The implantable cardioverter: Patient and family education. Dimensions of Critical Care Nursing 12(6):328–334, 1993

Sneed NV, Finch NJ, Leman RB: The impact of device recall on patients and family members of patients with automatic implantable cardioverter defibrillators. Heart Lung 23(4):317–322, 1994

Sorenson ER, Manna D, McCourt K: Use of epicardial pacing wires after coronary artery bypass surgery. Heart Lung 23(6):487–492, 1994

Strichberger S, Hummel J, Daoud E, Niebauer M, Williamson B, Man K, Horwood L et al: Implantation by electrophysiologists of 100 consecutive cardioverter defibrillators with non-thoracotomy lead systems. Circulation 90(2):868–872, 1994

Wever EF, Hauer RN, van Capelle FJ, Tijsen JG, Crijns HG, Algra A, Wisefeld AC, Bakker PF, de Medina EO: Randomized study of implantable defibrillator as first-choice therapy versus conventional strategy in postinfarct sudden death survivors. Circulation 91(8):2195–2203, 1995

Witherell C: Cardiac rhythm control devices. Critical Care Nursing Clinics of North America 6(1):85–101, 1994

Radiofrequency Catheter Ablation

Bubien R, Knotts S, McLaughlin S, George P: What you need to know about radiofrequency ablation. Am J Nurs 93(7):30–37, 1993

Bubien R, Knotts S, Kay G: Radiofrequency catheter ablation: Concepts and nursing implications. Cardiovascular Nursing 31(3):17–23, 1995

Calkins H, Kalbfleisch S, El-Atassi R, Langberg J, Morady F: Relations between efficacy of radiofrequency catheter ablation and site of origin of idiopathic ventricular tachycardia. Am J Cardiol 71(10):827–833 1993

Cliff D, Blazewicz P: Radiofrequency catheter ablation—part 1: Pre- and post-procedure nursing responsibilities. Dimensions of Critical Care Nursing 12(6):313–318, 1993

Craney J: Radiofrequency catheter ablation of supraventricular tachycardias: Clinical consideration and nursing care. Journal of Cardiovascular Nursing 7(3):26–39, 1993

Finkelmeier B: Ablative therapy in the treatment of tachyarrhythmias. Critical Care Nursing Clinics of North America 6(1):103–110, 1994

Flutterman L, Lemberg L: Radiofrequency catheter ablation for supraventricular tachycardias: Part I. American Journal of Critical Care 2(6):500–505, 1993

Flutterman L, Lemberg L: Radiofrequency catheter ablation for supraventricular tachycardias: Part II. American Journal of Critical Care 3(1):77–80, 1994

Guaglianone D, Tyndall A: Comfort issues in patients undergoing radiofrequency catheter ablation. Critical Care Nurse 15(1):47–50, 1995

Klein L, Miles W: Radiofrequency ablation of cardiac arrhythmias. Scientific American Science and Medicine 1(2):48–57, 1994

Lesh M: Interventional electrophysiology: State-of-the-art. Am Heart J 126(3, part 1):686–696, 1995

Moulton L, Grant J, Miller B, Moulton K: Radiofrequency catheter ablation for supraventricular tachycardia. Heart Lung 22(1):3–14, 1993

Porterfield L, Porterfield J: Radiofrequency ablation of a left-sided free-wall accessory pathway: A case study. Critical Care Nurse 13(2): 46–49, 1993

Teplitz L: Transcatheter ablation of tachyarrhythmias: An overview and case studies. Progress in Cardiovascular Nursing 9(3):16–31, 1994

Woods SJ, Froelicher ES, Halpenny CJ, Motzer SU: Cardiac Nursing (3rd Ed). Philadelphia, J.B. Lippincott, 1995

18

Common Cardiovascular Disorders

OBJECTIVES

Based on the content in this chapter, the reader should be able to:

- Differentiate between pericarditic and ischemic chest pain.
- Explain the underlying disease process in myocarditis.
- Explain the long-term effect of endocarditis on the heart valves.
- Differentiate dilated cardiomyopathy from hypertrophic cardiomyopathy.
- Analyze the similarities in clinical management between the three types of cardiomyopathies.
- Analyze the differences between arterial and venous peripheral vascular disease.
- Compare and contrast the clinical findings of aortic aneurysm with acute aortic dissection.
- Differentiate management of hypertension from hypertensive crisis.

*C*ardiovascular diseases remain the leading cause of death and disability in the United States. In addition to acute myocardial infarction, these disorders include inflammation and infections of the heart, pericardium, and valves and diseases involving the aorta and peripheral vascular system. This chapter reviews several common cardiovascular disorders, including pericarditis, myocarditis, endocarditis, cardiomyopathy, peripheral vascular disease, aortic diseases, and hypertensive crisis.

337

Infection and Inflammation of the Heart

Infectious and inflammatory diseases of the heart can cause acute pain and serious problems for the patient.

■ PERICARDITIS

Pathophysiological Principles

The heart muscle is surrounded by a membranous sac, the pericardium, which is composed of two layers: the outer parietal and inner visceral layers. Between these two layers is 10 to 50 mL of clear pericardial fluid, which acts as a lubricant. The pericardium helps to support the heart and to isolate it from infections in the surrounding structures.[1]

Pericarditis is an inflammation of the pericardial sac. This inflammation often involves the adjoining diaphragm. It can be a primary disease or occur secondarily as the result of some other disorder, such as an acute myocardial infarction. Causes of pericarditis are listed in the display. Infectious pericarditis is an increasing problem in the immunocompromised patient.[2]

Assessment

CLINICAL MANIFESTATIONS

The primary symptom in acute pericarditis is chest pain. This pain tends to be pleuritic in nature and classically is made worse by breathing deeply or lying supine. Because of pain from breathing, patients often complain of dyspnea. Relief is often obtained by sitting up, leaning forward, and taking shallow breaths. The chest pain of pericarditis may be difficult to distinguish from ischemic chest pain. Differential diagnoses are summarized in Table 18-1. One clue in the differentiation is that ischemic chest pain is not relieved by a change in the patient's position.

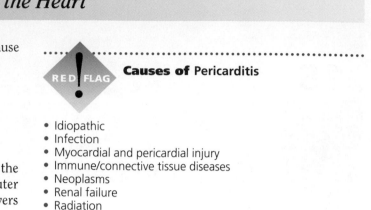

RED FLAG **Causes of** Pericarditis

- Idiopathic
- Infection
- Myocardial and pericardial injury
- Immune/connective tissue diseases
- Neoplasms
- Renal failure
- Radiation
- Drugs

There may also be general symptoms of an infection, such as a low-grade fever, cough, or malaise. The presence of a pericardial friction rub confirms the diagnosis.

DIAGNOSTIC STUDIES

The electrocardiogram (ECG) may show diffuse ST segment elevation with an upward concavity and PR segment depression (Fig. 18-1).[3] This contrasts with the ECG seen in acute myocardial injury, which typically shows upward convexity in leads facing the infarct zone (Fig. 18-2).

Management

Treatment for the patient with pericarditis includes the use of nonsteroidal anti-inflammatory agents, such as aspirin or ibuprofen. Steroids may be indicated in resistant cases in which infectious causes have been excluded. Anticoagulants should be avoided in the post–myocardial infarction patient. The goal of nursing management is pain relief.

TABLE 18-1   CLINICAL APPLICATION: Assessment Parameters
Differential Diagnosis of Chest Pain

Diagnosis	Onset of Pain	Quality of Pain	Relieved by
Angina pectoris	Sudden, after heavy meal or exertion	Crushing Squeezing Choking	Rest, nitrates
Acute myocardial infarction	Varies, may be associated with feeling of doom	Similar to angina, but more severe	No relief with rest
Pericarditis	Varies, may be preceded by "flulike" symptoms for several days to weeks	Pleuritic Sharp, stabbing	Sitting up Shallow breathing NSAIDs
Acute aortic dissection	Sudden, may be associated with syncope Intense from the onset	Ripping Tearing Worst pain in patient's life	No relief

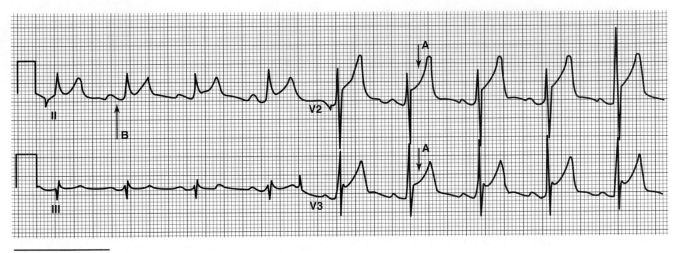

FIGURE 18-1
The 12-lead electrocardiogram in acute pericarditis. Note the diffuse upward concavity ST changes (**A**) and the PR segment depression (**B**).

Most episodes of pericarditis abate over 2 to 6 weeks. Rarely do patients develop recurrent episodes. Pericardial effusion with the potential for cardiac tamponade is a rare complication.

▬ MYOCARDITIS

Pathophysiological Principles

Myocarditis is an inflammation of the myocardium and the conduction system of the heart in the absence of myocardial infarction.[4] This relatively uncommon disease can be caused by many infectious agents, as listed in the display, and can occur in any age group. Myocarditis can be a devastating illness that evolves into a chronic, progressive disease with a poor prognosis. This disorder may result in dysrhythmias, congestive heart failure (CHF), or death.[4] In one study, mortality, defined as death or the need for cardiac transplantation, reached 56% at 4 years following diagnosis.[5]

Assessment

CLINICAL MANIFESTATIONS

Clinical presentation of myocarditis is variable, although unexplained heart failure is a common manifestation. Chest pain, often pleuritic in nature, is a frequent complaint. The presence of vague symptoms, such as fatigue, dyspnea, palpitations, and precordial discomfort, accompanied by a slight rise in serum enzymes and nonspecific ST-T wave changes in the ECG, may point to the diagnosis of myocarditis. Definitive diagnosis requires a positive endomyocardial biopsy.[5,6]

Management

Management of myocarditis depends on the etiology and clinical presentation. Although myocarditis evokes a severe inflammatory response, treatment with corticosteroids or immunosuppressive agents has not been effective in changing the clinical course.[4,5]

The display on the next page lists sample nursing diagnoses for a patient with myocarditis. Many of the skills re-

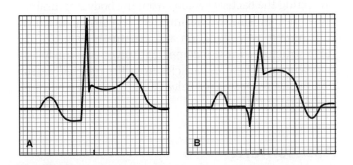

FIGURE 18-2
ST segment changes seen in acute pericarditis (**A**) and myocardial infarction (**B**).

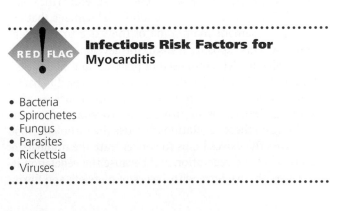

RED FLAG   **Infectious Risk Factors for** Myocarditis

- Bacteria
- Spirochetes
- Fungus
- Parasites
- Rickettsia
- Viruses

CLINICAL APPLICATION: Examples of Nursing Diagnoses for the Patient with Myocarditis

Fatigue related to acute myocarditis
Ineffective Individual or Family Coping related to sudden onset of a critical disease
Powerlessness related to medical regimen
Anticipatory Grieving related to loss of former lifestyle

quired by the nurse to care for the patient with myocarditis are similar to those needed in the care of the patient with CHF. In addition, the nurse must be prepared to help the patient and family deal with the unexpected reality of a potentially lethal disease that often has no cure and may require heart transplantation.

Some episodes of myocarditis will resolve on their own. Other patients will develop a subacute disease with persistent laboratory findings of inflammation, for example an increased white blood cell count or an elevated sedimentation rate. Idiopathic dilated cardiomyopathy may be the result of past episodes of viral myocarditis.

ENDOCARDITIS

Pathophysiological Principles

Endocarditis is an infection of the endocardial surface of the heart, including the valves. Infective endocarditis is a serious illness with mortality rates of 20% to 30%. These rates are higher in individuals over the age of 60.[7,8]

In the past, rheumatic heart disease caused the majority of cases of endocarditis. Currently, endocarditis is more likely to be found in patients with prosthetic valves, those who abuse intravenous drugs, or patients with mitral valve prolapse or other nonrheumatic abnormalities as detailed in the display. Common infectious organisms include *Streptococcus viridans*, *Staphylococcus epidermidis*, and *Staphylococcus aureus*.

The development of infective endocarditis is a complex process that requires the occurrence of several critical elements.[7,9] First, there must be endothelial damage that exposes the basement membrane of the valve to turbulent blood flow. This exposure leads to the development of a clot on the valve leaflet, composed of platelets and fibrin. Second, these clots, or vegetations, must be exposed to bacteria by way of bloodstream transport, such as occurs after dental manipulations or urological procedures. Bacteria proliferate on these vegetations because the turbulent blood flow across the valves helps to concentrate the numbers of bacteria near the vegetation and because the vegetation itself covers the bacteria with layers of platelets and fibrin,

RED FLAG ·

Risk Factors for Endocarditis

Native Valve Endocarditis
Adults:
- Mitral valve prolapse
- No underlying diseases
- Degenerative lesions of the mitral and aortic valves
- Congenital heart disease
- Rheumatic heart disease

Older People (age >60):
- Prosthetic valves
- Degenerative lesions

Diabetic Patients because of:
- Accelerated atherosclerosis
- Predisposition to infections

Pregnancy (rare) associated with:
- Underlying cardiac disease
- Dental procedures
- Premature labor
- Prolonged rupture of membranes
- Prolonged third stage of labor
- Manual removal of the placenta

Intravenous drug abusers:
- Risk varies with the type of drug, method of preparation, and route of administration

Prosthetic Valve Endocarditis
Early (within 60 days of surgery) usually due to:
- Nosocomial infections
- Central intravenous catheters
- Arterial catheters
- Cardiac pacing wires
- Endotracheal tubes

Late (after 60 days) usually due to:
- Dental, genitourinary, or gastrointestinal manipulations

Adapted from Karchmer AW: Infective endocarditis. In Braunwald E (ed): Heart Disease, pp 1077–1104 (5th Ed). Philadelphia, WB Saunders, 1997

· ·

protecting the bacterial colony from the body's natural defense mechanisms.[7,9] The infected vegetation interferes with normal valve function and eventually damages the valve structure. These incompetent valves eventually lead to severe heart failure. Particles from the infected vegetation or severely damaged valve can break loose and cause peripheral emboli.

Assessment

Symptoms of endocarditis usually occur within 2 weeks of the precipitating bacteremia and are outlined in the display. Nonspecific complaints, such as general malaise, anorexia,

Signs and Symptoms of
Endocarditis

- Fever
- Heart murmurs
- Splenomegaly
- Petechiae
    Splinter hemorrhages
    Osler's nodes (small, raised, tender nodules that occur on
      the fingers or toes)
    Janeway lesions (small erythematous or hemorrhagic
      lesions on the palms or soles)
- Musculoskeletal complaints
- Systemic or pulmonary emboli
- Neurological manifestations
    Headache
    Mycotic aneurysms

fatigue, weight loss, and night sweats, are common. Fevers and heart murmurs are present in almost all patients. Because symptoms are nonspecific, a careful history and physical examination are needed to alert the nurse to the potential diagnosis of endocarditis.

Management

Cure of infectious endocarditis is difficult and requires complete eradication of the bacterial colony from the vegetation. This usually involves a prolonged course of antibiotics. Treatment should not be delayed waiting for identification of the specific organism but should begin as soon as blood cultures are drawn. Antibiotic therapy is often continued in the home after discharge.

Immediate surgical intervention is indicated in the presence of severe CHF secondary to valve dysfunction, uncontrolled infections, and prosthetic valve dysfunction or dehiscence.

Considerations for Home Care
Endocarditis

- Stable, uncomplicated patient able to comply with medical regimen
- Daily nursing follow-up needed
- Intravenous administration of antibiotics preferred
- Care of vascular access site to avoid repeat infections
- Identification of original infectious source
- Future need for endocarditis prophylaxis

Cardiomyopathies

Cardiomyopathy refers to unknown etiological diseases involving heart muscle. Cardiomyopathies are of three types: dilated, hypertrophic, and restrictive (Table 18-2). Of the three types, dilated cardiomyopathy accounts for over 90% of cases.[10]

Pathophysiological Principles

Dilated cardiomyopathy (DCM) is characterized by increased ventricular size, impaired systolic function, and CHF.[11] In most instances, the cause is unknown. The clinical course is usually marked by progressive dilation of the heart chambers. As ventricular dilation increases, mitral and tricuspid insufficiency occur as the valve leaflets are stretched and separated. Dysrhythmias, such as ventricular tachycardia and fibrillation, make management of this condition difficult.

Hypertrophic cardiomyopathy (HCM), which rarely occurs, is distinguished by excessive myocardial hypertrophy usually involving the septal wall. The most characteristic feature of HCM is diastolic dysfunction. The heart is able to contract but is not able to relax and remains abnormally stiff in diastole. Sudden death is a catastrophic outcome of HCM. Death often occurs in young HCM patients, usually from a ventricular dysrhythmia.[12]

The least common of the three types in the United States is *restrictive cardiomyopathy* (RCM). Its hallmark is also a "stiff" ventricle, or diastolic dysfunction. Myocardial hypertrophy, fibrosis, or infiltration of the muscle can be the underlying pathological process. Classically, RCM presents as CHF with only a small or slightly enlarged heart.[13]

Assessment

Clinical findings will depend on the type of cardiomyopathy and the extent of the disease. Table 18-2 details the clinical manifestations and major management issues in cardiomyopathy.

Management

Nursing management is similar to the care of patients with severe CHF and their families. (Refer to Chapter 19 for a detailed discussion of heart failure and the associated medical and nursing management.) The nurse must incorporate the type of cardiomyopathy, the current level of physical functioning, and family needs into the plan of care. Psychosocial concerns are important as patients and families try to cope with this debilitating and potentially fatal illness. They must deal with feelings of uncertainty and loss of control and the financial impact of a serious chronic illness.

TABLE 18-2

Assessment and Management in Cardiomyopathy

Cardiomyopathy	Description	Clinical Manifestations	Management
Dilated (congestive)	Biventricular dilation	• Fatigue, weakness • Congestive heart failure (CHF) • Dysrhythmias • Tricuspid and mitral valve regurgitation	• Symptomatic treatment • Control CHF • Control dysrhythmias
Hypertrophic	Marked hypertrophy of left ventricle, occasionally also of right ventricle, and usually but not always, disproportionate hypertrophy of septum	• Dyspnea • Angina • Fatigue • Syncope • Palpitations • Atrial fibrillation • Ventricular dysrhythmias • CHF • Sudden death	• Symptomatic treatment • Beta-blockers • Pacemaker • Surgery
Restrictive	Reduced ventricular compliance; usually caused by infiltration of myocardium (eg, by amyloid, hemosiderin, or glycogen deposits); only mildly enlarged heart.	• Dyspnea • Fatigue • CHF • Tricuspid and mitral valve regurgitation • Heart blocks • Emboli	• Symptomatic treatment • Control hypertension • Exercise restrictions

Peripheral Vascular Disease

Peripheral vascular disease includes a group of distinct disorders involving the arteries, veins, and lymphatic vessels. Atherosclerosis is the most common cause. Risk factors include heredity, age, smoking, hypertension, elevated cholesterol, diabetes, obesity, and stress.[14]

ARTERIAL DISEASE

Pathophysiological Principles

ARTERIOSCLEROSIS OBLITERANS

Peripheral disease in the arteries involves the aorta and its branches, especially in the lower extremities. It typically affects men from age 50 to 70 and women after menopause. The most frequent cause of peripheral arterial disease is arteriosclerosis, with the most common form being arteriosclerosis obliterans (ASO). ASO is the result of progressive atherosclerosis, which results in insufficient blood supply to the tissues. ASO develops in major bifurcations and areas of acute angulations. In the diabetic patient, there is greater involvement of the smaller and more distal vessels.[14]

THROMBOANGIITIS OBLITERANS

Thromboangiitis obliterans, or Buerger's disease, is a severe, chronic, inflammatory disease affecting the intermediate and small arteries of the extremities. It may also involve adjacent veins and nerves. The etiology is unknown, but it is associated with heavy smoking. The chronic inflammatory process is often followed by thrombosis, with vascular lesions and fibrous obliteration of the vessel.[14]

Assessment

CLINICAL MANIFESTATIONS

Clinical signs of peripheral arterial disease reflect the blood's inability to circulate freely to an extremity. Symptoms depend on the extent of the disease and the presence of collateral circulation.[15] The most frequent symptom, intermittent claudication, is experienced as a cramping, burning, or aching pain in the legs or buttocks that is relieved with rest. Symptoms do not correlate with the extent of the disease. For example, patients may experience severe claudication but still have strong peripheral pulses. Patients will also experience trophic changes, such as hair loss on the extremities, thickening of the nails, and drying of the skin. Acute arterial obstruction, such as occurs with an embolism, results in the sudden onset of extreme pain and other signs of acute arterial obstruction as outlined in the display.

RED FLAG **Symptoms of** Vascular Obstruction

Acute Arterial Occlusion
- Pain
- Pulselessness
- Pallor
- Paresthesia
- Paralysis

Deep Venous Thrombosis
- Pain in calf with dorsiflexion of foot (Homans' sign)
- Pain when standing
- Inflammation
- Swelling
- Tenderness
- Redness, soreness

Management

Treatment of peripheral arterial disease is focused on modifying or eliminating risk factors, especially smoking. Medications, such as peripheral vasodilators, are controversial and have not been shown to improve clinical outcome.[16] Peripheral interventional procedures, such as balloon angioplasty, are successful in restoring circulation in many cases. Surgical bypass may be required when severe or diffuse arterial obstruction is present.

VENOUS DISEASE

Disease of the veins involves obstruction of blood flow or disruption of the venous valves.

Pathophysiological Principles

THROMBOPHLEBITIS

The most common form of venous disease is thrombophlebitis. Phlebitis is inflammation of the vessel wall as the result of direct injury to the vein or as a complication of varicose veins. Vessel wall injury, stasis of blood, and increased blood coagulability are known as Virchow's triad. These three conditions have been recognized as causative factors in the development of thrombophlebitis since 1846.[14] Two of the three factors must be present for phlebitis to develop.

VENOUS INSUFFICIENCY

The cause of venous insufficiency is incompetence of the valves. Veins become overstretched due to persistent excessive venous pressure, such as occurs with episodes of deep vein thrombosis. Over time, this condition may lead to stasis ulcers.

Assessment

CLINICAL MANIFESTATIONS

Clinical signs of peripheral venous disease reflect the inability of the blood to drain from the extremity. Patients with venous insufficiency complain of dull aching in the affected leg. Swelling increases throughout the day but is usually relieved by lying down or elevating the legs.

Deep vein thrombosis is characterized by pain, swelling, tenderness, and increased temperature over the affected area. The patient will also exhibit a positive Homans' sign (pain in the calf with passive dorsiflexion of the foot).

Management

The focus of care for the patient with venous disease is to increase blood flow and prevent complications. Patients with deep venous thrombosis are at high risk for the development of pulmonary emboli. Treatment strategies include anticoagulant therapy to prevent the formation of emboli, bed rest, and analgesics. Warm, moist compresses may be applied. Calf or thigh measurements should be obtained daily. Elastic stockings or ACE wraps may also be used.

Aortic Disease

◼◼ AORTIC ANEURYSM

Pathophysiological Principles

Aortic aneurysms are defined as a localized dilation of the aorta to a size greater than 1.5 times its normal diameter.[17] Most aneurysms are arteriosclerotic in origin. Other causes include syphilis, infection, inflammatory diseases, medial degeneration, aortic dissection, and trauma. Aneurysms tend to occur mostly in men. Frequently hypertension is present, and the majority of patients have a history of smoking.

Aneurysms are classified according to their shape. Fusiform aneurysms are diffuse dilations of the entire circumference of the artery. Saccular aneurysms are localized balloon-shaped outpouchings. True aneurysms involve the entire vessel wall. A false aneurysm is formed when blood leaks outside of the artery but is contained by the surrounding tissues, as illustrated in Figure 18-3.

Thoracic aneurysms occur relatively infrequently and are most often atherosclerotic and fusiform.[17] As with abdominal aneurysms, many thoracic aneurysms are asymptomatic at the time of diagnosis. Symptoms may include aortic insufficiency and signs of pericardial tamponade if the aneurysm involves the aortic root.

Assessment

In the majority of patients, aneurysms are asymptomatic. Improvements in noninvasive testing with ultrasound have led to the incidental discovery of many small (3–5 cm), asymptomatic aneurysms. Symptoms are usually related to expansion or rupture of the aneurysm.

Detection of aortic aneurysms by physical examination is difficult, especially in obese patients. The abdomen should be examined for the presence of bruits or masses, and peripheral pulses should be carefully evaluated.

Management

Management includes control of hypertension and elimination of risk factors such as smoking. The patient should be followed with serial noninvasive tests, such as ultrasound. Surgery is the only treatment for aneurysms and is usually indicated in aneurysms larger than 5 cm. Management of aneurysms between 4 and 5 cm remains controversial. Patients who are healthy with no other morbidity may elect to have 4-cm aneurysms repaired. Indications for surgical repair are listed in the accompanying display.

◼◼ AORTIC DISSECTION

Acute aortic dissection is the most common and the most lethal process involving the aorta. Mortality rates are very high with death usually occurring from rupture of the aorta.[18] The incidence is highest in men over the age of 40 with a history of hypertension.

Pathophysiological Principles

Dissection involves a longitudinal separation of the medial layers of the aorta by a column of blood as shown in Figure 18-4. The dissection begins at a tear in the aortic wall, usually at the proximal end of the dissection. Blood pumped through this tear creates a false channel, or lumen, that

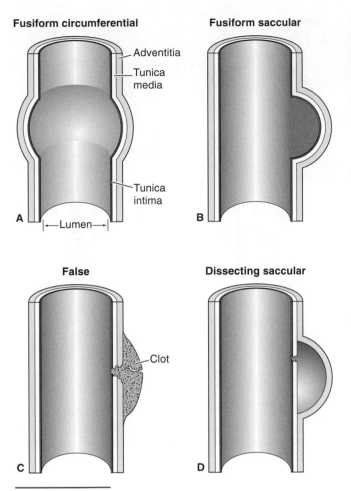

Fusiform circumferential

- Adventitia
- Tunica media
- Tunica intima

A |←Lumen→|

Fusiform saccular

B

False

- Clot

C

Dissecting saccular

D

FIGURE 18-3

Longitudinal sections of vessels showing types of aneurysms. True aneurysms are caused by vessel wall weakening and are illustrated in (**A**) fusiform circumferential and (**B**) fusiform saccular aneurysms. (**C**) False and (**D**) dissecting saccular aneurysms are usually caused by trauma and involve a break in the vessel wall.

> ### Insights Into Clinical Research
>
> *Bradbury A, P Bachoo, et al: Platelet count and the outcome of operation for ruptured abdominal aortic aneurysm. J Vasc Surg 21(3):484–491, 1995*
>
> The purpose of this retrospective chart review was to determine the relationship between platelet counts (PC) on admission and postsurgery and morbidity and mortality after emergency surgery for ruptured abdominal aortic aneurysm (AAA).
>
> Thirty-five patients (58%) survived and 25 did not (12 patients died intraoperatively and 13 died postoperatively). Those who survived ruptured AAA had a significantly higher systolic blood pressure at induction, shorter total clamp time, shorter total operative time, and smaller estimated blood loss during surgery than nonsurvivors. Survivors had a significantly higher PC preoperatively and postoperatively than did nonsurvivors. No patient with an admission PC $<100 \times 10^9/L$ survived, but all patients with a PC $>100 \times 10^9/L$ at the end of surgery survived. Fourteen of 15 patients with an admission PC $<150 \times 10^9/L$ died.
>
> This study established a direct relationship between admission and postoperative PC and mortality in patients who undergo surgery for a ruptured AAA. For the intensive care unit nurse and emergency department staff, these data are important for identifying people at risk for a poor outcome following ruptured AAA repair. While identifying prognostic indicators raises ethical questions, they also can assist the health care team in preparing families for a poor outcome and in making difficult decisions related to treatment.

the dissection involves the coronary arteries. Cardiac tamponade may be another complication of dissection involving the aortic root. Neurological deficits may occur if the aortic arch vessels are involved. Dissections involving the renal arteries will result in elevated serum creatinine, decreased urine output, and severe hypertension that is difficult to manage.

To confirm the diagnosis of acute aortic dissection, a transesophageal echocardiogram or contrast medium-enhanced computed tomography may be ordered.

rapidly becomes larger than the true aortic lumen. In the majority of patients, the plane of the dissection involves the ascending aorta. The false lumen typically extends all the way to the iliac bifurcation.

Assessment

CLINICAL MANIFESTATIONS

Over 90 percent of patients present with sudden, intense chest pain. Frequently the pain is described as ripping or tearing and may be accompanied by syncope (see Table 18-1). In most patients, the diagnosis can be determined with a careful history and physical examination. The clinician should look for the murmur of aortic regurgitation or alteration of the peripheral pulses in patients with known risk factors, such as hypertension. The chest x-ray may show a widened mediastinum. Cardiac ischemia may be present if

> ### CLINICAL APPLICATION: Diagnostic Studies
> *Indications for Surgical Repair of Aortic Aneurysms*
>
> - Aneurysms >5 cm
> - Aneurysms 4–5 cm in young patients in otherwise good health
> - Rapidly expanding aneurysms (growth rate >0.5 cm over a 6-month period)
> - Symptomatic aneurysm regardless of size

CLINICAL APPLICATION: Patient Care Study

Mr. Smith, a 57-year-old father of three, went to the local hospital emergency department (ED) complaining of "chest tightness progressing to my back." The ED nurse noted that Mr. Smith had a history of hypertension for which he was taking no medications and was a heavy smoker.

On admission to the ED, Mr. Smith appeared to be in moderate distress. His vital signs were BP 170/120 mmHg, equal in both arms; HR, 65 and regular; RR, 28; T, 37.2°C (99.0°F). Pulses were equal throughout. His skin was cool and diaphoretic.

While the ED staff was obtaining intravenous (IV) access, Mr. Smith suddenly complained of worsening chest pain and weakness in his legs. This weakness rapidly developed to paralysis of his lower extremities.

Mr. Smith was given morphine sulphate 2 mg IV to relieve his pain and placed on intravenous nitroglycerin to control his blood pressure. He was also started on oxygen 2 L by nasal cannula which increased his O_2 saturation to 95%. The bedside electrocardiogram (ECG) monitor displayed sinus tachycardia with no ectopy.

The ECG revealed nonspecific ST-T wave changes. The chest x-ray was nondiagnostic. A transesophageal echocardiogram (TEE) was suspicious for an aortic tear near the arch, but this was not confirmed by computerized tomography scan.

Mr. Smith was stabilized and transferred to a tertiary care hospital for further management and possible surgery for acute aortic dissection.

On arrival to the cardiac critical care unit, the paralysis had resolved. Mr. Smith's blood pressure remained 160 to 170/120 mmHg, so the decision was made to start nitroprusside. Labetalol was also started to decrease the stress on the aorta. Despite repeated reassurances and explanations of the procedures from the nurse, Mr. Smith became increasingly agitated. O_2 saturation remained normal. Lorazepam (Ativan) was administered intravenously to decrease Mr. Smith's agitation and help control his blood pressure.

A repeat TEE found no evidence of acute dissection. However, the TEE did find a bicuspid aortic valve and a diffusely dilated thoracic aorta, varying from 4.3 to 4.8 cm (normal is 2.5–3.5 cm). In addition, a 6.5-cm abdominal aortic aneurysm was noted. Because of the size of the aneurysm, urgent surgical repair was recommended.

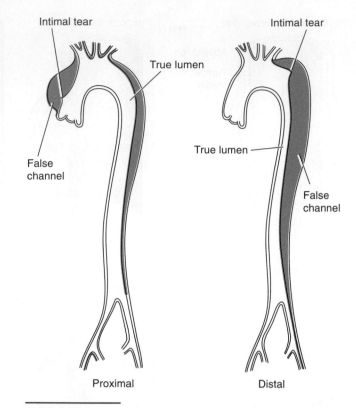

FIGURE 18-4
Two major patterns of aortic dissection. Blood pumps through a tear in the wall, creating a false channel or lumen. The false channel rapidly becomes larger than the true lumen.

Management

Survival of the acute phase depends on the location of the dissection, the severity of the complications, and the rapidity with which the diagnosis is confirmed. Clinical management focuses on controlling the blood pressure and on pain management. Surgery is the treatment of choice when the dissection involves the ascending aorta.

Hypertensive Crisis

Hypertension, defined as a sustained blood pressure in adults of greater than 140/90 mmHg, remains a major controllable risk factor for the development of cardiovascular diseases.[19] Over 90% of the time the etiology remains unknown (primary or essential hypertension). Hypertension is classified in stages, according to the systolic and diastolic pressures,[20] as detailed in Table 18-3.

Assessment

Although there may be a variety of causes, a hypertensive emergency or crisis rarely occurs. Possible causes and associated clinical situations are outlined in the accompanying display.

CLINICAL MANIFESTATIONS

A hypertensive crisis is characterized by the sudden onset of markedly increased diastolic pressure of 120 to 130 mmHg or greater, with the development of signs and symptoms indicating acute target organ vascular damage and the presence of retinal exudates and hemorrhages.[19] Once the diastolic pressure exceeds 120 mmHg, acute vascular damage and structural changes occur. Catecholamines are released,

TABLE 18-3
Classification of Blood Pressure

Category	Systolic (mmHg)	Diastolic (mmHg)
Normal	<130	<85
High normal	130–139	85–89
Hypertension		
Stage 1	140–159	90–99
Stage 2	160–179	100–109
Stage 3	180–209	110–119
Stage 4	≧210	≧120

Adapted from The Fifth report of the Joint National Commission on Detection, Evaluation, and Treatment of High Blood Pressure

the renin–angiotensin mechanism is activated, and the blood pressure is further exacerbated.

Management

The goal of treatment is to reduce the blood pressure within 1 hour of the crisis without sending the blood pressure too low.[20] Reducing the blood pressure too much can result in cerebral infarcts, myocardial infarction, or renal failure.[21] Because it is imperative to lower the blood pressure within minutes, intravenous medications are usually used (Table 18-4). Sodium nitroprusside remains the drug of choice in hypertensive crisis because of its almost instantaneous effects and short duration of action. Other medications include diazoxide and labetalol.

CONCLUSION

Cardiovascular disorders encompass a wide range of conditions that can be challenging in both establishing diagnosis and determining clinical management. Nursing care of these patients involves management of the acute episode and development of a plan for long-term care.

Clinical Applicability Challenges

Self-Challenge: Critical Thinking

1. Examine critical differences in clinical assessment between a patient with peripheral arterial disease and one with peripheral venous disease.

2. Compare and contrast the similarities and differences in the nursing management of the patient with acute myocarditis and dilated cardiomyopathy.

3. Management of patients, such as Mr. Smith, with a suspected acute aortic dissection requires rapid interventions from the health care team. Formulate a plan of care for these patients, classifying nursing actions in order of importance.

Study Questions

1. Three risk factors for the development of peripheral vascular disease are
   a. high blood pressure, diabetes, smoking.
   b. smoking, stress, infectious diseases.
   c. increased cholesterol, age, prior surgeries.
   d. increased cholesterol, gout, smoking.

2. Pain associated with pericarditis may be relieved by the
   a. prone position.
   b. supine position.
   c. side lying with knees bent position.
   d. sitting up and leaning forward position.

NURSING PERSPECTIVE
Summary of Hypertensive Crisis

Causes
- Acute or chronic renal disease
- Exacerbation of chronic hypertension
- Sudden withdrawal of antihypertensive medications
- Vasculitis

Associated Clinical Situations
- Eclampsia
- Hypertensive encephalopathy
- Acute aortic dissection
- Pulmonary edema
- Pheochromocytoma crisis
- Monoamine oxidase inhibitor and tyramine interaction
- Intracranial hemorrhage

Management
- Intravenous medications (see Table 18-4)

TABLE 18-4 CLINICAL APPLICATION: Drug Therapy
Intravenous Medications in Hypertensive Crisis

Drug	Dosage	Onset of Action	Adverse Effects
Nitroprusside	0.25–10 µg/kg/min	Instantaneous	Nausea, vomiting, muscle twitching, thiocyanate, and cyanide toxicity
Diazoxide	50–100 mg bolus repeated every 15–30 min	2–5 min	Nausea, hypotension, tachycardia, chest pain; not indicated in myocardial infarction, heart failure, or aortic dissection
Nicardipine	5–10 mg/h	10 min	Tachycardia, flushing, headache
Labetalol	20–80 mg bolus every 10–15 min 0.5–2 mg/min infusion	5–10 min	Nausea, vomiting, postural hypotension, dizziness
Esmolol	500 µg/kg/min for 4 min, then 150–300 µg/kg/min	1–2 min	Hypotension

3. *Key clinical findings in the assessment of the patient with suspected acute aortic dissection include*
   a. *high blood pressure, headache, sudden chest pain.*
   b. *unequal peripheral pulses, high blood pressure, nausea.*
   c. *unequal peripheral pulses; sudden onset of sharp, stabbing chest or back pain; new murmur of aortic insufficiency.*
   d. *high blood pressure, fever, absent distal pulses.*

REFERENCES

1. Lorell BH: Pericardial diseases. In Braunwald E (ed): Heart Disease, pp 1478–1534 (5th Ed). Philadelphia, WB Saunders, 1997
2. Dehmer GJ, O'Meara JJ III: Update on acute pericarditis. Hospital Medicine 31(1):39–44, 52–54, 1995
3. Dziadulewicz L, Shannon-Stone M: Postpericardiotomy syndrome: A complication of cardiac surgery. AACN Clinical Issues 6:464–470, 1995
4. Olinde KD, O'Connell JB: Inflammatory heart disease: Pathogenesis, clinical manifestations, and treatment of myocarditis. Annu Rev Med 45:481–490, 1994
5. Mason JW, O'Connell JB, Herskowitz A, et al: A clinical trial of immunosuppressive therapy for myocarditis. N Engl J Med 333:269–275, 1995
6. Wynne J, Braunwald E: The cardiomyopathies and myocarditides. In Braunwald E (ed): Heart Disease, pp 1404–1463 (5th Ed). Philadelphia, WB Saunders, 1997
7. Snelson C, Cline BA, Luby C: Infective Endocarditis: A challenging diagnosis. Dimensions of Critical Care Nursing 12:4–20, 1993
8. LeDoux D: Acquired valvular heart disease. In Woods SL, et al (eds): Cardiac Nursing, pp 798–819 (3rd Ed). Philadelphia, JB Lippincott, 1995
9. Karchmer AW: Infective endocarditis. In Braunwald E (ed): Heart Disease, pp 1077–1104 (5th Ed). Philadelphia, WB Saunders, 1997
10. Laurent-Bopp D: Cardiomyopathies and myocarditis. In Woods SL, et al (eds): Cardiac Nursing, pp 842–851 (3rd Ed). Philadelphia, JB Lippincott, 1995
11. Dec GW, Fuster V: Idiopathic dilated cardiomyopathy. N Engl J Med 331:1564–1575, 1994
12. Uszenski HJ, Booker SM, Goliash IB, et al: Hypertrophic cardiomyopathy: Medical, surgical, and nursing management. J Cardiovasc Nurs 7:13–22, 1993
13. Wynne J, Braunwald E: The cardiomyopathies and myocarditides. In Braunwald E (ed): Heart Disease, pp 1404-1463 (5th Ed). Philadelphia, WB Saunders, 1997
14. Wheeler EC, Brenner ZR: Peripheral vascular anatomy, physiology, and pathophysiology. AACN Clinical Issues 6:505–614, 1995
15. Krenzer ME: Peripheral vascular assessment: Finding your way through arteries and veins. AACN Clinical Issues 6:631–644, 1995
16. Karch AM: Pain, pills, and possibilities: Drug therapy in peripheral vascular disease. AACN Clinical Issues 6:614–630, 1995
17. Kent KC, Boyce SW: Aneurysms of the aorta. In Lindsay J (ed): Diseases of the Aorta, pp 109–125, Philadelphia, Lea & Febiger, 1994
18. House-Fancher MA: Aortic dissection: Pathophysiology, diagnosis, and acute care management. AACN Clinical Issues 6:602–613, 1995
19. Sollek MV: High blood pressure. In Woods SL, et al (eds): Cardiac Nursing, pp 766–767 (3rd Ed). Philadelphia, JB Lippincott, 1995
20. Joint National Committee on Detection, Evaluation, and Treatment of High Blood Pressure: The Fifth Report of the Joint National Committee on Detection, Evaluation, and Treatment of High Blood Pressure. National Institutes of Health, National Heart, Lung, and Blood Institute. March 1994; NIH Publication No. 93-1088
21. Porsche R: Hypertension: Diagnosis, acute antihypertension therapy, and long-term management. AACN Clinical Issues 6:515–525, 1995

BIBLIOGRAPHY

Braunwald E (ed): Heart Disease: A Textbook of Cardiovascular Medicine (5th Ed). Philadelphia, WB Saunders, 1997
Lindsay J (ed): Diseases of the Aorta. Philadelphia, Lea & Febiger, 1994

19

Heart Failure

OBJECTIVES

Based on the content in this chapter, the reader should be able to:

- Describe the four reserve mechanisms of the heart in response to stress.
- Explain the causes of heart failure and the physiological responses to failure.
- Compare and contrast the clinical manifestations of left ventricular failure versus right ventricular failure.
- Describe two classification systems used for heart failure patients.
- Explain the principles of management for a patient with heart failure.
- Identify nursing diagnoses for patients with heart failure.

*T*he heart, a complex structure composed of fibrous tissue, cardiac muscle, and electrical conducting tissue, has a single function: to pump blood. To do its job well, a good heart pump requires good functioning muscle, a good valve system, and an efficient pumping rhythm. An abnormality of sufficient severity of any component of the pump can affect its pumping efficiency and may cause the pump to fail.

■ PHYSIOLOGICAL PRINCIPLES

Reserve Mechanisms of the Heart in Response to Stress

When the heart is stressed, several reserve mechanisms can be called on to maintain good pumping function—that is, to provide a cardiac output sufficient to meet the demands of the body. These mechanisms are increased heart rate, dilation, hypertrophy, and increased stroke volume.

INCREASED HEART RATE

The first response is an increase in *heart rate*. This adjustment is rapid and has been experienced by everyone during periods of exercise or anxiety. Increasing the heart rate is an excellent way of quickly increasing the cardiac output and meeting the demands of the body for blood. Its utility and effectiveness, however, are functions of age, the functional state of the myocardium, and the amount of obstructive coronary artery disease (CAD).

The maximum heart rate that can be achieved is related to age (Table 19–1). For example, heart rate in a 20-year-old person will plateau at approximately 200 beats/min at maximum effort, whereas at 65 years of age, maximum heart rate is about 150 beats/min. After 25 years of age, maximum heart rate capability drops approximately 6 beats for each 5 years. There is, of course, considerable spread around these mean maximum heart rates for each age—some people will exceed the average value, whereas others will fail to achieve it. As heart rate increases, the time for diastolic ventricular filling decreases, and at high heart rates, the time available for ventricular filling may be so small that filling is inadequate and cardiac output starts to fall.

TABLE 19-1
Maximum Heart Rate According to Age

Age (y)	Maximum Heart Rate (Beats/Min)
20	200
22	198
24	196
26	194
28	192
30	190
32	189
34	187
36	186
38	184
40	182
45	179
50	175
55	171
60	160
65+	150

In addition to advancing age, the functional state of the heart muscle (how capable it is of maintaining repeated rapid contractions) and the state of the coronary circulation are important determinants of the effectiveness of heart rate as a response to stress. In people with CAD and significant obstruction to one or more coronary arteries, a substantial increase in heart rate can be a potentially dangerous event. Coronary artery blood flow to the left ventricle takes place primarily in diastole. With increasing heart rates, decreased diastolic filling time, and increased demands of the heart for oxygen (heart rate being one of the major determinants of myocardial oxygen demand), coronary blood flow may become critical, and angina pectoris, congestive failure, or occasionally myocardial infarction may result. Furthermore, if the heart muscle contracts poorly and cannot sustain strong contractions at moderate or rapid rates, heart failure may follow.

Heart rate, then, is an immediate response to stress that is effective in maintaining or increasing cardiac output but whose value depends on the patient's age, functional state of the myocardium, and amount of obstructive disease in the coronary arteries.

DILATION

The second reserve mechanism of the heart is *dilation*. With dilation, the muscle cell stretches. The relationship between the cardiac output (the amount of blood the heart pumps in each unit of time) and the length of the heart muscle cell at the end of diastole is expressed in the well-known *Starling relationship*, which states that as the end-diastolic fiber length increases, so does the cardiac output (Fig. 19–1).

Like heart rate, however, the usefulness of dilation is self-limiting. There is a point beyond which the stretching of the muscle cell leads not to an increase in cardiac output, but to a decrease. This is partly explained by the *Laplace relationship*, which states that the tension in the wall of a chamber, such as the left ventricle, is related directly to the pressure in that chamber and its radius. Put another way, as the radius of the chamber increases (dilation), so does the wall tension, as long as the pressure in the chamber rises or does not fall.

Because wall tension is directly related to the demand of the myocardium for oxygen, it is not difficult to see that eventually the radius will dilate to such a degree that the demand of the heart for oxygen cannot be met. In this instance, dilation has advanced to the point where it is no longer providing an increase in cardiac output, and the pump has started to fail.

HYPERTROPHY

The third reserve mechanism of the heart is the ability of the individual cardiac muscle cells to *hypertrophy*. The process of hypertrophy requires time and is not an acute adjustment to stress. If the stress is applied long enough, however, such as with systemic or pulmonary hypertension or

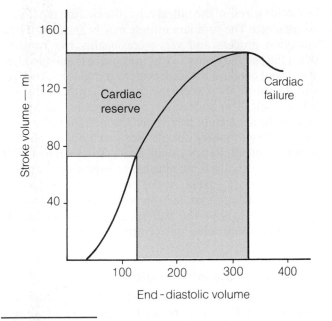

FIGURE 19-1
The Starling curve. As the end-diastolic fiber length increases, so does the cardiac output. At a self-limiting end point, further stretching results in a lessened cardiac output.

significant stenosis of the aortic or pulmonary valve (pressure loads), the muscle of the chamber pumping against the resistance may hypertrophy to such a degree that it effectively outgrows its blood supply and becomes ischemic. When this happens, hypertrophy ceases to be a useful compensatory mechanism, and the heart's pumping ability decreases. A similar situation may occur with the imposition of a volume load on the pumping ventricle, as occurs with mitral or aortic regurgitation.

INCREASED STROKE VOLUME

The fourth reserve mechanism of the heart is an increase in *stroke volume*, the amount of blood the heart ejects into the circulation with each systole. The heart can increase stroke volume either by increasing the percentage of the end-diastolic volume ejected with each beat (increase the ejection fraction through an increase in contractility) or by increasing the amount of blood presented to the heart (increased venous return). This increased venous return, known as preload, is usually accomplished by the reflexive increase of sympathetic nervous system activity, which increases venous tone. Venous pressure is then raised, and thus venous return to the heart is increased.

Venous return also is increased by elevated body temperature, which shortens the time required for blood to circulate completely through the body; by recumbence, in which case the volume of blood that is held in the legs as a result of gravity largely is returned to the central circulation and presented to the heart; or by taking a deep breath, which increases intrathoracic negativity, thereby "sucking"

more blood into the chest. Also, any increase in intravascular volume will increase venous return. By an increase in either ejection fraction (contractility) or venous return (volume), stroke volume and cardiac output will increase. As with other mechanisms of response to stress, increased venous return and increased contractility may not function to increase cardiac output. For example, the myocardium may be so fatigued (depressed contractility) that it cannot respond to further attempts to improve its force of contraction. Similarly, an increase in venous return may cause increased dilation and decrease, rather than improve, cardiac output.

■ PATHOPHYSIOLOGY OF HEART FAILURE

When the normal cardiac reserves for responding to stress are inadequate to meet the metabolic demands of the body, the heart fails to pump adequately, and heart failure results. Also, as stated previously, dysfunction of any of the components of the pump ultimately may result in failure. Heart failure was very simply and appropriately defined in 1933 by Lewis as "a condition in which the heart fails to discharge its contents adequately."[1] This definition is as good today as it was in the 1930s.

The Agency for Health Care Policy and Research (AHCPR) defines heart failure as "a clinical syndrome or condition characterized by (1) signs and symptoms of intravascular and interstitial volume overload including shortness of breath, rales, and edema, or (2) manifestations of inadequate tissue perfusion, such as fatigue or poor exercise tolerance."[2] More than 400,000 new cases of heart failure are diagnosed annually, and more than 2,000,000 Americans live with heart failure. About 10% of the population living with CHF die each year, and 1 million hospitalizations are the direct result of this condition. Five-year mortality is 50%.[2]

Causes of Failure

HEART MUSCLE ABNORMALITIES

Abnormalities of the *muscle* that cause ventricular failure include myocardial infarction, ventricular aneurysm, extensive myocardial fibrosis (usually from atherosclerotic coronary heart disease or prolonged hypertension), endocardial fibrosis, primary myocardial disease (cardiomyopathy), or excessive hypertrophy due to pulmonary hypertension, aortic stenosis, or systemic hypertension.

Ventricular dysfunction can be divided into two categories: *ventricular systolic dysfunction* is hallmarked by very low ejection fractions (less than 35%–40%) because of a decline in contractility. *Ventricular diastolic dysfunction* is when the ejection fraction is more than 40%, but heart failure exists because of stiffness of the left ventricle or valvular disease.

DYSRHYTHMIAS

Disorders of the cardiac *rhythm* can contribute to failure in several ways. *Bradycardia* allows for increased diastolic filling and myocardial fiber stretch with an associated increase in stroke volume (Starling relationship). Cardiac output therefore is preserved. This is well tolerated in healthy people; resting bradycardia is, in fact, a result of high levels of aerobic physical conditioning. In the diseased heart, however, contractility is decreased, the useful limits of the Starling relationship are exceeded, and cardiac output may be diminished.

With *tachycardia*, diastolic filling time is decreased, myocardial oxygen demand is increased, and the diseased myocardium or the heart with significant CAD may tolerate the burden poorly and fail or develop ischemia, injury, or infarction. Furthermore, frequent premature contractions may decrease the cardiac output, a circumstance that may be poorly tolerated in a patient with marginal pump function.

VALVE MALFUNCTION

Valve malfunction can lead to pump failure either by *pressure load* (obstruction to outflow of the pumping chamber, such as valvular aortic stenosis or pulmonary stenosis) or *volume load* (the valve may be regurgitant as with mitral and aortic insufficiency), which presents an increased volume of blood to the left ventricle.

Valve abnormalities that impose either a pressure load or a volume load on one or more chambers usually are slowly progressive conditions that cause the heart to use its long-term defense mechanisms of dilation and hypertrophy. Both of these mechanisms can be overcome, with resultant pump failure.

Less commonly, an acute volume load is imposed on the heart, causing a rapid onset of pump failure. Bacterial endocarditis of the aortic or mitral valves, rupture of a portion of the mitral valve apparatus (papillary muscle or chordae tendineae), or rupture of the intraventricular septum is the usual cause. In these cases, initial therapy is designed to support the heart during the period of acute insult so that the long-term compensatory mechanisms can be used. If initial therapy is not successful, however, emergency replacement of the abnormal valve or closure of the septal defect is indicated.

MYOCARDIAL RUPTURE

In acute myocardial infarction, *myocardial rupture* presents as a dramatic and often catastrophic onset of pump failure and is associated with a high mortality. Rupture usually occurs during the first 8 days after infarction, during the period of greatest softening of the damaged myocardium. Fortunately, myocardial rupture is a relatively rare complication of infarction. Rupture of a papillary muscle, of the interventricular septum, or of the free wall of the left ventricle may occur.

Rupture of a Papillary Muscle

There are two papillary muscles in the left ventricle that are thumblike projections of muscle to which the restrain-

ing "guide wires" of the mitral valve, the chordae tendineae, are attached. The papillary muscle may be involved in the infarction process and very occasionally may rupture. When the papillary muscle ruptures, there is a sudden loss of restraint of one of the leaflets of the mitral valve, and free mitral regurgitation occurs with each contraction of the left ventricle. This sudden profound pressure and volume load on the left atrium is reflected through the pulmonary veins to the pulmonary vascular bed, and the acute onset of symptoms of pulmonary vascular congestion is noted. This congestion usually is manifested as severe dyspnea and frank pulmonary edema. At the bedside, a loud murmur lasting throughout systole is present. Very often, nothing can be done to save the patient, although occasionally emergency mitral valve replacement can be accomplished successfully.

Rupture of the Interventricular Septum

Sudden heart failure is seen occasionally in acute myocardial infarction as a result of rupture of the interventricular septum. Like rupture of the papillary muscle, septal rupture is uncommon, but when it does appear, it also usually is noted in the first week after damage. Septal rupture is clinically characterized by chest pain, dyspnea, shock, and a rapid onset of evidence of pump failure. There is a loud murmur that lasts throughout systole at the lower left sternal border and often is accompanied by a thrill that one can feel by placing the hand over the precordium at the left sternal border. As with all myocardial ruptures, the prognosis of septal rupture is poor; however, it is occasionally possible to repair these ventricular septal defects by emergency surgery involving cardiopulmonary bypass.

Ruptures of a papillary muscle and the interventricular septum are virtually indistinguishable at the bedside, with both presenting as sudden onset of left ventricular failure, a new murmur, and occasionally a palpable thrill. The location of the infarction is not helpful, and the clinical course in each is rapidly downhill. Emergency cardiac catheterization is the only way to differentiate the two clearly.

Rupture of the Left Ventricle

Mechanical failure of the heart seen in acute myocardial infarction is another relatively rare event and is due to rupture of the free wall of the left ventricle and the spilling of blood into the pericardial cavity. This accumulation of blood results in acute compression of the heart or tamponade and the inability of both chambers to fill adequately. Very sudden pumping failure occurs with associated shock and death.

Rupture of the free wall may be preceded by or associated with a return of chest pain as the blood dissects through the necrotic myocardial wall. Sudden vascular collapse as occurs with ventricular fibrillation, but with an unchanged rhythm on the electrocardiogram (electromechanical dissociation), suggests rupture of the ventricular free wall. As with rupture of the papillary muscle and interventricular septum, rupture of the free wall of the left ventricle carries with it an extremely poor prognosis.

Responses to Failure

When the heart's normal reserves are overwhelmed and failure occurs, certain physiological responses to the decrease in cardiac output are important. All these responses represent the body's attempt to maintain a normal perfusion of vital organs.

INCREASED SYMPATHETIC TONE

The primary acute adjustment to heart failure is an increase in sympathetic nervous system influence on the arteries, veins, and heart. The sympathetic stimulation results in increased heart rate, increased venous return to the heart, and increased force of contraction; in addition, sympathetic tone helps maintain a normal blood pressure. The price extracted for this adjustment is an increase in myocardial oxygen demand and oxygen consumption, a request that may be met inadequately in the patient with significant obstructive CAD or poor pump contractility.

As a result of the autonomic nervous changes and other factors, the blood flow to the essential organs, especially the brain and heart, is maintained at the expense of less essential organs, such as the skin, gut, and kidneys. With severe heart failure, there is sufficient decrease in blood flow to the skeletal muscles to cause a *metabolic acidosis* (lactic acidosis from hypoxemia) that must be considered when a treatment program is planned.

SODIUM AND WATER RETENTION

When the kidneys sense a decreased volume of blood presented for filtration, they respond by retaining sodium and water and thereby try to do their part in increasing the central blood volume and venous return. With an increase in circulating blood volume and venous return to the heart, there is an increase in end-diastolic fiber length (dilation) and, within limits, an increase in stroke volume and cardiac output. With a failing heart, however, an increased circulatory volume may be too great a burden for the ventricle, and failure may be worsened.

In some patients with prolonged failure, the remaining heart cells increase the pumping efficiency through hypertrophy, and the clinical findings of heart failure may improve or disappear (Fig. 19–2).

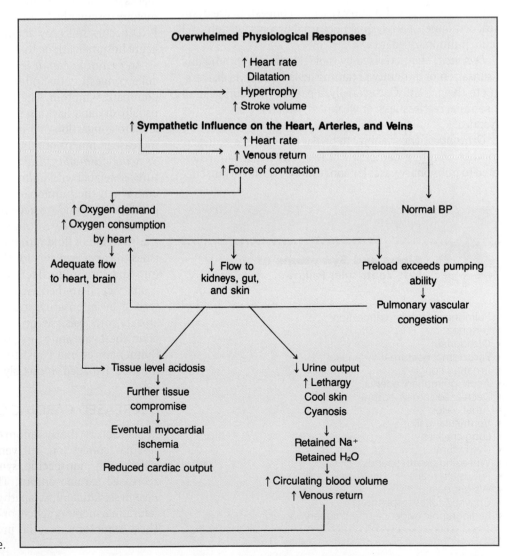

FIGURE 19-2
The vicious cycle of heart failure.

ASSESSMENT OF HEART FAILURE

Clinical Manifestations of Left Ventricular Failure

The clinical features of heart failure come from failure of either the left ventricle, the right ventricle, or both. When the *left ventricle* fails, its inability to discharge its contents adequately results in dilation, increased end-diastolic volume, and increased intraventricular pressure at the end of diastole. This results in the inability of the left atrium to empty its contents into the left ventricle adequately, and pressure in the left atrium rises. This pressure rise is reflected into the pulmonary veins, which bring blood from the lungs to the left atrium. The increased pressure in the pulmonary vessels results in pulmonary vascular congestion, which is the cause of the most specific symptoms of left ventricular failure.

The accompanying display summarizes signs and symptoms of left-sided heart failure.

PULMONARY VASCULAR CONGESTION

The symptoms of pulmonary vascular congestion are dyspnea, orthopnea, paroxysmal nocturnal dyspnea, cough, and acute pulmonary edema.

Dyspnea, characterized by rapid, shallow breathing and a sensation of difficulty obtaining adequate air, is distressing to the patient. Occasionally, a patient may complain of insomnia, restlessness, or weakness, which is caused by the dyspnea.

Orthopnea, the inability to lie flat because of dyspnea, is another common complaint of left ventricular failure related to pulmonary vascular congestion. The nurse must de-

---

RED FLAG **Signs and Symptoms of**
Left Ventricular Failure

- Pulmonary vascular congestion
- Dyspnea
- Orthopnea
- Paroxysmal nocturnal dyspnea
- Irritating cough
- Acute pulmonary edema
- Decreased cardiac output
- Atrial gallop—S_4
- Ventricular gallop—S_3
- Lung crackles
- Dysrhythmias
- Wheezing breath sounds
- Pulsus alternans
- Weight gain
- Cheyne-Stokes respirations
- Radiographic evidence of pulmonary vascular congestion

---

termine if the orthopnea is truly related to heart disease or whether elevating the head to sleep is merely the patient's custom. For example, if a patient requests three pillows, one might hasten to conclude that he or she is suffering from orthopnea. If, however, when asked the reason for sleeping on three pillows, the patient indicates a preference for sleeping at this elevation and has done so since before the symptomatic heart disease, the condition does not qualify as orthopnea.

Paroxysmal nocturnal dyspnea (PND) is a common complaint characterized by the patient's awakening in the middle of the night because of intense shortness of breath. PND is thought to be caused by a shift of fluid from the tissues into the intravascular compartment as a result of recumbence. During the day, the pressure in the veins is high, especially in the dependent portions of the body, due to gravity, increased fluid volume, and increased sympathetic tone. With this increase in hydrostatic pressure, some fluid escapes into the tissue space. With recumbence, the pressure in the dependent capillaries is decreased, and fluid is reabsorbed into the circulation. This increased volume represents an additional amount of blood that is presented to the heart to pump each minute (increased preload) and places an additional burden on an already congested pulmonary vascular bed, resulting in an acute onset of dyspnea. PND occurs not only at night, but also any time during acute hospitalizations that require bed rest.

An *irritating cough* is one symptom of pulmonary vascular congestion that often is overlooked but that may be a dominant symptom. The cough may be productive but is usually dry and hacking in character. This symptom is related to congestion of bronchial mucosa and an associated increase in mucus production.

Acute pulmonary edema is the most florid clinical picture associated with pulmonary vascular congestion. It occurs when the pulmonary capillary pressure exceeds the pressure that tends to keep fluid within the vascular channels (approximately 30 mmHg). At these pressures, there is transduction of fluid into the alveoli, which in turn diminishes the area available for the normal transport of oxygen into and carbon dioxide out of the blood within the pulmonary capillary bed. Acute pulmonary edema is characterized by intense dyspnea, cough, orthopnea, profound anxiety, cyanosis, sweating, noisy respirations, and very often chest pain and a pink, frothy sputum from the mouth. Pulmonary edema constitutes a medical emergency and must be managed vigorously and promptly.

DECREASED CARDIAC OUTPUT

In addition to the symptoms that result from pulmonary vascular congestion, left ventricular failure also is associated with nonspecific symptoms that are related to decreased cardiac output. The patient may complain of weakness, fatigability, apathy, lethargy, difficulty in concentrating, memory deficit, or diminished exercise tolerance. These symptoms may be present in chronic low-output

CLINICAL APPLICATION: Examples of Nursing Diagnoses and Collaborative Problems for the Patient With Heart Failure

Decreased Cardiac Output related to myocardial muscle damage or overwhelmed physiological responses of heart failure

Activity Intolerance related to decreased cardiac output

Decreased Tissue Perfusion related to decreased cardiac output

Impaired Gas Exchange related to pulmonary congestion

Fluid Volume Excess related to decreased cardiac output and sodium and water retention

Knowledge Deficit related to disease state, treatments, medications, complications, and lifestyle changes

Anxiety related to critical illness, fear of death, and lifestyle changes

states and may dominate the patient's complaints. Unfortunately, these symptoms are nonspecific and often are ascribed to depression, neurosis, or functional complaints. Therefore, these potentially important indicators of deteriorating pump function often are not recognized for their true import, and the patient is either inappropriately reassured or placed on a tranquilizer or mood-elevating preparation. The presence of the nonspecific symptoms of low cardiac output demands a careful evaluation of the heart as well as the psyche—an examination that will yield the information that will dictate proper management.

HEART AND BREATH SOUNDS

Physical signs associated with left ventricular failure that are easily recognized at the bedside include third and fourth heart sounds (S_3, S_4), a laterally displaced apical pulse, and crackles in the lungs.

S_4, or *atrial gallop*, is associated with and follows atrial contraction and is heard best with the bell of the stethoscope very lightly applied at the cardiac apex. The left lateral position may be required to elicit the sound. S_4 is heard just before the first heart sound (S_1) and is not always a definitive sign of congestive failure but may represent decreased compliance (increased stiffness) of the myocardium. (See Chapter 16 for a more detailed discussion of cardiac auscultation.) S_4 therefore may be an early, premonitory indication of impending failure. An S_4 is common in patients with acute myocardial infarction and likely does not have prognostic significance, but it may represent incipient failure.

S_3, or *ventricular gallop*, is an important sign of left ventricular failure and in adults almost never is present in the absence of significant heart disease. A third heart sound and a lateral displacement of the apical pulse are specific indicators of heart failure.

S_3 is heard in early diastole after the second heart sound (S_2) and is associated with the period of rapid passive ventricular filling. S_3 also is heard best with the bell of the

stethoscope applied lightly at the apex, with the patient in the left lateral position, and at the end of expiration.

The *crackles* or fine moist rales most commonly heard at the bases of the lungs posteriorly often are recognized as evidence of left ventricular failure, as indeed they may be. Before these crackles are ascribed to pump failure, the patient must be instructed to cough deeply to open any basilar alveoli that may be compressed as a result of recumbence, inactivity, and compression from the diaphragm beneath. Crackles that fail to clear after cough (post-tussic) need to be evaluated; those that clear after cough probably are clinically unimportant. The patient may have good evidence of left ventricular failure on the basis of a history of symptoms suggesting pulmonary vascular congestion or the finding of S_3 at the apex and yet have clear lung fields. Therefore, it is not appropriate to wait for the appearance of crackles in the lungs before instituting therapy for left ventricular failure.

OTHER SIGNS

Other signs of left ventricular failure that may be noted in addition to an S_3, lateral displacement of the apical pulse, crackles in the lungs, and supraventricular rhythms include wheezing breath sounds, pulsus alternans (an alternating greater and lesser volume of the arterial pulse), weight gain, and Cheyne-Stokes respirations. Indeed, patients may awaken at night during respiratory height of a Cheyne-Stokes cycle, a situation that may be interpreted falsely as PND but that may have the same pathophysiological significance. Weight gain resulting from retention of salt and water by the kidneys is a useful sign that the patient may follow at home. Daily weight should be recorded in the morning after voiding and before breakfast.

ELECTROCARDIOGRAPHIC FINDINGS

The electrocardiogram is nonspecific in heart failure but provides important information about the underlying rhythm and other cardiac abnormalities. Because an increase in heart rate is the heart's initial response to stress, sinus tachycardia might be expected and often is found in the examination of a patient with pump failure. Other rhythms associated with heart failure include atrial premature contractions, paroxysmal atrial tachycardia, atrial fibrillation, and ventricular premature beats. Whenever a rhythm abnormality is detected, attempts are made to define the underlying pathophysiological mechanism; therapy then can be properly planned and instituted. With left ventricular failure, evidence of left ventricular and left atrial enlargement patterns may be seen on the electrocardiogram. (See Chapter 16 for more information.)

RADIOGRAPHIC FINDINGS

Radiographic examination of the chest often helps the clinician diagnose heart failure and distinguish pulmonary from cardiac causes of dyspnea. Careful evaluation of the chest roentgenogram may demonstrate changes in the blood vessels of the lungs that result from an increase in pulmonary venous pressure. A common chest x-ray finding in heart failure is cardiomegaly with the cardiothoracic ratio increased by more than 0.50. Radiographic findings may be present in the absence of crackles, and careful examination of the chest film is necessary if left ventricular failure is suspected. Chest x-rays can also provide information about pulmonary disease, calcified heart valves, left atrial size, and left versus right ventricular enlargement.

LABORATORY FINDINGS

In addition to an electrocardiogram and chest radiograph, laboratory tests are performed as part of the assessment for a patient with heart failure. Laboratory tests include a complete blood count, urinalysis, serum creatinine, and serum albumin. A T_4 and thyroid-stimulating hormone (TSH) level should be checked in all patients over the age of 65 with heart failure and no obvious etiology and in patients who have atrial fibrillation or other signs or symptoms of thyroid disease.[2] Table 19–2 summarizes common laboratory findings in patients with heart failure.

Clinical Manifestations of Right Ventricular Failure

Failure of the *right ventricle* alone often is the result of severe underlying lung disease and such conditions as severe pulmonary hypertension (primary or secondary), stenosis of the pulmonary valve, and a massive pulmonary embolus. The right ventricle tolerates a volume load well, and pure right ventricular failure usually is due to resistance to outflow (pressure load). More commonly, however, right ventricular failure is the result of failure of the left ventricle. In this situation, signs and symptoms of both left and right ventricular failure are present. The accompanying display summarizes signs and symptoms of right ventricular failure.

DECREASED CARDIAC OUTPUT

In contrast to left ventricular failure, in which specific symptoms usually can be related to a single underlying mechanism—pulmonary vascular congestion—the symptoms of right heart failure are not so specific, and many are related to a low cardiac output. Fatigability, weakness, lethargy, or difficulty in concentrating may be prominent. Heaviness of the limbs (especially the legs), an increase in abdominal girth, inability to wear previously comfortable shoes, and weight gain reflect the ascites and edema associated with right ventricular failure.

In addition, symptoms of the underlying pulmonary disease usually dominate complaints if failure is due to a primary pulmonary problem, usually chronic bronchitis or emphysema. Occasionally, bronchiectasis or restrictive lung disease may be the primary pulmonary problem, but chronic bronchitis and emphysema are by far the most common pulmonary causes of right ventricular failure.

TABLE 19-2   CLINICAL APPLICATION: Diagnostic Studies
Suggested Laboratory Tests and Common Findings in Patients With Heart Failure

Laboratory Test	Finding in Heart Failure
Complete blood count	Anemia
Urinalysis	Proteinuria
	Red blood cells or cellular casts
Serum creatinine	Elevated
Serum albumin	Decreased
T_4 and thyroid-stimulating hormone (TSH)	Abnormal T_4 and TSH

Adapted from Konstam M, Dracup K, Baker D, et al: Heart Failure: Evaluation and Care of Patients with Left Ventricular Systolic Dysfunction, p 32. Clinical Practice Guideline No. 11. AHCPR Publication No. 94-0612. Rockville, MD. Agency for Heatlh Care Policy and Research, Public Health Service, U.S. Department of Health and Human Services, June 1994

JUGULAR VENOUS DISTENTION

When the right ventricle decompensates, there is dilation of the chamber, an increase in right ventricular end-diastolic volume and pressure, resistance to filling of the ventricle, and a subsequent rise in right atrial pressure. This increasing pressure is in turn reflected upstream in the venae cavae and can be recognized by an increase in the jugular venous pressure. The nurse assesses jugular venous distention by looking at the veins in the neck and noting the height of the column of blood. With the patient lying in bed and the head of the bed elevated between 30 and 60 degrees, the column of blood in the external jugular veins will be, in the normal person, only a few millimeters above the upper border of the clavicle, if it is seen at all (Fig. 19–3).

When an observation of venous pressure is recorded, the height of the column of blood above the sternal angle and

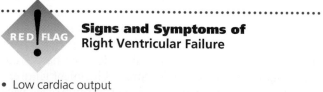

RED FLAG   **Signs and Symptoms of Right Ventricular Failure**

- Low cardiac output
- Jugular vein distension
- Dependent edema
- Dysrhythmias
- Right ventricular S_3 and S_4
- Hyperresonance with percussion
- Low immobile diaphragm
- Decreased breath sounds
- Increased anteroposterior chest diameter

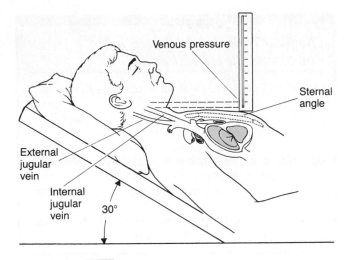

FIGURE 19-3
An assessment of jugular venous pressure. The highest point at which jugular vein pulsations can be seen is noted. The vertical distance between this point and the sternal angle is measured and recorded as centimeters "above or below" the sternal angle.

the elevation of the head of the bed should be included. This measurement will provide a useful basis for comparison of future observations.

EDEMA

Edema often is considered a reliable sign of heart failure, and indeed, it often is present when the right ventricle has failed. Edema is the least reliable sign of right ventricular dysfunction, however. Many people, particularly older adults, spend much of their time sitting in a chair with the legs dependent. As a result of this body position, the decreased turgor of subcutaneous tissue associated with old age, and perhaps primary venous disease, such as varicosities, ankle edema may be produced that reflects these factors rather than right ventricular failure.

When edema does appear related to failure of the right ventricle, it is dependent in location. If the patient is up and about, it will be noted primarily in the ankles and will ascend the legs as failure worsens. When the patient is put to bed, the dependent portion of the body becomes the sacral area, and edema should be looked for there. In addition, other signs of right ventricular failure should be present before the diagnosis is made. Dependent edema alone is inadequate documentation of the status of the right ventricle. With congestion of the liver, this organ may enlarge and become tender, ascites may be present, and jaundice may be noted.

HEART AND BREATH SOUNDS

As with left ventricular failure, S_3 and S_4 are common in patients with right ventricular failure. These sounds are heard best at the lower left sternal border, with the bell of the

stethoscope applied lightly to the chest. They can be recognized by an increase in intensity with inspiration.

A decrease in breath sounds may accompany right ventricular failure. Signs of any underlying cause of right ventricular failure also may be present, such as hyperresonance with percussion, low immobile diaphragms, increased anteroposterior chest diameter, and use of the accessory muscles of respiration in patients with severe pulmonary emphysema.

ELECTROCARDIOGRAPHIC FINDINGS

Although the electrocardiogram is nonspecific for heart failure, it provides information about the underlying cardiac rhythm and other cardiac abnormalities. As with left ventricular failure, the patient is likely to have a sinus tachycardia in response to sympathetic nervous system activation. Other rhythms associated with heart failure include atrial premature contractions, paroxysmal atrial tachycardia, atrial fibrillation, and ventricular premature beats. With right ventricular failure, evidence of right ventricular and right atrial enlargement patterns may be seen on the electrocardiogram. (See Chapter 16 for more information.)

RADIOGRAPHIC FINDINGS

As with left ventricular failure, the chest x-ray is an early diagnostic test for the patient with right ventricular failure. In addition to the presence of cardiomegaly, the chest x-ray may show indications of underlying pulmonary disease, calcified heart valves, and right versus left ventricular enlargement.

LABORATORY FINDINGS

Laboratory tests are the same for left and right ventricular failure and include a complete blood count, urinalysis, serum creatinine, and serum albumin. A T_4 and TSH level should be checked in all patients over the age of 65 with heart failure and no obvious etiology and in patients who have atrial fibrillation or other signs or symptoms of thyroid disease.[2] Table 19-2 summarizes common laboratory findings in patients with heart failure.

■ CLASSIFICATION OF HEART FAILURE

Heart failure may be present in varying degrees of severity. In acute myocardial infarction, heart failure has been simply and usefully classified by Killip into four classes: I, no failure; II, mild to moderate failure; III, acute pulmonary edema; and IV, cardiogenic shock (see display).

Early, moderate (Killip class II) failure and chronic failure often are characterized by an S_3, increased heart rate (usually sinus rhythm), and possibly fine post-tussic crackles (rales) at the lung bases. In addition, evidence of pul-

---

Killip Classification of Heart Failure

I: No failure
II: Mild to moderate failure
III: Acute pulmonary edema
IV: Cardiogenic shock

The New York Heart Association Functional Classification

Class I: Cardiac disease without resulting limitations of physical activity

Class II: Slight limitation of physical activity—comfortable at rest, but ordinary physical activity results in fatigue, palpitation, dyspnea, or anginal pain

Class III: Marked limitation in physical activity—comfortable at rest, but less than ordinary physical activity causes fatigue, palpitation, dyspnea, or anginal pain

Class IV: Inability to carry on any physical activity without discomfort or symptoms at rest

---

monary vascular congestion (often without pulmonary edema) often is seen on the chest roentgenogram, and dysrhythmias may be present: atrial premature contractions, atrial fibrillation, atrial flutter, paroxysmal atrial tachycardia, and junctional rhythms. The patient may be reasonably comfortable at rest or may have symptoms of low cardiac output or pulmonary vascular congestion. Symptoms are increased with activity.

Acute pulmonary edema (Killip class III) is a life-threatening situation characterized by transudation of fluid from the pulmonary capillary bed into the alveolar spaces, with associated extreme dyspnea and anxiety. Immediate care is required if the patient's life is to be saved.

Cardiogenic shock (Killip class IV) is the most ominous pump failure syndrome and is associated with the highest mortality, even with aggressive care. Cardiogenic shock is recognized clinically by the following:

- A systolic blood pressure less than 80 mmHg (often it cannot be measured)
- A thready pulse that often is rapid
- Pale, cool, and sweaty skin that frequently is cyanotic
- Restlessness, confusion, and apathy
- Possible alteration from usual mental status
- Decreased or absent urine output

These manifestations of shock are a reflection of the profound inadequacy of the heart as a pump and usually reflect a large amount of muscle damage (40% or more of the left ventricular mass).

Some patients with significant, long-standing arterial hypertension will have manifestations of cardiogenic shock at relatively normal pressures. These people require a higher pressure to perfuse vital organs and maintain viability. Knowledge of the preceding blood pressure history is of great importance in recognizing these people. Not all clinical circumstances of cardiogenic shock are associated with an inadequate cardiac output, however. Depending on modifying circumstances, such as fever, the cardiac output occasionally may be normal or even increased.

In addition to the Killip classification system for heart failure, the New York Heart Association functional classification system is used clinically for heart failure patients. This system classifies patients with heart disease on the basis of the activity level that initiates the onset of symptoms. The New York Heart Association classification system is shown in the display.

MANAGEMENT OF HEART FAILURE

The goals of the management of heart failure are to identify and eliminate the precipitating cause, promote optimal cardiac function, enhance patient comfort by relieving signs and symptoms, and help the patient and family cope with any lifestyle changes.

The AHCPR convened a multidisciplinary panel of professionals and consumers who established national guidelines for the evaluation and management of patients with heart failure due to reduced left ventricular systolic function. These guidelines are summarized in the algorithm seen in Figure 19–4.

Exercise

Bed rest has been an important part of the treatment of heart failure, especially in acute and refractory stages. In addition to decreasing the overall work demands made on the heart, bed rest assists in lowering the workload by decreasing the intravascular volume through a recumbence-induced diuresis.

Although many clinicians suggest bed rest and activity limitations for patients with heart failure, inactivity is associated with important risks and long-term detrimental ef-

---

Goals for Management of Heart Failure

- Identify and eliminate the precipitating cause.
- Promote optimal cardiac function.
- Enhance patient comfort by relieving signs and symptoms.
- Help the patient and family cope with any lifestyle changes.

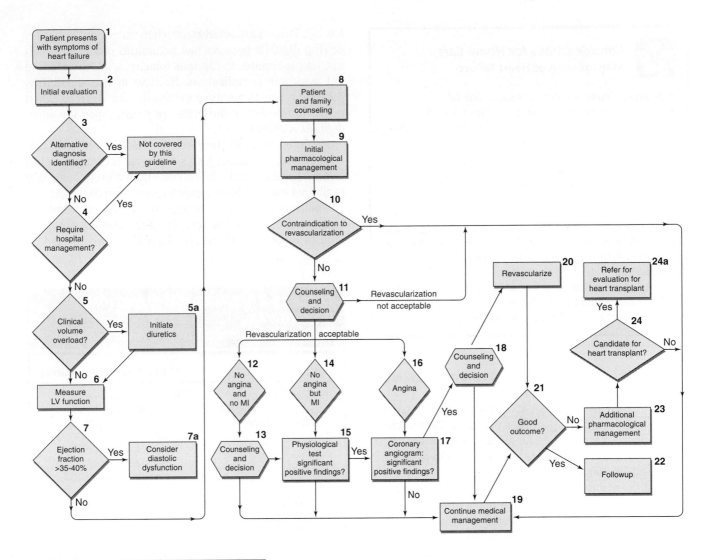

Note: LV = left-ventricular, MI = myocardial infarction

FIGURE 19-4
Clinical algorithm for evaluation and care of patients with heart failure. From Konstam M, Dracup K, Baker D, et al: Heart Failure: Evaluation and Care of Patients With Left-Ventricular Systolic Dysfunction. Clinical Practice Guideline No. 11. AHCPR Publication No. 94-0612. Rockville, MD. Agency for Health Care Policy and Research, Public Health Service, U.S. Department of Health and Human Services, June 1994.

fects on physical functioning. Even short periods of bed rest can result in reduced exercise tolerance and aerobic capacity and muscle atrophy and weakness.[2]

Rather than activity restriction, the AHCPR guidelines suggest a regular exercise program, such as walking or cycling, for all patients with stable New York Heart Class I through III heart failure.[2] Studies indicate that patients with heart failure are able to exercise safely, and regular exercise may actually improve functional status and decrease symptoms.[3-5] The benefit of exercise most likely results from effects on skeletal muscle rather than changes in myocardial function. Except for patients with a recent myocardial infarction or acute myocarditis, there is no evi-

dence that exercise negatively affects the natural history of heart failure.[2]

Diet

Dietary restrictions, especially sodium, are a fundamental part of the treatment plan for patients with heart failure. Reduction of sodium intake helps reduce fluid overload and increases the effectiveness of diuretic therapy. Dietary sodium should be restricted to as close to 2 g/d as possible, and in no case should sodium intake exceed 3 g/d.[2] Patients and family members may need education to avoid salty foods and to eliminate the addition of salt to foods. For ex-

Considerations for Home Care
Management of Heart Failure

- Begin discharge planning as soon as possible.
- Assess the home environment and family support systems. If the patient cannot care for himself or herself or if family cannot provide care, consider home care referral for registered nurse, home health aide, or homemaker as appropriate.
- Provide resources to take home, such as written materials about heart failure, information about medications, and person to contact for questions. Home care nurse will reinforce education and answer questions.
- Provide instruction about dietary sodium restriction and foods high in sodium. Home health nurse will assess patient for evidence of fluid retention and edema.
- Instruct the patient to record daily weights.
- Encourage patient to develop an exercise program at home. Start slowly and increase exercise gradually.

ample, avoiding processed foods and milk products can reduce sodium intake to about 1 g.

Heart failure patients should be discouraged from using alcohol because alcohol depresses myocardial contractility in patients with known cardiac disease. If abstinence from alcohol is unrealistic, patients are advised to have no more than one drink per day.

Good nutritional habits should be encouraged for the patient with heart failure because many of these patients experience a syndrome of chronic wasting known as "cardiac cachexia." Vitamin supplements may be advisable because of water-soluble vitamin loss associated with diuretic therapy.

Pharmacological Management

DIURETICS

Diuretic therapy (Table 19–3) is one of the mainstays of management for patients with heart failure. Sodium and water retention is a physiological response to the low cardiac output state. This retention results in severe volume overload. Patients with mild volume overload are managed on thiazide diuretics, whereas patients with more severe volume overload are placed on a loop diuretic.[2] The dose of the drug depends on the patient's size, age, renal function, compliance with dietary sodium restriction, and amount of edema.[2] Generally, the patient will feel symptomatic relief with diuretic therapy. Unfortunately, diuretics have not shown a slowing of the disease process or improved survival.[6]

All diuretics, regardless of the route of administration, may cause significant changes in the serum electrolytes, especially potassium and chloride. Therefore, regular determination of serum electrolytes is important in patient fol-

low-up. This is particularly true when the patient also is receiving digitalis because low potassium produced by diuretics predisposes to digitalis toxicity, a life-threatening but avoidable complication. Because of this possibility, potassium supplements customarily are ordered when potassium-depleting diuretics are given, especially when digitalis is given as well.

Angiotensin-converting enzyme (ACE) inhibitors decrease renal potassium losses and raise serum potassium levels. Therefore, patients who take both diuretics and ACE inhibitors may not be as prone to potassium depletion.

The choice of route of administration of the diuretic is largely a function of the severity of the clinical situation. Mild to moderate left ventricular failure (manifested by

TABLE 19-3   CLINICAL APPLICATION: Drug Therapy
Medications Commonly Used for Heart Failure

Drug	Major Adverse Reactions
Thiazide diuretics Hydrochlorothiazide Chlorthalidone	Postural hypotension, hypokalemia, hyperglycemia, hyperuricemia, rash Rare severe reaction—pancreatitis, bone marrow suppression and anaphylaxis
Loop diuretics Furosemide Bumetanide Ethacrynic acid	Same as thiazide diuretics
Thiazide-related diuretic Metolazone	Same as thiazide diuretics
Potassium-sparing diuretics Spironolactone Triamterene Amiloride	Hyperkalemia, especially if administered with ACE inhibitor, rash; gynecomastia (spironolactone only)
ACE inhibitors Enalapril Captopril Lisinopril Quinapril	Hypotension, hyperkalemia, renal insufficiency, cough, skin rash, angioedema, neutropenia
Digoxin	Cardiotoxicity, confusion, nausea, anorexia, visual disturbances
Hydralazine	Headache, nausea, dizziness, tachycardia, lupus-like syndrome
Isosorbide dinitrate	Headache, hypotension, flushing

Adapted from Konstam M, Dracup K, Baker D, et al: Heart Failure: Evaluation and Care of Patients with Left Ventricular Systolic Dysfunction, pp 52–53. Clinical Practice Guideline No. 11. AHCPR Publication No. 94-0612. Rockville, MD. Agency for Health Care Policy and Research, Public Health Service, U.S. Department of Health and Human Services, June 1994

Insights Into Clinical Research

Shimon I, Almog S, Vered Z, et al: Improved left ventricular function after thiamine supplementation in patients with congestive heart failure receiving long-term furosemide therapy. Am J Med 98(5): 485–490, 1995

The purpose of this study was to examine the hemodynamic and clinical effects of thiamine (Vitamin B_1) supplementation in 30 patients with chronic CHF (functional class II to IV) who had received daily doses of furosemide ($\geq$ 80 mg) for at least 3 months. A randomly chosen group of the patients received 100 mg of IV thiamine or placebo twice daily for 1 week. After the first week, all patients received 200 mg/day of oral thiamine for 6 weeks. At baseline and 1 week, two-dimensional echocardiograms of the left ventricular function, functional class, and thiamine levels were determined. Left ventricular function was determined again at 7 weeks.

Patients receiving the IV thiamine showed increased plasma thiamine levels, urine output, and urine sodium compared to baseline values. No changes in blood pressure, heart rate, or body weight occurred during the first week in either group; however, mean LVEF increased in the IV thiamine group, but not the placebo group. Following 6 weeks of oral thiamine dosing, LVEF increased 22% from baseline. At 7 weeks, functional class decreased from 2.6 (baseline) to 2.2 and plasma thiamine levels were increased.

Given the frequency of CHF as an admitting diagnosis, and the associated high inpatient costs and lifetime expenditures associated with chronic illness, a cheap medication, free from serious side effects, that can improve functional status is extremely beneficial.

sinus tachycardia, post-tussic crackles, and S_3) usually can be managed with oral preparations; however, acute pulmonary edema, a life-threatening situation, demands more drastic approaches, and the parenteral route should be chosen.

ANGIOTENSIN-CONVERTING ENZYME INHIBITORS

Heart failure is defined by the vicious cycle of both increased preload and afterload. Vasodilator therapy allows improved cardiac filling (preload) and reduces resistance to emptying (afterload). The vasodilator of choice in managing patients with mild, moderate, or severe heart failure is an ACE inhibitor. These drugs reduce the vasoconstrictor substance angiotensin II. A reduction in angiotensin II will decrease peripheral arterial resistance, lowering the blood pressure and reducing aldosterone secretion (which will reduce salt and water).

In cases of severe CHF, ACE inhibitors were first demonstrated to reduce mortality by 40% at 6 months and 31% at 1 year. Then ACE inhibitors were tested on moderate CHF in hospitalized patients, and fewer patients died or worsened their CHF.

As ACE inhibitor doses reach the ideal dose, adjustments to diuretic and other vasodilator therapies can be made. Some of the adverse reactions to ACE inhibitors include hypotension, azotemia, dizziness, cough, angioedema, proteinuria, and hyperkalemia. Hypotension and azotemia are more common in the older patient.

DIGOXIN

For more than 200 years, cardiac glycosides such as digoxin have been used to treat heart failure. The value of digoxin in heart failure patients with atrial fibrillation and a rapid ventricular response has been well documented. However, the use of cardiac glycosides in heart failure patients with normal sinus rhythm is controversial.[2] Recent clinical trials have shown that digoxin improves physical function and decreases symptoms in heart failure patients.[7] However, the effect of digoxin on mortality of heart failure patients is not known and is under investigation. Based on these findings, the AHCPR guidelines recommend initiation of digoxin with ACE inhibitors and diuretics in patients with severe heart failure and the addition of digoxin in patients who remain symptomatic despite optimal management with ACE inhibitors and diuretics.[2]

Digoxin is a positive inotropic agent that increases the intracellular calcium available for excitation–contraction coupling, resulting in improved contractility of the heart muscle. In the failing heart, digitalis slows the ventricular rate and increases the force of contraction, increasing cardiac efficiency. As cardiac output increases, a greater volume of fluid is presented to the kidneys for filtration and excretion, and intravascular volume decreases.

In early failure with acute myocardial infarction, digitalis may increase the potential amount of damaged myocardium by causing increased contractility and therefore increased myocardial oxygen demand. Treatment of failure in this circumstance probably is best if preload or afterload is decreased through the use of diuretics or nitrates. Patients with more severe heart failure are likely to benefit from long-term digitalis therapy. Careful monitoring of

Considerations for the Older Patient Pharmacological Therapy

Adding to the risk of the pharmacological therapy used to treat heart failure is the varying status of the fluid balance and renal function in the older person. Mild changes in renal filtration will vary clearance and lead to toxicity in many medications, including digoxin. Polydrug ingestion (by prescription) can lead to harmful side effects. Many hospital pharmacies offer a service of checking medications (including over-the-counter) for drug interactions. Fluid status and renal function can be watched by observing for any weight gain over 2 lb. If a weight gain or loss occurs, the serum blood urea nitrogen and creatinine may be drawn.

serum drug levels in indicated, and a serum drug level of 0.7 to 1.5 ng/mL is generally considered therapeutic.[2]

DRUG THERAPY IN ACUTE EXACERBATIONS OF HEART FAILURE

During acute exacerbations of heart failure, additional drugs may be indicated to reduce preload and afterload and to increase myocardial contractility. The aim of preload-reducing agents is to decrease intravascular volume, increase venous capacitance, and improve ventricular compliance. Intravenous diuretic therapy is used to reduce preload, and in an acute situation, multiple diuretic agents may be indicated. During rapid diuresis, the nurse must closely monitor the patient's potassium and magnesium levels.

In addition to diuretic therapy, nitrates can be used to attain a further reduction in preload. Nitrates increase venous capacitance, thus reducing the venous return to the heart. Additionally, nitrates lower pulmonary artery wedge pressures and dilate nonstenotic coronary arteries.

Afterload reduction is another important goal in the acute exacerbation of heart failure. Afterload-reducing agents decrease systemic vascular resistance, thus improving forward cardiac output. The drug of choice to achieve rapid reduction in afterload is sodium nitroprusside. Use of sodium nitroprusside results in a decreased pulmonary artery wedge pressure and a decreased systemic vascular resistance, resulting in an increased cardiac output.

Positive inotropic drugs, such as dopamine, dobutamine, and amrinone, may be used to increase contractility during an exacerbation of heart failure. These drugs improve systolic function by enhancing myocardial contractility. As a result, the patient experiences an increased stroke volume and cardiac output.

At low doses of 2.5 to 5.0 μg/kg, dopamine will stimulate α-adrenergic, β-adrenergic, and dopamine receptors. This results in a release of catecholamines from nerve storage sites, improving contractility and dilating renal, splanchnic, cerebral, and coronary vessels. A small reduction in systemic vascular resistance may be noted. At higher doses (5–10 μg/kg), a positive inotropic (force of contraction), chronotropic (heart rate), and dromotropic (speed of conduction) response occurs. This increases heart rate, cardiac output, and stroke volume. At maximal doses (10–20 μg/kg), vasoconstriction occurs, increasing cardiac workload.

Dobutamine stimulates only β-adrenergic receptors and results in less vasoconstriction. Dosing is similar to that with dopamine, but the synthetic dobutamine will improve stroke volume and cardiac output with less vasoconstriction and tachycardia.

Amrinone will reduce cardiac filling pressures and systemic vascular resistance to improve cardiac output. The clinical trials of amrinone produced variable results, but arterial and venous dilation had a positive inotropic impact. Amrinone is most likely to be used for patients with markedly elevated filling pressures.

Mechanical Measures

Patients who do not respond to pharmacological therapy during an acute exacerbation of heart failure may be placed on assistive mechanical device therapy. Mechanical support of the left ventricle began in 1967 with *intra-aortic balloon counterpulsation* or pumping. This temporary support enhances coronary blood flow, improves stroke volume, and reduces left ventricular preload and afterload. (See chapter 17 for a more detailed discussion.)

During the 1970s, mechanical support expanded. The use of *extracorporeal membrane oxygenation* (ECMO) emerged. This device replaces cardiac/lung function, resulting in a forward flow of blood and gas exchange. Extracorporeal membrane oxygenation may be used to buy time until definitive treatment, such as coronary artery bypass surgery, septal repair, or heart transplantation, can occur.

Left ventricular assist devices have been used as "bridge" therapy to maintain life until surgery or transplantation can be performed. These devices provide forward flow to maintain coronary artery and systemic circulation (see Chapter 17).

Cardiac Transplantation

Advances in cardiac transplantation have made this a viable option for patients with end-stage heart failure. Survival after heart transplant is 80% at 1 year, 70% at 5 years, and 50% at 10 years for patients on concurrent immunosuppressive therapy.[8] The successful use of cardiac transplant is severely limited, however, by the number of available organs. The number of patients needing a heart transplant far exceeds the amount of available organs, and as a result, many end-stage heart failure patients will die while waiting for a heart.

Patient and Family Counseling

It is important for patients and their families to understand heart failure and to take an active part in designing a plan of care. Patients and their families should be counseled regarding the nature of heart failure, drug regimens, dietary restrictions, symptoms of worsening heart failure, what to do if these symptoms occur, and prognosis.[2] The accompanying display suggests topics for patient, family, and caregiver education and counseling.

CLINICAL APPLICATION: Patient Care Study

Bob White, a white, 56-year-old man, did well in the intensive care unit for about 12 hours after the onset of his acute anterior lateral MI. His pain was controllable, and his rhythm was NSR at 85. During the night, his nurse noted a steady increase in heart rate. By morning, bibasilar crackles developed. His weight increased by 1.3 kg. He was short of breath, and his oxygen was increased from 2 L per nasal cannula to 6 L per nasal cannula and 40% by face mask to keep his pulse oximetry ≥ 92%. Furosemide (Lasix) was given with poor results (urine 200 mL/2 hours). Mr. White's color had been pale, but now his skin was cool and diaphoretic. An S_3 and S_4 had been present since admission. Bob was frightened and could get comfortable only with the head of his bed elevated 60 degrees. His jugular venous distention was elevated.

A Swan-Ganz catheter was placed using a right subclavian approach. Initially his readings were as follows:

PAS/PAD = 42/22 mmHg
PAWP = 20 mmHg
CO = 3.4 L/min
CI = 1.84 L/min/BSA
SVR = 1250 dynes/sec/cm^{-5}
BP = 90/50 mmHg
HR = 120/min

Dobutamine was initiated at 5 μg/kg. After the completion of the Swan-Ganz insertion, Mr. White developed chest pain. This moderate pain radiated down his left arm and was relieved by nitroglycerin 0.4 mg (1/150 gr) sublingually × 2. Unfortunately, his BP could not withstand the nitroglycerin, and fell to 80/50.

It was decided that an intra-aortic balloon pump (IABP) would be placed. Using a right femoral approach, the IABP was placed successfully and 1:1 counterpulsation was begun. After 2 hours his readings were as follows:

PAS/PAD = 28/16 mmHg
PAWP = 16 mmHg
CO = 4.32
CI = 2.34 L/min/BSA
SVR = 1080 dynes/sec/cm^5

BP = 100/56 mmHg
HR = 105/min

A serum potassium was verified as 4.2 and another furosemide 20-mg dose was given because the bibasilar crackles continued. Within 2 hours, a diuresis of 540 mL occurred.

Although close monitoring and assessment were required, this patient's outcome had been influenced positively by rapid assessment and intervention to reverse left ventricular heart failure.

■ CONCLUSION

Heart failure, with its accompanying symptoms of low cardiac output, pulmonary vascular congestion, or both, is one of the major sources of disability in cardiovascular disease. Its recognition and pathophysiologically based management are of paramount importance if a patient's functional capacity and vocational and community viability are to be optimized and maintained. A collaborative plan of care based on new developments in the management of heart failure is key in optimizing physiological and psychological function for patients with heart failure.

PATIENT TEACHING
Suggested Topics for Patient, Family, and Caregiver Education and Counseling

General Counseling

- Explanation of heart failure and the reason for symptoms
- Cause or probable cause of heart failure
- Expected symptoms
- Symptoms of worsening heart failure
- What to do if symptoms worsen
- Self-monitoring with daily weights
- Explanation of treatment/care plan
- Clarification of patient's responsibilities
- Importance of cessation of tobacco use
- Role of family members or other caregivers in the treatment/care plan
- Availability and value of qualified local support group
- Importance of obtaining vaccinations against influenza and pneumococcal disease

Prognosis

- Life expectancy
- Advance directives
- Advice for family members in the event of sudden death

Activity Recommendations

- Recreation, leisure, and work activity
- Exercise
- Sex, sexual difficulties, and coping strategies

Dietary Recommendations

- Sodium restriction
- Avoidance of excessive fluid intake
- Fluid restriction (if required)
- Alcohol restriction

Medication

- Effects of medications on quality of life and survival
- Dosing
- Likely side effects and what to do if they occur
- Coping mechanisms for complicated medical regimens
- Availability of lower cost medications or financial assistance

Importance of Compliance With the Treatment/ Care Plan

From Konstam M, Dracup K, Baker D, et al: Heart Failure: Evaluation and Care of Patients with Left Ventricular Systolic Dysfunction, p 42. Clinical Practice Guideline No. 11. AHCPR Publication No. 94-0612. Rockville, MD. Agency for Health Care Policy and Research, Public Health Service, U.S. Department of Health and Human Services, June 1994

COLLABORATIVE CARE GUIDE
for the Patient in Heart Failure

OUTCOMES	INTERVENTIONS
Oxygenation/Ventilation	
Patient has arterial blood gases within normal limits and pulse oximeter value > 90%.	• Assess respiratory rate, effort, and breath sounds q2–4h. • Obtain arterial blood gases per order or signs of respiratory distress. • Monitor arterial saturation by pulse oximeter. • Provide supplemental oxygen by nasal cannula or face mask as indicated. • Provide intubation and mechanical ventilation as necessary (refer to Mechanical Ventilation Care Guide, Chapter 24).
Patient demonstrates no evidence of pulmonary edema on chest x-ray and by clear breath sounds.	• Obtain chest x-ray qd. • Administer diuretics per order. • Provide measures to enhance cardiac output as described below. • Monitor signs of fluid overload as described below.
Patient demonstrates no evidence of atelectasis.	• Encourage nonintubated patients to use incentive spirometer, cough, and deep breathe q4h and PRN. • Turn side to side q2h. • Mobilize out of bed to chair.
Circulation/Perfusion	
Vital signs are within normal limits, including MAP > 70 mmHg and CI > 2.2 L/min/m².	• Monitor HR and BP q1–2h and PRN during acute failure phase. • Assist with pulmonary artery catheter insertion. • Monitor PAP and PAWP, CVP, or right atrial pressure q1h and cardiac output, SVR, and PVR q6–12h if pulmonary artery catheter is in place. • Maintain patent IV access. • Administer positive inotropic, vasodilator, or vasopressor agents guided by hemodynamic parameters and physician orders. • Evaluate effect of medications on BP, HR, and hemodynamic parameters. • Prepare patient for intra-aortic balloon pump assist if necessary.
There is no evidence of intravascular volume overload due to decreased cardiac output.	• Restrict volume administration as indicated by PAWP or CVP values. • Assess for neck vein distension, pulmonary crackles, S_3 or S_4, peripheral edema, increased preload parameters, elevated "a" wave of CVP, RAP, or PAWP waveform.
There is no evidence of further myocardial dysfunction, such as altered ECG or cardiac enzymes.	• Monitor 12-lead ECG qd and PRN. • Monitor cardiac enzymes, magnesium, phosphorus, calcium, and potassium as ordered. • Report and treat abnormalities per protocols or orders.
Serum lactate will be within normal limits.	• Monitor lactate qd until it is within normal limits. • Administer red blood cells, positive inotropic agents, colloid infusion as ordered to increase oxygen delivery.
Fluids/Electrolytes	
Renal function is maintained as evidenced by urine output > 30 mL/h, normal laboratory values.	• Monitor intake and output q1–2h. • Monitor BUN, creatinine, electrolytes qd and PRN. • Weigh daily. • Administer fluid volume and diuretics as ordered.
Mobility/Safety	
Patient maintains or improves mobility and activity tolerance.	• Assess activity tolerance and current ability of patient to conduct ADLs. • Encourage self-care, allowing frequent rest periods between activities.

(continued)

COLLABORATIVE CARE GUIDE
for the Patient in Heart Failure (Continued)

OUTCOMES	INTERVENTIONS
There is no evidence of DVT related to immobility and decreased cardiac output.	• Monitor cardiopulmonary signs of activity intolerance (tachycardia, ectopy, tachypnea, hypotension, hypertension). • Initiate DVT prophylaxis within 24 h of admission. • Avoid sustained hip flexion and reposition q2h. • Assess for signs and symptoms of DVT.
Skin Integrity Patient demonstrates no evidence of skin breakdown.	• Turn side to side q2h. • Evaluate skin for signs of pressure areas when turning. • Consider pressure relief/reduction mattress for high-risk patients. • Use Braden scale to monitor risk of skin breakdown. • Remove self-protective devices from wrists and monitor/document per hospital policy, if devices are in use.
Nutrition Caloric and nutrient intake meet metabolic requirements per calculation (eg, basal energy expenditure). Cholesterol and triglyceride levels are normal or reduced. Normal laboratory values reflect nutritional status.	• Provide appropriate diet: oral, parenteral, or enteral feeding. • Consult dietitian or nutritional support service. • Teach sodium, fat, cholesterol, fluid, and caloric restriction if indicated. • Administer potassium supplements if patient is on chronic diuretic therapy. • Monitor albumin, prealbumin, transferrin, cholesterol, triglycerides, total protein.
Comfort/Pain Control Patient does not complain of pain/discomfort. Patient demonstrates no evidence of pain, such as increased HR, BP, RR, or agitation during activity or procedures.	• Use visual analogue scale to assess pain. • Provide a calm, quiet environment. • Elevate head of bed and reposition patient. • Administer analgesics appropriately for chest pain.
Psychosocial Patient demonstrates decreased anxiety by calm demeanor and vital signs during procedures, discussions.	• Assess vital signs during treatments, discussions, and so forth. • Provide explanations and stable reassurance in calm and caring manner. • Cautiously administer sedatives and monitor response. • Consult social services, clergy as appropriate. • Provide blocks of time for adequate rest and sleep.
Teaching/Discharge Planning Family demonstrates appropriate coping during the acute/critical phase of congestive heart failure. In preparation for discharge to home, patient understands activity levels, dietary restrictions, medication regimen. Support services are in place prior to discharge.	• Provide frequent explanations and information to family. • Encourage family to ask questions regarding treatment plan, patient response to therapy, prognosis, and so forth. • Make appropriate referrals and consults early during hospitalization. • Initiate family education regarding activity, diet, rehabilitation after crisis phase has passed.

Clinical Applicability Challenges

Self-Challenge: Critical Thinking

1. *Create a discharge plan for a patient recovering from moderate heart failure.*

2. *Develop a plan of care for the heart failure patient who is at home.*

3. *Compare the nursing plan of care/critical pathway at a hospital with the national guidelines developed by the AHCPR. Suggest any revisions.*

Study Questions

1. *Which of the following mechanisms is not one of the reserve mechanisms of the heart?*
   a. *Dilation as described by the Starling relationship*
   b. *Decreased heart rate with increased filling time*
   c. *Hypertrophy—in chronic conditions*
   d. *Stroke volume, which increases the percentage of diastolic volume ejected*

2. *When physiological responses become overwhelmed, as in the vicious cycle of heart failure, all of the following occur except*
   a. *tissue alkalosis and ischemia.*
   b. *increased oxygen consumption by the heart.*
   c. *reduced cardiac output.*
   d. *preload that exceeds pumping ability of the heart.*

3. *Which dose of dopamine may be indicated in heart failure?*
   a. *2–5 μg/kg*
   b. *10–20 μg/kg*
   c. *> 20 μg/kg*
   d. *Any dose, because dopamine is titrated for the desired effect*

4. *The management of CHF is recommended to include ACE inhibitors because*
   a. *ACE inhibitors help the myocardium adjust to ventricular remodeling.*
   b. *ACE inhibitors act as a diuretic for the failing heart.*
   c. *ACE inhibitors reduce preload and afterload.*
   d. *national studies show that ACE inhibitors will eliminate postinfarct angina.*

REFERENCES

1. Lewis T: Diseases of the Heart. New York, Macmillan, 1933
2. Konstam M, Dracup K, Baker D, et al: Heart Failure: Evaluation and Care of Patients with Left Ventricular Systolic Dysfunction. Clinical Practice Guideline No. 11. AHCPR Publication No. 94-0612. Rockville, MD. Agency for Health Care Policy and Research, Public Health Service, U.S. Department of Health and Human Services, June 1994
3. Coats AJ, Adanopoulos S, Meyer TE, et al: Effects of physical training in chronic heart failure. Lancet 335(8681):63–66, 1990
4. Kellermann JJ, Shemesh J, Fisman EZ, et al: Arm exercise training in the rehabilitation of patients with impaired ventricular function and heart failure. Cardiology 77:130–138, 1990
5. Meyer TE, Casadei B, Coates AJ, et al: Angiotensin-converting enzyme inhibition and physical training in heart failure. Journal of Internal Medicine 230:407–413, 1991
6. Wright JM: Pharmacologic management of congestive heart failure. Critical Care Nursing Quarterly 18(1):32–44, 1995
7. Packer M, Gheorghiade M, Young D, et al: Withdrawal of digoxin from patients with chronic heart failure treated with angiotensin-converting-enzyme inhibitors. N Engl J Med 329:1–7, 1993
8. Kaye MP: The registry of the International Society for Heart and Lung Transplantation: Tenth official report—1993. Journal of Heart and Lung Transplantation 12:541–548, 1993

BIBLIOGRAPHY

Cash L: Heart failure from diastolic dysfunction. Dimensions of Critical Care Nursing 15(4):170–177, 1996

Dahlen R, Roberts SL: Nursing management of congestive heart failure. Intensive and Critical Care Nursing 11(6):322–328, 1995

Dahlen R, Roberts S: Acute congestive heart failure: Preventing complications. Dimensions of Critical Care Nursing 15(5):226–241, 1996

Dracup K, Dunbar SB, Baker DW: Rethinking heart failure. AJN 95(7):22–28, 1995

Funk M, Krumholz H: Epidemiologic and economic impact on advanced heart failure. Journal of Cardiovascular Nursing 10(2):1–10, 1996

Grady K: When to transplant: Recipient selection for heart transplantation. Journal of Cardiovascular Nursing 10(2):58–70, 1996

Jaarsma T, Dracup K, Walden J, Stevenson L: Sexual function in patients with advanced heart failure. Heart Lung 25(4):262–270, 1996

Moser D: Maximizing therapy in the advanced heart failure patient. Journal of Cardiovascular Nursing 10(2):29–46, 1996

Oka R: Physiologic changes in heart failure—"What's new." Journal of Cardiovascular Nursing 10(2):11–28, 1996

Paul S: The pathophysiologic process of ventricular remodeling: From infarct to failure. Critical Care Nursing Quarterly 18(1):7–21, 1995

Singh P: Managing congestive heart failure in the home. Home Healthcare Nurse 13(2):11–15, 1995

Sullivan M, Hawthorne M: Nonpharmacologic interventions in the treatment of heart failure. Journal of Cardiovascular Nursing 10(2):47–57, 1996

Yacone-Morton LA: Cardiovascular drugs: First-line therapy for CHF. RN 58(2):38–43, 1995

Yontz LL: Congestive heart failure: Early recognition of congestive heart failure in the primary care setting. Journal of the American Academy of Nurse Practitioners 6(6):273–279, 1994

20

Acute Myocardial Infarction

OBJECTIVES

Based on the content in this chapter, the reader should be able to:

- Explain the pathophysiology and risk factors for atherosclerosis.
- Describe the classification, assessment, and management of angina pectoris.
- Compare and contrast the pathophysiological principles and assessment findings of a patient with angina pectoris versus a patient with a myocardial infarction.
- Discuss the diagnostic tests used for a patient with a myocardial infarction.
- Summarize principles of patient management in the early phase, intensive care phase, and intermediate care phase of management.
- Describe the complications for a patient with a myocardial infarction.
- Explain the principles of cardiac rehabilitation and patient education.

*O*f the current United States population of approximately 255 million people, nearly 59 million (about one in four) have some form of cardiovascular disease. Although death rates from cardiovascular disease have declined during the last decade, cardiovascular disease remains the number one killer with more than 925,000 people dying annually.[1] About every 20 seconds, an American will have a heart attack, and about every minute, a person will die from one. More than 42% of all deaths every year are caused by cardiovascular disease, whereas cancer accounts for 23.9% of all deaths.[2] Of those people killed by cardiovascular disease, more than one sixth are under the age of 65. At all ages, cardiovascular disease is the leading cause of death for African Americans. African American men have a 3.5% higher death rate from coronary heart disease than white men. African American women have a 33% higher death rate from coronary artery disease than white women. If all forms of cardiovascular disease were eliminated, total life expectancy would increase by 9.78 years.[3]

As overwhelming as the mortality and morbidity statistics appear, much progress has been made in the prevention, diagnosis, and management of cardiovascular disease. As a result, the death rates from cardiovascular disease declined 24.5% from 1982 to 1992. During that same decade, the death rate from myocardial infarction (MI) declined 31.4%.[3]

Since the Framingham study of risk factors in 1951 and the development of coronary care units in the 1960s, the critical care nurse has played a major role in helping to reduce the mortality associated with heart disease. The critical care nurse uses advanced assessment skills, rapid decision making, and therapeutic interventions to treat the patient in the acute phase of cardiovascular disease. Patient education and psychological support provided by the nurse have enabled patients and their families to return home and maximize their health status.

ATHEROSCLEROSIS

Atherosclerosis is a major cause of cardiovascular disease. The term "atherosclerosis" comes from the Greek word *athere*, meaning gruel or paste, and *sclerosis*, meaning hardness.

Pathophysiological Principles

Atherosclerosis is a complex, insidious process, beginning long before symptoms occur. Although the process is not completely understood, scientific evidence suggests that it begins when the inner, protective layer of the artery (endothelium) is damaged. Three possible causes of the damage include elevated levels of cholesterol and triglycerides in the blood, hypertension, and cigarette smoking.[1]

Gradually, as fatty substances, cholesterol, cellular waste products, calcium, and fibrin pass through the vessel, they are deposited in the inner lining of an artery. As a result of the deposition of these materials, a lipid plaque with a fibrous covering, also known as an atheroma, builds up, and blood flow in the artery becomes partially or completely blocked.[1]

The injury to the vessel and the resulting accumulation of these substances in the inner lining of the artery cause white blood cells, smooth muscle cells, and platelets to aggregate at the site. As a result, a matrix of collagen and elastic fibers form, and the endothelium becomes much thicker. The core of the fibrous plaque can become necrotic, and hemorrhage and calcification may result. A thrombosis may also occur, thus contributing even more to the blockage of the vessel lumen (Fig. 20–1). These fibrous plaques are most often found in the coronary, popliteal, and internal carotid arteries and in the abdominal aorta.

Because of the fibrous plaque, the amount of blood flow through the artery is reduced, resulting in decreased sup-

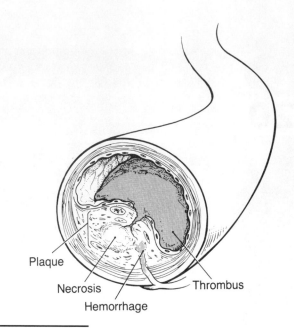

FIGURE 20-1

Thrombosis of an atherosclerotic plaque. It may partially or completely occlude the lumen of the vessel. (Source: Bullock BL: Pathophysiology: Adaptations and Alterations in Function [4th Ed]. Philadelphia, Lippincott-Raven 1996)

ply of oxygen to tissues. Symptoms often do not occur, however, until 75% or more of the blood supply to the area is occluded. The occurrence of symptoms may depend to an extent on the development of collateral circulation. Collateral vessels are small arteries that connect two larger arteries or different segments of the same artery. Under normal conditions, these collateral arteries carry very little of the blood flow. As the larger artery gradually occludes, pressure builds on the proximal side of the occlusion. As a result, flow is redirected through the collateral vessels, which enlarge and dilate over time (Fig. 20–2). Blood is then allowed to flow around an area of blockage through these alternate routes.[1]

Risk Factors

The cause of atherosclerosis is not clearly known. Through epidemiological studies, risk factors for the development of atherosclerosis have been identified. These risk factors are generally classified into two groups: major risk factors and contributing risk factors. Major risk factors are further divided into those that cannot be altered and those that can be altered.

MAJOR RISK FACTORS THAT CANNOT BE ALTERED

Age is a well-known risk factor. There is an increased incidence of all types of atherosclerotic disease with aging. Although 50% of all MIs occur in people under the age of 65, 80% of people who die from the MI are 65 years or older.[1]

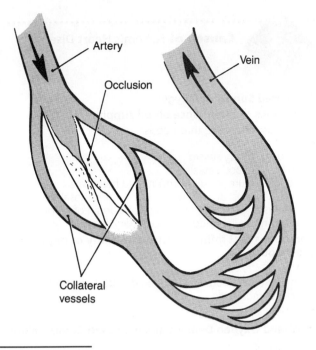

FIGURE 20-2
Collateral circulation can develop for slowly developing lesions to provide myocardial blood flow until the atherosclerosis progresses beyond the limits of collateral supply. (Source: Bullock BL: Pathophysiology: Adaptations and Alterations in Function [4th Ed]. Philadelphia, Lippincott-Raven, 1996)

Heredity is another important risk factor. The tendency to develop atherosclerosis seems to run in families, although the risk is presumed to be a combination of environmental and genetic influences. Even when other risk factors are controlled, the chance of developing coronary artery disease increases when there is a familial tendency. People with a parent or sibling who developed cardiovascular disease before 55 years of age generally have two to six times the risk of developing cardiovascular disease as those without a family history.[4,5]

Gender is another unalterable risk factor for atherosclerosis. Men have a greater risk for developing coronary artery disease than woman at earlier ages. After menopause, however, women's death rate from coronary disease rises.[1]

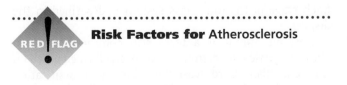

Risk Factors for Atherosclerosis

RED FLAG

- Major risk factors that cannot be altered: age, heredity, gender
- Major risk factors that can be altered: cigarette smoking, high blood cholesterol, hypertension, physical inactivity
- Contributing risk factors: diabetes mellitus, obesity, psychosocial factors, such as stress, anxiety, social resources, depression, cardiovascular reactivity

MAJOR RISK FACTORS THAT CAN BE ALTERED

Cigarette smoking is the biggest risk factor for peripheral vascular disease and sudden cardiac death. A smoker's risk of sudden death is two to four times greater than the nonsmoker's risk. Smokers have twice the risk of having an MI than nonsmokers. Smokers are more likely to die from the infarction. Exposure to environmental smoke also increases the risk of heart disease.[1]

High blood cholesterol increases the risk of coronary artery disease. Middle-aged adults with a blood cholesterol level below 200 mg/dL have a relatively low risk of coronary artery disease. A blood cholesterol level in the range of 200 to 239 mg/dL represents a moderate but increasing risk. When the level rises above 240 mg/dL, the risk of coronary artery disease is about double.[1]

For patients at risk, a further analysis of their high-density lipoprotein (HDL) and low-density lipoprotein (LDL) forms of cholesterol should be checked. The LDL form of cholesterol is associated with an increased risk of coronary artery disease. The HDL form of cholesterol tends to have a protective effect in preventing coronary artery disease. This protection occurs because the HDL form of cholesterol is a carrier that removes cholesterol from tissues and transports it to the liver where it is metabolized.[5]

Hypertension is a major risk factor that is termed the "silent killer" because it has no specific symptoms and no early warning signs. Men have a greater risk for hypertension than women until the age of 55. Between 55 and 75 years, the risk of developing hypertension is about the same for men and women. After the age of 75, women are more likely to develop hypertension than men.[1] African Americans, Puerto Ricans, Cuban Americans, and Mexican Americans are more likely to have hypertension than white Americans.[3]

Physical inactivity plays a significant role in the development of heart disease. When lack of regular exercise is combined with overeating and obesity, high cholesterol can result and further increase the risk of heart disease. Even moderate levels of regular low-intensity exercise have been shown to be beneficial in the prevention of heart disease.[1]

CONTRIBUTING RISK FACTORS

Diabetes mellitus doubles the likelihood of cardiovascular disease. The associated risk is greater for women than for men.[4] More than 80% of people with diabetes die of some form of heart or blood vessel disease.[1] Although there is no conclusive evidence that improved glucose tolerance lowers cardiovascular disease risk, more recent data indicate that close glucose control for insulin-dependent diabetics has a favorable effect on vascular changes.[4]

Obesity is associated with an increased mortality from coronary artery disease and stroke. Excess weight is also linked with an increased incidence of hypertension, insulin resistance, diabetes, and dyslipidemia.[4] Central obesity (intra-abdominal fat) appears to be a stronger predictor of cardiovascular disease than peripheral or subcutaneous obesity. Abdominal obesity has been defined as a waist/hip ratio greater than 1.0 for men and 0.8 for women. For men this means their waist measurement should not exceed their hip measurement. For women this means their waist measurement should not be more than 80% of their hip measurement.[1]

Psychosocial factors are also associated with the risk of cardiovascular disease. A relationship has been noted between cardiovascular disease and stress, anxiety, social resources, depression, and cardiovascular reactivity.[4] These psychosocial factors may not be the cause of heart disease but contribute to its development because they affect established risk factors. For example, under stress, a person may be more likely to overeat or smoke.

ANGINA PECTORIS

The term angina comes from the Latin word meaning to choke. "Angina is characterized as a deep, poorly localized chest or arm discomfort that is reproducibly associated with physical exertion or emotional stress and relieved promptly by rest or sublingual [nitroglycerin]."[6]

Pathophysiological Principles

Angina pectoris is caused by transient, reversible myocardial ischemia precipitated by an imbalance between myocardial oxygen demand and myocardial oxygen supply. The accompanying display summarizes causes of imbalances in oxygen supply and demand. In most cases, angina pectoris is the result of atherosclerotic narrowing of the coronary arteries. As blood flow to the myocardium decreases, autoregulation of coronary blood flow occurs as a compensatory mechanism. The smooth muscles of the arterioles relax, thus decreasing resistance to blood flow in the arteriolar bed. When this compensatory mechanism can no longer meet the metabolic demands, myocardial ischemia occurs, and the person feels pain.

As arterial blood flow is decreased, the myocardial tissue's need for oxygen and nutrients continues. The same work of pumping blood must be accomplished with less available energy and oxygen. The tissue that depends on the blood supply becomes ischemic as it functions with less oxygenated blood. Anaerobic metabolism can provide only 6% of the total energy needed. Glucose uptake by the cells is markedly increased as glycogen and adenosine triphosphate stores are depleted. Potassium rapidly moves out of the myocardial cells during ischemia. An acidotic cellular bath develops, further compromising cellular metabolism.

Classification of Angina

Many terms are used clinically to describe angina. Stable angina, classic angina, or exertional angina are terms used to describe paroxysmal substernal pain relieved by rest or

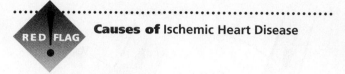

Causes of Ischemic Heart Disease

Decreased Supply of Oxygen
Conditions that influence blood supply:
- Atherosclerosis and thrombosis
- Thromboemboli
- Coronary artery spasm
- Collateral blood vessels
- Blood pressure, cardiac output, and heart rate
- Miscellaneous: arteritis (eg, periarteritis nodosa), dissecting aneurysm, luetic aortitis, anomalous origin of coronary artery, muscular bridging of coronary artery

Conditions that influence the availability of oxygen in the blood:
- Anemia
- Shift in the hemoglobin–oxygen dissociation curve
- Carbon monoxide
- Cyanide

Increased Oxygen Demand (ie, Increased Cardiac Work)
- Hypertension
- Valvular stenosis or insufficiency
- Hyperthyroidism
- Fever
- Thiamine deficiency
- Catecholamines

Source: Rubin E, Farber JL. Pathology (2nd Ed). Philadelphia, J.B. Lippincott, 1994

nitroglycerin. Prinzmetal's angina, also known as variant angina or vasospastic angina, refers to substernal pain caused by coronary artery spasm. Unstable angina, also called preinfarction angina or crescendo angina, implies a more severe form of angina with pain occurring more frequently, even at rest.

Use of these terms has resulted in confusion and a lack of a clear understanding of their differences. As a result, the Agency for Health Care Policy and Research (AHCPR) in their clinical practice guideline titled Unstable Angina: Diagnosis and Management encourages clinicians to use the Canadian Cardiovascular Society Classification System for Grading Angina Pectoris. Each stage of the four-class system is described in the display.

Unstable angina is a term still commonly used in clinical practice. Its definition has been clarified based on the Canadian Cardiovascular Society Classification System. According to the AHCPR guidelines, unstable angina is defined as having three possible presentations, which are described in another display. In most patients, symptoms are caused by significant coronary artery disease. Variant angina, non–Q-wave MI, and post-MI (> 24 hours) angina are part of the spectrum of unstable angina.[6]

Assessment

CLINICAL MANIFESTATIONS

Patients with angina typically present with chest discomfort described as a heaviness, squeezing, choking, or smothering sensation. The nurse uses the P, Q, R, S, T method of pain assessment when taking the patient's history. This method is described in the display on page 372. The patient often describes the pain as radiating to the left arm, neck, and jaw. The pain is often brought on by exertion or emotion. It may also occur after meals, exposure to cold, and at rest. As the angina becomes more severe (unstable angina) the pain is no longer relieved with rest. Patients may also have dyspnea related to inadequate cardiac output and anxiety. On physical examination, patients have an S_3 heart sound. The older patient who experiences angina may have a different presentation because of changes in neuroreceptors. Considerations for the older patient are described in the display on page 372.

DIAGNOSTIC TESTS

During the anginal episode, the electrocardiogram (ECG) may show T-wave inversions and ST segment depressions in the electrocardiographic leads associated with the anatomical region of myocardial ischemia (Fig. 20–3). Ectopic beats may also be present during an anginal episode. The ECG should be compared with previous ECGs. Between anginal episodes, the ECG may appear normal.

Other diagnostic tests include exercise stress testing in which the ECG and blood pressure are monitored before, during, and after exercise. The exercise stress test is especially useful in risk stratification of patients.[4] A thallium-201 perfusion exercise stress test or a persantine exercise stress test can be useful adjuncts in diagnosing angina pectoris. Coronary angiography is an invasive diagnostic test that provides a definitive diagnosis of coronary artery disease. (See Chapter 16 for a more detailed discussion of diagnostic tests.)

Management

The goal of therapy for the patient with angina pectoris is to restore the balance between oxygen supply and oxygen demand. An initial evaluation of the patient should include a systematic investigation of precipitating causes. A 12-lead ECG is recorded, and the patient is placed on a cardiac monitor for ischemia and dysrhythmia detection. A history focusing on precipitating factors and physical examination are completed. Blood is drawn for chemistry, hemoglobin, and hematocrit. The patient is placed on bed rest until stabilized to minimize oxygen demands. Supplemental oxygen may be given to unstable patients to increase oxygen supply. A pulse oximeter and arterial blood gases are used to evaluate oxygenation status.[6]

PHARMACOLOGICAL THERAPY

Pharmacological therapy is an important component in the management of patients with angina pectoris. The severity of symptoms, hemodynamic status of the patient, and medication history will guide the drug regimen.

Nitroglycerin is a mainstay of therapy and is used sublingually for acute anginal attacks. If oral and sublingual administration do not relieve the pain of angina, intravenous (IV) use is indicated. IV nitroglycerin should be started at a

The P, Q, R, S, T Characteristics of Chest Pain due to Myocardial Ischemia

P—Precipitating and Palliative Factors

PRECIPITATING

- Exercise
- Exercise after a large meal
- Exertion
- Walking on a cold or windy day
- Cold weather
- Stress or anxiety
- Anger
- Fear

PALLIATIVE

- Stop exercise.
- Sit down and rest.
- Use sublingual nitroglycerin.

Q—Quality

- Heaviness
- Tightness
- Squeezing
- Choking
- Suffocating
- Vise-like

R—Region and Radiation

- Substernal with radiation to the neck, left arm, or jaw
- Upper chest
- Epigastric
- Left shoulder
- Intrascapular

S—Severity

- Pain rated on a scale of 1 to 10, with 10 being the worst pain ever experienced, often rated as 5 or above

T—Time

- Pain lasts from 30 seconds to 30 minutes.
- Pain can last longer than 30 minutes for unstable angina or myocardial infarction.

dose of 5 to 10 µg/min by continuous infusion and titrated up to 10 µg/min every 5 to 10 minutes until symptoms are relieved or administration is limited by side effects. Patients on IV nitroglycerin should be switched to oral or topical nitrate therapy once they have been symptom free for 24 hours.[6] Nitroglycerin patches may be worn for up to 12 hours per day for the prevention of future anginal episodes.

Morphine sulfate is indicated for patients whose symptoms are not relieved after three serial sublingual nitroglycerin tablets or whose symptoms recur with adequate anti-ischemic therapy. A dose of 2 to 5 mg IV is recommended and may be repeated every 5 to 30 minutes as needed to relieve symptoms and maintain comfort.[6]

All patients diagnosed in the emergency department with unstable angina should receive regular aspirin 160 to 324 mg as soon as possible unless a definite contraindication exists. Patients with intermediate or high-risk unstable angina should be started immediately on IV heparin at an initial dose of 80 U/kg IV bolus followed by a continuous

infusion of 18 U/kg/h to maintain the activated partial thromboplastin time at 1.5 to 2.5 times control.[6]

Beta-blockers may be used to decrease myocardial oxygen consumption by blocking sympathetic response. In the absence of contraindications, IV beta-blockers are used for high-risk, unstable angina patients, and oral beta-blockers are used for intermediate and low-risk patients.[6] Patients who may not tolerate beta-blocker therapy include asthmatics and those with poor left ventricular function.

Calcium channel blockers cause arteriolar dilation, thus reducing afterload. Some calcium channel blockers decrease the inotropic state of the heart. Calcium channel blockers can be given in conjunction with nitrates and beta-blockers or can be given alone for patients who cannot tolerate adequate doses of nitrates or beta-blockers. Calcium channel blockers have been especially useful in preventing and treating angina caused by coronary artery spasms.[4,6]

INVASIVE THERAPY

Invasive therapy may be indicated for the management of patients with angina pectoris. Intra-aortic balloon pump

Considerations for the Older Patient
Angina Pectoris

Because of changes in neuroreceptors, older patients may not describe the typical pain profile associated with angina. Rather than substernal pain, the older patient may describe a sense of weakness or fainting. Because of differences in body composition of subcutaneous fat, the older person may develop anginal symptoms more quickly when exposed to cold. The older person should be taught to dress in warm clothing and to recognize feelings of weakness or fainting as possible indicators of angina.

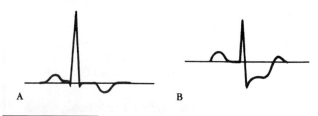

FIGURE 20-3
Inversion of T wave (**A**) and depression of ST segment (**B**). (Source: Bullock BL: Pathophysiology: Adaptations and Alterations in Function [4th Ed]. Philadelphia, Lippincott-Raven, 1996)

support may be used in a critically ill patient to provide increased coronary artery perfusion and to decrease afterload. Balloon angioplasty or coronary artery bypass grafting (CABG) are other invasive options for treatment. CABG has been shown to prolong life in patients with left main coronary artery disease and in patients with three-vessel disease with an ejection fraction less than 50%.[4] Overall success for angioplasty is 80% to 90% with restenosis occurring in about 30% to 40% of patients within 6 months.

RISK FACTOR MODIFICATION

Risk factor modification may help prevent an anginal episode or delay the worsening of existing angina. Patients should be encouraged to stop smoking and reduce their weight if obese.

Diet and medications may be prescribed to control hypertension, diabetes, and hyperlipidemia. Patient education, including home care considerations, is essential for patients with angina pectoris. Patient education guidelines and home care considerations are described in the accompanying display.

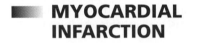

MYOCARDIAL INFARCTION

Prolonged ischemia caused by an imbalance between oxygen supply and oxygen demand causes MI. The prolonged ischemia causes irreversible cell damage and muscle death.

Although multiple factors can contribute to the imbalance between oxygen supply and oxygen demand, the presence of a coronary artery thrombosis characterizes most MIs. In a classic investigation, DeWood and colleagues demonstrated that 87% of patients studied in the first 4 hours after onset of MI symptoms had a thrombotic occlusion. The incidence of thrombotic occlusion decreases to 65% at 12 to 24 hours.[7]

Pathophysiological Principles

Most patients who sustain a MI have coronary atherosclerosis. The thrombus formation occurs most often at the site of an atherosclerotic lesion, thus obstructing blood flow to the myocardial tissues. Plaque rupture is believed to be the triggering mechanism for the development of the thrombus in most patients with an MI.[8]

Irreversible damage to the myocardium can begin as early as 20 to 40 minutes following interruption of blood flow. The dynamic process of infarction may not be completed, however, for several hours. Necrosis of tissue appears to occur in a sequential fashion. Reimer and associates demonstrated that cellular death occurs first in the subendocardial layer and spreads like a "wavefront" throughout the thickness of the wall of the heart. Using dogs, they showed that the shorter the time between coronary occlusion and coronary reperfusion, the greater the amount of myocardial tissue that could be salvaged. Their work indicates that a substantial amount of myocardial tissue can be salvaged if flow is restored within 6 hours after

---

PATIENT TEACHING
Home Care Considerations in Angina Pectoris

Activity and Exercise
- Participate in a daily program of exercise that does not precipitate pain.
- Alternate activity with periods of rest and moderate activity level as needed.

Diet
- Eat a well-balanced diet with an appropriate caloric intake.
- If obese, participate in a supervised weight-reduction program.
- Avoid activity directly following meals.
- Restrict intake of caffeine because it can increase heart rate.
- Maintain a diet low in fat.

Smoking
- Participate in a smoking cessation program. Smoking can increase heart rate, blood pressure, and blood carbon monoxide levels.
- Avoid smoke-filled environments.

Cold Weather
- Avoid exposure to cold and windy weather. Exercise indoors when necessary.
- When outdoors, dress in warm clothing, and cover mouth and nose with a scarf.
- Use a moderate pace of walking in cold weather.

Medications
- Carry sublingual nitroglycerin at all times.
- Keep the pills in a dark-colored glass bottle to protect them from sunlight.
- Do not place cotton in the bottle because the active ingredients of the medication will be absorbed by the cotton.
- If pain occurs, place tablet under the tongue, stop activity, and wait for medication to dissolve. Take another tablet in 3 to 5 minutes if pain is not resolved.
- If pain continues, seek immediate care.
- Be aware of side effects of nitroglycerin, including headache, flushing, and dizziness.

the onset of coronary occlusion.[9] For the clinician, this means time is muscle.

The cellular changes associated with an MI can be followed by the development of infarct extension (new myocardial necrosis), infarct expansion (a disproportionate thinning and dilation of the infarct zone), or ventricular remodeling (a disproportionate thinning and dilation of the ventricle).[10]

SIZE OF THE INFARCTION

Several factors determine the size of the resulting MI. These factors include the extent, severity, and duration of the ischemic episode; the amount of collateral circulation; and the metabolic demands of the myocardium at the time of the event.[5] MIs most often result in damage to the left ventricle, leading to an alteration in left ventricular function. Infarctions can also occur in the right ventricle or in both ventricles.

The term "transmural infarction" is used to imply an infarction process that has resulted in necrosis of the tissue in all the layers of the myocardium. Because the heart functions as a squeezing pump, systolic and diastolic efforts can be significantly altered when a segment of the heart muscle is dead and nonfunctional. If the area of the transmural infarction is small, the necrotic wall may be dyskinetic, a term meaning difficulty in moving. If the damage to the myocardial tissue is more extensive, the myocardial muscle may become akinetic, meaning without motion.

The normal myocardial muscle contracts with systole and relaxes with diastole. When normal motion is not possible because of infarction, diastolic filling and systolic pumping are altered. As a result, cardiac output is compromised. The larger the area of infarction, the greater the impact on ventricular function.

LOCATION OF THE INFARCTION

In addition to size, location of the infarction is an important determinant of ventricular function. MIs can be located in the anterior, lateral, posterior, or inferior walls of the left ventricle. In more recent years, clinicians have acknowledged the presence and clinical significance of MIs occurring in the right ventricle.

Anterior Left Ventricle

Infarctions of the anterior wall of the left ventricle and the interventricular septum result from occlusion of the left anterior descending (LAD) coronary artery. The LAD coronary artery supplies oxygenated blood to the anterior wall of the left ventricle, the interventricular septum, and the ventricular conducting tissue. (See Chapter 15 for a more detailed discussion of coronary artery anatomy and physiology.) Anteroseptal wall MIs are the most frequent type of infarction and have the potential for causing a significant amount of left ventricular dysfunction. Patients with an anteroseptal MI are at high risk for congestive heart failure, pulmonary edema, cardiogenic shock, and mortality be-

Insights Into Clinical Research

Karlson BW, Herlitz J, Hjalmarson A: In consecutive patients hospitalized with acute myocardial infarction, infarct location according to routine ECG is of minor importance for the outcome. Clin Cardiol 18(7):385–391, 1995

The objective of this study was to compare the mortality and morbidity of patients with an anterior wall infarction versus those with an inferior wall infarction. Most literature suggests that the anterior wall infarction has an adverse prognosis. A total of 921 patients admitted within 21 months were studied. Clinical management of each patient was similar, and care was provided by a single institution. Anterior wall infarction patients (n = 312) had a 1-year mortality of 26%, whereas inferior wall infarction patients (n = 219) had a 24% mortality at 1 year. If the patients had never had a previous infarction and now had a transmural, Q-wave infarction of the anterior wall, the patients had a mortality of 27%, and the patients with an inferior wall infarction had a mortality rate of 21%. Morbidity of reinfarction, thromboembolic events, and long-term complications appeared similar. This study suggests that when all patients are managed similarly, there is little difference between anterior and inferior myocardial infarction mortality rates. If the infarct is the patient's first infarct, the trend toward a higher mortality rate may exist with patients who infarct the anterior wall.

cause of an inadequate pump. Anteroseptal wall MIs are also associated with increased risk of intraventricular conduction disturbances, such as bundle branch blocks and fascicular blocks.

Lateral and Posterior Left Ventricle

Infarctions of the lateral and posterior walls of the left ventricle result from occlusion of the left circumflex vessel. In addition to supplying oxygenated blood to the lateral and posterior walls, the left circumflex vessel is the source of blood supply to the sinoatrial (SA) node in about 50% of the population and to the atrioventricular (AV) node in about 10% of the population. Infarctions of the lateral and posterior walls are less common than infarctions of the anteroseptal wall. Although muscle necrosis occurs with lateral and posterior wall MIs, the impact on left ventricular function is usually less than for patients with anteroseptal MI. Patients with a lateral or posterior wall MI are also at risk for dysrhythmias associated with dysfunction of the SA or AV nodes. Examples include sinus arrest, wandering atrial pacemaker, sinus pause, or junction rhythm.

Inferior Left Ventricle

Infarctions of the inferior wall result from occlusion of the right coronary artery. The right coronary artery supplies oxygenated blood to the inferior wall and the right ventricle. In addition, it is the source of blood supply to the SA node in about 50% of the population and the AV node in about 90% of the population. Infarctions of the inferior wall are less common than anteroseptal MIs but occur more frequently than MIs of the lateral or posterior walls. The potential impact on left ventricular function usually is less for a patient with an inferior wall MI than for a patient with an anteroseptal wall infarct. Because the right coronary artery supplies oxygenated blood to much of the conducting tissue, patients are at frequent risk for dysrhythmias related to altered function of the SA and AV nodes.

Right Ventricle

The right coronary artery provides the blood supply to the inferior wall and the right ventricle. Consequently, right coronary artery disease causing an inferior wall MI is likely to be associated with concomitant right ventricular infarction. Approximately 33% to 50% of patients with an inferior wall MI will have associated right ventricular involvement.[11,12] Patients may experience significant hemodynamic compromise due to biventricular dysfunction. Associated dysrhythmias involve dysfunction of the SA and AV nodes.

Q-Wave and Non–Q-Wave Infarctions

The terms Q-wave infarction and non–Q-wave infarction are often used to classify MIs. A Q wave is a portion of the QRS complex on the ECG. Specifically, the Q wave is the initial downward deflection of the QRS complex. A Q wave is not present on the normal ECG. The presence of significant Q waves indicates an MI. A Q wave is evident in about 60% of patients with an infarction and typically indicates a larger infarction. Q waves are associated with increased pathophysiological findings. A Q wave is not evident on the ECG in approximately 25% to 40% of patients with an MI. Non–Q-wave infarctions are smaller in terms of gram weight of necrotic tissue. Non–Q-wave infarctions are associated with a lower incidence of congestive heart failure, fewer pulmonary complications, lower cardiac enzyme levels, and a lower hospital mortality rate.[10]

Assessment

The nursing assessment of a patient with a probable MI must be organized and thorough. It is best to start with the history because this establishes rapport and provides valuable data. The history is followed by the physical examination and evaluation of diagnostic tests. Based on the data, a management plan is developed initially for the acute phase. Once stabilized, plans for cardiac rehabilitation are initiated.

HISTORY

The most common presenting complaint of a patient with an MI is the presence of chest discomfort or pain. Like patients with angina, MI patients describe a heaviness, squeezing, choking, or smothering sensation. Patients will often describe the sensation as "someone sitting on my chest." The substernal pain can radiate to the neck, left arm, or jaw. Unlike the pain of angina, the pain of an MI is often more prolonged and unrelieved by rest or sublingual nitroglyc-

erin. The P, Q, R, S, T assessment guide display outlined earlier in the chapter can be used to guide a comprehensive assessment of the pain.

Associated findings on history include nausea and vomiting, especially for the patient with an inferior wall MI. These gastrointestinal complaints are believed to be related to the severity of the pain and the resulting vagal stimulation. Patients may initially seek relief of the gastrointestinal symptoms through antacids and other home remedies, thus delaying their decision to go the the hospital. Additional complaints described during the history include diaphoresis, dyspnea, weakness, fatigue, anxiety, restlessness, and a sense of impending death.

After the patient is stabilized, a more comprehensive history is obtained. Information about risk factors, previous cardiac illnesses and surgeries, and family history is important to acquire. This information will be useful in guiding patient education, cardiac rehabilitation, and care at home.

PHYSICAL EXAMINATION

On physical examination, patients generally appear restless and in distress. They often assume a position to promote breathing and alleviate pain. The skin is warm and moist. Breathing may be labored and rapid. Fine crackles, coarse crackles, or rhonchi may be heard when auscultating the lungs. These sounds may indicate the presence of heart failure or pulmonary edema.

The cardiovascular examination may reveal an increased blood pressure related to anxiety or a decreased blood pressure caused by heart failure. The heart rate may vary from bradycardia to tachycardia. Sinus tachycardia that persists more than 24 hours after the infarction is associated with high mortality rates.[4] When the patient is placed in the left lateral decubitus position, abnormalities of the precordial pulsations can be felt. These abnormalities include a lack of a point of maximal impulse or the presence of diffuse contraction. On auscultation, the first heart sound may be diminished as a result of decreased contractility. A fourth heart sound is heard in almost all MI patients, whereas a third heart sound is detected in only about 10% to 20% of patients. Transient systolic murmurs may be heard because of papillary muscle dysfunction. After about 48 to 72 hours, many patients will develop a pericardial friction rub. Additional findings on physical examination may be related to the development of complications.

Patients with right ventricular infarcts may present with jugular vein distention, peripheral edema, and an elevated central venous pressure. Their lungs may be clear because the failing right ventricle has not provided adequate forward flow.

DIAGNOSTIC TESTS

The Electrocardiogram

When a coronary artery becomes about 70% occluded and oxygen demand exceeds oxygen supply, myocardial ischemia may result. If the ischemic state is not corrected, injury to the myocardium may occur. Eventually, if adequate blood flow to the myocardium is not restored, an MI may result. Ischemia and injury are reversible processes; however, infarction is not.

An ECG can be used to detect patterns of ischemia, injury, and infarction. When the heart muscle becomes ischemic, injured, or infarcted, depolarization and repolarization of the cardiac cells are altered, causing changes in the QRS complex, ST segment, and T wave in the ECG leads overlying the affected area of the heart.[13] Table 20–1 shows location of the MI, the artery affected, findings from the ECG, and clinical implications.

Ischemia. Myocardial ischemia may be a transient finding on ECG, or ischemic patterns may be more prolonged due to the presence of ischemic tissue surrounding a region of infarcted tissue. On the ECG, myocardial ischemia results in T-wave inversion or ST-segment depression in the leads facing the ischemic area. The inverted T wave representative of ischemia is symmetrical in shape, relatively narrow, and somewhat pointed. In contrast, asymmetric inversion of the T wave usually does not indicate ischemia. Instead, it may signify ventricular hypertrophy or bundle branch block (Fig. 20–4). ST segment depressions of 1 to 2 mm or more for a duration of 0.08 seconds may indicate myocardial ischemia. Ischemia also should be suspected when a flat or depressed ST segment makes a sharp angle when joining an upright T wave rather than merging smoothly and imperceptibly with the T wave (Fig. 20–5).

Injury. ECG patterns of myocardial injury indicate a state of cellular damage beyond ischemia. Like ischemia, myocardial injury is a reversible process if interventions are instituted rapidly. As described previously, the injury process begins in the subendocardial layer and moves throughout the thickness of the wall of the heart like a wave. If the injury process is not interrupted, it eventually results in a transmural MI.

On ECG, the hallmark of acute myocardial injury is the presence of ST segment elevations. In the normal ECG, the ST segment should not be elevated more than 1 mm in

TABLE 20-1
Location of Myocardial Infarction, Electrocardiographic (ECG) Findings, and Clinical Implications

Anatomical Location	Coronary Artery	ECG Evidence	Clinical Implications
Anteroseptal wall	Left anterior descending: Supplies blood to the anterior wall of left ventricle, the interventricular septum, and the ventricular conducting tissue	V_1 through V_4, Q waves and ST segment elevations	Potential for significant hemodynamic compromise; congestive heart failure, pulmonary edema, cardiogenic shock; intraventricular conduction disturbances
Lateral wall	Left circumflex: Supplies blood to the left lateral and left posterior walls and to the SA node in 45% of people and AV node in 10% of people	I, aVL, V_5, and V_6, Q waves and ST segment elevations	Evaluation for posterior wall involvement; some hemodynamic changes; dysrhythmias caused by SA and AV node dysfunction
Posterior wall	Left circumflex: Supplies blood to the left lateral and left posterior walls and to the SA node in 45% of people and AV node in 10% of people	V_1 and V_2, tall upright R waves with ST segment depression; Q waves and ST segment elevation in V_7 through V_9	Evaluation for lateral wall involvement; some hemodynamic changes; dysrhythmias caused by SA and AV node dysfunction
Inferior wall	Right coronary artery: Supplies blood to the inferior wall of the left ventricle, the right ventricle, and the SA node in 55% of people and the AV node in 90% of people	Q waves and ST segment elevation in II, III, aVF	Evaluation for right ventricular wall involvement; some hemodynamic changes; potential for significant arrhythmias caused by SA and AV node dysfunction
Right ventricular wall	Right coronary artery: Supplies blood to the inferior wall of the left ventricle, the right ventricle, and the SA node in 55% of people and the AV node in 90% of people	Q waves and ST segment elevations in right precordial chest leads (RV_1 through RV_6)	Evaluation for inferior wall involvement; some hemodynamic changes; potential for significant dysrhythmias caused by SA and AV node dysfunction

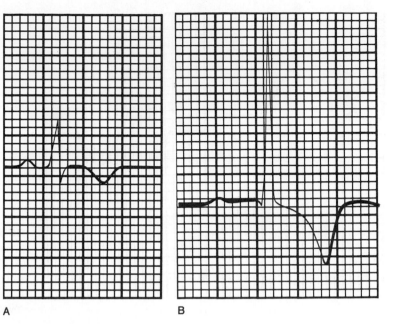

FIGURE 20-4

T-wave inversion seen with ischemia (**A**) versus T-wave inversion seen with left ventricular hypertrophy (**B**).

A   B

the standard leads or more than 2 mm in the precordial leads. With an acute injury, the ST segments in the leads facing the injured area are elevated. The elevated ST segments also have a downward concave or coved shape and merge unnoticed with the T wave (Fig. 20–6).

Infarction.   When myocardial injury persists, MI is the result. The pattern of the ECG indicative of an MI is seen on the ECG in stages and involves changes in the T wave, the ST segment, and the Q wave in the leads overlying the infarcted area. Figure 20–7 shows the evolution of the ECG in an MI. During the earliest stage of MI, known as the hyperacute phase, the T waves become tall and narrow. This configuration is referred to as hyperacute or peaked T waves. Within a few hours, these hyperacute T waves invert.

Next, the ST segments elevate, a pattern that generally lasts from several hours to several days. In addition to the ST segment elevations in the leads of the ECG facing the in-

jured heart, the leads facing away from the injured area may show ST segment depression. This finding is known as reciprocal ST segment changes. The clinical significance of the reciprocal changes is unclear. Reciprocal ST segment depressions may simply be a mirror image of the ST segment elevations and are not clinically significant. However, others have suggested that reciprocal changes may reflect ischemia due to narrowing of another coronary artery in other areas of the heart.[14]

The last stage in the ECG evolution of an MI is the development of Q waves, an initial downward deflection of the QRS complex. Q waves represent the flow of electrical forces toward the septum. Small narrow Q waves may be seen in the normal ECG in leads I, II, III, aVR, aVL, V$_5$, and V$_6$. Q waves compatible with an MI are usually 0.04 seconds or more in width or one-fourth to one-third the height of the R wave. Q waves indicative of infarction usually develop within several hours of the onset of the infarction, but in some patients, may not appear until 24 to 48 hours after the infarction.

Within a few days after the MI, the ST segments return to baseline. Persistent elevation of the ST segment may indicate the presence of a ventricular aneurysm. The T waves may remain inverted for several weeks, indicating areas of ischemia near the infarct region. Eventually, the T waves should return to their upright configuration. The Q waves do not disappear and therefore will always provide ECG evidence of a previous MI.

The ECG pattern can be used to distinguish acute MIs from "old" MIs. Abnormal Q waves accompanied by ST segment elevations indicate an acute MI. Abnormal Q waves accompanied by a normal ST segment indicate a previous MI. How long ago the infarction occurred cannot be determined by the ECG. The pattern could signify an infarction that occurred 2 weeks or 20 years before.

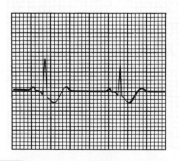

FIGURE 20-5

An ST segment pattern consistent with myocardial ischemia. Notice how the ST segment forms a sharp angle when joining an upright T wave rather than merging smoothly and imperceptibly with the T wave.

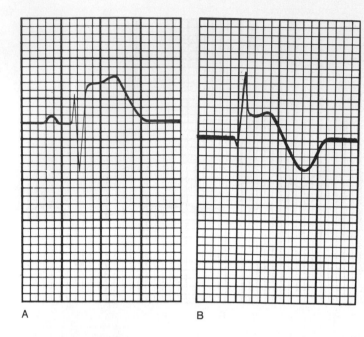

A   B

FIGURE 20-6

ST segment pattern consistent with acute myocardial injury. (**A**) shows ST segment elevation without T-wave inversion; and (**B**) shows ST segment elevation with T-wave inversion. The elevated ST segments have a downward concave or coved shape and merge unnoticed with the T wave.

The ECG is helpful not only in determining patterns of ischemia, injury, and infarction, but also in revealing the anatomical region of the heart where the abnormality has occurred. ECG leads V_1 through V_4 show the anteroseptal wall of the left ventricle. The inferior wall is seen in leads II, III, and aVF. Leads I, aVL, V_5, and V_6 reveal the lateral wall of the left ventricle.

The routine 12-lead ECG does not provide an adequate view of the right ventricle or of the posterior wall of the left ventricle. As a result, additional leads are needed to view these anatomical areas. To attain an accurate view of the right ventricle, right sided chest leads are recorded by placing the six chest electrodes on the right side of the chest using landmarks analogous to those used on the left side (see Fig. 16–13). These six right sided views are examined for patterns of ischemia, injury, and infarction in the same way left sided chest leads are evaluated.

Detection of posterior wall abnormalities is also difficult on the standard 12-lead ECG because none of the six chest leads provides an adequate view of the posterior wall. To detect posterior wall abnormalities, one of the precordial electrodes is placed posteriorly over the heart, a view known as V_7. The recording is examined for evidence of ischemia, injury, or infarction using the same criteria as described previously. If a V_7 lead was not recorded, it may still be possible to detect posterior wall abnormalities. To do so, the principle of reciprocal change is used. When an infarction in the posterior wall is suspected, the leads anatomically opposite the posterior wall are examined. These include V_1 and V_2 because the anterior wall is anatomically opposite the poste-

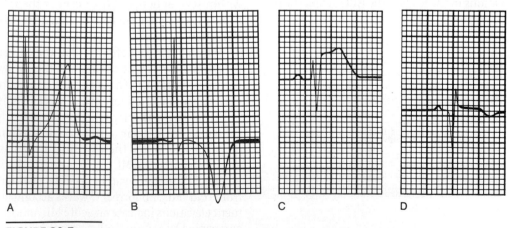

A   B   C   D

FIGURE 20-7

Evolution of the electrocardiogram in a patient with a myocardial infarction. (**A**) Tall peak T waves known as hyperacute T waves; (**B**) symmetrical T wave inversions; (**C**) ST segment elevation; (**D**) development of the Q wave.

rior wall. If tall R waves with ST segment depressions are noted in V_1 and V_2, the pattern is consistent with a posterior wall MI.

Figures 20–8, 20–9, and 20–10 show the 12-lead ECGs of patients with MIs.

Laboratory Tests

When myocardial cells are damaged by an infarction, biochemical markers are released into the bloodstream and can be detected by laboratory tests. The presence of abnormally high levels of biochemical markers, their distribution, and the time pattern for their appearance and disappearance make them very useful in the diagnosis of acute MI. For a more detailed discussion of laboratory tests, see Chapter 16.

Creatine Kinase. Creatine kinase (CK) is an enzyme found mainly in heart and skeletal muscles. When heart muscle is damaged, CK is released into the blood. The level of CK becomes abnormal within 6 to 8 hours after the onset of infarction and peaks within about 24 hours. The isoenzymes of CK are measured to determine if the CK came from the heart (MB) or the skeletal muscle. Elevation of CK-MB offers a more definitive indication of myocardial cell damage than total CK alone. For the patient with an MI, the CK-MB appears in the serum in 6 to 12 hours, peaks between 12 and 28 hours, and returns to normal levels in about 72 to 96 hours.[4] Serial samplings are performed every 4 to 6 hours for the first 24 to 48 hours after the onset of symptoms. If the CK-MB value is negative for 48 hours or more following chest pain, the chest pain is not due to an MI.[15]

New assay techniques to measure CK-MB based on monoclonal antibodies offer greater sensitivity and specificity than conventional means. Additionally, the results can be available in 30 minutes, which provides a distinct advantage in the diagnosis of a MI, especially in the emergency department.

Creatine Kinase Isoforms. When CK-MB is released by the myocardial cells, it is quickly transformed into two isoforms, also known as subforms. CK-MB$_1$ is the isoform found in the plasma, and CK-MB$_2$ is found in the tissues. In the normal person, these two isoforms are found in about equal amounts, resulting in a ratio of approximately one. In the patient with an MI, the CK-MB$_2$ level rises, resulting in a CK-MB$_2$ to CK-MB$_1$ ratio greater than one. This ratio can be rapidly measured in the laboratory and provides an ex-

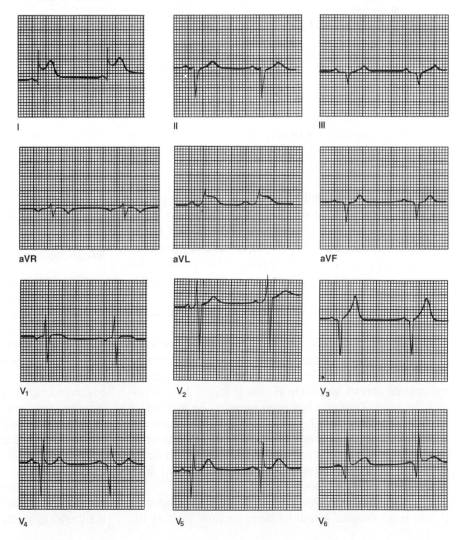

FIGURE 20-8

Twelve-lead ECG showing an acute lateral wall myocardial infarction. ST segment elevations can be seen in leads I, aVL, V_5, and V_6. Note also the deep Q waves in II, III, and aVF and normal ST segments, indicating a previous inferior wall myocardial infarction.

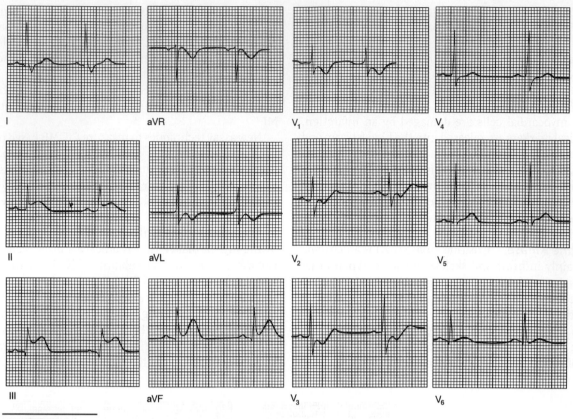

FIGURE 20-9

Twelve-lead ECG showing an acute inferior wall myocardial infarction. Note the ST segment elevations in II, III, and aVF. The posterior wall infarction is evidenced by a tall R wave, ST segment depression, and inverted T wave in V1 and V2.

cellent diagnostic marker for acute MI. Isoform CK-MB$_2$ is also a sensitive test for detecting an early extension of an MI during the first 24 hours.[4]

Myoglobin. Myoglobin is an oxygen-binding protein found in skeletal and cardiac muscle. Myoglobin's release from ischemic muscle occurs earlier than the release of CK. As a result, elevation of serum levels of myoglobin can be detected soon after the onset of symptoms. The myoglobin level can elevate in the first hour of acute MI and peaks approximately 4 hours later.[16] Because myoglobin is also present in skeletal muscle, an elevated myoglobin level is not specific for the diagnosis of MI. Consequently, its diagnostic value in detecting an MI is controversial.[15]

Troponin. Troponin is a contractile protein with two subforms (troponin T and troponin I) that are highly specific for cardiac muscle. Troponin levels are not detected in the normal person, and skeletal muscle injury does not affect the level. Troponin has been found to be a sensitive marker during the early hours following an MI. Levels rise within the first 3 to 4 hours and peak in 10 to 24 hours.[16] Unlike CK-MB, troponin remains elevated after AMI for up to several weeks and therefore provides an excellent diagnostic marker for early and late diagnosis of AMI.[4,17]

Lactase Dehydrogenase. Lactase dehydrogenase (LDH) is an enzyme found in many organs, such as the heart, liver, kidney, and lung. LDH levels are not as useful as CK levels in diagnosing an acute MI because it is not specific for cardiac muscle. Additionally, it takes about 12 to 24 hours after an acute MI before LDH can be detected in the blood. Peak LDH levels are reached in about 2 to 3 days and levels remain elevated for 7 to 10 days.[16]

RADIONUCLIDE IMAGING

Nuclear imaging techniques involve IV injection of radioactive substances and are considered noninvasive tests. A scintillation camera records the radiation emitted from the radioactive substance. These diagnostic tests are helpful in determining the location and size of an MI. (For a more detailed discussion, see Chapter 16.)

Technetium pyrophosphate is the agent frequently used to detect an area of infarction. The agent localizes in acute infarcted myocardium and forms an area known as a "hot spot." This hot spot image aids in locating the infarction and in determining its size.

Because thallium-201 accumulates rapidly in viable myocardial cells, it is commonly used. When myocardial perfusion is normal, the radioactive substance is distributed equally throughout the myocardium. If coronary blood flow is significantly reduced, thallium fails to accumulate in the

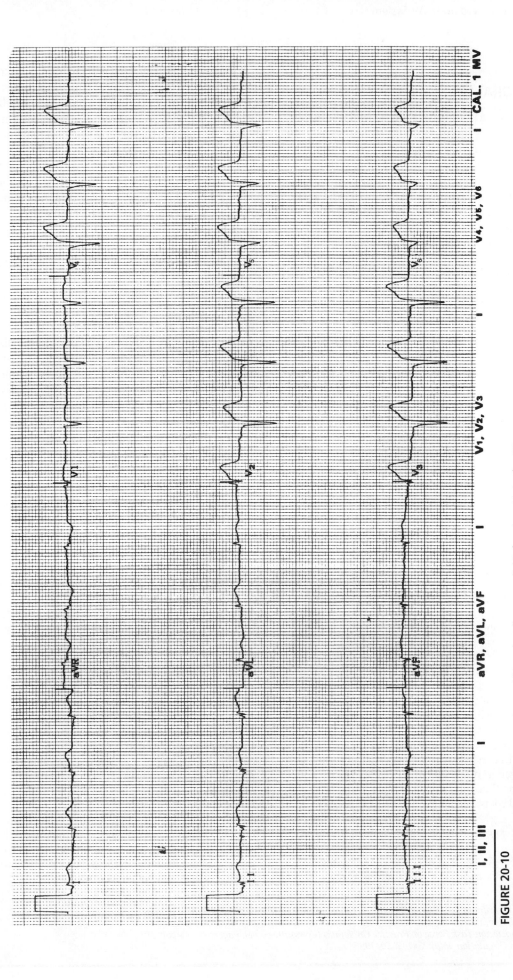

FIGURE 20-10

Twelve-lead ECG showing an acute anterior and lateral wall myocardial infarction. Note the ST segment elevations and Q waves in I, aVL, V5 and V6 (lateral), and V2, V3, and V4 (anterior).

area and forms an area known as a "cold spot" or perfusion defect.

ECHOCARDIOGRAM

An echocardiogram is a noninvasive ultrasound test involving the transmission of high-frequency sound waves into the heart. This commonly used diagnostic test helps determine ejection fraction, segmental wall motion, systolic and diastolic ventricular volumes, valve function, mural thrombi, pericardial fluid, intracardiac tumors, and aortic dissection. Two-dimensional and transesophageal echocardiograms are the most frequently used types of echocardiograms for patients with an MI (see Chapter 16).

Management

EARLY MANAGEMENT

When a patient with a possible MI arrives in the emergency department, the diagnosis and initial management of the patient must be rapid because the benefit of reperfusion therapy is greatest if therapy is initiated quickly.[18] An initial evaluation of the patient should occur within the first 10 to 20 minutes after arrival. If the initial history and physical examination suggest an MI, the interventions listed in the display are initiated. Vital signs are checked frequently, and the patient's cardiac rhythm is continuously assessed. A chest x-ray and stat echocardiogram are useful in ruling out an aortic dissection and acute pericarditis. During the initial evaluation, the patient and family may be anxious, necessitating brief and clear explanations of the interventions. Reassurance and support are essential components of the nurse's responsibilities.

Thrombolytic Therapy

If the patient is diagnosed with an MI, thrombolytic therapy may be used to establish reperfusion if there are no contraindications for its use. The accompanying display lists absolute and relative contraindications for thrombolytic therapy. Thrombolytic therapy provides maximal benefit if given within the first 2 to 3 hours after the onset of symptoms. Significant benefit does occur if given up to 6 hours after onset of symptoms, and some benefit has been shown up to 12 hours.[4] No benefit is realized, however, if thrombolytics are given more than 12 hours after the onset of symptoms. In addition to the thrombolytic agent, the patient should receive heparin and aspirin.

Thrombolytic drugs lyse coronary thrombi by converting plasminogen to plasmin. This conversion causes the degradation of fibrin and fibrinogen, resulting in clot lysis. Currently available thrombolytic agents for coronary occlusion include streptokinase, anisoylated plasminogen streptokinase activator complex (APSAC), and recombinant tissue plasminogen activator (rt-PA). Each has a similar mechanisms of action, although rt-PA is more fibrin selective in its plasminogen activation, resulting in a decreased risk of systemic lysis.

For the patient receiving thrombolytic therapy, two to three 18-gauge peripheral IV lines are usually started. One line is for the thrombolytic, and one to two lines are for the administration of other drugs. Subclavian and jugular sites are avoided because they are noncompressible, and blood could be lost into the chest or neck. Some type of blood sampling device is also inserted so that peripheral venous punctures can be avoided. With this device, blood is drawn for a complete blood count with differential, electrolytes,

---

Initial Management of the Patient With a Suspected Myocardial Infarction

Action: Give oxygen by nasal cannula.

Rationale: Hypoxemia often occurs in patients with a myocardial infarction because of pulmonary edema. If severe pulmonary edema is present and the patient is in respiratory distress, intubation may be necessary. A pulse oximeter is often applied, and when time permits, an arterial blood gas may be drawn.

Action: Administer sublingual nitroglycerin (unless the systolic blood pressure is less than 90 mmHg or the heart rate is less than 50 or greater than 100 beats/min).

Rationale: Nitroglycerin helps to promote vasodilation but is relatively ineffective in relieving pain in the early stages of a myocardial infarction. Intravenous nitroglycerin may also be initiated and continued for the first 24 to 48 hours of hospitalization.

Action: Provide adequate analgesia with morphine sulfate or meperidine.

Rationale: Morphine is the drug of choice to relieve the pain of a myocardial infarction. The drug is given intravenously in small doses (2–4 mg) and can be repeated every 5 minutes until the pain is relieved. Close respiratory monitoring is indicated because morphine can depress respirations. If necessary, meperidine can be substituted for morphine.

Action: Administer aspirin, 160 to 325 mg orally.

Rationale: Aspirin is used because it diminishes platelet aggregation. This effect is important because platelets are one of the main components in thrombus formation when a coronary plaque is disrupted. Aspirin has been shown to reduce mortality independently in patients with acute myocardial infarction.

Action: Record a 12-lead electrocardiogram (ECG).

Rationale: The ECG is examined for the presence of ST segment elevations of 1 mV or greater in contiguous leads. This pattern provides evidence of thrombotic coronary arterial occlusion. The patient is placed on a continuous cardiac monitor after the 12-lead ECG is recorded.

Ryan TJ, Anderson JL, Antman EM, Braniff BA et al: ACC/AHA guidelines for the management of patients with acute myocardial infarction: Executive summary. A report of the American College of Cardiology/American Heart Association Task Force on Practice Guidelines (Committee on Management of Acute Myocardial Infarction). Circulation 94(9):2341–2350, 1996

bleeding and clotting times, cardiac enzymes, partial thromboplastin time, blood urea nitrogen, and creatine.

The patient is closely monitored during and after the infusion of a thrombolytic agent. The nurse assesses the patient for resolution of chest pain, normalization of elevated ST segments, development of reperfusion dysrhythmias, any allergic reactions, evidence of bleeding, and the onset of hypotension. Commonly seen reperfusion dysrhythmias include an accelerated idioventricular rhythm, ventricular tachycardia, and AV heart block. Table 20–2 lists possible adverse effects of thrombolytic agents.

TABLE 20-2
Possible Adverse Effects of Thrombolytic Therapy

Effect	Streptokinase	rt-PA	APSAC
Allergic response	+	−	+
Bleeding	+	+	+
Dysrhythmias	+	+	+
Hypotension (unrelated to bleeding)	+	−	+

+, moderate to high risk of occurrence; −, minimal to no risk of occurrence

Evaluation of complications remains a key nursing intervention. The patient is closely monitored for evidence of reocclusion of the coronary artery. Indicators of reocclusion include chest pain, ST segment elevation, and hemodynamic instability. Close observation for evidence of bleeding also is essential. The patient is carefully assessed for indications of subcutaneous or mucous membrane bleeding. The nurse also monitors the patient for signs of internal bleeding, including positive results of urine and stool for blood or altered levels of consciousness due to intracranial bleeding.

Primary Angioplasty

Early reperfusion of myocardial tissue is essential to preserve myocardial function. In addition to pharmacological therapy, primary coronary angioplasty is an effective alternative to reestablish blood flow to ischemic myocardium. Primary coronary angioplasty is an invasive procedure in which the infarct-related coronary artery is dilated during the acute phase of an MI without prior administration of thrombolytic agents.[19] This therapeutic intervention necessitates the availability of a cardiac catheterization laboratory and skilled personnel at all times. (See Chapter 17 for a more detailed discussion of the angioplasty procedure.)

Evaluation of patients for this procedure is similar to that of thrombolytic therapy. The accessibility of the lesion in the coronary artery is an additional factor that must be considered. Primary angioplasty may be an excellent reperfusion alternative for patients ineligible for thrombolytic therapy.

Long-term survival rates for primary angioplasty patients, as determined by the length of follow-up and the severity of coronary artery disease, ranges from 84% to 95%.[20] In a large clinical trial comparing the use of rt-PA with primary coronary angioplasty, the overall mortality rates were not significantly different. However, myocardial ischemia recurred more often in the rt-PA group than in the primary coronary angioplasty group.[21] Additionally, primary coronary angioplasty is associated with less recurrent ischemia, fewer deaths, fewer recurrent MIs, and a decreased need for further revascularization.[22]

The nurse must carefully monitor the patient after a primary angioplasty for evidence of complications. These complications can include retroperitoneal or vascular hemorrhage, other evidence of bleeding, early acute reocclusion, and late restenosis.[19]

INTENSIVE AND INTERMEDIATE CARE MANAGEMENT

The management goal for the patient in the intensive care unit and intermediate care unit continues to be maximizing cardiac output while carefully minimizing cardiac workload. To achieve this goal, the patient will have frequent vital signs and continue on a cardiac monitor with ST segment monitoring. The lead selected for monitoring should be based on the infarct location and underlying rhythm. Serial ECGs and serial evaluations of serum chemical markers of infarction are recorded. Blood is also drawn for a lipid profile and serum electrolytes. For the first 12 hours of hospitalization, the patient remains on bedrest. Activity level increases gradually in hemodynamically stable patients. Pain relief takes on special significance. Nitroglycerin is not an appropriate substitute for analgesics. Daily weights are recorded and intake and output are measured to detect fluid retention.[18]

Prophylactic antiarrhythmics during the first 24 hours of hospitalization are not recommended. However, easy access to atropine, lidocaine, transcutaneous pacing patches, transvenous pacing wires, a defibrillator, and epinephrine are essential for management of dysrhythmias. IV nitroglycerin is continued for 24 to 48 hours. Daily aspirin is continued on an indefinite basis. Early IV beta-blocker therapy followed by oral therapy is recommended provided there are no contraindications. Beta-blockers are one of the few pharmacological agents that have been shown to reduce morbidity and mortality in the patient with an MI. Calcium channel blockers may be given to patients in whom beta-blocker therapy is ineffective or contraindicated. An angiotensin-converting enzyme (ACE) inhibitor should be initiated within hours of hospitalization and continued indefinitely in patients with impaired left ventricular function (ejection fraction < 40%) or congestive heart failure. In patients without complications and no evidence of symptomatic or asymptomatic left ventricular dysfunction by 6 weeks, ACE inhibitors can be stopped. If a magnesium deficit is detected, magnesium sulfate is administered.[18]

Hemodynamic monitoring is indicated in the MI patient who has severe or progressive congestive heart failure or pulmonary edema, cardiogenic shock, progressive hypotension and suspected mechanical complications, such as ventricular septal defect, papillary muscle rupture, or pericardial tamponade.[18] The pulmonary artery wedge pressure (PAWP) is closely followed for assessment of left ventricular filling pressures. A PAWP below 18 mmHg may indicate volume depletion, whereas a PAWP greater than 18 mmHg indicates pulmonary congestion or cardiogenic shock. Using the thermodilution technique, frequent measurements of cardiac output and cardiac index can be made to evaluate hemodynamic status further. In some situations, monitoring venous oxygen saturation may also be useful. For a more detailed discussion of hemodynamic monitoring, see Chapter 16. The Collaborative Care Guide for the Patient with a Myocardial Infarction provides further information about the care of these patients.

During the course of hospitalization, patients may be further evaluated by coronary angiography. Results of the angiography will help the physician determine if a percutaneous transluminal coronary angioplasty (PTCA) is indicated or if the patient is a candidate for CABG. (A more detailed discussion of PTCA can be found in Chapter 17, and a more detailed discussion of CABG can be found in Chapter 21.)

Complications

The nurse closely monitors the MI patient for evidence of complications. Prompt recognition and management of complications are essential in reducing mortality and morbidity.

CARDIOGENIC SHOCK

Cardiogenic shock is a complication of MI that occurs because of the loss of contractile forces in the heart. About 5% to 10% of hospitalized patients post-MI will develop cardiogenic shock, which is the most common cause of death.[4] Cardiogenic shock is more likely to occur when ventricular damage exceeds 40% and the ejection fraction is less than 35%. For a more detailed discussion of cardiogenic shock, see Chapter 49.

Clinical manifestations of cardiogenic shock include a rapid, thready pulse; a narrow pulse pressure; dyspnea; tachypnea; inspiratory crackles; distended neck veins; chest pain; cool, moist skin; oliguria; and decreased mentation. Arterial blood gas analysis reveals a decreased PaO_2 and respiratory alkalosis. Hemodynamic findings include a systolic blood pressure less than 85 mmHg, a mean arterial blood pressure less than 65 mmHg, a cardiac index less than 2.2 $L/min/m^2$, and a PAWP greater than 18 mmHg. Cardiac enzymes may show an additional rise or a delay in reaching peak values.

The goal of treatment for cardiogenic shock is to minimize myocardial workload and maximize myocardial oxygen delivery. Immediate actions must be taken to improve tissue perfusion and preserve viable myocardium. To improve oxygenation, supplemental oxygen is given to the patient, and if necessary, the patient may need to be intubated and placed on a mechanical ventilator. Efforts are aimed toward restoring blood pressure. This may require

CLINICAL APPLICATION:
Examples of Nursing Diagnoses and Collaborative Problems for Acute Myocardial Infarction Patients

Chest Pain related to MI, angina
Decreased Cardiac Output: Electrical factors affecting rate, rhythm or conduction
Decreased Cardiac Output: Mechanical factors related to preload, afterload, or left ventricular failure
Knowledge Deficit related to illness and impact on patient's future
Anxiety, stress related to fear of illness, death, and critical care environment
Activity Intolerance related to decreased cardiac output or alterations in myocardial tissue perfusion
Risk for Altered Tissue Perfusion related to thrombolytic therapy impact on myocardial tissue

COLLABORATIVE CARE GUIDE
for the Patient With Myocardial Infarction

OUTCOMES	INTERVENTIONS

Oxygenation/Ventilation

Patient has arterial blood gases within normal limits and pulse oximeter value >90%.

- Assess respiratory rate, effort, and breath sounds q2–4h.
- Obtain arterial blood gases per order or signs of respiratory distress.
- Monitor arterial saturation by pulse oximeter.
- Provide supplemental oxygen by nasal cannula or face mask for the first 6 h, then as needed.
- Provide intubation and mechanical ventilation as necessary. (Refer to Chapter 24, Mechanical Ventilation Care Guide.)

There is no evidence of pulmonary edema on chest x-ray and by clear breath sounds.

- Obtain chest x-ray qd.
- Administer diuretics per order.
- Monitor signs of fluid overload as described below.

There is no evidence of atelectasis.

- Encourage nonintubated patients to use incentive spirometer, cough, and deep breath q4h and PRN.
- While on bed rest, turn side to side q2h.

Circulation/Perfusion

Vital signs are within normal limits, including MAP >70 mmHg and cardiac index >2.2 L/min/m².

- Monitor HR and BP q1–2h and PRN during acute failure phase.
- Assist with pulmonary artery catheter insertion.
- Monitor PAP and PAWP, CVP, or right atrial pressure (RAP) q1h and cardiac output, SVR, and PVR q6–12h if pulmonary artery catheter is in place.
- Maintain patent IV access.
- Administer positive inotropic agents, and reduce afterload with vasodilating agents guided by hemodynamic parameters and physician orders.
- Evaluate effect of medications on BP, HR, and hemodynamic parameters.
- Prepare patient for intra-aortic balloon pump assist if necessary.

Patient has no evidence of congestive heart failure due to decreased cardiac output.

- Restrict volume administration as indicated by PAWP or CVP values.
- Assess for neck vein distension, pulmonary crackles, S_3 or S_4, peripheral edema, increased preload parameters, elevated "a" wave of CVP, RAP, or PAWP waveform.

Patient has no evidence of further myocardial dysfunction, such as altered ECG or cardiac enzymes.

- Monitor 12-lead ECG qd and PRN.
- Monitor cardiac enzymes, magnesium, phosphorus, calcium, and potassium as ordered.
- Monitor ECG for changes consistent with evolving MI.
- Consider obtaining right precordial chest leads, 12-lead ECG, if inferior wall/right ventricle is involved.
- Report and treat abnormalities per protocols or orders.
- Provide continuous ECG monitoring in the appropriate lead.

Dysrhythmias are controlled.

- Document rhythm strips every shift.
- Anticipate need for/administer pharmacological agents to control dysrhythmias.

Following thrombolytic therapy, patient will have relief of pain; no evidence of bleeding; no evidence of allergic reaction.

- Assess, monitor, and treat pain as described below.
- Monitor signs of reperfusion, such as dysrhythmias, ST segment return to baseline, early rise and peak in CK.
- Monitor for signs of bleeding, including neurological, GI, and GU assessment.
- Monitor PT, aPTT, ACT per protocol.
- Have anticoagulant antidotes available.
- Assess for itching, hives, sudden onset of hypotension or tachycardia.

(continued)

COLLABORATIVE CARE GUIDE
for the Patient With Myocardial Infarction (Continued)

OUTCOMES	INTERVENTIONS
There is no evidence of cardiogenic shock, cardiac valve dysfunction, or ventricular septal defect.	• Administer hydrocortisone or diphenhydramine (Benadryl) per protocol. • Monitor ECG, heart sounds, hemodynamic parameters, level of consciousness, and breath sounds for changes. • Report and treat deleterious changes as indicated.
Fluids/Electrolytes Renal function is maintained as evidenced by urine output >30 mL/h, normal laboratory values.	• Monitor intake and output q1–2h. • Monitor BUN, creatinine, electrolytes qd and PRN. Take daily weights. • Administer fluid volume and diuretics as ordered.
Mobility/Safety Patient will comply with ADL limitations. Patient will not fall or accidentally harm self.	• Provide clear explanation of limitations. • Provide bed rest with bed side commode privileges first 6 hours. • Progress to chair for meals, bathing self, bathroom privileges. Continually assess patient response to all activities. • Provide environment to prevent falls, bruising, or injury. • Use self-protective devices as indicated and per hospital policy.
Skin Integrity Patient has no evidence of skin breakdown.	• Turn side to side q2h while patient is on bed rest. • Evaluate skin for signs of pressure areas when turning. • Consider pressure relief/reduction mattress for high-risk patients. • Use Braden Scale to monitor risk of skin breakdown.
Nutrition Caloric and nutrient intake meet metabolic requirements per calculation (eg, Basal Energy Expenditure). Patient has normal laboratory values reflective of nutritional status.	• Provide appropriate diet: PO, parenteral, or enteral feeding. • Provide clear or full liquids the first 24 hours. • Restrict sodium, fat, cholesterol, fluid, and calories if indicated. • Consult dietitian or nutritional support services. • Monitor albumin, prealbumin, transferrin, cholesterol, triglycerides, total protein.
Comfort/Pain Control Patient has relief of chest pain. There is no evidence of pain, such as increased HR, BP, RR, or agitation during activity or procedures.	• Use visual analog scale to assess pain quantity. • Assess quality, duration, location of pain. • Administer IV nitroglycerin, and monitor pain and hemodynamic response. • Administer analgesics appropriately for chest pain and assess response. • Monitor physiological response to pain during procedures or after administration of pain medication. • Provide a calm, quiet environment.
Psychosocial Patient demonstrates decreased anxiety by calm demeanor and vital signs during, for example, procedures, discussions.	• Assess vital signs during treatments, discussions, and so forth. • Provide explanations and stable reassurance in calm and caring manner.

(continued)

COLLABORATIVE CARE GUIDE
for the Patient With Myocardial Infarction (Continued)

OUTCOMES	INTERVENTIONS
Patient/family demonstrate understanding of MI and treatment plan by asking questions and participating in care.	• Cautiously administer sedatives and monitor response. • Consult social services and clergy as appropriate. • Assess coping mechanism history. • Allow free expression of feelings. • Encourage patient/family participation in care as soon as feasible. • Provide blocks of time for adequate rest and sleep.
Teaching/Discharge Planning Patient reports occurrence of chest pain or discomfort. Family demonstrates appropriate coping during the critical phase of an acute MI. In preparation for discharge to home, patient understands activity levels, dietary restrictions, medication regimen, what to do if pain recurs.	• Explain importance of reporting all episodes of chest pain. • Provide frequent explanations and information to family. • Encourage family to ask questions regarding treatment plan, patient response to therapy, prognosis, and so forth. • Make appropriate referrals and consults early during hospitalization. • Initiate family education regarding heart-healthy diet, cardiac rehabilitation program, stress-reduction strategies, management of chest pain, after crisis phase has passed.

discontinuation of vasodilator drugs and drugs with negative inotropic effects. An IV dopamine drip may be initiated to improve the patient's blood pressure and improve myocardial contractility. Dobutamine may be used to improve contractility, especially in low cardiac output states. Nitroprusside, a vasodilator, may be used with a vasopressor to improve cardiac output by decreasing peripheral vascular resistance and reducing left ventricular preload. Treatment may also require the use of an intra-aortic balloon pump (IABP). This invasive device helps improve coronary artery perfusion and decrease left ventricular afterload. For a more detailed discussion of IABP therapy, see Chapter 17.

PERICARDITIS

Pericarditis occurs at the 48- to 72-hour postinfarct period. The patient reports chest pain that may be confused with ischemic pain. The precordial pain of pericarditis intensifies with deep breathing, and a friction rub often can be heard. Some friction rubs are transient; therefore, the absence of such a rub is not conclusive. Anti-inflammatory agents, such as aspirin, indomethacin, and corticosteroids, given in usual dosages, can bring dramatic relief.

DYSRHYTHMIAS

Dysrhythmias often accompany acute infarcts. Frequently the dysrhythmia is caused by a failing left ventricle rather than being a direct consequence of conduction system ischemia.

The pulse should be assessed ideally by an apical auscultation and simultaneous radial palpation. Apical–radial pulse assessment will document whether extrasystoles perfuse to the radial artery. Extrasystoles on a rhythm strip may be electrical events without a mechanical response, resulting in a decreased cardiac output.

Dysrhythmias must be treated and minimized in the presence of an acute MI. Ischemic myocardium has a lower fibrillatory threshold, and few ventricular dysrhythmias are considered benign after an infarct. The therapeutic goal of dysrhythmia control is to maintain cardiac output while reducing cardiac workload. This can be assessed by monitoring hemodynamics, blood pressure, urine output, general appearance, and level of consciousness.

Supraventricular Dysrhythmias

Supraventricular rhythms may be the result of high left atrial pressures caused by left ventricular failure. Although most rhythm disturbances are manageable with drugs or cardioversion, adequate response to therapy may be delayed until the ventricle heals or heart failure is treated. Synchronized cardioversion may convert atrial fibrillation, atrial flutter, and nonparoxysmal atrial tachycardias. Paroxysmal atrial tachycardia will respond to adenosine or verapamil. Digitalis can be effective but does not work promptly in the ischemic heart. Propranolol often is used if heart failure is not severe.

Ventricular Dysrhythmias

The most effective therapy for the treatment of ventricular dysrhythmias is lidocaine. After a bolus loading dose of 1 mg/kg IV push, a continuous infusion of 1 to 4 mg/min is begun. Lidocaine will decrease the automaticity of the Purkinje fibers and prevent a reentry circuit of tachydysrhythmias by depressing the action potential duration.

Some ventricular dysrhythmias will not respond to lidocaine. Hypoxia, electrolyte imbalances, and drug toxicities may be contributing factors that must be investigated and corrected. If ventricular dysrhythmias persist or recur despite the use of lidocaine, an additional antiarrhythmic agent must be used. Procainamide is often selected in this situation. An IV bolus of 1 to 2 mg/kg is given over 5 to 10 minutes, followed by an IV infusion of 20 to 80 mg/kg/min. Bretylium, given with a loading dose of 5 mg/kg and followed by a maintenance infusion of 1 to 2 mg/min, is another effective therapy for recurrent ventricular tachycardia or fibrillation. Bretylium produces a slow initial response (often 20–25 minutes after the loading bolus), so supportive resuscitative measures should be maintained during this time. Orthostatic hypotension may become a problem during continuous infusion.

Intraventricular Conduction Dysrhythmias

The right coronary artery is the source of oxygenated blood for the AV node in about 90% of people. Therefore, patients with inferior, posterior, or right ventricular wall infarctions due to right coronary artery occlusion are at risk for AV nodal conduction disturbances. First-degree heart block and Mobitz I (Wenckebach) block may appear but often are transient. These rhythm disturbances may progress to complete heart block and require pacing therapy.

The LAD coronary artery is the source of blood supply to the bundle of His and bundle branches. Therefore, patients with an anterior wall MI caused by an LAD occlusion are at risk of ventricular conduction defects. Conduction defects, such as right bundle branch block, left bundle branch block, anterior fascicular block, posterior fascicular block, bifascicular block, or trifascicular block, may occur. Transvenous pacing may be indicated to support ventricular conduction.

Catastrophic Complications

The most catastrophic complications of an infarct are intraventricular septal rupture, papillary muscle dysfunction or rupture, and cardiac rupture. These clinical situations develop rapidly and result in almost immediate physiological deterioration.

Insights Into Clinical Research

Cole FL, Slocomb EM: Myocardial infarction mortality in the hospital: An exploration of time of death and age. American Journal of Critical Care 3(1):65–69, 1994

Little information about patterns associated with myocardial deaths and any factors related to the patterns is known. University of Texas, Health Science Center in Houston studied time periods with greater than expected mortality in hospitalized patients. The researchers examined the relationship between time of death and age. Using death certificates of 1,045 cardiac patients, time of death was evaluated by log-linear analysis. Periods of greater than expected mortality rates were found to occur at three times: 0600–0659, 0900–0959, and 1700–1759 (5:00 PM to 5:59 PM). These times coincide with time periods when nurses are occupied with care functions. It is not known if these times coincide with patterns of physiological events. A relationship between age and time of death can be drawn for those in the less than 60 year old group. For those patients, the increased incidence of death occurred between 0800 and 0959, which coincides with the physiological rise in adrenalin.

VENTRICULAR SEPTAL RUPTURE

Intraventricular septal rupture is rare and is most often associated with an anterior wall MI. The patient presents with a new, loud, holosystolic murmur associated with a thrill felt in the parasternal area. Additionally, the patient has progressive dyspnea, tachycardia, and pulmonary congestion. Oxygen samples taken from the right atrium, right ventricle, and pulmonary artery will show higher PaO_2 in the right ventricle than in the right atrium because the oxygenated left ventricular blood is shunted to the right ventricle. This testing can be accomplished during pulmonary artery catheterization. Urgent cardiac catheterization and surgical correction are needed. The patient can be supported with afterload reducers (nitroprusside) and diuretics until emergency surgery is possible. Some fibrosis of the tissue is needed for suturing. Often it is impossible to maintain the patient medically until this occurs.

PAPILLARY MUSCLE RUPTURE

Papillary muscle rupture is rare and occurs most likely on the second to seventh day post-MI. The patient presents with a sudden onset of pulmonary edema secondary to pulmonary hypertension and cardiogenic shock. On physical examination, the patient has a new onset, low-pitched, holosystolic decrescendo murmur heard over the precordium with radiation to the axilla. Additionally, S_3 and S_4 heart sounds may be heard. Papillary muscle rupture carries a 95% fatality rate. Clinical presentation of sudden-onset valvular failure is similar to that of septal rupture, except that progressive oxygen testing will show equal PaO_2 levels in the right atrium, right ventricle, and pulmonary artery. Pulmonary artery pressures will be high, and the waveform will reflect a large V wave. Emergency surgery is required within hours of the onset of symptoms.[4]

CARDIAC RUPTURE

Cardiac rupture is also rare, occurs most likely within the first 5 days post-MI, and is more commonly seen in women older than 65 years.[4] The patient experiences prolonged chest pain, dyspnea, hypotension, neck vein distention, tamponade, and ECG evidence of electrical–mechanical dissociation. This event occurs so suddenly and with such severity that life-saving efforts are futile.

Cardiac Rehabilitation

Preparation for discharge must begin early in the patient's course of hospitalization. Patient and family education are an essential component of the process. A severely compromised critically ill patient may lack the ability to process and retain new information but usually is moti-vated to learn after the life-threatening event. Guidelines for patient and family education after an acute MI are described in Table 20–3. Almost 1 million people will survive an MI each year and are candidates for cardiac rehabilitation, yet only 11% to 20% of survivors have participated in cardiac rehabilitation programs.[23] "Cardiac rehabilitation is characterized by long-term services involving medical evaluation; prescribed exercise; cardiac risk factor modification; and education, counseling, and behavioral interventions."[23] The goals of cardiac rehabilitation are to limit the adverse physiological and psychological effects of heart disease, reduce the risk of sudden death or reinfarction, control cardiac symptoms, stabilize or reverse the atherosclerotic process, and enhance the patient's psychosocial and vocational status.[23] The display on page 390 outlines the recommended components of a cardiac rehabilitation program.

■■■ CONCLUSION

Cardiovascular disease continues to be the leading cause of death in the United States. Critical care nurses play a pivotal role in the prevention, treatment, and rehabilitation of patients with cardiovascular disease. Patient education and psychosocial support are an integral part of the manage-

---

TABLE 20-3
Patient Teaching: Goals After Acute Myocardial Infarction

Content	When Mastery of Content Is To Be Expected:		
	Acute Phase	*Before ICU Discharge*	*At Hospital Discharge*
Pathophysiology of heart disease	Can identify angina, using 1–10 scale for reference	Can initiate treatment of angina (rest, NTG, O_2 use)	Knowledgeable about medications, when to seek medical assistance
Environment of hospital	Understands procedures	Asks appropriate questions	Knowledgeable about disease process and therapy
Lifestyle modifications	Complies with activity limitations Complies with dietary limitations	Can state relationship between activity and cardiac workload Begins light activity States risk factors Selects appropriate meals	Can progress activity as tolerated Placement in cardiac rehabilitation program Can state dietary restrictions
Treatment of disease	Accepts medications as ordered	Can identify medications Can identify risk factors	Knowledgeable about medications, dose, timing, action, and side effects Plans for risk factor reduction Begins cardiac rehabilitation program
Emotional adaptation	Able to define support system	Begins to communicate about lifestyle changes Becomes involved with resolving emotions related to surviving a critical illness	Involves self and loved ones in plans for lifestyle changes Expresses feelings Participates in group recovery program

---

Recommended Components of a Cardiac Rehabilitation Program

Exercise

Exercise tolerance: Appropriately described and conducted exercise training is recommended as an integral component of cardiac rehabilitation services, particularly for patients with decreased exercise tolerance.

Strength training: Training measures designed to increase skeletal muscle strength should be included in the exercise-based rehabilitation of clinically stable coronary patients when appropriate instruction and surveillance are provided.

Exercise habits: Long-term cardiac rehabilitation exercise training is recommended to provide the benefit of enhanced exercise tolerance and exercise habits.

Symptom management: Exercise rehabilitation decreases angina pectoris in patients with coronary heart disease. Therefore, exercise training is recommended as an integral part of the symptomatic management of patients.

Smoking Cessation

Smoking cessation and relapse prevention programs should be offered to patients who are smokers to reduce their risk of subsequent coronary events.

Lipid Management

Education, counseling, and behavioral interventions about nutrition are recommended as a component of cardiac rehabilitation.

Body Weight Control

The optimal management recommended for overweight patients to promote maintenance of weight loss requires multifactorial rehabilitation, including nutrition education, counseling, and behavioral modification, in addition to exercise training.

Blood Pressure Control

A multifactorial approach, including education, counseling, behavioral modification, and pharmacological agents, is recommended for the control of hypertension.

Psychological Well-Being

Education, counseling, or psychological interventions are recommended to complement the psychosocial benefits of exercise training.

Social Adjustment and Functioning

Cardiac rehabilitation exercise training improves social adjustment and functioning and is recommended to improve social outcomes.

Return to Work

In selected patients, formal cardiac rehabilitation vocational counseling may improve rates of return to work.

Morbidity, Mortality, and Safety Issues

The safety of exercise rehabilitation is well established. Education, counseling, and behavioral interventions as components of multifactorial rehabilitation may decrease progression of coronary atherosclerosis, lower recurrent coronary event rates, and reduce cardiac and overall mortality rates.

Wenger NK, Froelicher ES, Smith LK et al: Cardiac Rehabilitation as Secondary Prevention. Clinical Practice Guidelines. Quick Reference Guide for Clinicians No. 17. Rockville, MD, U.S. Department of Health and Human Services, Public Health Service, Agency for Health Care Policy and Research and National Heart, Lung, and Blood Institute. AHCPR Pub. No. 96-0673. October, 1995

---

ment of the more than 1 million people who survive an MI each year.

CLINICAL APPLICATION: Patient Care Study

Mrs. Jones, a 62-year-old white woman, was brought to the emergency department (ED) by a 911 ambulance at 10:30 PM. While unloading groceries at 9:00 AM, she experienced nausea and left chest heaviness. The discomfort subsided when she sat down. She avoided activity that day and went to bed early that night. She awoke at 10:00 PM to intense jaw pain, chest heaviness, and nausea. Mrs. Jones called 911.

Her findings on admission to the ED included awake, alert, oriented, and cooperative but in a moderate amount of distress. Skin was pale, cool, and diaphoretic. Blood pressure was 92/40; HR, 105 and irregular; RR, 26 on 2 L/nasal cannula; T, 36.6°C (98.0°F); HT, 5′4″; WT, 60 kg.

The ED staff started a left forearm 20-gauge IV and a right antecubital 18-gauge IV. Her monitor displayed ST segment elevation with frequent PVCs. A lidocaine bolus of 60 mg was given IV push, and a lidocaine infusion at 2 mg/min was started. She rated her chest pain at an 8 on 1–10 scale. A nitroglycerin (NTG) infusion was started and titrated up to 20 mg. Morphine sulfate was given to relieve her pain to 0. A thorough history revealed no other illness, and hospitalization only for childbirth three times. She had no allergies to medications or foods.

On physical examination, neurological findings were normal. Heart examination showed S_1, S_2, no rubs, no murmurs. Peripheral pulses were present but thready. No edema or increased JVD were noted. Lungs had bilateral basilar crackles with no cyanosis or clubbing. Respiratory pattern was regular but tachypneic. Abdomen was not tender in spite of nausea, with active bowel sounds. No emesis was noted. GU examination was deferred.

Admission workup included the following:

ECG: ST segment elevation II, III, aVF; PR, 0.26 sec; QRS, 0.06 sec; RR, regular except for 4 PVCs/min; HR, 105. Right sided chest leads recorded and showed ST segment elevation in V_4R, V_5R, V_6R

LABS: SMA 22, CK-MB, Troponin, Hg and HCT, WBC, PT, PTT

X-ray: Portable chest radiograph—bilateral fluffy infiltrates consistent with CHF, no cardiac enlargement

Mrs. Jones was admitted to the intensive care unit with the diagnosis of acute myocardial infarction. Her status was unchanged except for nausea relief with inapsine, ½ mL IV push. Her vital signs were BP, 98/44; HR, 100; first-degree AV block; no PVCs; RR, 26; T, 36.6°C (98.0°F).

About 90 minutes after admission, the registered nurse noticed a Wenckebach rhythm. Mrs. Jones was sleeping but awakened when the nurse took her BP. It was 84/40. She stated her pain had returned, and was a 4 on the 1–10 scale. The nurse administered morphine sulfate 2 mg, IV push and increased the NTG to 25 µg, with complete relief. A dobutamine infusion was started at 5 µg/kg/min. Within 30 minutes, her BP was 100/48. The Wenckebach rhythm persisted, and the lidocaine infusion was discontinued.

Mrs. Jones' laboratory work returned within normal limits except for CK, 784; myocardial band, +; Troponin, elevated; K, 3.4. Her diagnosis was confirmed as an acute inferior wall infarction. Mrs. Jones also had an infarcted right ventricle. An IV of 5% dextrose with .45 normal saline was hung at 75 mL/h.

Mrs. Jones was anxious but cooperative. With her husband at the bedside, the cardiologist suggested that a heart catheterization could be performed safely in 48 hours. It was explained that her delay from initial symptoms to hospitalization precluded the use of thrombolytic therapy. The following orders were written:

Heparin 5,000 U SQ, q12h
Enteric-coated acetylsalicylic acid (ASA), qd
KCl 10 mEq/50 mL over 1 h × 3 IVPB
Colace i, po bid
Dobutamine 2–5 µg/kg/min to keep systolic pressure ≥95 mmHg
Titrate NTG gtt to relieve pain, keep BP ≥95 mmHg systolic
MSO₄ 2 mg IV push q30min for pain unrelieved with NTG
D₅ half normal saline at 75 mL per minute
Bed rest
O₂ 2–4 LPM, nasal cannula
Low-cholesterol, low-fat diet; start as clear liquids
Weight now and qd
I&O
Cardiac enzymes q8h × 3
ECG q AM × 3
Portable chest radiograph in AM
SMA 22, PTT in AM × 2

Mrs. Jones slept through the night except when awakened for vital signs q2h and assessments. Her skin was pale, warm, and dry. The nausea subsided. Both the Wenckebach rhythm and the bibasilar crackles persisted.

The AM labs revealed CK, 1,136; MB, +; K, 4.2. Lasix was given, 20 mg IV push. The 12-lead ECG with right sided chest leads was unchanged, except the rhythm was Wenckebach. The IV fluid infusion was stopped. By noon, she had diuresed 850 mL, and the crackles were diminishing. At approximately 2 PM, the Wenckebach rhythm converted to first-degree AV block. Vital signs were BP, 110/54; HR, 92; RR, 22; T, 36.5°C (97.8°F). No rubs or murmurs developed. With her nausea gone, her appetite returned, and she remained pain free.

During the afternoon visit with her husband, cardiac rehabilitation began with a booklet, video, and the nurse explaining heart disease. The Jones' questions were appropriate and demonstrated an understanding of the content presented. Mrs. Jones decided to have the heart catheterization, and plans were made to cover that educational content at 6 PM when her husband returned.

At bedtime, the nurse noted her lungs were clear, but the heart block was still present. Mrs. Jones slept all night except for vital signs q4h and assessments. She was NPO for the heart catheterization. At 8 AM, she received her pre-catheterization diphenhydramine 50 mg, PO. She went to the catheterization laboratory pain free.

Returning from the catheterization laboratory at 11 AM, she was kept flat in bed. A pressure dressing was on the right femoral area, and distal circulation to the right leg and vital signs were assessed q15min. The dobutamine and NTG were slowly weaned off. She was stable. Her preliminary report from the catheterization laboratory described a 90% occlusion of the proximal RCA. Surgery was offered as an option.

In her sleep that night, Mrs. Jones converted into an NSR at a rate of 88 beats/min. While bathing in the morning, Mrs. Jones found that she fatigued easily. This lack of energy frightened her, and she described it to the nursing staff as "feeling pooped out." When these data were communicated to the cardiologist, it was suggested that although her strength would return over time, surgical bypass of the right coronary artery would improve her fatigue and minimize her potential for heart failure.

Mrs. Jones had been worried about taking a vein from her leg, because this had caused severe pain and scarring for her sister. Once the surgeon consulted and suggested an internal mammary graft, Mrs. Jones agreed to have the bypass performed.

Clinical Applicability Challenges

Self-Challenge: Critical Thinking

1. Obtain a plan for nursing care or a critical pathway for a patient with a MI. Critique the plan based on recommendations from the Guidelines for the Management of Patients with Acute Myocardial Infarction published by the American College of Cardiology and the American Heart Association (see reference 18).

2. Analyze the discharge instructions and teaching materials available in your institution for post-MI patients. What is the reading level of the material? Is the information comprehensive and accurate? Are adaptations needed for patients with visual defects? What changes and improvements would you suggest?

Study Questions

1. A right ventricular wall MI is most likely to occur with which of the following types of infarctions?
   a. Anterior wall
   b. Posterior wall
   c. Inferior wall
   d. lateral wall

2. Mr. Lopez was admitted to the coronary care unit yesterday with a diagnosis of an acute anterior wall MI. His blood pressure is 80/52; mean arterial pressure, 60 mmHg; cardiac index, 1.8 L/min/m²; and PAWP, 25 mmHg. About which of the following complications are you most concerned?
   a. Pericarditis
   b. Cardiogenic shock
   c. Papillary muscle rupture
   d. Cardiac rupture

3. *Mrs. Martin is a patient in the coronary care unit with a diagnosis of acute lateral wall MI. Her heart rate is 128 beats/min, rhythm is sinus tachycardia, and blood pressure is 90/50 mmHg. She has a pulmonary artery catheter showing a wedge pressure of 6 mmHg. Her cardiac index is 1.8 L/min/m², and her urine output is 25 mL/h. The most likely intervention for Mrs. Martin would be*
   a. *a dopamine infusion.*
   b. *a positive inotropic agent.*
   c. *an intra-aortic balloon pump.*
   d. *volume replacement.*

4. *Which ECG changes are you most likely to see for a patient with angina pectoris?*
   a. *Q waves with ST segment elevations*
   b. *ST-segment elevations*
   c. *ST-segment depressions with T-wave inversions*
   d. *Q waves with normal ST segments*

5. *Risk factor modification is an important component of patient education and rehabilitation post-MI. Which of the following risk factors is considered a major risk factor that can be altered?*
   a. *Hypertension*
   b. *Obesity*
   c. *Diabetes mellitus*
   d. *Stress*

REFERENCES

1. American Heart Association: Heart and Stroke Facts. Dallas, American Heart Association, 1994
2. American Heart Association: Still Number One 1995. Dallas, American Heart Association, 1995
3. American Heart Association: Heart and Stroke Facts: 1995 Statistical Supplement. Dallas, American Heart Association, 1995
4. Roberts R: Acute myocardial infarction. In Kelley WN (eds): Textbook of Internal Medicine (3rd Ed), pp 385–398. Philadelphia, Lippincott-Raven, 1997
5. Bullock B: Coronary artery disease. In Bullock B (ed): Pathophysiology: Adaptations and Alterations in Function (4th Ed), pp 457–472. Philadelphia, Lippincott-Raven, 1996
6. Braunwald E, Mark DD, Jones RH et al: Unstable Angina: Diagnosis and Management. Clinical Practice Guideline Number 10. AHCPR Publication No. 94-0602. Rockville, MD: Agency for Health Care Policy and Research and the National Heart Lung and Blood Institute, Public Health Service, U.S. Department of Health and Human Services, March 1994
7. DeWood MA, Spores J, Notske R et al: Prevalence of total coronary occlusion during the early hours of transmural myocardial infarction. N Engl J Med 303:897–902, 1980
8. Stewart SL: Acute MI: A review of pathophysiology, treatment, and complications. Journal of Cardiovascular Nursing 6(4):1–25, 1992
9. Reimer KA, Lower JE, Rasmussen MM, Jennings RB: The wave front phenomenon of ischemic cell death 1. Myocardial infarct size versus duration of coronary occlusion in dogs. Circulation 56:786–794, 1977
10. Williams K, Morton PG: Diagnosis and treatment of acute myocardial infarction. AACN Clinical Issues: Advanced Practice in Acute and Critical Care 6(3):375–386, 1995
11. Kinch J, Ryan T: Right ventricular infarction. N Engl J Med 330(17):1211–1216, 1994
12. Levin T, Samaha F, Follman D, Feldman T: Right ventricular MI: When to suspect, what to do. The Journal of Critical Illness 10(1):14–22, 1995
13. Morton PG: Using the 12-lead ECG to detect ischemia, injury and infarction. Critical Care Nurse 16(2):85–95, 1996
14. Grauer K: A Practical Guide to ECG Interpretation. St. Louis, Mosby-Year Book, 1992
15. Fischbach F: A Manual of Laboratory Diagnostic Tests (5th Ed). Philadelphia, Lippincott-Raven, 1996
16. Levy DB, Hanlon DP, Katko JD: Advances in emergency department evaluation of acute chest pain. Topics in Emergency Medicine 16(2):14–33, 1994
17. Baker AJ, Koelemay MJ, Gorgels JP, van Vlies B, Smits R, Tussen JG, Haagen FD: Troponin T and myoglobin at admission: Value of early diagnosis of acute myocardial infarction. Eur Heart J 15:45–55, 1994
18. Ryan TJ, Anderson JL, Antman EM, Braniff BA et al: ACC/AHA guidelines for the management of patients with acute myocardial infarction: Executive summary. A report of the American College of Cardiology/American Heart Association Task Force on Practice Guidelines (Committee on Management of Acute Myocardial Infarction). Circulation 94(9):2341–2350, 1996
19. Coombs VJ, Brinker JA: Primary angioplasty in the acute myocardial infarction setting. AACN Clinical Issues: Advanced Practice in Acute and Critical Care 6(3):387–397, 1995
20. Michaels KB, Yauf S: Does PTCA in acute myocardial infarction affect mortality and re-infarction rates? Circulation 91:476–485, 1995
21. Grimes CL, Browne KF, Marco J et al: A comparison of immediate angioplasty with thrombolytic therapy for acute myocardial infarction. N Engl J Med 328:673–679, 1993
22. Simari RD, Berger PD, Bell MR et al: Coronary angioplasty in acute myocardial infarction. Primary, immediate adjunctive, rescue or deferred adjunctive approach? Mayo Clin Proc 69:346–358, 1994
23. Wenger NK, Froelicher ES, Smith LK et al: Cardiac Rehabilitation as Secondary Prevention. Clinical Practice Guideline. Quick Reference Guide for Clinicians N0. 17. Rockville, MD, U.S. Department of Health and Human Services, Public Health Service, Agency for Health Care Policy and Research and National Heart, Lung, and Blood Institute. AHCPR Pub. No. 96-0673. October, 1995

BIBLIOGRAPHY

Burns D: Review of Thrombolytic use in acute myocardial infarction, pulmonary embolism and cerebral thrombosis. Critical Care Nursing Quarterly 15(4):1–12, 1993

Cole FL, Slocomb EM: Myocardial infarction mortality in the hospital: An exploration of time of death and age. American Journal of Critical Care 3(1):65–69, 1994

Fothergill-Bourbonnais F et al: Nursing criteria for patient progression post myocardial infarction. Canadian Journal of Cardiovascular Nursing 6(1-2):22–32, 1995

Gullum RF: Trends in acute myocardial infarction and coronary heart disease death in the United States. J Am Coll Cardiol 23(6):1273–1277, 1994

Karlson BW, Herlitz J, Hjalmarson A: In consecutive patients hospitalized with acute myocardial infarction, infarct location according to routine electrocardiogram is of minor importance for the outcome. Clin Cardiol 18(7):385–391, 1995

Kernicki J: Differentiating chest pain: Advanced assessment techniques. Dimensions of Critical Care Nursing 12(2):66–76, 1993

Lieberman KS: Markers of reperfusion after thrombolytic therapy for acute myocardial infarction. Journal of Emergency Nursing 21(2):112–115, 1995

McGovern PG et al: Recent trends in acute coronary heart disease-mortality, morbidity, medical care and risk factors. N Engl J Med 334(14):884–890, 1996

Sadaniantz BT, Sadaniantz A, Garber CE: Coronary care unit requirements of patients with acute myocardial infarction treated with or without thrombolytic therapy: A pilot study. Heart and Lung: Journal of Critical Care 23(4):328–332, 1994

Turner DM, Turner LA: Right ventricular myocardial infarction: Detection, treatment and nursing implications. Critical Care Nurse 15(1):22–29, 1995

Yacone-Morton LA: Inotropic agents and nitrates. RN 58(3):22–29, 1995

21

Cardiac Surgery

OBJECTIVES

Based on the content in this chapter, the reader should be able to:

- Compare and contrast the pathophysiological impacts of stenosis and insufficiency in the mitral and aortic valves.
- Explain the cardiopulmonary bypass process.
- Describe five key assessment areas in the early postoperative period.
- Discuss causes, assessments, and interventions for the hypotensive postoperative cardiac surgery patient.
- Describe the indications, assessment, and management principles for a patient with a dynamic cardiomyoplasty.
- Explain the indications, assessment, and management principles for a patient with a carotid endarterectomy.
- Relate changes in blood pressure and ventilation following carotid endarterectomy to the pathophysiological cause.

*D*espite emphasis on modifying and preventing risk factors, cardiovascular disease remains a leading cause of disability and death in the United States. Development of new treatments, such as thrombolytic therapy, balloon and laser angioplasty, and directional and transluminal extraction atherectomy, have improved medical management of cardiac disease. These nonsurgical approaches are discussed in Chapter 17. Surgical intervention, however, remains the treatment of choice for some patients and is the subject of this chapter.

Two common situations requiring cardiac surgery are coronary artery disease (CAD) and acquired valvular disease. A discussion of these two and their management through open heart surgery begins this chapter. The major portion of the chapter discusses in detail the general procedure of open heart surgery and subsequent postoperative assessment and nursing care. Finally, cardiomyoplasty and carotid endarterectomy are discussed.

Coronary Artery Disease

Chapter 20 discusses CAD, Acute Myocardial Infarction, in detail. This section provides information about coronary artery bypass grafts (CABG).

▰▰ CORONARY ARTERY BYPASS GRAFTS

The first saphenous vein aortocoronary bypass graft was performed in 1964. Since then, the procedure has become an acceptable treatment for CAD. Compared to medical treatment, CABG has proven effective in relieving angina and improving exercise tolerance, and it prolongs life in patients with left main CAD and three-vessel disease with poor left ventricular function.

Increased use of percutaneous transluminal coronary angioplasty and atherectomy has eliminated the need for the CABG procedure in many cases. Patients selected for CABG today are older, have more advanced coronary disease and worse left ventricular function, and many have had previous CABG. CABG is now considered a reasonable alternative to transplantation or medical treatment alone for ischemic cardiomyopathy in patients with ejection fractions less than 25%.[1] Postoperatively, care of these high-risk patients is complex.

Saphenous Vein Grafts

Either the saphenous vein or the internal mammary artery (IMA) can be used for CABG. The saphenous vein can be taken from above or below the knee, but vein from below the knee is generally preferred because it is close in diameter to the size of the coronary artery. The vein is removed from an incision made along the inner aspect of the leg.

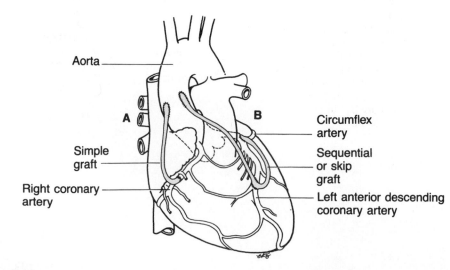

FIGURE 21-1

Aortocoronary bypass grafts using saphenous vein. (**A**) Simple graft from aorta to right coronary artery. (**B**) Sequential graft from aorta to left anterior descending coronary artery to diagonal or circumflex artery.

The obstruction in the coronary artery is bypassed by anastomosing one end of the vein graft to the aorta (proximal anastomosis) and the other end to the coronary artery just past the obstruction (distal anastomosis). Saphenous vein grafts can be *simple*, with an end-to-side anastomosis to the aorta and the coronary artery, or *sequential* (also called *skip*), with an end-to-side anastomosis to the aorta, a side-to-side anastomosis to one coronary artery, and an end-to-side anastomosis to another coronary artery (Fig. 21–1).

After 10 years, 50% of saphenous vein grafts are occluded.[2] Three main processes account for saphenous vein failure; thrombosis, fibrointimal hyperplasia, and atherosclerosis. Thrombosis is most common in the first month but may continue for as long as 1 year. Fibrointimal hyperplasia occurs predominantly between 1 month and 5 years and can result in a 25% decrease in luminal vessel diameter. Saphenous vein graft atherosclerosis begins as early as 1 year postoperatively and is fully developed after 5 years. To decrease the incidence of bypass graft occlusion, vessels other than the saphenous vein are being used.

Internal Mammary Artery Grafts

The IMA is one alternative to the saphenous vein for myocardial revascularization. The IMA is the second branch of the subclavian artery and descends down the anterior chest wall just lateral to the sternum behind the costal cartilage.

Grafts of IMA have shown a lesser degree of atherosclerosis over time and superior early and late graft patency rates compared with saphenous vein grafts. Ninety percent of IMA grafts were patent 10 years postoperatively, and IMA grafts were associated with lower long-term morbidity and improved long-term survival.[2] Other advantages and disadvantages of myocardial revascularization using the IMA are shown in the accompanying display.

To isolate the IMA, the pleural space is entered, the IMA is dissected free, and the intercostal artery branches from the IMA are cauterized. The IMA is used as a pedicle graft (ie, the proximal end remains attached to the subclavian artery), and both the left and the right IMA can be used. Because the left IMA is longer and larger than the right, it is usually used to bypass the left anterior descending coronary

---

Advantages and Disadvantages of Internal Mammary Artery for Myocardial Revascularization

Advantages

- Improved short- and long-term patency rates over saphenous vein grafts
- Diameter close to diameter of coronary arteries
- Aortic anastomosis not required
- Internal mammary artery (IMA) retains its nervous system innervation and thus has the ability to adapt size to provide blood flow according to myocardial demands
- No leg incision if only IMA used
- Vascular endothelium adapted to arterial pressure and high flow, resulting in decreased intimal hyperplasia and atherosclerosis

Disadvantages

- Dissection of IMA takes longer, resulting in longer cardiopulmonary bypass time.
- Extensive dissection may increase risk of postoperative bleeding.
- Pleural space is entered, so pleural chest tube is required postoperatively.
- Postoperative pain may be increased due to entry into pleural space and extensive dissection.
- In patients with diabetes mellitus or advanced age, use of bilateral IMAs can increase the risk of infection and sternal nonunion.

---

artery. The right IMA is anastomosed to the right coronary artery (RCA) or the circumflex coronary artery (CIRC).

Gastroepiploic Artery Grafts

Patients with severe peripheral vascular disease or repeat CABG where the IMAs have already been used may be candidates for gastroepiploic artery (GEA) use. This artery supplies blood to the greater curvature of the stomach. The GEA is resected, used as a pedicle graft, and pulled up into the pericardial cavity through a hole created in the diaphragm by electrocautery. Most frequently, the right GEA is used to bypass the distal RCA and CIRC.[3] When the GEA is used, the surgical incision is extended downward to midway between the xiphoid and the umbilicus.

Acquired Valvular Heart Disease

Cardiac valves maintain the unidirectional flow of blood. If structural changes occur as a result of disease, this function is disrupted. Abnormalities can affect the tricuspid, pulmonic, mitral, and aortic valves. Least common are pulmonic and tricuspid valve abnormalities. Pulmonic valve changes usually result from congenital anomalies. Tricuspid valve disease can be caused by endocarditis, rheumatic fever, or left-sided heart failure. Because of the lower pressures on the right side of the heart, the hemodynamic effects of tricuspid abnormalities are usually less significant than the effects of left-sided valvular heart disease; therefore, this discussion focuses on mitral and aortic abnormalities, which are more common and produce profound hemodynamic changes.

Disease causes either valvular stenosis or insufficiency (regurgitation). The stenotic valve has a narrowed orifice that creates a partial obstruction to blood flow, resulting in increasing pressure behind the valve and decreasing forward blood flow. The insufficient valve is incompetent or leaky; blood flows backward, increasing the pressure and volume behind the valve. Stenosis and insufficiency can occur alone or in combination, in the same valve, or in more than one valve.

Assessment and Diagnosis

The diagnosis of valvular disease is suggested by the history, clinical signs and symptoms, physical examination, and auscultation of the characteristic murmur (see Chapter 16). Diagnosis is confirmed by echocardiography and right and left heart catheterization. Echocardiography shows abnormal movement or thickening of the valve leaflets, valve area, and changes in the chamber size behind the diseased valve. Doppler echo reveals abnormal blood flow patterns. During cardiac catheterization, valvular gradients are measured. Normally there is no gradient; however, with stenotic valves, a pressure difference develops.

To determine the gradient across the mitral valve, left atrial and left ventricular pressures are measured during diastole. If there is a gradient of more than 15 to 20 mmHg (ie, left atrial diastolic pressure is 15–20 mmHg higher than left ventricular diastolic pressure), severe mitral stenosis exists. Valve area is also calculated during cardiac catheterization. The normal mitral valve area is 4 to 6 cm². An area less than 1.5 cm² signifies critical mitral stenosis, and surgery is indicated.

To determine the gradient across the aortic valve, left ventricular and aortic root pressures are measured during systole. A gradient of more than 50 mmHg (ie, left ventricular systolic pressure is 50 mmHg higher than aortic root systolic pressure) is associated with clinically significant aortic stenosis. Normal aortic valve area is 2.6 to 3.5 cm². Hemodynamically significant aortic stenosis occurs if the valve area is less than 1 cm².

Valvular insufficiency is diagnosed by regurgitation of the contrast medium backward through the incompetent valve. Mitral insufficiency causes the dye to flow from the left ventricle to the left atrium during ventricular systole. Aortic insufficiency produces regurgitation of contrast medium from the aortic root into the left ventricle during ventricular diastole.

▮▮▮ MITRAL STENOSIS

Pathophysiology

Mitral stenosis occurs most frequently as a result of rheumatic heart disease. The disease process causes fusion of the commissures and fibrotic contraction of valve leaflets, commissures, and chordae tendineae. Forward blood flow is impeded as the valve orifice becomes smaller.

As forward flow from the left atrium to the left ventricle decreases, cardiac output drops, creating a decrease in systemic perfusion. Blood backed up behind the stenotic valve causes left atrial dilation and increased left atrial pressure. This is reflected backward into the pulmonary circulation, and with prolonged high pressures, fluid moves from the pulmonary capillaries into the interstitial space and eventually the alveoli. Pulmonary hypertension develops, with thickening of the pulmonary arterial walls. If the process is not interrupted, right heart failure develops when the right ventricle is unable to pump against the high pulmonary vascular resistance.

Clinical Manifestations

Patients with mitral stenosis complain of fatigue, exertional dyspnea, orthopnea, or even pulmonary edema; they can develop hemoptysis as a result of pulmonary hypertension. Left atrial dilation causes atrial fibrillation in 40% to 50% of the patients (Fig. 21–2).

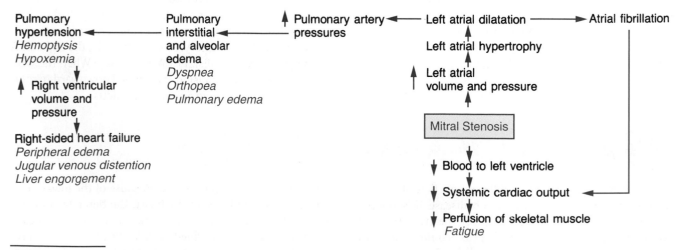

FIGURE 21-2

Hemodynamic and physiological effects of mitral stenosis. The resulting clinical signs and symptoms are noted in color.

■ MITRAL INSUFFICIENCY

Pathophysiology of Chronic Insufficiency

Chronic mitral insufficiency can result from rheumatic heart disease, myxomatous degeneration of the mitral valve, degenerative changes associated with aging, myocardial ischemia, or left ventricular dilatation. Rheumatic disease causes valve cusps to become thickened and contracted, preventing valve closure. Myxomatous changes cause enlarged leaflets or stretched or ruptured chordae, which allow the leaflets to balloon backward into the left atrium during ventricular systole. Left ventricular dilation stretches the mitral valve annulus, pulling the leaflet edges apart so they no longer approximate. Regardless of cause, the result is backward blood flow.

During ventricular systole, some of the left ventricular blood regurgitates into the atrium rather than being ejected through the aortic valve. This regurgitation decreases the forward cardiac output. Left ventricular hypertrophy occurs in an attempt to improve the cardiac output, but the hypertrophy can actually worsen the regurgitation. Left ventricular volume overload causes left ventricular dilation. Regurgitant flow into the left atrium causes increased left atrial pressure and dilation. This volume overload can be reflected backward to the pulmonary circulation; however, pulmonary and right heart symptoms usually do not occur until late in the disease process.

Clinical Manifestations

Patients with mitral regurgitation commonly complain of fatigue, palpitations, and sometimes shortness of breath (Fig. 21–3).

Pathophysiology of Acute Insufficiency

Endocarditis, chest trauma, or myocardial infarction can result in acute mitral insufficiency. Endocarditis erodes or perforates the valve leaflets or chordae. Trauma can rupture the chordae, and myocardial infarction can cause papillary muscle rupture (see Chapter 20), allowing blood to flow backward into the left atrium during ventricular systole.

In acute mitral regurgitation, there is insufficient time for dilation or hypertrophy to compensate. Cardiac output decreases dramatically, shock ensues, and pulmonary edema develops rapidly. Treatment of choice for acute mitral regurgitation with hemodynamic compromise is emergent mitral valve replacement.

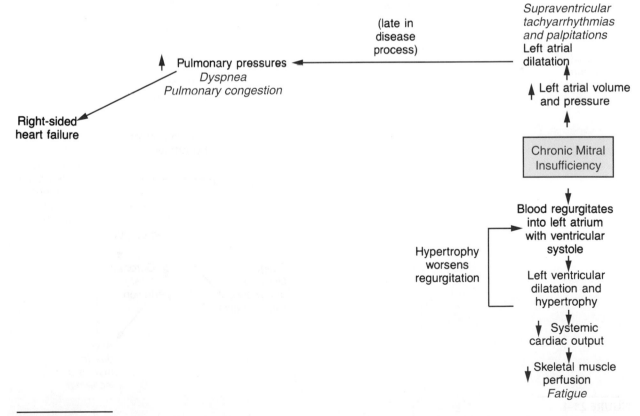

FIGURE 21-3

Hemodynamic and physiological effects of chronic mitral insufficiency. The resulting clinical signs and symptoms are noted in color.

◼◼◼ AORTIC STENOSIS

Pathophysiology

Aortic stenosis can develop as a result of rheumatic fever, calcification of a congenital bicuspid valve, or calcific degeneration, especially in older people. The disease process causes fusion of the commissures and fibrous contractures of the cusps, obstructing left ventricular outflow.

Forward cardiac output is diminished, and the left ventricle hypertrophies to maintain the cardiac output. As the stenosis worsens, compensation fails, and volume and pressure overload in the left ventricle cause left ventricular dilation. Increased left ventricular pressures are reflected backward through the left atrium and pulmonary vasculature.

Clinical Manifestations

Diminished cardiac output in the person with aortic stenosis can lead to two major problems—angina and syncope. Extreme left ventricular hypertrophy increases myocardial oxygen demand at the same time that cardiac output and coronary artery perfusion are decreased, creating ischemic myocardium evidenced by angina. Syncope

occurs in the late stages of aortic stenosis when the forward cardiac output cannot increase to meet the body demands of exercise. As the patient with severe aortic stenosis exercises, blood vessels to skeletal muscles dilate to increase the blood supply. The normal response is to increase the cardiac output to meet this demand; however, the patient with aortic stenosis is unable to do so. The vasodilation without a concomitant increase in cardiac output results in insufficient cerebral perfusion and syncope. Patients with aortic stenosis also experience exertional dyspnea, orthopnea, and paroxysmal nocturnal dyspnea (Fig. 21–4).

◼◼◼ AORTIC INSUFFICIENCY

Pathophysiology of Chronic Insufficiency

Rheumatic fever and aneurysm of the ascending aorta are common causes of chronic aortic insufficiency. Rheumatic disease results in thickened and retracted valve cusps, whereas aortic aneurysm causes annular dilation. Both problems prevent the edges of the valve leaflets from approximating, allowing blood to regurgitate backward from

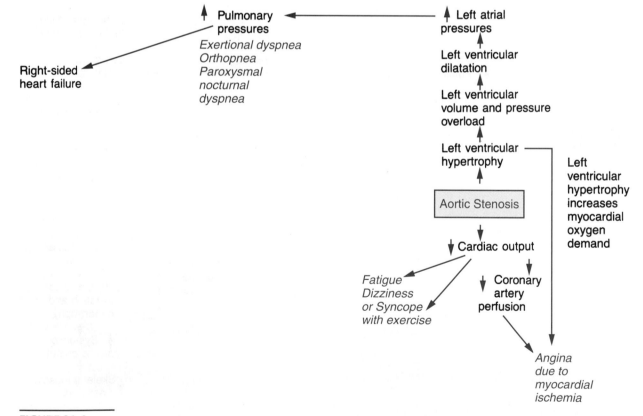

FIGURE 21-4

Hemodynamic and physiological effects of aortic stenosis. The resulting clinical signs and symptoms are noted in color.

the aorta into the left ventricle during ventricular diastole. Forward cardiac output decreases, and left ventricular volume and pressure increase. Left ventricular hypertrophy ensues. Eventually, the increase in left ventricular pressure is reflected backward into the left atrium and pulmonary circulation.

Clinical Manifestations

Patients with aortic insufficiency experience fatigue, low diastolic blood pressure, and a widened pulse pressure. Their pulse may be characterized by a rapid rise and sudden collapse (water-hammer or Corrigan's pulse) due to the forceful ventricular contraction and subsequent diastolic regurgitation from the aortic root into the left ventricle. They may also complain of angina, because aortic insufficiency creates an imbalance between left ventricular myocardial oxygen supply and demand. As left ventricular hypertrophy worsens, the oxygen demand increases, but regurgitant flow from the aortic root during diastole decreases coronary artery perfusion. Angina with aortic insufficiency is less common than with aortic stenosis (Fig. 21–5).

Pathophysiology of Acute Insufficiency

Acute aortic insufficiency can be caused by blunt chest trauma, ruptured ascending aortic aneurysm, or infective endocarditis. The patient with acute aortic insufficiency rapidly develops left heart failure and pulmonary edema because compensatory left ventricular hypertrophy does not have time to develop. In response to the diminished cardiac output, systemic vascular resistance (SVR) increases to maintain the blood pressure. The elevated SVR increases the degree of regurgitation and worsens the situation. Treatment for acute aortic insufficiency is emergent aortic valve replacement.

◼ SURGERY IN VALVULAR HEART DISEASE

The goals of valvular surgery are to relieve symptoms and restore normal hemodynamics. Surgery is indicated before left ventricular function deteriorates significantly and the patient becomes severely limited in activity or before severe

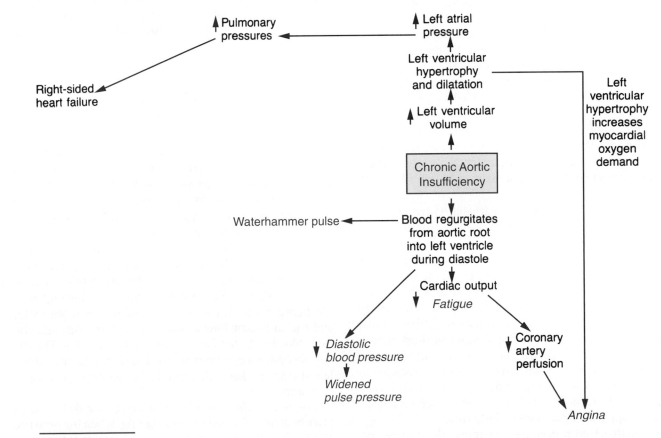

FIGURE 21-5
Hemodynamic and physiological effects of chronic aortic insufficiency. The resulting clinical signs and symptoms are noted in color.

symptoms, such as angina or syncope from aortic stenosis or pulmonary hypertension from mitral stenosis, develop. Intervention consists of either valve reconstruction or valve replacement. (See Chapter 17 for a discussion of percutaneous balloon valvuloplasty, which is indicated primarily for patients considered too high risk for surgery.) Because reconstruction is associated with decreased operative mortality and fewer thromboembolic and anticoagulation-related complications than valve replacement, reconstruction is gaining popularity.

Valve Reconstruction

With the development of transesophageal echocardiography to assess the effectiveness of repair intraoperatively, the use of valve reconstruction is increasing. Most valve reconstruction procedures are performed on the mitral valve. Although it is not as successful for mitral stenosis, approximately 69% of valves with degenerative mitral insufficiency can be reconstructed.[4] Compared with mitral valve replacement, reconstruction eliminates the need for long-term anticoagulation, decreases the risks of thromboembolism and endocarditis, decreases the need for reoperation, and increases survival. For aortic valve disorders, however, most attempts at reconstruction have not been successful because of late insufficiency and restenosis. Aortic valve reconstruction is considered an experimental procedure.

A common reconstruction technique for mitral stenosis is *commissurotomy*. Although not indicated for patients with severe mitral stenosis, commissurotomy can be effective for those with moderate stenosis with minimal calcification and regurgitation. During commissurotomy, the fused commissures are surgically divided. Calcified tissue is débrided and fused, and shortened chordae are incised. This procedure improves leaflet mobility and increases the mitral valve area, decreasing the degree of stenosis. Following mitral commissurotomy, the occurrence of restenosis and need for repeat surgery are approximately 10% of patients at 5 years.[5]

Mitral insufficiency can also be treated with *reconstruction*. If annular dilation causes the regurgitation, annuloplasty can be performed using sutures or a prosthetic ring (eg, Carpentier-Edwards annuloplasty ring). The ring is sewn around the mitral annulus so that excess annular tissue is drawn up. Suturing and the ring reduce the circumference of the enlarged annulus so that the edges of the leaflets coapt, diminishing regurgitation. If the chordae tendineae are stretched or ruptured, surgical shortening or transposition of chordae to substitute for ruptured chordae can be effective. Redundant mitral leaflets are repaired by resecting a portion of the leaflet, and perforated valve leaflets can be reconstructed by patching. Such repairs are usually supported by an annuloplasty ring.

Reconstruction procedures are more likely to be successful if performed early in the course of the disease, before left ventricular function deteriorates and irreparable damage occurs. Statistics speak strongly in favor of valve repair rather than replacement. At 10 years, the survival rate for valve repair is 90%; incidence of reoperation, only 8%; and freedom from thromboembolism, anticoagulant-related hemorrhage, and endocarditis, between 93% and 97%.[4] Anticoagulation is not usually needed following valve repair unless an annuloplasty ring is used. If so, anticoagulants are given for only 3 months until the ring is endothelialized. If reconstruction cannot be accomplished, valves are replaced.

Valve Replacement

The first valve replacement was performed by Harken and Starr in 1960 with a caged ball prosthesis. Since then, many new valve designs have evolved. The ideal prosthetic valve would be durable and last for the patient's life. The valve would have normal hemodynamics with unimpeded, non-turbulent blood flow through a central opening, no transvalvular gradient, and no regurgitation when closed. It would be nonthrombogenic and not damaging to blood components and acceptable to the patient in terms of noise and the need for anticoagulation. In other words, the replacement valve would perform exactly as a normal human valve. Unfortunately, no artificial valve currently meets these criteria, so research continues.

Two major types of prosthetic valves are available—mechanical and biological. Mechanical valves are made entirely of synthetic materials, whereas biological valves combine synthetic materials with chemically treated biological tissues.

MECHANICAL VALVES

Mechanical valves include the caged ball, tilting disk, and bileaflet designs.

The *caged ball valve* consists of a plastic or metal ball inside of a metal cage attached to a sewing ring. When pressure behind the valve increases, the ball is forced down into the cage, and blood flows around it. When pressure in front of the valve increases, the ball is forced upward against the sewing ring, preventing regurgitant flow. An example of the caged ball valve is the Starr-Edwards.

Hemodynamically, the ball in the cage produces a central obstruction to blood flow, which can result in a small stenotic pressure gradient, and ventricular outflow may be partially obstructed because of the cage's size and high profile. Because of the thrombogenicity of the plastic and metal and the turbulent flow around the ball and through the cage, blood clots can form on or around the valve. Thromboembolism is a common problem, and chronic anticoagulant therapy is essential. Caged ball valves have good long-term durability.

The *tilting disk valve* is constructed of a disk held in place by struts attached to a sewing ring. When the pressure behind the valve increases, the disk tilts open approximately 60 to 80 degrees, allowing blood to flow around it. When the pressure in front of the valve increases, the disk tilts back flat with the sewing ring to close. Because of its semi-centralized flow and lower profile, the tilting disk valve produces less obstruction to blood flow and has better hemodynamic characteristics than the caged ball valve. The tilting disk valve has good long-term durability, but the risk of thromboembolism requires long-term anticoagulant therapy. Examples of the tilting disk valve are the Medtronic-Hall and the Omniscience.

The newest type of mechanical prosthesis is the *bileaflet tilting disk valve*, which consists of two pyrolytic carbon semicircular disks or leaflets hinged to a sewing ring. When the pressure behind the valve increases, the leaflets open perpendicular to the sewing ring, and blood flows through the central opening with minimal obstruction. When pressure in front of the valve increases, the leaflets return to their flat position against the sewing ring, preventing insufficiency. An example of the bileaflet tilting disk valve is the St. Jude Medical. This type of valve has good hemodynamic characteristics and durability, but it is thrombogenic and requires long-term anticoagulation.

BIOLOGICAL VALVES

Biological prostheses, or tissue valves, offer another alternative for valve replacement. The *porcine heterograft* is constructed of an excised pig aortic valve preserved in glutaraldehyde and mounted on a frame attached to a sewing ring. Examples of porcine valves are the Hancock and the Carpentier-Edwards.

Biological prostheses provide good hemodynamics except in smaller sizes where obstruction to flow and a gradient can occur. Their main advantage is the lower risk of thromboembolism compared with mechanical valves. Because most thromboembolic events occur during the first 3 months after implant before the sewing ring is endothelialized, most patients with biological valves receive anticoagulants during that time only and none subsequently. However, the decision for anticoagulation must be based on the patient's condition. Patients in chronic atrial fibrillation undergoing mitral valve replacement frequently receive long-term anticoagulation therapy even with a biological prosthesis because of stagnant blood flow in the atria, which predisposes to clot formation.

A disadvantage to biological valves is their lack of durability. Valves studied at autopsy have shown structural deterioration beginning as early as 6 years after implant, and their durability is usually considered to be less than 10 years. However, less calcification and structural deterioration occur when the valves are placed in older patients.

Human aortic homografts are another alternative for biological valve replacement. The cadaver aortic valve is excised and frozen. For implant, it is trimmed to the correct size and sewn into place. Homografts have excellent hemodynamic characteristics and are nonthrombogenic, so anticoagulation is not needed; however, their availability is limited.

ADVANTAGES AND DISADVANTAGES

Because no "ideal" prosthetic valve has been developed, advantages and disadvantages must be weighed when choosing the appropriate valve for each patient. Mechanical valves offer the benefits of good long-term durability but pose a significant risk of thromboembolism and require long-term anticoagulation. Biological valves decrease the risk of thromboembolism and can obviate the need for long-term anticoagulation; however, their durability is not as good as that of mechanical valves.

Mechanical valves are generally placed in patients whose life expectancy is long. Biological valves are indicated for patients who are unable to comply with an anticoagulation regimen, for those in whom a long-term anticoagulation regimen is contraindicated, and for women of childbearing age who plan pregnancy (warfarin crosses the placental barrier). Frequently, older patients receive a bioprosthesis because these valves deteriorate more slowly in older people, the need for long-term durability of the valve is less, and the risk of anticoagulation may increase with advancing age.

SURGICAL PROCEDURE

The surgical approach for valve replacement is by the median sternotomy incision, using cardiopulmonary bypass and myocardial preservation techniques. The mitral valve is approached through the left atrium. Rather than excising the native valve, the chordae and papillary muscles are preserved when the prosthetic valve is sutured in place. This technique helps maintain left ventricular function and ejection fraction. The aortic valve is approached through the ascending aorta. The native aortic valve is excised, the annulus is sized, and the prosthetic valve of correct size is sutured to the annulus. Once the surgery is completed, the patient is transferred to the intensive care unit (ICU).

Advantages and Disadvantages of Prosthetic Cardiac Valves

Mechanical Valves
- Good long-term durability
- Adequate hemodynamics
- High risk of thromboembolism; long-term anticoagulation required
- Increased risk of bleeding complications

Biological Valves
- Poor long-term durability
- Better hemodynamics than mechanical valves except in small sizes
- No hemolysis
- Low incidence of thromboembolism; anticoagulation possibly not required
- Fewer bleeding complications

Cardiac Surgery

Cardiac surgery as it is known today was made possible by the development and practical application of cardiopulmonary bypass by Gibbon in 1953. This section presents general aspects of CABG and valvular heart disease surgery.

PREOPERATIVE PREPARATION

Preoperative preparation for cardiac surgery has physiological and psychological components. The physiological preparation is similar to that for any preoperative patient and includes a history, physical examination, chest x-ray, and electrocardiogram. Pulmonary function tests may be done to identify patients with underlying pulmonary problems. Laboratory tests include complete blood count, electrolytes, prothrombin time, partial thromboplastin time, blood urea nitrogen, and creatinine.

An important aspect of psychological preparation is effective preoperative teaching, which reduces anxiety and physiological responses to stress before and after surgery. An explanation of the surgical procedure and the intraoperative and postoperative experiences should be included. Because the patient is generally not in the ICU preoperatively, a tour of the unit helps familiarize the patient and family with the specialized equipment and environment. Seeing a patient who is successfully recovering from cardiac surgery helps instill confidence and allay anxiety. Specific teaching topics related to the patient's stay in the ICU are shown in the display.

Numerous invasive lines are placed in the patient before surgery and are used for monitoring during and after surgery. These include a thermodilution catheter, arterial line, and Foley catheter. The patient is intubated, and a nasogastric tube and additional intravenous lines may also be inserted. As long as the hemoglobin is > 11 g/dL, 2 to 3 U of whole blood may be withdrawn from the patient at the beginning of surgery. Plasma volume expanders are given to maintain the patient's volume and produce hemodilution. Infusion of this blood at the end of the procedure decreases the need for banked blood.

PATIENT TEACHING
Preoperative Teaching Regarding the Intensive Care Unit Experience for the Patient Undergoing Cardiac Surgery

Equipment
- Cardiac monitor
- Arterial line
- Thermodilution catheter
- IVs and IV infusion pumps
- Endotracheal tube and ventilator
    —Suctioning
    —Inability to talk
    —How to communicate when intubated
    —When extubation can be anticipated
- Foley catheter
- Chest tubes
- Pacing wires
- Nasogastric tube
- Soft-hand restraints

Incisions and dressings
- Median sternotomy incision
- Leg incision (if saphenous vein is used)

Patient's immediate postoperative appearance
- Skin yellow due to use of Betadine solution in operating room
- Skin pale and cool to touch due to hypothermia during surgery

- Generalized "puffiness" especially noticeable in neck, face, and hands due to third spacing of fluid given during cardiopulmonary bypass

Awakening from anesthesia
- Patient recovers in the intensive care unit; does not go to the postanesthesia care unit
- Sensations patient will feel
- Noises patient will hear
- May be aware or able to hear but unable to respond

Discomfort
- Amount of discomfort to be expected
- When pain might be expected
- Relief mechanisms
    —Positioning/splinting
    —Medications

Postoperative respiratory care
- Turning
- Use of pillow to splint median sternotomy incision
- Effective coughing and deep breathing after extubation
- Incentive spirometry
- Have patient practice above exercises preoperatively

Postoperative activity progression

Visiting policy in intensive care area

■ SURGICAL PROCEDURE

Median Sternotomy Incision

The surgical approach most commonly used for myocardial revascularization and valve surgery is the median sternotomy incision. The sternum is split with a sternal saw from the manubrium to below the xiphoid process. The ribs are spread to expose the anterior mediastinum and pericardium. Once the pericardium is opened and the heart and aorta are exposed, the patient is placed on cardiopulmonary bypass.

Cardiopulmonary Bypass

Because the heart must be still (not beating) and empty during the surgery, a cardiopulmonary bypass machine is used. This machine, also called a pump oxygenator, assumes the job of oxygenating the patient's blood and circulating it throughout the body.

Before implementation of the bypass, the pump tubing is primed with a balanced electrolyte solution; blood is not used. The patient's deoxygenated venous blood is brought to the pump either through one cannula that is placed in the right atrial appendage or by two cannulas, one of which is placed directly in the inferior vena cava and the other directly into the superior vena cava. Another cannula is placed in the ascending aorta to return oxygenated blood to the patient's systemic circulation (Fig. 21–6). Heparin is administered throughout cardiopulmonary bypass to prevent massive extravascular coagulation as the blood circulates through the mechanical parts of the bypass system. After bypass is established, the blood is pumped through the circuit by a series of roller-type pumps, which, unlike normal heart function, produce a nonpulsatile flow. Venous blood from the patient flows through the venous cannula to the cardiotomy reservoir and then into the oxygenator where exchange of oxygen and carbon dioxide occurs. The blood then travels through the heat exchanger, where it is cooled initially and later rewarmed.

COLD TECHNIQUE

During bypass, the patient's core body temperature is lowered to 28° to 32°C (82.4° to 89.6°F) to decrease metabolism. For each 1°C drop of body temperature, the metabolic demands of the body decrease by 7%. This reduction in metabolic demands helps protect the major organ systems from possible ischemic injury and adverse effects of nonpulsatile perfusion during cardiopulmonary bypass.

Oxygenated blood is filtered and returned to the patient's ascending aorta by way of the arterial cannula (see Fig. 21–6). Once extracorporeal circulation is established and systemic hypothermia is achieved, the aorta is cross-clamped just above the coronary arteries, and either crystalloid or blood cardioplegia solution is infused into the aortic root. The formula varies, but cardioplegia solution

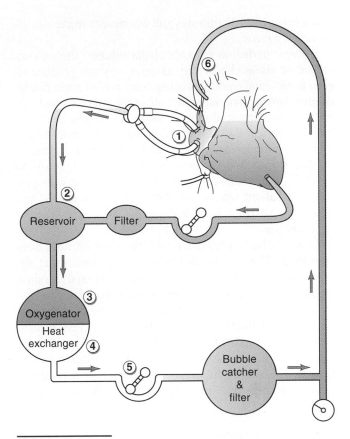

FIGURE 21-6
Blood flow through the circuit of the cardiopulmonary bypass machine: 1) Patient's deoxygenated blood enters the bypass circuit from the venous cannulas in the superior and inferior vena cavae. 2) The reservoir holds the blood temporarily. 3) The oxygenator removes carbon dioxide from and adds oxygen to the patient's blood. 4) The heat exchanger initially cools the blood and then rewarms the blood. 5) Roller pumps pump the blood through the circuit and back to the patient. 6) Oxygenated blood is returned to the ascending aorta by way of the aortic cannula.

is a balanced electrolyte solution high in potassium. Oxygenated blood from the bypass circuit or oxygenated crystalloid can be added to the cardioplegia solution.

After the aorta is cross-clamped, no blood circulates through the coronary arteries, so the myocardium becomes ischemic. Cold cardioplegia solution at 4°C (39.2°F) is infused into the aortic root under pressure. As it circulates through the coronary arteries, the high potassium concentration causes immediate asystole and relaxation, and the cold produces myocardial hypothermia. Asystole and hypothermia protect against myocardial ischemia by decreasing the metabolic need of myocardial tissue. Cardioplegia provides a substrate for ongoing cellular metabolism and ensures appropriate pH and calcium ion levels for myocardial preservation.[6] The inclusion of blood or oxygenated crystalloid in the cardioplegia solution lessens myocardial ischemia by supplying oxygen. Cardioplegia solution may be infused into the aortic root continuously or intermittently every 15 to 30 minutes and whenever cardiac electrical activity recurs.

Because perfusion of cardioplegia solution through occluded or diseased coronary arteries may not produce an even myocardial cooling, inadequately cooled areas risk ischemic damage. Therefore, hypothermia is also applied topically by pouring iced normal saline slush over the heart into the pericardial well. Cardioplegia with concomitant topical hypothermia cools the heart evenly while maintaining the myocardial temperature at 8° to 15°C (46.4° to 59°F). Thus, throughout surgery, a threefold approach protects the patient against possible detrimental effects: systemic hypothermia, cold cardioplegia, and topical cardiac hypothermia.

Several disadvantages to cold cardioplegia have been identified. These include postoperative myocardial depression, ventricular arrhythmias, decreased cerebral blood flow, irreversible platelet dysfunction, and shifts of the oxygen–hemoglobin dissociation curve to the left so that blood delivers oxygen to the tissues less readily. Hearts receiving cold crystalloid cardioplegia must have blood reintroduced into the coronary circulation (reperfusion). This reintroduction of oxygen can cause release of toxic substances that injure myocardial cells (reperfusion injury).

WARM TECHNIQUE

To avoid these disadvantages, some cardiac surgeons are using normothermic blood cardioplegia delivered at 37°C (98.6°F) so the heart is maintained at normal temperature. With the warm technique, topical cardiac hypothermia is not used, and systemic hypothermia may or may not be used.

Advantages of warm cardioplegia include more frequent spontaneous return of normal sinus rhythm postoperatively, better postoperative left ventricular function and cardiac index, less use of inotropic agents, and less postoperative bleeding. Warm cardioplegia patients require less time on the ventilator and almost no rewarming technology in the ICU.

While these advantages confer a cost saving, studies have shown an increased incidence of neurological events and perioperative cerebrovascular accidents in patients who have had warm surgery.[7] The majority of cardiac surgery is still done with cold techniques.

REWARMING THE BLOOD

After surgery is completed, the heat exchanger rewarms the blood to return the patient's core temperature to 37°C (98.6°F) if hypothermic techniques were used. After air is vented from the heart chambers and the aortic root, the aortic cross-clamp is removed so that blood again perfuses the coronary arteries, warming the myocardium. As perfusion and rewarming continue, a spontaneous cardiac rhythm can resume, ventricular fibrillation can develop (necessitating internal defibrillation), or pacing can be used

to initiate a rhythm. After a reliable rhythm with a rate adequate to maintain the cardiac output and blood pressure is established, total cardiopulmonary bypass is reduced to partial bypass. During partial bypass, some of the patient's blood circulates through the heart and lungs while some continues to circulate through the pump. If adequate arterial pressures are maintained, the patient's heart assumes total responsibility for the cardiac output, and bypass is discontinued. After the heart can maintain an adequate cardiac output, the cannulas are removed from the right atrium and aorta. Heparinization is reversed by the administration of protamine sulfate. If the patient cannot maintain adequate cardiac output during the weaning process, positive inotropic agents or intra-aortic balloon counterpulsation can be instituted (see Chapter 17).

Completion of Surgery

If the need for cardiac pacing is anticipated postoperatively, temporary pacing electrodes are placed on the epicardial surface of the heart and brought out through the chest wall on either side of the median sternotomy incision. Ventricular pacing electrodes are typically located to the left and atrial wires to the right (Fig. 21–7).

Chest tubes placed in the mediastinum and pericardial space for drainage are brought out through stab wounds just below the median sternotomy. If the pleural space has been entered, pleural tubes are also placed. After adequate hemostasis is obtained, the edges of the sternum are approximated with stainless steel wires, the incision is closed, and dressings are applied.

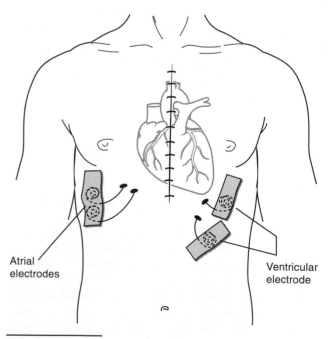

Atrial electrodes

Ventricular electrode

FIGURE 21-7

Temporary epicardial pacing wires: position of atrial and ventricular wires on chest wall.

◼ POSTOPERATIVE CARE

Assessment and Management

IMMEDIATE POSTOPERATIVE PERIOD

Patients are transported directly to the ICU, where they recover from anesthesia and usually remain for 24 hours postoperatively. Patients arrive with numerous lines and tubes attached (Fig. 21–8). Immediate postoperative nursing goals include maintenance of adequate ventilation, oxygenation, and hemodynamic stability. Rapid recognition of and intervention for changes in the patient's condition are imperative, because the person undergoing cardiac surgery is often more unstable than other surgical patients due to the effects of cardiopulmonary bypass and cardiac manipulation.

Nursing care of the postcardiac surgery patient is guided by the preoperative assessment, type of procedure done, and postoperative assessment. To achieve successful patient outcomes, the critical care nurse must possess advanced assessment, problem-solving, and technical skills. Additionally, the critical care nurse must work in collaboration with other members of the health care team in planning and implementing care.

VENTILATION AND OXYGENATION

The patient is ventilated by a volume ventilator on intermittent mandatory ventilation or assist-control mode (see Chapter 24). In some centers, 5 cm of positive end-expiratory pressure (PEEP) is used to decrease atelectasis and postoperative bleeding. The nurse auscultates breath sounds immediately to assess for endotracheal tube placement, pneumothorax, and secretions; applies the arterial blood oxygen saturation (SaO_2) monitor; and obtains a chest x-ray and arterial blood gases (ABGs) within the first 15 to 30 minutes after admission. The nurse suctions the patient as needed and intervenes as ordered for any abnormalities in the SaO_2 or ABGs.

CARDIAC RHYTHM

On admission of the patient to the ICU, the nurse connects the cardiac monitor, assesses the rate and rhythm, and obtains apical and radial pulses. If a pacemaker is present, the

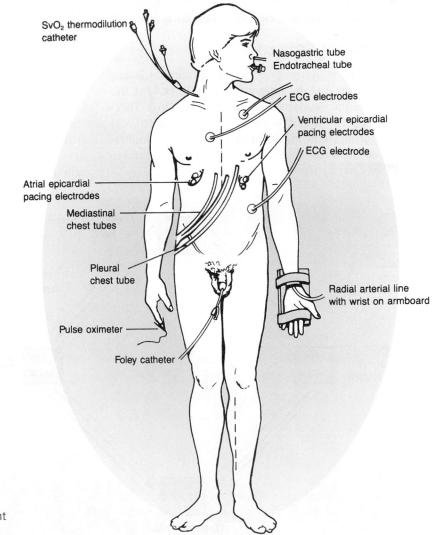

FIGURE 21-8

Typical postoperative appearance of a patient after cardiac surgery.

Decreased Cardiac Output related to changes in left ventricular preload, afterload, and contractility
Decreased Cardiac Output related to cardiac dysrhythmias
Altered Tissue Perfusion related to cardiopulmonary bypass, decreased cardiac output, hypotension
Impaired Gas Exchange related to cardiopulmonary bypass, anesthesia, poor chest expansion, atelectasis, retained secretions
Altered Comfort related to endotracheal tube, surgical incision, chest tubes, rib spreading
Anxiety related to fear of death, intensive care unit environment
Risk for Fluid Volume Deficit related to abnormal bleeding
Risk for Infection related to surgical procedure, invasive lines, drainage tubes, hypoventilation, retained secretions

nurse assesses its capture and sensing and the percent of paced rhythm and notes the settings. The critical care nurse obtains a potassium level within the first 30 minutes and treats as necessary. A 12-lead electrocardiogram is recorded.

HEMODYNAMIC STABILITY

As part of the admission process, the nurse connects, levels, and zeroes the arterial and pulmonary artery lines. Next, the nurse assesses the waveforms and records the values. Thermodilution cardiac output measurements are obtained, and vasoactive or inotropic medications or volume is administered as needed to maintain the blood pressure and cardiac output (see Chapter 16).

MIXED VENOUS OXYGEN SATURATION (S$\bar{v}$O$_2$) MONITORING

Mixed venous oxygen saturation (S$\bar{v}$O$_2$), the amount of oxygen in the blood returning to the right side of the heart, depends on three factors—oxygen supply, oxygen delivery, and oxygen consumption. Oxygen supply (amount of oxygen in the arterial blood) is dependent on the amount of hemoglobin and the oxygen saturation of that hemoglobin (SaO$_2$). Pulmonary dysfunction or bleeding can decrease the arterial oxygen concentration. Oxygen delivery to the tissues is determined by the cardiac output (CO). The greater the CO, the more oxygen delivered; the lower the CO, the less oxygen delivered. Oxygen consumption (the amount of oxygen used by the tissues) increases if the tissues' metabolic demand increases (eg, hyperthermia, shivering, and activity) and decreases if metabolic needs decrease (eg, hypothermia, anesthesia, and use of neuromuscular blocking agents). The oxygen left over after tissue use is the S$\bar{v}$O$_2$. Normal S$\bar{v}$O$_2$ ranges from 60% to 80% (Fig. 21–9).

The postoperative cardiac surgical patient with adequate SaO$_2$, hemoglobin, and CO often has a high S$\bar{v}$O$_2$ initially, because hypothermia and the effects of anesthesia and neuromuscular blockade decrease the tissue demand for oxygen. As rewarming occurs and the patient awakens from anesthesia, tissue demand increases; the S$\bar{v}$O$_2$ decreases but should remain above 60%.

The S$\bar{v}$O$_2$ is intended to reflect the interaction of all aspects of oxygenation rather than a single parameter. It can help in early detection of abnormalities in oxygen supply, delivery, or consumption and in assessing the effectiveness of interventions, such as titration of vasoactive or inotropic drugs or ventilator changes. However, S$\bar{v}$O$_2$ should never substitute for careful monitoring of each parameter individually. For example, the nurse must continue to assess cardiac

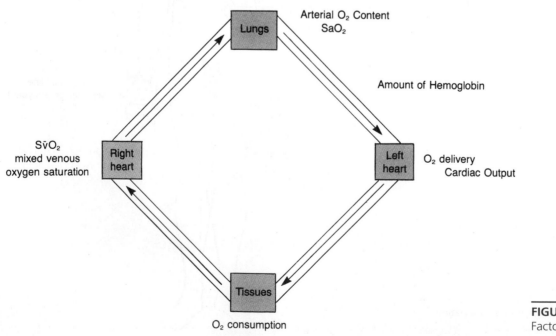

FIGURE 21-9
Factors affecting S$\bar{v}$O$_2$.

output measurements in the open heart surgery patient, even if SaO_2, hemoglobin, and oxygen consumption remain stable.

CHEST DRAINAGE AND BLEEDING

As soon as the patient is admitted to the ICU, the nurse connects the chest drainage container to suction (usually 20 cm H_2O) and positions the drainage tubes without loops or kinks. The nurse measures and records the amount and character of the drainage initially and then hourly. Continuous assessment of chest tube patency is done by observing for free-flowing drainage or the presence of clots in the tubing. Air leaks are assessed by watching for bubbling in the water seal chamber. If an air leak is present, the nurse implements troubleshooting techniques (see Chapter 24). A hemoglobin and hematocrit also are obtained within the first 30 minutes.

URINE OUTPUT

The nurse measures and records the urine output initially and hourly thereafter. Because of hemodilution during cardiopulmonary bypass, an obligatory postoperative diuresis should ensue. Frequently, the urine output exceeds 100 to 200 mL/h, and the specific gravity is low. It is important to note any cloudy, pink, or red urine, which could indicate hemoglobinuria.

HYPOTHERMIA

During rewarming on cardiopulmonary bypass, the patient's core temperature is returned to 37°C (98.6°F). However, as this warmed blood begins to circulate to the periphery, heat transfer to the surrounding tissues causes the core temperature to drop again. Patients frequently enter the ICU with a temperature in the 35° to 36°C (95° to 96.8°F) range. Hypothermia causes peripheral vasoconstriction and a shift of the oxygen–hemoglobin dissociation curve to the left, so less oxygen is released from the hemoglobin to the tissues. See discussion of hypothermia in Chapter 33.

The nurse assesses the patient's temperature on admission using pulmonary artery or tympanic membrane temperature; these are considered accurate indicators of core temperature. Rectal temperatures do not correlate with core temperature measurements until 8 hours postoperatively, and bladder temperature differs significantly from core temperature with rapid cooling and rewarming. Increasing the room temperature and using radiant heat and blankets or a warming blanket are effective techniques to increase core temperature. Rewarming should be accomplished slowly to prevent hemodynamic instability due to rapid vasodilation. It is important to prevent shivering, which occurs most often between 90 and 180 minutes after ICU admission, because it increases metabolic rate, oxygen consumption, carbon dioxide production, and myocardial workload. If shivering occurs, it is usually controlled with narcotics, midazolam, or in rare instances, neuromuscular blockade.

Many patients experience overshoot in body temperature following rewarming. One etiological theory is that narcotics and anesthetics received intraoperatively reset the hypothalamic regulatory center, altering peripheral blood flow and feedback.[8] A cold, constricted peripheral vascular bed may also be a factor in preventing heat dissipation.

Insights into Clinical Research

Stevens T, Fitzsimmons L: Effect of a standardized rewarming protocol and acetaminophen on core temperature after cardiopulmonary bypass. American Journal of Critical Care 4:189–197, 1995

Patients undergoing hypothermic cardiopulmonary bypass return to the intensive care unit (ICU) hypothermic. Rewarming produces normothermia and then, in many patients, hyperthermia. The purpose of this study was to investigate the effects of acetaminophen on core temperature and to determine the effects of a standardized rewarming protocol on core temperature, peak core temperature, rewarming time, and hyperthermia.

Sixty patients undergoing hypothermic cardiopulmonary bypass were assigned to one of three acetaminophen groups: Group 1 received 650 mg rectally at 38.1°C, group 2 received 650 mg rectally at 37°C and 650 mg at 38.1°C, and group 3 received 1300 mg rectally at 37°C and 650 mg at 38.1°C. All patients experienced the same rewarming protocol. Patients with core temperature < 36°C were placed on an electric heating blanket until core temperature reached 36°C. At this point, patients were covered with three room-temperature bath blankets: one around the head, one over the torso and arms, and one over the lower extremities and feet. Patients whose core temperature was equal to or greater than 36°C on arrival in the ICU received only the bath blankets. Blankets were removed from the head and upper torso at 37°C.

Core temperature was measured by PA catheter thermistor every 15 minutes for 2 hours, every 30 minutes for 4 hours, then every hour for 16 hours.

Rewarming time was significantly related to age, number of leg incisions, weight, and body surface area (BSA). Older patients and those with two leg incisions rewarmed more slowly. Larger patients rewarmed more rapidly. Peak core temperature was higher for patients rewarmed by cotton bath blankets as compared to electric heating blanket, and patients rewarmed with electric heating blankets took significantly longer (2.3 hours longer) to reach normothermia than those with cotton bath blankets. The onset of hyperthermia was unaffected by method of rewarming or acetaminophen.

This study suggests that further research is needed to determine the "ideal" core temperature at which to discontinue active rewarming to prevent hyperthermia and to determine if individual rewarming protocols based on weight, BSA, or age are indicated.

NEUROLOGICAL STATUS

The nurse performs a neurological assessment, including level of consciousness, pupillary reaction, ability to follow commands, and strength and movement of extremities, initially, hourly, and whenever a change is noticed until the patient is fully recovered from the anesthesia. The patient must be oriented and reassured frequently.

Postoperative Complications

Cardiac surgery patients risk developing problems because of their underlying disease and the surgical trauma. In addition, the nurse caring for these people must confront problems caused by cardiopulmonary bypass and intraoperative hypothermia. Because of abnormal blood interface and altered blood flow patterns, cardiopulmonary bypass produces profound physiological effects (Table 21–1) that make the postoperative course and care of the cardiac surgery patient unique and challenging. This discussion focuses on problems encountered early in the postoperative course of CABG and valve surgery patients while they are in the ICU. The Collaborative Care Guide defines the specific outcomes and interventions.

ALTERED FLUID AND ELECTROLYTE BALANCE

After cardiopulmonary bypass, total body fluid volume increases as a result of hemodilution, increased vasopressin levels, and nonpulsatile renal perfusion that activates the renin–angiotensin–aldosterone mechanism. Patients can return to the ICU with a positive fluid balance of 2 to 3 L or more, and extracellular fluid volume can increase by as much as 20% over preoperative levels. The amount of increase is directly proportional to the amount of time on bypass, and up to 15 lb of body water can be gained. Because of hemodilution, the colloid osmotic pressure of the plasma is decreased.

In addition to fluid retention, capillary permeability is markedly increased because vasoactive substances are released during cardiopulmonary bypass. Increased fluid volume, increased capillary permeability, and decreased plasma colloid osmotic pressure cause large amounts of fluid to move from the intravascular to the interstitial space during and up to 6 hours after surgery. The patient appears edematous (especially the face, neck, and hands) and often develops an intravascular volume deficit.

Intravascular hypovolemia is manifested clinically by decreased central venous pressure (CVP), decreased pulmonary artery diastolic (PAD) pressure, and decreased pulmonary artery wedge pressure (PAWP). If left untreated, low cardiac output and hypotension can occur. Abnormal postoperative bleeding and vasodilation as the body's temperature normalizes can contribute to the hypovolemia.

Initial treatment is aimed at restoring adequate intravascular volume by administering fluids. Colloids (hetastarch or Plasmanate) provide more effective volume expansion than crystalloids because they increase colloid osmotic pressure, drawing interstitial fluid back into the vasculature. Adequacy of fluid administration should be determined by PAD, PAWP, cardiac output, and blood pressure measurements.

Fluid usually shifts back into the vascular space during the first several postoperative days as capillary membrane integrity improves and plasma colloid osmotic pressure normalizes. Renal excretion of excess body fluid results in spontaneous diuresis and weight loss. Fluid and sodium restriction may be ordered until body weight and fluid balance return to normal.

The most common postoperative electrolyte imbalance is an abnormal potassium level. Hypokalemia can result from hemodilution, diuretics, and the effects of aldosterone, which causes potassium secretion into the urine at the distal renal tubule as sodium is retained. Hyperkalemia can occur as a result of large amounts of cardioplegia solution or acute renal failure. Potassium levels should be checked on admission to ICU, every 2 to 4 hours for the first 8 hours postoperatively, and daily for several days. Based on these laboratory values, potassium supplements are given as ordered.

DECREASED CARDIAC OUTPUT

Cardiac output (CO) is the product of heart rate (HR) and stroke volume:

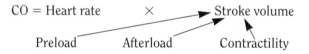

Decreased cardiac output can result from alterations in heart rate, stroke volume, or both. Abnormalities in heart rate are discussed as a separate postoperative problem under "Cardiac Dysrhythmias."

Stroke volume is dependent on preload, afterload, and contractility. An abnormality in one or more of these parameters can cause a decrease in output (see Chapter 16).

LOW PRELOAD

Left ventricular preload is the volume of blood in the left ventricle at the end of diastole. It reflects the volume status of the patient and is measured by the PAWP using the thermodilution catheter or by the left atrial mean pressure (LAMP) using a catheter placed directly into the left atrium and brought out through the chest wall at the end of surgery. Normal LAMP is approximately equal to the normal PAWP.

Because postoperative cardiac surgery patients frequently experience intravascular hypovolemia, the assessment of PAWP or LAMP is imperative to optimize cardiac output.

What should be considered "normal" PAWP must be related to the individual patient. For example, normal PAWP

TABLE 21-1
Effects of Cardiopulmonary Bypass

Causes	Clinical Implications
Increased Capillary Permeability Interface between blood and nonphysiological surfaces or bypass circuit leads to • Complement activation that increases capillary permeability • Platelet activation—platelets secrete vasoactive substances that increase capillary permeability • Release of other vasoactive substances that increase capillary permeability	Large amounts of fluid move from the intravascular to the interstitial space during and up to 6 h after cardiopulmonary bypass. Patient becomes edematous.
Hemodilution Solution used to prime extracorporeal circuit dilutes patient's blood. Secretion of vasopressin (ADH) is increased. Levels of renin–angiotensin–aldosterone are increased because of nonpulsatile renal perfusion. Total body water is increased.	Decreased blood viscosity improves capillary perfusion during nonpulsatile flow and hypothermia. Hgb and Hct decrease. Levels of coagulation factors are decreased because of dilution. Intravascular colloid osmotic pressure is decreased, contributing to movement of fluid from intravascular to interstitial spaces. Water is retained at collecting tubule of kidney. Aldosterone causes retention of sodium and water at renal tubule. Weight gain occurs.
Altered Coagulation Procoagulant effects: • Interface between blood and nonendothelial surfaces of bypass circuit activates intrinsic coagulation cascade. • Platelet damage activates intrinsic pathway. Anticoagulant effects: • Interface between blood and nonendothelial surfaces of bypass circuit causes platelets to adhere to tubing and to clump; abnormal platelet function; activation of coagulation cascade, which depletes clotting factors; denaturization of plasma proteins, including coagulation factors. • Coagulation factors are decreased as a result of hemodilution.	Risk of microemboli is increased. Platelet count decreases by 50% to 70% of baseline. Abnormal postoperative bleeding occurs. Possibility of bleeding diathesis exists.
Damage to Blood Cells Exposure of blood to nonendothelial surfaces causes mechanical trauma and shear stress. • Platelet damage occurs. • Red blood cell hemolysis occurs. • Leukocytes are damaged.	Platelet count is decreased. Free hemoglobin and hemoglobinuria are increased. Hct is decreased. Immune response is diminished.
Microembolization Emboli form from tissue debris, air bubbles, platelet aggregation.	Microemboli to body organs (brain, lungs, kidney) are possible.
Increased Systemic Vascular Resistance (SVR) Catecholamine secretion is increased when cardiopulmonary bypass is initiated. Renin secretion is due to nonpulsatile flow to kidney. Hypothermia develops.	Hypertension is possible. Increased SVR may decrease cardiac output.
Increased Capillary Permeability Interface between blood and nonphysiological surfaces or bypass circuit leads to • Complement activation that increases capillary permeability • Platelet activation—platelets secrete vasoactive substances that increase capillary permeability	Large amounts of fluid move from the intravascular to the interstitial space during and up to 6 h after cardiopulmonary bypass. Patient becomes edematous.

usually ranges from 6 to 12 mmHg. Because of surgical manipulation and cardiopulmonary bypass, the PAWP in patients undergoing cardiac surgery usually must be maintained above 10 mmHg. If the patient has valve disease, even higher filling pressures may be required. Valvular stenosis or insufficiency causes volume and pressure overload, which in turn cause hypertrophy and dilation of the chamber behind the valve. Valve replacement corrects the flow obstruction or leak; however, the myocardial changes of hypertrophy and dilation take months to improve. It can be thought of as a balloon that has been left inflated for several weeks. If the air is let out, it has little elastic recoil. To maximize cardiac output, the filling volume is increased (increased PAWP or LAMP) to stretch this dilated myocardium for optimal contractility (Starling's principle). Clinically, a PAWP of 10 mmHg is usually the low limit of "normal" for a valve patient, and a PAWP as high as 18 to 20 mmHg can be considered "normal" and necessary to maintain adequate output. Patients with poor left ventricular function due to a large infarction or left ventricular aneurysm also need a higher PAWP for optimal stretch and contractility according to Starling's principle. If the patient is on PEEP to decrease postoperative bleeding, the PAWP may not truly reflect the left ventricular preload. By increasing intrathoracic pressure, PEEP falsely elevates the PAWP.

Low preload is treated by administering Plasmanate, hetastarch, crystalloids, autotransfusion, or blood (if the hematocrit is low). The goal of fluid replacement is a PAWP or LAMP that produces an adequate output and blood pressure for each patient.

INCREASED LEFT VENTRICULAR AFTERLOAD

Afterload is the resistance to ejection of blood from the left ventricle and is determined in part by the degree of constriction or dilation of the arterial circulation. It is measured by SVR, which is calculated by the formula

$$SVR = \frac{MAP - CVP}{CO} \times 80$$

where MAP is mean arterial pressure, CVP is central venous pressure, and CO is cardiac output. Normal values are 800 to 1,200 dynes/sec/cm^{-5}.

Afterload can be elevated after cardiac surgery as a result of hypothermia; release of vasoactive substances during bypass; increase in catecholamines, renin, and angiotensin; or a history of hypertension. High afterload increases myocardial workload and oxygen demand and decreases output. If the cause is hypothermia, warming the patient with blankets and radiant heat or a heating blanket can lower the SVR. Care should be taken not to rewarm the patient too quickly, because rapid vasodilation could cause hypotension.

Increased afterload can also be treated by administering vasodilating drugs, such as nitroprusside. If the blood pressure seems low to administer nitroprusside, the drug can be started at very low doses. Often the vasodilation produced by a low dose of nitroprusside increases the output enough that there is no change in blood pressure.

DECREASED CONTRACTILITY

Contractility is the ability of the myocardial muscle fibers to shorten independent of preload and afterload. Contractility is measured by left ventricular stroke work index (LVSWI), which is calculated by the formula

$$LVSWI = SVI(MAP - PAWP) \times 0.0136$$

where MAP is mean arterial pressure, PAD is pulmonary artery diastolic pressure, SV is stroke volume.

The normal range for LVSWI is 35 to 85 g/m^2 per beat, but a "normal" postoperative LVSWI in a patient after cardiac surgery can be lower than 35 because of the effects of surgical manipulation of the myocardium, cardiopulmonary bypass, cardioplegia, ischemia during the aortic cross-clamping, and reperfusion injury. Abnormal decreases in LVSWI can be caused by myocardial infarction, changes in the ventricular muscle as a result of valve disease, or abnormalities of myocardial pH, electrolytes, or oxygenation.

If the underlying cause can be identified, it should be corrected. Positive inotropic medications, such as dopamine, dobutamine, or amrinone, can also be effective. Because postsurgical depression of myocardial function lasts only 6 to 18 hours postoperatively, attempts to wean these drugs can begin as soon as possible.

ALTERED BLOOD PRESSURE

After cardiac surgery, it is not unusual for hypotension or hypertension to develop quickly. Nursing interventions should be directed toward anticipating such changes and intervening to prevent them or to restore the blood pressure rapidly to a normotensive range. Generally, the systolic pressure should be kept in the 90 to 150 mmHg range. These parameters can vary depending on the patient and events in the operating room.

Hypotension

The patient is usually considered hypotensive if the systolic blood pressure is less than 90 mmHg. In CABG, the saphenous vein grafts can collapse if the perfusion pressure is too low (veins do not have the muscular walls that arteries do), resulting in myocardial ischemia. Inadequate tissue and organ perfusion can result from a systolic blood pressure lower than 90 mmHg, especially in the previously hypertensive patient.

Hypotension can be caused by decreased intravascular volume, vasodilation as a result of rewarming, poor left ventricular contractility, or dysrhythmias. If the patient is hypovolemic, rapid infusion of volume expanders as ordered by the physician should increase the blood pressure.

If the volume expansion alone does not correct the hypotension or if the low blood pressure is caused by decreased contractility, a vasopressor drug can be ordered. For example, dopamine started at 2 to 10 µg/kg/min has a primarily β-stimulating effect to increase contractility and blood pressure. If the hypotension is caused by dysrhythmia, interventions are aimed at correcting the dysrhythmia or obtaining a ventricular rate adequate to maintain the output (see discussion of cardiac dysrhythmias Chapter 16).

Hypertension

Hypertension is particularly dangerous in the postoperative cardiac surgery patient because it can cause rupture or leakage of suture lines and increase bleeding. Postoperative hypertension can result from a history of hypertension, increased levels of catecholamines or renin, hypothermia, or pain. Some patients are hypertensive postoperatively without an obvious cause.

A systolic blood pressure of 150 mmHg or more is usually considered hypertensive and should be treated. Nitroprusside, a vasodilator, can be titrated to bring the blood pressure into an acceptable range. Sometimes the blood pressure increases when the patient is stimulated by noise or nursing care procedures but returns to normal levels when the patient sleeps. This hypertension can often be controlled by intravenous analgesics or sedatives. Pain may also cause hypertension that can be managed by analgesics.

Unless the patient was hypertensive preoperatively, postoperative hypertension is usually transient, and the nitroprusside dose can be decreased within 24 hours. If this is not possible, oral antihypertensives can be started to facilitate discontinuation of the nitroprusside.

POSTOPERATIVE BLEEDING

Although bleeding from the chest tubes after cardiac surgery is expected, the nurse must differentiate between normal and excessive drainage. Normal chest tube drainage is dark red, thin, serosanguineous, and does not clot in the chest tubes because it is defibrinated. Usually, the amount of drainage is not more than 200 mL/h for the first 1 to 2 hours, with the amount decreasing subsequently. The actual amount of drainage is important, but the hourly trend must also be considered. If the drainage amount is excessive initially, but the trend is decreasing, this is less worrisome than a trend of increasing drainage.

Some patients normally bleed more than others. Patients who have had the IMA used for one of the grafts can have increased bleeding initially because of dissection of the chest wall to isolate the IMA. Those undergoing cardiac surgery for a second or third time may also bleed more because of the dissection of scar tissue and adhesions created by previous surgeries.

Arterial Bleeding

Although rare, arterial bleeding is a life-threatening emergency that usually results from rupture or leakage of suture lines at one of three sites: the proximal anastomosis of the vein graft to the aorta, the distal anastomosis of the vein graft to the coronary artery, or the aortic cannulation site where oxygenated blood is returned to the patient during cardiopulmonary bypass.

With an arterial bleed, the chest drainage container fills up with bright red blood within minutes, and the patient becomes hypovolemic and hypotensive extremely rapidly. Lost blood must be replaced as quickly as possible with blood or volume expanders until the chest can be reopened and surgical repair accomplished.

Venous Bleeding

Venous bleeding is more common than arterial bleeding and is caused by surgical problems or coagulopathy. Faulty hemostasis of one or more vessels results in abnormal bleeding. Coagulopathy can have multiple causes. Coagulation factors may be used during cardiopulmonary bypass more quickly than the body can replace them, and they are diluted by the pump prime solution. Thrombocytopenia can be present because of platelet destruction or loss of platelets by adherence to the bypass circuit tubing. Platelets may not work effectively because of damage from cardiopulmonary bypass or preoperative antiplatelet medication (eg, A.S.A.). The fibrinolytic system responsible for clot breakdown can be abnormally activated by surgery, increased levels of catecholamines, or stress.

Heparin "rebound" can also cause postoperative bleeding. After the patient is taken off cardiopulmonary bypass, intravascular heparin is neutralized by protamine. As the body temperature increases and the peripheral circulation improves, non-neutralized heparin shifts or "rebounds" from the interstitial spaces, resulting in a reanticoagulation.

Treatment of Bleeding

Controlling hypertension, maintaining chest tube patency to prevent cardiac tamponade, and maintaining adequate intravascular volume are essential actions while caring for a bleeding patient. Whether chest tubes should be milked or stripped routinely is controversial. Negative intrathoracic pressures up to −400 cm water can be generated with vigorous stripping. This can entrap intrathoracic tissue in the chest tube drainage holes and increase bleeding. However, if the tubes become occluded, life-threatening cardiac tamponade can develop. More research is needed to determine the effect of chest tube stripping on postoperative bleeding. Gentle milking when clots are evident should be implemented to ensure patency.

To maintain normovolemia, adequate cardiac output, and sufficient blood pressure, the blood loss must be replaced. Autotransfusion of the chest drainage (see Chapter 17) is an excellent way to accomplish this without the risks of heterologous blood transfusion. If the hematocrit is low, fresh whole blood or packed red cells can be given. Usually, transfusion is indicated only if the hematocrit is below 28% to 30% because as excess volume is excreted, the hematocrit increases. Plasmanate or hetastarch can be given if the hematocrit is adequate.

Treatment is also aimed at decreasing the amount of bleeding and correcting the underlying cause. PEEP of 5 to

10 cm added to the ventilator can decrease venous oozing by increasing intrathoracic pressure. Vital signs must be observed closely if PEEP is used, because the increased intrathoracic pressure can decrease venous return, causing low cardiac output and hypotension.

Laboratory work, including activated clotting time (ACT), prothrombin time (PT), partial thromboplastin time (PTT), fibrinogen, bleeding time, and platelet counts, helps determine appropriate treatment. The ACT, PT, and PTT assess the time required for the patient's blood to clot and are prolonged in the presence of heparin. If the results are abnormally prolonged, heparin "rebound" may be the cause of bleeding, and intravenous protamine can be given.

Bleeding time measures the ability of platelets to adhere to the blood vessel wall and aggregate to form a platelet plug. The bleeding time can be prolonged even when the platelet count is adequate, if platelet function is abnormal.

Thrombocytopenia can also cause abnormal bleeding. Normally, the platelet count drops to 50% to 70% of baseline when cardiopulmonary bypass is initiated. If the postoperative platelet count is less than 50,000/mm^3 or the patient's platelets are not functioning normally, platelet concentrate can be administered. Desmopressin acetate (DDAVP), an analog of vasopressin that lacks vasopressor activity, can also be given. DDAVP is thought to increase platelet aggregation. The platelet count usually returns to normal within 24 hours postoperatively as platelets sequestered in the spleen are released to the general circulation.

If the PT, PTT, or fibrinogen is abnormal, fresh frozen plasma or cryoprecipitate can be used. Fresh frozen plasma is rich in fibrinogen and factors V and VII; cryoprecipitate supplies factors VIII and XIII. These replace clotting factors diminished as a result of cardiopulmonary bypass and hemodilution.

If the bleeding is not stopped by these interventions and the chest tube drainage is more than 400 mL/h for longer than 3 hours or more than 100 mL/h for longer than 6 hours, surgical reexploration is indicated.

EARLY CARDIAC TAMPONADE

Cardiac tamponade can occur if blood accumulates around the heart and compresses the myocardium. This compression impedes venous return, decreasing cardiac output and blood pressure. Tamponade is an uncommon complication if the chest tubes are kept patent; however, if it does occur, it is dangerous and must be recognized and treated quickly.

Signs and symptoms include decreasing blood pressure accompanied by rising CVP and PAWP. CVP and PAWP values can become closer to one another (ie, they equalize) as blood surrounding the heart compresses the right and left ventricular chambers. A paradoxical pulse can be present (greater than 10 mmHg decrease in systolic pressure with inspiration). This can be a clue to tamponade, but paradoxical pulse does not always occur with tamponade after cardiac surgery. Patients with pulmonary disease and those on

ventilators can have a decrease in systolic pressure with inspiration when they do not have tamponade. Another clue can be an abrupt decrease in chest tube drainage that has been initially brisk, suggesting an acute chest tube occlusion. Definitive diagnosis is made by chest x-ray, which shows mediastinal widening, or by echocardiography, which demonstrates fluid in the pericardial space.

Treatment for postoperative tamponade includes fluids and vasopressors to maintain the cardiac output and blood pressure until surgical decompression is done. Generally, pericardiocentesis is not used for postoperative cardiac tamponade, because pericardial blood is usually clotted and cannot be aspirated with a needle.

CARDIAC DYSRHYTHMIAS

Bradyarrhythmias and tachyarrhythmias are common postoperatively and can decrease cardiac output. They are treated similarly to dysrhythmias occurring in any cardiac patient (see Chapter 16). (Cardiovascular problems of the older patient are discussed in Table 21-2.)

Tachyarrhythmias can be dangerous because they compromise cardiac output by decreasing ventricular diastolic filling time. They also decrease coronary artery perfusion and increase myocardial oxygen demand.

Sinus tachycardia can be caused by hypovolemia or side effects of inotropic drugs (especially dopamine). Catecholamine release during surgery, pain, anxiety, or fever may be a contributing factor. Treatment is directed toward correcting the underlying cause.

Premature ventricular contractions (PVCs) occur in 17% to 50% of patients following CABG, usually as a result of surgical trauma and manipulation, electrolyte imbalances (especially hypokalemia), changes in pH and PaO$_2$, and catecholamine release due to pain or anxiety.[9] Occasionally tactile irritation from the thermodilution catheter or mediastinal chest tubes also causes PVCs. Antiarrhythmic agents, such as lidocaine, are given for PVCs only if the arrhythmia compromises the patient's hemodynamic status.[9] The underlying cause should be identified and treated. If ventricular tachycardia or ventricular fibrillation develops, aggressive treatment with lidocaine or defibrillation according to accepted protocols must be initiated.

Of cardiac surgery patients, 20% to 35% develop supraventricular tachycardias (SVT), including paroxysmal atrial tachycardia, atrial fibrillation, and atrial flutter.[10] Most often these dysrhythmias develop 24 to 72 hours postoperatively with peak incidence on the second postoperative day.[9] They are thought to develop secondary to atrial ischemia during aortic cross-clamping and a postoperative inflammatory response to surgical trauma.[11] If the ventricular rate associated with the SVT is rapid, cardiac output can fall. Loss of atrial kick (contribution to cardiac output by atrial contraction) with atrial fibrillation and flutter can contribute to this decrease. If hemodynamic compromise ensues, SVT can be managed by intravenous verapamil,

❀	**Table 21-2** *Considerations for the Older Patient*

Management of the Cardiac Surgery Patient

Physiology	Clinical Effect
Cardiovascular System	
• Increased stiffness of myocardial muscle	• Higher filling pressures (PAD and PAWP)
• Increased stiffness of peripheral vasculature and decreased ability to adjust to changes in blood volume	• Decreased ability for vasoconstriction with position change leading to orthostatic hypotension
• Replacement of cells in conduction system with collagen and elastin	• Increased hemodynamic instability
• Decreasing number of pacemaker cells in the sinoatrial (SA) and atrioventricular (AV) nodes	• SA and AV node impairment, conduction blocks
• Decreased cardiac responsiveness to beta adrenergic stimulation	• Decreased heart rate
	• Cardiac output maintained by increase in stroke volume
Pulmonary System	
• Breakdown of elastin and collagen, which impairs elastic recoil of lung	• May lead to prolonged intubation
• Thoracic cage less compliant	• Less effective coughing
• Decreased expiratory muscle strength and mucociliary clearance decrease	• Increased risk of atelectasis, hypoxemia, and pulmonary infection
Renal System	
• Progressive loss of cortical nephrons and decrease in corticomedullary concentration gradient	• Slowing of renal response to dehydration
• Impaired renal concentrating ability	• Decreased effectiveness of fluid conservation
• Decreased clearance of renally excreted medications (may be reduced by up to 40% by age 80)[16]	• Toxic medication levels or abnormally prolonged duration of action
Gastrointestinal System	
• GI absorption of medications decreased and more variable	• Especially important with drugs with narrow therapeutic range, such as lanoxin
• Decline in liver function, resulting in decreased hepatic breakdown of medications	• More intense medication effect and longer duration of action for medications broken down in liver (eg, diazepam)
Musculoskeletal System	
• Skeletal osteoporosis	• May lead to impaired sternal healing and increased risk of sternal dehiscence
Immune Response	
• May be decreased, especially if concomitant malnutrition and decrease in serum proteins	• Increased potential for infection
Neurological System	
• Decline in neurotransmitters	• Increased risk for acute confusion
Response to Medications	
• Decreased percentage of lean body tissue	• As a result of decreased body water, water-soluble medications concentrated in the bloodstream resulting in higher serum drug levels
• Increased percentage of body fat	
• Decrease in body water	• Fat-soluble medications stored in fat; increase in fat tissue may result in slower therapeutic response and longer duration of action as drug is released slowly from fat (eg, diazepam—Because initial therapeutic response may be slower, dose is frequently increased to obtain expected therapeutic response. Elimination half-life may increase from 24 to 90 hours in older adults as drug slowly released from fat.[16,17] Toxic effects may result.

(continued)

❀ Table 21-2 *Considerations for the Older Patient*
Management of the Cardiac Surgery Patient (Continued)

Patient Teaching

- Accommodate sensory deficits.
  —Ensure hearing aides are in and on.
  —Speak loudly and face patient.
  —Use large print, easy to read materials.
- Teach one thing at a time, and ensure patient understands before moving on.
- Start with simple and progress to more complex information.
- Teach both patient and caregiver.

---

adenosine (Adenocard), synchronized cardioversion, or several seconds of rapid atrial pacing by the temporary atrial epicardial pacing electrodes.

In postoperative valve patients (especially mitral valve patients), atrial fibrillation is common because of long-standing atrial dilation and stretching. Many of these patients have had chronic atrial fibrillation preoperatively. If the ventricular response to the fibrillation is controlled, treatment may include digitalization or in patients who are already digitalized, adding quinidine. If the ventricular response is rapid, intravenous verapamil may slow it. Cardioversion is not usually indicated if the fibrillation has been chronic.

Bradyarrhythmias (sinus bradycardia, idiojunctional) and blocks (bundle branch block, second and third degree atrioventricular block) occur postoperatively because of depression of the conduction system cells by cardioplegia or injury to nodes and conduction pathways by surgical manipulation, sutures, or local edema. Valve surgery patients are particularly at risk because of the proximity of the cardiac conduction system to the mitral and aortic valves.

In most patients, bradyarrhythmias and blocks resolve as the effects of cardioplegia diminish and the surgical edema subsides. If the cardiac output is decreased as a result of a bradyarrhythmia, temporary atrioventricular or ventricular pacing is indicated to maintain an adequate heart rate. Atropine can be used for temporary treatment. Less than 1% of patients require treatment with a permanent pacemaker.[9]

PULMONARY DYSFUNCTION

Cardiac surgery patients are more at risk for developing pulmonary complications than other surgical patients because of the effects of cardiopulmonary bypass. During bypass, pulmonary ventilation is halted or diminished because the oxygenator, not the lungs, oxygenates the blood. This alteration in pulmonary ventilation results in pulmonary at-

electasis. (Table 21-2 summarizes pulmonary problems in the older patient.)

When the pulmonary circulation is restored, perfusion of nonventilated alveoli occurs, shunting nonoxygenated blood into the systemic circulation. Because of increased capillary permeability, fluid may move into the pulmonary interstitium and alveoli. This movement hampers gaseous diffusion and can increase secretions. Hypoxemia can develop. Large tidal volumes and PEEP are often used to prevent alveolar collapse, treat atelectasis, and improve oxygenation. Secretions are removed by endotracheal suctioning, and ventilatory status is assessed by SaO_2 monitoring and ABG determination. Patients are usually weaned from the ventilator the evening of surgery when extubation criteria are met (see Chapter 24), hemodynamic parameters are stable, and the chest tube drainage is within normal limits. Patients with preexisting pulmonary disease may remain on the ventilator longer.

After extubation, coughing and deep breathing are done every 1 to 2 hours with incentive spirometry every 2 hours. Mobilization should begin as soon as possible. Because the median sternotomy incision and chest tubes cause pain, they can interfere with coughing and deep breathing. Splinting the chest incision with a small pillow and providing pain medications before incentive spirometry and coughing can facilitate pulmonary hygiene.

RENAL FAILURE

Although renal failure is an uncommon complication, cardiac surgery patients are more at risk than others because of cardiopulmonary bypass. (Renal problems of the older patient are discussed in Table 21-2.) Renal blood flow is decreased during bypass, blood cells are damaged, and free hemoglobin is released from red blood cell destruction. Cellular debris and free hemoglobin can damage renal tubules. This risk accelerates with increasing time on bypass and with preexisting renal dysfunction.

Hematuria can occur because of renal filtration of hemoglobin. Maintaining adequate urinary output is imperative to prevent renal tubular damage and obstruction from cellular debris and hemoglobin. furosemide (Lasix) or mannitol can be given to promote urine flow.

Prerenal factors also cause postoperative renal failure. Decreased cardiac output, hypotension, and hypovolemia decrease renal blood flow and should be treated aggressively. Renal dose dopamine can improve renal blood flow.

NEUROLOGICAL DYSFUNCTION

Postoperative neurological dysfunction can vary in severity from mild temporary impairments in concentration to periods of agitation and confusion to major cerebrovascular accident or coma. The risk of neurological complications increases with increasing age, prolonged cardiopulmonary bypass time, preexisting carotid or cerebrovascular disease, and valve disease, especially if atrial fibrillation is present.

Altered cerebral perfusion and microembolization of fat, fibrin, or platelet aggregates during cardiopulmonary bypass and embolization of clots, particulate matter, or air can all be causes of neurological sequelae. Atrial clots occur commonly in patients with atrial fibrillation because of sluggish atrial blood flow. When a rhythm is reestablished after bypass, these clots can embolize. During manipulation of diseased valves, calcified material can break loose. Atheromatous plaque in the ascending aorta can also embolize when the aorta is manipulated during cannulation or proximal vein graft anastomosis. Air embolism arising from air trapped in the cardiopulmonary bypass system or from inadequate venting of air from the heart and aortic root can also cause neurological deficits.

Frank stroke occurs in 1% to 3% of patients undergoing heart surgery.[12] Although not always obvious to health care professionals on neurological examination, a substantial number of patients report minor cognitive impairments in their daily functioning. For example, they report statements like "I'm not as sharp as I used to be" or "I cannot remember things well." These abnormalities may occur in as many as 75% of patients and may be present in up to one third of patients 1 year after surgery.[13]

Identifying those at increased risk and assessing neurological status frequently can facilitate recognition of potential problems early so that intervention can begin. Maintaining adequate cardiac output, blood pressure, and ABGs ensures normal cerebral perfusion and oxygenation.

Brachial plexus injury is another potential postoperative neurological complication. This condition occurs in 5% to 25% of patients due to sternal retraction and is more common with IMA use.[11]

WOUND INFECTION

Postoperative wound infection can develop in the leg or median sternotomy incision or in chest tube insertion sites. Infection risk is increased by obesity, diabetes mellitus, mal-nutrition, operative time greater than 6 hours, and more than one surgery in a single admission (eg, reoperation for postoperative bleeding).

An ongoing assessment for signs of wound infection should be conducted. These include erythema, drainage, and temperature elevation that persists more than 72 hours postoperatively. Early temperature elevation as high as 38.9°C (102°F) during the first 48 hours after surgery is a normal response to cardiopulmonary bypass and is usually not a sign of infection.

Wound infection is not an early postoperative problem and is usually not evident until after the patient leaves the ICU. However, meticulous care should be taken to prevent infection by keeping incisions clean and dry and changing soiled dressings with aseptic technique.

POSTOPERATIVE PAIN

After cardiac surgery, the patient can experience pain resulting from the chest or leg incision, the chest tubes, rib spreading during surgery, endotracheal suctioning, and care activities. The ICU environment may accentuate the pain experience physiologically because of light and noise and psychologically through separation and fear.

Although pain perception varies from person to person, the median sternotomy incision is usually less painful than a thoracotomy incision, and most people report that the pain is the worst the first 3 to 4 days postoperatively. Discomfort from the leg incision often worsens after the patient is ambulatory, especially if leg swelling occurs. Stretching of back and neck muscles as the ribs are spread and immobilization for several hours during surgery can cause back and neck discomfort. Patients with IMA grafting can have increased pain because of more stretching of the intercostal muscles and because of incision into the parietal pleura, which is richly innervated. Meehan and colleagues report a pain score of 4.42 on the Visual Analogue Pain Scale (VAS) (scale range = 0–5, with zero being no pain and 5 the worst possible pain) for patients with IMA versus 3.36 for patients with saphenous vein grafts alone.[14]

Angina after CABG can indicate graft failure; therefore, the nurse must be able to differentiate angina from incisional pain. Typical median sternotomy pain is localized, does not radiate, and can be sharp, dull, aching, or burning. It is often worse with deep breathing, coughing, or movement. Angina is usually precordial or substernal, not well localized, and frequently radiates to arms, neck, or jaw. It is often described as a pressure sensation and is not affected by respiration or movement.

Pain often stimulates the sympathetic nervous system, increasing heart rate and blood pressure, which can be detrimental to the patient's hemodynamics. Discomfort can also result in diminished chest expansion, increased atelectasis, and retention of secretions.

Maxam-Moore and associates describe current practice in analgesic use for cardiac surgery patients in critical care.[15] At least 43% and as high as 90% of subjects continued to report moderate to severe pain despite treatment with analgesics, and 42% of patients received no analgesics on the day of surgery. Women were prescribed significantly smaller analgesic doses of morphine than men and had higher VAS scores then men (4.57 versus 3.70).

The goals of nursing management should be a thorough assessment of the patient's pain, administration of analgesics based on the patient's report of pain intensity, provision of pain relief reported as adequate by the patient, and alleviation of factors that enhance pain perception, such as anxiety and fear.

The Collaborative Care Guide outlines the care for the patient after cardiac surgery.

CLINICAL APPLICATION: Patient Care Study

Mr. C is a 62-year-old man with a history of an anterior myocardial infarction (MI) 2 years ago and hypertension controlled by medication. Preoperatively, he was taking aspirin (325 mg orally q.d.) and had stopped smoking 10 years ago. He has just returned to the ICU after CABG with an IMA graft to the LAD and saphenous vein graft to the RCA and diagonal.

Mr. C is mechanically ventilated on 50% FIO_2 with 5 cm PEEP. His breath sounds are clear and equal bilaterally, and the SaO_2 is 98%. Neurologically, he is unresponsive with pinpoint pupils. The monitor shows sinus tachycardia at 110 with occasional PVCs. He has atrial and ventricular epicardial pacing wires, but they are not connected to the pacemaker. His BP is 90/60; core temperature, 35.9°C; cardiac index (CI), 1.6 L/min/M; PAWP, 8 mmHg; SVR, 1,800; LVSWI, 25; and $S\bar{v}O_2$, 55%. The chest tubes have drained 250 mL, and the urine output is 100 mL.

Based on her assessment, the nurse knows that Mr. C's neurological and respiratory status are as expected immediately postoperatively. His BP is adequate, but the CI and SvO_2 are low. The PAWP of 8 indicates that Mr. C is hypovolemic. The nurse understands that the high SVR, indicating vasoconstriction, is most likely elevated because of the low core temperature and as a compensatory mechanism for hypovolemia. Both the low PAD (preload) and high SVR (afterload) contribute to Mr. C's low CI. His BP is probably low because of hypovolemia. The chest tube drainage of 250 mL is probably normal this early postoperatively, but the trend should be watched.

After his nurse consults with the physician, Mr. C receives 500 mL hetastarch over 30 minutes, autotransfusion of the chest tube drainage, and radiant heat and blankets to increase the core temperature.

Two hours postoperatively, the nurse notes that Mr. C is starting to arouse. He opens his eyes and moves all extremities weakly. His parameters are as follows: BP, 170/90; core temperature, 36.2°C; CI, 2.1 L/min/M; PAWP, 10; SVR, 1,600; LVSWI, 30; $S\bar{v}O_2$, 60%; urine output, 50 mL/h; and chest tube drainage 400 mL/h for the last 2 hours with few clots forming in the tubing. CI, PAWP, and LVSWI have all improved; however, the PAWP is still low for Mr. C, who is on 5 cm PEEP and has a history of MI. The core temperature, which is increasing slowly, is still low and may still be contributing to the increased SVR. Mr. C's nurse determines that the chest drainage of 800 mL over 2 hours is excessive, and Mr. C's BP is now too high. Hypertension is not unexpected, because Mr. C was hypertensive preoperatively.

After reporting her assessments to Mr. C's physician, the 800 mL of chest drainage is autotransfused rapidly, and a nitroprusside drip is started to control the hypertension. Lowering the BP should also help decrease the bleeding. Mr. C's physician orders an activated clotting time (ACT), bleeding time, and platelet count.

In evaluating the results of the blood work, the nurse recognizes that the ACT is normal, the bleeding time is prolonged, and the platelet count is 105,000/mm³. Because the ACT is normal, his nurse knows that adequate protamine was given to neutralize the heparin. The platelet count of 105,000/mm³ is low but expected at this time because of the effects of cardiopulmonary bypass. Prolonged bleeding time indicates that Mr. C's platelets are not functioning properly. This could be a result of the aspirin he was taking preoperatively and of the cardiopulmonary bypass. The physician orders transfusion of 5 U of platelet concentrate.

Four hours postoperatively, Mr. C is on a nitroprusside drip at 3 µg/kg/min. His BP is 136/85; CI, 2.5 L/min/M; PAWP, 12; SVR, 1,050; LVSWI, 32; SaO_2, 62%; core temperature, 36.8°C; and urine output, 75 mL/h. The chest tube drainage has been 350 and 200 mL for the last 2 hours, respectively. Mr. C is responding appropriately to commands and moves all extremities.

Mr. C's hemodynamic profile is normal, and his BP and SVR have decreased as a result of the vasodilating effects of nitroprusside. The chest tube drainage is still high but decreasing hourly, indicating that the bleeding is now under control. The nurse's assessments and interventions were critical in stabilizing Mr. C's condition.

COLLABORATIVE CARE GUIDE
for the Patient Following Cardiac Surgery

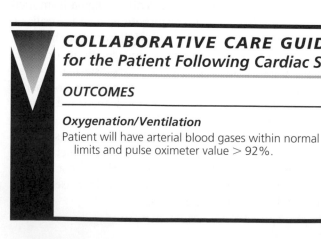

OUTCOMES	INTERVENTIONS
Oxygenation/Ventilation	
Patient will have arterial blood gases within normal limits and pulse oximeter value > 92%.	• Monitor arterial blood gases by pulse oximeter and end tidal CO_2. • Obtain arterial blood gases per order. • Wean from mechanical ventilation per protocol. • Provide supplemental oxygen after extubation.

(continued)

COLLABORATIVE CARE GUIDE
for the Patient Following Cardiac Surgery

OUTCOMES	INTERVENTIONS
There will be no evidence of pulmonary edema on chest x-ray and demonstrated by clear breath sounds. There will be no evidence of atelectasis.	• Obtain postoperative chest x-ray. • Administer diuretics per order. • Encourage use of incentive spirometer, cough and deep breath q 2–4 h after extubation. • Turn patient side to side q 2 h while on bedrest. • Mobilize out of bed after extubation.
Chest tubes will remain patent.	• Monitor drainage and air leaks q 1 h for 24 h. • Maintain tubing position to prevent pooling of drainage. • Milk chest tubes if necessary to facilitate forward clot movement.

Circulation/Perfusion

OUTCOMES	INTERVENTIONS
Vital signs will be within normal limits including MAP >70 mmHg, cardiac index >2.2 L/min/m², S$\bar{\text{v}}$O$_2$ between 60%–80%.	• Monitor vital signs q 1 h and PRN for first 12 h post-operatively or per protocol. • Monitor PA and PAWP, CVP or right atrial pressure q 1 h and cardiac output, SVR, and PVR q 6–12 h if pulmonary artery catheter is in place. • Monitor ECG, BP and S$\bar{\text{v}}$O$_2$ continuously. • Administer positive inotropic agents and reduce afterload with vasodilating agents guided by hemodynamic parameters and physician orders. • Evaluate effect of medications on BP, HR, and hemodynamic parameters. • Monitor and treat dysrhythmias. • Anticipate need for temporary cardiac pacing. • Prepare patient for intra-aortic balloon pump assist if necessary.
There will be no evidence of congestive heart failure due to decreased cardiac output and/or perioperative MI.	• Regulate volume administration as indicated PAWP and/or CVP values. • Assess for neck vein distension, pulmonary crackles, S$_3$ or S$_4$, peripheral edema, increased preload parameters, elevated "a" wave of CVP, RAP, or PAWP waveform. • Monitor cardiac enzymes and 12 lead ECG.
There will be no evidence of bleeding. Chest tube drainage will be <100 mL/h.	• Monitor chest tube drainage. • Monitor for signs of cardiac tamponade (eg, hypotension, pulsus paradoxus, tachycardia, PA pressure equalization). • Evaluate chest x-ray for widened mediastinum. • Monitor PT, PTT, ACT, CBC per protocol. • Autotransfuse shed blood if appropriate. • Administer blood products and protamine per order or protocol.
Patient will be euthermic.	• Assess temperature q 1 h. • Warm patient 1 degree C per h by using warming blankets and lights, fluid warmer.

Fluids/Electrolytes

OUTCOMES	INTERVENTIONS
Renal function will be maintained as evidenced by urine output >30 mL/h, normal laboratory values.	• Monitor intake and output q 1–2 h. • Monitor BUN, creatinine, electrolytes, Mg, PO$_4$. • Replace potassium, magnesium and phosphorous per order or protocol. • Take daily weights. • Administer fluid volume and diuretics as ordered.

Mobility/Safety

OUTCOMES	INTERVENTIONS
Patient will maintain range of motion and muscle strength.	• Keep patient on bed rest until extubated. • Provide range of motion exercises. • Turn, reposition q 2 h. • Progress activity to chair for meals, bathroom privileges, increase distance walking. • Monitor vital signs, respiratory effort during activity.

(continued)

COLLABORATIVE CARE GUIDE
for the Patient Following Cardiac Surgery (Continued)

OUTCOMES	INTERVENTIONS
Patient will not fall or accidentally harm self.	• Assess for orthostatic hypotension. • Utilize self-protective devices as indicated and per hospital policy. • Isolate epicardial pacing wires.
Skin Integrity Patient will have no evidence of skin breakdown. Incisions will heal without evidence of infection.	• Turn side to side q 2 h while patient is on bed rest. • Evaluate skin for signs of pressure areas immediately postoperatively and when turning. • Assess sternotomy and leg incision for redness, swelling, drainage. • Apply TED hose and elevate legs to reduce edema.
Nutrition Caloric and nutrient intake meet metabolic requirements per calculation (eg, Basal Energy Expenditure). Patient will have normal laboratory values reflective of nutritional status.	• Keep NPO while patient is intubated. • Remove NG tube after extubation. • Give clear, then full liquids, advance to heart healthy diet. • Use sodium, fat, cholesterol, fluid, and caloric restriction if indicated. • Consult dietitian or nutritional support services. • Monitor albumin, prealbumin, transferrin, cholesterol, triglycerides, total protein.
Comfort/Pain Control Patient will have relief of surgical pain. Patient will demonstrate no evidence of pain such as increased HR, BP, RR, or agitation during activity or procedures.	• Use visual analogue scale to assess pain quantity. • Assess quality, duration, location of pain. • Administer analgesics and monitor pain and hemodynamic response. • Assess effect of pain medication on weaning from mechanical ventilation.
Psychosocial Patient will have decreased anxiety evidenced by stable vital signs, cooperation with procedures and treatments.	• Provide a calm environment. • Explain all activities to patient. • Administer sedation cautiously and assess effect on ventilator weaning parameters. • Provide for adequate periods of rest and sleep.
Teaching/Discharge Planning Patient and family will understand need for tests, procedures, treatments. In preparation for discharge to home, patient will understand: activity levels, dietary restrictions, medication regimen, incision care.	• Provide clear explanations and descriptions of tests, procedures, etc. • Make appropriate referrals and consults early during hospitalization. • Initiate family education regarding heart healthy diet, physical activity limitations (eg, lifting over 10–15 lbs. and driving, stress reduction strategies, management of pain, incision care).

THROMBOSIS AND EMBOLISM AFTER VALVE REPLACEMENT

The risk of thromboembolism is present in all patients undergoing valve replacement, but it is greatest with a mechanical valve in the mitral position and in patients with atrial fibrillation. Anticoagulation reduces but does not eliminate the risk of these complications, and it increases the risk of significant hemorrhage.

Clots can form on the mechanical valve, obstructing blood flow through it or preventing proper valve closure, which results in regurgitant flow. Hemodynamic deterioration, development of a new murmur, or change in the normal valve sound may suggest these complications.

INFECTIVE ENDOCARDITIS AFTER VALVE SURGERY

Patients undergoing valve reconstruction or replacement are at risk for developing valvular endocarditis. Early postoperative endocarditis is usually associated with median sternotomy infection or sepsis from urinary tract infection or invasive lines. Because endocarditis takes time to develop, the critical care nurse's role is primarily prevention. Early removal of the Foley catheter, invasive intravenous and arterial lines, and early recognition and treatment of wound infections can prevent this complication.

▆▆ CONCLUSION

With managed care, capitation, rising costs, and limited resources, the usual length of stay for a cardiac surgery patient has decreased to 4 to 7 days. The unique challenge for the critical care nurse is to integrate theoretical knowledge, assessment skills, and problem-solving ability to provide optimal nursing care and maintain high quality outcomes and customer satisfaction while decreasing costs, resource consumption, and length of stay.

Considerations for Home Care
Home Care Following Cardiac Surgery

- Discharge planning that begins at admission is imperative because of short length of stay.
- Assessment of home environment and family support system are essential to planning. If patient cannot care for self, or family cannot provide convalescent care, consider home care referral for RN, home health aide, or homemaker as appropriate.
- Transient cognitive dysfunction, common after cardiac surgery, results in poor concentration, confusion, memory loss, and emotional instability at the time when patient must assimilate a vast amount of information about postoperative care. Provide resources to take home (eg, written materials, video discharge instructions). Teach both patient and caregiver. Caregivers are

often instrumental in ensuring that the patient follows the plan of care, they can identify unexpected complications that require medical attention and they may be responsible for transporting the patient to follow-up appointments.
- Information/skills needed for postoperative self-care are provided (see Patient Teaching display).
- Many patients benefit from referral to cardiac rehabilitation programs.
- Prior to discharge, the patient should be able to verbalize: disease process and surgical procedure; rehabilitation and treatment goals and how to achieve these goals; and signs, symptoms, and complications to report.

PATIENT TEACHING
Instructions Regarding Cardiac Postoperative Self-Care

General Instructions

- Avoid lifting heavy objects >10–15 lbs. for first 3 months.
- Avoid strenuous arm movement such as golf or tennis. When getting in and out of chair or bed use legs. Arms should not bear weight and should be used only for balance.
- Do not drive for 6 weeks postop. (May ride in car)
- Follow physician's instructions for activity progression.
- Resume sexual activity when you can climb 2 flights of stairs without stopping (with physician's recommendations).
- Use alternative positions for 3 to 4 months to decrease stress on sternum.
- Inspect and cleanse surgical incisions daily with soap and water.
- Use antiembolism hose on venectomy limb during the day for several weeks.
- Medication indications, including reason for taking, dosage, frequency, and side effects.
- Follow dietary restrictions.

Pain

- How much pain to expect and how to manage it.

Risk Factors

- Instruction on individual risk factors
- Their impact on health following cardiac surgery

- How to modify them
- Referrals should be made as appropriate (eg, weight loss program, stop smoking program).

Follow-up Appointments

- How and when to schedule follow-up appointments

What to Report to Physician

- Signs and symptoms of infection such as fever, increased redness, tenderness, drainage, or swelling of incisions
- Palpitations, tachycardia, irregular pulse (if normally regular)
- Dizziness or increased fatigue
- Sudden weight gain or peripheral edema
- Shortness of breath
- Chest pain

Valve Patients

- Information about anticoagulants if patient on warfarin including:
  a. Signs of covert bleeding and what to report to physician
  b. Importance of follow-up lab work to measure degree of anticoagulation and adjust dose
  c. Food/warfarin interactions
- Endocarditis prophylaxis before dental, surgical, GI, and GU procedures

Dynamic Cardiomyoplasty

Congestive heart failure (CHF) continues to be a major cause of morbidity and mortality in the United States despite continuing advances in medical and pharmacological therapy.[18] For end-stage heart failure, cardiac transplantation is the most viable long-term treatment option, but as the number of patients with end-stage failure increases, donor availability remains limited, and the wait for a heart is long. Dynamic cardiomyoplasty (DCMP) is an investigational surgical treatment for end-stage heart failure treatment. The first clinical trials were started by Carpentier and Chachques in France in 1955. DCMP involves wrapping the heart with skeletal muscle, which is electrically stimulated by a device called a cardiomyostimulator to contract in synchrony with the cardiac cycle. This contraction augments left ventricular function and improves cardiac output. The left latissimus dorsi muscle is the muscle of choice for this procedure because of its size and proximity to the heart and its single neurovascular bundle. The skeletal muscle must be trained to contract appropriately. Training is started about 2 weeks postoperatively and continues over 7 to 8 weeks. Operative survival after DCMP is 75% at 1 month and 70% at 5 years.[18]

Indications and Diagnosis

Patients with refractory end-stage heart failure resulting from ischemic or idiopathic dilated cardiomyopathy who are unsatisfactory candidates for heart transplantation because of age, associated medical problems, lack of compatible donor, or personal preference are candidates for DCMP. Suitable candidates are identified by a large variety of diagnostic tests. Echocardiogram and multiple-gated acquisition scan assess left ventricular ejection fraction (LVEF). Left and right heart catheterization measure hemodynamic parameters and allow visualization of the coronary arteries. Posterior-anterior and lateral chest x-rays assess heart size and cardiothoracic ratio. Computed tomography scan of the chest confirms cardiothoracic ratio and determines the thickness of the latissimus dorsi muscle. The presence and severity of arrhythmias with normal activity are assessed with 24-hour Holter monitoring.

Appropriate candidates for DCMP are Hew York Heart Association (NYHA) functional class III or intermittent class IV patients with LVEF less than 40% but greater than 15%, left ventricular end diastolic pressure (LVEDP) less than 35 mmHg, and in sinus rhythm with adequate neuromuscular, pulmonary, renal, and hepatic function.[18,19]

Contraindications

Because hemodynamic benefits of DCMP do not begin until completion of several months of postoperative muscle training, preoperative ventricular function must be adequate to survive the surgical procedure and muscle training period. Patients who are fixed NYHA functional class IV, are hemodynamically unstable, and require pharmacological or mechanical support before DCMP are not suitable candidates. Ejection fraction < 10%, cardiac index < 1.5 L/min/M², LVEDP > 40 mmHg, biventricular failure, and pulmonary hypertension are also contraindications.[18] Because muscle wrap stimulation cannot be adequately synchronized, DCMP is not done in patients with severe intractable ventricular arrhythmias or pacemakers. In patients with severe mitral insufficiency, increased left ventricular contractility will worsen the insufficiency. Patients younger than 18 years or older than 80 years and those with hypertrophic cardiomyopathy are also excluded.

Surgical Procedure

During the surgical procedure, the patient is positioned in the right lateral decubitus position, and a longitudinal incision is made from the axilla to the iliac crest. The left latissimus dorsi muscle is dissected, preserving the neurovascular bundle (Fig. 21-10A). Muscle-stimulating electrodes are placed at the thoracodorsal nerve. The muscle is then brought into the thorax through the resected third or fourth rib. The incision is closed, the patient is moved to the dorsal recumbent position, and a median sternotomy is performed. The latissimus dorsi muscle is wrapped around both ventricles and sutured in place. Cardiopulmonary bypass is not required. The epicardial sensing electrode is then screwed into the ventricular myocardium. Stimulating and sensing electrodes are connected to the cardiomyostimulator, which is placed in a subfascial pocket in the upper abdominal wall (see Fig. 21-10B).

Postoperative Management

Postoperative assessment, monitoring, nursing care, and complications of the DCMP patient are similar to that of the cardiac surgery patient except that problems related to cardiopulmonary bypass, such as hypothermia, rewarming, fluid shifts, and coagulopathy do not occur. Postoperative bleeding is less frequent. Initial care priorities include stabilization of oxygenation, blood pressure, rhythm, and hemodynamics.

Most DCMP patients have decreased cardiac output and hypotension because already poor left ventricular function deteriorates further from surgical manipulation and insult. Immediately after surgery, the muscle wrap may actually impair ventricular function, decreasing cardiac output even more. Vasodilators are often used to minimize cardiac workload along with inotropic agents titrated to maintain CI > 2 L/min/M² and systolic blood pressure > 80 mmHg.

Fluid management is guided by pulmonary artery pressures, keeping in mind that the muscle wrap decreases ven-

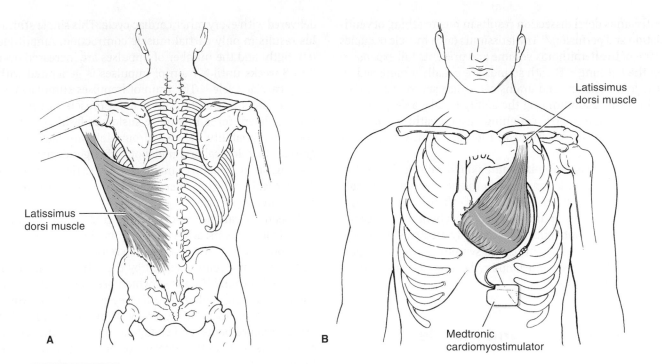

A

B

Latissimus
dorsi muscle

Latissimus
dorsi muscle

Medtronic
cardiomyostimulator

FIGURE 21-10

Two stages of cardiomyoplasty. (**A**) With the patient in a right lateral decubitus position, the surgeon detaches one of the latissimus dorsi muscles. (**B**) In the second stage, with the patient in a dorsal recumbent position, the surgeon lifts the heart. The posterior ventricular area is sutured to the larger border of the latissimus dorsi muscle flap. The heart is wrapped with the lateral and anterior walls of the left and right ventricles sutured to the borders of the latissimus dorsi muscle. A muscle stimulating device is attached, and the chest wall is closed.

tricular compliance. This decreased compliance results in higher PAWPs for any given volume; therefore, patients may require higher filling pressures to ensure adequate preload. However, when administering volume, care must be taken to prevent worsening of failure.

Prophylactic lidocaine may be used to prevent ventricular arrhythmias and to avoid the need for defibrillation, which can injure the muscle wrap or damage the cardiomyostimulator.[20] Supraventricular arrhythmias are also managed aggressively with medications or rapid atrial stimulation so cardioversion can be avoided.

Chest tubes are placed for drainage and lung expansion. A bulb suction device drains fluid from the dead space in the area of the latissimus dorsi muscle. Drainage is usually serosanguineous and should not exceed 50 to 100 mL/h for the first 24 hours. Wound drains are removed when drainage is < 30 mL/24 h.

Proper positioning is important to prevent injury to the latissimus dorsi neurovascular pedicle. Because the pedicle lies directly under the skin of the axilla, repositioning should always be done with a draw sheet—not by lifting under the axilla. Patients should not lie on their left side. In the early postoperative period, careful monitoring should be done with position changes between the right side and back to identify and lessen hemodynamic instability that is common early after surgery. Strenuous left arm activity should be limited, but gradual use of left arm and shoulder

is encouraged. Physical therapy may assist with range of motion and arm and shoulder mobilization.

In addition to the postoperative pain experienced by all cardiac surgery patients, DCMP patients have additional discomfort due to the muscle site incision, dissection, and drains. Pain management is critical to facilitate adequate turning, coughing, deep breathing, use of incentive spirometry, and early ambulation.

Many DCMP patients are debilitated with poor preoperative nutrition. Postoperative nutritional evaluation and intervention are imperative for wound healing and adequate immune function to decrease infection risk.

Postoperative Complications

One of the most common postoperative complications is the formation of a seroma in the area of latissimus dorsi dissection. A seroma is a mass caused by the localized accumulation of serum within a tissue or organ. A compression dressing is kept in place to help decrease fluid accumulation, and drains are emptied frequently and suction maintained. If a seroma develops, it usually reabsorbs spontaneously.

Pulmonary complications, such as atelectasis and decreased oxygenation, occur for several reasons. Preexisting pulmonary edema due to left ventricular failure is common. Positioning in the right lateral decubitus position during latissimus dorsi dissection results in mismatching of ventilation and perfusion.[21] The latissimus dorsi muscle occupies 10% of the hemithorax volume and prevents full expansion of the left lung.[22] Breath sounds are usually diminished on the left. Incisions and drains can cause severe discomfort with inspiration limiting the ability to take a deep breath. Incentive spirometry, coughing, deep breathing, and adequate, well-timed pain medication are critical to prevent pulmonary infection.

Myonecrosis of the latissimus dorsi muscle due to impairment of circulation through the neurovascular bundle is another complication of DCMP. Diabetes, advanced age, and low cardiac output with use of peripheral vasoconstrictors may be contributing factors. Myonecrosis is usually manifested by mediastinitis and symptoms such as hyperthermia, increased white blood cell count, and unexplained feelings of malaise.[21]

Follow-up Care and Muscle Training

Following DCMP, the patient remains in the ICU for 2 to 3 days until extubated and hemodynamically stable off intravenous (IV) inotropes and vasodilators. Preoperative oral medications to manage failure are restarted as soon as possible, including angiotensin-converting enzyme inhibitors, diuretics, and oral inotropes.

For the first 2 weeks following DCMP, the latissimus dorsi muscle is not stimulated. Due to extensive dissection and manipulation at surgery, the muscle is somewhat ischemic, and it takes 2 to 3 weeks to restore its blood supply partially and develop collateral blood flow.[21] Time is also necessary for the muscle wrap to develop adhesion to the heart muscle and pericardium so it does not become dislodged when stimulated to contract. After 2 weeks, the gradual muscle stimulation routine begins, usually after the patient has been discharged.

Because skeletal muscle is physiologically different from cardiac muscle, the skeletal muscle used in DCMP must be trained to work in synchrony with the heart. Cardiac muscle is fatigue resistant and can be stimulated to contract as a whole with one stimulus of sufficient strength (the "all or none" phenomenon). Skeletal muscle is randomly organized into separate motor units with slow and fast twitch myofibrils.[21] Slow twitch fibers are similar to cardiac muscle and resist fatigue, but fast twitch fibers are prone to fatigue with repetitive stimulation. The conditioning of skeletal muscle to behave like cardiac muscle is a long, gradual process. Progressive, sequential stimulation is initiated over a 7- to 8-week period using the cardiomyostimulator. The cardiomyostimulator has the ability to sense the patient's intrinsic ventricular activity and to deliver stimuli, either singly or in a series called a burst or pulse train. Stimulation is timed to occur with mitral valve closure and ventricular systole. Initially, a single stimulus is

delivered with every other cardiac cycle. This single stimulus results in only partial muscle contraction. Amplitude (strength) and the number of impulses are increased over 7 to 8 weeks until a train of impulses is generated with every cardiac cycle.[18] The train of impulses stimulates all muscle fibers in the latissimus dorsi muscle to contract with sufficient force in a more sustained fashion and decreases fatiguability. When appropriately stimulated, progressive histological and metabolic changes occur within the muscle so it acquires many characteristics of myocardial tissue. Fast-twitch fibers are actually transformed into slow-twitch myofibrils.[21]

Enhanced cardiac function following DCMP involves several mechanisms: active reinforcement in which the systolic contraction of the muscle wrap reinforces cardiac contraction; passive reinforcement by the intrinsic tension of the muscle around the heart, which prevents further ventricular dilation; biological effect by reducing the workload of the myocardium, thereby decreasing myocardial oxygen requirements; and change in the shape and length of the muscle wrap to conform to the shape of the myocardium.[18,21]

Because of the muscle training time and gradual change in the shape on the muscle wrap, benefit is not seen until 6 to 12 months postoperatively. Hemodynamic measurements improve somewhat, but the major benefits for 80% to 90% of hospital survivors include improved exercise capacity, a significant reduction in the need for drugs and hospital admissions for CHF, and a significant decrease in financial resource use.[18]

Home Care Considerations

Education is extremely important in enabling the patient to comply with postdischarge routines. These include multiple follow-up visits as the muscle-stimulating protocol progresses. At 6 weeks, an electrocardiogram, chest x-ray, echocardiogram, and 24-hour Holter monitoring are done to evaluate efficacy of the DCMP.

The patient and family must understand that improvement in cardiac function should not be expected for at least 6 months. Continuing fatigue and diminished activity tolerance frequently make it difficult to participate in follow-up care. This can be discouraging, so the nurse must teach families how they can support the patient during this time.

Conclusion

DCMP is one of several treatment alternatives for patients with end-stage CHF. It results in increased life expectancy and improved quality of life. Because the effectiveness of this procedure is not apparent for 6 months or more, the ICU nurse plays a significant role not only in the immediate unstable postoperative period, but also in preparing patients and families to cope with the long, slow period of muscle training when no improvement is seen.

Carotid Endarterectomy

The right carotid artery is a branch of the innominate artery that arises from the right side of the aortic arch. The left common carotid artery arises directly from the aortic arch. At the level of the thyroid the common carotids bifurcate into the external and internal carotids. Located near this bifurcation, in the carotid sinus, are the carotid chemoreceptors, which are sensitive to blood CO_2 and O_2 levels, and the baroreceptors, which help regulate the blood pressure. The external carotids supply blood to the structures in the head and neck, excluding the eyes and brain. The internal carotids give rise to the ophthalmic arteries and the posterior communicating, anterior cerebral, and middle cerebral arteries, which help supply blood to the brain.

Stenosis or occlusion of the carotid arteries is usually due to atherosclerotic disease and may cause stroke, a leading cause of morbidity and mortality in the United States. Carotid endarterectomy is a prophylactic operation designed to decrease the risk of stroke and stroke-related death.

Indications

Carotid endarterectomy is indicated for patients with transient ischemic attacks or transient monocular visual loss due to severe stenosis (> 70% or lumen < 2 mm in diameter) in the common carotid artery bifurcation region or proximal internal carotid artery.[23] Patients with acute stroke less then 6 weeks old may also be candidates for carotid endarterectomy because their chance for subsequent stroke within 5 years is 25% to 45%.[24,25] Use of carotid endarterectomy for asymptomatic stenosis < 70% remains controversial.

Because carotid artery occlusive disease is a part of the systemic atherosclerotic process, patients often exhibit signs of vascular disease in other places in the body, such as the heart (CAD) or peripheral arterial disease in the legs. Risk factors, such as hyperlipidemia, hypertension, smoking, and diabetes, are frequently present. A bruit can usually be auscultated in the neck due to turbulent flow though the narrowed carotid artery. Carotid ultrasound is usually done to estimate the presence and amount of stenosis, but angiography is the most reliable method to determine the precise degree.

Surgical Procedure

A skin incision is made along the lower anterior border of the sternocleidomastoid muscle just below the angle of the jaw, and the common, internal, and external carotid arteries are isolated. The carotid arteries on the operative side must be clamped. A heparin bolus may be given prior to clamping to prevent thromboembolus formation while the arteries are clamped. Clamping puts the ipsilateral cerebral hemisphere and eye at risk of ischemia and infarct because the only perfusion to these areas occurs through the circle of Willis and collaterals, which may be inadequate. Adequacy of circulation is determined by continuous electroencephalogram monitoring in the operating room. If determined to be inadequate, a temporary bypass or shunt may be placed from the common carotid artery to the distal portion of the internal carotid to provide continued intraoperative perfusion. Patients treated with shunts often include those with contralateral carotid stenosis, neurological deficits, history of cerebrovascular accidents, and stroke in evolution. However, shunt use is controversial because it carries a possible risk of embolization and injury to the arterial intima.[23]

Endarterectomy or removal of the ulcerated or stenotic atheromatous plaque is then performed, and the artery is closed. If primary closure will cause a narrowing, a patch may be used.

Postoperative Management

Following recovery, patients are transferred to the ICU with electrocardiogram monitoring, arterial line, CVP, and oxygen. The stay in the ICU is usually 24 hours.

BLOOD PRESSURE REGULATION

Blood pressure is commonly labile due to surgical manipulation of the carotid sinus and transient baroreceptor dysfunction. It is postulated that atheromatous plaques dampen the pressure wave reaching the carotid sinus baroreceptors, and after removal of the plaques, increased baroreceptor stimulation results in bradycardia and hypotension.[26] On the other hand, hypertension may occur as a result of damage to the carotid sinus itself or the carotid sinus nerve, which sends signals to the medulla. Interruption of these signals leads to tachycardia and hypertension.[26] The risk of hypertension is greatest during the first 3 postoperative hours, and patients who develop hypertension are at a much higher risk of developing neurological deficits (10.2% versus 3.4%).[26] In a circulation unable to autoregulate, hypertension may cause excessive cerebral perfusion, resulting in hyperperfusion syndrome and intracerebral hemorrhage.[26] Increased blood pressure may also increase the risk of wound bleeding. Hypotension increases the risk of brain infarct.

The goal of blood pressure regulation is a systolic blood pressure between 120 and 170 mmHg. Blood pressure >170 mmHg should be treated with IV medications, such as nitroprusside, while hypotension may be resolved with IV fluid if the CVP is low or with a phenylephrine drip.

CARE OF OPERATIVE SITE

If hemodynamically stable, the head of the bed is kept elevated 25 to 35 degrees to minimize venous oozing.[27] The patient's head and neck are kept in alignment to minimize stress on the operative site. The dressing and the area behind the patient's neck and shoulders are assessed for the presence of blood. Persistent oozing from deep tissue, coughing or straining during extubation, and disruption of suture lines may all lead to bleeding into the operative site. The risk of bleeding can be further aggravated by anticoagulation with heparin or aspirin. The nurse assesses the neck size, comparing the operative side with the nonoperative side. Swelling could indicate hematoma formation. The nurse should notify the physician immediately if a hematoma is suspected because tracheal compression by the hematoma could require surgical evacuation. Wound hematomas occur in about 5% of patients.[28]

VENTILATION AND OXYGENATION

Most carotid endarterectomy patients receive oxygen through a nasal cannula. The nurse assesses the respiratory rate, depth, oxygen saturation, and ABGs as appropriate. Carotid endarterectomy may result in chemoreceptor dysfunction with reduced ventilatory response, hypoxemia, and hypercapnia. In patients with coexisting pulmonary disease, this dysfunction is further exaggerated, increasing the patient's risk of respiratory compromise.[26] The nurse also encourages deep breathing and incentive spirometry use to prevent atelectasis.

NEUROLOGICAL INJURY

Neurological complications can involve both brain injury and local nerve injury.

Brain Injury

Perioperative stroke occurs in about 4% of patients and may be due to embolization of atheromatous debris, air from the operative site, or low flow during carotid artery clamping.[26] Neurological assessment includes level of con-

sciousness, pupils, eyes in midline, orientation, appropriateness of response, and motor function (flexion, extension, and hand grips) hourly for the first 24 hours. Abnormalities should be reported to the physician immediately.

Cranial Nerve Injury

Several cranial nerves (CNs) traverse the surgical area and can be exposed to trauma. CN injury occurs in 5% to 15% of patients undergoing carotid endarterectomy.[28] The most commonly affected are the facial (CN VII), vagus (CN X), hypoglossal (CN XII), and spinal accessory (CN XI). Specific functional assessment for each nerve should be performed postoperatively, including those listed in Table 21–3. If a deficit is present, the nurse notifies the physician and explains to the patient how it occurred and that the deficit is usually temporary.

HOME CARE CONSIDERATIONS

Patients are usually discharged on the second postoperative day. Education should include the items listed in the patient teaching display.

■ CONCLUSION

The critical care nurse plays an essential role in the care of the patient who has had an endarterectomy. Although considered a vascular surgical procedure, postoperative complications of carotid endarterectomy usually manifest as neurological symptoms, and the nurse must assess the patient for subtle neurological changes. Patient education is also a key component of care. Patients and their families need to understand that the patient has an underlying cardiovascular disease, and risk factor modification is necessary.

TABLE 21-3 CLINICAL APPLICATION: *Assessment Parameters*
Postoperative Functional Assessment of Cranial Nerves Following Carotid Endarterectomy

Nerve	Nerve Intervention	Functional Assessment	Functional Damage
Facial nerve (VII)	Motor function of facial muscles	Ability to smile and frown	Asymmetrical contraction of the mouth
Vagus nerve (X)	Motor and sensory function of larynx and throat	Quality and tone of voice and ability to swallow	Difficult swallowing, hoarseness, speech problems, loss of gag reflex
Hypoglossal nerve (XII)	Muscles to tongue	Movement of tongue	Difficult swallowing, speech problems, deviation of tongue, sometimes airway damage
Spinal accessory nerve (XI)	Trapezius and sternocleidomastoid muscles	Ability to shrug shoulders and raise arm to horizontal position	Shoulder may sag, difficulty raising shoulder against resistance, difficulty raising arm to horizontal position

PATIENT TEACHING
Discharge Teaching After Carotid Endarterectomy

Risk Factor Reduction

- Stop smoking.
- Eat a low-fat diet.
- Control hypertension if present.

Activity

- Usually no restrictions exist.
- Move neck in a normal manner.

Incision Care

- Bruising and discoloration are common.
- Wash neck and incision with soap and water.

General

- Be familiar with signs and symptoms of incisional infection.
- Notify physician of recurrent neurological symptoms or visual defects.
- Be knowledgeable about medication indications, including reason for taking, dosage, frequency, and side effects.
- Follow up on your physician appointments.

Clinical Applicability Challenges

Self-Challenge: Critical Thinking

1. You are assigned to admit Mr. L., who has just been wheeled into the ICU from the operating room following cardiac surgery. The transport monitor shows a systolic blood pressure of 70 mmHg, and the cardiac rhythm is atrial fibrillation with a ventricular response of 180. The Swan-Ganz catheter was not connected for transport, so no pulmonary artery pressures are available. The patient is on a dobutamine drip at 5 µg/kg/min and is being ventilated with 100% FIO_2 using an Ambu bag. There is 600 mL sanguineous drainage in the chest drainage container. Prioritize your interventions, and provide rationales for your decisions.

2. Compare and contrast your nursing care of the postoperative CABG patient with the postcardiomyoplasty patient.

3. Your cardiac surgery patient suddenly develops chest pain. Formulate assessment criteria to distinguish among the different causes of chest pain.

Study Questions

1. Effects of cardiopulmonary bypass include all of the following except
   a. damage to red blood cells.
   b. hemodilution.
   c. decreased capillary permeability.
   d. changes in coagulation.

2. Compared with mechanical valves, biological valves
   a. require life long anticoagulation.
   b. have poor durability.
   c. are the valve of choice for patients younger than 50 years.
   d. have a higher incidence of thromboembolism.

3. Postoperative bleeding in the cardiac surgery patient can be treated by
   a. protamine.
   b. PEEP.
   c. autotransfusion.
   d. All of the above

4. Interventions for decreased cardiac index caused by increased afterload soon after cardiac surgery include
   a. autotransfusion.
   b. dopamine drip.
   c. volume expansion with hetastarch.
   d. blankets and radiant heat.

5. The best way to assess the alert patient's postoperative pain level is to
   a. assess physiological parameters, such as heart rate and blood pressure.
   b. determine if the patient is able to sleep.
   c. ask the patient his or her intensity of pain on the 0 to 10 scale.
   d. look for nonverbal clues, such as grimacing and fist clenching.

6. Which of the following is the correct comparison between skeletal muscle and cardiac muscle?
   a. Skeletal muscle is composed of separate motor units, so it must be stimulated by a pulse train, while cardiac muscle can be stimulated to contract as a whole with one stimulus of sufficient strength.
   b. Both cardiac and skeletal muscle are resistant to fatigue.
   c. Initial stimulation of both cardiac and skeletal muscle produces a strong, synchronized contraction.
   d. Both cardiac and skeletal muscle must be conditioned to resist fatigue.

7. *Following right-sided carotid endarterectomy, you assess that the patient has an uneven smile. One side of the mouth turns up, and one does not. The most likely cause is*
   a. *a stroke affecting the left side of the brain.*
   b. *a stroke affecting the right side of the brain.*
   c. *surgical damage to the facial nerve (CN VII).*
   d. *surgical damage to the vagus nerve (CN X).*

REFERENCES

1. Langenburg S, Buchanan S, Blackbourne L, Scheri R, Sinclair K, Martinez J, Spotnitz W, Tribble C, Kron I: Predicting survival after coronary revascularization for ischemic cardiomyopathy. Ann Thorac Surg 60:1193–1196, 1995
2. Nwasokwa O: Coronary artery bypass graft disease. Ann Intern Med 123:528–545, 1995
3. Earp J: The gastroepiploic arteries a alternative coronary artery bypass conduits. Critical Care Nurse 14: 24-30, 1994
4. Strong M, Brockman S: Mitral valve reconstruction. Cardiovasc Clin 23:255–263, 1993
5. Gray R, Hefant R: Timing of surgery for valvular heart disease. Cardiovasc Clin 23:209–231, 1993
6. Spaniol S, Bond E, Brengelmann G, Savage M, Pozos R: Shivering following cardiac surgery: Predictive factors, consequences and characteristics. American Journal of Critical Care 3:356–367, 1994
7. Barden C, Hansen M: Cold Vs. Warm cardioplegia: Recognizing hemodynamic variations. Dimensions in Critical Care Nursing 14: 114–123, 1995
8. Stevens T, Fitzsimmons L: Effect of a standardized rewarming protocol and acetaminophen on core temperature after coronary artery bypass grafting. American Journal of Critical Care 4:189–197, 1995
9. Pires L, Wagshal A, Lancey R, Huang S: Arrhythmia and conduction disturbances after coronary artery bypass graft surgery: Epidemiology, management and prognosis. Am Heart J 129:799–808, 1995
10. Riddle M, Dunstan J, Castanis J: A rapid recovery program for cardiac surgery patients. American Journal of Critical Care 5:152–159, 1996
11. Ayres S: Textbook of Critical Care. Philadelphia, WB Saunders, 1995
12. Sotaniemi K: Long term neurological outcome after cardiac surgery. Ann Thorac Surg 59:1336–1339, 1995
13. Brillman J: Central Nervous system complications in coronary artery bypass graft surgery. Neurol Clin 11:475–495, 1993
14. Meehan D, Mcrae M, Rourke D, Eisenring C, Imperial F: Analgesic administration, pain intensity and patient satisfaction in cardiac surgical patients. American Journal of Critical Care 4:435–442, 1995
15. Maxam-Moore V, Wilkie D, Woods S: Analgesics for cardiac surgery patients in critical care: Describing current practice. American Journal of Critical Care 3:31–39, 1994
16. Loughran S: Medication use in the elderly: A population at risk. Medical Surgical Nursing 5:121–124, 1996
17. Hirsch C: When your patient needs surgery: Weighing risks vs. benefits. Geriatrics 50:26–31, 1995
18. Futterman L, Lemberg L: Cardiomyoplasty: A potential alternative to cardiac transplantation. American Journal of Critical Care 5:80–86, 1996
19. English M: Dynamic cardiomyoplasty. Critical Care Nurse 18:56–64, 1995
20. Bove L, Mancini M, Duris L, Terracino G, Paschal D, Babin S, Hammet B: Nursing care of patients undergoing dynamic cardiomyoplasty. Critical Care Nurse 15:96–104, 1995
21. Pettrey L, Leflar-DiLeva K: Preparing for cardiomyoplasty: A new horizon in cardiac surgery. Dimensions of Critical Care Nursing 13: 226–236, 1994
22. Stewart J, Hicks S, Leflar K, Kaempf G, Bove L, Dimarzio D: Cardiomyoplasty: Treatment of failing heart muscle using the skeletal muscle wrap. J Cardiovasc Nurs 7:23–31, 1993
23. Ojemann R, Ogilvy C, Cromwell R: Surgical Management of Neurovascular Disease. Baltimore, Williams and Wilkins, 1995
24. Berman S, Bernhard V, Erly W, McIntyre K, Erdoes L, Hunter G: Critical carotid artery stenosis: Diagnosis, timing of surgery and outcome. J Vasc Surg 20:499–508, 1994
25. Moore W, Barnett H, Beebe H, Bernstein E, Brenner B, Brott T, Caplan L, Day A, Goldstone J, Hobson R, Kempczinski R, Matchar D, Mayberg M, Nicholaides A, Norris J, Ricotta J, Robertson J, Rutherford R, Thomas D, Toole J, Trout H Wiebers D: Guidelines for carotid endarterectomy. Circulation 91:566–579, 1995
26. Zierler R: Surgical Management of Cerebrovascular Disease. New York, McGraw Hill, 1995
27. Drain C: The Post Anesthesia Care Unit. Philadelphia, WB Saunders, 1994
28. Hankey G, Warlow C: Transient Ischemic Attacks of the Brain and Eye. Philadelphia, WB Saunders, 1994

BIBLIOGRAPHY

Beattie S: CAB surgery: The second time around. Am J Nurs 93:42–45, 1993

Black J, Matassarian-Jacobs E: Luckmann and Sorensen's Medical Surgical Nursing. Philadelphia, WB Saunders, 1993

Clochesy J, Breu C, Cardin S, Rudy E, Whittaker A: Critical Care Nursing. Philadelphia, WB Saunders, 1993

Cotton P: Fast track improves CABG outcomes. JAMA 70:2023, 1993

Earp J, Mallia G: Myocardial protection for cardiac surgery: The nursing perspective. AACN Clinical Issues 8(1):20–32, 1997

Fahey V: Vascular Nursing. Philadelphia, WB Saunders, 1994

Gaw-Ens B: Informational support for families immediately after CABG surgery. Critical Care Nurse 14:41–50, 1994

Gilski D: Controversies in patient management after cardiac surgery. J Cardiovasc Nurs 7:1–13, 1993

Gross S: Early extubation: Preliminary experience in the cardiothoracic patient population. American Journal of Critical Care 4:262–266, 1995

Halm M: Acute gastrointestinal complications after cardiac surgery. American Journal of Critical Care 5:109–118, 1996

Kelly T: The evolving health-care environment: New arguments for closer collaboration between cardiac surgical intensive-care nurses and clinical engineers. AACN Clinical Issues 8(1):71–77, 1997

Martin T, Crater J, Gott J, Weintraub W, Ramsay J, Mora C, Guyton R: Prospective randomized trial of retrograde warm blood cardioplegia: Myocardial benefit and neurologic threat. Ann Thorac Surg 57: 298–304, 1994

Staples J, Ramsay J: Advances in anesthesia for cardiac surgery: An overview for the 1990s. AACN Clinical Issues 8(1):41–49, 1997

Stovsky B, Dehner S: Patient education after valve surgery. Critical Care Nurse 14:117–123, 1994

Vaca K, Lohmann D, Moskoff M: Cardiac Surgery in the octogenarian: Nursing implications. Heart Lung 23:413–422, 1994

Respiratory System

22

Anatomy and Physiology of the Respiratory System

OBJECTIVES

Based on the content in this chapter, the reader should be able to:

- Describe the anatomical structures of the upper and lower respiratory tracts.
- Explain the principles of pulmonary circulation.
- Describe five properties that influence the mechanics of ventilation.
- Compare and contrast volume, capacity, and dynamic measurements of pulmonary function testing.
- Explain the normal ventilation perfusion ratio and ventilation perfusion mismatches due to altered ventilation or perfusion.
- Describe the role of the pulmonary membrane and diffusion in the transport of gas.
- Describe the key features of the oxygen dissociation curve and the meaning of shifts to the right or left.
- Explain mechanisms controlling respiration.

The respiratory system provides the body with oxygen that is essential for life and removes carbon dioxide, a waste product of cellular metabolism. The respiratory system also helps regulate acid–base balance for the body. Intact respi-

ratory structures and proper functioning of the respiratory system are necessary for transport of these gases in and out of the body. This chapter offers a review of structures and functions of the respiratory system. Knowledge of normal respiratory structures and functions helps the nurse understand respiratory assessment techniques, principles of respiratory system management, and common disorders of the respiratory system.

STRUCTURES OF THE RESPIRATORY SYSTEM

The Upper Respiratory Tract

The respiratory system is composed of the upper and lower respiratory tracts. Composed of the structures outside of the chest cavity, the upper respiratory tract includes the nose, mouth, nasopharynx, oropharynx, laryngopharynx, larynx, and upper trachea (Fig. 22–1). Air enters the body through the nose and mouth and then passes to the pharynx, which is a muscular tube posterior to the nasal and oral cavities and anterior to the cervical vertebrae. The

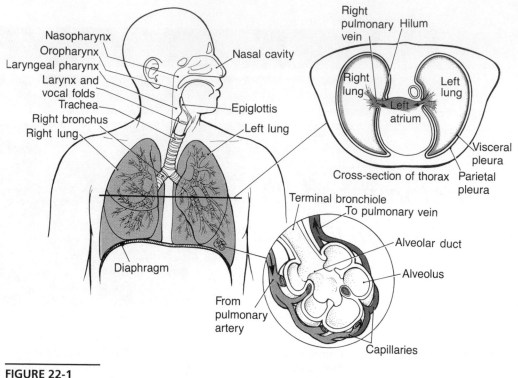

FIGURE 22-1

The respiratory system showing the upper and lower respiratory tracts. Insets show the alveoli and a horizontal cross-section of the lungs. (Source: Bullock BL: Pathophysiology: Adaptations and Alteration in Function [4th Ed], p. 545. Philadelphia, Lippincott-Raven, 1996)

pharynx is composed of three parts: the nasopharynx, the oropharynx, and the laryngopharynx. Positioned posterior to the nasal cavities, the nasopharynx is the upper portion of the pharynx and contains the adenoids and the eustachian tubes. Only air moves through the nasopharynx, whereas both air and food pass through the oropharynx and the laryngopharynx. The oropharynx, located posterior to the mouth, contains the palatine tonsils and the uvula. The laryngopharynx is the most inferior portion of the pharynx and opens anteriorly into the larynx and posteriorly into the esophagus. The larynx, commonly called the voice box, includes the epiglottis, the vocal cords, and the glottis. The larynx is composed of nine pieces of cartilage connected by ligaments that keep the air passage open at all times, allowing air to move from the pharynx to the trachea.

The upper respiratory tract furnishes a passageway for airflow; warms, humidifies, and filters the air; provides for taste, smell, and mastication; and supplies involuntary responses and defense mechanisms. Sneezing, coughing, gagging, and spasm are examples of defense mechanisms that protect the respiratory system from infection and inhalation of foreign bodies.

The Lower Respiratory Tract

The lower respiratory tract contains the respiratory structures found within the chest cavity, including the lower trachea, the bronchial tubes, the lungs, and the alveoli (see

Fig. 22–1). Like the larynx, the trachea contains cartilage, which keeps the trachea open. The right and left main bronchi branch off the trachea and enter the lungs. Within the lungs, the bronchi divide into many branches, known as the bronchial tree. The smaller branches of the bronchial tree are called bronchioles. The bronchioles end in the alveoli, the air sacs of the lungs.

Positioned within the protection of the thoracic cage, the lungs are located on either side of the chest. These air-filled spongy structures are attached to the body only at the pulmonary ligament at the mediastinum. The right lung contains three lobes, and the left lung contains only two lobes because of the space limitation imposed by the heart. The base of each lung rests anteriorly at the level of the sixth rib at the midclavicular line and at the eighth rib at the midaxillary line. The apices extend 2 to 4 cm above the inner aspects of the clavicles.

The lung is composed of about 300 million alveoli, which are arranged in clusters of 15 to 20.[1] The alveoli are the functional units of the lung and are only one cell layer thick (Fig. 22–2). Each alveolus is surrounded by a network of pulmonary capillaries, which also are only one cell layer thick. As a result, gases are efficiently diffused across the alveolocapillary interspace. For this diffusion of gas to occur, the gas must first dissolve in a liquid. A thin layer of fluid lines each alveolus, thus providing the liquid medium in which the gas can dissolve.

Pleural membranes surround the lungs and line the thoracic wall. The parietal pleura is the membrane lining

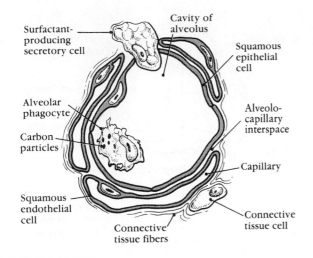

FIGURE 22-2

Representation of a single alveolus with surrounding capillaries and other cells. Note alveolar capillary interspace. (Source: Bullock BL: Pathophysiology: Adaptations and Alteration in Function [4th Ed], p. 547. Philadelphia, Lippincott-Raven, 1996)

the chest wall, and the visceral pleura overlays the lung parenchyma. The parietal and visceral pleurae slide over each other with each inspiration and expiration, lubricated by a thin layer of serous fluid in the intrapleural space.

Pulmonary Circulation

The right and left pulmonary arteries bring deoxygenated blood from the right side of the heart to the lungs, as shown in Figure 22–3. The pulmonary arteries divide into distal branches known as arterioles that eventually terminate as a capillary network in the alveolar sacs where oxygen and carbon dioxide diffusion occurs. The capillary network joins to form venules that collect the oxygenated blood from the capillaries and transport it into larger veins. The oxygenated blood then flows through the right and left pulmonary veins, returning the blood to the left atrium. This process of blood moving through the pulmonary capillary system to the alveoli for the purpose of gas exchange is known as perfusion.

FUNCTIONS OF THE RESPIRATORY SYSTEM

Ventilation

Ventilation refers to the movement of air into and out of the alveoli. Air flows from a region of higher pressure to a region of lower pressure. Therefore, when there is no airflow in or out of the lungs, alveolar and atmospheric pressure have equilibrated. To initiate a breath, airflow into the lungs

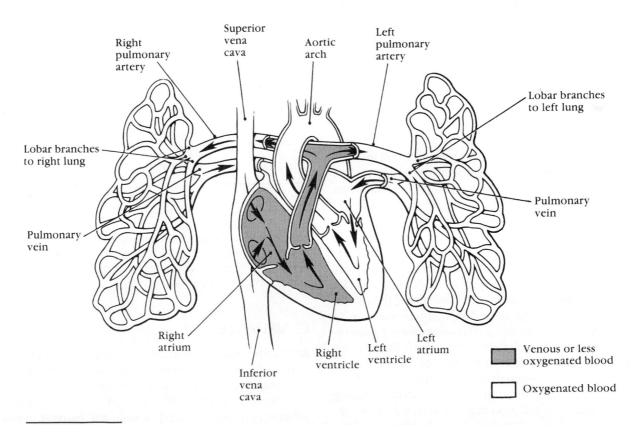

FIGURE 22-3

Circulation from the right heart to the lungs to the left heart. (Source: Bullock BL: Pathophysiology: Adaptations and Alteration in Function [4th Ed], p. 548. Philadelphia, Lippincott-Raven, 1996)

must be precipitated by a drop in pressure within the alveoli. This involves a complex process of multiple variables, referred to as the *mechanics of ventilation* and includes the properties of elasticity, compliance, resistance, pressure, and gravity.

ELASTICITY

Elasticity is the return of the original shape of matter after alteration by an outside force. Elastic forces are those promoting the return to the normal position or original shape. The lungs and the chest are elastic, requiring energy to move but quickly returning to their original shape when the energy is not actively applied.

The downward and upward movement of the diaphragm, which lengthens and shortens the chest cavity, combined with the elevation and depression of the ribs, which increases and decreases the anteroposterior diameter of the cavity, causes the expansion and contraction of the lungs. These actions are illustrated in Figure 22–4. Approximately 70% of the expansion and contraction of the lungs is accomplished by the change in anteroposterior measurement, and about 30% is achieved by the change in length due to movement of the diaphragm.

During inspiration, the diaphragm and intercostal muscles contract, increasing the volume of the chest cavity. The lungs are expanded, and the pressure within the alveolar sacs, the intra-alveolar pressure, becomes slightly negative (−3 mmHg) with regard to the atmosphere. This slightly negative pressure sucks air into the alveolar sacs through the respiratory passage.

After inspiration, the muscles used for inspiration relax, and the chest cavity returns to its resting position. With this decrease in chest size and resultant compression of the lungs, the intra-alveolar pressure builds to about +3 mmHg and forces air out of the respiratory passages. During maximum respiratory efforts, the intra-alveolar pressure can vary from −80 mmHg during inspiration to +100 mmHg during expiration. One respiratory cycle consists of one inhalation and one exhalation. At rest, inhalation normally requires about 1 second, which is less than that required for exhalation. Exhalation lasts about 2 seconds.

The lungs continually tend to collapse. Two factors are responsible for this phenomenon. First, the many elastic fibers contained within the lung tissue itself are constantly attempting to shorten. The second and more important factor is the high surface tension of the fluid lining the alveoli. If surface tension is high, the moist interior surfaces of an alveolus are difficult to separate from one another. This increases the energy required to open and fill the alveolus with air during inspiration. If surface tension is low, the alveoli walls more easily separate, requiring less effort for alveolar filling during inspiration. A lipoprotein substance called surfactant, which is constantly secreted by the epithelial alveolar lining, decreases the surface tension of the fluids of the respiratory passages 7- to 14-fold. The inability to secrete surfactant in the newborn is called hyaline membrane disease or respiratory distress syndrome.[2]

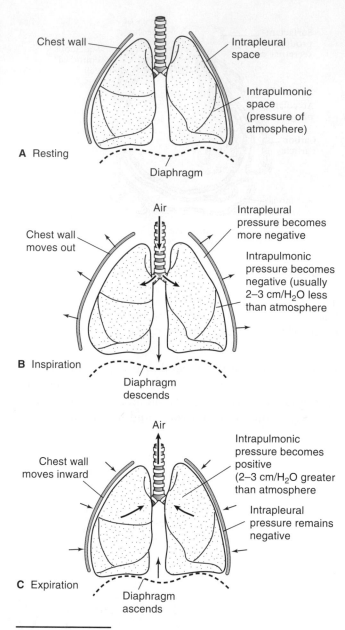

FIGURE 22-4

Phases of ventilation. (**A**) No air movement (resting). (**B**) Air moves from the environment to the intrapulmonic space (inspiration). (**C**) Air moves from the intrapulmonic space to the environment (expiration). (Source: Bullock BL: Pathophysiology: Adaptations and Alteration in Function [4th Ed], p. 551. Philadelphia, Lippincott-Raven, 1996)

COMPLIANCE

Another property of the lungs is compliance. Compliance is a measurement of distensibility or how easily a tissue is stretched. The more compliant a tissue is, the less the pressure required to stretch it. Compliance is expressed as the volume increase in the lung for each unit increase in intra-alveolar pressure.

$$\text{Compliance} = \frac{\text{Change in lung volume (liters)}}{\text{Change in lung pressure (cm } H_2O)}$$

Normal total pulmonary compliance, that is, both lungs and thorax, is 0.13 L/cm water pressure. In other words, every time alveolar pressure is increased by an amount necessary to raise a column of water 1 cm in height, the lungs expand 130 mL in volume.

Because inspiration requires muscle contraction, it is an active process requiring energy. Energy is also required to overcome two other factors that tend to prevent expansion of the lungs: nonelastic tissue resistance and airway resistance, meaning that energy is required to rearrange the large molecules of viscous tissues of the lung itself so that they slip past one another during respiratory movements. Under normal conditions, exhalation is a passive process that requires no energy. The lungs, with the chest wall, simply recoil to their original position.

A normal person at rest expends less than 6% of his or her total bodily oxygen consumption on the work of breathing. This percentage increases as the airway diameters decrease or compliance decreases.

Pulmonary compliance is reduced by conditions or situations that destroy lung tissue, cause it to become fibrotic, produce pulmonary edema, block alveoli, or in any way impede lung expansion and expansibility of the thoracic cage. If compliance is reduced, it is more difficult to expand the lungs for inspiration. (If compliance is increased, it is easier to expand lung tissue.) In the presence of tissue edema, the lungs lose many of their elastic qualities, and increased viscosity of the tissues and fluids increases the nonelastic resistance. The work of breathing is increased, and the energy expended to accomplish the task is also greatly increased. Energy can be required for exhalation if elasticity is lost (emphysema) or air passages are obstructed (asthma).

RESISTANCE

Airways offer resistance to airflow. The amount of airway resistance directly affects the amount of pressure required to move air in and out of the lungs. Airway resistance is determined mainly by the radius or size of the airway through which the air is flowing. When resistance is increased, the effort required to achieve ventilation increases. Conditions that cause an increased airway pressure include asthma, thickening of bronchial mucosa, increased mucus in the airway, a tumor, or a foreign body in the airway.

PRESSURE

The air that is taken into the respiratory passages is a mixture of primarily nitrogen and oxygen (99.5%) and a small amount of carbon dioxide and water vapor (0.5%). The molecules of the various gases behave as they do in solution and exhibit brownian movement. Therefore, in a mixture of gases such as air, all molecules are evenly distributed throughout the given volume. Because of this constant molecular bombardment, the volume of gases exerts pressure against the walls of the container. This pressure can be defined as the force with which a gas or mixture of gases attempts to move from the confines of the present environment. Each of the components of a mixture such as air accounts for part of the total pressure of the entire mixture. Consequently, if 100 volumes of air are placed in a container under 1 atmosphere of pressure (760 mmHg), an analysis would reveal that nitrogen constitutes 79 of the 100 volumes, and oxygen accounts for 21 volumes, or 79% and 21% concentration, respectively.

Both oxygen and nitrogen are contained at 760 mmHg pressure in this container. If the same volume of nitrogen is moved to a container of the same volume and allowed to expand until it completely fills all of the volume (100%), the pressure in the second container drops from 760 to 600 mmHg. If the 21 volumes of oxygen are moved to a container of the same volume and allowed to expand to 100% of the volume, the pressure in the third container drops from 760 to 160 mmHg. Therefore, in the original container the *part* of the total pressure due to nitrogen was 600 mmHg and the *part* due to oxygen was 160 mmHg. This pressure of nitrogen is called the *partial pressure* of nitrogen (PN_2) and that of oxygen, the *partial pressure* of oxygen (PO_2).

The partial pressure of a gas in a given volume is the force it exerts against the walls of the container. If the walls of the container are permeable, like the pulmonary membrane, the penetrating or diffusing power of a gas is directly proportional to its partial pressure.

Atmospheric air differs from alveolar air in partial pressures of the components. There is increased concentration of carbon dioxide and water in alveolar air. There are two reasons for these differences. First, the air is humidified as it is inspired by the moisture of the epithelial lining of the respiratory tract. At normal body temperature, water vapor has a partial pressure of 47 mmHg and mixes with and dilutes the other gases, decreasing their partial pressures. Second, molecules in a given volume of gas behave like molecules in a solution and diffuse from an area of high concentration to one of lower concentration.

Abbreviations Used for Partial Pressure of Gas

P	= Pressure
PO_2	= Partial pressure of oxygen
PCO_2	= Partial pressure of carbon dioxide
PaO_2	= Partial pressure of alveolar oxygen
$PaCO_2$	= Partial pressure of alveolar carbon dioxide
PaO_2	= Partial pressure of arterial oxygen
$PaCO_2$	= Partial pressure of arterial carbon dioxide
PvO_2	= Partial pressure of venous oxygen
$PvCO_2$	= Partial pressure of venous carbon dioxide
P_{50}	= Partial pressure of oxygen when the hemoglobin is 50% saturated

GRAVITY

In an erect adult, the force of gravity increases the intrapleural pressure (and therefore the intra-alveolar pressure) at the base of the lungs. Consequently, more air exchange occurs in the upper regions of the lungs than at the bases. Similarly, in any other body position, gravitational forces increase the amount of effort required to ventilate dependent portions of the lungs. This causes a shift in ventilation wherein ventilation of these portions is decreased and ventilation of other, less dependent areas is increased.

Pulmonary Function Tests

The flow of air in and out of the lungs provides tangible measures of lung volumes. Although referred to as "pulmonary function" measures, in reality these volumes represent *pulmonary anatomy* measures. In the evaluation of ventilation, structure or anatomy often determines function.

Ventilatory or pulmonary function tests measure the ability of the chest and lungs to move air into and out of the alveoli. Pulmonary function tests include volume measurements, capacity measurements, and dynamic measurements. These measurements are influenced by exercise and disease. Age, sex, body size, and posture are other variables that are taken into consideration when the test results are interpreted. Figure 22–5 illustrates pulmonary function tests showing normal lung volumes and capacity.

VOLUME MEASUREMENTS

Volume measurements show the amount of air contained in the lungs during various parts of the respiratory cycle. Measures of lung volume include tidal volume, inspiratory re-

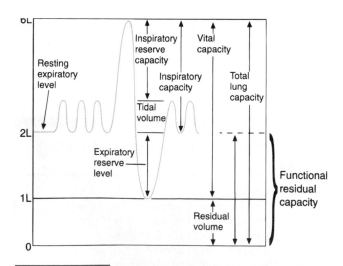

FIGURE 22-5
Pulmonary function tests showing normal lung volumes and capacity. (Source: Bullock BL: Pathophysiology: Adaptations and Alteration in Function [4th Ed], p. 566. Philadelphia, Lippincott-Raven, 1996)

serve volume, expiratory reserve volume, and residual volume, as shown in Table 22–1.

CAPACITY MEASUREMENTS

Capacity measurements quantify a part of the pulmonary cycle. They are measured as a combination of the previous volumes and include inspiratory capacity, functional residual capacity, vital capacity, and total lung capacity (see Table 22–1).

DYNAMIC MEASUREMENTS

The following measurements, called dynamic measurements, provide data about airway resistance and the energy expended in breathing (work of breathing).

- *Respiratory rate or frequency* (f) is the number of breaths per minute. At rest, f equals about 15.
- *Minute volume*, sometimes called minute ventilation ($\dot{V}_E$), is the volume of air inhaled and exhaled per minute. It is calculated by multiplying tidal volume (V_T) by f. At rest, $\dot{V}_E$ equals approximately 7,500 mL/min.
- *Dead space* (V_D) is the part of the V_T that does not participate in alveolar gas exchange. V_D (measured in milliliters) is the air contained in the airways (anatomical dead space) plus the volume of alveolar air that is not involved in gas exchange (physiological dead space; eg, air in an unperfused alveolus due to pulmonary embolism or, more commonly, air in underperfused alveoli).

  Adult anatomical dead space is usually equal to the body weight in pounds (eg, 140 mL in a 140-lb person). In the healthy person, V_D is composed only of anatomical dead space. Physiological dead space occurs in certain disease states.

  V_D is calculated by subtracting the partial pressure of arterial carbon dioxide ($PaCO_2$) from the partial pressure of the carbon dioxide of alveolar air (P_ACO_2). The normal value of V_D in healthy adults is typically less than 40% of the V_T. The V_D/V_T ratio is used to follow the effectiveness of mechanical ventilation.
- *Alveolar ventilation,* the complement of V_D, is expressed as the *volume of tidal air that is involved in alveolar gas exchange.* This volume is represented as volume per minute by the symbol $\dot{V}_A$. $\dot{V}_A$ indicates effective ventilation. It is more relevant to the blood gas values than either V_D or V_T because these last two measures include physiological dead space. $\dot{V}_A$ is calculated by subtracting V_D from V_T and multiplying the result by the respiratory rate per minute:

$$\dot{V}_A = (V_T - V_D) \times f$$

About 2,300 mL of air (functional residual capacity [FRC]) remains in the lung at the end of expiration. Each new breath introduces about 350 mL of air into the alveoli.

TABLE 22-1
Lung Volumes and Lung Capacities

Term Used	Symbol	Description	Remarks	Normal Values
Lung Volumes				
Tidal volume	VT or TV	Volume of air inhaled and exhaled with each breath	Tidal volume may not vary, even with severe disease.	500 mL
Inspiratory reserve volume	IRV	Maximum volume of air that can be inhaled after a normal inhalation		3,000 mL
Expiratory reserve volume	ERV	Maximum volume of air that can be exhaled forcibly after a normal exhalation	Expiratory reserve volume is decreased with restrictive disorders, such as obesity, ascites, pregnancy.	1,100 mL
Residual volume	RV	Volume of air remaining in the lungs after a maximum exhalation	Residual volume may be increased with obstructive diseases.	1,200 mL
Lung Capacities				
Vital capacity	VC	Maximum volume of air exhaled from the point of maximum inspiration	Decrease in vital capacity may be found in neuromuscular disease, generalized fatigue, atelectasis, pulmonary edema, and chronic obstructive pulmonary disease (COPD).	4,600 mL
Inspiratory capacity	IC	Maximum volume of air inhaled after normal expiration	Decrease in inspiratory capacity may indicate restrictive disease.	3,500 mL
Functional residual capacity	FRC	Volume of air remaining in lungs after a normal expiration	Functional residual capacity may be increased with COPD and decreased in adult respiratory distress syndrome.	2,300 mL
Total lung capacity	TLC	Volume of air in lungs after a maximum inspiration and equal to the sum of all four volumes (VT, IRV, ERV, RV)	Total lung capacity may be decreased with restrictive disease (atelectasis, pneumonia) and increased in COPD.	5,800 mL

The ratio of new alveoli air to total volume of air remaining in the lungs is

$$\frac{350 \text{ mL}}{2,300 \text{ mL}}$$

Therefore, new air is only about one seventh of the total volume contained within the lungs. The normal $\dot{V}_A$ is 5,250 mL/min (350 mL/breath $\times$ 15 breaths/min = 5,250 mL/min).

A normal breath (V_T) can replace 7,500 mL of air per minute (500 mL/breath $\times$ 15 breaths/min = 7,500 mL/min), requiring a time of .008 sec/mL:

$$\left(\frac{1 \text{ min}}{7,500 \text{ mL}} \times \frac{60 \text{ sec}}{1 \text{ min}} = 0.008 \text{ sec/mL} \right)$$

Therefore, the FRC of the lungs can be completely replaced in 18.4 seconds (2,300 mL $\times$ .008 s/mL = 18.4 seconds), if there is uniform air diffusion. This slow turnover rate prevents rapid fluctuations of gas concentrations in the alveoli with each breath.

Perfusion

The pulmonary circulation provides mixed venous blood exiting the right ventricle of the heart a chance to exchange gas before returning to the left atrium (see Fig. 22–3). The pulmonary circulation is unique and differs from other organ-specific circulatory beds.

Anatomically, the pulmonary vascular bed has no thick-walled muscular vasculature similar to arterioles. This results in a very distensible vascular bed with low resistance to flow. Although the pulmonary circulation receives the same volume of blood as the systemic system, the pulmonary vascular resistance (PVR) is one-sixth the systemic vascular resistance.[4]

If systemic pressures rise, PVR decreases. Using recruitment, previously low or nonperfused pulmonary vessels are opened, and low perfused vessels are dilated.

Most of the PVR, at least 50%, is believed to be generated at the level of the capillaries. The size of the capillaries can be influenced by the nearby intra-alveolar pressures. The capillaries not near alveolar surfaces are subject to pressure generated by motion in the connective tissue of the lung. Chemical stimulation (by catecholamines, histamine, angiotensin II, and prostaglandins) results in vasoconstriction. For unknown reasons, hypoxia increases PVR.

A major force in perfusion distribution in the lung is gravity. Low pressures systems, like the pulmonary vasculature, are subject to hydrostatic pressure created by gravity. In an upright position, the dependent base of the lung distends the vasculature, offering very low PVR. The apex vasculature has little perfusion and higher PVR as constriction occurs.

Ventilation and Perfusion

Maximal efficiency in the exchange of gases between blood and alveolus results when ventilation (movement of air in alveoli = $\dot{V}$) and perfusion (movement of blood around alveoli = $\dot{Q}$) correspon3d equally (Fig. 22–6A). Alterations in perfusion may be the result of changes in pulmonary artery pressure, alveolar pressure, or gravity. Alterations in ventilation may be due to airway obstruction, changes in lung compliance, and gravity.

A ventilation–perfusion imbalance, known as a ventilation–perfusion mismatch, occurs when there is inadequate ventilation, inadequate perfusion, or both. Three types of ventilation–perfusion imbalances may occur: low, high, and silent:

- *Low ventilation–perfusion ratio:* When perfusion exceeds ventilation, the ratio is low and a shunt is present. A shunt means that blood passes by an alveolus without gas exchange occurring. Severe hypoxia results when the amount of shunted blood exceeds 20%. A low ventilation–perfusion ratio is seen with pneumonia, atelectasis, tumor, or mucous plug (see Fig. 22–6B).
- *High ventilation–perfusion ratio:* When ventilation exceeds perfusion, dead space develops. The alveolus has inadequate perfusion available, and gas exchange cannot occur. A high ventilation–perfusion ratio is seen with a pulmonary embolus, pulmonary infarction, and cardiogenic shock (see Fig. 22–6C).
- *Silent unit:* When both ventilation and perfusion are decreased, a silent unit occurs. A silent unit is seen with pneumothorax and severe adult respiratory distress syndrome (see Fig. 22–6D).

Gas Transportation

PULMONARY MEMBRANE

The pulmonary membrane is composed of all the surfaces in the respiratory wall that are thin enough to permit the exchange of gases between the lungs and the blood. The total area of this membrane in the average normal adult male is about 60 m², or about the size of a moderate-sized classroom. It is 0.2 to 0.4 μ thick, or less than the thickness of the average red blood cell. These two outstanding fea-

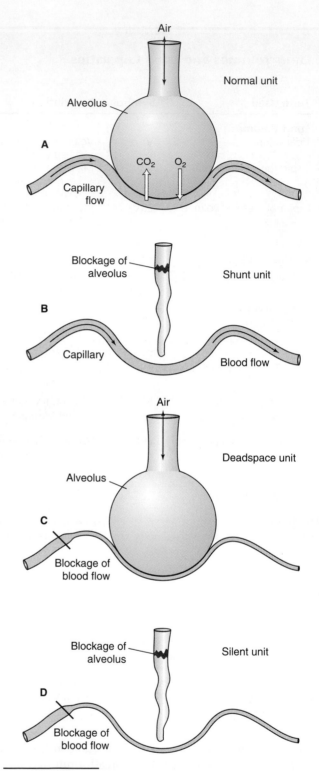

FIGURE 22-6

A schematic representation of various respiratory units showing ventilation–perfusion situations in (**A**) a normal unit with normal ventilation, normal perfusion; (**B**) a shunt unit with no ventilation, normal perfusion; (**C**) a dead space unit with normal ventilation, no perfusion, and (**D**) a silent unit with normal ventilation and no perfusion. (Source: Smeltzer SC, Bare BG: Brunner and Suddarth's Textbook of Medical-Surgical Nursing [8th Ed], p. 437. Philadelphia, Lippincott-Raven, 1996)

tures combine to allow large quantities of gases to diffuse across the pulmonary membrane in a very short time.

DIFFUSION

The factors that govern the rate of diffusion of the gases through the pulmonary membrane are as follows:

- The greater the pressure difference across the membrane, the faster the rate of diffusion.
- The larger the area of the pulmonary membrane, the larger the quantity of gas that can diffuse across the membrane in a given period.
- The thinner the membrane, the more rapid the diffusion of gases through it to the compartment on the opposite side.
- The diffusion coefficient is directly proportional to the solubility of the gas in the fluid of the pulmonary membrane and inversely proportional to molecular size. Therefore, small molecules that are highly soluble diffuse more rapidly than do large-molecular gases that are less soluble.

The diffusion coefficients are as follows:

- Oxygen: 1
- Carbon dioxide: 20.3
- Nitrogen: 0.53

The coefficients indicate that carbon dioxide is the most soluble and nitrogen the least soluble of these three gases. They are similar to one another with regard to molecular size but have quite different solubilities in the fluids of the pulmonary membrane. These differences account for the difference in the rate of diffusion of the gases through the pulmonary membrane.

TISSUE OXYGEN AND CARBON DIOXIDE

As oxygen diffuses from the lungs to the blood, a small portion of it becomes dissolved in the plasma and cell fluids, but more than 60 times as much combines immediately with hemoglobin. At a PO_2 of 100 mmHg, almost 96% of all hemoglobin molecules have combined with oxygen. This percentage represents the *saturation* of hemoglobin. Saturation is important because it reflects the oxygen available to tissues more accurately than the PaO_2. It is the oxygen carried on hemoglobin molecules that tissues can access, not the oxygen dissolved in the blood. Hemoglobin carries oxygen to the tissues. Here the oxygen is used by the cells, and carbon dioxide is formed.

As the carbon dioxide diffuses into the interstitial fluids, about 5% is dissolved in the blood, and the remainder diffuses into the red blood cells where one of two things occurs:

- Carbon dioxide combines with water to form carbonic acid and then reacts with the acid–base buffer and is transported as the bicarbonate ion.
- A small portion of the carbon dioxide combines with hemoglobin at a different bonding site from that of oxygen and is transported as carbaminohemoglobin.

Nitrogen diffuses from the alveolus into the blood. Because there is no carrier mechanism and under standard conditions nitrogen has only slight solubility in tissue fluid, it quickly establishes an equilibrium state on either side of the membrane and therefore is essentially inert. Concentration gradients are established that then foster the diffusion of these gases in the direction that is physiologically advantageous.

Factors affecting alveolar–capillary gas exchange are summarized in Table 22–2.

TABLE 22-2
Factors Affecting Alveolar–Capillary Gas Exchange

Factors Affecting Gas Exchange	Examples
Surface area available for diffusion	Removal of a lung or diseases such as emphysema and chronic bronchitis, which destroy lung tissue or cause mismatching of ventilation and perfusion
Thickness of the alveolar–capillary membrane	Conditions such as pneumonia, interstitial lung disease, and pulmonary edema, which increase membrane thickness
Partial pressure of alveolar gases	Ascent to high altitudes where the partial pressure of oxygen is reduced; in the opposite direction, increasing the partial pressure of a gas in the inspired air (eg, oxygen therapy) increases the gradient for diffusion.
Solubility and molecular weight of the gas	Carbon dioxide, which is more soluble in the cell membranes, diffuses across the alveolar–capillary membrane more rapidly than oxygen

Source: Porth CM: Pathophysiology: Concepts of Altered Health Studies (4th Ed), p 514. Philadelphia, JB Lippincott, 1994

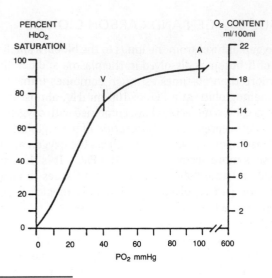

FIGURE 22-7

Normal oxyhemoglobin dissociation curve. Point *A* illustrates the relationship between the partial pressure of oxygen (PO_2) and the percentage of oxyhemoglobin saturation (SaO_2) in the lungs. Point *V* illustrates the same relationship in venous blood returning from the tissues.)

OXYHEMOGLOBIN DISSOCIATION CURVE

Adequate oxygenation of the tissues depends on the ability of the hemoglobin molecule to bind oxygen in the lungs and to release the oxygen as it is needed in the tissues. The term *affinity* is used to refer to the capacity of hemoglobin to combine with oxygen. Thus, when affinity is high, hemoglobin binds readily with oxygen. When affinity is low, hemoglobin releases oxygen more readily.

The oxyhemoglobin dissociation curve is a graphic depiction of the relationship between oxyhemoglobin saturation (the percent of hemoglobin combined with oxygen, SaO_2) and the oxygen tension (PaO_2) to which it is exposed. The influence of PaO_2 on saturation, or the attachment of oxygen to hemoglobin, is not a straight-line function. In other words, the relationship is not directly proportioned on a 1:1 basis. The initial part of the curve is very steep and then flattens at the top (Fig. 22–7). The flat portion represents the binding of oxygen to hemoglobin in the lungs. The steep portion of the curve (between 40 and 60 mmHg) represents the release of oxygen from the hemoglobin that occurs in the capillaries. At a PO_2 of 40, hemoglobin molecules are still about 70% to 75% saturated with oxygen. This provides a reserve supply of oxygen that can be given to the tissues in cases of emergency or strenuous exercise. Only about 25% to 30% of the arterial oxygen supply is used to meet tissue needs.

When the oxyhemoglobin dissociation curve shifts to the right (Fig. 22–8), there is reduced affinity of the hemoglobin for oxygen at any given PaO_2, resulting in more oxygen released to the tissues. Causes of a shift of the curve to the right include fever, acidosis, an increased $PaCO_2$ and a rise in 2,3-Diphosphoglycerate (2,3-DPG). 2,3-DPG is plentiful in red blood cells.

When the oxyhemoglobin dissociation curve shifts to the left (see Fig. 22–8), there is increased affinity of the hemoglobin for oxygen at any given PaO_2, resulting in less oxygen released to the tissues. This could cause tissue hypoxia even with an adequate PaO_2. Causes of a shift of the curve to the left include hypothermia, alkalosis, a decreased $PaCO_2$, and a drop in 2,3-DPG. In blood obtained from a blood bank, 2,3-DPG levels are low, thus reducing the ability of transfused blood to release O_2 to the tissues.

Regulation of Respiration

Breathing is controlled by both nervous system and chemical regulation. Nervous system regulation is achieved by the respiratory centers located in the medulla and pons that are part of the brain stem. Chemical regulation of breathing occurs due to the effect of blood pH and blood levels of oxygen and carbon dioxide.

BRAIN STEM CENTERS AND THE RESPIRATORY CYCLE

Unlike the heart, the lungs have no spontaneous rhythm. Ventilations depend on rhythmic operation of brain stem centers and intact pathways from there to the respiratory muscles. There are two centers in the medulla: a center that stimulates inspiration by diaphragmatic contraction (by way of phrenic nerves) and another center that innervates both inspiratory and expiratory intercostal and accessory muscles (Fig. 22–9).

The phrenic and intercostal nerves exit the spinal cord at C6, whereas motor nerves that supply accessory muscles

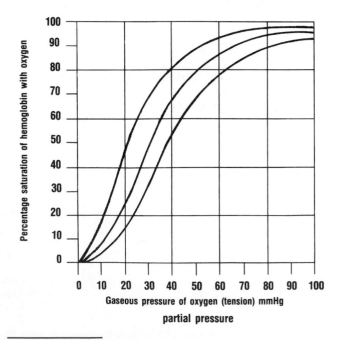

FIGURE 22-8

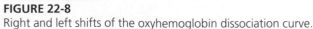

Right and left shifts of the oxyhemoglobin dissociation curve.

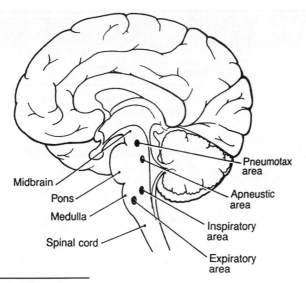

FIGURE 22-9

Location of respiratory centers in the brain. (Source: Bullock BL: Pathophysiology: Adaptations and Alteration in Function [4th Ed], p. 548. Philadelphia, Lippincott-Raven, 1996)

exit higher. This has implications for respiratory drive and efficacy in people with spinal cord injury.

The pons also contains two centers included in respiration. One is called the pneumotaxic center. The other, the apneustic center, produces sustained inspiration if stimulated. Voluntary control and involuntary control are further established by descending fibers from other brain centers. (These facilitate the alterations in respiration seen, for example, during swallowing, coughing, yawning, and willed action.)

In breathing at rest, the following sequence is thought to occur. The neurons innervating the inspiratory muscles fire bursts of impulses to these muscles, leading to inspiration. These neurons also stimulate the pneumotaxic center. This center, in turn, fires inhibitory impulses back to the inspiratory neurons, causing a halt in inspiration. Expiration follows passively. After expiration, the inspiratory neurons are again stimulated to fire automatically. During exercise or other occasions when more vigorous ventilation occurs, the expiratory neurons of the medulla are postulated to participate in this sequence, causing active exhalation.[3] A more comprehensive picture of the breathing process awaits further data.

CHEMICAL REGULATION

Respiratory centers in the medulla and pons and specialized sensory tissues in the aorta and carotids, called the aortic and carotid bodies, adjust respiratory rates and volumes (Fig. 22–10). Changes in PaO_2, $PaCO_2$, and pH stimulate all these areas.

Carbon dioxide in the blood dissociates into carbonic acid and then into hydrogen ion and bicarbonate. Hydrogen ion is a strong acid. Practitioners may find it most useful to think of carbon dioxide as an acid, regulated rapidly by the respiratory system.

If the blood carbon dioxide level rises (hypercapnia), the blood pH drops to acidic levels. Because carbon dioxide diffuses rapidly in fluids, it crosses to cerebrospinal fluid (CSF), and the CSF pH drops. Central chemoreceptors located in the medulla respond to the low pH by increasing, through medullary stimuli to the muscles of inspiration, both rate and volume. Cerebral vasodilation also occurs during acidosis, increasing the carbon dioxide supply to the CSF.

Low blood pH is most commonly due to hypercapnia, although blood pH can drop because of lactic acid production during anaerobic metabolism, or with renal disease causing hydrogen ion, potassium, and bicarbonate imbalances. A low blood pH is rapidly toxic to all chemical reactions of the body. This principle and the strength of the medullary response to hypercapnia illustrate the importance of carbon dioxide and hydrogen ion regulation to life processes.

Although aortic and carotid bodies respond to hypercapnia and low pH by increasing ventilation, their response is weak compared to medullary actions. Instead, these bodies respond strongly to hypoxia (decreased PaO_2). Hypoxia stimulates the carotid bodies, which signal the carotid sinus

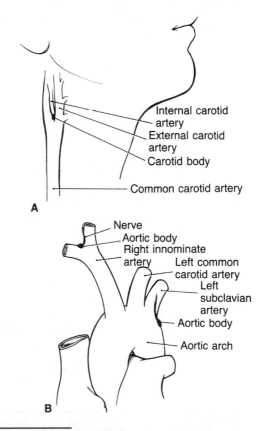

FIGURE 22-10

Location of peripheral chemoreceptors. (Source: Bullock BL: Pathophysiology: Adaptations and Alteration in Function [4th Ed], p. 549. Philadelphia, Lippincott-Raven, 1996)

TABLE 22-3
Peripheral Receptors and Their Regulatory Effect in Ventilation

Peripheral Receptor	Stimulus	Response
Pulmonary stretch receptors (Hering–Breuer reflex)	Lung distention	Vagal stimulus to medulla, causing increased expiratory time, leading to slowed rate
Irritant receptors in upper airways	Antigens such as pollen, histamine, and cold air	Vagal stimulus to bronchioles, causing bronchiolar constriction; important in asthma
Juxtacapillary receptors in alveolar walls	Pulmonary capillary distention, inhaled antigens, such as anesthetics	Vagal stimulus to medulla, causing increased rate and decreased depth; may lead to apnea
Gamma system receptors in intercostals and diaphragm	Muscle stretch	Increased stretch leads to increased contraction
Gamma receptors in joints and muscles	Muscle stretch	Afferent stimuli to medulla, causing increased rate and depth; important in exercise
Receptors in nose, nasopharynx, larynx	Antigens or mechanical irritants	Sneezing, coughing, laryngeal spasm, bronchoconstriction; important in airway defense

nerve. This nerve causes the medulla to increase ventilatory rate and depth. The aortic bodies respond somewhat more weakly than the carotid bodies but in the same way. Low PaO_2 stimulates the aortic bodies, which activate the vagus nerve, leading to the medullary increase in ventilation.

For people with chronically high levels of carbon dioxide, the hypercapnic drive to adjust carbon dioxide can be lost due to accommodation. In such people, changes in PaO_2, and the response of the carotid and aortic bodies, can provide the only stimulus to adjust ventilation. In people with chronically high $PaCO_2$ and low PaO_2, the medulla is depressed by hypercarbia. Therefore, the only stimulus for respirations is hypoxia. Administering oxygen to long-term hypercapnic and hypoxic patients can result in respiratory standstill or apnea.

Table 22–3 shows peripheral receptors and their regulatory effects on ventilation. Normally, peripheral receptors play a minor role in ventilation. Emotional stimuli commonly increase ventilation. Ventilatory rate and depth have been shown to increase before exercise, leading to the hypothesis that cognition of impending exercise affects the medulla.

The compensatory mechanisms discussed in this chapter illustrate the rapidity of the respiratory response to alterations in blood chemistry.

Clinical Applicability Challenges

Self-Challenge: Critical Thinking

1. Analyze the pulmonary function test results of a patient.
2. Interpret the patient's lung volume status and lung capacity status.

Study Questions

1. Which of the following is most likely to reduce lung compliance?
   a. Fibrotic lung disease
   b. Decreased pulmonary perfusion
   c. Increased oxygen consumption
   d. High levels of $PaCO_2$

2. Dead space in the lungs develops when
   a. the ventilation perfusion ratio is 1.
   b. the ventilation perfusion ratio is less than 1.
   c. the ventilation perfusion ratio is greater than 1.
   d. neither ventilation nor perfusion is normal.

3. The oxygen dissociation curve describes several factors that shift the curve to the right, decreasing the oxygen affinity for hemoglobin. These factors are
   a. tidal volume, functional residual volume, and anatomical dead space.
   b. pH, $PaCO_2$, and temperature.
   c. alveolar perfusion and diffusion gradients.
   d. alterations in barometric pressure.

4. The aortic and carotid bodies respond to hypercapnia by
   a. vasodilation of the pulmonary vasculature.
   b. vasoconstriction of the pulmonary vasculature.
   c. decreasing respiratory rate and depth.
   d. increasing respiratory rate and depth.

REFERENCES

1. Smeltzer SC, Bare BG: Brunner and Suddarth's Textbook of Medical-Surgical Nursing (8th Ed). Philadelphia, Lippincott-Raven, 1996
2. Bullock BL: Pathophysiology: Adaptations and Alteration in Function (4th Ed). Philadelphia, Lippincott-Raven, 1996
3. Scanlon VC, Sanders T: Essentials of Anatomy and Physiology. Philadelphia, FA Davis, 1995

BIBLIOGRAPHY

Applegate EJ: The Anatomy and Physiology Learning System. Philadelphia, WB Saunders, 1995

Guyton AC: Textbook of Medical Physiology (9th Ed). Philadelphia, WB Saunders, 1996

Hall-Craggs EC: Anatomy as a Basis for Clinical Medicine (3rd Ed). Baltimore, Williams and Wilkins, 1995

Huether SE, McCance KL: Understanding Pathophysiology. St. Louis, Mosby, 1996

Lindsay DT: Functional Human Anatomy. St. Louis, Mosby-Year Book, 1996

Memmler RL: Human Body in Health and Disease (8th Ed). Philadelphia, Lippincott-Raven, 1996

Porth CM: Pathophysiology: Concepts of Altered Health States (4th Ed). Philadelphia, JB Lippincott, 1994

Seeley RR, Stephens TD, Tate P: Essentials of Anatomy and Physiology (2nd Ed). St Louis, Mosby, 1996

Thibodeau GA, Patton KT: Anatomy and Physiology (2nd Ed). St. Louis, Mosby, 1993

Patient Assessment: Respiratory System

OBJECTIVES

Based on the content in this chapter, the reader should be able to:

- Describe the components of the history for respiratory assessment.
- Explain the use of inspection, palpation, percussion, and auscultation for respiratory assessment.
- Discuss the purpose of pulse oximetry.
- Compare and contrast the arterial oxygen saturation and the partial pressure of oxygen dissolved in arterial blood.
- Describe the purpose of end-tidal carbon dioxide monitoring.
- Explain the components of an arterial blood gas and the normal values for each component.
- Compare and contrast the causes, signs, and symptoms of respiratory acidosis, respiratory alkalosis, metabolic acidosis, and metabolic alkalosis.
- Analyze examples of an arterial blood gas result.
- Describe the purpose of mixed venous oxygen saturation monitoring.
- Discuss the purpose of respiratory diagnostic tests and associated nursing implications.

*N*urses contribute significantly to the care of patients with respiratory problems by taking a comprehensive history and performing a thorough physical examination. This information allows the nurse to establish a baseline level of assessment of the patient's status and provides a framework for detection of rapid changes in the patient's condition. Assessments are valuable if made before, during, and after interventions that are likely to alter or improve respiratory status. Because the nurse is with the patient more consistently than most other health care professionals, it is often the nurse who detects the patient's changing condition. Quality assessments often uncover complications or changes that precede the information provided by other diagnostic tests.

■■■■ HISTORY

The patient's history starts with information about the present illness. Often, if the patient is very ill, a relative or friend provides more information. Data about the present illness should include onset of the problem, its manifestations, and the outcomes of any attempts to treat the problem. Principle symptoms should be investigated in more detail and commonly include dyspnea, chest pain, sputum production, and cough.

DYSPNEA

If dyspnea is present, information about the onset of symptoms gives clues as to the source and duration of the problem. The nurse asks questions such as the following:

- Does the dyspnea occur when the patient is lying flat (therefore requiring the patient to sit up, as is seen more commonly in heart failure)?
- Does the dyspnea awaken the patient at night (paroxysmal nocturnal dyspnea)?
- Does the dyspnea occur only with exertion?

Paroxysmal nocturnal dyspnea and orthopnea often signify heart failure but can be seen in a variety of pulmonary disorders. The entire course of dyspnea should be described, including exacerbating factors, length of episodes, and relief measures attempted thus far.

CHEST PAIN

Dyspnea that occurs with primary lung disease is associated with an anterior chest discomfort that must be distinguished from angina. First, the nurse determines if the patient experiences more than one type of pain. For each type of chest pain, the nurse asks the patient to describe what makes the pain better or worse. For example, the pain may be worsened by breathing or movement (eg, in pleurisy) or be relieved by position changes or movement. The nurse inquires about the outcome of relief measures that have been used (eg, over-the-counter drugs, prescription drugs, rest, nitroglycerin, antacids, or belching). In addition, the nurse asks about the quality of the pain, where the pain radiates, the severity of the pain, the duration of the pain, and other associated symptoms.

SPUTUM PRODUCTION

A pulmonary illness often results in the production (or a change in the production) of sputum. The nurse questions the patient about the amount (eg, a tablespoonful, one-half cup) and color of the sputum produced in 24 hours. The color of the sputum provides important information about infection. Yellow, green, or brown sputum typically signifies bacterial infection; clear or white sputum may indicate absence of bacterial infection. The color comes from white blood cells in the sputum. However, a yellow color can occur if there are many eosinophils in the sputum, thereby signifying allergy rather than infection. An increase in either the color or the amount of sputum often means infection.

Sometimes in infections, the patient is unable to cough up the sputum; a decrease in sputum production associated with worsening hypoxemia can signify bronchiolitis. Usually, though, cough without sputum production means that the problem is not bacterial in origin. It is important to know if the mucus production comes from the nose, the chest, or sinus postnasal drainage.

Sometimes the patient is afraid to mention if there has been blood in the sputum, so it is essential to ask the patient, family members, or caregivers about the presence of blood. The amount of blood should be evaluated. Was it just streaks or specks, blood-colored mucus, or pure blood (bright red or dark)? Through careful questioning, the nurse determines if the blood is associated with retching and vomiting or sputum production, as it often is in bronchitis and pneumonia, or whether it occurs alone, as is often the case with a pulmonary embolus.

COUGH

A cough is a frequent respiratory symptom with varying significance. A cough can be stimulated by external agents, from inflammation of the respiratory mucosa, or from pressure on an airway caused by a tumor. Information obtained from the patient about the cough should include onset, precipitating factors, timing, frequency, and whether the cough is productive.

HEALTH HISTORY

Information obtained from the health history is also important in the comprehensive assessment of the patient. These data should include environmental exposure and risk factors, past surgical and medical history, and family history. The patient's use of tobacco should be quantified by amount and how long the patient smoked.

◼ PHYSICAL EXAMINATION

Physical assessment of the respiratory system is a reliable means of gathering essential data and is guided by the information obtained through the history. A thorough physical assessment includes inspection, palpation, percussion, and auscultation.

Inspection

Inspection of the patient involves checking for the presence or absence of several factors.

Cyanosis refers to a bluish discoloration of the skin or mucous membranes. Cyanosis is notoriously hard to detect if the patient is anemic. The patient who is polycythemic can have cyanosis in the extremities even if oxygen tension is normal. Peripheral cyanosis occurs in the extremities or on the tip of the nose or ears. Even with normal oxygen tensions, peripheral cyanosis may appear if there is diminished blood flow to these areas, particularly if they are cold or in a dependent position. Central cyanosis is observed on the tongue or lips and usually means the patient has low oxygen tension. Unfortunately, the presence of cyanosis is a late and often ominous sign.

Labored breathing is an important marker of respiratory distress. As part of the inspection, the nurse determines if the patient is using the accessory muscles of respiration (the scalene and sternomastoid muscles). *Intercostal retractions* (ie, sucking in of the muscles and skin between the ribs during inspiration) usually means that the patient is making a larger effort at inspiration than normal. The nurse also observes the patient for use of the abdominal muscles during the usually passive expiratory phase. Labored breathing may be accompanied by staccato speech, in which the patient's speech pattern is frequently interrupted as the patient gulps for air. Sometimes, the number of words a patient can say before having to gasp for another breath is a good measure of the amount of labored breathing.

An increase in the anteroposterior (AP) diameter of the chest (ie, an increase in the size of the chest from front to back) also is checked. An increased AP diameter often is caused by overexpansion of the lungs from obstructive pulmonary disease; an increase in AP diameter also can be found in patients with kyphosis (curvature of the spine).

Chest deformities and scars are important in helping determine the reason for respiratory distress. A chest deformity, such as kyphoscoliosis or flail chest from trauma, can indicate why the patient has respiratory distress. A scar may signify recent or old injuries to the chest and provide clues to possible sources of distress. For example, there may be evidence of recent trauma to the chest, such as a stabbing or compression injuries from an automobile collision, which could be responsible for the present distress.

The patient's posture must be observed. Patients with obstructive pulmonary disease often sit and prop themselves up on outstretched arms or lean forward with their elbows on a table in an effort to elevate their clavicles. This posture gives the patient a slightly greater ability to expand the chest.

The position of the trachea is important to observe. The nurse determines if the trachea is in the midline as it should be, or if it is deviated off to one side. Pleural effusion, hemothorax, pneumothorax, or a tension pneumothorax can deviate the trachea away from the affected side (toward the opposite side). With atelectasis, fibrosis, and phrenic nerve paralysis, however, the trachea often is pulled toward the affected side. Table 23–1 summarizes significant signs during physical examination.

The respiratory rate is an important parameter to follow. It should be counted over at least a 15-second period for stable patients and over a full minute for critically ill patients. The patient's rate must be compared with his or her usual rate. Breathing 24 to 26 times a minute may be normal for one patient, but it may be abnormal for another patient. The patient's family or friends may provide additional important information about the patient's usual rate of breathing.

The depth of respiration often is as meaningful as the respiratory rate. For instance, if a patient is breathing 40 times per minute, the nurse might think a severe respiratory problem is the source of patient distress. However, the rate may be the result of Kussmaul respirations caused by diabetic acidosis. If a patient's respiration is shallow at a rate of 40 times per minute, the indication may be severe respiratory distress from a primary pulmonary problem. Deep and rapid respirations may indicate compensation for acidosis. The pattern of respirations is also noted because the pattern may correlate with various disease processes.

The duration of inspiration versus the duration of expiration helps determine the presence of obstructive lung disease. In patients with any of the obstructive lung diseases, expiration is more than 1½ times as long as inspiration.

Observation of *general chest expansion* is an integral part of examining a patient. Normally, about a 3-inch expansion of the chest occurs from maximal expiration to maximal inspiration. Motion of the abdomen in breathing efforts (normal in men more than women) may be observed. Ankylosing spondylitis is a condition in which general chest expansion is limited. During the inspection, the nurse compares the expansion of the upper chest with that of the lower chest. The nurse also observes the movement of the diaphragm to determine whether the patient with obstructive pulmonary disease is concentrating on expanding the lower chest and using the diaphragm properly. Expansion of one side of the chest versus the other side is important to note because atelectasis, especially that caused by a mucous plug, can cause unilaterally diminished chest expansion because the air is unable to move equally through the pulmonary bed. Abnormal chest expansion can also occur with flail chest, where the chest collapses instead of expanding during inspiration. Flail chest can result from broken or fractured ribs that are unable to maintain the integrity of the chest wall during respiration. The nurse also notes the patient's symmetry of respiratory effort by observing if the abdomen and chest rise and fall together as they should or if the effort is not coordinated. Asynchronous respiratory effort decreases the quality of respiration at the cost of increased work of breathing. Asynchronous respiratory effort often precedes the need for ventilatory support.

A pulmonary embolus, pneumonia, pleural effusion, pneumothorax, or any problem associated with chest pain, such as fractured ribs, can lead to diminished chest expansion. An endotracheal or nasotracheal tube positioned beyond the trachea into one of the main stem bronchi (usually the right) is a serious cause of diminished expansion of one side of the chest. If the tube slips into the right main stem bronchus, the left lung is not expanded, and the patient may develop atelectasis on the left side and hypoxemia.

Palpation

Chest palpation can indicate lung or chest abnormalities. Palpation of the chest is done by placing the hand flat against the patient's chest. Sounds are generated by the larynx when a patient speaks, and these sounds travel along the bronchial tree, resulting in a resonant motion of the chest wall. *Tactile fremitus* is the ability to feel the sound on the chest wall. Tactile fremitus is more easily palpated

TABLE 23-1
Physical Examination Signs in Selected Respiratory Disorders

Condition	Trachea	Percussion Note	Breath Sounds	Tactile Fremitus and Transmitted Voice Sounds	Adventitious Sounds
Normal	Midline	Resonant	Vesicular, except perhaps bronchovesicular and bronchial sounds over the large bronchi and trachea, respectively	Normal	None, except perhaps a few transient inspiratory crackles at the bases of the lungs
Chronic bronchitis	Midline	Resonant	Normal	Normal	None or scattered coarse crackles in early inspiration and perhaps expiration; or wheezes or rhonchi
Consolidation	Midline	Dull over the airless area	Bronchial over the involved area	Increased over the involved area with bronchophony, egophony, and whispered pectoriloquy	Late inspiratory crackles over the involved area
Atelectasis	May be shifted toward the involved side	Dull over the airless area	Usually absent when the bronchial plug persists; exceptions—right upper lobe atelectasis, where adjacent tracheal sounds may be transmitted	Usually absent when the bronchial plug persists; exceptions (eg, right upper lobe atelectasis), may be increased	None
Pleural effusion	Toward the opposite side in a large effusion	Dull to flat over the fluid	Decreased to absent, but bronchial breath sounds possibly heard near the top of a large effusion	Decreased to absent, but may be increased toward the top of a large effusion	None, except a possible pleural rub
Pneumothorax	Toward the opposite side if much air	Hyper-resonant or tympanitic over the pleural air	Decreased to absent over the pleural air	Decreased to absent over the pleural air	None, except a possible pleural rub
Emphysema	Midline	Diffusely hyper-resonant	Decreased to absent	Decreased	None, or the crackles, wheezes, and rhonchi of associated chronic bronchitis
Asthma	Midline	Normal to diffusely hyper-resonant	Often obscured by wheezes	Decreased	Wheezes, possibly crackles

Adapted from Bates B: A Guide to Physical Examination and History Taking (6th Ed), pp 256–257. Philadelphia, Lippincott-Raven, 1995

over the large bronchi and is more difficult to palpate over the distant lung fields.

To assess tactile fremitus, the nurse asks the patient to say "ninety-nine" as the nurse moves his or her hands over the posterior surfaces of the chest wall. Tactile fremitus should be symmetrical. Tactile fremitus can be diminished or absent if there is an increase in air per unit volume of lung because air impedes the transmission of sound. For example, patients with emphysema will have little or no tactile fremitus on physical examination. Tactile fremitus is slightly increased by the presence of solid substances, such as the consolidation of a lung due to pneumonia. Other respiratory conditions causing an alteration in tactile fremitus are listed in Table 23–1.

Palpation is also used to assess for subcutaneous emphysema, a condition in which air "leaks" out of the alveolus and moves through the subcutaneous tissue. By moving the fingers in a gentle rolling motion across the chest and neck, it is possible to feel the pockets of air underneath the skin. Feeling subcutaneous emphysema is often likened to the "crunch" of Rice Krispies under the skin. Subcutaneous emphysema may result from a pneumothorax, small pockets of alveoli that have burst with increased pulmonary pressure, or the use of positive end-expiratory pressure. In severe cases, the subcutaneous emphysema may spread into the lower thorax, arms, and face.

Percussion

Percussion of the chest results in slight motion of the chest wall and underlying structures resulting in audible and tactile vibrations. When percussing a patient's chest, one finger is pressed flat against the chest, and a fingertip from the dominant hand is used to strike the knuckle pressed against the chest. Normally, the chest has a resonant or hollow percussion note. In diseases in which there is increased air in the chest or lungs, such as pneumothorax and emphysema, there can be hyper-resonant percussion notes. These loud, low-pitched sounds, however, are sometimes hard to detect.

More important is a flat percussion note (such as is heard when percussing over a part of the body that contains no air). A flat percussion note is a soft, high-pitched sound that is more obvious in its presentation. If the lung underneath the examining hand has a large pleural effusion, a flat to dull percussion note is likely to be heard. A dull percussion note is medium in intensity and pitch, and is heard with atelectasis or consolidation from pneumonia, pulmonary edema, or pulmonary hemorrhage. A tympanic drumlike sound is a high-pitched noise heard with asthma or a large pneumothorax. See Table 23–1 for a description of percussion sounds associated with various respiratory pathologies.

Auscultation

In chest auscultation, the diaphragm of the stethoscope is pressed firmly against the chest wall. The nurse listens to the intensity or loudness of breath sounds. Normally there is a fourfold increase in loudness of breath sounds when a patient takes a maximum deep breath as opposed to quiet breathing. Sounds are louder in the upper and central chest when listening to the larger bronchus and become quieter as the smaller airways are auscultated. The intensity of the breath sounds can be diminished because of decreased flow through the airways or the presence of substances between the lungs and the stethoscope. In pleural thickening, pleural effusion, pneumothorax, and obesity, there is an abnormal substance (fibrous tissue, fluid, air, or fat) between the stethoscope and the underlying lung; this substance insulates the breath sounds from the stethoscope, making the breath sounds seem less loud. In airway obstruction, such as chronic obstructive pulmonary disease or atelectasis, the intensity of breath sounds is diminished. With shallow breathing, there is diminished air movement through the airways, and the breath sounds are not as loud. With restricted movement of the thorax or diaphragm, there will be diminished breath sounds in the restricted areas.

Generally, four types of sounds are heard in the normal chest:

- Vesicular breath sounds, which are heard over most of the lung fields
- Bronchovesicular breath sounds, which are heard over the bronchi on either side of the sternum and between the scapulae posteriorly
- Bronchial breath sounds, which are heard over the manubrium
- Tracheal breath sounds, which are heard over the trachea in the neck

Vesicular breath sounds are quiet, low-pitched sounds and have an inspiratory phase that is longer than the expiratory phase. *Bronchovesicular breath sounds* are medium in pitch and have equal inspiratory and expiratory phases. *Bronchial breath sounds* are higher pitched and louder when compared with vesicular sounds. Bronchial sounds have a longer expiratory than inspiratory phase. *Tracheal breath sounds* are loud, high-pitched sounds with about equal inspiratory and expiratory phases. Table 23–2 explains the characteristics of breath sounds.

Not only are bronchial breath sounds heard over the manubrium of the normal person, but they are also heard when there is consolidation, as seen with pneumonia. Bronchial breath sounds are also heard above a pleural effusion in which the normal lung is compressed and sounds are transmitted through the tissue, which is not participating in airflow. Wherever there is bronchial breathing, there may be two associated changes also: E to A changes and whispered pectoriloquy.

An *E to A change* means that when the nurse listens with a stethoscope and the patient says "E," what is heard is actually an A sound rather than an E sound. This occurs if there is consolidation. Egophony is the term used to describe voice sounds that are distorted.

Whispered pectoriloquy is the presence of loud, clear sounds heard through the stethoscope when the patient

TABLE 23-2
Characteristics of Breath Sounds

	Duration of Sounds	Intensity of Expiratory Sound	Pitch of Expiratory Sound	Locations Where Heard Normally
Vesicular*	Inspiratory sounds last longer than expiratory ones.	Soft	Relatively low	Over most of both lungs
Bronchovesicular	Inspiratory and expiratory sounds are about equal.	Intermediate	Intermediate	Often in the first and second interspaces anteriorly and between the scapulae
Bronchial	Expiratory sounds last longer than inspiratory ones.	Loud	Relatively high	Over the manubrium, if heard at all
Tracheal	Inspiratory and expiratory sounds are about equal.	Very loud	Relatively high	Over the trachea in the neck

*The thickness of the bars indicates intensity; the steeper their incline, the higher the pitch.
Source: Bates B: A Guide to Physical Examination and History Taking (6th Ed), p 245. Philadelphia, Lippincott-Raven, 1995

whispers. Normally the whispered voice is heard faintly and indistinctly through the stethoscope. The increased transmission of voice sounds indicates that air in the lungs has been replaced by fluid as a result of pneumonia, pulmonary edema, or hemorrhage.

Additional breath sounds heard with auscultation are known as *adventitious sounds* and include discontinuous sounds, continuous sounds, and rubs. Discontinuous sounds are brief, nonmusical, intermittent sounds and include fine and course crackles. Crackles were formerly known as rales. Fine crackles are soft, high-pitched very brief popping sounds that occur most commonly during inspiration. Crackles result from fluid in the airways or alveoli, or from the opening of collapsed alveoli. Restrictive pulmonary disease results in crackles during late inspiration, whereas obstructive pulmonary disease results in crackles during early inspiration. Crackles become more coarse as the air moves through larger fluid accumulations, such as in bronchitis or pneumonia. Crackles that clear with coughing are not associated with significant pulmonary pathology. When assessing crackles, the nurse also notes their loudness, pitch, duration, amount, location, and timing in the respiratory cycle.[1] Continuous adventitious breath sounds are longer in duration than crackles, and include wheezes and rhonchi. Wheezes are continuous musical sounds that are longer than crackles in duration and persist throughout the respiratory cycle. Wheezes (also known as sibilant wheezes) are a continuous adventitious sound that are high pitched and have a shrill quality. Wheezes are caused by the movement of air through a narrowed or partially obstructed airway, as in asthma, chronic obstructive pulmonary disease, or bronchitis.[1]

Rhonchi, another type of continuous adventitious breath sound, are deep, low-pitched rumbling noises that are sometimes referred to as sonorous wheezes or gurgles. The presence of rhonchi indicate the presence of secretions in the large airways.[1]

A friction rub is a crackling, grating sound heard in both inspiration and expiration that results from the visceral and parietal pleura rubbing against each other. A friction rub can be heard with pleural effusion, pneumothorax, or pleurisy.

RESPIRATORY MONITORING

Pulse Oximetry

Approximately 3% of oxygen is dissolved in the plasma. The partial pressure of oxygen dissolved in the arterial blood is measured by the PaO_2. The normal PaO_2 is 80 to 100 mmHg at sea level. The remaining 97% of oxygen is attached to hemoglobin molecules in red blood cells. Each gram of hemoglobin can carry a maximum of 1.34 mL of oxygen. The percentage of saturation of hemoglobin is defined as the amount of oxygen that hemoglobin is carrying compared with the amount of oxygen that hemoglobin (Hgb) can carry, expressed as a percentage:

Percentage O_2 saturation of Hgb =
$$\frac{\text{Amount } O_2 \text{ Hgb is carrying}}{\text{Amount } O_2 \text{ Hgb can carry}} \times 100$$

Because the amount of oxygen that Hgb can carry is a constant 1.34 mL/g,

$$1.34 \text{ mL/g} \times \text{g Hgb} \times \% \text{ saturation Hgb}$$
$$= \text{No. of mL of O}_2 \text{ that Hgb is carrying}$$

The arterial oxygen saturation of hemoglobin is known as the SaO_2. The normal SaO_2 ranges from 93% to 99% (Table 23–3).

The relationship between PO_2 and SaO_2 is depicted by the oxyhemoglobin dissociation curve (Fig. 23–1). The initial part of the curve is very steep and flattens at the top. The flattened part means that large changes in the PO_2 result in only small changes in SaO_2. A critical point of the curve occurs when the PO_2 drops below 60 mmHg. At this point, the curve drops sharply, meaning that a small decrease in PO_2 is associated with a large decrease in SaO_2.

When the curve shifts to the right, there is a reduced capacity for hemoglobin to combine with oxygen, resulting in more oxygen released to the tissues. When the curve shifts to the left, there is an increased capacity for hemoglobin to combine with oxygen, resulting in less oxygen released to the tissues. For a more detailed discussion of the oxyhemoglobin dissociation curve, see Chapter 22.

A pulse oximeter is a device used to measure a value known as SpO_2 and reflects the arterial oxygen saturation of hemoglobin (Fig. 23–2). Through oximetry, light-emitting and light-receiving sensors quantify the amount of light absorbed by oxygenated/deoxygenated hemoglobin in arterial blood. Usually, the sensors are in a clip placed on a finger or ear lobe, and allow for evaluation of the quality of the pulsatile waveform. An oximeter reading should not be used to replace arterial blood gas (ABG) monitoring. Instead, pulse oximetry may be used as a trending device when the correlation between arterial blood and pulse oximetry reading has been established. Values obtained by pulse oximetry are unreliable when using vasoconstricting medications or intravenous administration of dyes and in people with shock, cardiac arrest, severe anemia, and high carbon monoxide levels.

End-Tidal Carbon Dioxide Monitoring

At the end of exhalation, the percentage of arterial carbon dioxide dissolved in the blood ($PaCO_2$) approximates the percentage of alveolar CO_2. Therefore, samples of exhaled

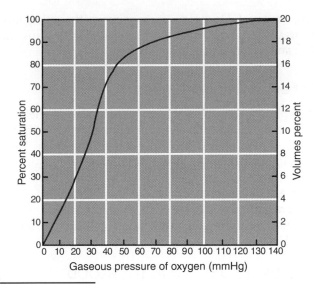

FIGURE 23-1
The oxyhemoglobin dissociation curve.

CO_2 measured at the end of exhalation ($PETCO_2$) can be used to approximate levels of alveolar CO_2. Levels of alveolar CO_2 and arterial CO_2 are similar; therefore, samples of exhaled CO_2 measured at the end of expiration ($PETCO_2$) can be used to estimate $PaCO_2$.

Although the values are similar, $PETCO_2$ values are usually lower than the $PaCO_2$ levels. Research also indicates that the two values tend to move in opposite directions about 22% of the time.[2] $PETCO_2$ values are obtained by monitoring samples of expired gas from an endotracheal tube, an oral airway, or a nasopharyngeal airway. Because $PETCO_2$ provides continuous estimates of alveolar ventila-

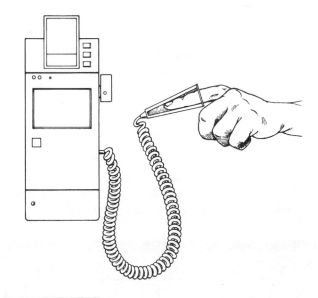

FIGURE 23-2
Pulse oximetry monitor. (Source: Fuller J, Schaller-Ayres J: Health Assessment: A Nursing Approach [2nd Ed]. Philadelphia, JB Lippincott, 1994)

TABLE 23-3
How Oxygen Is Carried in the Blood

Oxygen dissolved in the plasma measured as PaO_2	0.3 mL/100 mL of blood
Oxygen combined with hemoglobin measured as SaO_2	19.4 mL/100 mL of blood
Total oxygen in blood	19.7 mL/100 mL of blood

tion, it is a useful technique for monitoring the patient during weaning from a ventilator, cardiopulmonary resuscitation, and endotracheal intubation.

Arterial Blood Gases

A sample of arterial blood is drawn and analyzed to help determine the quality and extent of pulmonary gas exchange and acid–base status. The ABG test measures the PaO_2, SaO_2, $PaCO_2$, pH, and bicarbonate (HCO_3).

The procedure involves obtaining arterial blood from a direct arterial puncture or from an arterial line often placed in the radial artery. More recent technology allows the continuous monitoring of ABGs using a fiberoptic sensor placed in the artery.

MEASURING OXYGEN IN THE BLOOD

Oxygenation can be evaluated through an ABG by evaluating the partial pressure of oxygen dissolved in the arterial blood (PaO_2) and the arterial oxygen saturation of hemoglobin (SaO_2). As mentioned previously, only 3% of oxygen is dissolved in the arterial blood, and the remaining 97% is attached to hemoglobin in the red blood cells. The normal PaO_2 is 80 to 100 mmHg at sea level (barometric pressure 760 mmHg). For people living at higher altitudes, the normal PaO_2 is lower because of a lower barometric pressure. The PaO_2 value tends to decrease with age. For patients who are 60 to 80 years old, it is normal to have a PaO_2 of 60 to 80 mmHg. An abnormally low PaO_2 is referred to as hypoxemia. Hypoxemia may result from many conditions, which are most commonly grouped according to their origin: intrapulmonary (disturbances within the lung), intracardiac (disturbance of flow to or from the heart, which impedes pulmonary flow or function), or perfusion deficits (inadequate perfusion of the lung tissues, which causes decreased oxygen uptake from the alveoli).

The normal SaO_2 ranges between 93% to 97%. SaO_2 is an important oxygenation value to assess because most oxygen supplied to tissues is carried by hemoglobin. Normal values are given in the accompanying display.

MEASURING PH IN THE BLOOD

The pH is a measure of the hydrogen ion concentration in the blood and provides information about the acidity or alkalinity of the blood. A normal pH is 7.35 to 7.45. As hydrogen ions accumulate, the pH drops, resulting in acidemia. Acid*emia*

> **Normal Values for an Arterial Blood Gas**
>
> PaO_2: 80–100 mmHg
> SaO_2: 93%–99%
> pH: 7.35–7.45
> $PaCO_2$: 35–45 mmHg
> HCO_3: 22–26 mEq/L

> ## Clinical Terminology: Acid–Base
>
> Acid: A substance that can donate hydrogen ions (H^+).
> Example: H_2CO_3 (an acid) $\rightarrow H^+ + HCO_3$
> Base: A substance that can accept hydrogen ions, H^+; All bases are alkaline substances. Example: HCO_3 (base) $+ H^+ \rightarrow H_2CO_3$
> Acidemia: Acid condition of the blood in which the pH is <7.35
> Alkalemia: Alkaline condition of the blood in which the pH is >7.45
> Acidosis: The process causing acidemia
> Alkalosis: The process causing alkalemia

---

refers to a condition in which the *blood* is too acidic. Acido*sis* refers to the *process* that caused the acidemia.

A decrease in hydrogen ions results in an elevation of the pH and alkalemia. Alkalemia refers to a condition in which the blood is too alkaline. Alkal*osis* refers to the *process* that causes the alkal*emia*. The display lists terms in acid–base balance.

Acids

An acid is a substance that can donate a hydrogen ion (H^+) to a solution. There are two different types of acids: volatile acids and nonvolatile acids.

Volatile acids are those that can move between the liquid and gaseous states. Once in the gaseous state, these acids can be removed by the lungs. The major acid in the blood serum is carbonic acid (H_2CO_3). This acid is broken down into CO_2 and H_2O by an enzyme produced in the kidneys.

Nonvolatile acids are those that cannot change into a gaseous form and therefore cannot be excreted by the lungs. They can only be excreted by the kidneys (a metabolic process). Examples of nonvolatile acids are lactic acid and ketoacids.

An acid–base disorder can be either respiratory or metabolic in origin. An excess of either kind of acid results in acidemia. If CO_2 accumulates, then respiratory acidosis exists. If nonvolatile acids accumulate, then metabolic acidosis exists.

Alkalemia may be the result of losing too many acids from the serum. If too much CO_2 is lost, the result is respiratory alkalosis. If there are less than normal amounts of nonvolatile acids, the result is metabolic alkalosis.

Bases

A base is a substance that can accept a hydrogen ion, thereby removing it from the circulating serum. The main base found within the serum is bicarbonate (HCO_3). The amount of bicarbonate that is available in the serum is regulated by the kidney (a metabolic process). If there is too little bicarbonate within the serum, the result is metabolic acidosis. If there is too much bicarbonate in the serum, the result is metabolic alkalosis.

Conditions leading to acidemia or alkalemia are influenced by a multitude of physiological processes. Some of these processes include respiratory and renal function or dysfunction, tissue oxygenation, circulation, lactic acid production, substance ingestion, and electrolyte loss from the gastrointestinal tract. The identification of a pH variance should lead to the investigation of possible contributing factors. Table 23–4 lists the possible causes and signs and symptoms of acid–base imbalances.

MEASURING CARBON DIOXIDE IN THE BLOOD

The $PaCO_2$ refers to the pressure or tension exerted by dissolved CO_2 gas in arterial blood. CO_2 is the natural byproduct of cellular metabolism. CO_2 levels are regulated pri-

RED FLAG **Table 23-4** Possible Causes and Signs and Symptoms of Acid–Base Disorders

Condition	Possible Causes	Signs and Symptoms

Respiratory Acidosis
$PaCO_2 > 45$ mmHg
pH < 7.35
	Central nervous system depression
	  Head trauma
	  Oversedation
	  Anesthesia
	  High cord injury
	Pneumothorax
	Hypoventilation
	Bronchial obstruction and atelectasis
	Severe pulmonary infections
	Heart failure and pulmonary edema
	Massive pulmonary embolus
	Myasthenia gravis
	Multiple sclerosis
		Dyspnea
		Restlessness
		Headache
		Tachycardia
		Confusion
		Lethargy
		Dysrhythmias
		Respiratory distress
		Drowsiness
		Decreased responsiveness

Respiratory Alkalosis $PaCO_2 < 35$ mmHg pH > 7.45	Anxiety and nervousness Fear Pain Hyperventilation Fever Thyrotoxicosis Central nervous system lesions Salicylates Gram-negative septicemia Pregnancy	Light-headedness Confusion Decreased concentration Paresthesias Tenatic spasms in the arms and legs Cardiac dysrhythmias Palpitations Sweating Dry mouth Blurred vision

Metabolic Acidosis
$HCO_3 < 22$ mEq/L
pH < 7.35
	Increased acids
	  Renal failure
	  Ketoacidosis
	  Anaerobic metabolism
	  Starvation
	  Salicylate intoxication
	Loss of base
	  Diarrhea
	  Intestinal fistulas
		Headache
		Confusion
		Restlessness
		Lethargy
		Weakness
		Stupor/coma
		Kussmaul respiration
		Nausea and vomiting
		Dysrhythmias
		Warm flushed skin

Metabolic Alkalosis
$HCO_3 > 26$ mEq/L
pH > 7.45
	Gain of base
	  Excess use of bicarbonate
	  Lactate administration in dialysis
	  Excess ingestion of antacids
	Loss of acids
	  Vomiting
	  Nasogastric suctioning
	  Hypokalemia
	  Hypochloremia
	  Administration of diuretics
	  Increased levels of aldosterone
		Muscle twitching and
		  cramps
		Tetany
		Dizziness
		Lethargy
		Weakness
		Disorientation
		Convulsions
		Coma
		Nausea and vomiting
		Depressed respiration

marily by the ventilatory function of the lung. The normal $PaCO_2$ is 35 to 45 mmHg. In interpretation of ABGs, $PaCO_2$ is thought of as an "acid." Elimination of CO_2 from the body is one of the main functions of the lungs, and an important relationship exists between the amount of ventilation and the amount of CO_2 in blood.

If a patient hypoventilates, CO_2 will accumulate, and the $PaCO_2$ value will rise above the upper limit of 45 mmHg. The retention of CO_2 results in respiratory acidosis. Respiratory acidosis can occur even with normal lungs if the respiratory center is depressed and the respiratory rate or quality is insufficient to maintain normal carbon dioxide concentrations.

If a patient hyperventilates, CO_2 will be eliminated from the body, and the $PaCO_2$ value will drop below the lower limit of 35 mmHg. The loss of CO_2 results in respiratory alkalosis.

MEASURING BICARBONATE IN THE BLOOD

Bicarbonate (HCO_3), the main base found within the serum, helps the body to regulate pH because of its ability to accept a hydrogen ion (H^+). The concentration of HCO_3 is regulated by the kidneys and is referred to as a metabolic process of regulation. The normal HCO_3 level is 22 to 26 mEq/L. HCO_3 can be thought of as a "base" (alkaline). When the HCO_3 level increases above 26 mEq/L, a metabolic alkalosis exists. Metabolic alkalosis results from a gain of base (alkaline) substances or a loss of metabolic acids. When the HCO_3 level decreases below 22 mEq/L, a metabolic acidosis exits. Metabolic acidosis results from a loss of base (alkaline) substances or a gain of metabolic acids.

ALTERATIONS IN ACID–BASE BALANCE

Disturbances in acid–base balance result from an abnormality of the metabolic or respiratory system. If the respiratory system is responsible, it is detected by the CO_2 in the serum. If the metabolic system is responsible, it is detected by the HCO_3 in the serum.

Respiratory Acidosis

Respiratory acidosis is defined as a $PaCO_2$ greater than 45 mmHg with a pH of less than 7.35. Respiratory acidosis is characterized by inadequate elimination of CO_2 by the lungs and may be the result of inefficient pulmonary function or excessive production of CO_2.

Respiratory Alkalosis

Respiratory alkalosis is defined as a $PaCO_2$ less than 35 mmHg with a pH of greater than 7.45. Respiratory alkalosis is characterized by excessive elimination of CO_2 from the serum.

Metabolic Acidosis

Metabolic acidosis is defined as an HCO_3 of less than 22 mEq/L with a pH of less than 7.35. Metabolic acidosis is characterized by an excessive production of nonvolatile acids or an inadequate concentration of HCO_3 for the concentration of acid within the serum.

Metabolic Alkalosis

Metabolic alkalosis is defined as an HCO_3 of greater than 26 mEq/L with a pH of greater than 7.45. Metabolic al-

CLINICAL APPLICATION:
Nursing Intervention Guidelines
Interpretation of an Arterial Blood Gas

1. Evaluate oxygenation by examining the PaO_2 and the SaO_2.
2. Evaluate the pH. Is it acidotic, alkalotic, or normal?
3. Evaluate the $PaCO_2$. Is it high, low, or normal?
4. Evaluate the HCO_3. Is it high, low, or normal?
5. Determine if compensation is occurring. Is it complete, partial, or uncompensated?

kalosis is characterized by excessive loss of nonvolatile acids or excessive production of HCO_3.

INTERPRETING ARTERIAL BLOOD GAS RESULTS

Evaluate Oxygenation

The first step in ABG analysis is to examine the patient's oxygenation status by evaluating the PaO_2 and the SaO_2. If the PaO_2 value is less than the patient's norm, hypoxemia exists. If the SaO_2 is less than 93%, inadequate amounts of oxygen are bound to hemoglobin.

Evaluate Acid–Base Status

An examination of the arterial pH is the first step in evaluating the acid–base status. If the pH is less than 7.35, acidemia exists. If the pH is greater than 7.45, alkalemia exists.

The second step in measuring acid–base balance is an evaluation of the $PaCO_2$. A $PaCO_2$ of less than 35 mmHg indicates a respiratory acidosis, whereas a $PaCO_2$ of greater than 45 mmHg signifies a respiratory alkalosis.

An evaluation of the HCO_3 level is the third step in acid–base analysis. If the HCO_3 value is less than 22 mEq/L, metabolic acidosis is present. If the HCO_3 value is greater than 26 mEq/L, metabolic alkalosis exists. ABG examples are given in the display.

Examples of Arterial Blood Gases

Sample blood gas: Case 1

PaO_2	80 mmHg	Normal
SaO_2	95%	Normal
pH	7.30	Acidemia
$PaCO_2$	55 mmHg	Increased (respiratory cause)
HCO_3	25 mEq/L	Normal

Conclusion: Respiratory acidosis (uncompensated)

Sample blood gas: Case 2

PaO_2	85 mmHg	Normal
SaO_2	90%	Low saturation
pH	7.49	Alkalemia
$PaCO_2$	40	Normal
HCO_3	29 mEq/L	Increased (metabolic cause)

Conclusion: Metabolic alkalosis with a low saturation (uncompensated)

Occasionally, patients will present with both respiratory and metabolic disorders that *together* cause an acidemia or alkalemia. For example, alkalosis could result from an increase in bicarbonate and a decrease in CO_2, or an acidosis could result from a decrease in bicarbonate and an increase in CO_2. A patient with metabolic acidosis from acute renal failure could also have a very slow respiratory rate that causes the patient to retain CO_2, creating a respiratory acidosis. Therefore, the ABG would reflect a *mixed respiratory and metabolic acidosis*. Examples of mixed gases are the following:

Mixed Acidosis	Mixed Alkalosis
pH: 7.25	pH: 7.55
$PaCO_2$: 56	$PaCO_2$: 26
PaO_2: 80	PaO_2: 80
HCO_3: 15	HCO_3: 28

Determine Compensation

If the patient presents with an alkalemia or acidemia, it is important to determine if the body has tried to compensate for the abnormality. If the buffer systems within the body are unable to maintain normal pH, then the renal or respiratory systems attempt to compensate. *If the problem is respiratory in origin, the kidneys will work to correct it. If the problem is renal in origin, the lungs will try to correct it.* It may take as little as 5 to 15 minutes for the lungs to recognize a metabolic presentation and start to correct it. It may take up to a day for the kidneys to correct the respiratory-induced problem. One system will not overcompensate; that is, an acidotic patient will never be made alkalotic by a compensatory mechanism, and an alkalotic patient will never be made acidotic.

The respiratory system responds to metabolic-based pH imbalances in the following manner:

- *Metabolic acidosis:* increase in respiratory rate/depth
- *Metabolic alkalosis:* decrease in respiratory rate/depth

The renal system responds to respiratory-based pH imbalances in the following manner:

- *Respiratory acidosis:* increase in hydrogen secretion and bicarbonate reabsorption
- *Respiratory alkalosis:* decrease in hydrogen secretion and bicarbonate reabsorption

---

Arterial blood gases are defined by their degree of compensation: they are either uncompensated, partially compensated, or completely compensated. To determine the level of compensation in the ABG, the pH, CO_2, and HCO_3 are examined. First it is determined whether the pH is acidotic or alkalotic. In some cases, the pH will be out of the normal range, indicating an acidosis or alkalosis. If it is

within the normal range, on which side of 7.40 (the midpoint of the normal pH range) does the pH fall? For example, if the pH is 7.38, then the blood gas pH value is *tending toward* acidosis, while a value of 7.41 is *tending toward* alkalosis. Next, an evaluation is made to see which one (CO_2 or HCO_3) has changed to account for the acidosis or alkalosis. Then it is determined if the opposite system (metabolic or respiratory) has worked to try to move the patient back toward a normal pH. The primary abnormality (metabolic or respiratory) is correlated with the abnormal pH (acidotic or alkalotic). The secondary abnormality is an attempt to correct the primary disorder. Using the rules for defining compensation in the display, it is possible to determine the compensatory status of the patient's ABGs.

Mixed Venous Oxygen Saturation

Mixed venous oxygen saturation ($S\overline{v}O_2$) is a parameter that can be measured to evaluate the balance between oxygen supply and oxygen demand. Blood obtained from a vein in an extremity gives information mostly about that extremity and can be quite misleading if the metabolism in the extremity differs from the metabolism of the body as a whole. This difference is accentuated if the extremity is cold or underperfused, as in a patient in shock; if the patient has done local exercises with the extremity, such as opening and closing the fist; if there is local infection in the extremity; and so forth.

Sometimes blood is sampled through a central venous line (CVP catheter) in the hope of getting mixed venous blood, but even in the superior vena cava or right atrium where a CVP catheter ends, there is usually incomplete mixing of venous return from various parts of the body. For complete mixing of the blood, one would have to obtain a blood sample from a pulmonary artery catheter. Use of the pulmonary artery catheter provides a sample of blood that has returned from the extremities and has been mixed in the right ventricle.

Oxygen measurements of mixed venous blood indicate whether the tissues are being oxygenated, but the value cannot separate the independent contributions of the heart and the lungs. $S\overline{v}O_2$ indicates the adequacy of the supply of oxygen relative to the demand for oxygen at the tissue levels. Normal mixed venous oxygen saturation is 60% to 80%. A normal $S\overline{v}O_2$ means that supply of oxygen to the tissues is adequate to meed the tissue's demand. However, a normal value does not indicate if compensatory mechanisms were needed to maintain the perfusion. In some patients, for example, an increase in cardiac output is needed to compensate for a low supply of oxygen.

A low $S\overline{v}O_2$ reading can be caused by a decrease in oxygen supply to the tissues or an increase in oxygen use because of a high demand. A decrease in oxygen supply results from low hemoglobin, hemorrhage, or low cardiac output. Causes of increased oxygen demand include hyperthermia, pain, stress, shivering, or seizures. $S\overline{v}O_2$ of 40% to 60% can

Uncompensated: pH is *abnormal,* and *either* the CO_2 or HCO_3 is also abnormal. There is no indication that the opposite system has tried to correct for the other.

In the example below, the patient's pH is alkalotic as a result of the low (below the normal range of 35–45 mmHg) CO_2 concentration. The renal system value (HCO_3) has not moved out its normal range (22–26 mEq/L) to compensate for the primary respiratory disorder.

PaO_2:	94 mmHg	Normal
pH:	7.52	Alkalotic
$PaCO_2$:	25 mmHg	Decreased
HCO_3:	24 mEq/L	Normal

Partially compensated: pH is *abnormal,* and *both* the CO_2 and HCO_3 are also abnormal; this indicates that one system has attempted to correct for the other but has not been completely successful.

In the example below, the patient's pH remains alkalotic as a result of the low CO_2 concentration. The renal system value (HCO_3) has moved out its normal range (22–26 mEq/L) to compensate for the primary respiratory disorder but has not been able to bring the pH back within the normal range.

PaO_2:	94 mmHg	Normal
pH:	7.48	Alkalotic
$PaCO_2$:	25 mmHg	Decreased
HCO_3:	20 mEq/L	Decreased

Completely compensated: pH is *normal* and *both* the CO_2 and HCO_3 are abnormal; the normal pH indicates that one system has been able to compensate for the other.

In the example below, the patient's pH is normal but is tending toward alkalosis (>7.40). The primary abnormality is respiratory because the $PaCO_2$ is low (decreased acid concentration). The bicarbonate value of 18 mEq/L reflects decreased concentration of base and is associated with acidosis, not alkalosis. In this case, the decreased bicarbonate has completely compensated for the respiratory alkalosis.

PaO_2:	94 mmHg	Normal
pH:	7.44	Normal, tending toward alkalosis
$PaCO_2$:	25 mmHg	Decreased, primary problem
HCO_3:	18 mEq/L	Decreased, compensatory response

be found with heart failure, and values less than 40% may indicate profound shock. A decrease in $S\overline{v}O_2$ often occurs before other hemodynamic changes and therefore is an excellent clinical tool in the assessment and management of critically ill patients. The goals of interventions for a low $S\overline{v}O_2$ include increasing the oxygen supply by blood trans-

fusions or by increasing cardiac output. Treatment could also be aimed at eliminating the cause of the high demand.

A high $S\overline{v}O_2$ value indicates that oxygen supply exceeds demand or a decrease in the demand. Elevated $S\overline{v}O_2$ values are associated with increased delivery of oxygen (high FIO_2) or with decreased demand from hypothermia, hypothyroidism, or anesthesia. An elevated value also is seen in the early stages of septic shock when the tissues are unable to use the oxygen. Table 23-5 summarizes possible causes of abnormalities in $S\overline{v}O_2$.

A pulmonary artery catheter that allows continuous monitoring of $S\overline{v}O_2$ with an oximeter built into its tip provides ongoing assessment of oxygen supply and demand imbalances. If a catheter with a built in oximeter is not available, the nurse can draw blood from the pulmonary artery through a regular pulmonary artery catheter, send the sample to the laboratory for blood gas and $S\overline{v}O_2$ analysis, and use the information in the same way.

RESPIRATORY DIAGNOSTIC TESTS

Chest Radiography

Chest radiography is a valuable diagnostic tool frequently used to assess anatomical and physiological features of the chest and to detect pathologies. As x-rays are passed

RED!FLAG **Table 23-5** Possible Causes of Abnormalities in Mixed Venous Oxygen Saturation ($S\overline{v}O_2$)

Abnormality	Possible Cause
Low $S\overline{v}O_2$ < 60%	***Decreased oxygen supply*** Low hematocrit from anemia or hemorrhage Low arterial saturation and hypoxemia from lung disease, ventilation–perfusion mismatches Low cardiac output from hypovolemia, heart failure, cardiogenic shock, myocardial infarction ***Increased oxygen demand*** Increased metabolic demand, such as hyperthermia, seizures, shivering, pain, anxiety, stress, strenuous exercise
High $S\overline{v}O_2$ > 80%	***Increased oxygen supply*** Supplemental oxygen ***Decreased oxygen demand*** Anesthesia, hypothermia, early stages of sepsis ***Technical problems*** False high reading because of wedged pulmonary artery catheter Fibrin clot at end of catheter

through the chest wall, various structures are visualized. Dense tissues, such as bones, absorb the x-ray beam and appear as opaque or white on the radiograph. Blood vessels and blood-filled organs, such as the heart, are moderately dense structures and appear as grey areas on the radiograph. During inspiration, the normal lung is filled with air and appears black on the radiograph. When areas of the lungs are filled with fluid, which is a more dense material, the lungs appear white.

The radiograph is used by the nurse as an assessment parameter to validate clinical findings and suspected abnormalities. Using a systematic approach, the nurse examines the radiograph by comparing the film with previous films. One recommended approach is to examine the film by moving from external to internal, side to side, and top to bottom.[3] The nurse scrutinizes the soft-tissue areas, the bony structures, the inner layers just under the bone, and the internal structures.

Soft tissues are examined on the radiograph by looking for homogeneity, beginning with lateral areas and moving medially. Air visualized in the lateral soft tissue may indicate the presence of a pneumothorax.

Bony structures inspected on the chest film include the ribs, clavicles, sternum, manubrium, spine, and vertebrae. Approximately eight to nine ribs should overlie lung tissue on the normal chest film. The ribs are examined for the presence of fractures by following the curve of each rib beginning anteriorly and moving around posteriorly. Like the ribs, the other bony structures are examined for correct position and intactness.

The contour of the diaphragm also is examined on the radiograph. Normally, the diaphragm is rounded with sharp, pointed costophrenic angles. Pleural effusions may cause the angles to become blunted. The top of the diaphragm is visualized at about the sixth rib. A lowered diaphragm may indicate hyperinflation caused by emphysema.

The lung parenchyma is assessed by comparing right and left sides moving top to bottom. Normal air-filled lungs should appear black or very dark compared to the bones and heart. It is important in the evaluation to look for symmetry. Abnormally high density on one side of the chest may indicate edema, a mass, pleural effusion, or pneumonia.[4]

Interlobar fissures separate the lobes of the lungs. The minor fissure in the right lung is usually visible in the frontal film. Displacement of the normal fissures seen on the film may indicate the presence of atelectasis or lobar collapse.

The trachea should appear midline over the thoracic vertebrae. The trachea can shift toward areas of atelectasis and away from areas of pneumothorax, pleural effusion, or tumors.

Ventilation–Perfusion Scanning

Ventilation–perfusion scanning is a type of nuclear imaging test used to evaluate a suspected alteration in the ventilation–perfusion (V/Q) relationship. (See Chapter 22 for a discussion of ventilation–perfusion relationships.) A V/Q scan is helpful in detecting the percentage of each lung that is functioning normally, diagnosing and locating pulmonary emboli, and assessing the pulmonary vascular supply.[5]

The test consists of two parts: ventilation scan and perfusion scan. For the ventilation scan, the patient inhales radioactive gas, which follows the same pathway as air in normal breathing. In pathological conditions, the diminished areas of ventilation will be noted on the scan. For the perfusion scan, a radioisotope is injected intravenously, and the blood supply to the lungs can be visualized. When a pulmonary embolus is present, the blood supply beyond the embolus is restricted, and the test will reveal poor or no visualization of the affected area.

Ventilation–perfusion scans are often not useful on patients dependent on mechanical ventilation because the ventilation component of the scan is hard to perform. Because of ventilation perfusion mismatches, interpretation of ventilation–perfusion scans is difficult in patients with lung diseases, such as pneumonia. As a result of these limitations, the critically ill patient may have a pulmonary angiography test performed, especially if a pulmonary embolus is suspected.[3]

Pulmonary Angiography

Pulmonary angiography involves the rapid injection of a radiopaque substance for radiographic studies of the pulmonary vasculature. Suspected pulmonary embolus is the most common indication for a pulmonary angiogram. A radiopaque substance is injected into one or both arms or the femoral vein. Another alternative is to inject the substance through a catheter that has been placed in the pulmonary artery. A positive test result is indicated by the flow of the radiopaque substance through a narrowed vessel or by the abrupt cessation of flow of the substance in a vessel.

Bronchoscopy

Bronchoscopy involves the direct visualization of the larynx, trachea, and bronchi through a flexible fiberoptic bronchoscope. When used for diagnostic purposes, bronchoscopy provides a means to examine tissues, collect secretions, determine the extent and location of pathology, and obtain a biopsy. When used for therapeutic purposes, bronchoscopy offers a means to remove foreign bodies or secretions from the tracheobronchial tree, treat postoperative atelectasis, and excise lesions.

In preparation for a bronchoscopy, a history and physical examination are performed. A chest x-ray, clotting studies, and ABGs also are obtained. The patient often receives intravenous sedation or analgesia before the procedure. If the purpose of the bronchoscopy is therapeutic, medications that suppress a cough or diminish secretions are avoided. These medications include intratracheal topical anesthetics, atropine, and codeine.

Careful monitoring of the patient is indicated after a bronchoscopy. The nurse assesses the patient for any evidence of complications, which may include laryngospasm, fever, hemodynamic changes, cardiac dysrhythmias, pneumothorax, hemorrhage, or cardiopulmonary arrest.

■ CONCLUSION

Comprehensive respiratory assessment is an essential component of the care of critically ill patients. A thorough history and physical examination, combined with continuous monitoring and evaluation of results of diagnostic tests, provide the nurse with a wealth of data. These data are used to develop appropriate nursing interventions and to guide a collaborative plan of care.

Clinical Applicability Challenges

Self-Challenge: Critical Thinking

1. *Formulate the rationale for the acid–base disturbance that may occur with continuous nasogastric suctioning, head trauma, renal failure, and malnutrition.*

2. *Your patient has been admitted to the intensive care unit with a diagnosis of pleural effusion. Describe the physical assessment findings you would anticipate in this patient.*

3. *Interpret the following ABGs: PaO_2, 80 mmHg; pH, 7.42; $PaCO_2$, 26 mmHg; HCO_3, 18 mEq/L. Discuss possible causes of the ABG value.*

Study Questions

1. *Normal breath sounds that are heard over the periphery of the lung are called*
   a. *bronchial breath sounds.*
   b. *bronchovesicular breath sounds.*
   c. *vesicular breath sounds.*
   d. *loud crackles.*

2. *Mixed venous blood has an oxygen saturation that is*
   a. *60% to 80%, which is lower than arterial blood.*
   b. *80% to 90%, which is lower than arterial blood.*
   c. *30% to 40%, which is lower than arterial blood.*
   d. *95% or greater, which is the same as arterial blood.*

3. *This ABG analysis indicates which of the following conditions?*
   PaO_2, 86 mmHg
   pH, 7.31
   $PaCO_2$, 52 mmHg
   HCO_3, 24 mEq/L
   a. *Respiratory alkalosis*
   b. *Metabolic alkalosis*
   c. *Metabolic acidosis*
   d. *Respiratory acidosis*

4. *The primary abnormality in respiratory alkalosis is*
   a. *decreased $PaCO_2$.*
   b. *increased $PaCO_2$.*
   c. *decreased HCO_3.*
   d. *increased HCO_3.*

5. *A high SvO_2 level may be the result of*
   a. *pain and anxiety.*
   b. *anemia.*
   c. *hypothermia.*
   d. *hyperthermia.*

REFERENCES

1. Bates B: A Guide to Physical Examination and History Taking (6th Ed). Philadelphia, JB Lippincott, 1995
2. Christensen MA, Bloom J, Sutton KR: Comparing arterial and end-tidal carbon dioxide values in hyperventilated neurosurgical patients. American Journal of Critical Care 4:116–121, 1995
3. Dettenmeier PA: Radiographic Assessment for Nurses. St. Louis, Mosby, 1995
4. Kelley WN: Textbook of Internal Medicine (3rd Ed). Philadelphia, Lippincott-Raven, 1997
5. Fischbach FT: A Manual of Laboratory and Diagnostic Tests (5th Ed). Philadelphia, Lippincott-Raven, 1996

BIBLIOGRAPHY

Ahrens T: Changing perspectives in the assessment of oxygenation. Critical Care Nurse 13(4):78–83, 1993
Dickson SL: Understanding the oxyhemoglobin dissociation curve. Critical Care Nurse 15(5):54–58, 1995
Mays DA: Turn ABGs into child's play . . . arterial blood gas. RN 58(1):36–40, 1995
Misasi RS, Keyes J: Matching and mismatching ventilation and perfusion in the lung. Critical Care Nurse 16(3):23–401, 1996
Shapiro BA: Evaluation of blood gas monitors: performance criteria, clinical impact and cost/benefit. Critical Care Medicine 22(4):546–548, 1994
Shapiro BA, Peruzzi W, Kozelowski-Templin R: Clinical Application of Blood Gases. Chicago, Mosby-Year Book, 1994
Tasota FJ, Wesmiller SW: Assessing ABGs: maintaining the delicate balance. Nursing 24(5):34–46, 1994
Tonnessen TI: Intracellular pH and electrolyte regulation. In Shoemaker W (ed): Textbook of Critical Care. Philadelphia, WB Saunders, 1995

24

Patient Management: Respiratory System

457

OBJECTIVES

Based on the content in this chapter, the reader should be able to:

- Summarize the desired outcomes of the various bronchial hygiene techniques.
- Compare and contrast situations in which chest physiotherapy (including postural drainage) is useful with those in which it is contraindicated.
- Compare and contrast indications for and complications of orotracheal intubation versus nasotracheal intubation.
- Summarize procedures commonly performed in the intensive care unit that can precipitate pneumothorax.
- Compare and contrast the principles governing one-, two-, and three-bottle chest tube drainage systems.
- Discuss nursing interventions necessary to prevent complications in a patient with a chest tube drainage system.
- Discuss the use of bronchodilators in the treatment of bronchospasm.
- Explain causes of agitation in critically ill patients.
- Analyze the process by which each of the following conditions can cause respiratory failure: benzodiazepine overdose, asthma, pulmonary embolus.
- Differentiate between the principles of negative pressure ventilation and positive pressure ventilation. In positive pressure ventilation, differentiate between pressure-cycled and volume-cycled ventilators.
- Compare and contrast intermittent mandatory, assist-control, pressure-support, and pressure-controlled ventilation.
- Summarize strategies to maximize oxygen delivery with the goal of achieving a nontoxic FiO_2 setting.
- Summarize adverse effects of positive end-expiratory pressure, how they are identified, and appropriate treatment for each.
- Compare and contrast the advantages and disadvantages of tracheostomy versus endotracheal intubation.
- Name four nursing interventions for the ventilated patient, and explain how each impacts on decreasing length of mechanical ventilation.

Respiration is necessary to sustaining life, and the nurse plays an important role in helping the critically ill patient breathe. The nurse must be knowledgeable and skilled in assessing patient needs, providing quick and efficient care, evaluating results, and supporting, teaching, and preparing the patient and family. Techniques, equipment, and procedures vary according to the patient's respiratory status. Bronchial hygiene, artificial airways, chest tubes, pharmacological agents, and various types of ventilatory support are discussed in this chapter.

Bronchial Hygiene

Bronchial hygiene is helpful in preventing and treating pulmonary complications. The primary phases of lung function that most bronchial hygiene aims to improve are ventilation and diffusion (Fig. 24–1). These are accomplished through the therapeutic goals of mobilization and removal of secretions and improved gas exchange.

Specific bronchial hygiene depends on existing pulmonary dysfunction. Assessment of the need for and the effectiveness of various methods of bronchial hygiene are based on physical assessment, chest radiograph, measurement of arterial blood gases (ABGs), and additional sources of information as indicated. Any one or a combination of the following measures may be used: coughing and deep-breathing maneuvers, chest physiotherapy (CPT), and bronchodilator aerosol therapy.

METHODS OF BRONCHIAL HYGIENE

Effective Coughing and Deep Breathing

Effective coughing is necessary to the patient's ability to clear secretions. The objectives of deep breathing and coughing are to promote lung expansion, mobilize secretions, and prevent the side effects of retained secretions (which are atelectasis and pneumonia). The efficacy of these techniques is limited to patients who are able to cooperate.

Ideally the patient is positioned upright on the edge of the bed or chair with the feet supported. He or she is instructed to take a slow, deep breath; hold it for at least 3

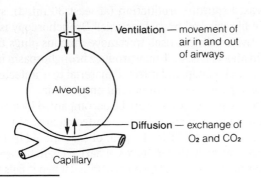

FIGURE 24-1
Primary lung functions: ventilation and diffusion.

Chest Physiotherapy

Postural drainage, chest percussion, and chest vibration are methods of CPT. These may be used in sequence in different lung drainage positions and should be preceded by bronchodilator therapy and followed by deep breathing and coughing.

POSTURAL DRAINAGE

Postural drainage positions facilitate gravitational drainage of pulmonary secretions into the main bronchi and trachea based on anatomy of the lung segments, as shown in Figure 24–2.

Postural drainage is not appropriate or tolerated in all positions in critically ill patients. Contraindications are listed in the display. The nurse must closely monitor the patient in a head-down position for aspiration, respiratory distress, and dysrhythmias.

seconds; and exhale slowly. If secretions are auscultated, then a cough is initiated on maximum inspiration. Incentive spirometers are available to encourage and quantify deep breathing by giving immediate visual feedback to the patient.

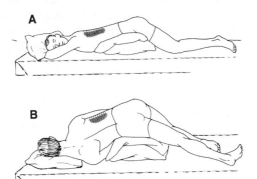

A. Face-lying–hips elevated 16–18 inches on pillows, making a 30°–45° angle.
Purpose: to drain the posterior lower lobes.

B. Lying on the left side—hips elevated 16–18 inches on pillows.
Purpose: to drain the right lateral lower lung segments.

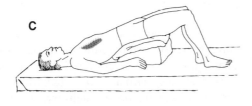

C. Back lying—hips elevated 16–18 inches on pillows.
Purpose: to drain the anterior lower lung segments.

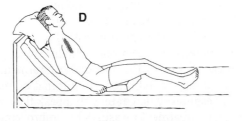

D. Sitting upright or semireclining.
Purpose: to drain the upper lung field and allow more forceful coughing.

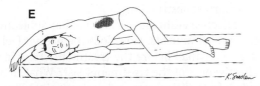

E. Lying on the right side—hips elevated on pillows forming a 30°–45° angle.
Purpose: to drain the left lower lobes.

FIGURE 24-2
Positions used in lung drainage.

Contraindications for Chest Physiotherapy

Contraindications to Postural Drainage
- Increased intracranial pressure
- After meals/during tube feeding
- Inability to cough
- Hypoxia/respiratory instability
- Hemodynamic instability
- Decreased mental status
- Recent eye surgery
- Hiatal hernia
- Obesity

Contraindications to Percussion/Vibration
- Fractured ribs/osteoporosis
- Chest/abdominal trauma
- Pulmonary hemorrhage or embolus
- Chest malignancy/mastectomy
- Pneumothorax/subcutaneous emphysema
- Cervical cord trauma
- Tuberculosis
- Pleural effusions/empyema
- Asthma

CHEST PERCUSSION AND VIBRATION

Chest percussion and vibration are used to dislodge secretions. Neither method has been shown to be superior; there are many contraindications to using either technique. Contraindications are listed in the display.

Percussion involves striking the chest wall with the hands formed into a cupped shape by flexing the fingers and placing the thumb tightly against the index finger. The patient's position depends on the segment of lung to be percussed. A towel or pillow case is draped over the area to be percussed, and percussion is performed for 3 to 5 minutes per position. Percussion is never performed over the spine, over the sternum, or below the thoracic cage. If performed correctly, percussion does not hurt the patient or redden the skin. A clapping sound (as opposed to slapping) indicates correct hand position. Mechanical percussors are also available.

Vibration increases the velocity and turbulence of exhaled air to loosen secretions. This technique is accomplished by placing the hands side by side with fingers extended over the chest area. The patient inhales deeply, and then slowly exhales. While the patient exhales, the nurse vibrates the patient's chest by quickly contracting and relaxing arm and shoulder muscles. Vibration is used instead of percussion if the chest wall is extremely painful.

CONTRAINDICATIONS AND ADAPTATIONS

Contraindications to CPT are listed in the accompanying display. Recent studies have questioned the efficacy of CPT except in segmental atelectasis and diseases that result in

increased sputum production (at least 30 mL/d), such as cystic fibrosis and bronchiectasis.[1] Bronchoscopy is an alternative treatment used to remove mucous plugs that result in atelectasis. CPT may produce bronchospasm in asthmatics and may spread infected material to uninfected lung tissue in patients with unilateral pneumonia.

To be effective, CPT must be accompanied by a postural drainage position specific to the affected area of the lung. The inclusion of CPT in the plan of care should be individualized and evaluated in terms of derived benefit versus potential risks and should be discontinued when it fails to promote treatment goals.

In patients who cannot tolerate CPT, turning the patient every 2 hours aids in draining the lungs and prevents stagnation of secretions. Patients with an artificial airway or an ineffective cough may require suctioning after CPT.

Patients with unilateral disease are positioned with the healthy lung down for better ventilation and perfusion.[2] Positioning the patient with the diseased lung down is likely to cause hypoxemia with ventilation–perfusion mismatching and shunting. Positioning, however, is changed if the patient has a lung abscess. In such case, the preferred position is with the diseased lung down, because the abscessed lung in a gravity-dependent position can drain its purulent contents into the opposite lung. The healthy lung would then be contaminated by the abscessed lung, and gas exchange would most likely be affected.

Recent studies have demonstrated improved oxygenation in patients with acute respiratory failure who were placed in the prone position. This enhanced oxygenation was attributed to recruitment of collapsed lung areas.[3]

Bronchodilator Aerosol Therapy

The goals of bronchodilator therapy are to relax the airways, mobilize secretions, and reduce mucosal edema. Bronchodilator therapy can be delivered through metered dose inhalers, preferably with a spacer attachment, or nebulization. Regardless of the mode of delivery, assessment before, during, and after the therapy is essential.

Assessment before and after treatment includes breath sounds, pulse, and respiratory rate (RR). The last two commonly increase during bronchodilator therapy and can remain elevated up to 1½ hours after treatment. ABG measurement may be indicated. (In asthmatics, measurement of peak expiratory flow rate with a peak flow meter before and after a treatment measures the improvement in severity of airway obstruction.)

Objective evaluation is crucial, but subjective information is also valuable. How does the patient feel? Is breathing better than before the treatment? How long does the effectiveness of the treatments last? What, if any, are the side effects (jitteriness, palpitations, inability to concentrate, increased heart rate), and how long do these symptoms last?

Artificial Airways

Rigorous bronchial hygiene and carefully monitored oxygen therapy may eliminate the need for an artificial airway or ventilatory support. An artificial airway and ventilatory support become mandatory if these measures fail to provide adequate oxygenation and removal of carbon dioxide. Artificial airways have a fourfold purpose:

- Establishment of an airway
- Protection of the airway, with the cuff inflated
- Provision of continuous ventilatory assistance
- Facilitation of airway clearance

Knowledgeable, aggressive nursing care is required to maintain airway patency, maximize therapeutic effects, and minimize damage to the patient's natural airway.

■■■ EQUIPMENT FEATURES

The selection of the appropriate artificial airway is important. Because all artificial airways increase airway resistance, it is essential that the largest tube possible be used

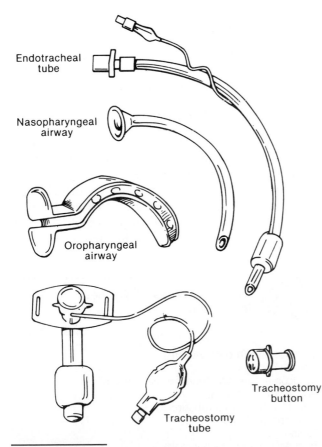

FIGURE 24-3
Five frequently used artificial airways.

Endotracheal tube

Nasopharyngeal airway

Oropharyngeal airway

Tracheostomy tube

Tracheostomy button

for intubation. The cuff on the endotracheal or tracheostomy tube must be of low compliance (soft) so that trauma to the trachea, vocal cords, and subglottic area is minimized. The competency of the cuff must be established before intubation. Approximately 10 cc of air is injected into the cuff before use.

Airways

If a patient is sedated and lying supine or becomes unconscious, innervation of the genioglossal muscle is decreased, causing the tongue to occlude the airway. Although an oropharyngeal or nasopharyngeal airway will maintain the air passage, it will not eliminate the potential for aspiration. Figure 24–3 illustrates some frequently used artificial airways.

The nasopharyngeal airway (nasal trumpet) is a flexible tube that is inserted nasally past the base of the tongue to maintain airway patency. Nasal airways are frequently used to prevent patient discomfort and airway trauma from repeated introduction of the suction catheter through the nare in patients who require frequent nasotracheal suctioning.

Endotracheal Tubes

An endotracheal tube (ETT) is inserted if the patient needs ventilation or protection of the airway from aspiration. Equipment listed in the accompanying display is assembled before intubation.

The ETT can be inserted nasally or orally. Advantages and disadvantages of each placement are listed in Table 24–1.

CLINICAL APPLICATION:
Equipment for Tracheal Intubation

- Laryngoscope with blades and intact bulb
- Suction setup
- Correct size endotracheal tube* (Stylet)
- 10-mL syringe for cuff inflation
- Adhesive tape
- Magill forceps
- Pulse oximetry
- Oxygen source
- Manual resuscitation bag with mask

---

* *In adults, tube size usually ranges from 7.0 to 8.0 mm. Larger diameter tubes are recommended for patients with reactive airways or when bronchoscopy is anticipated.*

TABLE 24-1
Airway Placement

Type	Advantages	Disadvantages
Nasal endotracheal	Patient comfort Prevents tube obstruction from biting Easily anchored Used in patients with maxillo-facial trauma or cervical spine injuries	Can kink and obstruct airway Predisposes to acute sinusitis, which may result in bacteremia Tube and cuff can cause tracheal damage High risk for shearing off nasal polyps in asthmatics
Oral endotracheal	Less trauma during intubation than nasal route Permits use of a larger endotracheal tube	Predisposes to mouth sores Uncomfortable for patient Easily obstructed by biting Tube and cuff can cause tracheal damage Complicates effective oral hygiene Difficult to secure Makes communication difficult

▬▬ PROCEDURES

Techniques

INSERTION OF OROPHARYNGEAL AIRWAY

An oropharyngeal airway is never placed in a conscious patient, because it stimulates the gag reflex and can cause vomiting and aspiration. Before placing an artificial airway, the nurse makes sure any possible obstruction is cleared. Insertion of an oropharyngeal airway follows three steps:

1. Gently open the patient's mouth using a crossed finger technique or a modified jaw thrust.
2. Hold down the tongue with a depressor and guide the airway over the back of the tongue. (An optional method is to position the tip of the airway toward the roof of the mouth and gently advance the airway by rotating it 180 degrees.)
3. Monitor the patient frequently for airway patency; suction as needed.

INSERTION OF NASOPHARYNGEAL AIRWAY

Insertion of a nasopharyngeal airway involves the following steps:

1. Determine and select the correct tube length by measuring from the tip of the nose to the earlobe. Use a tube with the largest outer diameter that will fit the patient's nostril.
2. Lubricate the tube with water or a soluble jelly.
3. Reassure patient and familiarize him or her with the procedure.
4. Insert the airway into the nostril up to the end of the nasal trumpet.

5. Have the patient exhale with the mouth closed. (If the tube is in the correct position, air can be felt exiting from the tube opening.
6. Open the patient's mouth, depress the tongue, and look for the tube's tip just behind the uvula.

REMOVAL OF PHARYNGEAL AIRWAY

To remove the pharyngeal airway, the oropharynx is suctioned, and the airway is gently removed. The nasal airway may have to be gently rotated to withdraw it from the nares.

INSERTION OF ENDOTRACHEAL TUBES

To reduce the incidence of complications, such as those listed in the display, tracheal intubation must be performed by rigorously credentialed personnel.

The nurse explains the procedure to the patient. The patient is positioned on his or her back with a small blanket under the shoulder blades. This hyperextends the neck and opens the airway. Air is injected into the endotracheal

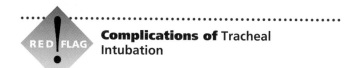

Complications of Tracheal Intubation

- Laryngospasm/bronchospasm
- Trauma/bleeding
- Nosocomial infection (pneumonia, sinusitis)
- Displacement of tube:
    Right main stem intubation
    Gastric intubation
- Aspiration
- Tracheal stenosis/tracheomalacia
- Laryngeal damage and necrosis
- Hypoxemia during intubation

RED FLAG **Complications of** Suctioning

- Hypoxemia
- Dysrhythmias
- Vagal stimulation (bradycardia, hypotension)
- Bronchospasm
- Elevated intracranial pressure
- Atelectasis
- Tracheal mucosal trauma
- Bleeding
- Nosocomial infection

cuff before insertion to ensure an intact cuff. The cuff then is deflated.

Prior to the procedure, the nurse confirms that the suction is working properly. Using a manual resuscitation bag (MRB) and mask, the nurse preoxygenates the patient. The physician may use topical anesthetics, sedatives, or a short-acting neuromuscular blocking agent (NMBA) to facilitate rapid and nontraumatic intubation.

The nurse assists during intubation by providing suction as necessary and monitoring the patient's oxygen saturation (SaO$_2$) by pulse oximetry. Intubation attempts should be held and the patient oxygenated with the MRB if SaO$_2$ falls below 90%.

Following placement, the cuff is inflated. The chest is auscultated bilaterally for equal breath sounds, and the abdomen is auscultated for evidence of esophageal intubation. Waterproof tape is used to secure the ETT. A portable chest x-ray is used immediately following the insertion to confirm proper tube placement, which is about 3 to 7 cm above the

carina. ETT care is discussed later in the chapter under Assessment and Management of the Ventilated Patient.

SUCTIONING

The presence of an artificial tube prevents glottic closure. As a result, the patient is unable to use the normal clearing mechanism (ie, effective coughing). Additionally, the foreign object increases production of secretions. Suctioning, therefore, becomes paramount for removing secretions and maintaining patency.

Suctioning is not without risks and should be done only when needed.[4] Complications of suctioning are listed in the display. Indications for suctioning include visual observation of secretions, determination of the presence of secretions or mucous plugs by chest auscultation, coughing, an increase in peak airway pressure, a decrease in tidal volume during pressure ventilation, or deterioration of the patient's oxygenation.

The procedure for suctioning is given in the display. The nurse performs suctioning as a sterile procedure, using practices recommended by the Centers for Disease Control and Prevention.

In-line suction catheters are available for use in patients on high levels of positive end-expiratory pressure (PEEP), those with copious secretions requiring frequent suctioning, or those with grossly bloody secretions.

Hyperoxygenation and Salination

The patient must be hyperoxygenated using the ventilator method if an in-line system is used. Patients not on ventilators also need to be hyperoxygenated before suctioning. The patient should be instructed to take deep breaths while connected to a 100% O$_2$ source. Patients incapable of tak-

---

CLINICAL APPLICATION: Nursing Intervention Guidelines
Procedure for Suctioning

Equipment
Sterile suction catheter
Sterile gloves
Sterile normal saline for irrigation, when indicated
Sterile disposable container

Technique
1. Perform routine procedures prior to suctioning: Administer medication, assemble equipment, explain the procedure to the patient, adjust bed to comfortable working position, prepare suction pressure, wash hands, and don gloves.
2. Hyperoxygenate the patient with 100% O$_2$ using an MRB or the ventilator. If the ventilator method is used, preoxygenation must last at least 2 minutes, and the nurse must return to the previous oxygen setting after suctioning is completed. (Clinical research shows that the use of the patient's ventilator for preoxygenation delivers higher oxygen concentrations and lower peak pressures than those generated with an MRB.)[5]

3. Quickly but gently insert the catheter as far as possible into the artificial airway without application of suction.
4. Withdraw the catheter 1 to 2 cm, and apply intermittent suction while rotating and removing the catheter. Limit suction pressure to −80 to −120 mmHg. Aspiration should not exceed 10 to 15 seconds. (Prolonged aspiration can lead to severe hypoxia, hemodynamic instability, and ultimately cardiac arrest.)
5. Hyperoxygenate the patient between each subsequent pass of the catheter and at the end of the procedure before reconnection to the ventilator.
6. Monitor heart rate and rhythm and pulse oximetry during suctioning.
7. Discontinue the procedure if the patient does not tolerate it as evidenced by dysrhythmias, bradycardia, or a drop in SaO$_2$.
8. Remove equipment. Wash your hands.
9. Document procedure.
10. Offer oral hygiene.

ing a deep breath should be assisted by an MRB with mask. The presence of epiglottitis or croup is an absolute contraindication to nasotracheal suctioning of patients without an artificial airway.

The routine instillation of normal saline has become increasingly questionable. In a test tube, saline and sputum act like oil and water; they do not form a mixture. Therefore, it is unlikely that saline instillation liquefies or increases the amount of sputum obtained during suction. In addition, saline instillation causes oxygenation to decrease and may predispose patients to nosocomial infection by transporting bacteria to lower airways. To illustrate how nursing research can change nursing

---

Insights Into Clinical Research

Ackerman MH: The effect of saline lavage prior to suctioning. American Journal of Critical Care 2:326–330, 1993

Forty mechanically ventilated men, all over the age of 40, were studied to determine the effect that instillation of normal saline prior to suctioning would have on oxygenation as measured by pulse oximetry. The subjects served as their own controls. They were alternately suctioned with and without saline for 24 hours with oxygen saturation recorded immediately before, immediately after, and at 1-minute intervals for 5 minutes after suctioning. The instillation of saline had an adverse effect on oxygenation that worsened over time with significant desaturation at 2, 3, 4, and 5 minutes after suctioning. Nurses should curtail the practice of routine instillation of saline during suctioning.

Insights Into Clinical Research

Hagler DA, Traver GA: Endotracheal saline and suction catheters: Sources of lower airway contamination. American Journal of Critical Care 3:444–447, 1994

Normal saline (NS) instillation prior to endotracheal suctioning is a common practice. Endotracheal tubes are made of polyvinyl chloride, which supports the colonization of local bacteria, protecting bacterial colonies from natural and pharmacological bacterial agents, thereby increasing their virulence. The ETTs of 10 patients who were intubated for at least 48 hours were studied at the time of extubation to determine the extent to which NS irrigation and suction catheter insertion dislodge viable bacteria into the lower airway. Each suction catheter was used in random order to test for number of bacteria dislodged by catheter insertion and by saline instillation. Viable bacteria in numbers large enough to be reported as 4+ were dislodged by both actions; the number of bacteria dislodged by saline was significantly larger than that dislodged by catheter insertion. Nurses should curtail the practice of routine instillation of NS during suctioning.

---

practice, the results of two studies demonstrating the effects of saline instillation during suctioning are summarized here.

Assessment and Management

Care of the patient with an airway and ETT is discussed later in this chapter under Assessment and Management of the Ventilated Patient.

Chest Tubes

The chest tube is a drain. Its purposes are to remove air, fluid, or blood from the pleural space; restore negative pressure to the pleural space; re-expand a collapsed or partially collapsed lung; and prevent reflux of drainage back into the chest.

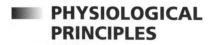

PHYSIOLOGICAL PRINCIPLES

A short review of chest anatomy and pleural pressures is provided for understanding of chest tubes and drainage systems.

Chest Anatomy

The chest is composed of three compartments: the mediastinum, a right pleural cavity, and a left pleural cavity. Each pleural cavity is lined with a thin, slippery membrane called the parietal pleura. A similar membrane covers the

lung and is called the visceral pleura. A thin layer of fluid with a total volume of 5 to 15 mL acts as a lubricant between the visceral and parietal pleurae, allowing them to slide smoothly over each other during breathing.

Because the two pleurae lie in contact with each other, the pleural space is a "potential" space only. If the area between these membranes becomes an actual space, the lung collapses.

Pleural Pressures

The lung is supported within the chest cavity by intrapleural negative pressure. The negative pressure is created by two opposing forces. The first is the tendency of the chest wall to spring upward and outward. The second is the tendency of the elastic alveolar tissue to contract.

An analogy is two microscopic slides held together by a drop of water placed between them. One is not able to pull the slides apart because of the surface tension of the fluid.

Compare the lung to the two slides. One slide is the visceral pleura; the other is the parietal pleura. The drop of water is pleural fluid. As in the analogy of the slides, the opposing forces attempt to pull the pleurae in different directions. A negative pressure is generated, which holds the lung tightly to the chest wall, preventing lung collapse. During inspiration, the intrapleural pressures become more negative, favoring the flow of gas into the lungs. On expiration, the pressures become less negative (increase), and gas flows out of the lungs (Table 24–2).

All gases move from an area of higher pressure to an area of lower pressure. During inspiration, the chest cavity enlarges through diaphragmatic contraction. This increases lung space and causes intrapleural pressure to fall below atmospheric pressure. Air flows from the relatively high atmospheric pressure into the area of low pressure in the lungs.

During expiration, this process is reversed. The diaphragm recoils, decreasing the space in the chest cavity and compressing the lungs. Intrapleural pressure is now higher than atmospheric pressure, causing air to move out of the lungs.

After the respiratory muscles relax, the pressure between the outside air and the lungs is equalized (760 mmHg at sea level). Because the pressure is equalized, there is no air movement.

EQUIPMENT FEATURES

Equipment needed for chest tube insertion is listed in the accompanying display.

CHEST TUBES

Most chest tubes are multifenestrated, transparent tubes with distance and radiopaque markers. This enables the physician to visualize the tube on chest x-ray and position it correctly in the pleural space. All openings in the tube must reside within the rib cage to ensure that air leaks do not develop either in subcutaneous tissue or outside the chest wall.

Chest tubes are categorized as pleural or mediastinal, depending on the location of the tube's tip. Patients can have more than one tube in different locations, depending on the purposes of the tubes.

TABLE 24-2 **The Effect of Breathing on Intrapleural Pressure**	
Ventilation Cycle	Intrapleural Pressures
At rest	−5 cm H_2O
Inspiration	−6 to −12 cm H_2O
Expiration	−4 to −8 cm H_2O

CLINICAL APPLICATION:
Equipment for Chest Tube Insertion

- Chest tube tray or thoracotomy tray (with scalpel)
- Chest tube
- 1% lidocaine
- Antiseptic (povidone–iodine)
- Sterile gloves
- Large hemostats
- Suture material (0-0 or 2-0 silk)
- Cutting needle
- Bacteriostatic ointment or petroleum gauze
- Sterile gauze with a slit
- Tape
- Chest tube drainage system and suction

Larger tubes (20–36 French) are used to drain blood or thick pleural drainage. Smaller tubes (16–20 French) are used to remove air.

DRAINAGE SYSTEMS

The chest tube is a drain for air or fluid. To reestablish intrapleural negative pressure, a seal for the chest tube that prevents outside air from entering the system is required. The simplest way to accomplish this is to use an underwater system of drainage.

A review of the one-, two-, and three-bottle systems can provide a basis for understanding all of the commonly used disposable drainage units. Knowledge of these systems enables the nurse to manage safely the most complex chest tube drainage setup.

One-Bottle System

The simplest chest drainage system is the one-bottle system (Fig. 24–4). This system consists of a bottle with a sealed cap. The cap has two openings. One is for an air vent, and the other allows a tube to pass through, which extends almost to the bottom of the bottle.

Sterile water is poured into the bottle until the tip of the rigid tube is submerged 2 cm. This creates a water seal by closing the system to outside air. A fluid level higher than 1 cm of water can make breathing more difficult because the patient has a longer column of fluid to move during respiration. More positive pressure is then required to drive drainage out through the water seal.

The top of the tube is connected to about 6 ft of latex rubber tubing that is in turn attached to the open end of the patient's chest tube. The vent in the bottle stays open to allow air from the pleural space to escape. This prevents pressure from building up in the pleural space. Except for the vented cap, the entire drainage system from the chest tube insertion site to the bottle must be airtight.

The fluid level in the water seal fluctuates during respiration. During inspiration, pleural pressures become more negative, causing the fluid level in the submerged tube to rise. During expiration, pleural pressures become more positive, causing the fluid level to descend.

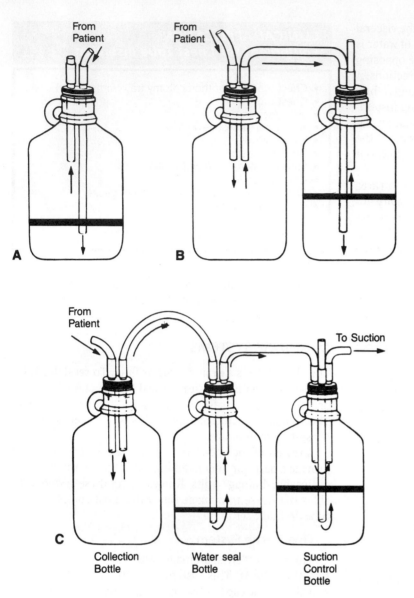

From Patient

From Patient

A

B

From Patient

To Suction

C

Collection Bottle

Water seal Bottle

Suction Control Bottle

FIGURE 24-4
(**A**) One-bottle system underwater seal drainage.
(**B**) Two-bottle system underwater seal drainage.
(**C**) Underwater seal drainage with suction.

If the patient is being mechanically ventilated, this process is reversed. Bubbling should only be seen in the underwater seal chamber during expiration as air and fluid drain from the pleural cavity. Constant bubbling indicates either an air leak in the system or a bronchopleural fistula. This is discussed further under Nursing Management.

Two-Bottle System

In a two-bottle system (see Fig. 24–4), the first bottle is the collection receptacle, and the second bottle is the water seal. In a two-bottle system, suction can be applied to the underwater seal bottle by connecting it to the air vent.

Three-Bottle System

In the three-bottle system, a suction control bottle is added to the two-bottle system (see Fig. 24–4). This is the safest way to regulate the amount of suction. The third bottle is configured similarly to the underwater seal bottle.

In this system, it is the depth of the submerged tube in the third bottle and not the amount of wall suction that determines the amount of suction applied to the chest tube,

most commonly -20 cm H_2O. The amount of wall suction applied to the third bottle should be sufficient to create a gently rolling bubble in the bottle. Vigorous bubbling results in water loss, changing suction pressure and increasing the noise level in the patient's unit.

To check for chest tube patency and respiratory cycle fluctuations, the suction must be momentarily disconnected.

Disposable Drainage Units

Disposable chest tube drainage systems mirror, in physiological principles, the bottle setups described previously (Fig. 24–5). Dry suction uses a spring mechanism to control suction level and can provide higher levels of suction with easier setup.[6]

EMERSON PLEURAL SUCTION PUMP

The Emerson Pleural Suction Pump is commonly used instead of wall suction. It can be set up using a two- or three-bottle system. In contrast to the wall unit, the pressure con-

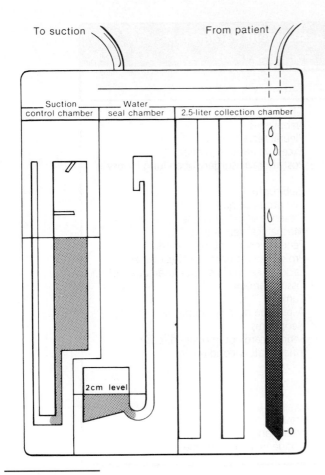

FIGURE 24-5
Disposable chest tube drainage system.

trol knob on the front of the pump controls the suction generated. The amount of pressure is registered on the suction dial.

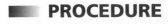

INDICATIONS FOR CHEST TUBE PLACEMENT

If injury, surgery, or any disruption in the integrity of the lungs and chest cavity occurs, placement of a chest tube is warranted. In addition, iatrogenic pneumothorax can occur in the intensive care unit (ICU) during thoracic central line placement, during thoracentesis, or after transbronchial lung biopsy. Indications for chest tube placement are listed in Table 24–3.

PROCEDURE

CHEST TUBE INSERTION

Chest tube insertion can be accomplished in the operating room, in the emergency room, or at the bedside. Placement is based on the principle that because of their different densities and weights, air rises and liquid sinks. The insertion site

for air removal is near the second intercostal space along the midclavicular line. The insertion site for liquid drainage is near the fifth or sixth intercostal space on the midaxillary line. After heart surgery, placement can be in the mediastinum to drain blood from in front of and beneath the heart.

The nurse prepares the patient and family for the procedure, answering any questions they may have. The nurse also prepares the patient physically. Because parietal pleurae are innervated from the intercostal and phrenic nerves, this is a painful procedure, and administration of analgesics is indicated. The patient is positioned in Fowler's or semi-Fowler's position.

After the skin has been cleaned and anesthetized, the physician makes a small skin incision. A hemostat is used to penetrate the pleural space (Fig. 24–6). The tract made by the hemostat is then dilated with a finger. The proximal end of the tube is clamped with the hemostat and then inserted into the pleural space. If the placement is difficult, a metal trocar can be used to penetrate the chest wall, leaving the tube in place and removing the trocar.

After insertion, the external end of the tube is connected to a chest drainage unit. To prevent the tube from dislodging, the skin around the tube is sutured. The ends of the suture are wrapped around the tube and tied off.

Bacteriostatic ointment or petroleum gauze can be applied to the incision site. Petroleum gauze has been preferred, because it is thought to prevent air leaks; however, it also has the potential to macerate the skin and predispose the site to infection. A gauze 4×4 with a split is positioned over the tube and taped occlusively to the chest. All connections from the insertion site to the drainage collection system are securely taped to prevent air leaks. The tube is taped to the chest to prevent traction on the tube and sutures if the patient moves.

A postinsertion chest x-ray is always ordered to confirm proper positioning. The lungs are auscultated, and the condition of the tissue around the insertion site is evaluated for the presence of subcutaneous air. This assessment provides a baseline for determining improvement or worsening of the patient's condition. Pain management continues to be an issue throughout the duration of chest tube use.

CHEST TUBE REMOVAL

Chest tubes are removed after drainage is minimal and 12 to 24 hours after clamping or placing the chest tube to water seal. This identifies persistent air leaks or reaccumulation of fluid on repeat chest x-ray. Other indications for removal of the chest tube are listed in the accompanying display. When the tube is to water seal, disconnect the suction tube to facilitate atmospheric venting.

The patient is placed in a Fowler's or semi-Fowler's position. Premedication is recommended to alleviate pain and discomfort. The dressing over the insertion site is removed and the area is cleaned. The suture is clipped. The tube is removed in one quick movement at peak inspiration or during expiration to prevent entraining air back into the pleural cavity through the chest tube eyelets.

TABLE 24-3 CLINICAL APPLICATION: Assessment Parameters
Indications for Chest Tube Placement

Indication	Cause
Hemothorax	Chest trauma
	Neoplasms
	Pleural tears
	Excessive anticoagulation
	Post-thoracic surgery/open lung biopsy
Pneumothorax	
Spontaneous: >20%	Bleb rupture
	Symptomatic patient
	Presence of lung disease
Tension	Mechanical ventilation
	Penetrating puncture wound
	Prolonged clamping of chest tubes
	Lack of seal in chest tube drainage system
Bronchopleural fistula	Tissue damage
	Tumor
	Aspiration of toxic chemicals
Pleural effusion	Neoplasms
Complicated parapneumonia:	Serious cardiopulmonary disease
Gross pus (empyema)	Inflammatory conditions
Gram-positive stain or bacterial culture	
Glucose <40 mg/dL	
pH <7.0	
pH 7.0–7.2 and LDH >1,000 IU/L	
Chylothorax	Trauma
	Malignancy
	Congenital abnormalities

Immediately after removal, lung fields are auscultated, and a dressing is applied over the site. A chest x-ray is obtained several hours later to assess the presence of residual air or fluid.

ASSESSMENT AND MANAGEMENT

Nursing care is directed at maintaining patency and proper functioning of the chest tube drainage system. Vigilant and expert nursing care can prevent serious complications in a patient with a chest tube and drainage system.

Positioning

The ideal position for a patient with a chest tube is semi-Fowler's. Turning the patient every 2 hours enhances air and fluid evacuation. The nurse teaches the patient how to support the chest wall near the tube insertion site. Coughing, deep breathing, and ambulation are encouraged. Administration of pain medication before these exercises decreases pain and enhances lung expansion.

Maintenance of System Patency

The latex tubing should be lifted frequently to drain the fluid into the collection container. Coiling the latex tubing loosely on the bed will prevent kinks and pooling of blood in a dependent loop hanging on the floor. The chest tube

drainage system is never raised above the chest or the drainage will back up into the chest. At frequent intervals, the chest tube drainage system is checked for drainage and water seal integrity.

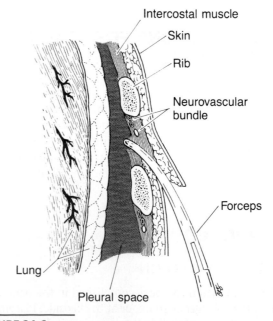

FIGURE 24-6
Forceps penetrates the pleural space to create a track for the chest tube.

- One day after cessation of air leak
- Drainage of <50–100 mL of fluid per day
- 1–3 days post cardiac surgery
- 2–6 days post thoracic surgery
- Obliteration of empyema cavity
- Serosanguineous drainage from around the chest tube insertion site

Drainage Monitoring

The nurse assesses and documents the color, consistency, and amount of drainage, remaining alert to sudden changes. A sudden increase indicates hemorrhage or sudden patency of a previously obstructed tube. A sudden decrease indicates chest tube obstruction or failure of the chest tube or drainage system.

The following nursing actions are recommended to reestablish chest patency:

- Attempt to alleviate the obstruction by repositioning the patient.
- If the clot is visible, straighten the tubing between the chest and drainage unit and raise the tube to enhance the effect of gravity.

Studies have suggested that milking and stripping techniques may not be beneficial for maintenance of chest tube patency.[6] These techniques may excessively increase intrapleural and intrapulmonary pressures, affecting ventricular function or causing trauma from aspiration of lung tissue into chest tube eyelets.

Water Seal Monitoring

Monitoring the water seal of the chest tube drainage system is as important as observing the drainage. Visual checks are made to ensure water seal chambers are filled to the 2-cm water line. If suction is applied, the nurse ensures the water line in the suction chamber is at the ordered level, because water evaporates over time, decreasing the amount of suction being applied. If an Emerson Pleural Suction Pump is used, the suction gauge is checked. The air vent opening must never be occluded.

Respiratory fluctuations are observed in the underwater seal. The absence of fluctuations can indicate that the lung is re-expanded or that there is an obstruction in the system. Continuous vigorous bubbling in the water seal without suction indicates continued pneumothorax or can indicate the tube has been displaced or disconnected. The entire system has to be checked for disconnections and the chest tube inspected to see if it is displaced outside the chest.

Bubbling that occurs 24 hours after chest tube insertion in conjunction with a resolved pneumothorax indicates the presence of a bronchopleural fistula. This usually occurs in the setting of mechanical ventilation at high tidal volumes and pressures and can require surgical intervention.

COMPLICATIONS

The most serious complication of a chest tube is tension pneumothorax, which can develop if there is any obstruction in the chest tube drainage system. Clamping chest tubes as a routine practice predisposes patients to this complication. Clamping of chest tubes is recommended in only two situations:

- To locate the source of an air leak if bubbling occurs in the water seal chamber
- To replace the chest tube drainage unit (Clamping is done only momentarily.)

If the tube must be clamped, padded hemostats are used to avoid cutting the vinyl chest tube.

Occasionally the chest tube may fall out or be accidentally pulled out. In such a circumstance, the insertion site is quickly sealed off to prevent air from entering the pleural cavity.

Pharmacological Agents

Bronchospasm is an important component of reversible obstructive airway disease (asthma). Other important characteristics of asthma include airway inflammation and increased responsiveness to a variety of stimuli (noxious fumes and gases, air pollutants, animal dander, extreme cold, and exercise). Bronchospasm may also be present in chronic obstructive pulmonary disease (COPD).

Pharmacological therapy is used to treat reversible airflow obstruction and airway hyper-responsiveness. This includes bronchodilators and anti-inflammatory agents, listed in Table 24–4.

BRONCHODILATORS

Bronchodilators act principally to dilate the airways by relaxing bronchial smooth muscles. They may be divided into three categories based on their mechanism and site of action. These are beta$_2$ adrenergic agonists, anticholinergic agents, and methylxanthines.

BETA$_2$ ADRENERGIC AGONISTS

The bronchodilatory effects of beta adrenergic agonists result from the stimulation of beta$_2$ adrenergic receptors in

TABLE 24-4 CLINICAL APPLICATION: Drug Therapy
Action, Dosage, and Side Effects of Pulmonary Drugs

Agent	Usual Dose	Common Adverse Effects	Comments
Albuterol (Proventil, Ventolin)	*Aerosol* 1–2 inhalations every 4–6 h *Solution for inhalation* 2.5 mg tid–qid	Palpitations, tachycardia, anxiety, irritability, tremor, GI upset, cough, dry mouth, hoarseness, flushing, headache	Shake well before using; allow 1 full minute between inhalations.
Metaproterenol (Alupent, Metaprel)	*Inhaler* 2–3 inhalations every 3–4 h Maximum dose: 12 inhalations daily *Solution for inhalation* One treatment every 4–6 h	Palpitations, tachycardia, anxiety, irritability, tremor, GI upset, cough, dry mouth, hoarseness, flushing, headache	Shake well before using; allow 1 full minute between inhalations.
Salmeterol (Serevent)	*Asthma/bronchospasm* 1–2 inhalations every 12 h Maximum dose: 4 inhalations daily	Palpitations, tachycardia, anxiety, irritability, tremor, GI upset, cough, dry mouth, hoarseness, flushing, headache	Shake well before using; allow 1 full minute between inhalations; should not be used for relief of acute asthmatic symptoms.
Terbutaline (Brethine, Bricanyl)	*Asthma/bronchospasm Aerosol* 1–2 inhalations every 4–6 h	Palpitations, tachycardia, anxiety, irritability, tremor, GI upset, cough, dry mouth, hoarseness, flushing, headache	Shake well before using; allow 1 full minute between inhalations.
Beclomethasone (Beclovent, Vanceril)	2 inhalations tid–qid or 4 inhalations bid Maximum dose: 20 inhalations daily	Throat irritation, hoarseness, coughing, dry mouth, oral thrush; adrenal suppression with large doses over a prolonged period; rare cases of immediate and delayed hypersensitivity reactions	Use bronchodilator therapy several minutes before using inhaled steroid therapy to enhance penetration.
Methylprednisolone (Solu-Medrol)	125 mg IV every 6 h initially; dose tapered according to patient response; may switch to oral prednisone when tapering	Hyperglycemia, impaired immune response, hypertension, fluid retention, psychosis, steroid myopathy, fragile skin	Long-term use should be avoided due to adverse effects.
Prednisone (Deltasone)	40–60 mg qid initially then taper based on patient response	Hyperglycemia, impaired immune response, hypertension, fluid retention, osteoporosis, hyperkalemia	Long-term oral therapy should be avoided if possible; inhaled therapy is preferred for chronic use if necessary.
Triamcinolone (Azmacort)	2 inhalations tid–qid Maximum dose: 16 inhalations daily	Throat irritation, hoarseness, coughing, dry mouth, oral thrush; adrenal suppression with large doses over a prolonged period	Use bronchodilator therapy several minutes before using inhaled steroid therapy to enhance penetration.
Ipratropium (Atrovent)	Initial dose: 2 inhalations qid Maximum dose: 12 inhalations daily	*Aerosol/inhalation solution* Cough, dry mouth, nervousness, agitation, dizziness, headache, GI upset, palpitations, urinary retention, constipation, worsening narrow angle glaucoma	Must be used regularly to achieve benefit in patients with COPD.

(continued)

TABLE 24-4 CLINICAL APPLICATION: Drug Therapy
Action, Dosage, and Side Effects of Pulmonary Drugs (Continued)

Agent	Usual Dose	Common Adverse Effects	Comments
Cromolyn (Intal, Gastrocrom, Nasalcrom)	20 mg inhaled capsule or nebulizer solution or 2 sprays of aerosol qid	Lacrimation, urinary frequency, dizziness, headache, rash, cough, wheezing, nasal irritation, sneezing, epistaxis, unpleasant taste	Must be used regularly to achieve benefit.
Nedocromil (Tilade)	2 inhalations qid	Cough, pharyngitis, rhinitis, bronchospasm, dry mouth, unpleasant taste, GI upset, dizziness, headache	Must be used regularly to achieve benefit.
Theophylline (Aerolate, Bronkodyl, Elixophyllin, Quibron-T, Slo-bid, Slo-Phyllin, Theo-Dur, Theolair, Uniphyl)	*Asthma/bronchospasm* *Regular release preparations* Initial dose: 16 mg/kg (up to 400 mg) in three to four divided doses *Time-release preparations* Initial dose: 12 mg/kg (up to 400 mg) in two to three divided doses Maximum dose: 13 mg/kg daily	GI irritation, diarrhea, increased gastroesophageal reflux, palpitations, tachycardia, potentiation of diuresis Toxic levels—possible cardiac dysrhythmias, convulsions, and death *Theophylline therapeutic range: 5–15 µg/mL*	Do not chew or crush enteric-coated or sustained-release capsules or tablets; take at the same time, with or without food each day; do not change from one brand to another without consulting a physician. *Drug–drug interactions:* Agents that may decrease theophylline concentrations include **phenobarbital, phenytoin, ketoconazole, rifampin,** and **smoking**. Agents that may increase theophylline concentrations include **allopurinol, cimetidine, corticosteroids, erythromycin,** and **ciprofloxacin.**

the bronchial smooth muscle. In addition, these agents may decrease the release of mediators from mast cells and basophils. Beta$_1$ adrenergic receptors in the heart may also be stimulated and lead to undesired cardiac effects. Newer beta agonists are more specific for the beta$_2$ receptor, although they still retain some beta$_1$ activity.

Beta agonists may be administered orally or inhaled. Aerosolized or inhaled therapy is preferred. It has been shown to produce comparable bronchodilation and fewer systemic adverse effects.

Beta agonists are the bronchodilators of choice for the treatment of acute exacerbations of asthma because of their rapid onset of action. Beta agonists produce less bronchodilation in patients with COPD than in those with asthma. Until recently, all available inhaled beta agonists had short durations of action (4–6 hours). Salmeterol is the first long-acting beta agonist and has a duration of action of 12 hours. Salmeterol cannot be used for acute exacerbations of asthma because of its slow onset of action.

ANTICHOLINERGIC AGENTS

Anticholinergic agents produce bronchodilation by reducing intrinsic vagal tone to the airways. They also block reflex bronchoconstriction caused by inhaled irritants.

Atropine is the prototype anticholinergic agent but is used infrequently. It is readily absorbed from the respiratory tract but produces unwanted systemic effects (blurred vision, drying of respiratory secretions, tachycardia, anxiety).

Ipratropium, a quaternary amine, which is not well absorbed from the respiratory tract, produces fewer systemic adverse effects and has taken the place of atropine. It is most effective in patients with COPD when used on a regular basis. Ipratropium should not be used alone in acute exacerbations because of its slower onset of effect compared to beta agonists. It has been shown to be effective during status asthmaticus when administered through a nebulizer in combination with beta agonists.

METHYLXANTHINES

The use of methylxanthines in the treatment of bronchospastic airway disease is controversial. The mechanism of action of these agents is poorly understood. They inhibit phosphodiesterase, an enzyme that catalyzes the breakdown of cyclic adenosine monophosphate. They may also possess some degree of anti-inflammatory activity and may augment respiratory muscle contractility.

Theophylline, the prototype methylxanthine, may be used chronically in the treatment of bronchospastic disease but is usually considered third- or fourth-line therapy. Some patients with severe disease who are not controlled with beta agonists, anticholinergics, or anti-inflammatory agents may benefit from theophylline. Aminophylline, the intravenous form of theophylline is rarely used in acute exacerbations because of the lack of evidence that it is beneficial in this situation.

Theophylline has a narrow therapeutic index. Depending on the clinical situation, serum drug concentration should be monitored to ensure efficacy and prevent toxicity. The accepted therapeutic range is 5 to 15 µg/mL. Theophylline interacts with a variety of other medications that may alter its serum concentration. These include erythromycin, ciprofloxacin, and cimetidine. Patients with liver disease or congestive heart failure eliminate theophylline more slowly and may be at an increased risk of developing toxicity.

ANTI-INFLAMMATORY AGENTS

Anti-inflammatory agents interrupt the development of bronchial inflammation and have a prophylactic or preventive action. They may also reduce or terminate ongoing inflammation in the airway. Anti-inflammatory agents include corticosteroids and mast cell stabilizers.

CORTICOSTEROIDS

Corticosteroids are the most effective anti-inflammatory agents for the treatment of reversible airflow obstruction. They may be administered parenterally, orally, or as aerosols. In acute exacerbations, high-dose parenteral steroids are used and then tapered as the patient tolerates. Short courses of oral therapy may be used to prevent the progression of acute attacks. Long-term oral therapy is associated with systemic adverse effects and should be avoided if possible. If necessary, the chronic use of inhaled corticosteroids is preferred because of the decreased risk of systemic adverse effects.

MAST CELL STABILIZERS

The two available mast cell stabilizers are cromolyn and nedocromil. They are thought to stabilize the membrane and prevent the release of mediators from mast cells. These agents are not indicated for acute exacerbations of asthma but are used prophylactically to prevent acute airway narrowing after exposure to allergens (eg, exercise, cold air). A 4- to 6-week trial may be required to determine the efficacy in individual patients. The desired endpoint is to reduce the frequency and severity of asthma attacks and enhance the effects of concomitantly administered bronchodilator and steroid therapy. As a result, it may be possible to decrease the dose of bronchodilators or corticosteroids in patients who respond to mast cell stabilizers.

ANTIBIOTICS

Pneumonia is often treated empirically until the results of cultures and sensitivities are available. Then, the antibiotic regimen should be tailored to eradicate the pathogenic organism (Table 24–5). Commonly, broad-spectrum antibiotics or combination therapy is used. The critically ill patient is at increased risk for developing pneumonia due to mechanical ventilation, decreased immune responses, use of corticosteroids, debilitated general health, and cross-infection by health care workers.

Empiric therapy for community-acquired pneumonia should include therapy directed toward the most common organisms associated with this type of pneumonia. These organisms include *Streptococcus pneumoniae* and *Haemophilus influenzae*. Methacillin-resistant *Staphylococcus aureus* should be suspected in patients admitted to the hospital from a nursing home. *Legionella* should be suspected in patients with severe multilobar pneumonia, and patients infected with the human immunodeficiency virus should be empirically treated for *Pneumocystis carinii* pneumonia.

Nosocomial pneumonia is often associated with gram-negative bacilli, such as *Pseudomonas aeruginosa*, or it may be polymicrobial. Aspiration is a concern in mechanically ventilated patients or patients unable to protect their airway. Aspiration pneumonia is associated with anaerobic organisms. Atypical organisms (*Mycoplasma pneumoniae*, *Chlamydia pneumoniae*) should also be considered, as should viral infection.

SEDATION IN CRITICAL ILLNESS

Critically ill patients frequently require pharmacological intervention for analgesia, sedation, control of anxiety, and facilitation of mechanical ventilation. The selection of appropriate pharmacological agents is based on the etiology of the agitation (see display), underlying illness, possible adverse effects, history of previous drug use, and cost. Agents most commonly used in the ICU include opiates, benzodiazepines, haloperidol, and propofol (Diprivan) (Table 24–6).

These agents can be given as bolus doses, by continuous infusion, or using a combination of the two approaches. When administering these agents by continuous infusion,

TABLE 24-5   CLINICAL APPLICATION: Drug Therapy
Antibiotic Therapy in Pulmonary Disease

Pulmonary Infection	Empiric Therapy
Community-acquired pneumonia	Ceftriaxone 1–2 g qd or cefotaxime 2 g every 8 h (Adjust dose for renal function.)
Methicillin-resistant *Staphylococcus aureus* (MRSA) pneumonia	Vancomycin 750–1,500 mg every 12 h (Adjust dose for weight and renal function.)
Legionella pneumonia	Erythromycin 1 g every 6 h
Pneumocystis carinii pneumonia	Trimethoprim/sulfamethoxazole (TMP/SMZ) 5 mg/kg (as TMP) every 6 h (Adjust dose for renal function.)
Nosocomial pneumonia	Ceftazidime 2 g every 8 h (Adjust for renal function; if pseudomonas is suspected, ceftriaxone 1–2 g qd.)
	Cefotaxime 2 g every 8 hours (Adjust for renal function.)
Aspiration pneumonia	Clindamycin 600 mg every 6 h or 900 mg every 8 h
	Ampicillin/sulbactam 1.5–3 g every 6 h (Adjust for renal function.)
	Ticarcillin/clavulanate 3.1 g every 4–6 h (Adjust for renal function.)
Mycoplasma pneumoniae	Erythromycin 500 mg every 6 h
Chlamydia pneumoniae	Doxycycline 100 mg every 12 h
	Erythromycin 500 mg every 6 h

it is important to establish an objective protocol for adjusting the dose to meet the need of each individual patient. Such a protocol can help prevent the prolonged use of these agents and can lower the cumulative amount required for the control of agitation. This can contribute to a decreased length of hospital stay.

When using a continuous infusion, if an increase in dosage is necessary, an additional small bolus dose should be given to facilitate rapid increase to the new desired blood level. Patients who have received large amounts of opiates or benzodiazepines for 2 or more weeks must have their dosage tapered gradually to prevent symptoms of with-

drawal. As a general rule, the dose may be decreased by 20% to 25% a day.

■ NEUROMUSCULAR BLOCKING AGENTS

If metabolic demands and work of breathing continue to compromise ventilatory or hemodynamic stability after maximization of sedation, NMBAs may be required. The goal of therapy with NMBAs is to maximize oxygenation and prevent complications, such as barotrauma, that can be caused by high ventilatory pressures.

The use of NMBAs is almost always required if the pressure-controlled inverse ratio mode of ventilation is used. NMBAs do *not* possess analgesic or sedative properties. When NMBAs are used, sedation and analgesia are required, along with patient and family education. A chemically paralyzed patient should never be left unattended.

Commonly used NMBAs are vecuronium (Norcuron), atracurium (Tracrium), and cisatracurium (Nimbex). Each has advantages and disadvantages related to concomitant drug effects, underlying illness, and cost.

Many recent reports of prolonged paralysis following NMBA use have prompted many institutions to initiate protocols for instituting, monitoring, and withdrawing NMBAs. These range from the use of peripheral nerve stimulators to assess the level of neuromuscular blockade to the routine daily discontinuation of NMBAs to assess neurological status and the need for continued administration.

Etiologies of Agitation in Critically Ill Patients

Pain
Mechanical ventilation
Dyspnea
Hypoxia
Metabolic disarray
Withdrawal from alcohol or drugs
Anxiety
Sleep deprivation
Immobility
Sepsis
Age
Steroid administration

° TABLE 24-6 CLINICAL APPLICATION: Drug Therapy
Pharmacological Options in Critically Ill Patients

Agents	Comments	Antagonist
Opiates	Can cause hypotension and respiratory distress	Naloxone
Morphine sulfate		
Fentanyl		
Benzodiazepines		
Midazolam	Shorter acting	Flumazenil
Lorazepam	Lower cost	Flumazenil
Haloperidol	Monitoring for prolongation of Q–T interval, ex-	
(Haldol)	trapyramidal symptoms needed	
Propofol	For short-term use; may cause hypotension, brady-	
(Diprivan)	cardia, myocardial depression; lipid-based: in-	
	cluded in nutritional assessment to prevent over-	
	feeding; no analgesic effects	

Ventilatory Support

When the patient has been intubated and resuscitated successfully, a commitment has been made to mechanical ventilation. This commitment poses a financial and psychological burden on the patient and family. Every effort and consideration must be given to avoid mechanical ventilation, because ventilatory support reduces mortality very little.

Two approaches can eliminate the need for mechanical ventilation:

- Identification of high-risk patients
- Institution of appropriate measures to forestall or prevent respiratory failure

Patients are predisposed to developing respiratory failure if any of the systems involved in respiration are compromised or overwhelmed (Table 24–7). The degree of risk for developing respiratory failure depends on the patient's ability to move air, secretions, and blood. Inability to do the latter is reflected clinically as pulmonary edema due to poor cardiac output.

▬ PHYSIOLOGICAL PRINCIPLES

Effects of Mechanical Ventilation

To understand the effects of mechanical ventilation, the reader is encouraged to review the physiology of normal respirations and lung compliance, as discussed in Chapter 22. The relationship between pressures in inspiration and expiration is reversed during mechanical ventilation. The ventilator delivers air by virtually pumping it into the patient; therefore, pressures during inspiration are positive. The positive pressures pumped into the lungs result in in-

creased intrathoracic pressures and decreased venous return during inspiration. With the institution of PEEP, even greater pressures are generated during inspiration. During expiration, pressures decrease to PEEP level and continue to be positive throughout expiration. Most patients com-

TABLE 24-7
Body Systems and Possible Events Leading to Respiratory Failure

Systems	Events
Nervous system	Head trauma
Brain stem	Poliomyelitis
Spinal cord and nerves	Cervical (C1–C6) fractures
	Overdose
Muscular system	Myasthenia gravis
Primary—diaphragm	Guillain-Barré
Secondary—respiratory	
Skeletal system	Flail chest
Thorax	Kyphoscoliosis
Respiratory system	Obstruction
Airways	Laryngeal edema
	Bronchitis
	Asthma
Alveoli	Emphysema
	Pneumonia
	Fibrosis
Pulmonary circulation	Pulmonary embolus
Cardiovascular system	Congestive heart failure
	Fluid overload
	Cardiac surgery
	Myocardial infarction
Gastrointestinal system	Aspiration
Hematological system	Disseminated intravascular
	coagulation
Genitourinary system	Renal failure

pensate by increasing peripheral venous tone. If conditions of decreased sympathetic response (eg, hypovolemia, drugs, older age) are present, hypotension develops. In addition, a large tidal volume (VT), greater than 10 to 12 mL/kg, which generates pressures greater than or equal to 35 cm H_2O, can not only influence cardiac output, but also increase the risk of pneumothorax.

The movement of air through the airways creates friction and turbulence: the more flow, the more friction. If the airway is narrowed, the friction increases even more. Therefore, with spontaneously generated inspiration, more negative pressure must be generated for a given flow of air to occur. With mechanical ventilation, more positive pressure is needed to deliver air through the narrowed airway. This is one of the reasons for a high mortality rate in patients with status asthmaticus requiring mechanical ventilation.

Compliance

Compliance is an expression of the elastic properties of the lung, its tendency to want to collapse. In terms of its compliance, the lung is frequently compared with a balloon. Initially it is hard to inflate, until it is stretched. After repeated inflations, the elasticity is lost, and the balloon becomes very easy to blow up.

As the volume of gas is delivered to a patient on a mechanical ventilator, the ventilator's pressure gauge slowly rises from zero to peak inspiratory pressure (PIP). The rise in pressure is caused by resistance to flow or resistance to lung and chest wall inflation (see display). A graph of pressure over time, depicting inspiration, would look like that shown in Figure 24–7. Dynamic pressures and PIP can give an indication of flow properties of the airways.

Factors Decreasing Compliance

Airway Factors
Peak flow
Size of airways
Airway obstructions
External obstructions (kinked ventilator tubing or water in the tubing)

Lung Factors
Elasticity (stiffness) of the lung
Presence of auto-PEEP
Shunt (ARDS)

Chest Wall Factors
Chest wall deformities
Position of patient
External compression of chest wall or diaphragm (distended abdomen, obesity)

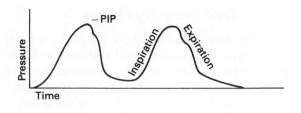

FIGURE 24-7
Graph displaying peak respiratory pressure (PIP).

STATIC PRESSURE

One of the measurements used to obtain compliance is static pressure or plateau pressure.[7] Plateau pressure is obtained by occluding the exhalation valve when the patient is in maximum inspiration. This holds the volume of delivered air in the patient's chest by preventing exhalation. The pressure recorded at this moment is plateau pressure and reflects the force necessary to deliver the preset volume of air to the patient and hold the airways open. Graphically, it would appear as in Figure 24–8. Static compliance is determined by dividing the effective tidal volume by plateau pressure minus total PEEP:

$$\frac{V_T}{\text{Plateau pressure} - \text{PEEP}} = \text{Static compliance}$$

A higher compliance means that the lung is more easily distended; a lower compliance means that the lung is stiff and difficult to distend. In other words, a higher compliance is better. Low compliance may be due to stiff lungs, a stiff chest wall (kyphoscoliosis), or ventilation of only a small portion of lung (acute respiratory distress syndrome [ARDS]). Serial measurements of compliance can alert the nurse to sudden decreases, which may be due to pneumothorax, mucous plugging, or pulmonary edema.

■ EQUIPMENT FEATURES

Many different oxygen delivery systems are available. Manual resuscitators are used in emergencies in acute respiratory failure. Several mechanical ventilators can be used, and they offer a variety of modes.

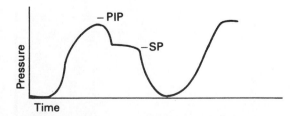

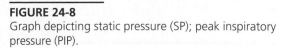

FIGURE 24-8
Graph depicting static pressure (SP); peak inspiratory pressure (PIP).

Oxygen Delivery Systems

If external or internal respiration is impaired, supplemental oxygen is vital to maintain the patient's cellular function. Oxygen therapy corrects hypoxemia, decreases the work of breathing, and decreases myocardial work. Oxygen delivery systems are traditionally divided into high-flow and low-flow systems. These are listed in the accompanying display.

Low-flow oxygen devices work by supplying oxygen at flow rates less than the patient's inspiratory volume. The rest of the volume is pulled from room air (entrained). Because of this oxygen and room air mixing, the actual FIO_2 delivered to the patient is unknown. Low-flow oxygen devices are suitable for patients with normal respiratory patterns, rates, and ventilation volumes.

High-flow oxygen devices supply flow rates high enough to accommodate two to three times the patient's inspiratory volume. These devices are suitable for patients with shallow breathing patterns and COPD patients. The latter patients are "sensitive" to oxygen; a small increment increases their PaO_2 and dramatically increases their $PaCO_2$, resulting in respiratory depression.

If lower concentrations of oxygen are needed, the system selected is usually the nasal cannula. The cannula can be used even with mouth breathers, because movement of air through the oropharynx creates the Bernoulli effect, pulling oxygen from the nasopharynx. The exact concentration of oxygen depends on the patient's V_T. If the patient hypoventilates, the oxygen concentration increases in the upper airway. In contrast, if hyperventilation occurs, the concentration of oxygen decreases owing to large amounts of room air diluting the oxygen delivered.

If the oxygen concentration must be constant, the system used is the Venturi mask. It delivers an exact percentage of oxygen regardless of the patient's V_T. Patients with COPD may require oxygen delivery by the Venturi system. They can be detected through serial ABG monitoring, which reveals large increases in $PaCO_2$ with small increases in oxygen flow.

Oxygen Delivery Devices

Low-Flow
- Nasal cannula
- Simple mask
- Rebreather
- Non-rebreather

High-Flow
- Venturi mask
- Aerosol mask
- Tracheostomy collar
- T-piece
- Face tent

As higher concentrations of oxygen are needed, the nasal cannula is replaced by a mask system. A simple mask delivers the lowest concentrations of oxygen, and a non-rebreather, the highest. If a patient's PaO_2 cannot be maintained using the non-rebreather, respiratory failure with the need for intubation and mechanical ventilation is imminent.

Manual Resuscitator

The nurse's first line of defense for acute respiratory failure is the MRB. During artificial resuscitation, hyperinflation before suctioning, or "bagging" of any mechanically ventilated patient, MRBs with reservoirs must be used and connected to an oxygen source to deliver 0.74 to 1.00 concentrations of oxygen.

Knowledge of the bag and skill in using it are vital. The function of this simple ventilator can be compared with that of the more sophisticated models. The following pertain to the manual resuscitator:

- The force of squeezing the bag determines tidal volume delivered to the patient.
- The number of hand squeezes per minute determines the rate.
- The force and rate that the bag is squeezed determine the peak flow.

While the bag is being used, one must carefully observe the patient's chest to determine whether the bag is performing properly and whether any gastric distension is developing. In addition, the ease or resistance encountered can roughly indicate lung compliance. If a patient becomes progressively harder to "bag," an increase in secretions, pneumothorax, worsening bronchospasms, or other condition that might decrease the patient's compliance must be considered.

When delivering breaths with an MRB, the nurse allows time for complete exhalation between breaths to prevent auto-PEEP, which can cause hypotension and barotrauma, especially in patients with obstructive airway disease.

Mechanical Ventilators

The goal of mechanical ventilation is to maintain an alveolar ventilation appropriate for the patient's metabolic needs and to correct hypoxemia and maximize oxygen transport. Most ventilators can be divided into two categories—volume-cycled and pressure-cycled. Regardless of which type or model is used, the nurse must be familiar with the ventilator's function and limitations. A mechanical device used to sustain life is only as good as its design and the medical team using it.

The following discussion of ventilators is in order of evolution and use.

NEGATIVE PRESSURE VENTILATOR

Early negative pressure ventilators were known as "iron lungs." The patient's body was encased in an iron cylinder and negative pressures were generated to enlarge the thoracic cage. This caused alveolar pressures to fall, and a pressure gradient was formed so that air flowed into the lungs. The iron lung was used most frequently during the poliomyelitis epidemics of the 1930s and 1940s,[8] but iron lungs are infrequently used today. Intermittent short-term negative pressure ventilation can sometimes be used in patients with chronic diseases that predispose them to episodes of acute hypercapnic ventilatory failure, such as COPD, diseases of the chest wall (kyphoscoliosis), and neuromuscular diseases (Duchenne's muscular dystrophy, amyotrophic lateral sclerosis), preventing the need for intubation and conventional ventilatory support.

Normally, negative pressure ventilation uses a mobile ventilator. It fits like a tortoise shell, forming a seal over the chest, and a hose connects the shell to a negative pressure generator. The thoracic cage is literally "sucked up" to initiate inspiration, which is preset manually with a trigger. Negative pressure ventilators are advantageous in that they mimic normal respiration. Their use is restricted, however, because of their limitations on positioning and movement and their lack of adaptability to large or small body torsos.

POSITIVE PRESSURE VENTILATOR

Pressure-Cycled Ventilator

The pressure-cycled ventilator works on the basic principle that once a preset pressure is reached, inspiration is terminated. At this pressure point, the inspiratory valve closes, and exhalation occurs passively. Ultimately this means that if a patient's lung compliance or resistance to flow changes, the volume of air delivered varies.

Clinically, as a patient's lungs become stiffer (less compliant), the volume of air delivered to the patient drops—sometimes drastically. Consequently, to ensure adequate minute ventilation (MV) and to detect any changes in lung compliance and resistance, one must frequently monitor inspiratory pressure, rate, and tidal volume. In a patient whose pulmonary status is unstable, the use of a pressure ventilator is not recommended. However, in a very stable patient with compliant lungs, pressure ventilators are adequate and can be used as a weaning tool in selected patients.

Time-Cycled Ventilator

The time-cycled ventilator works on the basic principle that once a preset time is finished, inspiration is terminated. Expiratory time is determined by inspiratory time and rate (number of breaths per minute). Normal inspiratory–expiratory ratio is 1:2.

Volume-Cycled Ventilator

The volume ventilator is the most frequently used type in critical care settings. The basic principle of this ventilator is that once a designated volume of air is delivered to the patient, inspiration is terminated. A piston or bellows pushes a predetermined volume (V_T) into the patient's lungs at a set rate. The advantage of a volume ventilator is that despite a change in patient lung compliance, a consistent V_T is delivered.

HIGH-FREQUENCY VENTILATOR

Because of the complications associated with positive pressure ventilation, other methods that may be more physiologically compatible are being investigated. The technique of high-frequency ventilation (HFV) is one such method. HFV accomplishes oxygenation by the diffusion of oxygen and carbon dioxide from high to low gradients of concentration. This diffusion movement is increased if the kinetic energy of the gas molecules is increased. HFV uses small V_T (1–3 mL/kg) at frequencies greater than 100/min.[9] (A patient experiencing HFV is somewhat analogous to a panting dog; the dog moves small volumes of air at a very fast rate.)

Theoretically, HFV would be used to achieve lower peak ventilatory pressures, thus lowering the risk of barotrauma and improving ventilation–perfusion matching because of its different flow delivery characteristics. Clinical data are lacking to show that HFV improves outcomes. Potential adverse effects of HFV include gas trapping and necrotizing tracheobronchitis when used in the absence of adequate humidification.[10]

THE CURRENT GENERATION OF MECHANICAL VENTILATOR

Ventilators today are complex, incorporating every known cycling mode, pressure wave, and monitoring feature. The most technologically advanced ventilator has a computer and a microprocessor system. Pulse oximetry and end-tidal CO_2 sensors have also been added to the latest generation of ventilators. They provide visual feedback to the respiratory care team as to what the ventilator is doing. The more complex the ventilator, the higher the cost and the greater the margin for error. These ventilators are most appropriate for the patient with high MV requirements that frequently outstrip conventional ventilators.

Careful monitoring by the nurse is still the essence of therapy. All types of mechanical ventilation require attention to patient care.

Ventilatory Modes

Several different modes of ventilatory control can be found on ventilators. Figure 24–9 and Table 24–8 compare these modes. Ventilatory modes include assist-control, intermittent mandatory ventilation, pressure support ventilation, pressure-controlled ventilation, inverse ratio ventilation, volume-assured pressure support, continuous positive airway pressure, and noninvasive positive pressure ventilation.

ASSIST-CONTROL MODE

In the assist-control mode (A/C), basic rate is set. If the patient wishes to breathe faster, he or she can trigger the ventilator. If the patient's drive to breathe is negated, the ventilator "kicks in" at the preset rate. In the A/C mode, all breaths—whether triggered by the patient or delivered at a

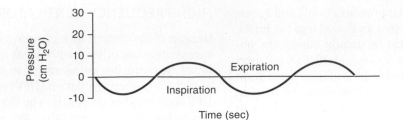

Spontaneous breathing

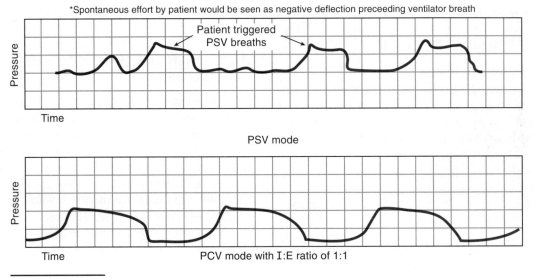

FIGURE 24-9

Comparison of ventilatory modes using continuous airway pressure monitoring.

set rate—are at the same V_T. Because of this, hyperventilation (reflected in the ABGs as a respiratory alkalosis) can occur, as can air trapping in patients with obstructive airway disease.

INTERMITTENT MANDATORY VENTILATION MODE

The intermittent mandatory ventilation (IMV) mode allows intermittent mandatory ventilation. The rate and V_T are preset. If the patient wants to breathe above this rate, he or she may. However, unlike the A/C mode, any breaths taken above the set rate are spontaneous breaths taken through the ventilator circuit. The V_T of these breaths can vary drastically from the V_T set on the ventilator, because they are determined by the patient's ability to generate negative pressure in the chest. The risk of increased work of breathing

because of inappropriate flow delivery during spontaneous breaths can be minimized by applying pressure support during spontaneous breaths. IMV has been used as a weaning mode by gradually decreasing the set number of breaths, thereby allowing the patient to assume more and more of the work of breathing.

PRESSURE SUPPORT VENTILATION

The pressure support ventilation (PSV) mode augments or assists spontaneous breathing efforts to a point where the preset pressure is reached in patients who have an intact respiratory drive. Pressure support is used at low pressure levels (5–10 cm H_2O) to aid the patient in breathing during the spontaneous breaths in the IMV mode. When PSV is used as a stand-alone mode of ventilation, the pressure support level is adjusted to achieve the targeted V_T and RR. At

TABLE 24-8
Comparison of Modes of Ventilation

Ventilatory Mode	Indications	Advantages/Disadvantages	Special Monitoring
A/C	Often used as initial mode of ventilation	A: Ensures vent support during every breath Each breath same VT D: Hyperventilation, air trapping	Work of breathing may be increased if sensitivity or flow rate is too low.
IMV	Often used as initial mode of ventilation	A: Allows spontaneous breaths (VT determined by patient) between vent breaths D: Patient–ventilator asynchrony possible	
PSV	Intact respiratory drive in patient necessary Used as a weaning mode	A: Decreases work of breathing, increases patient comfort D: Should not be used in patients with acute bronchospasm	Adjust PSV level to maintain desired respiratory rate and VT. Monitor for changes in compliance, which can cause VT to change. Monitor respiratory rate and VT at least hourly.
PCV	Used to limit airway pressures that can cause barotrauma Severe ARDS	D: Patient–ventilator asynchrony possible, necessitating sedation/paralysis	Monitor VT at least hourly. Monitor for barotrauma, hemodynamic instability.
IRV	Usually used in conjunction with PCV Increases ratio I:E to allow for recruitment of alveoli and improve oxygenation	D: Almost always requires paralysis	Monitor for auto-PEEP, barotrauma, hemodynamic instability.
VAPS	Combines comfort of PSV with guaranteed VT	A: Decrease in work of breathing D: Increase in peak airway pressure	
CPAP	Constant positive airway pressure for patients who breathe spontaneously	A: Used in intubated or nonintubated patients D: Some systems, no alarm if respiratory rate falls	Monitor for increased work of breathing if system uses a demand valve.
Noninvasive	Nocturnal hypoventilation in patients with neuromuscular disease, chest wall deformity, obstructive sleep apnea, and COPD	A: Decreased cost when patients can be cared for at home; no need for artificial airway D: Patient discomfort or claustrophobia Aspiration risk	Monitor for gastric distension, air leaks from mouth.

high pressure levels, PSV provides nearly total ventilatory support.

Specific uses of PSV are to promote patient comfort and synchrony with the ventilator, to decrease the work of breathing necessary to overcome the resistance of the ETT, and for weaning. ETT resistance can be related to the effort needed in breathing through a straw if one is submerged under water. The smaller the straw, the larger the effort to move air from the atmosphere into the lungs. Pressure support reduces this work. As a weaning tool, PSV is thought to increase the endurance of the respiratory muscles by decreasing the physical work and oxygen demands during spontaneous breathing.

During PSV, inspired VT and RR must be constantly monitored to detect changes in lung compliance. PSV should not be used in patients experiencing bronchospasm.

PRESSURE-CONTROLLED VENTILATION

The pressure-controlled ventilation (PCV) mode is used to limit peak airway pressures when low compliance and high airway resistance produce high ventilating pressures with the risk of barotrauma. PCV is most often used in patients with ARDS. Pressure and RR are parameters that must be set. Tidal volume varies with compliance and airway resistance and must be closely monitored. Sedation and the use of NMBAs is frequently indicated, because the discomfort associated with this mode of ventilation often results in patient–ventilator asynchrony.

INVERSE RATIO VENTILATION

Most ventilators operate with a short inspiratory time and a long expiratory time (1:2 or 1:3); this promotes venous return and allows time for air to exit the lungs. Inverse ratio ventilation (IRV) mode reverses this ratio so that inspiratory time is equal to or longer than expiratory time (1:1 to 4:1).

The IRV mode is used to improve oxygenation in ARDS by expanding stiff alveoli using longer distending time and preventing alveolar collapse during shorter expiratory time. IRV predisposes to auto-PEEP with the associated complications of hypotension and barotrauma. In addition, because this method of ventilation feels so unnatural to the patient, it is very uncomfortable, usually necessitating heavy sedation (often with paralysis) to ensure patient–ventilator synchrony.

With this inverse ratio, intrathoracic pressure is often higher, so IRV is usually combined with PCV (PC-IRV). Inspiratory VT must be monitored in this mode of ventilation.

VOLUME-ASSURED PRESSURE SUPPORT

The volume-assured pressure support (VAPS) mode (ie, pressure augmentation, Bear 2 ventilator) combines the patient comfort of PSV with the guaranteed tidal volume of a volume ventilator. VAPS can be used with A/C or IMV. If the set VT is not delivered by the end of a pressure support breath, flow will continue until the VT is reached. VAPS results in an increase in peak airway pressure but an overall decrease in work of breathing.

CONTINUOUS POSITIVE AIRWAY PRESSURE

The CPAP mode assists spontaneously breathing patients to improve their oxygenation by elevating end-expiratory pressure in the lungs throughout the respiratory cycle. CPAP can be used for intubated and nonintubated patients. It is used as a weaning mode and for nocturnal ventilation (nasal or mask CPAP) to splint open the upper airway, preventing upper airway obstruction in patients with obstructive sleep apnea.

NONINVASIVE POSITIVE PRESSURE VENTILATION

Noninvasive positive pressure ventilation uses either nasal or face mask. It is used in the treatment of patients with chronic respiratory insufficiency to manage acute or chronic respiratory failure without intubation and conventional mechanical ventilation, as an aid in weaning patients from mechanical ventilation, and as an alternative to conventional mechanical ventilation in patients who are ventilated in their homes.[11] The advantages of noninvasive ventilation over conventional ventilation include decreased costs when hospitalization is not required, increased patient satisfaction when patients receive care in their homes, easier administration, and controlled nocturnal hypoventilation.

Noninvasive ventilation is used to control central alveolar hypoventilation, which contributes to nocturnal hypoventilation in patients with neuromuscular disease, chest wall deformity, obstructive sleep apnea, and COPD. Its success largely depends on patient motivation. Noninvasive ventilation is not successful in all patients; these will usually progress to tracheostomy for nocturnal ventilation.

Noninvasive ventilation operates on the principle that gas flow from the machine ceases when the predetermined pressure is reached. The expiratory pathway is then opened, and exhalation occurs.

Disadvantages and complications of noninvasive ventilation include inability of claustrophobic patients to tolerate the mask or headgear, painful gastric distension, mouth leaking in patients who are unable to close their mouths when mask ventilation is used, skin necrosis caused by the tightly fitting equipment, aspiration, and secretion retention.

BiPAP ventilation[11] permits independent control of inspiratory (IPAP) and expiratory (EPAP) pressures and provides nasal PSV.

■ INDICATIONS FOR VENTILATORY SUPPORT

Respiratory failure is defined as an inability to maintain an adequate pH, $PaCO_2$, and PaO_2. Adequate means a pH greater than 7.25, a $PaCO_2$ less than 50 mmHg, and a PaO_2 greater than 50 mmHg with the patient on oxygen. If the ABGs deteriorate and the patient fatigues, mechanical ventilatory support is indicated.

Often it is the nurse who initially recognizes the onset of respiratory failure. Identification of high-risk patients, serial monitoring and evaluation of progressive respiratory status, and institution of appropriate measures may forestall or negate the need for mechanical ventilation.

The objective of mechanical ventilation is to support the patient through an illness. Clinical goals of mechanical ventilation include reversal of hypoxemia, reversal of acute respiratory acidosis, relief of respiratory distress, prevention or reversal of atelectasis, resting of ventilatory muscles, decrease in systemic or myocardial oxygen consumption, reduction in intracranial pressure, and stabilization of the chest wall.

Mechanical ventilation is not curative and can actually cause complications.

■ PROCEDURE

Setting Ventilator Controls

The nurse must be adept at handling the various ventilator systems, modes, and controls before giving mechanical ventilatory support to a patient. The following section discusses the various controls and settings and their implications in nursing care.

FRACTION OF INSPIRED OXYGEN

Most ventilators allow for easy adjustment of oxygen percentage (fraction of inspired oxygen, FIO_2) by means of a dial. Oxygen analyzers, either in-circuit or external, allow the nurse to ascertain the FIO_2 that is being delivered. Initially a patient is placed on a high level of FIO_2 (.60 or higher). Subsequent changes in FIO_2 are based on ABG and SaO_2. Usually FIO_2 is adjusted to maintain an $SaO_2 > 90\%$ (roughly equivalent to a $PaO_2 > 60$ mmHg). Oxygen toxicity is a concern when FIO_2 of greater than .60 is required for 12 to 24 hours; therefore, most clinicians attempt to use strategies to allow for maintenance of FIO_2 of .60 or less.

RESPIRATORY RATE

The number of breaths per minute delivered to the patient can be directly dialed on most ventilator models. The nurse should double-check the functioning of the ventilator with a watch that has a second hand.

In the pressure ventilator, the inspiratory time determines the duration of inspiration by regulating the velocity of gas flow. The higher the flow rate, the faster peak airway pressure is reached and the shorter the inspiration; the lower the flow rate, the longer the inspiration. A high flow rate produces turbulence, shallow inspirations, and uneven distribution of volume.

Respiratory rate times tidal volume equals minute ventilation ($RR \times VT = MV$). In turn, MV determines alveolar ventilation. These two parameters are adjusted according to the $PaCO_2$. Increasing MV decreases $PaCO_2$; conversely, decreasing MV increases $PaCO_2$. In special cases, hypoventilation or hyperventilation is desired. For example, in a head injury, a respiratory alkalosis may be required to promote cerebral vasoconstriction, with a resultant decrease in intracranial pressure. In this case, the VT and RR are increased to achieve the desired alkalotic pH by $PaCO_2$ manipulation. In contrast, COPD patients whose baseline ABGs have elevated $PaCO_2$ should not be hyperventilated. Instead, the goal should be restoration of baseline $PaCO_2$. These patients usually have a large acid load, and lowering their carbon dioxide levels rapidly may result in seizures. Rate adjustments may also be necessary to enhance patient comfort or when rapid rates cause air trapping that results in auto-PEEP.

TIDAL VOLUME

In the volume ventilator, a dial is turned to the number of cubic centimeters of air to be delivered with each breath. Tidal volumes of 10 to 15 mL/kg of body weight have traditionally been used. Research has identified a phenomenon of iatrogenic lung injury that has been dubbed "volutrauma,"[12] in which forces produced on the lungs by the ventilator may aggravate the damage inflicted on the lungs by the pathological process that necessitated mechanical ventilation. For this reason, lower VT targets (8–10 mL/kg) are recommended.

PEAK FLOW

Peak flow is the velocity of air flow per unit of time and is expressed as liters per minute. On most ventilators, this is a separate dial. In the pressure ventilator, this is manipulated with the inspiratory time flow-rate control. If MV is high, peak flow may need to be increased to provide time for exhalation before a new inhalation is triggered. However, increasing peak flow increases turbulence, which is reflected in increasing airway pressures.

PRESSURE LIMIT

On volume-cycled ventilators, the pressure limit dial limits the highest pressure allowed in the ventilator circuit. Once the high pressure limit is reached, inspiration is terminated. Therefore, if the pressure limit is being constantly reached, the designated VT is not being delivered to the patient. The cause of this can be coughing, accumulation of secretions, kinked ventilator tubing, pneumothorax, decreasing compliance, or a pressure limit set too low.

POSITIVE END-EXPIRATORY PRESSURE

The PEEP knob adjusts the pressure that is maintained in the lungs at the end of expiration. PEEP is the term used to describe positive end-expiratory pressure with positive pressure (machine) breaths. CPAP is the term used when PEEP is supplied during spontaneous breathing. PEEP and CPAP can be visualized on the respiratory pressure gauge. Instead of returning to zero at the end of expiration, the pressure needle drops to PEEP/CPAP level.

Oxygenation is improved when PEEP is used to recruit alveolar units that are totally or partially collapsed. It holds the alveoli open by maintaining a pressure greater than atmospheric pressure in the alveoli at the end of expiration. This end-expiratory pressure increases functional residual capacity by reinflating collapsed alveoli, keeping the alveoli open, and decreasing the pressure needed to ventilate them. In addition, there is some evidence that keeping the alveoli open enhances surfactant regeneration. It is used for patients who require FIO_2 levels greater than .50 for more than several hours to achieve adequate arterial oxygen levels. Most often, this is a patient who develops ARDS with refractory hypoxemia in which the PaO_2 deteriorates rapidly despite greater concentrations of oxygen administration.

In the patient who does not have adequate circulating blood volume, institution of PEEP decreases blood return to the heart, decreases cardiac output, and decreases oxygen to the tissues. If hypotension or decreased cardiac output results from PEEP application, restoring circulating intravascular volume with administration of intravenous fluids may correct the hypotension.

Another serious complication of PEEP is barotrauma, alveolar rupture that can result in death. It can occur in any mechanically ventilated patient but is most common when high levels of PEEP are used (10–20 cm H_2O), in lungs with high ventilating pressures and low compliance, and in patients with obstructive airway disease. The development of barotrauma is an emergency and usually requires placement of a chest tube.

To evaluate whether the effects of PEEP are beneficial, monitoring of ABGs, SaO_2, and hemodynamic pressures (to include cardiac output, compliance, and blood pressure) is necessary. Baseline values are obtained before changes in PEEP. PEEP is usually increased in increments of 2.5 to 5 cm of water pressure. The patient is monitored for adverse effects, such as hypotension and dysrhythmias. If these occur, the PEEP is removed. If PEEP is tolerated, the patient is stabilized on the new PEEP settings for approximately 15 minutes. The monitored parameters are then repeated. Because the goal of PEEP therapy is to increase oxygen delivery to the tissues, a calculation using the following formula can determine its effectiveness:

$$O_2 \text{ delivery} = SaO_2 \times CO \times Hgb \times 1.34 \times 10$$

where SaO_2 is oxygen saturation, CO is cardiac output, Hgb is hemoglobin, 1.34 is the amount of oxygen in milliliters with which 1 g of hemoglobin can combine when maximally saturated, and 10 is a conversion factor. Strategies that enhance O_2 delivery are based on manipulation of these elements: increasing FIO_2 to increase SaO_2, using dobutamine (when appropriate) to increase cardiac output, and red blood cell transfusion to increase hemoglobin. Normal oxygen delivery is between 800 and 1,200 mL/min.

During PEEP trials, compliance is calculated and monitored. "Best PEEP" is the point at which compliance begins to decrease, indicating that increases in PEEP are not opening collapsed alveoli but merely overinflating those that are already open. Reduction of PEEP is considered if the patient has a PaO_2 of 80 to 100 mmHg on an FIO_2 of .50 or less, is hemodynamically stable, and has stabilization or improvement of the underlying illness. Oximetry is recommended to monitor reduction of PEEP level. If saturation falls dramatically in the first 3 minutes, the PEEP level is returned to the previous setting. If oxygenation is maintained at an adequate level, PEEP is reduced, monitoring the parameters discussed above at appropriate intervals. If a patient requires high levels of PEEP for a prolonged period, PEEP must be decreased slowly. Within 4 hours after PEEP is decreased, alveolar units may again collapse and result in hypoxemia.

Hemodynamic measurements (pulmonary artery pressures and pulmonary artery wedge pressure) are taken at end-expiration with the patient on PEEP. Accuracy in selecting the point of end-expiration on the waveform tracing is facilitated by using continuous airway monitoring[13] (Fig. 24–10). PEEP does not need to be discontinued before obtaining hemodynamic measurements. Hemodynamic measurements can be inaccurate indicators of oxygen delivery to the tissues if a patient is on PEEP and the position of the catheter is not below the left atrium. The position of the catheter should be verified on a lateral chest x-ray.

Attempts should be made to minimize removing the patient from the ventilator when using high levels of PEEP. Oxygenation can deteriorate and be slow to rebound, because it takes a significant amount of time for the effects of PEEP to be reestablished. Therefore, if the patient is being oxygenated using an MRB, it must be equipped with a valve that allows levels of PEEP to be dialed in. In-line suction may be helpful to prevent breaking the PEEP circuit to suction the patient.

SENSITIVITY

The sensitivity knob controls the amount of patient effort needed to initiate an inspiration, as expressed by required negative inspiratory effort. Increasing the sensitivity decreases the amount of work the patient must do to initiate a ventilatory breath. Likewise, decreasing the sensitivity increases the amount of negative pressure that the patient needs to initiate inspiration and increases the work of breathing.

ALARMS

Mechanical ventilators are used to support life. Alarm systems are necessary to warn the nurse of developing problems. Alarm systems can be categorized according to volume, pressure, high, and low. Low-pressure alarms warn of disconnection of the patient from the ventilator. High-pressure alarms warn of rising pressures. Low-volume alarms warn of leaks.

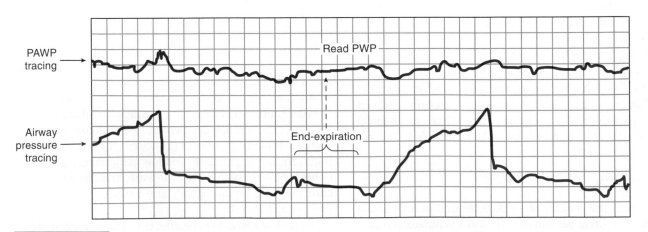

FIGURE 24-10

Use of continuous airway pressure monitoring to assist in identifying point of end-expiration

Electrical failure alarms are a must for all ventilators. A nurse or respiratory therapist must respond to every ventilator alarm. Alarms must never be ignored or disarmed. Some trouble-shooting guidelines are presented in Table 24–9.

HUMIDIFICATION AND THERMOREGULATION

Mechanical ventilation bypasses the upper airway, thus negating the body's protective mechanism for humidification and warming. These two processes must be added to

the ventilator circuit in the form of a humidifier with a temperature control. All air delivered by the ventilator passes through the water in the humidifier, being warmed and saturated. Because of this, insensible water loss is decreased. In most instances, the temperature of the air is about body temperature. In some rare instances (severe hypothermia), the air temperatures can be increased. Caution is advised, because prolonged high inhaled temperatures can cause tracheal burns. A dry humidifier contributes to drying the

TABLE 24-9
Troubleshooting the Ventilator

Problem	Possible Causes	Action
Volume or pressure alarm	*Patient related*	
	Patient disconnected from ventilator	Reconnect STAT.
	Loss of delivered VT	Auscultate neck for possible leak around ETT cuff. Review chest film for endotracheal tube placement—may be too high. Check for loss of VT through chest tube.
	Decrease in patient-initiated breaths	Evaluate patient for cause: check respiratory rate, ABGs, last sedation.
	Increased compliance	May be due to clearing of secretions or relief of bronchospasms.
	Ventilator related	
	Leaks	Check all tubing for loss of connection, starting at patient and moving toward humidifier. Check for change in ventilator settings. (*Note:* If problem is not corrected STAT, bag-breathe patient until ventilator problem is corrected.)
High-pressure or peak-pressure alarm	*Patient related* Decreased compliance	
	Increased dynamic pressures	Suction patient. Administer inhaled β-agonists. If sudden, evaluate for pneumothorax. Evaluate chest film for ETT placement in right main stem bronchus. Sedate if patient is bucking the ventilator or biting the ETT.
	Increased static pressure	Evaluate ABGs for hypoxia, fluids for overload, chest film for atelectasis. Auscultate breath sounds.
	Ventilator related	
	Tubing kinked	Check tubing.
	Tubing filled with water	Empty water into a receptacle: Do not drain back into the humidifier. (*Note:* Water in tubing will increase PEEP levels.)
	Patient–ventilator asynchrony	Recheck sensitivity and peak flow settings. Provide sedation/paralysis if indicated.
Abnormal ABGs	*Patient related*	
Hypoxia	Secretions	Suction.
	Increase in disease pathology	Evaluate patient and chest film.
	Positive fluid balance	Evaluate I & O.
Hypocapnia	Hypoxia	Evaluate ABGs and patient.
	Increased lung compliance	Evaluate for wean potential.
Hypercapnia	Sedation	Increase respiratory rate or VT settings.
	Fatigue	
	Ventilator related	
Hypoxia	FiO₂ drift	Check ventilator with oxygen analyzer.
Hypocapnia	Settings not correct	Decrease respiratory rate, VT, or MV.
Hypercapnia	Settings not correct	Increase respiratory rate, VT, or MV.
Heater alarm	Adding cold water to humidifier	Wait.
	Altered setting	Reset.
	Cold air blowing on humidifier	Redirect air flow.

airway, with resultant mucous plugging and an inability to suction out secretions.

As air passes through the ventilator to the patient, water condenses in the corrugated tubing. This moisture is considered contaminated and must be drained into a receptacle and not back into the sterile humidifier. If the water is allowed to build up, resistance is developed in the circuit, and PEEP is generated. In addition, if left unchecked, the water can be aspirated by the patient. Attention to this is a nursing responsibility.

The humidifier is an ideal medium for bacterial growth. Institutional policies guide timing of ventilator circuit changes.

■ COMPLICATIONS OF MECHANICAL SUPPORT

Complications that can occur with mechanical ventilation are listed in the accompanying display. These complications can be minimized by prevention.

Aspiration

Aspiration can occur before, during, or after intubation. The potential for developing ARDS is increased if aspiration occurs.

Complications of Mechanical Ventilation

Airway
Aspiration
Decreased clearance of secretions
Predisposition to infection

Endotracheal Tube
Tube kinked
Tube plugged
Rupture of pyriform sinus
Tracheal stenosis
Tracheal malacia
Right main stem intubation
Cuff failure
Sinusitis
Otitis media
Laryngeal edema

Mechanical
Ventilator malfunction
Hypoventilation
Hyperventilation
Tension pneumothorax

Physiological
Water and NaCl retention
Left ventricular dysfunction → hypotension
Stress ulcers
Paralytic ileus
Gastric distention
Starvation

Methods and nursing care in prevention of aspiration are discussed under Assessment and Management.

Ventilator Malfunction

Ventilator malfunction is a potentially serious problem. Ventilator checks are performed by nursing or respiratory therapists every 2 to 4 hours. Table 24–9 summarizes common mechanical problems and troubleshooting techniques. While a second person manually ventilates the patient during suspected mechanical problems, the nurse troubleshoots.

Iatrogenically induced complications include overventilation, which causes respiratory alkalosis, and underventilation, which causes respiratory acidosis or hypoxemia. ABG studies determine the effectiveness of mechanical ventilation. COPD patients, however, are ventilated at their normal ABG values, which can involve high carbon dioxide levels.

Barotrauma

Mechanical ventilation involves "pumping" air into the chest, creating positive pressures during inspiration. If PEEP is added, the pressures are increased and continued throughout expiration. These positive pressures can rupture an alveolus or emphysematous bleb. Air then escapes into and is trapped in the pleural space, accumulating until it begins to collapse the lung. Eventually the collapsing lung impinges on the mediastinal structures, compressing the trachea and eventually the heart; this is called tension pneumothorax. Signs and symptoms of tension pneumothorax are listed in the display. Signs of pneumothorax include extreme dyspnea, hypoxia (indicated by a decrease in oxygen saturation), and an abrupt increase in PIP. Breath sounds may be decreased or absent on the affected side; however, this sign may not be reliable in the patient on positive pressure ventilation. Observation of the patient may reveal a tracheal deviation or the sudden development of subcutaneous emphysema. The most ominous signs of tension pneumothorax are hypotension and bradycardia that

Signs and Symptoms of Tension Pneumothorax

- Tachycardia
- Tachypnea
- Agitation
- Diaphoresis
- Midline tracheal shift
- Muffled heart tones
- Absent breath sounds over affected lung
- Hyper-resonance to percussion over affected lung
- Elevation in peak airway pressures in ventilated patients
- Decrease in oxygen saturation or PaO₂
- Hypotension
- Cardiac arrest

can deteriorate into a cardiac arrest without timely medical intervention. The physician may decompress the chest with a needle until a chest tube can be inserted.

Decreased Cardiac Output

Although decreased cardiac output reflected by hypotension at the initiation of mechanical ventilation is often attributed to the drugs used for intubation, the most important contribution to this phenomenon is lack of sympathetic tone and decreased venous return. In addition to hypotension, other signs and symptoms can include unexplained restlessness, decreased levels of consciousness, decreased urine output, weak peripheral pulses, slow capillary refill, pallor, fatigue, and chest pain. Hypotension is usually corrected by increasing fluids to correct the hypovolemia.

Water Imbalance

The decreased venous return to the heart is sensed by the vagal stretch receptors located in the right atrium. This sensed hypovolemia stimulates the release of antidiuretic hormone from the posterior pituitary. The decreased cardiac output leading to decreased urine output compounds the problem by stimulating the renin–angiotensin–aldosterone response. The patient who is mechanically ventilated, hemodynamically unstable, and requiring large amounts of fluid resuscitation can experience extensive edema, including scleral and facial edema.

Immobility

Many complications that contribute to the morbidity and mortality of mechanically ventilated patients are the result of immobility. These include muscle wasting and weakness, contractures, loss of skin integrity, pneumonia, deep vein thrombosis that can result in pulmonary embolus, constipation, and ileus.

Gastrointestinal Problems

Nosocomial pneumonia is the second most common hospital-acquired infection and the leading cause of death from nosocomial infections. Intubated patients have a 10-fold increase of nosocomial pneumonia. Factors that lead to nosocomial pneumonia are oropharyngeal colonization, gastric colonization, aspiration, and compromised lung defenses. Maintenance of the natural gastric acid barrier in the stomach plays a major role in decreasing incidence and mortality from nosocomial pneumonia.

The widespread use of antacids or histamine H_2 blockers can predispose the patient to nosocomial infections also. Used to guard against stress bleeding, these medications can increase colonization of the upper gastrointestinal tract owing to decreased gastric acidity.

Other gastrointestinal complications associated with mechanical ventilation include distension (secondary to air

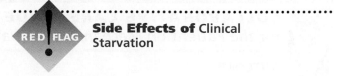

Side Effects of Clinical Starvation

- Atrophy of respiratory muscles
- Decreased protein
- Decreased albumin
- Decreased cell-mediated immunity
- Decreased surfactant production
- Decreased replication of respiratory epithelium
- Intracellular depletion of ATP
- Impaired cellular oxygenation
- Central respiratory depression

swallowing), hypomotility and ileus (secondary to immobility and the use of narcotic analgesics), vomiting, and translocation of bacteria from the gut into the bloodstream, leading to bacteremia in patients who are unable to be fed enterally. Attention to maintenance of stooling is necessary to prevent abdominal distension with resulting impingement on diaphragmatic excursion.

Many mechanically ventilated patients are already malnourished due to underlying chronic disease. Research verifies that the many side effects of clinical starvation can lead to pulmonary complications and death, as listed in the accompanying display.

Muscle Weakness

Respiratory muscles, like all other body muscles, need energy to work. If energy needs are not met, muscle fatigue occurs, leading to discoordination of respiratory muscles and a decrease in V_T. Hypomagnesemia and hypophosphatemia have been implicated in muscle fatigue caused by depleted levels of adenosine triphosphate.

In prolonged starvation, the body cannibalizes the intercostal and diaphragmatic muscles for energy. In addition, the respiratory muscles of a patient on long-term ventilation atrophy from inactivity and passive movement by the ventilator. The patient's potential for infection is increased, because immunological competence is impaired.

ASSESSMENT AND MANAGEMENT OF THE VENTILATED PATIENT

The patient who needs ventilatory support also needs primary nursing care. One of the greatest contributions the nurse can make to decreasing costs, length of stay, and mortality in patients with respiratory problems is to implement interventions that will prevent or minimize complications (discussed above). Because mechanical ventilation is supportive rather than curative, focus of care for the mechanically ventilated patient is holistic. The accompanying collaborative care guide summarizes care of the patient on

COLLABORATIVE CARE GUIDE
for the Patient on Mechanical Ventilation

OUTCOMES	INTERVENTIONS

Oxygenation/Ventilation

A patent airway is maintained.
Lung is clear on auscultation.
There is no evidence of atelectasis.

- Auscultate breath sounds q2–4h and PRN.
- Suction only when rhonchi are present or secretions are visible in endotracheal tube.
- Hyperoxygenate and hyperventilate before and after each suction pass.

Peak, mean, and plateau pressures are within normal limits.

- Monitor airway pressures q1–2h.
- Monitor airway pressures after suctioning.
- Administer bronchodilators and mucolytics.
- Perform chest physiotherapy.
- Monitor airway pressures for decrease after interventions.
- Turn side to side q2h.
- Consider kinetic therapy or prone positioning.
- Mobilize to standing position and chair whenever possible.

Arterial blood gases (ABGs) are within normal limits.

- Monitor pulse oximetry and end tidal CO_2.
- Monitor ABGs as indicated by changes in noninvasive parameters, patient status, or weaning protocol.

Circulation/Perfusion

Blood pressure, cardiac output, CVP, and pulmonary artery pressures remain stable related to mechanical ventilation.

- Assess hemodynamic effects of initiation of mechanical ventilation (eg, decreased venous return and cardiac output).
- Monitor ECG for dysrhythmias related to hypoxemia.
- Assess hemodynamic effects of changes in inspiratory pressure settings, tidal volume, and PEEP.
- Assess effects of ventilator setting changes on cardiac output and oxygen delivery.
- Administer intravascular volume as ordered to maintain preload.

Fluids/Electrolytes

Intake and output measurements are balanced.

- Monitor hydration status to reduce viscosity of lung secretions.
- Assess urine specific gravity or serum osmolality to evaluate hydration.

Mobility/Safety

There is no evidence of or minimal muscle wasting.

Endotracheal tube will remain in proper position.

- Promote standing at bedside, sitting up in chair, ambulating with assistance as soon as possible.
- Securely stabilize endotracheal tube into position.
- Note and record the "cm" line on endotracheal tube position at lip.
- Use patient self-protective devices per hospital protocol.
- Evaluate endotracheal tube position on chest x-ray.
- Keep emergency airway equipment and manual resuscitation bag readily available, and check each shift.

Proper inflation of endotracheal tube cuff is maintained.

- Inflate cuff using minimal leak technique, or pressure <25 mmHg.
- Monitor cuff inflation/leak q2–4h.
- Protect pilot balloon from damage.

Ventilator alarm system remains activated.
Joint range of motion is maintained while patient receives neuromuscular blocking and sedation/analgesia.

- Perform ventilator setting and alarm checks q1–2h.
- Perform range-of-motion exercises q2–4h.
- Reposition extremities frequently.

(continued)

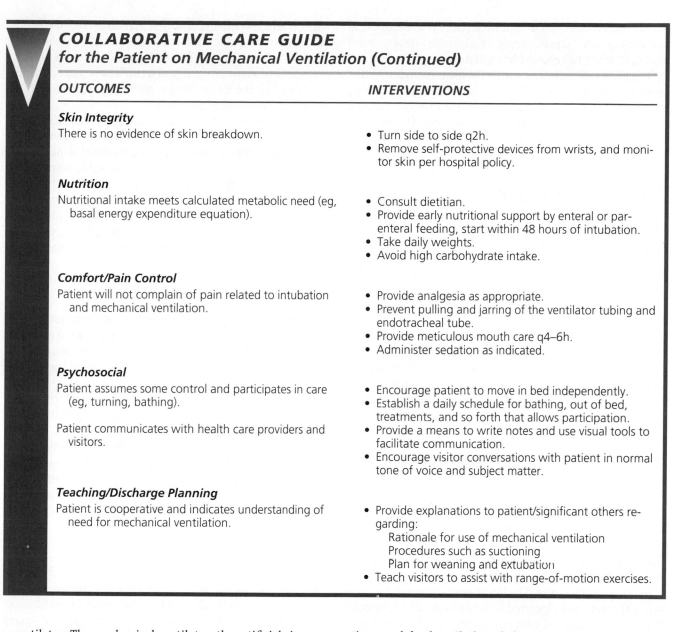

COLLABORATIVE CARE GUIDE
for the Patient on Mechanical Ventilation (Continued)

OUTCOMES	INTERVENTIONS
Skin Integrity There is no evidence of skin breakdown.	• Turn side to side q2h. • Remove self-protective devices from wrists, and monitor skin per hospital policy.
Nutrition Nutritional intake meets calculated metabolic need (eg, basal energy expenditure equation).	• Consult dietitian. • Provide early nutritional support by enteral or parenteral feeding, start within 48 hours of intubation. • Take daily weights. • Avoid high carbohydrate intake.
Comfort/Pain Control Patient will not complain of pain related to intubation and mechanical ventilation.	• Provide analgesia as appropriate. • Prevent pulling and jarring of the ventilator tubing and endotracheal tube. • Provide meticulous mouth care q4–6h. • Administer sedation as indicated.
Psychosocial Patient assumes some control and participates in care (eg, turning, bathing). Patient communicates with health care providers and visitors.	• Encourage patient to move in bed independently. • Establish a daily schedule for bathing, out of bed, treatments, and so forth that allows participation. • Provide a means to write notes and use visual tools to facilitate communication. • Encourage visitor conversations with patient in normal tone of voice and subject matter.

Teaching/Discharge Planning
Patient is cooperative and indicates understanding of need for mechanical ventilation.
	• Provide explanations to patient/significant others regarding:
	    Rationale for use of mechanical ventilation
	    Procedures such as suctioning
	    Plan for weaning and extubation
	• Teach visitors to assist with range-of-motion exercises.

a ventilator. The mechanical ventilator, the artificial airway, and the care that is required to maintain mechanical ventilation require specialized nursing knowledge and skills that are discussed in the following sections.

Endotracheal Tube Care

To prevent tube movement, tube migration, or inadvertent extubation, ETTs must be anchored securely. Anchoring can be accomplished with adhesive tape or with specially manufactured tube immobilization appliances. Usual practice is to retape the ETT every 1 to 2 days or when soiled or insecure. In orally intubated patients, the position of the ETT should be changed from side to side to facilitate mouth care and to prevent areas of pressure necrosis. The disadvantage of frequent retaping is that patients with fragile skin or prolonged intubation may incur skin breakdown; twill tape can be substituted for adhesive tape in these situations and for heavily bearded patients. Retaping by two people is desirable to prevent tube displacement.

The final step in retaping is to check tube placement in comparison to placement before retaping. Placement of an oral bite block can prevent biting on the tube, which can cause airway narrowing (high pressure alarm on the ventilator) or tube displacement. Oral inspection and hygiene are of paramount importance when a bite block is used. The use of a swivel connector (connecting the tube to the ventilator circuit), along with anchoring a large loop of tubing to the bed, facilitates patient movement without tube movement.

ETT placement is verified by x-ray following initial intubation. The position in cm at the lips or nare is recorded; this placement is verified every shift to detect inadvertent position changes. Persistent coughing may suggest that the ETT has migrated to touch the carina, requiring the tube to be withdrawn to an appropriate level.

Sinusitis is common in intubated patients and can cause bacteremia and sepsis. Signs of sinusitis (fever, nasal drainage) must be reported immediately.

The pilot cuff balloon is protected from inadvertent disruption; cuff rupture or ETT occlusion with a mucous plug requires reintubation. If a patient is prematurely extubated for any reason, the airway must be kept patent. Oxygenation and ventilation may be provided with an MRB and mask until reintubation can be accomplished.

Tracheostomy Care

In patients requiring long-term mechanical ventilation, the airway is converted to tracheostomy at some point to prevent complications of endotracheal intubation, such as tracheal stenosis and vocal cord paralysis. A review of the literature reveals no consensus as to optimal timing for tracheostomy; the most common time seems to be about 21 days after intubation.[14]

The advantages of tracheostomy over endotracheal intubation include faster weaning (at least in part because of decreased dead space), enhanced patient comfort, enhanced communication, and the possibility of oral feeding. Tracheostomy is not without disadvantages. These include hemorrhage, pneumothorax, and the need for an operative procedure. Recently, the practice of bedside percutaneous tracheostomy using a progressive dilation technique has been touted to decrease the morbidity and cost incurred with an operative procedure. Less infection and bleeding have also been given as advantages over the standard procedure.[15]

Tracheostomy care includes frequent changing of tracheostomy ties and dressing, although initial ties are not changed until at least 24 hours after placement. As with retaping of the ETT, changing of tracheostomy ties should be a two-person procedure. The ties should be tied so that one to two fingers can be inserted between the ties and the skin. The stoma is cleansed with half-strength hydrogen peroxide and observed for wound healing, bleeding, and signs of infection. The routine practice of inner cannula cleaning or changes may not be necessary according to a recent study.[16] It is mandatory to maintain a midline position for the tracheostomy to prevent pressure on surrounding tissue, the most serious complication of which is erosion into the innominate artery, which can result in exsanguination.

If decannulation occurs within the first 7 days after tracheostomy insertion, the patient should be reintubated with an ETT. An obturator and a new, appropriately sized tracheostomy tube are kept at the bedside. If inadvertent decannulation occurs after a tract has developed, the tube is carefully replaced using the obturator.

TUBE CUFF PRESSURE MONITORING

Tube cuff pressures are monitored every shift to prevent overdistension and excess pressure on the tracheal wall that can cause complications such as tracheal stenosis. If a patient is on the ventilator, the best pressure is the lowest possible pressure without having a leak of V_T. Physiologically, arterial circulation to the tracheal wall is obliterated by pressures of about 30 mmHg. If a cuff leak is suspected, auscultation at the neck for air turbulence can determine whether the seal is adequate.

One method used to inflate a cuff is called the minimal occluding volume. Air is injected slowly during ventilator inspiration. During this time, auscultation is performed over the trachea. When the harsh "rhonchi" sound is no longer audible, the minimal occluding volume has been reached, and the tube cuff is occluding the airway without excessive pressure on the trachea. Extra air should not be added. A manometer can also be attached to the pilot balloon to measure cuff pressure, which should be maintained at less than 20 mmHg.

PREVENTION OF ASPIRATION

The risk of aspiration after intubation can be minimized by maintaining appropriate cuff inflation; evacuation of gastric distension with suction; suctioning of the oropharynx, especially before cuff deflations; and elevation of the head of the patient's bed during tube feeding.

Patients must be individually assessed to determine the need for physical restraints to prevent self-extubation. If restraints are needed, a physician's order is required, with regular review of continued need. Patients must be closely monitored for potential injury, and circulatory checks with removal of restraints must be performed frequently. Self-extubation result in aspiration and vocal cord damage because of the inflated cuff.

Nutritional Support

Metabolic needs in critically ill patients are much higher than in normal subjects. Basic caloric requirements are usually increased by 25% for hospital activity and stress associated with treatment. Adequate nutrition is a necessary prerequisite for weaning from mechanical ventilation; nutritional support should be instituted early.

If the gastrointestinal tract is intact, enteral nutrition is preferred, and can be provided through a feeding tube. Many chronically ill patients, such as those with COPD, have longstanding protein and calorie malnutrition. Initial tube feeding is started slowly. The nurse observes the patient for signs of intolerance, such as diarrhea and hyperosmolar dehydration. Blood glucose determinations are monitored. If the patient tolerates feedings, the rate is gradually increased until the desired rate is achieved. If tube feedings cannot be tolerated, parenteral hyperalimentation is considered (see Chapter 39).

Patients who require long-term mechanical ventilation need 2,000 to 2,500 calories per day. Large caloric loads increase carbon dioxide production and can precipitate respiratory failure in a compromised patient. When available, metabolic chart determinations can guide nutritional requirements.

Eye Care

Eye care of the ventilator patient is important. Many ICU patients are comatose, sedated, or chemically paralyzed and therefore have lost the blink reflex or ability to close their eyelids completely. This can lead to corneal dryness and ulceration.

Few studies have established the efficacy of one eye care measure over another. Current practices include instillation of lubricating drops or ointment, taping the eyes, applying eye shields, or applying a moisture chamber.[17] Scleral edema is common in the ventilated patient. Raising the head of the bed may reduce scleral edema.

Mouth Care

Frequent mouth care must be performed for all mechanically ventilated patients. Mouth care not only increases comfort and decreases thirst, but also preserves the integrity of the oropharyngeal mucosa. An intact mucosa helps prevent infection and colonization of organisms that may lead to systemic, possibly life-threatening infection.

Psychological Care

The ventilated patient is subjected to extreme physical and emotional stress in the ICU. Psychological distress can be caused by sleep deprivation, sensory overstimulation, pain, fear, the inability to communicate, and commonly used pharmacological agents. Treatments can often seem dehumanizing. In many cases, the prognosis is poor, and the possibility of death is ever-present.

Feelings of helplessness and lack of control can be overwhelming. The patient may attempt to gain some element of control through constant demanding or exhibition of other "inappropriate" behavior. If the patient is incapable of dealing with stress through coping mechanisms, he or she may exhibit depression, apathy, and lack of emotional involvement. These reactions may be exacerbated in patients with a history of psychiatric problems or drug or alcohol abuse.

Assisted ventilation can precipitate a psychological dependence. If for the first time in years, a patient is receiving enough oxygen to meet metabolic needs and does not have to struggle for air, he or she may be reluctant to give up the ventilator. Weaning can become even more stressful for this patient.

This is also a stressful time for the family of a patient in the ICU. Family members must deal with a strange environment, a critically ill loved one, and the financial strain imposed by the illness. Nursing support is given by familiarizing the family with the physical surroundings, supplying information about visitation policies, and providing frequent progress reports on the patient's condition.

Studies show improvement in patient outcomes from increased presence of loved ones during hospitalization. Based on these findings and on increased patient and family satisfaction, many ICUs have instituted open visitation policies and increased involvement of family members in patient care.

Weaning From Mechanical Ventilation

As soon as the patient is placed on mechanical ventilation, plans are made for weaning the patient from mechanical support. The process to achieve this goal includes the following:

- Correction of the cause of respiratory failure
- Maintenance of muscle strength
- Proper nutrition
- Psychological preparation

Patients can be categorized into two groups: those requiring short-term ventilation (3 days or less) and those requiring long-term ventilation (more than 3 days).[18]

Each patient is evaluated daily for readiness to wean. Criteria are listed in the display. Many weaning indices have been advocated for use in predicting weaning readiness. Some look exclusively at respiratory factors, such as muscle strength and endurance (eg, negative inspiratory pressure [NIP], Weaning Index, ratio of frequency to tidal volume). Others are integrated indices that look at a broad range of physiological factors that influence weaning readiness; these are not only predictors, but also tools to assist in identifying and improving on factors that influence the weaning process.[19]

In addition to controversy concerning weaning indices, there is disagreement and lack of evidence regarding which approach to weaning is best. Some clinicians maintain total ventilatory support up until the time of weaning trials; others use intermittent trials of increasing frequency and duration. Regardless of the mode or approach, certain factors have been found to influence weaning success positively. These include the use of collaborative, multidisciplinary teams to formulate comprehensive plans of care based on assessment of individual patients; the use of standardized weaning protocols that are assigned to each patient on the basis of individual assessment; and the use of critical pathways.

Respiratory muscle fatigue impedes weaning. It may take as long as 24 hours of complete rest (the mechanical ventilator assumes all of the work of breathing for the patient)

CLINICAL APPLICATION: Assessment Parameters
Criteria for Weaning

Weaning Tests

Vital capacity (VC): 10–15 mL/kg
Tidal volume (VT): 4–5 mL/kg
Minute ventilation (MV): * <10 L
Negative inspiratory pressure (NIP): ** < −20 cm H_2O
RR: <25/min

Ventilator Settings

FiO_2: <.50
PEEP: <5 cm H_2O
VT: Average for the patient

ABGs

$PaCO_2$: Normal for the patient
PaO_2: 60–mid 70s or normal for the patient
pH: Normal with all electrolyte imbalances corrected

Airway

Secretions: Thin and minimal
Bronchospasm: Controlled
Position: Up in chair, semi-Fowler's, or positioned for maximizing air exchange and diaphragm movement

Drugs

Sedatives and paralytics off more than 24 hours. Patient may require mild sedation if anxiety impedes weaning.

Emotional

"Psyched up" for the wean

Physical

Stable; no new acute process; rested
Good nutritional status

---

* If MV is higher than 20 L, the work of breathing is high. The patient may well wean, but after a couple of hours may fatigue and need to be reintubated.

** NIP gives an indication of inspiratory muscle strength. A pressure less than −30 mL/cm H_2O pressure indicates muscle weakness. The work of breathing will be costly, and fatigue will result.

for recovery of fatigued respiratory muscles. Therefore, it is common practice to increase ventilatory support at night to ensure rest.

In addition, weaning trials should be discontinued if signs of fatigue or respiratory distress develop. These are summarized in the display.

CLINICAL APPLICATION:
Assessment Parameters
Criteria That May Terminate Weaning From Mechanical Ventilation

Physiological Data

Pulse: Increase or decrease of 20% of baseline (sustained)
BP: Systolic increase or decrease of 20 mmHg (sustained)
RR: Respiratory rate >35 breaths/min (sustained)

Psychological/Subjective Data

Dyspnea
Panic
Pain (chest)
Fatigue

Objective Observations

ECG changes: development of dysrhythmias, ST changes
Increased accessory muscle use
Increased intercostal retractions
Increased flaring of nostrils
Erratic breathing pattern (paradoxical breathing)
Neurological changes (increased restlessness, increased drowsiness)
Diaphoresis
ABG deterioration: Increased $PaCO_2$ resulting in pH <7.3 or oxygen desaturation using oximetry

SHORT-TERM WEANING

Patients typically intubated for a short time include those who are intubated for surgical procedures, for an acute exacerbation of an underlying lung disease that can be easily reversed (eg, asthma), and for airway protection during an acute neurological event (eg, drug overdose). Weaning within a short period of time is desirable, because physiological changes caused by the mechanical ventilation begin within 72 hours.

Two frequently used predictive criteria for short-term weaning success are a negative inspiratory pressure of < −20 cm H_2O and spontaneous MV of < 10 L/min. The choice of weaning method does not seem to be important.

Weaning procedures may vary slightly from hospital to hospital, but general guidelines remain the same. For instance, weaning should be started in the morning when the patient is rested. The patient is made comfortable, and the nurse elevates the head of the bed. Pharmacological agents for comfort, such as bronchodilators or sedatives, are administered. By explaining the procedure, the nurse helps the patient through some of the discomfort and apprehension. Weaning is begun with suctioning, which clears the lungs and breathing passages. The nurse obtains weaning indices.

Support and reassurance help the patient through the discomfort and apprehension as the nurse remains with the patient following initiation of the weaning process. The nurse also evaluates and documents the patient's response to weaning.

LONG-TERM WEANING

The process of long-term weaning often takes weeks. Usually this process is complicated and involves delays and setbacks. The accompanying display lists several adjuncts that may be

Adjuncts to Weaning

Fenestrated Trach*

- Provides for communication during weaning periods

Kirshner Button

- Provides for communication during weaning periods
- Gives less resistance than with fenestrated trach

Large ETT (>7.0 mm)

- Decreases resistance to breathing; decreases work of breathing

Exercise

- Provides increased stimulation to breathing
- Increases and changes environmental stimuli
- Improves strength

Nutrition

- Provides energy for breathing
- Maintains protein balance
- Aids in resistance to infection

Pulse Oximetry

- Provides noninvasive monitoring of O_2 saturation

---

* The fenestrated trach tube has an opening in the outer cannula but not the inner cannula. With the inner cannula in place and the cuff inflated, the patient is easily mechanically ventilated. During the weaning process, the inner cannula is removed, the cuff deflated, the outer cannula capped, and supplemental oxygen supplied by nasal cannula. This system permits air to pass from the patient's nares through the hole in the outer cannula (fenestration in the trach tube) and past the vocal cords, allowing verbal communication on the part of the patient. Never inflate the cuff while the inner cannula is capped; the patient will be unable to breathe.

used to optimize weaning. Regular reevaluation of the plan of care by the multidisciplinary team coupled with continuous communication with the patient and family are necessary.

Procedure

METHODS

T-Piece Trial

The T-piece is connected to the patient at the desired FIO_2 (usually slightly higher than the previous ventilator setting). The patient's response and tolerance to the trial are continuously observed. The duration of T-piece trials is not standardized; some clinicians extubate if an initial trial of 30 minutes ends with acceptable ABGs and patient response. Some use trials of increasing frequency and duration to evaluate and build the patient's endurance with periods of rest on the ventilator between trials. When the latter method is used, the patient is generally deemed ready to be extubated after 24 successive hours on a T-piece.

Intermittent Mandatory Ventilation

The IMV mode was initially heralded as the optimal weaning mode, allowing for some spontaneous breathing (to prevent respiratory muscle atrophy) while providing a backup rate. Weaning with the IMV method entails a gradual reduction in the number of delivered breaths until a low rate is reached, usually 4 breaths/min. The patient is then extubated if all other weaning criteria are met. Because the demand valve of an IMV circuit can markedly increase the work of breathing, the superiority of IMV versus T-piece weaning has been questioned.

Continuous Positive Airway Pressure

Continuous positive airway pressure entails breathing through the ventilator circuit with a small amount (or zero amount) of positive pressure. The use of CPAP versus the use of T-piece for weaning is controversial. However, the use of 0-CPAP in COPD patients can prevent airway collapse, thereby decreasing work of breathing and sense of breathlessness.

Pressure Support Ventilation

Low levels of PSV decrease the work of breathing associated with ETTs and ventilator circuits. Weaning using the PSV mode entails a progressive decrease in pressure based on the patient maintaining an adequate VT and RR < 30 breaths/min. PSV can also be combined with IMV; the IMV rate is reduced while the patient's spontaneous breaths are augmented with low-level PSV.

EXTUBATION CRITERIA

Whichever mode or combination of modes is used for weaning, extubation cannot occur until several criteria are met. Before extubation, the patient must be able to maintain his or her own airway as evidenced by an appropriate level of consciousness and the presence of cough and gag reflexes. In all patients, but especially in those with a history of difficult intubation or reactive airways disease, the "cuff leak test" should be performed prior to extubation. This entails deflation of the tube cuff (after suctioning of the oropharynx) to demonstrate an air leak. Absence of a leak can indicate edema and may predict laryngeal edema postextubation.

TECHNIQUE

Extubation should never occur unless a qualified person is available to reintubate emergently if the patient does not tolerate extubation. After explaining the procedure and preparing the patient, the nurse suctions the patient's tube and oropharynx. Equipment includes an MRB and mask at bedside. After the nurse loosens the tape, the cuff is deflated. The ETT is removed quickly while the patient coughs. The patient's mouth is suctioned and humidified oxygen is applied immediately. The patient is evaluated for immediate signs of distress: stridor, dyspnea, and decrease in oxygen saturation. Treatment for stridor includes inhaled racemic epinephrine and administration of intravenous steroids. If these interventions fail, immediate reintubation is necessary.

Clinical Applicability Challenges

Self-Challenge: Critical Thinking

1. The respiratory therapy department in your institution has a policy that requires them to suction every ventilated patient every 2 hours, using normal saline instillation with each pass of the suction catheter. You want to change these clinical practices on your unit. Defend your rationale using clinical research findings.

2. Your patient has severe ARDS secondary to aspiration pneumonia. He has been on an FiO_2 of 1.00 for 3 days with PaO_2 of 50. His temperature is 40.0°C (104°F). His only medications are antibiotics. Any activity, including suctioning, causes profound and prolonged episodes of desaturation. Explore medical and nursing interventions designed to enhance the patient's oxygenation and decrease his oxygen consumption.

3. Formulate an assessment tool that incorporates both pulmonary and nonpulmonary factors that influence readiness to wean from mechanical ventilation. The tool should be useful for predicting weaning readiness and for formulating a plan of care to optimize factors that are identified as not optimal for weaning.

Study Questions

1. Which of the following would be an example of effective application of bronchial hygiene techniques?
   a. Positioning a patient with right middle and lower lobe pneumonia who is requiring an FiO_2 of .80 on his right side for the next 2 hours
   b. Performing CPT for a lower lobe process with the patient in a semireclining position
   c. Assisting the stable patient on long-term mechanical ventilation to sit in a chair and to ambulate
   d. Suctioning the patient immediately before administering bronchodilators

2. Which of the following is a contraindication to CPT?
   a. Lobar atelectasis
   b. Acute bronchospasm
   c. Cystic fibrosis
   d. Sputum production of at least 30 mL/d

3. Indications that the ETT is improperly positioned include all of the following except that
   a. the patient is able to talk.
   b. breath sounds are auscultated only over the right lung.
   c. on chest x-ray, the tip of the ETT is 5 cm above the carina.
   d. the patient has an incessant cough.

4. Which of the following could indicate the presence of a tension pneumothorax?
   a. Oxygen saturation of 98% in a patient with muffled heart tones
   b. Systolic blood pressure of 30 mmHg in a patient with a rapidly deteriorating level of consciousness
   c. Mediastinal structures in the midline on chest x-ray
   d. Hypokalemia, hyperglycemia, hypernatremia

5. Which of the following would alert the nurse to take emergency action?
   a. The patient's face and neck suddenly double in size and when palpated, exhibit crepitus.
   b. The water seal chamber of a chest tube system bubbles immediately after the chest tube is inserted.
   c. The water level in the water seal chamber fluctuates with the patient's respiratory excursions.
   d. The water level in the suction chamber has fallen 5 cm below the ordered level.

6. All of the following effects of steroid use are routinely encountered in the ICU except
   a. hyperglycemia requiring insulin coverage.
   b. masking of signs and symptoms of infection.
   c. psychotic behavior.
   d. reversal of ARDS.

7. One rationale for monitoring the degree of neuromuscular blockade when using NMBAs is
   a. because NMBAs do not possess sedative or analgesic properties.
   b. NMBA dosage should always be maintained at the highest limit of dosage range.
   c. to prevent prolonged hospitalization and rehabilitation.
   d. to observe for development of pneumothorax.

8. Which of the following are potential complications of mechanical ventilation?
   a. Oxygen toxicity, hyperventilation, and cardiac tamponade
   b. Barotrauma, volutrauma, and multiple trauma
   c. Hypotension, disseminated intravascular coagulation, and sepsis
   d. Pneumonia, pneumothorax, and respiratory acidosis

9. The ventilator's high pressure alarm sounds continuously. Which of the following could be the cause?
   a. The ventilator tubing is disconnected from the patient.
   b. The patient has developed a pneumothorax.
   c. The patient's initial dose of a paralytic drug has just kicked in.
   d. The FiO_2 level has been inadvertently left on 1.00 after an episode of hyperoxygenation with suctioning.

REFERENCES

1. Peruzzi WT, Smith B: Bronchial hygiene therapy. Crit Care Clin 11(1):79–96, 1995
2. Doering LV: The effect of positioning on hemodynamics and gas exchange in the critically ill: A review. Am J Crit Care 2:208–216, 1993
3. Pappert D, Rossaint R et al: Influence of positioning on ventilation-perfusion relationships in severe adult respiratory distress syndrome. Chest 106:1511–1516, 1994
4. AARC Clinical Practice Guideline: Endotracheal suctioning of mechanically ventilated adults and children with artificial airways. Respiratory Care 38(5):500–504, 1993
5. Grap MJ, Glass C et al: Endotracheal suctioning: Ventilator vs manual delivery of hyperoxygenation breaths. Am J Crit Care 5:192–197, 1996
6. Gross SB: Current challenges, concepts, and controversies in chest tube management. AACN Clinical Issues 4(2):260–275, 1993
7. Slutsky AS: Consensus conference on mechanical ventilation—January 28–30, 1993 at Northbrook, Illinois, USA. Intensive Care Med 20:64–79, 1994
8. Levine S, Henson D: Negative pressure ventilation. In Tobin MJ (ed): Principles and Practice of Mechanical Ventilation, pp 393–411. New York, McGraw-Hill, 1994
9. Slutsky AS: Consensus conference on mechanical ventilation—January 28–30, 1993 at Northbrook, Illinois, USA. Intensive Care Med 20:150–162, 1994
10. MacIntyre NR: High-frequency ventilation. In Tobin MJ (ed): Principles and Practice of Mechanical Ventilation, pp 455–460. New York, McGraw-Hill, 1994
11. Elliott M: Noninvasive mechanical ventilation by nasal or face mask. In Tobin MJ (ed): Principles and Practice of Mechanical Ventilation, pp 427–453. New York, McGraw-Hill, 1994

12. Bidani A, Tzouanakis AE et al: Permissive hypercapnia in acute respiratory failure. JAMA 272(12):957–962, 1994
13. Aloi A, Burns SM: Continuous airway pressure monitoring in the critical care setting. Crit Care Nurse 15(2):66–74, 1995
14. Heffner JE: Timing of tracheotomy in mechanically ventilated patients. Am Rev Respir Dis 147:768–771, 1993
15. Zavotsky KE, D'Amelio LF: Bedside percutaneous tracheostomy: Implications for critical care nurses. Crit Care Nurse 15(5):37–43, 1995
16. Fiorell M, Burns SM et al: Are frequent tracheostomy inner cannula changes necessary? NTI Research Abstract. Am J Crit Care 5(3):235, 1996
17. Cortese D, Capp L, McKinley S: Moisture chamber versus lubrication for the prevention of corneal epithelial breakdown. Am J Crit Care 4(6):425–428, 1995
18. Burns SM, Clochesy JM et al: Weaning from long-term mechanical ventilation. Am J Crit Care 4(1):4–22, 1995
19. Burns SM, Burns JE, Truwit JD: Comparison of five clinical weaning indices. Am J Crit Care 3(5):342–352, 1994

BIBLIOGRAPHY

Ackerman MH: The effect of saline lavage prior to suctioning. Am J Crit Care 2(4):326–330, 1993
American Thoracic Society: Guidelines for the initial management of adults with community-acquired pneumonia: Diagnosis, assessment of severity, and initial antimicrobial therapy. Am Rev Respir Dis 148:1418–1426,1993
American Thoracic Society: Hospital-acquired pneumonia in adults: Diagnosis, assessment of severity, initial antimicrobial therapy, and preventative strategies. Am J Respir Crit Care Med 153:1771–1725, 1995
American Thoracic Society: Standards for the diagnosis and care of patients with chronic obstructive pulmonary disease. Am J Respir Crit Care Med 152:S77–S120, 1995
Atkins PJ, Egloff ME, Willms DC: Respiratory consequences of multisystem crisis: The adult respiratory distress syndrome. Crit Car Nurs Q 16:27–38: 1994
Burns S: Understanding, applying, and evaluating pressure modes of ventilation. AACN Clinical Issues. 7(4):495–506, 1996

Chulay M: Caring for the mechanically ventilated patient: Changing your mindset. Proceedings of the Twenty-Second Annual National Teaching Institute of the American Association of Critical Care Nurses, 113–114, 1995
Clochesy JM, Daly BJ, Montenegro HD: Weaning chronically critically ill adults from mechanical ventilatory support: A descriptive study. Am J Crit Care 4:93–99, 1995
Corbridge TC, Hall JB: The assessment and management of adults with status asthmaticus. Am J Respir Crit Care Med 151:1296–1316, 1995
Hagler DA, Traver GA: Endotracheal saline and suction catheters: Sources of lower airway contamination. Am J Crit Care 3(6):444–447, 1994
Hanneman SKG, Ingersoll GL et al: Weaning from short-term mechanical ventilation: A review. Am J Crit Care 3(6):421–443, 1994
Harvey MA: Managing agitation in critically ill patients. Am J Crit Care 5(1):7–16, 1996
Karch AM: 1997 Lippincott's Nursing Drug Guide. Philadelphia, Lippincott-Raven, 1997
Kharasch M, Graff J: Emergency management of the airway. Crit Care Clin 11(1):53–66, 1995
Knebel A: Ventilator weaning protocols and techniques: Getting the job done. AACN Clinical Issues. 7(4):550–559, 1996
Harvey MA: Managing agitation in critically ill patients. Am J Crit Care 5(1):7–16, 1996
Karch AM: 1997 Lippincott's Nursing Drug Guide. Philadelphia, Lippincott-Raven, 1997
Luer JM: Sedation and chemical relaxation in critical pulmonary illness: Suggestions for patient assessment and drug monitoring. AACN Clinical Issues 6(2):333–343, 1995
Olin BR (ed): Facts & Comparisons. St. Louis, Facts & Comparison, 1996
Quigley RL: Thoracentesis and chest tube drainage. Crit Care Clin 11(1):111–126, 1995
Riker RR, Fraser GL, Cox PM: Continuous infusion of haloperidol controls agitation in critically ill patients. Crit Care Med 22:433–440, 1994
Watling SM, Dasta JF: Prolonged paralysis in intensive care unit patients after the use of neuromuscular blocking agents: A review of the literature. Crit Care Med 22:884–893, 1994
Wilmoth DF, Carpenter RM: Preventing complications of mechanical ventilation: Permissive hypercapnea. AACN Clinical Issues 7(4):473–481, 1996

25

Common Respiratory Disorders

OBJECTIVES

Based on the content in this chapter, the reader should be able to:

- Compare and contrast three causes of atelectasis.
- Discuss the signs and symptoms frequently seen with atelectasis and pneumonia.
- Describe the pathophysiology and anticipated management of various pulmonary disorders.
- Correlate the signs and symptoms of chronic obstructive pulmonary disease to the anticipated therapeutic management.
- Discuss nursing management of the patient with selected pulmonary disorders.

Critical care nurses face a continual challenge in meeting the needs of the patient with pulmonary disease. The ability of the nurse to anticipate, recognize, and intervene in the course of pulmonary disorders can modify or prevent the development of certain common lung problems. This chapter assists nurses in enhancing their knowledge of abnormal pulmonary function present in various common pulmonary disorders and in applying the information to the assessment, intervention, and evaluation of the patient with an abnormal pulmonary condition. Patient observation and recognition of the classic signs of pulmonary insufficiency—tachypnea, tachycardia, diaphoresis, and anxiety—are key to the nursing role.

Potentially Reversible Causes of Respiratory Insufficiency

ATELECTASIS

Atelectasis can be defined as a diminution of volume or collapse of lung units. It is a common postoperative problem.

Pathophysiological Principles

Several etiological factors can precipitate atelectasis.

Absorption atelectasis occurs if communications between the alveoli and trachea are obstructed, for example, by plugging of a bronchus with mucus. The alveolar gas is rapidly absorbed into the circulation and, because of the obstruction, cannot be replenished. When the critical closing volume (the amount of air needed to keep the alveoli open) is depleted, alveolar collapse ensues. Alveolar units require both volume and gases to maintain patency. When increased oxygen concentrations are given to the patient, the relative concentration of nitrogen is decreased. Nitrogen has a low solubility level and helps keep the alveoli open. As the oxygen is rapidly absorbed and nitrogen levels fall, atelectasis results.

Passive atelectasis occurs if air or fluid in the pleural space prevents normal alveolar filling.

Compression atelectasis occurs in the presence of a space-occupying lesion, such as a pulmonary mass. Atelectasis can also occur in patches, which can be caused by mucous plugging or altered compliance in the atelectatic area.

Atelectasis causes a pathological return of unoxygenated blood from the pulmonary circulation to the left side of the heart, resulting in partially desaturated blood entering the systemic circulation. The degree of shunt present depends on the severity of the atelectasis. In the normal patient, a small amount of unoxygenated blood enters the systemic circulation because the venous outflow of some vessels bypasses pulmonary capillaries. Shunting is increased by atelectasis because blood flow passes through the pulmonary capillaries that are in contact with nonventilated alveoli, resulting in increased amounts of unoxygenated blood in the left ventricle. (See Fig. 22–6 and Chapter 22 for a more detailed discussion of shunts.)

Assessment

CLINICAL MANIFESTATIONS

Signs and symptoms vary with the severity of atelectasis and degree of shunt present. With severe shunts (ie, large areas of atelectasis), cyanosis may become evident. In less severe shunts, cyanosis may become evident as atelectasis increases.

Large areas of atelectasis can cause a shift of the mediastinal structures toward the affected side, which can be demonstrated by x-ray. Auscultatory examination reveals decreased breath sounds over the atelectatic lung. There may be diminished chest expansion of the affected side. The patient may complain of shortness of breath, dyspnea on exertion, and weakness. Tachypnea, tachycardia, fever, anxiety, restlessness, and confusion may be present.

DIAGNOSTIC STUDIES

Arterial blood gases (ABGs) reflect the degree of hypoxemia and the adequacy of alveolar ventilation. Frequently there is evidence of atelectasis on x-ray. In compression atelectasis, there is x-ray evidence of air or fluid collection in the pleural space. All the radiographic signs are based on diminished volume of the affected lobe or segment.

Management

Treatment is based on the etiology of the atelectasis, but prevention should be the goal. Meticulous bronchial hygiene (see Chapter 24), mobilization of the patient if appropriate or frequent change of position in bed, and careful use of oxygen constitute the basic framework of therapy. Deep breathing on a scheduled, regular basis is important but may be hampered by decreased levels of consciousness, lessened mobility, and pain.[1] Bronchodilators and mucolytics, if indicated, and chest physiotherapy can be useful. Adequate ventilation may be improved with positioning, coughing, deep breathing, or incentive spirometry.

PNEUMONIA

Pneumonia is an inflammatory process in which alveolar compartments are filled with exudate. Pneumonia is a primary cause of death in the older adult.

Pathophysiological Principles

The cause of pneumonia can be viral, bacterial, fungal, protozoan, or rickettsial; hypersensitivity pneumonitis may produce the primary presenting illness. Pneumonia can also result from aspiration. Most markedly, in the intubated patient, colonization of the trachea and microaspiration of infected upper airway secretions occur.[2] Not all of these colonizations will result in pneumonia.

Assessment

CLINICAL MANIFESTATIONS

Signs and symptoms depend on the location and extent of involvement (ie, segmental or lobar), the cause of the pneumonia, and the overall condition of the patient.[1] Subjective findings include dyspnea, tachypnea, pleuritic chest pain, fever, chills, hemoptysis, and cough productive of rusty or purulent sputum. Objective findings include fever, splinting of involved hemithorax, hypoxemia, percussion dullness, coarse inspiratory crackles, and diminished breath sounds over the involved area. Chest x-rays may reveal infiltrates, consolidation, or opacification.

Management

Management of pneumonia depends on the cause. Although identification of a specific causative organism is ideal, often the patient's condition warrants empirical administration of antibiotics based on the most likely infectious agent. Broad-spectrum antibiotics effective against both gram-negative and gram-positive organisms are usually administered while testing continues to isolate the specific causative organism. The patient's response to the therapy is monitored for signs of improvement, such as return of an elevated white blood cell count to more normal levels and the absence of fever. Failure to respond, as evidenced by a worsening of the patient's condition, will require a change in the selection of antibiotics guided by the most recent testing data. Superinfection is always a concern with pharmacological therapy.

Supplemental oxygen therapy (humidified), adequate hydration, nutritional support, and mechanical ventilation if indicated for acute respiratory failure are also components of the treatment plan for pneumonia. Interventions to mobilize and clear secretions, such as the use of mucolytics, nasotracheal or endotracheal suctioning, chest physical therapy, and deep breathing and coughing should be instituted. Therapeutic bronchoscopy may be indicated for especially difficult secretion problems or to aid in diagnosis.

Preventing the development of nosocomial infections remains paramount. Nosocomial pneumonia is associated with high morbidity and a mortality rate in excess of 30%. Proper handwashing, aseptic handling of invasive lines and suctioning equipment, and proper disinfection of respiratory equipment and other supplies will reduce contamination and cross-spread of infection.

Complications of pneumonia include abscess formation, pleural effusion, empyema, bacteremia, and septicemia.

Insights Into Clinical Research

Malangoni M, Crafton R, Mocek F: Pneumonia in the surgical intensive care unit: Factors determining successful outcomes. Am J Surg 167(2):250–255, 1994

Through retrospective chart review of 1,027 patients, this study attempted to identify risk factors that predicted successful treatment of pneumonia that developed while in the surgical intensive care unit.

Eighty-three percent of the patients (85) developed pneumonia. Risk factors included smoking (31%), malnourishment (28%), COPD (13%), immunosuppression (4%), and aspiration (9%). Three variables associated with successful versus failed treatment were the duration of intubation (7.2 versus 29.3 days), duration of ventilation (6.7 versus 14.8 days), and the patient's alveolar–arterial oxygen gradient when diagnosed (215 versus 343 mmHg). Patients with pneumonia caused by Pseudomonas aeruginosa (56% failed) and Staphylococcus aureus (45% failed) were at greatest risk for treatment failure.

Because nosocomial pneumonia is associated with high morbidity and mortality, prevention is primary, along with vigilant nursing care. Given the high preponderance of treatment failure with P. aeruginosa and S. aureus, early identification assumes even greater importance.

■ PULMONARY EMBOLISM

Pulmonary emboli can occur as a complication of many medical conditions that predispose to venous thrombosis, including postoperative states, prolonged bed rest, and trauma. Deep venous thrombosis, particularly in the lower extremities, is the main predisposing factor, causing 90% to 95% of pulmonary emboli (PE). Fat, air, and amniotic fluid emboli can also cause a PE.

Pathophysiological Principles

Both pulmonary and hemodynamic changes occur as a result of occlusion of a pulmonary artery by an embolus. Alveoli are ventilated but not perfused, thereby producing areas of mismatched ventilation and perfusion. As a result, well-ventilated alveoli are underperfused, and gas exchange is compromised (increased respiratory dead space). If the embolus fills both branches of the pulmonary vascular bed it is known as a saddle embolus. Aptly named because on removal at autopsy, the clot hangs from the middle, appearing like a horse saddle. Very large emboli have a poor prognosis.

Pulmonary vascular constriction resulting from a lack of carbon dioxide normally present in pulmonary arterial blood shifts ventilation from the underperfused alveoli. The decrease in pulmonary blood flow due to an embolus results in deficient nutrients for surfactant production, ultimately resulting in atelectasis. The severity of hemodynamic changes depends on the size of the embolus. Increased pulmonary vascular resistance occurs, which, if pulmonary blood flow remains constant, can result in right ventricular failure and pulmonary hypertension (marked elevation of pulmonary catheter pressures). PE can resolve or infrequently can lead to death of tissue, that is, pulmonary infarction.

Assessment

CLINICAL MANIFESTATIONS

The symptom complex of a PE depends on its size. Dyspnea, one of the most frequent complaints, is often out of proportion to the physical findings. Tachypnea and tachycardia may be present in varying degrees. Mild fever may exist, although leukocytosis is rare. Pleuritic chest pain and hemoptysis are associated with pulmonary infarction rather than with PE. Hypoxemia and lowered oxygen saturations with low-dose supplemental oxygen therapy are common.

Massive pulmonary embolization (occlusion of > 50% of pulmonary artery blood flow) results in a more dramatic clinical manifestation of acute illness, as shown in the accompanying display. The patient develops pronounced tachypnea, usually with cyanosis, tachycardia, restlessness, confusion, and hypotension. The resulting shock state produces concomitant changes of decreased urinary output and cold, clammy skin.

DIAGNOSTIC STUDIES

Diagnostic studies that may be helpful in the diagnosis of PE are outlined in Table 25–1. Suspected PE is sometimes con-

· · · · · · · ! ·

RED FLAG   **Signs and Symptoms of Pulmonary Embolus**

Submassive embolus:

- Dyspnea
- Tachypnea
- Tachycardia
- Chest pain
- Mild fever
- Hypoxemia
- Apprehension
- Cough
- Diaphoresis
- Decreased breath sounds over affected area
- Rales
- Wheezing

Massive embolus (a more pronounced manifestation of the above signs and symptoms plus the following):

- Cyanosis
- Restlessness
- Anxiety
- Confusion
- Hypotension
- Cool, clammy skin
- Decreased urinary output
- Pleuritic chest pain ⎫
- Hemoptysis   ⎬ Associated with pulmonary infarction

· ·

TABLE 25-1   CLINICAL APPLICATION: Diagnostic Studies in Pulmonary Embolism

Diagnostic Study	Abnormal Findings
Electrocardiogram	May be normal; sinus tachycardia; transient ST-T wave changes
Chest x-ray	May be normal; infiltrates, atelectasis, elevated diaphragm on affected side
Arterial blood gases	Decreased PaO_2; decreased $PaCO_2$; increased pH (respiratory alkalosis)
Ventilation–perfusion lung scan	Large perfusion defect (>75% of a lung segment) associated with $\dot{V}/\dot{Q}$ mismatch (high probability scan)
Pulmonary angiography*	Intraluminal filling defect or abrupt termination of a vessel >2.5 mm in diameter in multiple films

Accepted diagnostic standard for pulmonary embolism.

firmed by ventilation–perfusion lung scanning ($\dot{V}/\dot{Q}$ scan) and positive pulmonary angiography findings. Lower extremity deep vein thrombosis studies may also assist in the diagnosis.

Management

Definitive treatment of PE is aimed at removing the clot and correcting the hypoxemia. Thrombolytic therapy, surgery to remove the clot, and respiratory modalities, such as oxygen administration, intubation, and mechanical ventilation, may be used.

Ongoing management of PE includes anticoagulation and correction of predisposing causes of venous thrombosis. Initially, heparin is given as an intravenous bolus of 5,000 to 10,000 U followed by a continuous intravenous infusion delivering 30,000 to 40,000 U each 24 hours as a maintenance dose. The activated partial thromboplastin time (aPTT) is checked 4 to 6 hours after the initial bolus and daily thereafter or more frequently if necessary. Because failure to achieve an adequate anticoagulant response (aPPT > 1.5 times normal) has been associated with a high risk of recurrent venous thromboembolism, the heparin dose should be sufficient to maintain the aPPT 2 to 2.5 times the patient's baseline.[3] Anticoagulant therapy usually is continued for 3 months for an initial episode of PE. Recurrent venous thromboembolism should be treated with a longer course, sometimes 6 months to 1 year, depending on the patient's risk factors.

The use of thrombolytic agents in the treatment of PE is less clear. They probably have a role in the management of patients with life-threatening PE, but their place in the treatment of acute venous thrombosis is still controversial.

For patients in whom anticoagulant therapy is absolutely contraindicated, transvenous placement of a filter in the inferior vena cava is the management of choice for preventing recurrent pulmonary embolism.

Patient education regarding anticoagulation therapy and measures to reduce deep vein thrombosis is critical.

■ PNEUMOTHORAX/ HEMOTHORAX

A pneumothorax occurs if air enters the pleural space between the visceral and parietal pleurae. Blood in this location is called a hemothorax. There are two types of pneumothorax: spontaneous pneumothorax and tension pneumothorax. (See Chapter 50 for a discussion of these disorders in relation to trauma.)

A spontaneous pneumothorax can result from the rupture of a subpleural alveolar cyst or an emphysematous bleb. The signs and symptoms vary with the size of the pneumothorax and can range from mild shortness of breath to chest pain and signs of increasing respiratory distress. Physical examination reveals decreased breath sounds and decreased respiratory movement on the affected side.[3] The diagnosis is confirmed by x-ray.

Chest trauma, intermittent positive pressure breathing, positive end-expiratory pressure, cardiopulmonary resuscitation, thoracic and high abdominal surgery, and thoracentesis can precipitate an iatrogenic pneumothorax or hemothorax. A pneumothorax, regardless of cause, becomes problematic and clinically significant when gas exchange is compromised and oxygen levels fall as tension in the pleural space occurs.

If a tension pneumothorax develops, the tear in lung bronchus or chest wall acts as a one-way valve that allows air to enter the pleural space on inspiration but not to escape on expiration.[4] If it is not immediately recognized and treated, massive atelectasis results. In addition, the mediastinal structures are displaced toward the unaffected side, and tracheal deviation can be especially prominent. This mediastinal shift results in a decreased venous return, decreased cardiac output, and ultimately, death.

Assessment

CLINICAL MANIFESTATIONS

Clinically, the patient with a pneumothorax or hemothorax manifests severe respiratory distress. Agitation, cyanosis, and tachypnea are severe. Tachycardia and the initial increase in blood pressure are followed by hypotension as cardiac output decreases. Tracheal deviation and movement of the point of maximal impulse are other indicators of tension pneumothorax. The diagnosis is based not only on the clinical manifestations, but on the clinical setting as well. Any patient who is being ventilated and suddenly develops acute respiratory distress during ventilation evidenced by markedly increased inspiratory pressures is possibly experiencing a tension pneumothorax.

Management

Treatment of a tension pneumothorax must be immediate. A 16- to 18-gauge needle is inserted into the second, third, or fourth intercostal space at the midclavicular line on the affected side to relieve pressure. Sucking chest wounds resulting from gunshot or stab wounds (air enters the pleural space from the outside through a hole in the chest wall) should be occluded with a sterile dressing. After pressure relief has been accomplished, measures to prevent any further development of tension and to allow for lung reexpansion must be instituted. Usually this is accomplished through the insertion a chest tube connected to underwater seal drainage, needle aspiration of the air, or placement of a catheter attached to a one-way valve or thoracic vent (see Chapter 24). Usually reexpansion of the lung is confirmed by chest x-ray.

■ PLEURAL EFFUSION

The pleural space is a potential space between the visceral and parietal pleurae that line the lungs and interior chest wall.

Pathophysiological Principles

This space normally contains a small amount of fluid. Excess fluid can accumulate with neoplastic, thromboembolic, cardiovascular, and infectious disease processes. This is caused by at least one of four basic mechanisms:

- Increased pressure in subpleural capillaries or lymphatics
- Decreased colloid osmotic pressure of the blood
- Increased intrapleural negative pressure
- Inflammatory or neoplastic involvement of the pleura

Congestive heart failure causes more pleural effusions than any other disease process.

Assessment

Subjective findings include shortness of breath and pleuritic chest pain, depending on the amount of fluid accumulation. Objective findings include tachypnea and hypoxemia if ventilation is impaired, dullness to percussion, and decreased breath sounds over the involved area. A lateral decubitus chest radiograph will best demonstrate free pleural fluid.

Management

Removal of the pleural effusion by thoracentesis or chest tube placement is palliative treatment. Major treatment is directed toward the underlying cause. Pleural fluid from an undiagnosed source should be tested for glucose, amylase, and lactate dehydrogenase levels; cytology; microorganisms; and differential cell count.

Bronchiectasis

Bronchiectasis refers to an irreversible dilation of the bronchi that can be caused by repeated or prolonged episodes of pneumonitis, foreign body aspiration, tuberculosis or fungal infections, or a neoplasm encroaching on the bronchial lumen with resultant obstruction. Rather than being a primary disease process, bronchiectasis is a sequela of many earlier pulmonary insults, usually occurring in childhood.

Assessment

A hallmark of the disease is the production of copious amounts of yellow-green, often foul-smelling, sputum that settles into three layers: cloudy mucus on top, clear saliva in the middle, and a cloudy purulent residue on the bottom. Hemoptysis may be significant, and clubbing of the fingers is common. The diagnosis is made largely from chest radiographic imaging procedures. Because a standard chest x-ray may miss up to 20% of bronchiectatic conditions, computed tomography, which is noninvasive and widely available, is the procedure of choice.[3] Patients with severe bronchiectasis will have a decreased forced expiratory volume (FEV) and functional residual capacity because of chronic inflammatory changes.

Management

A primary treatment modality is rigorous bronchial hygiene (postural drainage, percussion, and vibration) to clear retained secretions. This therapy is essential because effective secretion clearance is altered in these patients owing to the abnormal widening and loss of elasticity of the airways. Broad-spectrum antibiotics, beta$_2$ bronchodilators (eg, albuterol, terbutaline), and oral methylxanthines (eg, aminophylline, theophylline) may also be used. Surgical resection of segmental or isolated lobar bronchiectasis is a possibility.

Chronic Obstructive Pulmonary Disease

With the exception of bronchiectasis, the common pulmonary disorders discussed previously are potentially reversible causes of respiratory insufficiency, but several disease entities result in chronic obstructive pulmonary disease (COPD). These include chronic bronchitis, emphysema, and asthma. This group of disorders is characterized by progressively decreasing FEV$_1$ (forced expiratory volume in 1 second) chronic cough and expectoration, and exertional dyspnea. Smoking, family history, age, and male sex are major risk factors.

Death rates for COPD are rising in spite of a national trend toward decreased smoking. Probably this increase is a result of the insidious nature of the disease and the long latency period from onset of smoking to clinical disease. Although mortality still is higher in men than in women, prevalence rates are increasing in women and decreasing in men. The critical care clinician will be most aware of the even greater impact of COPD on morbidity—precipitating 13% of all hospitalizations and significantly reducing function and increasing disability in the patient.

Dyspnea is the classic symptom that leads to diagnosis. Productive cough, a history of frequent respiratory infections, reduced expiratory flow rate, and hypoxemia or hypercapnia are also clinical findings. A simple spirometry test will measure maximal airflow and is useful in staging the disease and monitoring clinical course. For measuring disease severity, FEV$_1$ is the parameter of choice. FEV$_1$ also correlates with survival rates (Fig. 25–1).

Intervention strategies are always aimed at prevention. First and foremost, the nurse encourages cessation of smoking. Patients with COPD are susceptible to lung infections. The severity of influenza and some bacterial pneumonias may be prevented or modified by immunization or chemoprophylaxis. Long-term, continuous oxygen therapy is the one modality that has been shown to increase survival in patients with COPD. Quality of life, exercise tolerance, and ability to perform activities of daily living can be improved by pulmonary rehabilitation programs.

At times, the health care provider may be uncertain whether the problem is asthma or chronic bronchitis. For the purpose of teaching and learning, distinct pathophysiological differences among emphysema, chronic bronchitis, and asthma are presented in this chapter.

Often the asthmatic person is a nonsmoker; gives a history of a nonproductive cough possibly associated with chest tightness; states that symptoms are frequently triggered by allergens, cold air, exercise, or irritants; and tends to hyperventilate (defined by a decreased PaCO$_2$) and blow off carbon dioxide in acute attacks.

The patient with chronic bronchitis usually gives a history of smoking; has experienced cough at least 2 months per year for 2 or more years with excessive sputum production; may have right heart failure secondary to hypoxemia; and tends to hypoventilate and retain carbon dioxide. Certain signs and symptoms may overlap. Some of these are

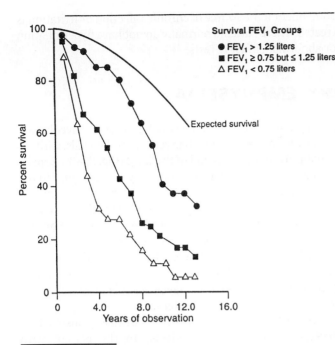

FIGURE 25-1
Long-term survival of 200 patients with COPD grouped by initial FEV$_1$. From Kelley WN: Textbook of Internal Medicine (3rd Ed), p 1981. Philadelphia, Lippincott-Raven, 1997.

chronic cough, shortness of breath, wheezing, airway obstruction, hyperinflation, and hypoxemia secondary to ventilation–perfusion mismatching and altered gas exchange.

▄▄▄ CHRONIC BRONCHITIS

Chronic infection or irritation of the bronchi can result in bronchitis. The mucus-secreting glands of the tracheobronchial tree become thickened and encroach on the diameter of the airway lumen (Fig. 25–2). In addition, there is increased mucus production in peripheral airways. By far the most common cause is tobacco smoking.

Considerations for Home Care
Oxygen Use

Many patients with chronic respiratory diseases will receive oxygen on a continual or intermittent basis. When these patients are admitted or visits made to their home, the nurse reviews oxygen safety. The nurse also verifies the patient's knowledge of the oxygen dose and checks his or her ability to read the reserve volume in the tank or oximizor. The patient is taught (if the patient can do this) to check a pulse oximetry reading at rest and with exercise. Nutritional counseling is necessary for patients too short of breath to eat solid foods.

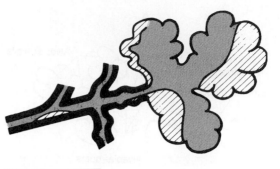

FIGURE 25-2
Bronchitis inflammation and thickening produce narrowing of airways. Lined areas indicate secretions.

The two most common bacterial organisms isolated from the secretions of the patient with chronic bronchitis are Haemophilus influenzae and Streptococcus pneumoniae. Occasionally, Mycoplasma and anaerobes are implicated also. Exacerbation of chronic bronchitis with resultant respiratory insufficiency most often is caused by an acute bacterial inflammation of the bronchial tree. Other manifestations are listed in the accompanying display. An essential prophylactic measure in preventing an acute inflammatory process is rigorous bronchial hygiene to promote clearance of secretions that provide an ideal medium for bacterial growth in the peripheral airways. In contrast to emphysema, chronic bronchitis can have a reversible

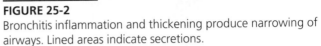

◆ RED FLAG **Manifestations of** Severe Exacerbations of Chronic Bronchitis

Constitutional Signs
Temperature frequently subnormal
WBC varies—may be slightly ↑, normal, or ↓

CNS Disturbances
Headache
Confusion
Hallucinations
Depression
Drowsiness
Somnolence
Coma
Papilledema

Cardiovascular Signs
Diaphoresis
Tachycardia
Blood pressure varies: normal, ↑, or ↓
Vasoconstriction initially followed by vasodilation

Neuromuscular Signs
Fine tremors
Asterixis
Flaccidity
Convulsions

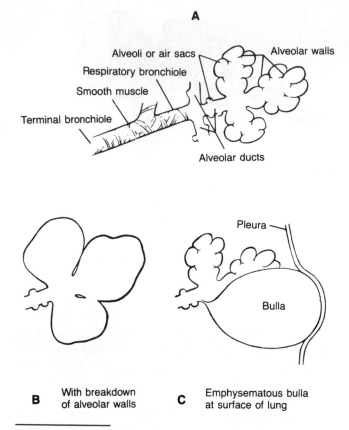

FIGURE 25-3
Emphysema. Airway showing normal primary lobule (**A**) and emphysematous lobule (**B** and **C**).

component if the source of chronic infection or irritation is treated. These patients normally do not have hyperinflation or abnormal diffusion tests.

EMPHYSEMA

Emphysema is an irreversible dilatation of the alveolus accompanied by destructive changes of alveolar walls, with resultant loss of elastic recoil of the lung (Fig. 25–3). Experimental studies have confirmed the key role of injury to the elastic fiber network in the structural changes of emphysema. Two possible sources of elastolytic activity are neutrophils and alveolar macrophages, both of which are increased in cigarette smokers. Cigarette smoking is a major factor in the development of emphysema. In addition, elastase can be released from neutrophils because of components of smoke. This factor may play a role in an imbalance of an elastase–antielastase system.

The destructive process resulting in airway obstruction develops insidiously. In contrast to the patient with chronic bronchitis, patients with emphysema usually have mild chronic hypoxemia because destruction of alveolar walls is accompanied by destruction of corresponding vasculature. The ratio of ventilated to perfused lung tissue remains stable.

The majority of patients with COPD have a mixture of chronic bronchitis and emphysema rather than "pure" bronchitis or emphysema (Table 25–2).

TABLE 25-2
COPD: Features That Distinguish Bronchitis and Emphysema

Features	Bronchitis	Emphysema
Primary location of pathology	Airways	Air sacs
Clinical Examination		
Subjective Data	Frequent recurrent chest infections	Frequently only insidious dyspnea—
	Sputum production	initially with exercise only, then
	Cough	progressing
Objective Data		
Appearance	"Blue bloaters" (type B COPD)	"Pink puffers" (type A COPD)
Chest examination	Noisy chest, *slight* overdistention	Quiet chest, marked overdistention
Sputum	Frequently copious and purulent	Usually scant and mucoid
Chronic cor pulmonale	Common—may occur relatively early	Infrequent until terminal stages
Dyspnea	Mild	Severe
Laboratory Tests		
ABGs		
Chronic hypoxemia	Often significant	Usually mild
Chronic hypercapnia	Common	Uncommon (normal to low $PaCO_2$)
Spirometry		
FEV_1/FVC	Decreased	Decreased
FEV_1	Decreased	Decreased
Therapeutic Modalities		
Bronchial hygiene (measures to enhance secretion clearance)	Very important	Less important unless patient has respiratory infection

> ### *Considerations for the Older Patient*
> #### Asthma
>
> Asthma may not develop until middle age. Symptoms of fatigue and exercise intolerance may go unrecognized or be camouflaged by other complications. The nurse must keep a level of suspicion when patients complain of "new allergies," frequent infections, exercise intolerance, and shortness of breath.

> **RED FLAG**   **Common Triggers of** Asthma
>
> * Inhaled irritants
> * Exercise
> * Cold air
> * Viral infections
> * Allergens
> * Medications
> * Food additives (sulfites)
> * Emotions

ASTHMA

Pathophysiological Principles

Compared with emphysema and, to a lesser extent, chronic bronchitis, asthma is an acute reversible airway disease. (It is not reversible, however, in all patients.) Asthma has the characteristics of airway obstruction that is usually reversible (spontaneously or with treatment), airway inflammation, and increased airway responsiveness.[4]

Bronchospasm occurs and includes smooth muscle constriction, mucosal edema, and excessive mucus with plugging of the conducting airways in the advanced stages. The accompanying display lists some of the common triggers for asthma.

Assessment

CLINICAL MANIFESTATIONS

Signs and symptoms vary with the degree of bronchospasm. The patient may complain of shortness of breath associated with wheezing respirations. Additional findings include tachycardia, tachypnea, retractions, restlessness, anxiety, inspiratory/expiratory wheezing, hypoxemia, hypercapnia, cyanosis, and cough. A decrease in wheezing does not necessarily mean decreased bronchospasm, but rather progression of airway narrowing and markedly decreased ventilation.

Figure 25–4 illustrates a series of events that can become a vicious cycle, resulting in life-threatening status asthmaticus unless bronchospasm is controlled.

Management

In spite of improved understanding of this disease, the death rate from acute asthma is increasing, perhaps because of lack of uniform intervention strategies. Treatment is directed at removing the cause of bronchospasm and initiating bronchodilator and other appropriate therapies. Table 25–3 provides a summary of current therapies recommended for managing the asthmatic patient with a severe exacerbation. The patient must be observed for increasing

FIGURE 25-4
Sequence of events leading from asthma to hypoxemia.

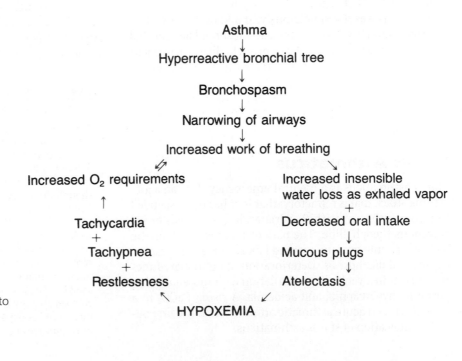

TABLE 25-3
Management of Severe Asthma*

These findings help assess the degree of bronchospasm and the patient's respiratory reserve in a crisis situation:

Clinical Findings	Interpretation
Pulsus paradoxus: >12 mmHg Low, normal, or decreasing	Severe respiratory compromise due to increased muscle force Patient improving or impending respiratory failure in patient with fatigue and poor air exchange
Peak expiratory flow: <150 L/min or <50% predicted values	Severe bronchospasm and respiratory failure

Treatment	Purpose
Aerosolized β_2-agonists IV corticosteroids	Mainstays of drug treatment Bronchodilation and anti-inflammatory therapy Side effects: vasodilation, hypotension, ↓ PaO_2, tolerance

Parenteral β_2-agonists (eg, epinephrine, terbutaline)
 Theophylline, atropine derivatives, magnesium
 Heliox (helium and O_2)
 Mechanical ventilation
   a. ↑ expiratory time by decreasing minute volume
   b. ↑ inspiratory flow rate
   c. Inspiratory waveform to minimize inspiratory time and maximize expiratory time
   d. Sedatives
	Used only in patients <30 y
	 Additional therapies; additive effect with β_2-agonists
	 May reduce work of breathing
	 Provide adequate alveolar ventilation while avoiding barotrauma or shock
	
	 To assist patient's synchrony with ventilation

If above measures fail: Anesthetics Heliox	May ↓ bronchial muscle spasm May ↓ airway pressure and barotrauma

* Based on: Manthous, C: Management of severe exacerbations of asthma. Am J Med 99(3):298–308, 1995

bronchospasm and deteriorating pulmonary function manifested by a rising $PaCO_2$.

The key to successful management of the asthmatic patient is identification and prevention of all possible factors that trigger bronchospasm. A display listing these trigger mechanisms was given previously. If a known cause of an asthmatic attack is exercise, the patient should be educated to take an inhaled quick-release bronchodilator treatment before starting exercise. The adult patient should always carry an inhaled bronchodilator (ie, metered dose) device, such as a metaproterenol inhaler or a dose of bronchodilator in a hand-powered nebulizer. (See Table 24–4 to review bronchodilator drugs.)

Status Asthmaticus

Status asthmaticus is a medical emergency. It is an acute asthma attack that is refractory; that is, it has not responded to rigorous therapy with β_2-adrenergic compounds or intravenous theophylline. The patient manifests a dramatic picture of acute anxiety, marked labored breathing, tachycardia, and diaphoresis. Deterioration of pulmonary function results in alveolar hypoventilation with subsequent hypoxemia, hypercapnia, and acidemia. A rising $PaCO_2$ in a patient with an acute asthmatic attack is often the first objective indication of status asthmaticus.

Multiple therapeutic modalities must be instituted. All patients in status asthmaticus demonstrate hypoxemia and require oxygen therapy. Dehydration usually exists and requires correction. Pharmacological agents consist of methylxanthines, sympathomimetic amines, and corticosteroids. If pulmonary function cannot be improved and respiratory failure ensues, the patient may require intubation and assisted ventilation (see Table 25–2).

CLINICAL APPLICATION: Patient Care Study

Tom Blair, a 58-year-old white man, was well known to the critical care nursing staff. His emphysema was brought on by a 32-year history of cigarette smoking. He was admitted 4 months ago for respiratory failure and received a tracheostomy during his 3 weeks of mechanical ventilation. Although discharged on home oxygen therapy, Tom continued to smoke one pack of cigarettes per day.

Six days ago, Mr. Blair presented in his physician's office with increasing shortness of breath, increased yellow-tinged secretions, and a very poor activity tolerance. He was sent home on erythromycin syrup, O_2 4 L/min by nasal cannula, and home care by respiratory therapy. Mr. Blair managed his care adequately until last night. At 9:00 PM, he developed shaking chills and severe shortness of breath. He increased his oxygen to 6 L/min. His daughter found him unresponsive at 10:35 PM and called the paramedics.

On presenting in the emergency department, he was orally intubated by the paramedics, had a liter of normal saline infusing through a left antecubital #18 gauge angiocath and was barely responsive to deep pain. His initial vital signs were BP, 98/52 mmHg; HR, 108/min; sinus tachycardia; RR, 20 per Ambu bag at 100% FiO_2; T, 102°F per rectum. Mr. Blair was once again admitted to the intensive care unit (ICU) on a mechanical ventilator with the diagnosis of COPD exacerbation and pneumonia.

After he was settled in the ICU, routine laboratory tests were done. This included serum chemistry tests, a complete blood count, ABG, urinalysis, serum toxicology screen, and coagulation studies. A portable chest film was completed. After performing a thorough bedside physical assessment, the critical care nurse reviewed all the pertinent findings. Mr. Blair was barely arousable. His weight had dropped 15 lb since his last admission. His breath sounds were very coarse, with rhonchi throughout all anterior and lateral lung fields. Thick yellow secretions were suctioned out of the endotracheal tube. His vital signs were similar to the findings in the emergency department.

The laboratory results were normal except for the following:

- ABG on 100% FiO_2, tidal volume 650 mL, assist–control rate of 14:
   - pH, 7.30
   - $PaCO_2$, 58
   - PaO_2, 81
   - O_2 saturation, 90%
   - HCO_3, 35
- Serum chemistry:
   - K, 3.4
   - Glucose, 154
- CBC:
   - Hemoglobin, 11.4
   - Hematocrit, 32%
- Toxicology screen:
   - Negative for sedatives, barbiturates, alcohol, and cocaine

The chest radiograph showed white fluffy infiltrates in all lung fields and confirmed correct endotracheal tube placement. The chest film showed rib changes consistent with COPD and a mild enlargement of the cardiac shadow. A comparison of this film to previous studies was not available.

The nurse medicated Mr. Blair with an acetaminophen (Tylenol) suppository (650 mg) and collected a sputum culture specimen. A Foley catheter and nasogastric tube (to low intermittent wall suction) were placed. The intravenous fluid was changed to 5% dextrose/.45% normal saline with 40 mEq KCl at 125 mL/h. Bilateral soft wrist restraints were placed and secured to the bed frame. Continuous oxygen saturation was monitored with a finger pulse oximeter. A rectal probe was placed for verification of body temperature, and a second intravenous site was initiated, although capped with a dead end plug. These interventions took about 1 hour to perform, and after they were completed, Mr. Blair was awake, alert, and cooperative with the care in progress.

The Gram stain of the sputum specimen showed gram-positive cocci, most likely Haemophilus influenzae. Amoxicillin (Augmentin) 500 mg was begun. Respiratory therapy began to titrate down the FiO_2 as long as the SaO_2 was equal to or greater than 92%. By morning, the FiO_2 was at 50%. His temperature responded to antipyretics and fell to 100°F per rectum.

By mid-morning, Mr. Blair was comfortable on the ventilator. His secretions remained thick and yellow but were decreasing in amount. He was cooperative with all of his care, communicating by writing notes. Whenever weaning from the ventilator was mentioned, Mr. Blair became frightened, tachypneic, and tachycardic. He did not want the support discontinued. It took extra time for the respiratory therapists to perform routine ventilator checks because Mr. Blair was so fearful that they were decreasing his support. Finally, the medical team chose not to increase his work of breathing by weaning the ventilator until he had rested thoroughly.

The next morning, all attempts to increase Mr. Blair's work of breathing failed. He would panic, rapidly increasing his respiratory and heart rates, while decreasing his SaO_2. His chest radiograph showed some response to antibiotic therapy. His supportive care included sitting in the chair, physical therapy exercises, occupational therapy for mental stimulation, intravenous aminophylline, maintenance intravenous fluids, ice chips for oral comfort, and aerosol treatments every 4 hours. Mr. Blair was comfortable and wrote notes that he was not short of breath for the first time since his discharge from the ICU months ago.

Recognizing the chronicity of Mr. Blair's disease, it was decided to provide nutrition through a feeding tube. A low, acid ash formula was started at half strength at 30 mL/h. This was to be advanced by 10 mL every 2 hours until at 75 mL/h. The nurses checked for gastric residual every 4 hours or if Mr. Blair complained of feeling full. He tolerated the tube feedings well. It seemed like another long stay was in order for Mr. Blair.

Mr. Blair's hospital course was unremarkable for several days. He was comfortable on the ventilator, and little progress was made in weaning attempts. The discharge planning team decided to meet with him and discuss placement in a nursing home. Mr. Blair found this idea totally unacceptable, and he agreed to participate in ventilator weans immediately.

Weans began with decreasing the FiO_2 to 35%. Because Mr. Blair's SaO_2 remained above 92%, the assist–control respiratory rate was slowly dropped to 8, and his total respiratory rate stayed in the low 20s. Mr. Blair was allowed to rest overnight, and weaning resumed in the morning. Again, the weaning process was tolerated well. By that evening, the sixth hospital day, Mr. Blair was performing all of his own work of breathing on a 35% T-piece adapter. Again he rested on the ventilator overnight.

Mr. Blair was extubated at 10:00 AM on the seventh day of his hospital stay. His antibiotic course was complete. His only request was to have some ice cream for lunch. His post-extubation ABG revealed:

- pH, 7.38
- $PaCO_2$, 52
- PaO_2, 78
- O_2 saturation, 91%
- HCO_3, 36

The nurses were confused about his sudden cooperation with the ventilator weans and decided to confront him about the radical behavior change. Mr. Blair revealed that the only thing that frightened him more than being short of breath was to lose his independence. He saw the nursing home as a place to go to die. He admitted that the ventilator and ICU setting provided him with confidence and a feeling of ease. He did not realize that this "service" could not be provided indefinitely.

The Collaborative Care Guide outlines care provided for the patient with COPD.

(text continues on page 508)

COLLABORATIVE CARE GUIDE
for the Patient With Chronic Obstructive Pulmonary Disease

OUTCOMES	INTERVENTIONS
Oxygenation/Ventilation	
Patient has arterial blood gases within normal limits and pulse oximeter value >90%.	• Assess respiratory rate, effort, and breath sounds q2–4h. • Obtain arterial blood gases per order or signs of respiratory distress. • Monitor arterial saturation by pulse oximeter. • Provide supplemental oxygen by nasal cannula or face mask using lowest possible FIO_2 and flow rate. • Provide humidification with oxygen. • Provide intubation and mechanical ventilation as necessary (refer to Collaborative Care Guide for the Patient on Mechanical Ventilation).
Patient maintains normal rate and depth of respiration.	• Monitor respiratory rate, pattern, and effort (eg, use of accessory muscles). • Assess respirations during sleep; note sleep apnea or Cheyne-Stokes patterns.
Patient has clear chest x-ray. Patient has clear breath sounds.	• Obtain chest x-ray qd. • Monitor breath sounds for crackles, wheezes, or rhonchi q2–4h. • Administer diuretics per order. • Administer bronchodilators and mucolytics as indicated.
There is no evidence of atelectasis or pneumonia.	• Encourage nonintubated patients to use incentive spirometer, cough, and deep breath q2–4h and PRN. • Assess quantity, color, and consistency of secretions. • Turn side to side q2h. • Mobilize out of bed to chair.
Circulation/Perfusion	
Blood pressure, heart rate, and hemodynamic parameters are within normal limits.	• Monitor vital signs q1–2h. • Monitor pulmonary artery pressures and right atrial pressure q1h and cardiac output, SVR, and PVR q6–12h if pulmonary artery catheter is in place. • Assess for signs of right ventricular dysfunction (eg, increased CVP, neck vein distension, peripheral edema). • Maintain patent IV access.
Patient is free of dysrhythmias.	• Monitor for atrial dysrhythmias due to right atrial dilation and ventricular dysrhythmias due to hypoxemia and hypoxia.
Serum lactate will be within normal limits.	• Monitor lactate qd until it is within normal limits. • Administer red blood cells, positive inotropic agents, colloid infusion as ordered to increase oxygen delivery.
Fluids/Electrolytes	
Renal function is maintained as evidenced by urine output >30 mL/h, normal laboratory values.	• Monitor intake and output q1–2h. • Monitor BUN, creatinine, electrolytes, Mg, PO_4. • Replace potassium, magnesium, and phosphorus per order or protocol.
Patient is euvolemic.	• Take daily weights. • Administer fluid volume and diuretics based on vital signs, physical assessment, secretion viscosity, as ordered.
Mobility/Safety	
There is no evidence of loss of muscle tone or strength.	• Promote standing at bedside, sitting up in chair, ambulating with assistance as soon as possible. • Establish activity program. • Monitor response to activity.

(continued)

COLLABORATIVE CARE GUIDE
for the Patient With Chronic Obstructive Pulmonary Disease (Continued)

OUTCOMES	INTERVENTIONS
Patient maintains joint flexibility.	• Consult with physical therapist. • Use passive and active ROM q4h while awake.
There is no evidence of infection. WBCs are within normal limits.	• Monitor systemic inflammatory response syndrome criteria: increased WBC, increased temperature, tachypnea, tachycardia. • Use strict aseptic technique during procedures and monitor others. • Maintain invasive catheter tube sterility. • Per hospital protocol, change invasive catheters, culture blood, line tips, or fluids.
There is no evidence of DVT.	• Initiate DVT prophylaxis within 24 hours of admission. • Monitor for leg pain, redness, or swelling.
Skin Integrity There is no evidence of skin breakdown.	• Turn side to side q2h. • Remove self-protective devices from wrists, and monitor skin per hospital policy. • Assess risk of skin breakdown using objective tool (eg, Braden Scale). Consider pressure relief/reduction mattress.
Nutrition Caloric and nutrient intake meet metabolic requirements per calculation (eg, Basal Energy Expenditure).	• Provide parenteral, enteral, or oral nutrition within 48 hours. • Consult dietitian or nutritional support service. • Avoid high-carbohydrate load if patient retains CO_2. • Monitor albumin, prealbumin, transferrin, cholesterol, triglycerides, glucose.
Comfort/Pain Control Patient is comfortable and evaluates pain as <4 on the pain scale.	• Assess pain/comfort q4h. • Administer analgesics and sedatives cautiously, closely monitoring respiratory rate, depth, and pattern. • Differentiate between agitation caused by discomfort or caused by hypoxia prior to medication administration. • Elevate head of bed to improve breathing comfort.
Psychosocial Patient demonstrates decreased anxiety.	• Assess vital signs during treatments, discussions, and so forth. • Cautiously administer sedatives. • Consult social services, clergy as appropriate. • Provide for adequate rest and sleep. • Provide support during periods of dyspnea.
Teaching/Discharge Planning Patient/significant others understand procedures and tests needed for treatment. Significant others understand the severity of the illness, ask appropriate questions, anticipate potential complications. In preparation for discharge, to home, patient understands activity levels, dietary restrictions, medication regimen, metered inhaler.	• Prepare patient/significant others for procedures such as CPT, bronchoscopy, pulmonary artery catheter insertion, or laboratory studies. • Explain the causes and effects of COPD and the potential for complications, such as pneumonia or cardiac dysfunction. • Encourage significant others to ask questions related to the ventilator, pathophysiology, monitoring, treatments, and so forth. • Make appropriate referrals and consults early during hospitalization. • Initiate family education regarding proper use of metered inhaler, signs and symptoms of respiratory failure, and appropriate actions.

Sleep Apnea Syndrome

A prevalent disorder in patients with COPD is sleep apnea syndrome (SAS). This condition is more common in men than in women, although the incidence increases in women after menopause, suggesting that female hormones are in some way protective. The patient's partner, if questioned directly, or the nurse in attendance for hospitalized patients, usually describes intermittent loud snoring followed by silence (apnea) lasting 10 to 100 seconds or longer.

Pathophysiological Principles

There are three classifications of apnea:

- Obstructive apnea—associated with absence of airflow despite ventilatory efforts
- Central apnea—associated with absence of both airflow and ventilatory efforts
- Mixed apnea—an initial period of central apnea followed by obstructive apnea

The site of obstruction in obstructive apnea is the oropharynx, and it is apparently related to an abrupt loss of tone in the muscles surrounding the oropharynx just before the onset of inspiration. It is believed that a decreased ventilatory drive exists, for unknown reasons, in central and obstructive apnea; ventilatory responsiveness to hypoxemia and hypercarbia is depressed.

In the obstructive type of sleep apnea caused by laryngeal obstruction by the tongue or other neck structures, the patient often has struggling respirations but no airflow, followed by loud snoring. However, in the central apneas, the reduced central nervous system drive to breathe is not associated with characteristic loud snoring. Obstructive apneas are more common.

Assessment

CLINICAL MANIFESTATIONS

Signs and symptoms of SAS are listed in the display. Most cases of SAS occur in middle-aged men between 40 and 60 years of age. Suspicion of SAS is based on a middle-aged man who gives a history of sleep disturbance that may be accompanied by the displayed signs and symptoms. A de-

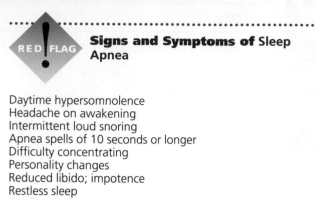

RED FLAG

Signs and Symptoms of Sleep Apnea

Daytime hypersomnolence
Headache on awakening
Intermittent loud snoring
Apnea spells of 10 seconds or longer
Difficulty concentrating
Personality changes
Reduced libido; impotence
Restless sleep
Cardiac rhythm disturbances
Systemic hypertension
Hypoxemia
Fatigue (chronic)

finitive diagnosis is based on the results of polysomnography and a detailed patient history.

Conditions that can predispose to secondary sleep apnea include obesity, myxedema, acromegaly, anatomical upper airway obstruction (ie, nasal deformity with resultant obstruction), brain stem lesions, cervical spine injury, encephalitis, and myotonic dystrophy.

Management

Treatment of SAS is based on the type of apnea and the severity of symptoms. For example, a tracheostomy for obstructive apnea may resolve all symptoms. Before this drastic measure is performed—unless the condition is life-threatening—a protriptyline trial is warranted. Protriptyline is a nonsedating tricyclic antidepressant that reduces the amount of rapid eye movement sleep in which most apnea occurs and decreases upper airway resistance. If successful, this agent decreases somnolence, but patients continue to have abnormal sleep patterns associated with many apneas and arousals. Other forms of treatment include medroxyprogesterone acetate (very useful in obesity–hypoventilation syndrome), continuous positive airway pressure, and surgical enlargement of the pharyngeal airway by resection of excessive mucosa. By far the simplest treatment is nocturnal oxygen administration, which often prevents the nocturnal desaturation and many of the other symptoms.

Interstitial Lung Disease

Many use the term pulmonary interstitium in reference to alveolar walls. However, the term interstitial lung disease (ILD), while somewhat misleading, is comprehensively defined as an inflammatory process involving each component of the alveolar and airway architecture. These components are the connective tissue of the pleura, the bronchi, and the respiratory airspace walls. The inflammatory process can heal completely or result in subsequent development of excess connective tissue (diffuse scarring or fibrosis), accompanied by significant distortion of lung structure.

> ## NURSING PERSPECTIVE
> ### *Summary of Interstitial Lung Disease*
>
> ### *Pathology of ILD*
>
> - Primary process—active inflammation (alveolitis)
> - Secondary process—fibrosis
>
> ### *Pathophysiology*
>
> - Alveolitis involving lymphocytes—exposure to an antigen is initiating event
> - Alveolitis involving neutrophils—production of chemical mediators potentially toxic to components of alveolar walls
>
> ### *Pathophysiology Basic to Majority of ILD*
>
> Inflammation and fibrosis of alveolar wall components and airway structures:
>
> - Decreased pulmonary compliance (increased stiffness) due to significant inflammatory and fibrotic process
> - Generalized decrease in lung volume due to change in compliance (stiffness) of the lung
> - Impaired diffusion of O_2 and CO_2 due to destruction of alveolar–capillary walls with resultant decrease of available surface area for gas exchange
> - Disturbances in gas exchange (primarily ↓PaO_2) secondary to disruption of normal matching of ventilation and perfusion
> - Pulmonary hypertension—ultimate sequelae with severe ILD secondary to:
>   (1) bronchoconstriction associated with hypoxemia and
>   (2) destruction of small pulmonary vessels by the alveolar wall fibrotic process
>
> ### *Clinical Features/Assessment*
>
> - Dyspnea on exertion progressing to dyspnea at rest
> - Cough—usually nonproductive
> - Velcro (dry) crackles—most prominent at base of lungs; end-inspiratory
> - Tachypnea
> - Reduced chest expansion
> - Finger clubbing (idiopathic pulmonary fibrosis)
> - Extrapulmonary findings suggestive of connective tissue disease (eg, erythema nodosum, subcutaneous nodules, uveitis)
>
> ### *Diagnosis*
>
> - Chest roentgenogram
> - Bronchoalveolar lavage
> - Lung biopsy as indicated/appropriate
> - High-resolution computed tomography
> - Pulmonary function tests
>
> ### *Management*
>
> - Corticosteroids to reduce inflammatory process
> - Immunosuppressive agents
> - Physical conditioning program
> - Supplemental oxygen

Hypersensitivity pneumonitis, asbestosis, pneumoconiosis, sarcoidosis, pulmonary vasculitis, idiopathic pulmonary fibrosis, and ILD associated with connective tissue diseases are all considered ILD. The etiological factors of most of these disorders remain unknown; however, occupational and environmental exposures (inorganic dust) are related to many ILDs.

Pathology, pathophysiology, clinical features, assessment, diagnostic approaches, and management of ILDs are summarized in the accompanying display.

Nonpulmonary Respiratory Complications

Patients can manifest respiratory complications in which the primary cause is not an underlying disorder of the lungs or respiratory system. Nonpulmonary causes of respiratory complications include abdominal and thoracic surgery, pharmacotherapy complications, disease states or trauma involving the neuromuscular system, and disorders restricting the chest.

Postoperative Pulmonary Compromise

Patients who have surgery, notably high abdominal thoracic and low abdominal resection, are especially susceptible to respiratory compromise. The mechanism of pulmonary compromise is a restrictive entity in which there is a reduction of vital capacity (VC), resulting in a limited ventilatory reserve. The major restrictive insult occurs in the first 24 hours postoperatively. Patients without complications gradually resume their preoperative ventilatory status.

Postoperative pulmonary complications can be avoided or minimized by adequate preoperative cardiopulmonary evaluation by the critical care nurse. The nurse can thereby institute measures to monitor pulmonary status and provide modalities aimed at improving VC.

Pharmacotherapy Complications

Appropriate administration of narcotics and sedatives is a necessary adjunct to pulmonary care. The use of these drugs must be guided by the patient's clinical status. The aim of pharmacological therapy is to minimize pain so the patient can tolerate respiratory therapy and other therapeutic modalities. However, overzealous use of these drugs can result in respiratory depression and acute respiratory failure.

The patient with a sedative or narcotic overdose presents with respiratory insufficiency. The severity of the respiratory insufficiency depends on the specific type and amount of drug(s) ingested, time of ingestion, and rate of metabolism of the drug(s).

Factors that can alter drug effects include multiple drug ingestion, hepatic or renal function abnormalities, and preexisting pulmonary disease, such as COPD.

Care of patients with drug overdose is guided by this information and by the knowledge that patients with certain types of drug ingestion (eg, glutethimide) can show a fluctuation in level of consciousness. This presents a problem in the maintenance of an adequate airway. It must not be assumed that a patient who at one time appears alert and able to maintain the airway will continue to do so.

There are also drugs that in normal pharmacological doses can cause neuromuscular blockage with resultant respiratory paralysis. These include kanamycin, gentamicin, streptomycin, neomycin, and polymyxin B.

Neuromuscular Involvement

Disease states or trauma involving the neuromuscular system can affect pulmonary function. The degree of dysfunction depends on the extent of respiratory muscle involvement.

In certain neurological diseases, gag and cough reflexes can be diminished, resulting in aspiration of food, fluid, or secretions. The aspirated contents can cause atelectasis and pneumonia, which, if not recognized, lead to progressive respiratory failure. As impairment of respiratory muscles progresses, there is a resultant decrease in VC.

Taking serial measurements of the VC is an important method of assessing adequacy of pulmonary function. This assessment can be done quite readily by the nurse. Cardinal signs of respiratory compromise, pulmonary function measurements, and ABG analysis must be correlated with the clinical status of the patient.

Long-term management of a patient with a neuromuscular disorder includes maintenance of a patent airway, rigorous clearance of secretions, treatment of infections, maximal mobilization of the patient, and ventilatory assistance if indicated.

Restrictive Disorders

Several entities restrict chest wall expansion, with resultant compromised pulmonary function. These include kyphoscoliosis, rheumatoid spondylitis, scleroderma, pectus excavatum, and use of orthopedic appliances, such as spica casts. Patients with these conditions can, in a stable environment, have normal pulmonary function. A crisis such as trauma or a major medical illness such as drug overdose can precipitate severe respiratory impairment. In the management of these patients, the nurse must use measures that maximize ventilation and minimize pulmonary complications.

◼ CONCLUSION

Common pulmonary disorders can test the skill of the critical care nurse in the assessment and intervention arenas. Many of these conditions are highly dependent on meticulous nursing care for prevention of complications and for uncompromised recovery. Advances in technology and understanding of disease mechanisms are no substitute for knowledgeable nursing management.

Clinical Applicability Challenges

Self-Challenge: Critical Thinking

1. *Using Tom Blair, the patient in the Patient Care Study, explore other options the staff could have used to help him psychologically prepare for the ventilator wean.*

2. *Develop a discharge plan for a patient with a chronic obstructive respiratory disease.*

Study Questions

1. *Which of the following is not a symptom of atelectasis?*
   a. Tachycardia and tachypnea
   b. Asymmetric chest expansion
   c. Pain on deep inspiration
   d. Shortness of breath or dyspnea on exertion

2. The best definition of PE is
   a. increased dead space from ventilation past a nonperfused alveolus.
   b. an expansion of the normal ventilation–perfusion mismatch.
   c. perfusion of a nonventilated alveolar area, causing an increased ventilation–perfusion mismatch.
   d. a showering of multiple small emboli to the distal pulmonary capillary beds.

3. All of the following statements are true except
   a. cor pulmonale occurs more often with bronchitis than with emphysema.
   b. bronchial hygiene is crucial to the management of emphysema.
   c. asthma management focuses on preventing the attack, and the cause of the attacks should be avoided.
   d. sleep apnea occurs most often in men between 40 and 60 years of age and in women past menopause.

4. Which of the following statements about sleep apnea syndrome is not true?
   a. It is more common in men than in women.
   b. Female hormones may be a protective factor in women.
   c. The apnea can be obstructive, central, or mixed.
   d. It occurs most commonly in men 60 to 70 years of age.

REFERENCES

1. Henneman E, Bellamy P: Preventing complications in the intensive care unit. In Shoemaker W, et al: Textbook of Critical Care. Philadelphia, WB Saunders, 1995
2. Christman JW: Pulmonary host defenses and inflammatory lung disease. In Shoemaker W, et al: Textbook of Critical Care. Philadelphia, WB Saunders, 1995
3. Kelley WN: Textbook of Internal Medicine (3rd Ed). Philadelphia, Lippincott-Raven, 1997
4. National Asthma Educational Program (NAEP): Expert Panel Report, Guidelines for the diagnosis and management of asthma. National Heart, Lung & Blood Institute. Allergy Clin. Immunology, 1991, 88–425.

BIBLIOGRAPHY

Grossbach I: The COPD patient in acute respiratory failure. Critical Care Nurse 14(6):32–40, 1994
Ketelaars CAJ, et al: Process standards of nursing care for patients with COPD: Validation of standards and criteria by the delphi technique. Journal of Nursing Care Quality 9(1):78–86, 1994
McKinney B: Under new management: Asthma and the elderly. Journal of Gerontological Nursing 21(11):39–45, 1995
Spenceley SM: The CNS in multidisciplinary pulmonary rehabilitation: A nursing science perspective. Clinical Nurse Specialist 9(4):192–198, 1995

26

Adult Respiratory Distress Syndrome

OBJECTIVES

Based on the content in this chapter, the reader should be able to:

- Relate the assessment and diagnostic findings of adult respiratory distress syndrome (ARDS) to the pathophysiological processes.
- Describe nursing and medical interventions related to management of ARDS.
- Anticipate potential complications of ARDS and the related interventions.

Adult respiratory distress syndrome (ARDS) was first described as a clinical syndrome in 1967 and was termed acute respiratory distress in adults. ARDS is an acute and severe form of respiratory failure, often occurring in previously healthy people who have been exposed to a pulmonary or nonpulmonary insult. Examples of common insults precipitating ARDS are sepsis, aspiration of gastric contents, trauma, and hemorrhagic shock.

Typically ARDS is manifested within 72 hours following the predisposing insult, resulting in direct or indirect lung injury. The 1994 American-European Consensus Conference on acute respiratory distress syndrome recommended the use of a common definition for acute lung injury and ARDS. These are listed in Table 26–1. ARDS is characterized by noncardiogenic pulmonary edema, collapsed and fluid-filled alveoli, and, subsequently, severe hypoxemia. The incidence of ARDS is estimated to be 200,000 to 250,000 cases per year and is associated with a mortality rate of 40% to 90%.[1]

PATHOPHYSIOLOGICAL PRINCIPLES

The pathological pulmonary alterations of ARDS are directly related to a cascade of events initiated by the systemic inflammatory response syndrome (SIRS), which is triggered by any of the various predisposing insults. SIRS initiates the release of multiple inflammatory mediators, which cause increased microvascular permeability, pulmonary hypertension, and pulmonary endothelial damage.[2] The activation, interactions, and multisystem actions of the inflammatory mediators are extremely complex. Table 26–2 lists some of the primary mediators responsible for lung damage in ARDS and their major actions as they relate to ARDS.

RED FLAG

Risk Factors for Adult Respiratory Distress Syndrome

Systemic Disorders
- Shock of any etiology
- Sepsis
- Hypothermia
- Hyperthermia
- Drug overdose
- Disseminated intravascular coagulation
- Massive transfusion
- Cardiopulmonary bypass
- Eclampsia
- Burns
- Pancreatitis
- Severe nonthoracic trauma

Pulmonary Disorders
- Pneumonia
- Inhalation injury
- Aspiration (gastric fluids/near-drowning)
- Pneumonitis

TABLE 26-2
Examples of Inflammatory Mediators and Pathological Responses

Response	SIRS Mediators
Persistent inflammatory response	Complement, thromboxane, interleukin, tumor necrosis factor
Endothelial membrane disruption	Complement, thromboxane, kinins, tumor necrosis factor, toxic oxygen metabolites, leukotrienes
Selective vasoconstriction	Thromboxane, tumor necrosis factor, platelet activating factor, toxic oxygen metabolites
Systemic vasodilation	Complement, prostaglandin, tumor necrosis factor, interleukin
Myocardial depression	Complement, leukotrienes, tumor necrosis factor, myocardial depressant factor
Bronchoconstriction	Complement, thromboxane, leukotrienes, platelet activating factor

---

Adequate pulmonary gas exchange is dependent on open, air-filled alveoli; intact alveolar–capillary membranes; and normal blood flow through the pulmonary vasculature. In ARDS, diffuse alveolar–capillary membrane damage occurs and increases membrane permeability. Alterations in alveolar–capillary membrane integrity allow fluids to move from the vascular space into the interstitial and alveolar space. The resultant interstitial and alveolar edema and eventual alveolar collapse impair both oxygenation and ventilation. The pathogenesis of ARDS is explained in Figure 26–1.

The diffusion of oxygen into the pulmonary capillary blood and the elimination of carbon dioxide are significantly reduced in ARDS. Ventilation is impaired because of a decrease in lung compliance and an increase in airway resistance. Decreased lung compliance is caused by the increased membrane permeability and secondary fluid-filled and collapsed alveoli and by a reduction in the production

of surfactant, a substance that decreases the surface tension of alveoli and prevents their collapse. Mediator-induced bronchoconstriction causes airway narrowing and increased airway resistance, restricting the flow of air into the lungs.

Several of the inflammatory mediators cause the pulmonary vascular bed to vasoconstrict. Pulmonary hypertension and reduced blood flow to portions of the lung result. Because of the reduction in blood flow, and therefore a decreased amount of hemoglobin in the capillaries, less oxygen is picked up by the hemoglobin, further impairing oxygenation. Figure 26–2 summarizes the pathophysiology of ARDS.

As endothelial damage progresses and tissue hypoxia ensues from the severely impaired gas exchange, the inflam-

---

TABLE 26-1
Recommended Criteria for Defining Acute Lung Injury and Adult Respiratory Distress Syndrome

Criteria	Acute Lung Injury	ARDS
Onset	Acute	Acute
PaO_2/FiO_2, regardless of PEEP level	< 300	< 200
Chest x-ray	Bilateral infiltrates	Bilateral infiltrates
PAWP	< 18 mmHg	< 18 mmHg

From: Bernard GR, Artigas A, Brigham KL et al: The American European Consensus Committee on ARDS: Definitions, mechanisms, relevant outcomes, and clinical trial coordination. Journal of Critical Care 9(1):72–81, 1994

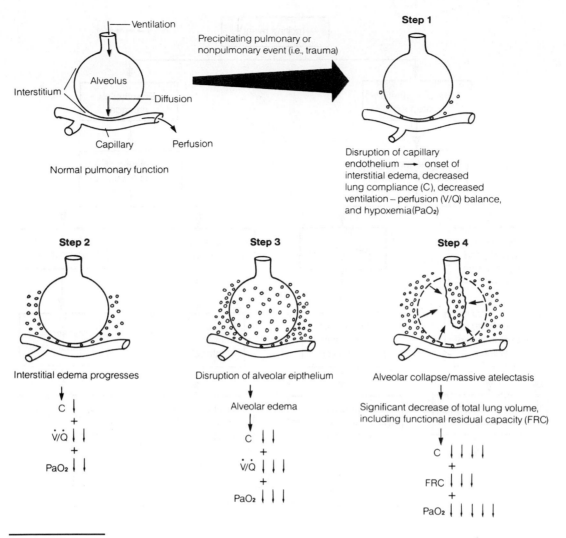

FIGURE 26-1
Pathogenesis of adult respiratory distress syndrome.

matory response is perpetuated and the SIRS cascade intensifies (upregulates) with the release of more mediators. ARDS and multiple organ system dysfunction (MODS) are therefore part of a vicious cycle and the continuum of SIRS.[3]

ASSESSMENT

Physical Examination

Acute respiratory failure initially may present within a few hours to several days, depending on the initial insult, and does not always progress to ARDS.[4] Monitoring patients who meet the SIRS criteria (listed in the accompanying display) may aid identification of those who are at risk for developing ARDS.

Early signs and symptoms of respiratory failure include tachypnea, dyspnea, and tachycardia. Breath sounds often are clear in this phase. As pathophysiological changes occur, lung auscultation may reveal crackles; however, the bubbling crackles of cardiogenic pulmonary edema may be minimal. Rhonchi, secondary to an increase in secretions and narrowed airways, may develop. Consolidation of the lungs with fluids reduces breath sounds, particularly in the dependent portions of the lungs.

Patients with acute respiratory failure may exhibit neurological changes, such as restlessness and agitation, associated with impaired oxygenation and decreased perfusion to the brain. Other signs of tissue hypoxia may become evident as organs become dysfunctional. Examples of signs of hypoxia are dysrhythmias, chest pain, decreased renal function, decreased bowel sounds, fatigue, and weakness.

Diagnostic Studies

BLOOD GAS ANALYSIS

Deterioration of arterial blood gases, despite interventions, is a hallmark of ARDS. Initially hypoxemia, $PaO_2 < 60$ mmHg, may improve with supplemental oxygen; however,

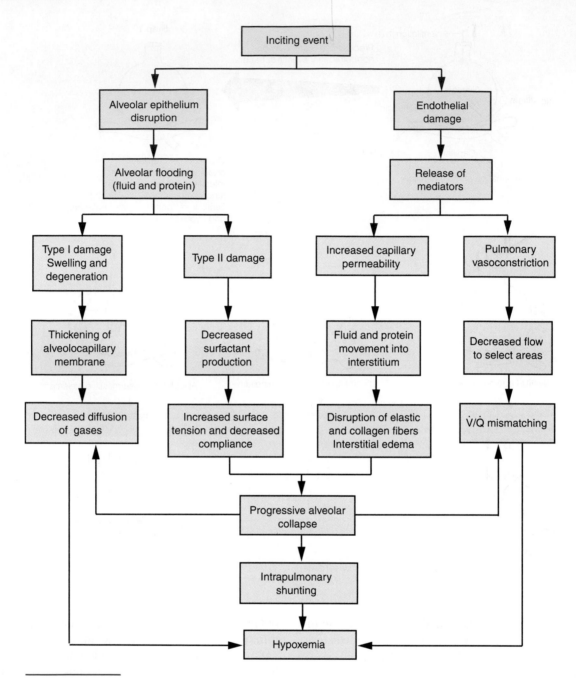

FIGURE 26-2
Pathophysiological cascade mechanism of adult respiratory distress syndrome. From Huddleston VB: Pulmonary problems. Critical Care Nursing Clinics of North America, 2:531, 1990.

SIRS Criteria

SIRS response is manifested by two or more of the following:
Temperature: > 38°C (100.4°F) or < 36°C (96.8°F)
Heart rate: > 90 beats/min
Respiratory rate: > 20 breaths/min or $PaCO_2$ < 32 mmHg
White blood cell count: > 12,000 cells/mm³ or < 4,000 cells/mm³ or > 10% immature (band) forms

From: ACCP/SCCM Consensus Conference Committee: Definitions of sepsis and organ failure and guidelines for use of innovative therapies in sepsis. Crit Care Med 20(6):864–874, 1992

refractory hypoxemia (no improvement of PaO_2 with supplemental oxygen) and persistently low SaO_2 eventually develop. Dyspnea and tachypnea are associated with decreased $PaCO_2$ early in acute respiratory failure. Hypercarbia develops as gas exchange and ventilation become increasingly impaired. Arterial pH in the early phase may be high, > 7.45, consistent with respiratory alkalosis secondary to rapid respirations and low $PaCO_2$. The arterial pH measurements in ARDS are typically lower because of respiratory and ventilatory failure and tissue hypoxia, anaerobic metabolism, and subsequent metabolic acidosis. Base excess and deficit follow a similar trend, depending on the degree of tissue and organ hypoxia.

INTRAPULMONARY SHUNT MEASUREMENT

An intrapulmonary shunt (Qs/Qt) is a type of ventilation–perfusion mismatch. It may be defined as the percent of cardiac output that is not oxygenated owing to pulmonary blood flowing past collapsed or fluid-filled and nonventilated alveoli (physiological shunt), absence of blood flow to ventilated alveoli (dead space ventilation), or a combination of both of these conditions (absolute shunt). Normally, an intrapulmonary shunt of 3% to 5% is present in all people. Advanced respiratory failure and ARDS are associated with a shunt of 15% or more due to the pathological changes in blood flow, endothelial disruption, and alveolar collapse. As the intrapulmonary shunt increases to 15% and greater, more aggressive interventions, including mechanical ventilation, are required because this level of shunt is associated with profound hypoxemia and may be life threatening.

Qs/Qt is calculated using the arterial (CaO_2), mixed venous (CvO_2), and capillary (CcO_2) oxygen contents by the following formula:

$$Qs/Qt = CcO_2 - CaO_2 \div (CcO_2 - CvO_2)$$

Oxygen content is determined by hemoglobin (Hgb), oxygen saturation (SO_2), and partial pressure of oxygen (PO_2), measured by calculating oxygen content in the pulmonary capillary bed, from the systemic arterial system, and from mixed venous blood from the pulmonary artery. The formulas to calculate oxygen content are:

$$CcO_2 = (Hgb \times 1.36 \times 1) + (100 \times 0.0031)$$

$$CaO_2 = (Hgb \times 1.36 \times SaO_2) + (PaO_2 \times 0.0031)$$

$$CvO_2 + (Hgb \times 1.36 \times S\overline{v}O_2) + (PvO_2 \times 0.0031)$$

The intrapulmonary shunt fraction may be estimated using a simple calculation, that is the PaO_2/FIO_2 ratio. Generally, a $PaO_2/FIO_2 > 300$ is normal, a value of 200 is associated with a 15% to 20% intrapulmonary shunt, and a PaO_2/FIO_2 of 100 is associated with $> 20\%$ shunt.

LUNG COMPLIANCE, AIRWAY RESISTANCE, AND PRESSURES

Lung mechanics are altered in ARDS and reduce alveolar ventilation and pulmonary gas exchange. Lung compliance, or distensibility, is decreased as the alveoli become fluid filled or collapsed. More effort and greater pressure are required to move air into the lungs as they become increasingly "stiff." In addition, the resistance to air flow into and out of the lungs increases with the accumulation of secretions and mediator-induced bronchoconstriction. Because the patient with ARDS requires mechanical ventilation to support oxygenation and ventilation, evaluation of lung compliance and airway resistance is possible by assessing ventilator pressures and tidal volume changes.

Precise measurement of airway resistance (Raw) involves measurement of air flow velocity and airway diameter; however, it may be estimated by comparing the ventilator peak inspiratory pressure (PIP) to the plateau (static) pressure (Pst) at end inspiration. A normal Raw is considered to be a value of 10 cm H_2O or less, whereas increased resistance is reflected by a greater difference. Although the Raw estimation using PIP-Pst is not an exact measurement of resistance, it is useful to trend changes and evaluate the effectiveness of interventions that are directed toward reducing airway resistance.

Lung compliance likewise may be estimated and trended. The static lung compliance (Cst) calculation uses the plateau pressure and requires use of a specific constant associated with different types of mechanical ventilators. Dynamic lung compliance (Cdyn) is less precise because its calculation uses PIP, which does not eliminate resistance factors; however, it is more simple and may be useful to trend through the course of ARDS. Cdyn = tidal volume ÷ (PIP − positive end-expiratory pressure [PEEP].) Normal Cdyn is approximately 100 mL/cm H_2O.

Close monitoring of airway pressures, including mean airway pressure, PIP, and plateau pressure, is an important component of patient assessment in ARDS. Increases in these pressures as tidal volumes are maintained to achieve normal levels of $PaCO_2$ indicate reduced compliance and increased resistance to airflow. As airway pressures rise, the lung epithelium is traumatized and results in further lung tissue damage. Volutrauma or barotrauma from persistently elevated airway pressures thus have additional deleterious effects on ventilation and oxygenation.[5]

RADIOGRAPHIC STUDIES

In the early phase of ARDS, the chest x-ray changes are usually negligible. Within a few days, the chest x-ray findings show scant alveolar infiltrates, usually in the dependent lung fields, progressing to diffuse infiltrates, consolidation, and air bronchograms in the later stages. Computed tomography of the chest also shows areas of infiltrates and consolidation of lung tissue. Daily chest x-rays are important in the continuing evaluation of the progression and resolution of ARDS.

■ MANAGEMENT

Therapeutic modalities for the treatment of ARDS have remained elusive. Treatment is supportive; that is, while contributing factors are corrected or reversed and the lungs heal, care is taken that treatment does no further damage. Figure 26–3 describes the current status of the management of ARDS.[4,6]

Oxygenation and Ventilation

MECHANICAL VENTILATION

Multiple modes of mechanical ventilation are available to support the patient with respiratory failure. Generally the principles of "do no harm" include use of the lowest FIO_2 to achieve adequate oxygenation and small tidal volumes (<10

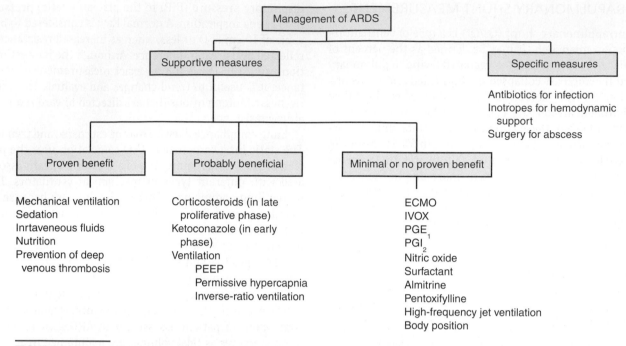

FIGURE 26-3
Status of various therapeutic modalities available for management of adult respiratory distress syndrome. ECMO, extracorporeal membrane oxygenation; IVOX, intravascular oxygenation.
From: Brandstetter RD, Sharma KC, DellaBadia M et al.: Adult respiratory distress syndrome: A disorder in need of improved outcome. Heart Lung 26(1): p. 9, 1997.

mL/kg) to minimize airway pressures, thus preventing or reducing lung damage (barotrauma and volutrauma) while maintaining $PaCO_2$ within a relatively normal range.[4,5,7] PEEP prevents collapse and opens alveolar sacs, allowing diffusion of gases across the alveolar capillary membrane. Levels of PEEP between 5 and 15 cm H_2O are usually sufficient to maintain open alveoli and oxygenation yet will not overinflate the lung and contribute to traumatizing the lung epithelium.

Permissive hypercapnea is a relatively recent strategy that allows the $PaCO_2$ to rise slowly above normal through reduction of tidal volume, therefore limiting the plateau and peak airway pressures. $PaCO_2$ in the 55 to 60 mmHg range and pH of 7.25 to 7.35 are tolerated when achieved in a gradual fashion.[6,7]

Several modes of mechanical ventilation are directed toward minimizing airway pressures and iatrogenic lung injury, historically associated with conventional volume-controlled mechanical ventilation.[4,6] Pressure-control ventilation limits the PIP to a set level as opposed to volume-controlled ventilation, which delivers a set tidal volume despite the pressure required to move the set volume into the lungs. Pressure-control ventilation also uses a decelerating inspiratory air flow pattern to minimize the peak pressure while delivering the necessary tidal volume. Patients on pressure-control ventilation mode typically require significant amounts of sedation and pharmacological paralysis to prevent attempts at breathing and dys-synchrony with the ventilator. Airway pressure release ventilation is similar to pressure-control ventilation but with the advantage of allowing the patient to initiate breaths; therefore, they do not require the same level of sedation or paralysis to achieve pressure-limited ventilation.

Reversal of the normal inspiratory–expiratory ratio to 2:1 or 3:1 is another strategy used to maintain open alveoli, reduce inspiratory air flow rate, and decrease peak airway pressures. Inverse I:E ratio is achieved through manipulation of the mechanical ventilator.

High-frequency ventilation (HFV) uses very low tidal volumes delivered at rates between 60 and 100 breaths/min, re-

---

CLINICAL APPLICATION:
Examples of Nursing Diagnoses and Collaborative Problems for the Patient With Adult Respiratory Distress Syndrome

Impaired Gas Exchange related to refractory hypoxemia and pulmonary interstitial/alveolar leaks found in alveolar capillary injury states
Ineffective Airway Clearance related to increased secretion production and decreased ciliary motion
Ineffective Breathing Patterns related to inadequate gas exchange, increased secretions, decreased ability to oxygenate adequately, fear, or exhaustion
Anxiety related to critical illness, fear of death, role changes, or permanent disability
Risk for Infection related to invasive monitoring devices and endotracheal tube

sulting in lower airway pressures and reduced barotrauma; however, this mode has not shown efficacy in the management of ARDS. Deleterious effects of HFV include increased trapping of air in the alveoli (auto-PEEP) and increased mean airway pressures to high levels in some patients.

EXTRACORPOREAL LUNG ASSIST

Extracorporeal lung-assist technology incorporates large vascular cannulas to remove blood from the patient; this pumping device and circuit circulate the blood, and one or two "artificial lungs" remove carbon dioxide and oxygenate the blood. Extracorporeal membrane oxygenation and extracorporeal carbon dioxide removal may potentially be effective in the management of ARDS but at present are controversial. These highly invasive, high-risk technologies allow the lungs to "rest" because near apneic ventilation or ventilation with small tidal volumes and slow respiratory rates greatly reduces airway pressures while gas exchange takes place in the artificial membrane lungs.

POSITIONING

Frequent position change is well established as a means to prevent and reverse atelectasis and facilitate removal of secretions from the airways.[8] Although not a treatment for ARDS, turning a patient side to side, sitting upright, and using Trendelenburg position for postural drainage are necessary interventions to prevent worsening of respiratory failure due to atelectasis and pneumonia. Continuous lateral rotation using a kinetic therapy bed turns patients slowly 60 degrees to each side over 11 minutes and is useful to enhance secretion removal.

Prone positioning, either in the patient's bed or using a Stryker frame, improves pulmonary gas exchange, facilitates secretion removal, and aids resolution of consolidation, particularly in the posterior lung regions. Prone positioning also improves access for chest percussion, an important adjunctive intervention in ARDS.

PHARMACOLOGICAL THERAPY

A majority of the pharmacological agents used in the ARDS population are supportive. Others, many still experimental, are used to interfere with SIRS and are directed toward specific mediators.

The use of corticosteroids to decrease the inflammatory response is not uncommon yet is controversial and not well supported by research.[4,5]

Antibiotic therapy is appropriate in the presence of a known microorganism but should not be used prophylactically.[4,5,7] Because SIRS is associated with the same symptoms as infection (tachycardia, fever, increased white blood cell count), isolation of specific bacteria through blood, wound, pulmonary, and other cultures is essential to identify a source of infection before initiation of antibiotics. Emphasis is on prevention of infection, especially as related

Insights Into Clinical Research

McHugh L, Milberg J, Whitcomb M et al: Recovery of function in survivors of the acute respiratory distress syndrome. Am J Resp Crit Care Med 150(1):90–94, 1994

This study examined when and to what extent perceived health and pulmonary function improved in patients who survived adult respiratory distress syndrome (ARDS). Pulmonary function parameters (FEV_1, FVC, TLC, DL_{co}) and a self-assessment of physical and psychological condition (sickness impact profile) were measured in 52 post-ARDS patients at 2 weeks, 3, 6, and 12 months postextubation.

Twenty patients were followed for the entire 12 months; data from 37 patients were obtained at least to the 3-month interval. The study concluded that the greatest improvement in perceived health status and pulmonary function occurred by 3 months postextubation. Only slight further improvement was noted at 6 months. More severe ARDS was associated with more reduced pulmonary function than was a milder form of the syndrome.

These research findings have implications for patient and family teaching.

to invasive vascular catheter maintenance and ventilator-associated nosocomial pneumonia.

Bronchodilators and mucolytics are useful in ARDS to assist in maintaining airway patency and reducing the inflammatory reaction and accumulation of secretions in the airways. The response to therapy is evaluated by monitoring airway resistance and pressures and lung compliance.

Exogenous surfactant replacement therapy has been used for several years in neonates with hyaline membrane disease to decrease alveolar surface tension and facilitate the maintenance of open alveoli. Administration of surfactant to adults with ARDS has shown some usefulness but requires further investigation.[5,7]

Newer pharmacological agents directed toward blocking mediators and the SIRS inflammatory cascade are in the clinical and experimental investigation phase and may prove efficacious in ARDS. Nitric oxide is an inhaled gas that causes selective pulmonary vasodilation and therefore reduces the deleterious effects of pulmonary hypertension. Antioxidants, such as *N*-acetylcysteine, which repletes a natural antioxidant, glucothione, may decrease endothelial damage caused by oxygen radicals. Antilipid mediators interact with the arachidonic acid cascade metabolites, which produce lung endothelial injury and inflammation. Examples are prostacylin (PGI_2), ketoconazole, and nonsteroidal anti-inflammatory drugs, such as ibuprofen or indomethacin. Monoclonal antibodies interfere with specific mediators that increase white blood cell (neutrophil) adhesion and activation, contribute to the inflammatory response, and cause endothelial injury. Pentoxifylline is a recently touted anticytokine agent with potential utility in ARDS and sepsis.[4,5,7]

Oxygen Delivery

Oxygen delivery is the amount of oxygen delivered to the tissues and organs every minute and is dependent on the flow of oxygenated blood through the tissue beds. Oxygen delivery (DaO_2) is determined by hemoglobin, arterial oxygenation, and cardiac output (CO) (or index; CI). It is calculated by the following formula:

$$DaO_2 = CO \times (Hgb \times SaO_2 \times 1.38) + (PaO_2 \times 0.0031)$$

Adequate oxygen delivery, $DaO_2 > 800$ mL O_2/min, is essential to meet tissue requirements for oxygen, thereby preventing anaerobic metabolism and hypoxia, which can trigger and perpetuate SIRS. Critically ill patients with ARDS have high demands for oxygen to maintain organ function.

Hemoglobin combines with oxygen to form oxyhemoglobin; therefore, sufficient amounts of hemoglobin are necessary to carry oxygen to the cells. Hemoglobin should be monitored routinely and be maintained at levels of at least 10.0 to 12.0 g/dL by administering packed red blood cells when indicated.[2]

Cardiac output is typically altered in ARDS due to the SIRS response, the effect of hypoxemia on the myocardium, and the decrease in venous return induced by mechanical ventilation.[2,3] Evaluation of CO is important to assess oxygen delivery and initiate appropriate interventions. Therapies to optimize CO are directed toward enhancing preload and contractility and normalizing afterload. Use of a thermodilution pulmonary artery catheter to assess oxygen delivery and consumption is routine in patients with ARDS to ensure that the appropriate interventions are instituted.

Fluid administration to ensure adequate intravascular volume and optimize preload is important before other interventions are initiated. Controversy exists regarding the administration of crystalloids or colloids in ARDS patients due to the increased permeability of capillaries and the risks of worsening pulmonary function. Generally, the pulmonary artery wedge pressure should be maintained at > 12 mmHg and breath sounds and blood gases closely monitored during fluid administration.[4]

Positive inotropic agents, such as dopamine or dobutamine, are used to enhance contractility and increase CO. Vasoconstrictors, such as norepinephrine, may be added to the therapies to counteract the SIRS-induced vasodilation. Vasoconstricting agents, however, must be administered cautiously because many vascular beds, especially in the lungs, are constricted, also as a result of SIRS mediators and hypoxia. Patients receiving inotropic or vasoactive drugs require regular evaluation of CO, systemic vascular resistance, and pulmonary artery wedge pressure, in addition to continuous arterial blood pressure monitoring.

Nutritional Support

Early initiation of nutritional support is essential in patients with ARDS. Balanced caloric, protein, carbohydrate, and fat intake are calculated based on metabolic needs, with particular attention to specific amino acids, lipid, and carbohydrate intake. These patients usually require 35 to 45 kcal/kg per day. High-carbohydrate solutions are avoided to prevent excess carbon dioxide production. Intralipids are judiciously administered to prevent further upregulation of the lipid mediators of SIRS, which contribute to inflammation and lung injury.[4,5]

Total parenteral nutrition and enteral feeding are acceptable routes of administration, providing that the patient receives adequate nutrients and calories. Current research suggests that enteral feeding is important to preserve gut function and protect the gut mucosal barrier from breakdown. Not uncommonly, a combination of parenteral and enteral nutrition is used.

An overview of management of the patient with ARDS is provided in the Collaborative Care Guide.

COLLABORATIVE CARE GUIDE
for the Patient With Adult Respiratory Distress Syndrome (ARDS)

OUTCOMES	INTERVENTIONS
Oxygenation/Ventilation	
Patent airway will be maintained. Lung is clear on auscultation.	• Auscultate breath sounds q2–4h and PRN.
	• Suction endotracheal airway when appropriate (see Collaborative Care Guide for Patient on Ventilator).
	• Hyperoxygenate and hyperventilate before and after each suction pass.
Peak, mean, and plateau pressures are within normal limits.	• Monitor airway pressures q1–2h.
	• Monitor airway pressures after suctioning.
	• Administer bronchodilators and mucolytics.
	• Perform chest physiotherapy q4h.
	• Monitor airway pressures and lung compliance for improvement after interventions.
	• Consider change in ventilator mode to pressure control or airway pressure release ventilation as mean and peak airway pressures increase to 1½ times normal.

(continued)

COLLABORATIVE CARE GUIDE
for the Patient With Adult Respiratory Distress Syndrome (ARDS) (Continued)

OUTCOMES	INTERVENTIONS
There is no evidence of atelectasis or infiltrates. Arterial blood gases are within normal limits.	• Turn side to side q2h. • Consider kinetic therapy or prone positioning. • Take chest x-ray daily. • Monitor pulse oximetry and end tidal CO_2. • Monitor arterial blood gases as indicated by changes in noninvasive parameters. • Monitor intrapulmonary shunt ($\dot{Q}s/\dot{Q}t$ and PaO_2/FiO_2). • Increase PEEP and FiO_2 to decrease intrapulmonary shunting, using lowest possible FiO_2. • Consider permissive hypercapnea to minimize airway pressures and barotrauma. • Monitor for signs of barotrauma, especially pneumothorax.
Circulation/Perfusion Blood pressure, cardiac output, CVP, and pulmonary artery pressures remain stable related to mechanical ventilation. Blood pressure, heart rate, and hemodynamic parameters are optimized to therapeutic goals (eg, DaO_2I >600 mL O_2/m^2). Serum lactate will be within normal limits.	• Assess hemodynamic effects of initiation of mechanical ventilation (eg, decreased venous return and cardiac output). • Monitor ECG for dysrhythmias related to hypoxemia. • Assess hemodynamic effects of changes in inspiratory pressure settings, tidal volume, PEEP and ventilatory modes. • Assess effects of ventilator setting changes on cardiac output and oxygen delivery. • Administer intravascular volume as ordered to maintain preload. • Monitor vital signs q1–2h. • Monitor pulmonary artery pressures and right atrial pressure q1h and cardiac output, SVR, PVR, DaO_2, and VO_2, q6–12h if pulmonary artery catheter is in place. • Administer intravascular volume as indicated by real or relative hypovolemia, and evaluate response. • Consider monitoring gastric mucosal pH as a guide to systemic perfusion. • Monitor lactate qd until it is within normal limits. • Administer red blood cells, positive inotropic agents, colloid infusion as ordered to increase oxygen delivery.
Fluids/Electrolytes Patient is euvolemic. Urine output is >30 mL/h (or >0.5 mL/kg/h). There is no evidence of electrolyte imbalance or renal dysfunction.	• Monitor hydration status to reduce viscosity of lung secretions. • Monitor intake and output q1h. • Administer fluids and diuretics to maintain intravascular volume and renal function, per order. • Monitor intake and output q1h. • Administer fluids and diuretics to maintain intravascular volume and renal function, per order. • Monitor electrolytes daily and PRN. • Replace electrolytes as ordered. • Monitor BUN, creatinine, serum osmolarity, and urine electrolytes daily.
Mobility/Safety There is no evidence of complications related to bed rest and immobility.	• Initiate deep vein thrombosis prophylaxis. • Reposition frequently. • Mobilize to chair when acute phase is past, hemodynamic stability and hemostasis achieved.

(continued)

COLLABORATIVE CARE GUIDE
for the Patient With Adult Respiratory Distress Syndrome (ARDS) (Continued)

OUTCOMES	INTERVENTIONS
Physiological changes are detected and treated without delay.	• Consult physical therapist. • Conduct range-of-motion and strengthening exercises. • Monitor mechanical ventilator alarms and settings, and patient parameters (eg, tidal volume pressures) q1–2h. • Ensure appropriate settings and narrow limits for hemodynamic, heart rate, and pulse oximetry alarms.
There is no evidence of infection; WBCs are within normal limits.	• Monitor systemic inflammatory response syndrome (SIRS) criteria: increased WBC, increased temperature, tachypnea, tachycardia. • Use strict aseptic technique during procedures, and monitor others. • Maintain sterility of invasive catheters and tubes. • Change chest tube and other dressings, invasive catheters, culture blood, line tips, or fluids per hospital protocol.
Skin Integrity Skin will remain intact.	• Assess skin q4h and each time patient is repositioned. • Turn q2h. • Consider pressure relief/reduction mattress. • Use Braden Scale to assess risk of skin breakdown.
Nutrition Caloric and nutrient intake meet metabolic requirements per calculation (eg, basal energy expenditure).	• Provide parenteral or enteral nutrition within 48 h. • Consult dietitian or nutritional support service. • Monitor lipid intake. • Monitor albumin, prealbumin, transferrin, cholesterol, triglycerides, glucose.

Comfort/Pain Control
Patient will be as comfortable as possible as evidenced by stable vital signs or cooperation with treatments or procedures.
	• Objectively assess comfort/pain using a pain scale.
	• Provide analgesia and sedation as indicated by assessment.
	• Monitor patient cardiopulmonary and pain response to medication.
	• If patient is receiving neuromuscular blockade for ventilatory control:
	  Use peripheral nerve stimulator to assess pharmacological paralysis.
	  Provide continuous or routine q1–2h IV sedation and analgesia.

Psychosocial Patient demonstrates decreased anxiety.	• Assess vital signs during treatments, discussions, etc. • Cautiously administer sedatives. • Consult social services, clergy, as appropriate. • Provide for adequate rest and sleep.
Teaching/Discharge Planning Patient/significant others understand procedures and tests needed for treatment. Significant others understand the severity of the illness, ask appropriate questions, anticipate potential complications.	• Prepare patient/significant others for procedures, such as bronchoscopy, pulmonary artery catheter insertion, or laboratory studies. • Explain the causes and effects of ARDS and the potential for complications, such as sepsis or barotrauma, or renal failure. • Encourage significant others to ask questions related to the ventilator, pathophysiology, monitoring, treatments.

■ PREVENTION OF COMPLICATIONS

Complications of ARDS are primarily related to SIRS, the interventions for ARDS, and immobility imposed by critical illness. The most serious of these is the development of MODS due to hypoxemia, hypoxia, and the persistent inflammatory response. The mortality rate of ARDS continues to be more than 60% when associated with MODS.[2]

Mechanical ventilation with high levels of PEEP, high tidal volumes, and volume-controlled modes predisposes the patient with ARDS to volutrauma (lung epithelial damage) and barotrauma as previously described. Barotrauma may present as a pneumothorax, pneumomediastinum, or subcutaneous or interstitial emphysema. Prompt chest tube insertion is required for the presence of a pneumothorax. Prevention of volutrauma and barotrauma by maintaining the lowest possible airway pressures, PEEP, and tidal volumes may be achieved through use of pressure-limiting modes of mechanical ventilation.

Immobility due to bed rest, sedation, or pharmacological paralysis has multisystem effects. Nosocomial pneumonia not infrequently is acquired from accumulation of secretions in the airways and atelectasis secondary to immobilization, and bacterial access through the endotracheal tube. As discussed, frequent repositioning and prone positioning accompanied by chest physiotherapy help to reduce stasis of secretions and facilitate removal. Endotracheal suctioning using the endotracheal tube to remove secretions is necessary but poses risks related to disconnecting the ventilator and introducing microorganisms. Suctioning only when indicated, using sterile technique, and avoiding use of saline instillation reduce the transmission of bacteria into the lungs.

Deep vein thrombosis (DVT) and subsequent pulmonary embolus may be life-threatening complications of immobility. Initiation of DVT prophylaxis within 48 hours of admission minimizes the risk of developing DVT. Low-dose heparin, graded elastic stockings, external pneumatic compression devices, frequent mobilization, and ambulation have shown utility in reducing DVT formation.

CLINICAL APPLICATION: Patient Care Study

A 21-year-old man involved in a motor vehicle crash sustained multiple extremity fractures, a closed head injury, and a right pneumothorax. He was admitted to the ICU following resuscitation and surgery. Three days after admission, he was diagnosed with ARDS. His chest x-ray showed bilateral infiltrates, and his peak airway pressures were 45 to 55 cm H_2O with a dynamic lung compliance of 20 cm H_2O. The volume-controlled ventilator settings were FiO_2, 1.0; V_T, 800; PEEP, 10. The nurse obtained blood gases and hemodynamic parameters. The PaO_2 was 50 mmHg; $PaCO_2$, 55 mmHg; SaO_2, 71%; and pH, 7.1. His cardiac output was 12 L/min; systemic vascular resistance, 324 dynes/s; PAWP, 18 mmHg; and a mean pulmonary artery pressure, 32 mmHg.

The patient was placed on pressure control, inverse ratio mode of mechanical ventilation, and a dopamine infusion, and pharmacological paralysis with morphine infusion were initiated. During the next 48 hours, the nurses obtained cardiac outputs and blood gases every 6 hours; conducted hourly assessment of respiratory parameters, vital signs, breath sounds, mental status, and urine output, and performed frequent side-to-side turning with chest physiotherapy every 4 hours. Drugs and fluids were collaboratively titrated based on the assessment parameters. The ventilator settings were adjusted to decrease the FiO_2 and minimize airway pressures. The peak inspiratory pressures were reduced to 35 cm H_2O, and the blood gases began to show improvement, although still abnormal. Cardiac output was increased to 14 L/min with fluid administration and dopamine. The patient also received 4 U of red blood cells to increase his hemoglobin to 12.5 g/dL.

The patient survived and did not develop MODS; however, he was mechanically ventilated for 15 days and in the ICU for 18 days. The aggressive interventions, attention to prevention of complications, and close monitoring by the critical care staff most likely resulted in this patient's positive outcome from ARDS.

■ CONCLUSION

On the continuum of SIRS, ARDS is a severe and complex form of respiratory dysfunction and failure. Nursing care of these patients requires constant vigilance of pulmonary, cardiac, and other organ system assessment parameters and the patient's response to supportive interventions. Management of ARDS continues to be supportive rather than curative, with emphasis on treatment of underlying diseases and prevention of further injury to the lungs, MODS, and complications, such as pneumonia, sepsis, and DVT.

Clinical Applicability Challenges

Self-Challenge: Critical Thinking

1. *Identify patient populations that may be at risk for developing ARDS and nursing interventions that may minimize that risk.*

2. *Discuss the rationale for minimizing mechanical ventilator inspiratory pressures and the assessment strategies appropriate for monitoring the ARDS patient's response to changes in ventilator parameters.*

3. *Formulate nursing diagnoses and appropriate interventions for the patient in the care study.*

Study Questions

1. *Increased permeability of the alveolar capillary membrane associated with ARDS may lead to all of the following except*
   a. *interstitial pulmonary edema.*
   b. *alveolar edema.*
   c. *decreased lung compliance.*
   d. *decreased pulmonary artery wedge pressure.*

2. *Pressure-limited mechanical ventilation is appropriate for patients with ARDS because it*
   a. *helps to reduce volutrauma and barotrauma.*
   b. *increases airway pressures.*
   c. *limits pulmonary artery pressures.*
   d. *limits lung compliance.*

3. *The pathophysiological changes associated with ARDS are primarily the result of*
   a. *pulmonary embolus associated with immobility.*
   b. *high levels of oxygen administered to the patient.*
   c. *high levels of carbon dioxide associated with respiratory distress.*
   d. *the release of inflammatory mediators.*

REFERENCES

1. Bernard GR, Artigas A, Brigham KL et al: The American European consensus on ARDS: Definitions, mechanisms, relevant outcomes, and clinical trial coordination. Journal of Critical Care 9(1):72–81, 1994
2. ACCP/SCCM Consensus Conference Committee: Definitions of sepsis and organ failure and guidelines for use of innovative therapies in sepsis. Crit Care Med 20(6):864–874, 1992
3. Vollman KM: ARDS: Mediators on the run. Critical Care Nursing Clinics of North America 6(2):341–358, 1994
4. Brandstetter RD, Sharma KC, DellaBadia M et al: Adult respiratory distress syndrome: A disorder in need of improved outcome. Heart Lung 26(1):3–14, 1997
5. Dellinger RP (ed) ARDS: Current considerations in future directions. New Horizons 1(4):463–650, 1993
6. Cottingham CA, Habashi NM: Extracorporeal lung assist in the adult trauma patient. AACN Clinical Issues 6(2):229–241, 1995
7. Morris MT: Adult respiratory distress syndrome. In Secor VH (ed): Multiple Organ Dysfunction and Failure, pp 167–195. St. Louis, Mosby, 1996
8. Hamner J: Challenging diagnosis: Adult respiratory distress syndrome. Crit Care Nurse 10(5):46–51, 1995

BIBLIOGRAPHY

Chillcott S, Sheridan P: ECCO2R: An experimental approach to treating ARDS . . . extracorporeal carbon dioxide removal. Crit Care Nurse 15(2):50–56, 1995

Dirkes S: Liquid ventilation: New frontiers in the treatment of ARDS. Crit Care Nurse 16(3):53–58, 1996

DiRusso S, Nelson L, Safcsak K, Miller R: Survival in patients with severe adult respiratory distress syndrome treated with high-level positive end expiratory pressure. Crit Care Med 23:1485–1496, 1995

Fulkerson W, MacIntyre N, Stamler J, Crapo J: Pathogenesis and treatment of the adult respiratory distress syndrome. Arch Intern Med 156:29–38, 1996

Jones M, Hoffman L, Delago E: ARDS revisited: New ways to fight an old enemy . . . acute respiratory distress syndrome. Nursing 24(12):34–45, 1994

Meduri G, Headley S, Kohler G, Strentz F, Tolley E, Umberger R et al: Persistent elevation of inflammatory cytokines predicts a poor outcome in ARDS. Chest 107:1062–1073, 1995

Moss M, Goodman P, Heinig M, Barkin S, Ackerson L, Parsons P: Establishing the relative accuracy of three new definitions of the adult respiratory distress syndrome. Crit Care Med 23:1629–1637, 1995

Rossaint R, Gerlach H, Schmidt-Ruhnke H, Pappert D, Lewandowski K, Stendel W et al: Efficacy of inhaled nitric oxide in patients with severe ARDS. Chest 107:1107–1115, 1995

Safcsak K, Nelson L: High-level positive and expiratory pressure management in the surgical patient with acute respiratory distress syndrome. AACN Clinical Issues 7(4):482–494, 1996

Renal System

27

Anatomy and Physiology of the Renal System

NORMAL STRUCTURE OF THE KIDNEY

NORMAL RENAL PHYSIOLOGY
Glomerular Filtration
Tubular Reabsorption and Secretion
OVERVIEW OF NEPHRON FUNCTION

HORMONAL INFLUENCES

CLEARANCE

RENAL REGULATORY FUNCTIONS
Electrolyte Concentration
pH Regulation

OTHER RENAL FUNCTIONS NOT ASSOCIATED WITH URINE FORMATION

OBJECTIVES

Based on the content in this chapter, the reader should be able to:

- Identify the structures comprising the nephron: glomerulus, proximal tubule, loop of Henle, distal and collecting tubules.
- Differentiate the functions of the nephron, including glomerular filtration, passive and active transport, tubular secretion, and clearance.
- Compare normal fluid pressures in the nephron and how they affect glomerular filtration rate.
- Explain the relationship of antidiuretic hormone, renin, and aldosterone to fluid regulation by the kidneys.
- Explain the mechanisms used by the kidneys to help maintain homeostasis.

*T*he regulation and concentration of solutes in the extracellular fluid (ECF) of the body are the primary functions of the kidney. The kidneys remove metabolic waste products and excess concentrations of constituents and conserve substances present in normal or low quantities.

NORMAL STRUCTURE OF THE KIDNEY

Urine, the end product of kidney function, is formed from the blood by the nephron. A nephron (Fig. 27–1) is composed of one glomerulus, proximal tubule, loop of Henle, and distal tubule. Several distal tubules drain into a collecting tubule. From the collecting tubules, urine flows to the pelvis of the kidney. From there, it leaves the kidney by way of the ureter and flows into the urinary bladder. Each human kidney (see Fig. 27–1) consists of about 1 million nephrons, all of which function identically; thus, kidney function can be explained by describing the function of one nephron.

The nephron is illustrated in Figure 27–2. Each nephron is made up of two major components: the glomerulus and Bowman's capsule, in which water and solutes are filtered from the blood, and the tubules, which reabsorb essential materials from the filtrate and permit waste substances and unneeded materials to remain in the filtrate and flow into the renal pelvis as urine.

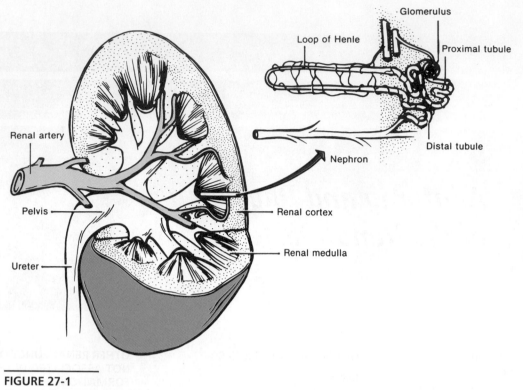

FIGURE 27-1

General characteristics of kidney structure. One nephron contains glomerulus, located in the renal cortex, and a proximal, distal, and collecting tubule, located in the renal medulla.

The glomerulus consists of a tuft of capillaries fed by the afferent arteriole, drained by the efferent arteriole. The glomerulus is surrounded by Bowman's capsule. The efferent arteriole supplies blood to the peritubular capillaries. Fluid that is filtered from the capillaries into this capsule then flows into the tubular system, which is divided into four sections: the proximal tubule, the loop of Henle, the distal tubule, and the collecting tubule.

Most of the water and electrolytes are reabsorbed into the blood in the peritubular capillaries that surround the tubular structures. The end products of metabolism remaining in the tubules pass into the urine.

The nephron is arranged so that the initial portion of the distal tubule lies at the juncture of the afferent and efferent arterioles, which is very near the glomerulus. Here, macula densa cells of the distal tubule lie in approximation to the juxtaglomerular cells of the wall of the afferent arteriole. Both these cell types plus some connective tissue cells constitute the juxtaglomerular apparatus.

NORMAL RENAL PHYSIOLOGY

Glomerular Filtration

Like other body capillaries, the glomerular capillaries are relatively impermeable to large plasma proteins and are permeable to water and smaller solutes, such as elec-

trolytes, amino acids, glucose, and nitrogenous waste. Unlike other capillaries in the body, the glomerular capillaries have an elevated blood pressure (90 mmHg versus 10–30 mmHg). This elevated pressure occurs because the afferent arteriole leading to the glomerular capillaries is larger in diameter than the efferent arteriole. The increased pressure in the glomerular capillaries results from blood squeezing into a smaller and smaller space. This forces the water and small-solute particles of the plasma to exude into Bowman's capsule. This pressure of blood against vessel walls is called *hydrostatic pressure* (HP). The movement of exudate into Bowman's capsule is termed *glomerular filtration*, and the material entering Bowman's capsule is called *filtrate*.

The HP of the glomerulus does not operate unopposed. Three other factors participate in filtration: the HP and osmotic pressure (OP) of the filtrate in Bowman's capsule and the plasma OP. Figure 27–3 illustrates the interaction of these factors. OP is the pressure exerted by water (or any solvent) on a semipermeable membrane as it attempts to cross the membrane into an area containing more molecules that cannot cross the semipermeable membrane. The pores in the glomerular capillary make it a semipermeable membrane that permits smaller molecules and water to cross but prevents larger molecules (eg, plasma proteins) from crossing. Filtrate HP, about 15 mmHg, results from the presence of filtrate in the capsule and opposes blood HP. The filtrate also exerts an OP of 1 to 3 mmHg, which opposes plasma OP. The difference between the OPs of the plasma and fluid in Bowman's capsule reflects a difference

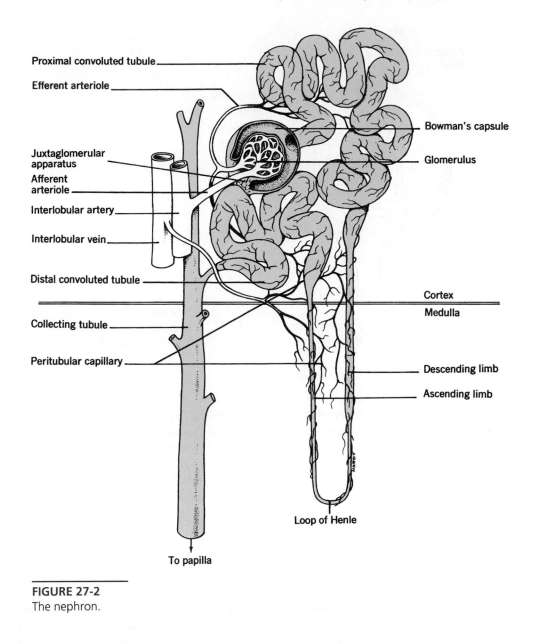

Proximal convoluted tubule

Efferent arteriole

Juxtaglomerular apparatus

Afferent arteriole

Interlobular artery

Interlobular vein

Distal convoluted tubule

Collecting tubule

Peritubular capillary

Bowman's capsule

Glomerulus

Cortex

Medulla

Descending limb

Ascending limb

Loop of Henle

To papilla

FIGURE 27-2
The nephron.

in protein concentrations. This difference occurs because the capillary pores prevent most plasma proteins from being filtered. Indeed, the filtrate in Bowman's capsule contains only 0.03% protein. Plasma HP (90 mmHg) and Bowman's capsule filtrate OP (1–3 mmHg) cooperate to promote the movement of water and small permeable molecules from the plasma into Bowman's capsule. Plasma OP (32 mmHg) and the HP of the filtrate (15 mmHg) within Bowman's capsule prompt the movement of water and permeable molecules from Bowman's capsule back into the capillary. The sum of these pressures is the net gradient of 46 mmHg ([90 + 3] − [32 + 15] = 46) that favors movement of filtrate from the bloodstream into Bowman's capsule.

The rate at which the filtrate is formed is termed the *glomerular filtration rate* (*GFR*). In the typical healthy person, this amounts to the formation of 125 mL of filtrate per minute. Major clinical factors that influence the GFR are the blood HP and filtrate OP. Hypoproteinemia, as in

starvation, will lower filtrate OP and increase the GFR. The GFR decreases with severe hypotension due to a drop in blood HP. Other factors that decrease the HP and thus the GFR are afferent arteriole constriction and renal artery stenosis.

Because of the influence of HP on the GFR, the kidneys long were thought to function in the normal homeostasis of systemic blood pressure. It is now known that the GFR is relatively stable over a wide range of arterial blood pressures. The reason for this stability is that the afferent arterioles adjust their diameter in response to the pressure of blood coming to them. If the blood pressure decreases, the smooth muscles of the afferent arterioles relax. This causes dilation of these arterioles, which increases the perfusion of the glomeruli and maintains the GFR at its normal rate; conversely, with an increase in blood pressure, these vessels constrict. There is a limit, however, to this autoregulatory mechanism. Below a mean arterial pressure of 90 mmHg

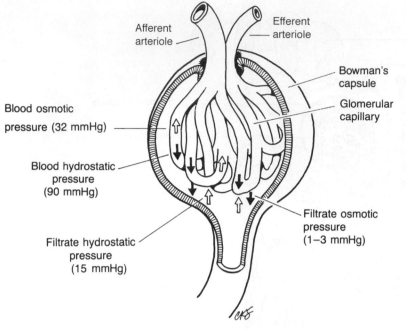

Afferent arteriole

Efferent arteriole

Bowman's capsule

Glomerular capillary

Blood osmotic pressure (32 mmHg)

Blood hydrostatic pressure (90 mmHg)

Filtrate osmotic pressure (1–3 mmHg)

Filtrate hydrostatic pressure (15 mmHg)

FIGURE 27-3

Opposing pressures in glomerular capillaries and Bowman's capsule that result in renal filtration.

and above a mean of 250 mmHg, GFR is proportional to perfusion pressure. For example, if the systemic blood pressure falls greatly, such as in shock, the GFR will fall to near zero, thereby producing near anuria.

Tubular Reabsorption and Secretion

Roughly 23% of the cardiac output goes to the kidneys in a resting adult. From this, about 125 mL of filtrate is produced each minute. This totals 180 L/d and is about 4.5 times the total amount of fluid in the body. Not all this filtrate is excreted as urine. As this filtrate passes from Bowman's capsule through the remainder of the nephrons, all but about 1.5 L/d will be returned to the bloodstream. Similarly, at plasma glucose levels of less than 200 mg/dL, none of the filtered glucose is found in the urine when it enters the collecting tubules. The volume and content of the urine are the result of tubular reabsorption and tubular secretion. Reabsorption is accomplished by active transport, osmosis, and diffusion. It occurs in all parts of the nephron. Secretion involves active transport and is performed only by distal tubule cells.

Active transport involves the binding of a molecule of a substance to a carrier, which then moves the molecule from one side of the membrane to the other against the concentration gradient of that substance. Because it helps molecules to move in a direction opposite the direction they would move by simple diffusion, the carrier acts like a pump. In tubular cells, the carrier is located in the cell membrane nearest the peritubular capillaries, and it transports material out of the tubular cell into the peritubular fluid. This lowers the intracellular concentration of the type of molecule being transported. The decreased concentra-

tion enables more of those molecules to diffuse from the urine (filtrate) into the tubule cell. These molecules, in turn, exit the cell and enter the peritubular fluid by active transport. The movement of molecules increases the peritubular fluid concentration of the molecule, and this increase stimulates the diffusion of the molecule into the peritubular capillaries. Thus, in the nephrons, active transport removes molecules from the filtrate (urine) back to the bloodstream.

Because active transport involves carrier molecules and energy exchanges, there is an upper limit to the number of molecules of a substance that can be transported at one time. This maximum limit for reabsorption rates is called T_{max}. Glucose is an example of a molecule that will appear in the same concentrations that it appears in the blood. As serum glucose rises, filtrate glucose also rises. The renal tubules will reabsorb the filtered glucose at faster and faster rates, until this molecule's active transport mechanisms all are being used. At this T_{max}, more glucose is appearing in the filtrate than can be reabsorbed, and glucose will be excreted in the urine. This "spilling" of glucose into the urine indicates serum levels higher than T_{max}.

Urea is an example of a molecule that is reabsorbed by diffusion. Under the high pressures in the glomerular capillaries, urea is filtered. In the tubules, as water is reabsorbed into the bloodstream, urea follows by simple diffusion. No selective permeability prevents its return to the bloodstream, and no transport mechanism is required. The reabsorption rates of urea range from 40% to 60% of what is filtered and depend entirely on water reabsorption rates.

The active transport of sodium is responsible for the osmotic reabsorption of water from the filtrate in the proximal and later in the distal tubule. As sodium ions are actively transported out of the cell and into the peritubular fluid, they make the OP of this peritubular fluid higher than that of the cellular or tubular fluid. Water is thus osmotically "pulled out" of the tubular fluid. Both water and sodium then diffuse into peritubular capillaries and thus are returned to the bloodstream. This movement of positively charged sodium ions also creates an electrochemical gradient that draws negatively charged ions—especially chloride—out of the tubular fluid and back into the bloodstream.

Tubular secretion involves the active transport of molecules from the bloodstream through tubule cells into the filtrate. Many substances that are secreted do not occur naturally in the body (eg, penicillin). Naturally occurring bodily substances that are secreted include uric acid and potassium and hydrogen ions.

In the distal tubule, the active transport of sodium uses a carrier system that also is involved in the tubular secretion of hydrogen and potassium ions (Fig. 27–4). In this relationship, every time the carrier transports sodium out of the tubular fluid, it carries *either* a hydrogen *or* a potassium ion into the tubular fluid on its "return trip." Thus, for every sodium ion reabsorbed, a hydrogen *or* potassium must be secreted, and *vice versa*. The choice of cation to be secreted depends on the ECF concentration of these ions (hydrogen and potassium).

Knowledge of this cation exchange system in the distal tubule helps to explain some of the relationships that these electrolytes have with one another. For example, it is clear why an aldosterone blocker may cause hyperkalemia or why there can be an initial fall in plasma potassium as severe acidosis is corrected therapeutically.*

OVERVIEW OF NEPHRON FUNCTION

Approximately 80% of the filtrate is returned to the bloodstream by reabsorption in the proximal tubule. In the normal healthy person, all the filtered glucose and amino acids; much sodium, chloride, and other electrolytes; and uric acid are reabsorbed here. The proximal tubule cells also secrete urea, creatinine, hydrogen, and ammonia into the urine (filtrate).

In the loop of Henle the filtrate (urine) becomes highly concentrated. This part of the nephron is composed of a thin-walled descending portion and a thick-walled ascend-

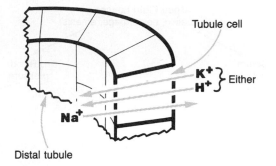

FIGURE 27-4
Cation exchange in the distal tubule.

ing portion. Loops of Henle belonging to juxtamedullary nephrons dip into the medulla of the kidney, which contains a highly concentrated interstitial fluid. (The thin walls of the descending portion are quite permeable.) This permeability, together with the high concentration of the interstitial fluid at this point, causes water to osmose from the filtrate into the interstitial fluid. This makes the filtrate quite concentrated by the time it reaches the ascending limb of the loop.

The thicker-walled ascending limb is relatively impermeable to water, but it contains ion carriers that actively transport chloride ions out of the filtrate. This creates an electrochemical gradient that "pulls" the positively charged sodium ions out of the filtrate as well. This exit of electrolytes without water now makes the filtrate more dilute than before.

In the distal tubule, sodium again is reabsorbed by active transport, and hydrogen, potassium, and uric acid can be added to the urine by tubular secretion.

The collecting ducts or collecting tubules receive the contents from many distal tubules. There is no further electrolyte reabsorption or secretion and in the well hydrated person, no further water reabsorption as well. Water reabsorption without electrolyte reabsorption can occur in the collecting ducts under the stimulus of antidiuretic hormone (ADH).

HORMONAL INFLUENCES

Through the reabsorption of sodium and the passive "following" of water and chloride, it is possible to make urine of the same osmolality as blood. Under conditions of dehydration, however, urine is very concentrated, whereas if a great deal of water is drunk, urine will be more dilute than blood. This final regulation of urine, and thus serum osmolality and volume, is regulated by three hormones.

Osmoreceptors in the hypothalamus are sensitive to serum osmolality (Fig. 27–5). During dehydration, when serum osmolality rises, osmoreceptors in the hypothalamus respond by stimulating the hypothalamus to secrete ADH, which increases the permeability of collecting tubule cells

---

The aldosterone blocker reduces sodium reabsorption. Such reduced reabsorption of sodium also reduces the tubular secretion of either hydrogen or potassium. The hydrogen excess can be buffered, but the potassium simply rises to above-normal levels. In severe acidosis, the nephrons have been attempting to compensate by increasing their hydrogen ion secretion rates. As acidosis is therapeutically corrected (eg, by sodium bicarbonate administration), one change is secretion of potassium ions (another concerns a shift of potassium into cells). As hydrogen ions no longer need to be secreted, potassium ions become the sole exchange for sodium ions, leading, it is thought, to a reduction in plasma potassium.

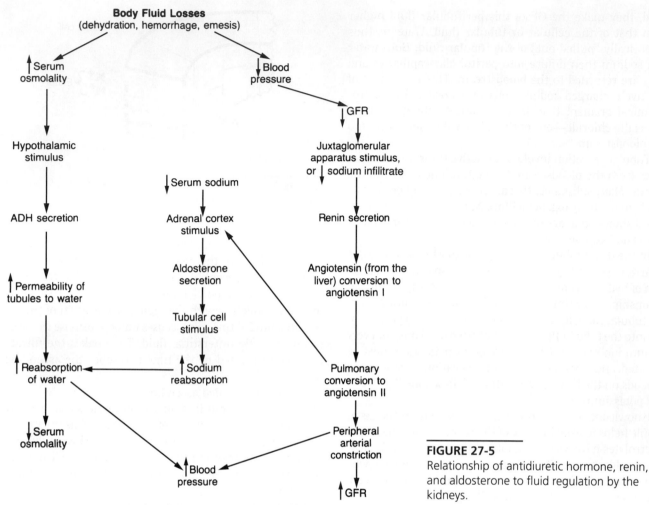

FIGURE 27-5

Relationship of antidiuretic hormone, renin, and aldosterone to fluid regulation by the kidneys.

to water. This permits the reabsorption of water alone (without electrolytes), which in turn will decrease the concentration of the ECF. Negative feedback loops regulate ADH secretion. This means that as the concentration of the ECF returns to normal, the stimulus for ADH secretion disappears, and ADH secretion is stopped.

Another hormone that influences urine concentration is renin. When GFR falls because of dehydration or blood loss, the juxtaglomerular apparatus will secrete renin. Subnormal sodium levels in the filtrate also stimulate renin secretion. Renin converts angiotensin, which is secreted by the liver, into angiotensin I. Pulmonary capillary cells, in turn, convert this into angiotensin II.

Angiotensin II constricts the smooth muscle surrounding arterioles. This increases blood pressure, which increases the GFR. Angiotensin II also triggers the secretion of aldosterone, the third hormone that influences urine osmolality. The adrenal cortex, when stimulated by angiotensin II, secretes aldosterone. By increasing sodium reabsorption in distal tubule cells, aldosterone causes an increase in renal water reabsorption. This increases blood pressure and decreases serum osmolality. Aldosterone also is secreted in response to subnormal serum sodium levels.

■ CLEARANCE

From the previous discussion, an important concept in renal function emerges—*clearance*. As the filtrate moves along the nephron, a large proportion of metabolic end products remains in it, unreabsorbed. These products thus are removed (cleared) from the blood and exit the body in the urine. Indeed, of each 125 mL of glomerular filtrate formed per minute, about one half, or 60 mL, returns to the blood without urea, and about one half is excreted with urea. Stated another way, 60 mL of plasma is "cleared" of urea each minute in normally functioning kidneys. In the same way, 125 mL of plasma is cleared of creatinine, 12 mL of uric acid, 12 mL of potassium, 25 mL of sulfate, 25 mL of phosphate, and so forth each minute.

It is possible to calculate renal clearance by simultaneously sampling urine and plasma. By dividing the quantity of substance found in each milliliter of plasma into the quantity found in the urine, the milliliters cleared per minute can be calculated. This method is used as one means of testing kidney function.

Other methods of assessing renal function involve chemicals that are known to be either filtered only or both filtered and secreted. *Inulin*, for example, is filtered only and neither absorbed nor secreted. Thus, the clearance of insulin provides a measure of glomerular filtration. *Mannitol* can be used similarly. Para-aminohippurate sodium (PAH) or iodopyracet (Diodrast) are drugs that are secreted in addition to being filtered. As such, their clearance provides an index of plasma flow through the kidneys. They also can be used together with a filtered-only drug in assessing tubular secretion and thus the health of tubular cells.

The sodium concentration in the urine also can serve as an index of tubular health in certain situations. For example, in acute renal failure, an increased clearance of sodium can indicate acute tubular necrosis. Accordingly, supernormal blood levels of filtered substances (creatinine and other nitrogenous wastes) indicate a fall in glomerular filtration and thus in nephron health.

RENAL REGULATORY FUNCTIONS

In addition to excreting nitrogenous wastes as urea and other by-products of metabolism, the kidneys can function in regulating the electrolyte concentration and the pH of the ECFs (blood and interstitial fluids) of the body.

Electrolyte Concentration

Decreased ECF sodium concentrations will stimulate aldosterone secretion directly from the adrenal cortex. Because decreased ECF sodium also can cause a decrease in tubular sodium, it may stimulate the juxtaglomerular secretion of renin, which will increase aldosterone levels indirectly. Aldosterone stimulates sodium reabsorption of the distal tubule cells. Thus, sodium homeostasis is restored. A rise in ECF sodium can cause the reverse.

The kidneys also function in the homeostasis of plasma potassium levels. If there are high levels of potassium in the face of normal sodium levels, the distal tubules and collecting ducts actively secrete (reverse of active reabsorption) potassium back into the urine. Specific reabsorption mechanisms exist for divalent ions, such as calcium, magnesium, and phosphates, and regulate the plasma concentrations of these ions as well.

The regulation of the monovalent anions, chloride and bicarbonate, is secondary to sodium ion regulation. As the positively charged cation, sodium, is reabsorbed, a negatively charged ion is carried along electrochemically. This maintains electroneutrality. Whether the negative ion is bicarbonate or chloride depends on the pH of the ECF, which also is regulated by buffers and respiratory and renal mechanisms.

pH Regulation

If buffers and the respiratory mechanism for pH homeostasis are insufficient, the kidneys then take part, although much more slowly than the respiratory system. Although respiratory control of carbon dioxide, and therefore hydrogen ion levels, can take only seconds to achieve, 48 to 72 hours may pass before the renal system can change serum acid–base balance significantly.

Alkalosis occurs as a result of too few hydrogen ions or too many bicarbonate ions. To compensate, the body must conserve hydrogen ions. In renal compensation for alkalosis, tubular reabsorption of hydrogen ions is increased, and secretion is decreased. This increases the hydrogen ion concentration of the ECF and thereby decreases the alkalosis.

Acidosis occurs as a result of too many hydrogen ions and too few bicarbonate ions. To compensate, the body must secrete hydrogen ions. Renal compensation for acidosis involves an increase in the hydrogen ion secretion of the tubule cells, especially in the distal tubule cells. Now, bicarbonate and sodium ions are continually being filtered from the glomerulus. Also, hydrogen ion secretion by distal tubule cells causes an increase in sodium reabsorption. Such sodium reabsorption can increase bicarbonate reabsorption electrochemically. Thus, as hydrogen ions are being eliminated from the ECF, sodium and bicarbonate ions are being added to it. Both will decrease the acidosis (Fig. 27–6).

Urine can be acidified (by hydrogen ion secretion) only to a pH level of 4.0 to 4.5. If the tubular secretion of hydrogen ions was the only mechanism operating, only a few hydrogen ions could be secreted before the critical shut-off level of 4.0 was reached, because hydrogen would combine with urinary chloride to make hydrochloric acid (HCl). Not many of these strong HCl molecules are needed to make the urine pH 4.0. The formation of HCl would then stop tubular hydrogen ion secretion before sufficient compensation for acidosis could be obtained. This does not occur because tubule cells deaminate certain amino acids and secrete the nitrogenous component as ammonia (NH_3). This ammonia combines with hydrogen in the urine to form ammonium

FIGURE 27-6
Renal compensation for acidosis. Hydrogen is moved from blood into filtrate by secretion and exits the body as ammonium and sodium hydrochloride. In exchange, sodium and bicarbonate enter the blood.

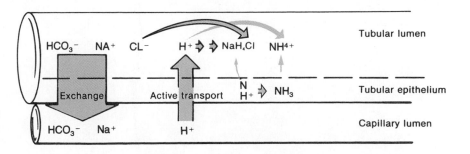

(NH_4^+). Because tubule membranes are not permeable to NH_4^+, much of it is secreted in this form. Some ammonia combines with chloride to form ammonium chloride (NH_4Cl).

OTHER RENAL FUNCTIONS NOT ASSOCIATED WITH URINE FORMATION

Renal interstitial (not nephron) cells manufacture and secrete two hormones, calcitriol and erythropoietin, the actions of which are unrelated to urine formation. These hormones are discussed in Chapter 41.

Clinical Applicability Challenges

Self-Challenge: Critical Thinking

1. Your postoperative patient is experiencing severe hypotension and increased blood urea nitrogen levels. Explain the effect of hypotension on GFR, renin secretion, and the kidney's attempt to maintain homeostasis.

Study Questions

1. In the glomerulus, urine is formed by
   a. secretion.
   b. filtration.
   c. reabsorption.
   d. b and c

2. Aldosterone stimulates increased sodium reabsorption by distal tubule cells. One consequence of elevated plasma aldosterone levels would be
   a. metabolic acidosis.
   b. hypokalemia.
   c. metabolic alkalosis.
   d. supernormal urine sodium levels.

3. Hyperglycemia increases the OP of the filtered urine in the nephron. This would cause
   a. increased sodium and water reabsorption, leading to oliguria.
   b. decreased sodium and water reabsorption, leading to diuresis.
   c. decreased glomerular filtration, leading to prerenal azotemia.
   d. increased glomerular secretion of proteins into the filtrate.

BIBLIOGRAPHY

Applegate EJ: The Anatomy and Physiology Learning System. Philadelphia, WB Saunders, 1995

Hole JW: Human Anatomy and Physiology (6th Ed). Debuque, IA, WC Brown Publishers, 1993

Huether SE, McCance KL: Understanding Pathophysiology. St. Louis, Mosby, 1996

LeVay DL: Human Anatomy and Physiology (3rd Ed). Lincolnwood, IL, NTC Publishing Group, 1993

Seeley RR, Stephens TD, Tate P: Essentials of Anatomy and Physiology (2nd Ed). St. Louis, Mosby, 1996

Sherwood L: Human Physiology: From Cells to Systems (2nd Ed). Minneapolis/St. Paul, West Publishing Company, 1993

Thibodeau GA, Patton KT: Anatomy and Physiology (2nd Ed). St. Louis Mosby, 1993

Valtin H, Schafer JA: Renal Function (3rd Ed). Boston, Little Brown, 1995

Patient Assessment: Renal System

OBJECTIVES

Based on the content in this chapter, the reader should be able to:

- Analyze the relationship between the physiological function of the kidneys and the signs and symptoms that indicate renal dysfunction.
- Formulate a plan for collecting assessment data for patients with renal disorders and fluid and electrolyte imbalance.
- Explain the basis for using serum electrolyte levels to assess renal function.
- Explore diagnostic tests used to evaluate renal status.
- Differentiate renal ultrasound, computerized axial tomography, and magnetic resonance imaging.
- Differentiate normal and abnormal findings for hypovolemia and hypervolemia and hyponatremia and hypernatremia.

*A*ssessment of the renal system involves determining how well the kidneys perform their many functions. It also includes gathering information about other systems. The nurse plays a vital role in assessing renal function and

fluid and electrolyte balance. A careful assessment of the history and physical findings, along with interpretation of laboratory results, can provide early clues to the diagnosis of disorders of water and volume imbalance and other complications of renal dysfunction in the critically ill patient.

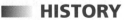 HISTORY

The patient history provides important information that helps determine the cause, severity, treatment, and management of renal dysfunction. It involves gathering information about the present illness, current signs and symptoms (system review), and significant past health history. A format for renal assessment is summarized in the accompanying display.

To begin, the patient should be asked about his or her perception of the chief complaint. The description should include the onset, duration, and frequency of the complaint;

CLINICAL APPLICATION:
Assessment Parameters
Factors in Renal Assessment

History
- Chief complaint
    Description
    Signs and symptoms
    Treatments and response to treatments
- Systems review
- Medical history
- Family history

Physical examination
- Skin: turgor, temperature, dryness/moisture, scratches, lesions
- Mucous membranes
- Presence of edema, ascites
- Respiratory rate, lung sounds
- Blood pressure, heart rate, rhythm, sounds
- Behavioral changes, mental status
- Test for tetany: Chvostek's, Trousseau's signs
- Paresthesias, numbness, weakness, tremors of extremities

Additional findings
- Laboratory values
    Serum creatinine, urea nitrogen, osmolality
    Urine specific gravity, sodium, osmolality
    Serum electrolytes
- Radiographic studies
- Electrocardiogram tracing
- Intake and output records
- Weight records

the setting in which it developed; and factors that lessen or aggravate the problem. The complaint's significance to the patient and its impact on the patient's life should be ascertained. The patient is asked if this is the first time it has occurred.

Once the patient has described the presenting problem, the nurse inquires about past medical history and family history. This information may offer clues to the underlying cause of the problem. A history of polycystic kidney disease, renal calculi, or hereditary nephritis is common in patients with kidney disease. Certain systemic diseases, such as the following, also may contribute to the development of renal failure:

- Diabetes mellitus
- Systemic lupus erythematosus
- Hypertension
- Sickle cell anemia
- Wegener's granulomatosis
- Goodpasture's syndrome

The patient should be asked if there is history of heart disease, because chronic congestive heart failure can affect renal function. Have there been problems with the liver,

such as hepatitis or cirrhosis? The patient should also identify any recent illnesses, including infections, surgeries, or severe injuries because endotoxins, severe hypotension, and skeletal muscle destruction can result in kidney damage. Some cellular contents that can be nephrotoxic at high levels include myoglobin, potassium, organic acids, and phosphorus. Because another common cause of kidney disease can be exposure to nephrotoxic agents, the nurse should ascertain whether the patient has been exposed to such agents as amino glycosides, furosemide, radiographic dyes, or other drugs and chemical agents. Is there possible exposure to environmental agents at home or work, such as cleaning products, pesticides, lead (such as paint or gas fumes), and mercury? Does the patient have serious allergic reactions?

When the patient has end-stage renal disease (ESRD) and is receiving dialysis, the nurse should ask about the following:

- Cause(s) of ESRD
- Date dialysis began
- Type of dialysis (hemodialysis or peritoneal dialysis)
- History of transplant
- Date, time, and place of last dialysis
- Common problems, complications, and management associated with treatments

When the patient is receiving hemodialysis, ask if there have been problems with the arteriovenous fistula or graft, such as scar tissue, aneurysms, redness, or infection.

The nurse will also need to know all current medications, including over-the-counter and home remedy drugs. This may also be the time to ask about alcohol intake and the use of (illicit) drugs.

Next, the nurse conducts a review of signs and symptoms to determine further the patient's health status. How has the person's health been in general? Have there been any changes in hearing or vision? Have activity levels changed? Is there fatigue, muscle weakness, or problems with walking? How has the person been sleeping? The gastrointestinal system review can include questions about diet, changes in appetite, bowel elimination, and abdominal tenderness or fullness.

The patient is questioned about fluid intake, thirst, and urination:

- Have you ever had any dysuria, nocturia, polyuria, or incontinence?
- Have you ever experienced any flank pain or hematuria? Can you describe it?
- Have you noticed a change in the amount, color, smell, or pattern of voiding?
- Have you had a recent change in weight? When and with what was it associated?
- Have you ever passed a renal stone?

- Have you ever had difficulty with starting urination (hesitancy), urgency, dribbling at end of urination, or stopping the stream?
- Have you ever experienced burning during urination?
- Do you have any history of urinary tract infections; if so, how were they treated?

The nurse explores factors such as shortness of breath, number of pillows used for sleep, and unusual tightness of shoes, waistband, or rings. Has there been puffiness around the eyes? The patient is asked to describe any skin problems, such as dryness, itching, bruising, rashes, or bumps. Has there been poor healing of cuts and scratches?

The patient's neurological status is addressed, including a history of fainting, seizures, localized weakness, numbness, tingling or burning sensations, asterixis (involuntary jerking commonly seen in the hands, tongue, or feet), tremors, paralysis, foot-drop, and restless leg syndrome. Has the patient or family noticed any memory loss, decreased interest in the environment, lethargy, or difficulty with usual activities?

PHYSICAL EXAMINATION

The physical examination provides objective data that are used to substantiate and clarify the history. The history guides the physical examination and helps determine areas of the examination that require more depth. If time permits, the nurse reviews the chart, including laboratory results, before beginning the physical examination. This can help identify data that require follow-up during the physical examination.

The nurse begins the physical examination by observing the patient's overall appearance, including facial expression, height and weight, position in bed, grooming, personal hygiene, and signs of distress. The nurse observes the patient's level of responsiveness, cognition, and interaction with people, including positive, negative, or unusual responses.

Because patients with renal problems usually have significant problems with fluid and electrolyte balance, the nurse evaluates the patient's volume status throughout the examination. The nurse may begin by taking the blood pressure (noting pulse pressure and a positive pulse paradoxus) and temperature. Patients with ESRD tend to have low temperatures because they are generally immunosuppressed.

The anterior and posterior chest is assessed for respiratory rate, rhythm, depth, and effort. Deformities of the thorax, shape of chest, or bulging of interspaces during expiration are noted. The precordial area is observed and palpated for heaves, pulsations, and thrills. The nurse listens for heart rate and rhythm, extra heart sounds, murmurs, clicks, and pericardial friction rub. The nurse also observes for jugular vein distention and determines the need to measure jugular venous pressure. Anterior and posterior lung fields are auscultated. The nurse notes the quality of vesicular breath sounds and the presence of adventitious breath sounds (crackles, wheezes, rubs). After auscultating the posterior chest, the nurse can assess kidney tenderness. This is done by the examiner placing one hand over the posterior costovertebral angle (CVA). Then, using the fist of the second hand, the examiner delivers a gentle percussion to the CVA and notes whether or not the patient has discomfort.

The nurse listens for bowel sounds, percusses and palpates the abdomen, and then palpates the liver border to determine enlargement. If ascites is suspected, the nurse measures abdominal girth and may check for a fluid wave or shifting dullness.

The nurse inspects the skin on the extremities and trunk for color, evidence of excoriation, bruising, or bleeding; palpates for moistness, dryness, temperature (using the back of the fingers), and edema; and checks mobility and turgor by lifting a fold of skin and noting the ease (mobility) and speed with which it returns into place (turgor). To assess hydration further, the nurse inspects the tongue and mucous membranes in the mouth and looks for a saliva pool under the tongue.

If the patient is at risk for excess vascular volume, the nurse will look for hypertension; pulmonary edema; rales; engorged, elevated neck veins; liver congestion and enlargement; congestive heart failure; and shortness of breath. Signs and symptoms related to excess extravascular volume include pitting edema of feet, ankles, hands, and fingers; periorbital edema; sacral edema; and ascites.

While examining the extremities, the nurse can check the quality of the peripheral pulses; observe for tremors; test for paresthesia, numbness, and weakness; and palpate fingernails and toenails, checking for color, shape, and capillary refill time.

The arteriovenous graft or fistula is assessed for patency in chronic ESRD patients and for adequate circulation to the extremity distal to the access. If the patient has a temporary access, the exit site is inspected for signs of inflammation or infection. The presence, direction, and quality of the access pulsation and bruit are checked.

If the patient is at risk for hypocalcemia, hypomagnesemia, or both, the nurse can also check for Chvostek's or Trousseau's signs. Chvostek's sign occurs when there is facial irritability after tapping the facial nerve in front of the auditory meatus with the finger. Trousseau's sign occurs then there is spasm of the hands and feet (carpopedal spasm) in response to arm compression.

During the history and examination, the nurse has observed the patient's level of consciousness and mental status. If more data are needed, the nurse may use tools such as the Glasgow Coma Scale and Folstein Mini Mental Examination.

◼◼ DIAGNOSTIC STUDIES

Laboratory Tests That Assess Renal Function

CREATININE AND CREATININE CLEARANCE

Creatinine is a by-product of normal muscle metabolism and is excreted in the urine primarily as the result of glomerular filtration with a small percentage secreted into the urine by the kidney tubules. Therefore, creatinine is the most important indicator of glomerular filtration rate (GFR). The amount of creatinine excreted in the urine is directly related to muscle mass and will normally remain constant unless significant muscle wasting (a catabolic state) occurs. The creatinine clearance can be defined as the amount of blood that is cleared of creatinine in 1 minute and is an excellent clinical indicator of renal function. As renal function diminishes, creatinine clearance decreases. To obtain an accurate creatinine clearance, the nurse needs to collect a 24-hour urine specimen and obtain a blood specimen at some point during the urine collection. For consistency, the blood sample is usually collected at the midpoint of the urine collection. It is important to note the exact beginning and ending time of the urine collection.

The actual creatinine clearance is calculated by the following formula:

$$\text{creatinine clearance} = \frac{UV}{PC}$$

where U is the urine creatinine concentration; V, the urine volume; and P, the plasma creatinine concentration.

The expression UV tells how much creatinine appears in the urine during the period of collection. This can be converted readily to milligrams per minute, which is the standard reference point. Dividing this value by the plasma creatinine concentration (which must be converted from mg/100 mL to mg/mL) tells the minimum number of milliliters of plasma that must have been filtered by the glomeruli to produce the measured amount of creatinine in the urine. The final result is usually expressed in milliliters per minute. The normal range varies between 80 and 120, depending on the person's size, age, and gender. The results can be adjusted to a standard body size of 1.73 m^2 (body surface area [BSA]), which can be derived from standard tables if the patient's height and weight are known; it averages between 120 and 125 mL/min/1.73 m^2 BSA. After age 40, normal creatinine clearance values generally decrease 6.5 mL/min per decade because of a decline in GFR.

There are also formulas that estimate creatinine clearance based on a single serum creatinine level. An estimate may be done when there is difficulty collecting a 24-hour urine sample or when it will assist prompt treatment as in the case of drug nephrotoxicity. The estimate may only be accurate in patients with chronic renal failure with stable renal function who are not edematous or extremely overweight.

Interpretation of Creatinine

When the kidneys are damaged by a disease process, the creatinine clearance will decrease, and the serum creatinine concentration will rise. The urine creatinine excretion will decrease initially until the blood level rises to a point at which the amount of creatinine appearing in the urine is equal to the amount being produced by the body. For example, a normal person with a serum creatinine concentration of 1 mg/dL and a creatinine excretion of 1 mg/min has a creatinine clearance of 100 mL/min. When the patient experiences a 50% loss of renal function, the serum creatinine will rise to 2 mg/dL, and the patient will continue to excrete 1 mg/min of creatinine in the urine when balance is restored. When the patient has rapidly changing renal function and oliguria (eg, acute renal failure [ARF]), the creatinine clearance is less reliable. Until renal function stabilizes, serum creatinine levels provide a better indication of the rate and direction of change. In patients with rhabdomyolysis, the serum creatinine will be elevated out of proportion to the reduction of GFR as the result of chemical conversion of muscle creatine to creatinine. In this situation, the serum creatinine is less reliable as an indicator of renal function.

BLOOD UREA NITROGEN

The blood urea nitrogen (BUN) has been used for numerous years as an indicator of kidney function, but unlike the serum creatinine, its level can be influenced by many factors. At low urine flow rates, more sodium and water, and consequently more urea, are reabsorbed. Therefore, when the patient is volume depleted, the BUN will tend to rise out of proportion to any change in renal function.

Interpretation of Blood Urea Nitrogen

Increased urea production can result from increased protein intake (tube feedings and some forms of hyperalimentation) or increased tissue breakdown, as with crush injuries, febrile illnesses, steroid or tetracycline administration, and reabsorption of blood from the intestine in a patient with intestinal hemorrhage. The BUN also may be elevated in the dehydrated patient because the lack of fluid volume causes a concentrated value. The patient in shock and the patient with congestive heart failure may have an elevated BUN secondary to decreased renal perfusion. The opposite is true for patients with decreased protein intake

---

Tests That Assess Renal Function

- Creatinine
- Blood urea nitrogen
- Specific gravity
- Osmolality (blood and urine)
- Urinary sodium concentration
- Fractional excretion of sodium

or liver disease (both of which reduce urea production) and for patients with large urine volumes secondary to excessive fluid intake.

The BUN can be of significant value, however, when used as a comparison to the serum creatinine concentration. Normally, there is a ratio of 10:1 (urea:creatinine). Discrepancies in this ratio might suggest a potentially correctable situation, as noted in the display.

SPECIFIC GRAVITY

The specific gravity of the urine tests the kidneys' ability to concentrate and dilute the urine. The specific gravity measures the buoyancy of a solution compared with water and depends on the number of particles in the solution and their size and weight. There are three methods used to obtain this measurement in clinical practice: a multiple test *dipstick* that has a reagent area for specific gravity, the *urinometer*, and the *refractometer* (TS meter). The urinometer has been in clinical use for many years and requires enough urine to float the urinometer. Its results are questionable. The refractometer gives highly reproducible results and only requires one drop of urine for the measurement. In addition, this instrument can be used to measure the total solids in plasma (hence the name, *TS* meter), which is a good indicator of the plasma protein concentration and can be a useful indicator of a patient's fluid balance (especially if serial determinations are done).

Interpretation of Specific Gravity

The normal kidney has the capacity to dilute the urine to a specific gravity of 1.001 and to concentrate the urine to at least 1.022. Normally, a person's water balance will determine whether the urine is concentrated or dilute; dilute urine is an indicator of water excess, and concentrated urine indicates water deficit. In many renal diseases, the ability of the kidneys to form a concentrated urine is lost, and the specific gravity can become "fixed" at 1.010. This finding is often be seen in acute tubular necrosis, acute nephritis, and chronic renal disease. A false high specific gravity can be seen when high–molecular-weight substances, such as protein, glucose, mannitol, and radiographic contrast material, are present in the urine. Therefore, a greater degree of accuracy can be obtained by checking the urine osmolality.

OSMOLALITY

The *osmolality* of a solution is an expression of the total number (concentration) of particles in solution and is independent of the size, molecular weight, and electrical charge of the molecules. All substances in solution contribute to the osmolality. For example, 1 mol (gram molecular weight) of sodium chloride dissociates incompletely into Na and Cl ions and produces 1.86 osm when dissolved in a kilogram of solvent (such as plasma). A mole of nonionic solute (eg, glucose or urea) produces only 1 osm when dissolved in 1 kg of solvent. The total concentration of particles in a solution equals the osmolality and is normally reported in units of osmoles per kilogram of solvent. In the clinical setting (because of much smaller concentrations), the osmolality is reported in milliosmoles (thousandth of an osmole, abbreviated mOsm) per kilogram of solvent (plasma or serum).

The normal *serum osmolality* consists primarily of sodium and its accompanying anions, with urea and glucose contributing about 5 mOsm each. Therefore, when the serum sodium, urea, and glucose concentrations are known, the osmolality of plasma can be calculated by the following formula:

$$\text{osmolality} = 2\,\text{Na} + \frac{\text{BUN}}{2.6} + \frac{\text{glucose}}{18}$$

The calculated osmolality normally is within 10 mOsm of the measured osmolality. The normal adult average is 290 ± 5 mOsm/kg and remains quite constant. Because water can move freely between the blood, interstitial fluid, and tissues, any change in the osmolality of one body compartment will produce a shift in body fluids. Therefore, the osmolality of the plasma is the same as that of other body compartments except in rapidly changing conditions when a slight lag may occur.

Normal urine osmolality ranges from 300 to 900 mOsm/kg/24 hours. Because of this wide range, more information about renal function is obtained when simultaneous serum and urine samples are collected and interpreted. In renal disease, one of the first functions to be lost is the ability to concentrate urine. This can result in the urine osmolality becoming fixed within +50 mOsm of the simultaneously determined serum osmolality.

A decrease in the serum osmolality can occur only when the serum sodium is decreased. An increase in the serum osmolality can occur whenever the serum sodium, urea, or glucose is elevated or when abnormal compounds are present in the blood, such as drugs, poisons, or metabolic waste products, such as lactic acid. Symptoms generally do not occur until the osmolality is greater than 350 mOsm. Coma can occur when the osmolality is 400 mOsm or greater.

CLINICAL APPLICATION: Diagnostic Studies
Facts Affecting Serum Urea: Creatinine Ratio

Decreased urea: creatinine (<10:1)
- Liver disease
- Protein restriction
- Excessive fluid intake

Increased urea: creatinine (>10:1)
- Volume depletion
- Decreased "effective" blood volume
- Catabolic states
- Excessive protein intake

URINARY SODIUM CONCENTRATION

The urinary sodium excretion is used as an indicator of renal function in differentiating the oliguria associated with ARF from other prerenal causes. States of underperfusion of the kidney are usually associated with a decrease in urinary sodium concentration (usually <10 mEq/L), whereas in ARF (because of damage to the tubular transport mechanisms), urine sodium concentration generally is above 30 to 40 mEq/L despite oliguria. However, when the urine pH is alkaline, urine sodium concentration will not reflect sodium balance accurately, and the chloride concentration becomes a better indicator of volume depletion.

FRACTIONAL EXCRETION OF SODIUM TEST

The sodium (FE_{Na}) test gives a more precise estimation of the amount of filtered sodium that remains in the urine and is more accurate in predicting tubular injury than the urinary sodium concentration. It can be calculated by using the following formula:

$$(U/P) \, Na/(U/P) \, Cr \times 100$$

in which U and P are the urinary and plasma concentrations of sodium and creatinine, respectively. (Although volume measurements are necessary to derive the absolute urinary excretion of both sodium and creatinine, these cancel out in deriving this formula.)

The test requires the determination of both serum and urinary sodium and creatinine concentrations on simultaneously obtained samples. Values less than 1% indicate prerenal azotemia, or underperfusion. Values greater than 1% (and frequently greater than 3%) are indicative of ARF.

Diagnostic Tests That Assess Renal Function

RADIOLOGICAL STUDIES

Radiological studies of the kidneys that may be useful in evaluating renal abnormalities include roentgenography, ultrasonography, and radionuclide studies. These studies and their purposes are summarized in Table 28–1.

RENAL BIOPSY

Renal biopsy is the most invasive but ultimate diagnostic tool used in the comprehensive renal evaluation. It is used to define the histological counterpart of the clinical picture, provide etiological clues for diagnosis, assess prognosis, and guide therapy. It is also used as an assessment tool for insurability, employment, or disability. Contraindications for

---

TABLE 28-1 CLINICAL APPLICATION: Diagnostic Studies
Radiological Study of Kidneys

Diagnostic Test	Purpose
Roentgenography	
• Radiograph of kidney–ureter–bladder (KUB)	Detect abnormal calcifications, renal size
• Tomography	Determine renal outlines and abnormalities
• Intravenous pyelography (IVP)	Detect anatomical abnormalities of the kidneys and ureters
• Retrograde pyelography	Assess renal size, evaluate ureteral obstruction, localize and diagnose tumors, obstructions
• Antegrade pyelography	Distinguish cysts from hydronephrosis
• Renal arteriography and venography	Evaluate possible renal arterial stenosis, renal mass lesions, renal vein thrombosis, and venous extension of renal cell carcinoma
• Digital subtraction angiography	Visualize major arterial vessels
Ultrasonography	
	Delineate renal outlines
	Measure longitudinal and transverse dimensions of the kidneys
	Evaluate mass lesions
	Examine perinephric area
	Detect and grade hydronephrosis
Radionuclide scintillation imaging (renal scan)	
• Static imaging	Evaluate location, size, and contour of functional renal tissue; may reveal areas of inhomogeneity or filling defects
• Dynamic imaging	Monitor the passage of a radiopharmaceutical agent through the vascular, renal parenchymal, and urinary tract compartments
Magnetic resonance imaging	Determine anatomical abnormalities

biopsy include serious bleeding disorders, excessive obesity, and severe hypertension (Table 28–2).

Procedure

Renal biopsies are generally performed percutaneously with a biopsy needle, but an open renal biopsy under general anesthesia still is performed.

Preparation for a renal biopsy includes obtaining informed consent, prebiopsy clotting studies, preoperative blood typing, and sedation (usually diazepam, 5–10 mg) and establishing intravenous access to prevent or treat complications. After the biopsy, the patient's vital signs are checked every 15 minutes for the first 2 hours, hourly for 4 hours, and then every 4 hours for the first 24 hours. The patient's urine should be examined for blood. The major complication is bleeding, which can occur either retroperitoneally or into the urinary tract. Other complications that can occur are biopsy of other abdominal viscera, such as bowel, pancreas, liver, spleen, and vessels, and tears in the diaphragm or pleura.

Laboratory Tests That Assess Electrolyte Balance

The role of the kidney is central in maintaining fluid volume and ionic composition of body fluids. When the kidneys properly regulate the excretion of water and ions,

homeostasis is achieved. When they fail to adapt adequately, imbalances occur. Electrolyte values and signs and symptoms of imbalance are listed in Tables 28–3 through 28–7.

ACID–BASE BALANCE

A normal acidity or alkalinity (pH of 7.35–7.45) of the body fluid is essential for life. The body maintains acid–base balance by the buffer system, the respiratory system, and the renal system. The buffer and respiratory systems are able to react quickly to changes in body pH. However, the kidneys take more time to adjust to changes in body pH.

Five major processes are associated with the regulation of acid–base balance by the renal system: hydrogen ion excretion; sodium ion reabsorption; bicarbonate ion generation and reabsorption; phosphate salt and titrateable acid excretion; and ammonia synthesis and ammonium excretion. Acid–base imbalances may result when the kidneys are unable to perform those processes adequately. Acid–base balances are summarized in Table 28–3.

THE ANION GAP

To maintain chemical neutrality, the total concentration of cations and anions in the blood (and other body fluids) must be equivalent in terms of milliequivalents per liter. However, because there are a number of anions and cations present in blood that are not routinely measured, a "gap" exists between the total concentration of cations and anions and the concentration normally measured in the plasma:

$$Na + K \text{ vs } Cl + HCO_3$$

The anion gap is composed primarily of an excess of unmeasured anions, including plasma proteins, inorganic phosphates and sulfates, and organic acids. The unmeasured cations that exist in smaller concentrations are primarily calcium and magnesium.

The anion gap generally is calculated by using the following formula:

$$Na - (Cl + HCO_3)$$

and has a normal mean of approximately 12 mEq/L (range, 8–16 mEq/L). Potassium is generally, but not always, omitted from the formula because of its relatively low concentration and narrow range of fluctuation. However, departures from this "normal" anion gap may have important diagnostic significance in acid–base disorders, especially metabolic acidoses.

The most common abnormality of the anion gap is an increase that is associated with increased concentrations of lactate, ketone bodies, or inorganic phosphate and sulfate that are found in lactic acidosis, ketoacidosis, and uremia, respectively. Other forms of acidosis associated with ingestion of toxins, such as ethylene glycol, methanol, paraldehyde, and salicylates, also may produce significant increases in the anion gap.

Decreases in the anion gap are less common but equally important. They can occur because of increases in unmea-

---

TABLE 28-2   CLINICAL APPLICATION:
Assessment Parameters
Indications for Renal Biopsy

Clinical Condition	Biopsy Indicated	Expected Gain
Orthostatic proteinuria	No	—
Isolated hematuria and/or proteinuria	No*	—
Hematuria and/or proteinuria with ↓ GFR	Yes	D,P,T
Nephrotic syndrome	Yes	D,P,T
Systemic disease with renal abnormalities	Yes†	D,P,T
Classic ARF	No	—
ARF with		
1. azotemia >3 wk	Yes	D,P
2. moderate proteinuria	Yes	D,T
3. anuria	Yes	D,T
4. eosinophilia or eosinophiluria	Yes	D,T
Post-transplant ↓ in GFR	Yes	D,P,T

GFR, glomerular filtration rate; D, diagnosis; P, prognosis; T, therapy; ARF, acute renal failure
* Biopsy may be indicated for insurance, administrative reasons, and so forth.
† Biopsy may or may not be indicated, depending on clinical picture.

TABLE 28-3   CLINICAL APPLICATION: Diagnostic Studies
Electrolyte Abnormalities: Acid–Base Balance

Electrolyte	Abnormality	Assessment Findings
Acid–base balance	Metabolic acidosis pH below 7.35 HCO_3 below 22 $PaCO_2$ normal	Tachypnea (Kussmaul's respiration), headache, confusion, drowsiness, cold, clammy skin; vasodilation, which leads to low cardiac output and hypotension
	Metabolic alkalosis pH above 7.45 HCO_3 above 26 $PaCO_2$ normal	Increased neuromuscular irritability, paresthesias; tetany, seizures; dysrhythmias; hypoventilation

sured cations or because of decreases in unmeasured anions, as listed in the display.

SODIUM BALANCE

Serum sodium concentration is normally 135 to 145 mEq/L. It is regulated by the kidneys and depends on the sodium concentration in the extracellular fluid. When the concentration rises, the kidneys retain water in response to antidiuretic hormone (ADH). When the concentration falls, aldosterone promotes sodium retention by the kidneys (see Fig. 27–5). When the kidneys malfunction, this balance is not maintained. A low serum sodium usually indicates water intake in excess of sodium and is characterized by an increase in body weight. A high serum sodium usually indicates water loss in excess of sodium and is reflected in weight loss. Table 28–4 lists sodium abnormalities. Sodium is essential for maintaining the osmolality of extracellular fluids, neuromuscular function, acid–base balance, and various other cellular chemical reactions.

POTASSIUM BALANCE

Potassium is essential for regulating nerve impulse conduction and muscle contraction and is involved in numerous other body functions, including intracellular osmolality and acid–base balance. The normal serum potassium concentration is 3.5 to 5.0 mEq/L. Potassium balance is maintained by dietary intake and renal excretion. Ninety-eight percent of potassium is located in the skeletal muscle; therefore, the balance of this electrolyte also is strongly tied to the exchanges between the intracellular and extracellular compartments in the body.

Hypokalemia can result from inadequate potassium intake, excessive potassium loss through the kidneys, gastrointestinal loss, and extracellular-to-intracellular potassium shifts. Also, diuretic therapy can contribute to potassium excretion, further compounding the problem.

Hyperkalemia may be caused by a decrease in the renal excretion of potassium or transcellular shifts of potassium. This is seen most often in acidosis, cell injury or destruction, and hyperglycemia. Potassium abnormalities are listed in Table 28–5.

CALCIUM AND PHOSPHATE BALANCE

Calcium and phosphate are regulated reciprocally in the body by vitamin D, parathyroid, and calcitonin. The calcium and phosphate salts are normally deposited in bone. When calcium levels are high, phosphate levels are low. Because in renal failure, the kidneys are unable to eliminate phosphate, renal failure patients often have high phosphate and low calcium levels.

CLINICAL APPLICATION: Diagnostic Studies
Causes of an Altered Anion Gap

Increased Anion Gap
Increased unmeasured anions
- Endogenous metabolic acidosis
  Lactic acidosis
  Ketoacidosis
  Uremic acidosis
- Exogenous anion ingestion
  Ethylene glycol
  Methanol
  Paraldehyde
  Salicylates
  Penicillin
  Carbenicillin
- Increased plasma proteins
  Hyperalbuminemia

Decreased unmeasured cations
- Hypokalemia
- Hypocalcemia
- Hypomagnesemia

Decreased Anion Gap
Increased unmeasured cations
- Normal cations
  Hypercalcemia
  Hyperkalemia
  Hypermagnesemia
- Abnormal cations
  Increased globulins (eg, myeloma)
  Lithium

Decreased unmeasured anions
- Hypoalbuminemia

TABLE 28-4   CLINICAL APPLICATION: Diagnostic Studies
Electrolyte Abnormalities: Sodium

Electrolyte	Abnormality	Assessment Findings
Sodium	Hypernatremia Na >145 mEq/L	Sticky or dry oral mucous membranes; thirst; hypotension; firm body tissues; tachycardia, oliguria or anuria, anxiety
	Hyponatremia Na <135 mEq/L	
	135–125 mEq/L	Generally none
	125–110 mEq/L	Headache, apathy, lethargy, weakness, disorientation
	110–100 mEq/L	Confusion, hostility; lethargy or violence; nausea and vomiting; areflexia
	100–95 mEq/L	Delirium, convulsions, coma, hypothermia; Cheyne-Stokes respiration; death

Calcium's primary function is maintenance of bone and tooth strength. It also plays an important role in myocardial and skeletal contractility. Calcium also maintains cellular permeability and assists in blood coagulation.

The normal serum concentration of calcium is 8.5 to 10.5 mg/dL. Serum calcium consists of ultrafilterable calcium and the calcium that is bound to protein, primarily albumin. Ultrafilterable calcium includes ionized calcium and the calcium complexed to bicarbonate, citrate, and phosphate.

Phosphate is essential for the formation of adenosine triphosphate. Phosphate also assists in the maintenance of cell membrane structure, oxygen delivery, and cellular immunity. The normal phosphate level is 3.0 to 4.5 mg/dL.

All of the electrolytes need to be monitored closely by the critical care nurse, because minor shifts can be lethal. Calcium and phosphate abnormalities are listed in Table 28–6.

MAGNESIUM BALANCE

The magnesium ion is the second major intracellular ion. The normal serum concentration is 1.4 to 2.1 mEq/L. Magnesium balance is necessary for the functional integrity of the neuromuscular system. The parathyroid glands regulate both magnesium and calcium. Sodium is necessary for magnesium reabsorption. Magnesium can accumulate in the serum, bone, and muscle in renal failure causing numerous problems. Table 28–7 lists abnormalities in magnesium.

Nonspecific Tests

HEMATOCRIT AND HEMOGLOBIN

The normal hemoglobin for men is 13.5 to 17.5 g/dL and 12 to 16 g/dL for women. The normal hematocrit should be 40% to 52% for adult men and 37% to 48% for adult women. False elevations of hematocrit can be seen with dehydration or after dialysis. Low hematocrits may be a dilutional value due to hypervolemia. The kidney is the primary site for the production of erythropoietin. It stimulates the bone marrow to release mature red blood cells. Many ESRD patients produce insufficient amounts of erythropoietin, which can result in chronic anemia. These patients can also have bleeding problems due to impaired platelet function and immunological abnormalities.

TABLE 28-5   CLINICAL APPLICATION: Diagnostic Studies
Electrolyte Abnormalities: Potassium

Electrolyte	Abnormality	Assessment Findings
Potassium	Hyperkalemia K > 5.0 mEq/L	Irritability and restlessness; anxiety; nausea, vomiting, and diarrhea; muscle cramps, weakness; paresthesias; ECG changes with cardiac irregularities; peaked T waves, ventricular fibrillation, cardiac arrest
	Hypokalemia K < 3.5 mEq/L	Fatigue that progresses to paralysis; paresthesias; nausea, vomiting, anorexia, dizziness; confusion; ventricular ectopy, cardiac arrest; increased sensitivity to digitalis

TABLE 28-6   CLINICAL APPLICATION: Diagnostic Studies
Electrolyte Abnormalities: Calcium and Phosphate

Electrolyte	Abnormality	Assessment Findings
Calcium	Hypercalcemia Ca > 10.5 mg/dL	Muscle weakness/atrophy; lethargy, coma; personality or behavioral changes; pathological fractures; bone pain; polyuria; excessive thirst; anorexia, nausea, vomiting, constipation; hypertension; ECG changes (ie, shortened QT, AV block)
	Hypocalcemia Ca < 8.5 mg/dL	Paresthesias, tetany, seizures, abdominal spasms, cramps; skeletal muscle cramps; laryngeal spasm; positive Chvostek's and Trousseau's signs, impaired memory, irritability; decreased cardiac output; bleeding
Phosphate	Hyperphosphatemia P > 4.5 mg/dL	Tachycardia; nausea, diarrhea, abdominal cramps; muscle weakness, paralysis, increased reflexes; decreased calcium
	Hypophosphatemia P < 3 mg/dL	Ataxia, paresthesias, confusion, coma, seizures; muscle weakness, joint stiffness, bone pain; anorexia, dysphagia; anemia, platelet dysfunction, impaired immunity

URIC ACID

The normal uric acid serum level is between 2 and 8.5 mg/dL. It is excreted primarily by the kidneys with some in the stool. Uric acid may be elevated because of excessive production from cell breakdown or because it is not adequately excreted by the kidney.

■ NURSING ASSESSMENT OF FLUID BALANCE

The nurse's role in the assessment of problems of fluid balance includes accurate measurement of intake and output, weight, and vital signs. The most sensitive indices of changes in body water content are serial weights and intake and output patterns. Although vital signs can provide supporting data, they may not be abnormal until significant volume or water deficits occur. Assessment of fluid imbalance needs to be based on keen observation and recognition of pertinent symptoms.

Intake and Output

An accurate intake and output record provides valuable data for evaluating and treating fluid and electrolyte imbalances. It is important that the nurse teach the patient or visitors to assist in this assessment. Intake and output is measured and recorded as it occurs and totaled at the end of every shift. In the presence of excessive losses or deterioration of cardiac, hepatic, renal, or respiratory function, more detailed recording of every source of fluid intake and output is necessary, and calculations may be required every 1 to 4 hours.

Intake should include all liquids, such as water, juices, or soup, and any foods that are high in water content (eg, oranges, grapefruit, gelatin, and ice cream). It is useful to keep a list of equivalents for fruits, ice cubes and chips, and other sources of fluid. Output should include urinary and intestinal losses and estimating respiratory and cutaneous losses when the patient's temperature or the ambient temperature is high. Also recorded are other sources of fluid loss that are present, such as ileostomy or other enteric drainage, wound, or thoracic drainage.

TABLE 28-7   CLINICAL APPLICATION: Diagnostic Studies
Electrolyte Abnormalities: Magnesium

Electrolyte	Abnormality	Assessment Findings
Magnesium	Hypermagnesemia Mg > 2.1 mEq/L	CNS depression, respiratory paralysis; lethargy, coma; bradycardia, hypotension
	Hypomagnesemia Mg < 1.4 mEq/L	Tremors, tetany, seizures; positive Chvostek's or Trousseau's signs; tachycardia, hypertension, ventricular dysrhythmias; personality changes

In severe electrolyte and fluid imbalances, the time and type of fluid intake and the time and amount of each voiding must be recorded. In the event that renal function decreases, this information may aid immeasurably in the diagnosis and possible prevention of prerenal azotemia or ARF. Some sources of excessive loss are given in the accompanying display.

Weight

Rapid daily gains and losses of weight usually are associated with changes in fluid volume. It is often difficult to obtain accurate figures for intake and output records because of

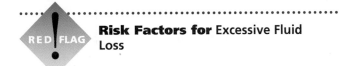

RED FLAG **Risk Factors for** Excessive Fluid Loss

- *Fever.* A patient with a fever of 40°C (104°F) and a respiratory rate of 40 breaths/min can lose as much as 2,500 mL of fluid in a 24-hour period from the respiratory tract and from the skin.
- *Environment.* Hot, dry climates can increase evaporative sweat losses to 1,500 mL/h to maintain body evaporative heat loss. This can increase to between 2 and 2.5 L/h for short times in acclimatized people exercising in hot climates.
- *Hyperventilation.* Hyperventilation can increase respiratory water losses as a result of either disease or use of nonhumidified respirators or oxygen delivery systems.
- *Gastrointestinal tract.* Vomiting, nasogastric suction, diarrhea, and enterocutaneous drainage or fistulas can increase gastrointestinal losses.
- *Third-spacing.* Formation of pleural or peritoneal effusions and edema from liver, renal, or hepatic disease or from the diffuse capillary leak syndrome can result in a loss of effective intravascular volume. Drainage of peritoneal or pleural fluid, when formation of these third spaces still is occurring, can result in further effective intravascular losses because of continued fluid shifts from the vascular compartment to the third space.
- *Burns.* Fluid loss into burned tissues can result in a significant decrease in effective intravascular volume. Because both evaporative and transudative losses through the burned skin can result in very large losses of fluid daily, the burned patient requires special attention to maintain fluid and electrolyte balance. Formulas for determining burn area and fluid resuscitation are discussed in Chapter 51.
- *Renal losses.* Inappropriate solute and fluid loss from the kidneys can occur because of renal salt wasting. This is seen in the diuretic phase of acute tubular necrosis, in some rare patients with true renal salt wasting, and as a result of excessive diuretic administration. It also may occur as a result of solute diuresis from high-protein or high-saline enteral and parenteral alimentation and from administration of osmotic agents, such as mannitol and radiocontrast agents. Finally, fluid can be lost during the generation phase of metabolic alkalosis, in which compensatory urinary bicarbonate excretion obligates renal sodium excretion. This frequently results in volume depletion.

the variables mentioned previously. Serial weights often are more reliable. In addition, *weight changes usually will pick up imbalances before any symptoms are apparent*.

As with intake and output records, the weighing procedure should be consistent. The patient should be weighed on the same scale with the same attire, preferably in the morning before breakfast and after voiding. Variations in the procedure should be noted and made known to the physician. A kilogram scale provides for greater accuracy because drug, fluid, and diet measurements can be calculated easily using the metric system.

A normal patient with a balanced nutritional intake should be able to maintain his or her weight. However, a patient whose protein intake is limited or who is catabolic can lose about 2.2 lb/d (1 kg/d). A weight gain of more than 2.2 lb/d (1 kg/d) usually suggests fluid retention. *A generally accepted guide is that 473 mL (1 pt) of fluid is reflected in 1.1 lb (0.5 kg) of weight gained.*

Hypovolemia and Hypervolemia

The critical care nurse must be continually on the alert to detect early changes in the patient's volume status. Seldom is the diagnosis made on the basis of one parameter. The first clue may be the patient's general appearance; after observing this, the nurse should seek and note more specific parameters.

Symptoms vary with the degree of imbalance; some are seen early in imbalance states, and others are not evident until severe imbalances have occurred. Table 28–8 lists the signs and symptoms of hypovolemia and hypervolemia.

In volume depletion, the patient may complain of orthostatic light-headedness when assuming the sitting or standing position (this also can occur from inactivity and autonomic dysfunction). Development of tachycardia on assuming the upright position and a decrease in blood pressure (orthostatic hypotension), as opposed to the normal rise, are frequent early findings. Later, the pulse may become rapid, weak, and thready. There may be early dryness of the skin, with loss of elasticity, sunken eyes, loss of axillary sweating, and a dry, coated tongue. When severe volume depletion occurs, thirst, decreased urine volume, and weight loss may be noted; however, weight loss and orthostatic blood pressure and pulse changes may be the only findings present.

Laboratory studies, such as a high urine osmolality and low urinary sodium, may facilitate the diagnosis. Other guidelines, such as elevated hematocrit, decreased central venous pressure, and decreased pulmonary wedge pressure, may corroborate the diagnosis.

In fluid overload, the patient, if alert, may complain of puffiness or stiffness in the hands and feet. Later, periorbital edema or puffiness, followed by pitting edema of the dependent parts (feet and ankles if upright; sacral area and posterior thighs if supine) will occur, followed by dyspnea or ascites, depending on etiology (ie, cardiac decompensation and systemic fluid overload versus hepatic disease). Urine volume and urine sodium may be normal, increased,

TABLE 28-8 CLINICAL APPLICATION: Assessment Parameters
Signs and Symptoms of Hypovolemia and Hypervolemia

Parameters	Hypovolemia	Hypervolemia
Skin and subcutaneous tissues	Dry, less elastic	Warm, moist, pitting edema over bony prominences; wrinkled skin from pressure of clothing
Face	Sunken eyes (late symptom)	Periorbital edema
Tongue	Dry, coated (early symptom); fissured (late symptom)	Moist
Saliva	Thick, scanty	Excessive, frothy
Thirst	Present	May not be significant
Temperature	May be elevated	May not be significant
Pulse	Rapid, weak, thready	Rapid
Respirations	Rapid, shallow	Rapid dyspnea, moist rales, cough
Blood pressure	Low, orthostatic hypotension; small pulse pressure	Normal to high
Weight	Loss	Gain

or decreased, depending on the etiology. In most diseases with fluid retention, except for the syndrome of inappropriate ADH secretion, urine sodium will be reduced. The hematocrit will be decreased, reflecting hemodilution.

The pulse may be rapid and auscultation of the heart may reveal the presence of S_3, S_4, or a murmur secondary to volume overload. Respirations may be increased because of pulmonary congestion, and auscultation of the chest may reveal rales. A chest film may reveal pulmonary vascular congestion, increased alveolar lung markings, cardiac dilation, frank pulmonary congestion, and pleural effusions.

All data should be evaluated in the light of other evidence. Trends usually are more significant than isolated values. For example, when a decrease in urine output is noted, a systematic assessment should be done to determine why this is happening and what nursing interventions are most appropriate. Factors affecting water balance are listed in Table 28–9.

Hyponatremia and Hypernatremia

Hyponatremia is important because it can produce a wide range of neurological symptoms, including death. The severity of symptoms depends on the degree of hyponatremia and the rate at which it has developed. Generally, symptoms do not occur until the serum sodium is below 120 mEq/L. Table 28–4 depicts the symptoms to be expected in several ranges of hyponatremia. For each level of sodium concentration, the severity of symptoms encountered will depend on how rapidly the sodium concentration was lowered.

Symptoms of hypernatremia generally are the same as those of hyperosmolality and result from CNS dehydration. Mental confusion, stupor, seizures, coma, and death may occur, in addition to other signs of dehydration, such as fatigue, muscle weakness and cramps, and anorexia. The serum osmolality generally is above 350 mOsm/L before

significant symptoms are noted. This corresponds to a serum sodium of 165 to 170 mEq/L.

CLINICAL APPLICATION: Patient Care Study

Mr. Ellis, a 46-year-old man, was admitted with a 48-hour history of jaundice and increasing mental confusion. Mr. Ellis indicated that he has a history of alcoholism and had been drinking heavily during the past few weeks. For 2 weeks he had noted increasing edema and increasing abdominal girth. During physical examination, he was moderately obtunded but arousable. Blood pressure was 98/68 mmHg, pulse was 92 beats/min, and temperature was 36.1°C (97°F). Mr. Ellis had marked scleral icterus, tense abdominal ascites, and diffuse pitting edema below the waist. Initial laboratory studies revealed the following:

Serum
- Na: 115 mEq/L
- Cl: 75 mEq/L
- K: 2.8 mEq/L
- CO_2: 30 mEq/L
- BUN: 10 mg/dL
- Creatinine: 0.8 mg/dL
- Albumin: 2.4 g/dL

Urine
- Specific gravity: 1.028; pH, 6.8
- U_{osm}: 890 mOsm/L
- U_{Na}: 8 mEq/L
- U_K: 33 mEq/L
- U_{Cl}: 2 mEq/L

The serum bilirubin, aspartate aminotransferase, alkaline phosphatase, and lactate dehydrogenase levels all were elevated, but the blood ammonium level was normal.

Discussion

Mr. Ellis had severe hyponatremia even though he had an increase in total body sodium and water, as reflected by the pronounced edema. His sodium retention is due to the combined effects of decreased renal perfusion secondary to hypovolemia from hypoalbuminemia and ascites formation,

TABLE 28-9   CLINICAL APPLICATION: Assessment Parameters
Factors Affecting Water Balance

	Water Excess	Water Deficiency
Intake		
Thirst	Decreased thirst threshold	Increased thirst threshold
	Increased osmolality	Decreased osmolality
	Potassium depletion	Lack of access
	Hypercalcemia	Psychiatric disorders
	Fever	
	Dry mucous membranes	
	Poor oral hygiene	
	Unmisted O_2 administration	
	Hypotension	
	Psychiatric disorders	
Parenteral fluids	Excessive D5W	Deficient replacement
		Osmotic loads
		Hyperalimentation
		Hyperglycemia
		Mannitol
		Radiographic contrast
		agents
Output		
Sweating		High ambient temperature
		High altitude
		Fever
Renal excretion	Inappropriate ADH release	Excess excretion
	Appropriate ADH release	Central
	Congestive failure	Nephrogenic
	Decompensated cirrhosis	Potassium depletion
	Volume depletion	Hypercalcemia
	Adrenal insufficiency	Lithium administration
	Renal salt wasting	Declomicin
	Hemorrhage	Methoxyflurane (Penthrane)
	Diuretics	
	Burns	
	Hypothyroidism	
	Renal disease	
	ARF	
	Chronic renal failure	
	Nephrotic syndrome	
	Acute glomerulonephritis	
	Nonsteroidal anti-inflammatory	
	agents	

D5W, Dextrose 5% in water; ADH, antidiuretic hormone; ARF, acute renal failure

alcoholic peripheral vasodilation, and secondary hypoaldosteronism. The hyponatremia is due to the combined effects of volume-mediated vasopressin release, as reflected in the high urine specific gravity and osmolality, and to decreased distal nephron sodium and water delivery due to renal underperfusion.

Mr. Ellis had acute alcoholic hepatitis and was treated with enteral feedings through a nasogastric tube. His hyponatremia was treated by restricting water initially and administering a thiazide diuretic and aldactone. This slowly corrected his serum sodium.

In addition to his hyponatremia, Mr. Ellis also had a hypokalemic metabolic alkalosis, probably resulting from the combined effects of volume and potassium depletion. His urinary sodium of 8 mEq/L was considerably higher than his urine chloride concentration of 2 mEq/L, probably due to bicarbonate spilling in the urine. This bicarbonaturia is accompanied by urinary sodium excretion, even when there is volume depletion. In this situation, the urinary chloride concentration is a better indication of volume depletion than the urinary sodium concentration.

CONCLUSION

The nurse plays a critical role in the assessment of patients with fluid and electrolyte disorders associated with chronic and acute renal disease in the intensive care unit. A thorough history can contribute valuable information that can be used by the critical care team to provide a holistic approach in the patient's care. Careful assessment of the patient's symptoms, general appearance, and changes in weight, blood pressure, and pulse may provide early clues to changes in volume status and to disorders of water balance. Knowledgeable application and interpretation of laboratory studies will facilitate the diagnosis and treatment of fluid and electrolyte disorders and other complications of renal dysfunction in the seriously ill patient.

Clinical Applicability Challenges

Self-Challenge: Critical Thinking

1. A 50-year-old manufacturing worker was brought to the hospital when he became increasingly difficult to arouse after having a "stomach virus." There is a risk of nephrotoxicity. Explore the assessment data that will further describe this illness.

2. Examine assessment parameters that will help differentiate a fluid volume excess from a fluid volume deficit.

3. Contrast the history, examination, and laboratory data for patients with a sodium excess and deficit.

Study Questions

1. Which laboratory value is most useful in assessing renal function?
   a. Potassium
   b. BUN
   c. Creatinine
   d. Uric acid

2. Which of the following laboratory values will be elevated in renal failure?
   a. Potassium, phosphate, and magnesium
   b. Calcium, potassium, and phosphate
   c. Calcium and magnesium
   d. Bicarbonate and chloride

3. Signs and symptoms of hypocalcemia include
   a. edema, dry skin, bradycardia.
   b. thirst, high specific gravity, hypotension.
   c. muscle weakness, bone pain, hypertension.
   d. cramps, tetany, positive Chvostek's and Trousseau's signs.

BIBLIOGRAPHY

Bates B: A guide to physical examination and history taking (6th Ed). Philadelphia, JB Lippincott, 1995

Brunier GM: Calcium/phosphate imbalances, aluminum toxicity, and renal osteodystrophy. ANNA Journal 21(4):171–179, 1994

Goshorn F: Kidney stones. Am J Nurs 96(9):40–41, 1996

Kirton CA: Assessing for ascites. Nursing 26(4):53, 1996

Metheny NM: Fluid and electrolyte balance: Nursing considerations. Philadelphia, Lippincott-Raven, 1996

Preisig P: Renal acidification. ANNA Journal 2(5):251–259 1994

O'Donnell ME: Assessing fluid and electrolyte balance in elders. Am J Nurs 95(11):40–46, 1995

Shoop KL: Pruritus in end stage renal disease. ANNA Journal 21(2): 147–153, 1994

29

Patient Management: Renal System

OBJECTIVES

Based on the content in this chapter, the reader should be able to:

- Explore the physiological principles involved in renal replacement therapy: hemodialysis, continuous renal replacement therapies, and peritoneal dialysis.
- Analyze the differences in equipment and procedures used in renal replacement therapy.
- Explain the types of vascular access used in hemodialysis and continuous renal replacement therapies.
- Compare and contrast the indications, assessment and management, and complications for each renal replacement therapy.
- Explore the psychosocial and teaching needs surrounding renal replacement therapy for patients and their families.

*R*enal function can be replaced by a process called dialysis. It is a life-maintaining therapy used in acute and chronic renal failure. Critical care nurses may encounter patients suffering from the effects of acute renal failure (ARF) or patients already on some form of chronic dialysis who subsequently become critically ill. Critical care nurses must be familiar with various dialysis therapies to help care for patients with complex illnesses. This chapter presents the three most common forms of renal replacement therapy: hemodialysis, continuous renal replacement therapies (CRRT), and peritoneal dialysis.

■ PHYSIOLOGICAL PRINCIPLES

All forms of dialysis use the principles of osmosis and diffusion to remove waste products and excess fluid from the blood. This is accomplished by placing a semipermeable membrane between the blood and a specially formulated solution called dialysate. Dissolved substances, such as urea and creatinine, diffuse across the membrane from an area of greater concentration (the blood) to an area of lesser concentration (the dialysate). Water molecules move across the membrane by osmosis to the solution that contains fewer water molecules. Dialysate is formulated with varying concentrations of dextrose or sodium to create an osmotic gradient and thus pull excess water from the circulatory system. This process of fluid moving across a semipermeable membrane in relation to forces created by osmotic and hydrostatic pressures is called ultrafiltration. These basic principles are the foundation of any dialysis therapy. The manner in which they are accomplished varies depending on the therapy.

■ THE EXTRACORPOREAL THERAPIES

Hemodialysis and the CRRTs use an extracorporeal (outside of the body) circuit. Therefore, they require access to the patient's circulation and anticoagulation of the circuit.

Access to Circulation

The three most common methods used to access a patient's circulation are through a vascular catheter, an arteriovenous (AV) fistula, and a synthetic vascular graft. Patients who suddenly need hemodialysis or CRRT will have a catheter placed in either the internal jugular, subclavian, or femoral vein. Patients already receiving chronic hemodialysis probably have either an AV fistula or a synthetic vascular graft. General guidelines for nursing care are summarized in the display.

VENOUS CATHETERS

Dual-lumen catheters inserted into large veins are used for acutely ill patients who need hemodialysis, continuous venovenous hemofiltration, or continuous venovenous he-

---

CLINICAL APPLICATION:
Nursing Intervention Guidelines
Dialysis Vascular Access

Dual-Lumen Venous Catheter
- Verify central line catheter placement radiographically before use.
- Do not inject IV fluids or medication into the catheter. Both lumens of the catheter usually are filled with concentrated heparin.
- Do not unclamp the catheter unless preparing for dialysis therapy. This can cause blood to fill the lumen and clot.
- Maintain sterile technique in handling vascular access.
- Observe catheter exit site for signs of inflammation or catheter kinking.

Arteriovenous Fistula or Graft
- Do not take blood pressure or draw blood from the access limb.
- Listen for bruit, and palpate for thrill q8h.
- Make sure there is no tight clothing or restraints on the access limb.
- Check access patency more frequently when patients are hypotensive. Hypotension can predispose to clotting.
- In the event of postdialysis bleeding from the needle site, apply just enough pressure to stop the flow of blood and hold until bleeding stops. Do not occlude the vessel.

---

mofiltration with dialysis. Venous catheters are also used for hemodialysis when there is no other means of access to the circulation. Veins commonly used are the femoral, internal jugular, or subclavian. The site chosen depends on the patient's anatomy and vein accessibility and the physician's experience and site preference.

Dual-lumen vein catheters, as shown in Figure 29–1, also are used temporarily for acute dialysis patients who are critically ill or chronic patients who are waiting for a more permanent access to mature. Tunnelled dual-lumen central venous catheters are often used as a permanent means of access in patients who have exhausted all other means of entry into their circulatory system. The tunnelled catheter has an implantable Dacron cuff around which tissue grows and acts as a barrier against infection. The catheter should be placed in the right or left internal jugular vein, if possible, because catheters placed in the subclavian vein can cause stenosis. The stenosis can cause increased venous pressure and edema that may thwart future efforts to create an AV fistula or place a graft.

Whenever venous catheters are used, care must be taken to avoid accidental slippage and dislodgement during hemodialysis. Femoral catheters usually are secured to the leg with tape, while central venous catheters in the upper body are sutured to the skin. The length of time catheters are left in place depends on catheter function and institution policy. Central vein catheters generally can be used for up to 3 to 4 weeks. Usually femoral catheters, to avoid infection, are

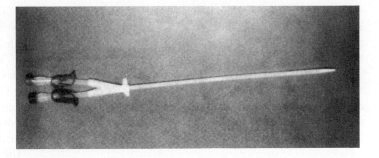

FIGURE 29-1
Dual-lumen venous catheter.

removed within 24 to 48 hours after insertion. More permanent internal jugular vein catheters often function for many months before problems force their removal. Catheters left in place between dialysis treatments usually are filled with a concentrated heparin–saline solution after dialysis and plugged to prevent clotting. These catheters should *never* be used for any purpose other than hemodialysis without first checking with dialysis unit personnel. Cleansing and dressing of the insertion site are the same as with other central lines.

If the catheters are removed at the end of dialysis, pressure is applied to the puncture sites until complete clotting occurs. The site is checked for several hours thereafter so that any recurrent bleeding can be detected. Removal of the more permanent tunnelled catheter requires use of local anesthetic at the exit site and careful dissection around the Dacron cuff to free it from the attached subcutaneous tissue.

Catheter patency must be maintained. Urokinase is used to dissolve clots in venous catheters. This enzyme, derived from streptococcal bacteria, is capable of activating the fibrinolytic system and dissolving intravascular thrombi. As a result, Urokinase can help preserve vascular access and reduce the need for surgery or catheter reinsertion. Despite these advantages, there are risks and side effects inherent in the use of urokinase. These include local pain, bleeding, and an allergic response, such as fever and chills.

In the early days of dialysis, vascular access was created every treatment by cannulating an artery to remove blood from the body and a vein to return dialyzed blood to the patient. Thus, the lines carrying blood to the dialyzer were labelled arterial lines and the lines returning blood to the body were called venous lines. The terms arterial and venous are still used in this manner today. As a result, the two lumens of the venous catheter used in dialysis are designated as arterial and venous. The arterial lumen is longer than the venous lumen so it can catch blood flowing by and allow it to be pumped out of the body. Blood is returned upstream from the arterial lumen to avoid pulling out the blood that has just been dialyzed and returned to the body. The lumens are distinguished by the presence of colored clamps: red on the arterial lumen and blue on the venous lumen.

ARTERIOVENOUS FISTULAS

The AV fistula technique was developed in 1966 by Cimino and Brescia in an effort to provide long-term use of an access for hemodialysis. To create the AV fistula, a surgeon anastomoses an artery and a vein, creating a fistula or artificial opening between them. Arterial blood flowing into the venous system results in a marked dilation of the vein, which can then be punctured easily with 15- or 16-gauge dialysis fistula needle. Two venipunctures are made at the time of dialysis, one for blood outflow and one for blood return.

After the AV fistula incision has healed, the site is cleansed by normal bathing or showering. To avoid scar formation, excessive bleeding, or hematoma of the AV fistula, care is taken to avoid traumatic venipuncture, excessive manipulation of the needles, and repeated use of the same site for venipuncture. Adequate pressure must be put on the puncture sites after the needles are removed. In addition, blood pressures and venipunctures should *not* be done on the arm with the fistula.

Most AV fistulas are developed and ready to use in 1 to 3 months after surgery. After initial healing has occurred, patients are taught to exercise the arm to assist in vessel maturation. They also are encouraged to become familiar with the quality of the "thrill" felt at the site of anastomosis so that they can report any change in its presence or strength. A loud, swishing sound termed the *bruit* indicates a functioning fistula.

Although AV fistulas usually have a long life, complications can occur. These include thrombosis, aneurysm or pseudoaneurysm, or arterial insufficiency causing a "steal syndrome." This syndrome occurs when shunting of blood from the artery to the vein produces ischemia of the hand, causing pain or coldness in the hand. Surgical intervention can remedy all of these problems and restore adequate fistula flow.

SYNTHETIC GRAFTS

The synthetic graft is made from polytetrafluoroethylene (PTFE), a material manufactured from an expanded, highly porous form of Teflon. The graft is anastomosed between an artery and a vein and is used in the same manner as an AV fistula.

For many patients whose own vessels are not adequate for fistula formation, PTFE grafts are extremely valuable. PTFE segments also are used to patch areas of AV grafts or fistulas that have stenosed or developed areas of aneurysm. It is best to avoid venipuncture in new PTFE grafts for 2 to

4 weeks while the patient's tissue grows into the graft. When tissue growth progresses satisfactorily, the graft has an endothelium and wall composition similar to the patient's own vessels.

The procedures for preventing complications in grafts are the same as those used for AV fistulas. However, certain complications are seen more frequently with grafts than with fistulas, including thrombosis, infection, aneurysm formation, and stenosis at the site of anastomosis.

Heparinization

Blood in the extracorporeal system, such as the dialyzer and blood lines, clots rapidly unless some method of anticoagulation is used. Heparin is the drug of choice because it is simple to administer, increases clotting time rapidly, is monitored easily, and may be reversed with protamine.

Specific heparinization procedures vary, but the primary goal in any method is to prevent clotting in the dialyzer with the least amount of heparin. Two methods commonly used are intermittent and constant infusion.

SYSTEMIC HEPARINIZATION

In both methods, an initial priming dose of heparin usually is given, followed by smaller doses at intervals or at a constant rate by an infusion pump. This results in systemic heparinization, in which the clotting times of the patient and the dialyzer essentially are the same.

Definitive guidelines are difficult to provide because methods and dialyzer requirements vary. The normal clotting time of 6 to 10 minutes may be increased to the range of 30 to 60 minutes. The effect of heparin usually is monitored at the bedside by the activated clotting time, prothrombin time (PT), or partial thromboplastin time (PTT). These tests can provide results in seconds, which gives the dialysis nurse the opportunity to make rapid adjustments in heparin administration.

The patient's need for heparinization and an appropriate beginning heparin dose should be assessed routinely before dialysis, especially in the critically ill patient who may be actively bleeding or at risk for bleeding. The patient's platelet count, serum calcium level, and results of coagulation studies are valuable in assessing current function of the clotting process. Often, little or no heparin can be used when the patient has serious alterations in one or more factors needed for effective clotting.

REGIONAL HEPARINIZATION

Systemic heparinization does not usually present a risk unless the patient has overt bleeding (eg, gastrointestinal bleeding, epistaxis, or hemoptysis), is 3 to 7 days postsurgery, or has uremic pericarditis. In these situations, other methods to prevent clotting of the extracorporeal system can be used. One method is regional heparinization, in which the patient's clotting time is kept normal while the clotting time of the dialyzer is increased. This is accomplished by infusing heparin at a constant rate into the dialyzer and simultaneously neutralizing its effects with protamine sulfate before the blood returns to the patient.

Like systemic heparinization, regional heparinization has no associated standard heparin–protamine ratio. Frequent monitoring of the clotting times is the best way to achieve effective regional heparinization. Because of the rebound phenomenon that has occurred after regional heparinization, low-dose heparinization may be used, even in the presence of overt bleeding. With this method, minimal heparin doses are used throughout dialysis. Although some clotting may take place in the dialyzer, the small blood loss is preferable to the risk of profound bleeding.

Bleeding problems occasionally occur because of accidental heparin overdose. This may be caused by infusion pump malfunction or an error in setting the delivery rate. Because of the hazards, heparin delivery must be monitored carefully and frequently.

Another way to prevent dialyzer clotting and reduce the risk of bleeding due to heparin is to infuse a small initial heparin dose (eg, 250 U) and use frequent normal saline flushes of the extracorporeal system or use saline flushes alone.

Some dialysis centers perform regional citrate anticoagulation in which citrate is infused into the system before the dialyzer binds calcium, obstructing the normal clotting pathway. The citrate–calcium complex is then cleared from the blood by the dialyzer, and the anticoagulant effect is reversed by infusing calcium chloride before the blood returns to the patient.

▆ PSYCHOLOGICAL ASPECTS

The psychological impact of short-term renal replacement therapy is different from that of lifelong therapy. Even though the patient depends on a machine in both situations, in short-term therapy there is usually hope that the patient may recover renal function. Thus, concerns usually focus on the discomfort associated with insertion of the temporary vascular access and the dialysis treatment. Once these situations are handled, the patient and family then must cope with the uncertainty of how long renal failure will last and how long dialysis will be necessary.

Patients who develop chronic renal failure must deal with the fact that renal replacement therapy will be necessary for the rest of their lives. At first, patients usually deny a great deal of what is happening to them. This may continue for some time and prevent some patients from accepting necessary aspects of their treatment regimen. Other patients who feel considerably better after starting dialysis may enter a "honeymoon phase" and appear quite euphoric for a while. Patients should progress through the normal grieving stages and develop healthy coping mechanisms to deal with their long-term treatment.

Hemodialysis

In hemodialysis, water and excess waste products are removed from the blood as it is pumped through an extracorporeal circuit into a device called a dialyzer, or artificial kidney. The blood is in one compartment, and the dialysate is in another compartment. There, the blood flows through a semipermeable membrane. The semipermeable membrane is a thin, porous sheet made of a cellulose or synthetic material. The pore size of the membrane permits diffusion of low–molecular-weight substances such as urea, creatinine, and uric acid. Water molecules also are small and move freely through the membrane, but most plasma proteins, bacteria, and blood cells are too large to pass through the pores of the membrane. The difference in the concentration of the substances in the two compartments is called the *concentration gradient*.

The blood, which contains waste products, such as urea and creatinine, flows into the blood compartment of the dialyzer where it comes into contact with the dialysate, which contains no urea or creatinine. A maximum gradient is established so that these substances move from the blood to the dialysate. These waste products fall to more normal levels as the blood passes through the dialyzer repeatedly at a rate ranging from 200 to 400 mL/min over 2 to 4 hours.

Excess water is removed by a pressure differential created between the blood and fluid compartments. This pressure differential is aided by the action of the dialyzer pump and usually consists of positive pressure in the blood path and negative pressure in the dialysate compartment. This is the process of *ultrafiltration*. Hemodialysis accomplishes the following:

- Removes the by-products of protein metabolism, such as urea, creatinine, and uric acid
- Removes excess water
- Maintains or restores the body buffer system
- Maintains or restores the level of electrolytes in the body

◼◼ EQUIPMENT FEATURES

DIALYZERS

Dialyzers are designed to provide a parallel path through which blood and dialysate flow and to have a maximal membrane surface area between the two. Dialyzers vary in size, physical structure, and type of membrane used to construct the blood compartment. All these factors determine the potential efficiency of the dialyzer, which refers to its ability to remove water (ultrafiltration) and waste products (clearance).

The hollow-fiber dialyzer is the most commonly used configuration. In this design, the blood path flows through hollow fibers composed of semipermeable membrane, and the dialysate path is encased in a rigid plastic tube. Dialysate surrounds each hollow fiber. This provides a large surface area to cleanse the blood. Blood and dialysate flow in opposite directions from each other (called countercurrent flow) so that as blood travels through the dialyzer, it is constantly exposed to a fresh flow of dialysate. This countercurrent flow maintains the concentration gradient between the two compartments and provides the most efficient dialysis.

Synthetic membranes are used most commonly because they are highly biocompatible. They remove waste products efficiently, and there is little reaction between the blood and the membrane material. Because the synthetic membranes are highly permeable to water, they should only be used with a machine that controls the amount of ultrafiltration.

The size, efficiency, and patient's metabolic needs are considered when choosing a dialyzer. A large patient who is highly catabolic will benefit from use of a larger and more efficient dialyzer, while someone with a smaller body surface area or lower metabolic needs will benefit from a smaller, less permeable dialyzer.

DIALYSATE

The dialysate, or "bath," is a solution composed of water and the major electrolytes of normal serum. It is made in a clean system with filtered tap water and chemicals. It is not a sterile system, because bacteria are too large to pass through the membrane, and the potential for infection of the patient is minimal. However, because bacteria by-

---

Insights Into Clinical Research

Wagner C: Family needs of chronic hemodialysis patients: A comparison of perceptions of nurses and families. ANNA J 23:19–26, 1996

The purpose of the study was to determine the psychosocial needs of families of end-stage renal disease patients receiving hemodialysis as perceived by nurses and family members and to compare the perception of needs between the two groups. The author modified the Norris and Grove questionnaire so that it contained 33 statements about psychosocial needs and administered it to 10 family members and nine registered nurses.

The results of the study suggest that family members and nurses differ in what they perceive as important family needs. Six statements were significantly different between the two groups. All of these need statements were perceived as more important by family members than by nurses. Family members identified the needs for information and comfort as being very important. Nurses will need to assess family needs and become sensitive to the suggestions of family members and patients regarding their own needs.

products can cause pyrogenic reactions, especially in highly permeable membranes, water used to make dialysate must be bacteriologically safe. Dialysate concentrates usually are provided by commercial manufacturers. A standard bath generally is used for patients receiving chronic dialysis, but variations may be made to meet specific patient needs.

DIALYSATE DELIVERY SYSTEM

A single delivery unit provides dialysate for one patient, while a multiple delivery system may supply as many as 20 patient units. In either system, an automatic proportioning device and metering and monitoring devices ensure precise control of the water–concentrate ratio.

The single delivery unit usually is used in acute dialysis patients. It is a mobile unit, and dialysate requirements are tailored easily to meet individual patient needs.

ACCESSORY EQUIPMENT

Hardware used in most dialysis systems includes a blood pump, infusion pumps for heparin delivery, and monitoring devices for detection of unsafe temperatures, dialysate concentration, pressure changes, air, and blood leaks. All dialysis delivery systems consist of a single compact unit that includes the dialysate delivery equipment and blood monitoring components (Fig. 29–2). Disposable items used in addition to the artificial kidney include dialysis tubing for transport of blood between the dialyzer and patient, pressure transducers for protection of monitoring devices from blood exposure, and a normal saline bag and tubing for priming the system before use.

THE HUMAN COMPONENT

Expertise in the use of highly technical equipment is gained through theoretical and practical training in the clinical setting. The operation and monitoring of various kinds of dialysis equipment will differ, however. Reference to the manufacturer's instruction manuals will give the nurse guidelines for the safe operation of equipment. Although the technical aspects of hemodialysis may at first seem overwhelming, they can be learned fairly rapidly. A more critical aspect that takes longer to achieve is the understanding and knowledge that the nurse will use when caring for patients during dialysis.

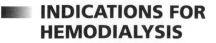

INDICATIONS FOR HEMODIALYSIS

Hemodialysis is indicated in chronic renal failure and for complications of ARF. These include uremia, fluid overload, acidosis, hyperkalemia, and drug overdose. Table 29–1 compares hemodialysis, continuous venovenous hemofiltration with dialysis (CVVH/D), and peritoneal dialysis.

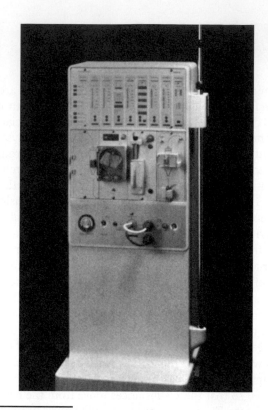

FIGURE 29-2
Hemodialysis delivery unit. Includes automatic blood pressure cuff, heparin infusion pump, and blood pump. Displays continuous readout of ultrafiltration goal, rate, and total fluid removed. Monitors dialysate temperature and conductivity; can vary dialysate sodium concentration. (Fresenius 2008E, Fresenius VSA, Inc., Concord, CA)

CONTRAINDICATIONS TO HEMODIALYSIS

Hemodialysis may be contraindicated in patients with coagulopathies because the extracorporeal circuit needs to be heparinized. It may also be difficult to perform when patients have extremely low cardiac output and are sensitive to changes in volume status. For critically ill patients such as these, peritoneal dialysis may be the therapy of choice, even though it is less efficient. In addition, intermittent hemodialysis may not keep up with the metabolic needs of a highly catabolic patient. In such a case, a CRRT would probably be chosen.

ASSESSMENT AND MANAGEMENT

The degree and complexity of problems arising during hemodialysis vary among patients and depend on many factors. Important variables are the patient's diagnosis, stage of illness, age, other medical problems, fluid and electrolyte balance, and emotional state. Because more older adults are receiving dialysis, it also is important to consider the nor-

TABLE 29-1
**Comparison of Hemodialysis, CVVH/D, and Peritoneal Dialysis
as Treatment for Acute Renal Failure**

	Hemodialysis	CVVH/D	Peritoneal
Access	AV fistula or graft; dual-lumen venous catheter	Same as hemodialysis	Temporary or permanent peritoneal catheter
Heparin requirements	Systemic heparinization or frequent saline flushes	Same as hemodialysis	May only need heparin intraperitoneally; is not absorbed systemically
Length of treatment	3–4 h, three to five times per week, depending on patient acuity	Continuous through the day; may last as many days as needed	Continuous (cycled) or intermittent exchanges; time between exchanges, 1–6 h
Advantages	Quick, efficient removal of metabolic wastes and excess fluid; useful for drug overdoses and poisonings	Best choice for the hypercatabolic patient who receives large amounts of IV fluids; good for patients with fragile cardiac status because less blood is outside the body than with hemodialysis	Continuous removal of wastes and fluid, better hemodynamic stability, fewer dietary restrictions
Disadvantages	May require frequent vascular access procedures; places strain on a compromised cardiovascular system; potential blood loss from bleeding or clotted lines	Requires vascular access procedures; potential blood loss from clotting or equipment leaks; uses an extra piece of equipment	Contraindicated after abdominal surgery or in presence of many scars; waste products may be removed too slowly in a catabolic patient; danger of peritonitis

mal decreases in cardiac function and other system changes due to the aging process.

Predialysis Phase

A predialysis assessment is the first step in managing the patient having hemodialysis. It consists of a review of the patient's history and clinical findings, response to previous dialysis treatment, laboratory results, consultation with other caregivers, and the nurse's direct assessment of the patient.

The nurse evaluates fluid balance before dialysis so that corrective measures may be initiated at the beginning of the procedure. Blood pressure, pulse, weight, intake and output, tissue turgor, and other symptoms will assist the nurse in estimating fluid overload or depletion. Monitoring tools, such as pulmonary artery pressure, also help determine cardiovascular fluid load.

The term dry or ideal weight is used to express the weight at which fluid volume is in a normal range for a patient who is free of the symptoms of fluid imbalance. It provides a guideline for fluid removal or replacement. The figure is not absolute. It requires frequent review and revision, especially in patients receiving dialysis in whom frequent changes in weight occur.

After reviewing the data and while consulting with the physician, the dialysis nurse will establish objectives for the dialysis treatment. The objectives will vary from one dialysis to the next in the patient whose condition may change rapidly. For example, fluid removal may take pre-

cedence over correction of an electrolyte imbalance or vice versa.

Anxiety and apprehension, especially during the first dialysis, may contribute to change in blood pressure, restlessness, and gastrointestinal upsets. The presence of a competent and caring nurse during dialysis may increase the patient's sense of security enough to avoid the need for an antianxiety drug that might precipitate changes in vital signs.

A basic explanation of the procedure and its place in the total care plan for the patient also may allay some of the anxiety experienced by the patient and family. They must understand that dialysis is being used to support normal body function rather than to "cure" the kidney problem.

Procedure Phase

The nurse begins the procedure with an equipment check, as outlined in the accompanying display. After the predialysis preparation and a safety check of equipment, the nurse is ready to begin hemodialysis. Access to the circulatory system is gained by one of several options: a dual-lumen catheter, an AV fistula, or graft. The dual-lumen catheter is opened under aseptic conditions according to institutional policy. Two large-gauge (15- or 16-gauge) needles are needed to cannulate a graft or fistula.

Figure 29–3 illustrates the hemodialysis circuit. After vascular access is established, blood begins to flow, assisted by the blood pump. The part of the disposable circuit before the dialyzer is designated the arterial line, both to distinguish the blood in it as blood that has not yet reached the dialyzer and in reference to needle placement. The arterial needle is placed closest to the AV anastomosis in a graft or fistula to maximize blood flow. A clamped saline bag always is attached to the circuit just before the blood pump. In episodes of hypotension, blood flow from the patient can be clamped while the saline is opened and allowed to infuse rapidly to correct blood pressure. Blood transfusions and plasma expanders also can be attached to the circuit at this point and allowed to drip in, assisted by the blood pump. Heparin infusions may be located either before or after the blood pump, depending on the equipment in use.

The dialyzer is the next important component of the circuit. Blood flows into the blood compartment of the dialyzer, where exchange of fluid and waste products takes place. Blood leaving the dialyzer passes through an air and foam detector that will clamp off and shut down the blood pump should any air be detected. At this point in the pathway, any medications that can be given during dialysis are infused through a medication port. However, unless otherwise ordered, most medications are held until after dialysis.

Blood that has passed through the dialyzer returns to the patient through the venous, or postdialyzer, line.

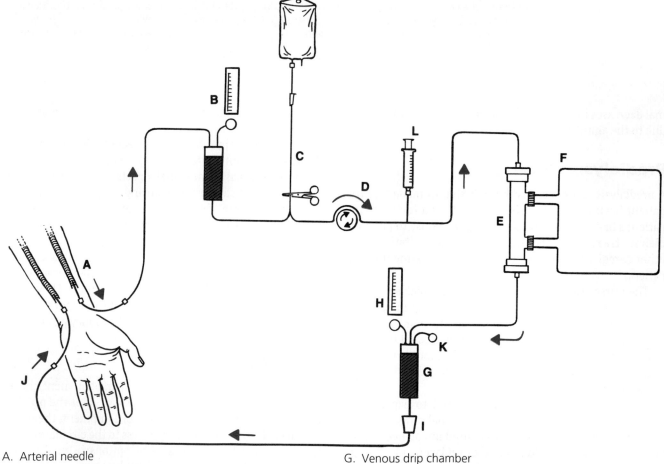

A. Arterial needle
B. Arterial pressure monitor
C. Saline line
D. Blood pump
E. Dialyzer
F. Dialysate delivery system
G. Venous drip chamber
H. Venous pressure monitor
I. Air and foam detector and clamp
J. Venous needle
K. Medication administration port
L. Heparin infusion

FIGURE 29-3
Hemodialysis circuit.

After the prescribed treatment time, dialysis is terminated by clamping off blood from the patient, opening the saline line, and rinsing the circuit to return the patient's blood.

A dialysis nurse is in constant attendance during acute hemodialysis. Blood pressure and pulse are recorded at least every half hour when the patient's condition is stable. All machine pressures and flow rates are checked and recorded on a regular basis. The nurse assesses the patient's responses to fluid and solute removal and the condition and function of the patient's vascular access. Standard Precautions, one tier of Centers for Disease Control and Prevention Isolation Guidelines, are followed. A protective face shield and gloves are worn by the nurse performing hemodialysis because of the risk of exposure to blood. The dialysis nurse and critical care nurse work together to care for the patient and therefore must coordinate their specific patient care responsibilities.

Postdialysis Phase

The results of a dialysis treatment can be determined by assessing the amount of fluid removed and the degree to which electrolyte and acid–base imbalances have been corrected. This includes postdialysis weight and laboratory results. Blood drawn immediately postdialysis may show falsely low levels of electrolytes, urea nitrogen, and creatinine. The process of equilibration is thought to continue for some time after dialysis, as these substances move from inside the cell to the plasma.

◼ HEMODIALYSIS APPLIED TO OTHER THERAPIES

The technical equipment and knowledge needed to perform hemodialysis often are applied to other therapies that involve an extracorporeal blood process, such as hemoperfusion and therapeutic apheresis. *Hemoperfusion* is used primarily for the treatment of drug overdose. Blood is pumped from the body and perfused through a column of charcoal or other absorbent materials that bind the drug. This leads to a rapid reduction in serum levels and avoids potential tissue damage caused by an abnormally high drug level. This therapy is particularly useful for drugs that are fat bound or whose molecular structure is too large to be removed by hemodialysis. A hemodialysis blood pump and air detector often are used with hemoperfusion cartridges and tubing.

Therapeutic plasma exchange, or *apheresis*, is another therapy that may be performed using standard hemodialysis equipment in conjunction with a plasma separator cell and replacement fluids. Apheresis is used to treat diseases caused or complicated by circulating immune complexes or their abnormal proteins. During the procedure, the patient's whole blood is separated into its major components, and the offending components are removed.

◼ COMPLICATIONS IN HEMODIALYSIS

DIALYSIS DISEQUILIBRIUM

Uremia must be corrected slowly to prevent disequilibrium syndrome, which is a set of signs and symptoms ranging from headache, nausea, restlessness, and mild mental impairment to vomiting, confusion, agitation, and seizures. This is thought to occur as the plasma concentration of solutes, such as urea nitrogen, is lowered. Because of the blood–brain barrier, solutes are removed much more slowly from brain cells. Therefore, plasma becomes hypotonic in relation to the brain cells. This results in a shift of water from plasma to the brain cells and causes cerebral edema and symptoms of disequilibrium syndrome. This syndrome can be avoided by dialyzing patients for short periods of time, such as 1 to 2 hours on 3 or 4 consecutive days.[1]

HYPOVOLEMIA

Fluid overload is treated during dialysis by removing excess water. Because this removal depends on shifting fluid from other body compartments to the vascular space, care must taken to avoid removing fluid so rapidly during dialysis that it leads to volume depletion. Excessive fluid removal may lead to hypotension, and little is gained if intravenous fluids are given to correct the problem. Thus, it is better to reduce the volume overload over two or three dialyses, unless pulmonary congestion is life threatening.

HYPOTENSION

Normal saline in bolus amounts of 100 to 200 mL is used to correct hypotension. Dialysis machines now aid in preventing hypotension because the amount of ultrafiltration is controlled at the push of a button. It is also possible to vary the sodium concentration of dialysate. A higher sodium level in the dialysate means that less sodium will be removed from the blood. A higher serum sodium will assist the body as it shifts fluid from the interstitial to the intravascular compartment. Blood volume expanders, such as albumin, sometimes are used in patients with a low serum protein.

The use of antihypertensive drugs in the dialysis patient may precipitate hypotension during dialysis. To avoid this, standard practice in many dialysis units is to omit antihypertensive drugs 4 to 6 hours before dialysis. Fluids and sodium restrictions are more desirable controls for hypertension. Sedatives and tranquilizers also may cause hypotension and should be avoided if possible.

HYPERTENSION

Fluid overload, disequilibrium syndrome, renin response to ultrafiltration, and anxiety are the most frequent causes of hypertension during dialysis. Hypertension during dialysis is usually caused by sodium and water excess. This can be confirmed by comparing the patient's present weight to ideal or dry weight. If fluid overload is the cause of hypertension, ultrafiltration usually will bring about a reduction in the blood pressure.

Some patients who may be normotensive before dialysis become hypertensive during dialysis. The rise may occur either gradually or abruptly. Although the cause is not well understood, it may be the result of renin production in response to ultrafiltration and an increase in renal ischemia. These patients must be carefully monitored because the vasoconstriction caused by the renin response is limited. Once a decrease in blood volume surpasses the ability to maintain blood pressure through vasoconstriction, hypotension can occur precipitously.

MUSCLE CRAMPS

Muscle cramps can occur during dialysis as a result of excess fluid removal, which results in diminished intravascular volume and reduced muscle perfusion. Cramps are treated by lowering the rate of ultrafiltration, giving a saline bolus of 100 to 200 mL, and either administering 10 mL of 23.4% saline or increasing the sodium content of the dialysate.[2]

DYSRHYTHMIAS AND ANGINA

Dysrhythmias and angina may occur in patients with underlying cardiac disease in response to fluid removal. Decreasing the rate of fluid removal may help. Medication may be needed to control the rhythm.

■ TROUBLESHOOTING RELATED TO HEMODIALYSIS

One of the major objectives of a dialysis unit is to prevent complications resulting from the treatment itself. Hemodialysis involves the use of highly technical equipment. The efficiency of the dialysis and the patient's comfort and safety are compromised if the patient and the equipment are not adequately monitored. Mechanical monitors provide a margin of safety but should not replace the observations and actions of the nurse. Monitoring devices are designed to monitor many parameters, the most important of which are flow, concentration, and temperature of the dialysate; flow and leakage of blood; and air in the dialysis circuit.

BLOOD FLOW

Changes in blood flow rate are the most common reason for alarms. An adequate rate of blood flow is essential to achieve the clearance goals for the dialysis. Hemodialysis blood flow rates range from 200 to 500 mL/min. Lower flow rates or a flow rate that is frequently interrupted because of a poorly functioning vascular access will prolong the treatment and make it less efficient.

Factors that influence blood flow rate are blood pressure, fistula and catheter function, and the extracorporeal circuit. A manometer connected to the drip chamber is used to measure the pressure in the blood lines. Changes in blood line pressures are transmitted to the drip chamber and register on the manometer as high- or low-pressure alarms.

A high-pressure alarm indicates a problem in the venous blood line, a clot in the venous needle or catheter, or a clotted vein. If clotting is suspected in any portion of the venous line or blood access, immediate flushing with normal saline solution may help to determine where the clot is and whether the clot can be removed, thereby reducing the pressure. A low-pressure alarm reflects an obstruction to blood flow from the patient. Arterial spasm, clotting, displacement of a fistula needle, and a drop in blood pressure are possible causes.

BLOOD LEAKS

A blood leak detector is invaluable when outflow dialysate is not visible, as in a single-pass delivery system. One type of blood leak detector is a color-sensitive photocell that picks up color variations in the outflow dialysate. Any foreign material, such as blood, will be detected, and an alarm will be set off. Because false alarms sometimes are set off by air bubbles, the nurse will check the dialysate visually for a gross leak and with a hemastick for smaller leaks.

Dialysis usually is discontinued immediately with a gross leak. Whether or not the blood is returned to the patient is either a matter of unit policy or a determination based on individual circumstances. If the patient is severely anemic, the risk of losing the blood in the dialyzer may outweigh the risk of a reaction to dialysate-contaminated blood. Sometimes minor leaks, in which there is no visible blood in the dialysate and only a small hemastick reaction, seal over, and dialysis is continued.

AIR IN THE CIRCUIT

The risk of air embolism is one of the most serious patient safety problems in the hemodialysis unit. Air can enter the patient's circulation through defective blood tubing, faulty blood line connections, vented intravenous fluid containers, or accidental displacement of the arterial needle.

The use of air and foam detectors and nonvented plastic fluid containers has minimized air embolus risks, but the emphasis is on preventing potential problems by attending to technical details and visual monitoring.

Continuous Renal Replacement Therapies

In CRRT, blood circulates outside the body through a highly porous filter. This process is similar to hemodialysis in that water, electrolytes, and small- to middle-sized molecules are removed by ultrafiltration. It is accompanied by a simultaneous reinfusion of a physiological solution. This process occurs continuously for an extended period.

Continuous renal replacement therapies include continuous AV hemofiltration, continuous AV hemofiltration with dialysis, continuous venovenous hemofiltration (CVVH), and CVVH/D. This discussion focuses on CVVH and primarily on CVVH/D because these therapies are replacing the AV procedures.

The same type of venous catheters as those used for short-term hemodialysis are used for CVVH and CVVH/D. The extracorporeal circuit is similar to the artificial kidney, although the hemofilter has somewhat different ultrafiltration properties. A pump is added to assist blood flow. Because of the ultrafiltration rate and the patient's hemodynamic status, the amount of replacement fluid generally is ordered based on an hourly fluid loss goal. The amount and composition of fluid replacement are usually customized for the patient and may be infused either before or after the filter, depending on institutional practice. When peritoneal dialysate is added to the CVVH process, it is called CVVH/D. Adding the dialysate increases the ability to remove wastes. Therefore, it is used when uremia must be aggressively managed, such as with the highly catabolic patient. CVVH and CVVH/D can be performed by critical care nurses who are not trained in hemodialysis.

Ideally, continuous renal replacement therapies are used for patients with a high risk for hemodynamic instability who would not tolerate the rapid fluid shifts that occur with hemodialysis and for those who require large amounts of hourly intravenous fluids or parenteral nutrition. It is also used when the patient needs more than the usual 3- to 4-hour hemodialysis treatment to correct the metabolic imbalances of ARF. CVVH is used when patients primarily need excess fluid removed, whereas CVVH/D is used when patients also need waste products removed due to uremia. Comparisons among hemodialysis, CVVH/D, and peritoneal dialysis are made earlier in the chapter in Table 29–1.

■ EQUIPMENT FEATURES

A typical CVVH/D setup is shown in Figure 29–4. Blood exits the body through the arterial limb of the vascular access. The first infusion line shown is for heparin. Located just prior to the blood pump is a line that measures pressure in the prefilter portion of the circuit, known as the arterial pressure. The next step in the path is the blood pump, which propels blood into the filter. An infusion port just after the blood pump is usually connected to normal saline for flushing the circuit. A bag of dialysate is shown flowing through the filter and surrounding the hollow fibers where the blood travels. As the dialysate exits the filter, it passes through a sensor that will detect microscopic amounts of blood, thus warning of filter rupture. The dialysate and excess fluid removed from the patient are collected in a graduated collection device for easy measurement. Meanwhile, the blood exits the filter and passes into a drip chamber, where air and foam will be trapped instead of entering the patient's circulation. The drip chamber also contains a line to which a syringe can be attached to raise and lower the blood level and another line that measures pressure in the postfilter section of the circuit, known as venous pressure. A clamp is located after the drip chamber and will automatically engage if air tries to pass through. The arterial and venous pressure transducers are protected by a disposable filter. As blood returns to the body, replacement fluid is infused. In some systems, the line for replacement fluid is placed before the blood pump so it can be infused before the blood reaches the filter. The total amount of blood in the circuit is about 150 mL.

■ ASSESSMENT AND MANAGEMENT

Preprocedure Phase

Before starting therapy, an inventory is taken of all intravascular lines. If it becomes necessary to administer other intravenous infusions through the same line, a pharmacist should be consulted regarding compatibilities. If the arterial port of the CVVH/D is too close to other infusion ports, a portion of the infused medication may be lost by being pulled out of the circulatory system and into the CVVH/D circuit. Because of this, certain medications may need dose adjustments and blood level monitoring. This may occur with vasopressors, such as epinephrine and dopamine, and with fentanyl. A pharmacist can assist with changing dosages.[3]

Because the filters used in the continuous therapies are much more porous than those used in hemodialysis and the circuit does not contain a mechanism to control the amount of fluid removed, the potential exists for uncontrolled losses of a large amount of fluid. Because of this, an hourly fluid balance goal is set by the nephrologist. Fluid will be replaced each hour in varying amounts to achieve the goal. An example is given in the accompanying display.

Procedure Phase

Equipment is checked as outlined in the display earlier in this chapter. Before therapy is initiated, the lines and filter

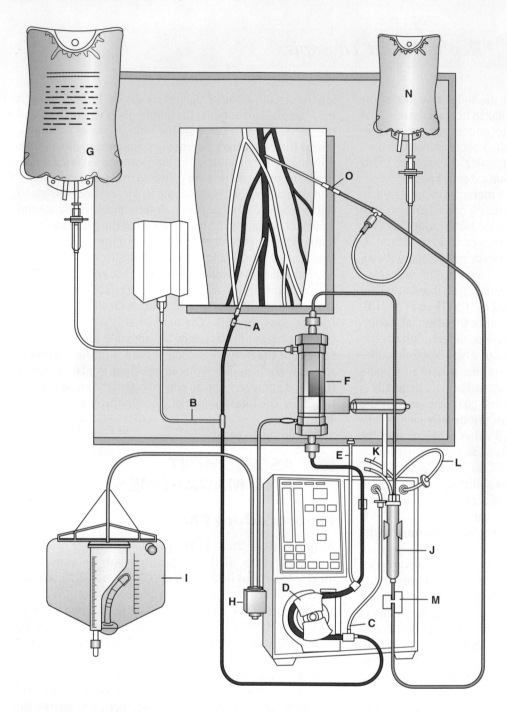

FIGURE 29-4
Continuous venovenous hemofiltration with dialysis (CVVH/D). (Baxter Health Care Corporation, Renal Division, McGaw Park, IL)

A. Blood exiting the body
B. Heparin infusion
C. Arterial pressure monitor (prefilter pressure)
D. Blood pump
E. Saline infusion line (saline not shown here)
F. Filter
G. Dialysate
H. Blood leak detector
I. Graduated collection device
J. Air and foam detector
K. Syringe line
L. Venous pressure monitor (postfilter pressure)
M. Clamp
N. Replacement fluid
O. Blood returns to body

are primed to expel air from the circuit. Arterial and venous lines are connected to the corresponding port of the access catheter, and the blood pump is turned on. Blood will start to flow through the tubing. Ultrafiltration will begin to produce plasma water (ultrafiltrate) that will start to flow into the collection device. Most experts recommend controlling the amount of ultrafiltrate by raising or lowering the collection device until the desired hourly rate of ultrafiltration is achieved. Blood flow rates through the circuit average 100 mL/h, and the standard dialysate flow rate is 1 L/h. Substances are adequately cleared when ultrafiltration produces 500 to 600 mL/h of ultrafiltrate.

Anticoagulation is administered as therapy begins. Low-dose heparin is the standard anticoagulant used in patients at low risk for bleeding. It may be used along with saline flushes to prevent circuit clotting. Saline flushes without low-dose heparin may be used when the patient has a low platelet count. A typical protocol is to flush 100 mL through the circuit every half hour. Another method of anticoagulation is to infuse 4% trisodium citrate before the filter. This will anticoagulate only the extracorporeal part of the circuit. It chelates calcium, which is then replaced through infusion in a central line. For this process to be effective, the dialysate solution must be calcium free. The patient will need to be closely monitored to prevent hypercalcemia or hypocalcemia.[3]

Hourly maintenance of the CVVH/D system includes measuring blood and dialysate flows, calculating net ultrafiltration and replacement fluid, titrating anticoagulants, assessing the integrity of the vascular access, and monitoring hemodynamic parameters and the blood circuit pressures. The nephrologist will set a goal for hourly fluid balance, and the critical care nurse is responsible to see that it is met. Interventions in monitoring fluid and electrolyte balance are listed in the accompanying display. By comparing total intake and output, the hourly net fluid balance is calculated. The amount of replacement fluid is determined by the difference between desired and net fluid balance. Fluid balance and replacement should be recorded on a bedside flow sheet.[3]

Replacement fluid may be infused prefilter or postfilter. Each system has advantages and disadvantages. When fluid is given prefilter, it decreases blood viscosity and increases blood flow through the filter. This enhances ultrafiltrate (plasma fluid) production and solute removal and decreases the frequency of clotting. The disadvantage is that this system increases the need for fluid replacement, and calculating fluid output is more complicated. If replacement fluid is given postfilter, there is less total fluid loss and less need for replacement fluid. There is an increased incidence of filter clotting and decreased filter life. The methods chosen will depend on the system used and institutional preference.[3]

Electrolytes, urea nitrogen, creatinine, and glucose levels are drawn before the procedure is started and then at a least twice daily. Electrolyte imbalances can be corrected by altering the composition of the replacement fluid or by custom mixing the dialysate.[3] Anticoagulation is monitored by checking activated clotting times or PT and PTT. Although frequency is determined by each institution, it is not unusual to check clotting times every 1 or 2 hours to prevent clotting of the filter and blood lines.[3]

There is no one policy that describes the optimal time to change the circuit. Many institutions put a 24- to 48-hour limit on circuit life, although there are reports of filters lasting an average of 4 days. System performance is monitored by checking the amount of urea nitrogen in the filtrate compared with the amount of urea nitrogen prefilter. A decreasing ratio indicates inadequate performance. A decreasing rate of ultrafiltration and increases in the circuit's venous pressure indicate clotting in the filter.[3]

Treatment may be terminated temporarily to transport the patient to a diagnostic test or surgery or fix a mechanical problem with the circuit or vascular access. Treatment may also be terminated if the patient shows signs of recovering renal function. When it is determined that continuous therapy can be terminated, the blood is returned to the patient. First, the ultrafiltrate outlet is clamped, and the dialysate is turned off. Then, anticoagulation is turned off, and the blood is returned to the patient through a saline flush. Once the lines are clear, they are disconnected from the vascular access. Then the vascular access is heparinized per unit policy. Documentation should include fluid balance, condition of the access, and the patient's response to treatment. The tubing and filter are disposable. When working with the circuit and ultrafiltrate, the nurse uses Universal Precautions.

TROUBLESHOOTING RELATED TO CONTINUOUS VENOVENOUS HEMOFILTRATION WITH DIALYSIS

HYPOTENSION

If blood pressure and intravascular filling pressures fall below optimal, the nurse can increase the infusion rate of replacement fluid or give a normal saline bolus of 100 to 200 mL. At the same time, the ultrafiltrate collection device should be raised to decrease ultrafiltration until pressures stabilize. An infusion of 5% albumin may also help stabilize blood pressure. If this situation persists, the nephrologist should be consulted to adjust the net ultrafiltration goal.

ACCESS PROBLEMS

Blood flows used in CVVH/D are much lower than for hemodialysis, making it more likely that a catheter will provide adequate flow. However, a poorly functioning access will jeopardize the entire CVVH/D procedure. Often, the position of the patient's extremity affects blood flow. If the access is in a limb, it should be gently immobilized. An obstruction, such as a clot or kink in the arterial lumen of the catheter, will result in less blood being delivered to the circuit and will manifest as lowered arterial and venous pressures. Clots or kinks in the venous lumen of the catheter will raise venous pressures as blood tries to return against an obstruction. The treatment may be temporarily halted while the nurse manually flushes each lumen to determine patency. If blood flow still cannot be established, the nephrologist should be notified immediately to replace the catheter.

CLOTTING

An early sign of filter clotting is a reduced rate of ultrafiltration, which cannot be corrected by increasing blood flow or by lowering the collection device. As clotting progresses, venous pressure rises, arterial pressure drops, and the blood lines appear dark. Clotting times will be low. A saline bolus can help to determine the location and extent of clotting. It may be possible to return some to the patient's blood before changing the circuit, but if clotting is extensive this should not be attempted.

AIR IN THE CIRCUIT

If the connections are loose, or a prefilter infusion line runs dry, air will disrupt the system by collecting in the drip chamber and setting off the air detector alarm and triggering the clamp to close on the venous line. The nurse should assess the circuit's integrity to correct the source of air. Before resetting the line clamp, the nurse should make sure all bubbles have been tapped out of the drip chamber, all connections are tight, and there is no danger of air getting into the patient's bloodstream.[3]

BLOOD LEAKS

Blood will appear in the ultrafiltrate if there is any rupture inside the filter. The blood leak alarm will sound and the blood pump will stop. Testing the ultrafiltrate with a dipstick can verify a microscopic leak. Blood can be safely returned to the patient as long as there is no gross blood in the ultrafiltrate. Then the circuit should be changed. A gross leak will be readily identifiable. Blood should not be returned to the patient, and the patient's hematocrit should be checked to determine the need for transfusion.

Some patients experience chills and lowered body temperature while their blood is circulating outside the body. If this happens, it may be advisable to use a blood warmer to warm either the dialysate or the replacement fluid.

CLINICAL APPLICATION:
Nursing Intervention Guidelines
Maintaining Blood Flow Through CVVH/D Circuit

- Check clotting times at initiation and at the prescribed intervals throughout treatment.
- Flush system as often as needed with saline to assess appearance of filter and circuit.
- Monitor ultrafiltration rates, venous and arterial pressure, and color of blood in circuit.
- If system is clotting, return as much blood as possible to the patient before changing the system.

Peritoneal Dialysis

Peritoneal dialysis and hemodialysis accomplish the same function and operate on the same principle of diffusion. In peritoneal dialysis, however, the peritoneum is the semipermeable membrane, and osmosis is used to remove fluid, rather than the pressure differentials used in hemodialysis.

Intermittent peritoneal dialysis is an effective alternative method of treating ARF when hemodialysis is not available or when access to the bloodstream is not possible. It sometimes is used as an initial treatment for renal failure while the patient is being evaluated for a hemodialysis program.

Table 29–1 earlier in the chapter compares hemodialysis, CVVH/D, and peritoneal dialysis.

Peritoneal dialysis has some advantages over hemodialysis:

- The required technical equipment and supplies are less complicated and more available.
- There is less need for highly skilled personnel.
- The adverse effects associated with the more efficient hemodialysis are minimized.

The latter may be important for patients with severe cardiac disease, who cannot tolerate rapid hemodynamic changes.

There also are a few disadvantages associated with peritoneal dialysis. It requires more time to remove metabolic wastes adequately and to restore electrolyte and fluid balance than does hemodialysis. In addition, repeated treatments may lead to peritonitis, and long periods of immobility may result in complications, such as pulmonary congestion and venous stasis. Because fluid is introduced into the peritoneal cavity, peritoneal dialysis is contraindicated in patients who have existing peritonitis, in those who have undergone recent or extensive abdominal surgery, and in those who have abdominal adhesions. In the event of a cardiac arrest, the patient's abdomen should be drained immediately to maximize the efficiency of chest compressions.

■ EQUIPMENT FEATURES

SOLUTIONS

As in hemodialysis, peritoneal dialysis solutions contain "ideal" concentrations of electrolytes but lack urea, creatinine, and other substances that are to be removed. Unlike dialysate used in hemodialysis, solutions must be sterile. Dextrose concentrations of the solutions vary; a 1.5%, 2.5%, or 4.25% dextrose solution can be used. Use of 2.5% or 4.25% solutions usually is reserved for more fluid removal and occasionally for better solute clearance. If peritoneal dialysate does not contain potassium, a small amount of potassium chloride may have to be added to the dialysate to prevent hypokalemia. The patient's serum potassium must be monitored closely to regulate the amount of potassium to be added.

AUTOMATED PERITONEAL DIALYSIS SYSTEMS

Automated peritoneal dialysis systems have built-in monitors and a system of automatic timing devices that cycle the infusion and removal of peritoneal fluid. For this reason, they are called cyclers. Cyclers may be used in the intensive care setting. They are convenient to use because they eliminate the need to change solution bags constantly. Most cyclers also have a log that retains cycle by cycle information on ultrafiltration. Setting up the cycler requires attaching the appropriate strength of large-volume (5 L) solution bags

to the cycler tubing, using aseptic technique. The cycler is programmed to deliver a set amount of dialysate per exchange for a certain length of time. When the time is up, the patient will automatically be drained and then filled again. Cyclers are usually used when patients have a permanent peritoneal access device.

■ ASSESSMENT AND MANAGEMENT

Preliminary Phase

1. Prepare the patient for catheter insertion and the dialysis procedure by giving a thorough explanation of the procedure. A consent form may be signed according to hospital policy.
2. Ask the patient to empty the bladder just prior to the procedure to avoid accidental puncture with the trocar.
3. Give a preoperative medication, as ordered, to enhance relaxation during the procedure.
4. Warm the dialyzing fluid to body temperature or slightly warmer, using a device manufactured solely for this purpose. It is not recommended that peritoneal dialysate be warmed in microwave ovens due to uneven heating of the fluid and inconsistency from one microwave to another.
5. Take and record baseline vital signs, such as temperature, pulse, respirations, and weight. An in-bed scale is ideal for frequent monitoring of the patient's weight.
6. Take the patient's history, identifying abdominal surgery or trauma.
7. Examine the abdomen before the catheter is inserted.
8. Follow specific orders, obtained before the procedure, regarding fluid removal, replacement, and drug administration.

Procedure Phase

The following items are needed for the procedure:

- Peritoneal dialysis administration set
- Peritoneal dialysis catheter set, which includes the catheter, a connecting tube for connecting the catheter to the administration set, and a metal stylet
- Trocar set of the physician's choice
- Ancillary drugs: local anesthetic solution—2% lidocaine, aqueous heparin—1,000 U/mL, potassium chloride, broad-spectrum antibiotics

The physician makes a small midline incision just below the umbilicus under sterile conditions. A trocar is inserted through the incision into the peritoneal cavity. The obturator is removed, and the catheter is inserted and secured.

The dialysis solution flows into the abdominal cavity by gravity as rapidly as possible (5–10 minutes). If it flows in too slowly, the catheter may need to be repositioned. When the solution is infused, the tubing is clamped, and the solution remains in the abdominal cavity for 30 to 45 minutes. Next, the solution bottles or bags are placed below the abdominal cavity, and the fluid is drained out of the peritoneal cavity by gravity. If the system is patent and the catheter well placed, the fluid will drain in a steady, forceful stream (Fig. 29–5). Drainage should take no more than 20 minutes.

This cycle is repeated continuously for the prescribed number of hours, which varies from 12 to 36, depending on the purpose of the treatment, the patient's condition, and the proper functioning of the system. Dialysis effluent is considered a contaminated fluid, and gloves should be worn while handling it.

Ongoing Phase

Following the procedure, the nurse continues the following interventions:

- Maintain accurate records of intake and output and weights obtained from the same scale for assessment of volume depletion or overload.
- Monitor blood pressure and pulse frequently. Orthostatic blood pressure changes and increased pulse rate are valuable clues that help the nurse evaluate the patient's volume status.

- Detect signs and symptoms of peritonitis early. Low-grade fever, abdominal pain, and cloudy peritoneal fluid all are possible signs of infection.
- Maintain sterility of the peritoneal system. Masks and sterile gloves must be worn while the abdominal dressing is being changed. Solution bags or bottles should be changed in as controlled a physical environment as possible to avoid contamination (eg, avoiding areas of high traffic and high air flow).
- Detect and correct technical difficulties early before they result in physiological problems. Slow outflow of the peritoneal fluid may indicate early problems with the patency of the peritoneal catheter.
- Prevent complications of bed rest and provide an environment that will assist the patient in accepting bed rest for prolonged periods.
- Prevent constipation. Difficult or infrequent defecation will decrease the clearance of waste products and cause the patient more discomfort and distention.

■■■ COMPLICATIONS

Complications arising from peritoneal dialysis may be technical or physiological.

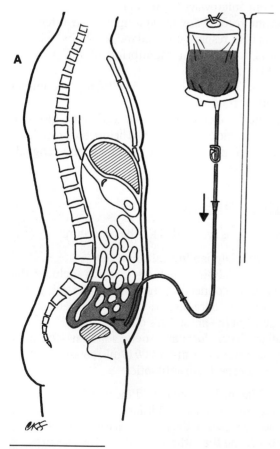

FIGURE 29-5
Periotoneal dialysis. (**A**) Dialysate flowing in. (**B**) Dialysate draining.

Technical Complications

Incomplete Recovery of Fluid

The fluid that is removed should equal or exceed the amount inserted. Commercially prepared dialysate contains approximately 1,000 to 2,000 mL of fluid. If after several exchanges, the volume drained is less (by 500 mL or more) than the amount inserted, an evaluation must be made. Signs of fluid retention include abdominal distention or complaints of fullness. The most accurate indication of the amount of unrecovered fluid is weight.

If the fluid drains slowly, the catheter tip may be buried in the omentum or clogged with fibrin. Turning the patient from side to side, elevating the head of the bed, and gently massaging the abdomen may facilitate drainage.

If fibrin or blood exists in the outflow drainage, heparin will need to be added to the dialysate. The specific dose, which is ordered by the physician, will be 500 to 1,000 U/L.

Leakage Around the Catheter

Superficial leakage after surgery may be controlled with extra sutures and a decrease in the amount of dialysate instilled into the peritoneum. Increases in intra-abdominal pressure also may cause dialysate leaks. Therefore, continued vomiting, coughing, and jarring movements should be avoided during the initial postoperative period. The abdominal dressing must be checked frequently to detect leakage. Dialysate leaks can be distinguished from other clear fluids by checking with a dextrose test strip. Dialysate will test positive because of its dextrose content. A leaking catheter should be corrected because it acts as a pathway for bacteria to enter the peritoneum.

Blood-Tinged Peritoneal Fluid

Blood-tinged peritoneal fluid is expected in the initial outflow but should clear after a few exchanges. Gross bleeding at any time is an indication of a more serious problem and should be investigated immediately.

Physiological Complications

Peritonitis

Peritonitis is a serious but manageable complication of peritoneal dialysis. Signs of peritonitis include low-grade fever, abdominal pain when fluid is being inserted, and cloudy peritoneal drainage fluid. Early detection and treatment will lessen the patient's discomfort and prevent more serious complications.

Treatment should begin as soon as a sample of peritoneal fluid is obtained for culture and sensitivity. The patient then should be started on a broad-spectrum antibiotic, which usually is added to the dialysate solution, although it also can be given intravenously. Depending on the severity of the infection, the patient's condition should improve dramatically after 8 hours of antibiotic therapy.

Catheter Infection

During the daily dressing change, the nurse examines the exit site closely for signs of infection, such as tenderness, redness, and drainage around the catheter. In the absence of peritonitis, a catheter infection generally is treated with an oral, broad-spectrum antibiotic.

Hypotension

Hypotension may occur if excessive fluid is removed. Vital signs are monitored frequently, especially if a hypertonic solution is used. Lying and sitting blood pressure readings are especially useful for evaluating fluid status. A progressive drop in blood pressure and weight are signs of fluid deficit.

Hypertension and Fluid Overload

If all the dialysate solution is not removed in each cycle, hypertension and fluid overload may occur. If there is hypertension and a weight increase, the nurse assesses catheter patency and notes the exact amount of fluid in the dialysate bottle. Some manufacturers add 50 mL to a 1,000-mL bottle. Over a period of hours, this can make a considerable difference.

The nurse also observes the patient for signs of respiratory distress and pulmonary congestion. In the absence of other symptoms of fluid overload, hypertension may be the result of anxiety and apprehension. Nonpharmacological measures to reduce anxiety are preferable to administering sedatives and tranquilizers.

Blood Urea Nitrogen and Creatinine

Blood urea nitrogen and creatinine levels are closely monitored because they help evaluate the effectiveness of the dialysis. When levels remain high, it indicates inadequate clearance of these waste products.

Hypokalemia

The serum potassium is monitored closely, because hypokalemia is a common complication of peritoneal dialysis. When the serum potassium level is low, potassium chloride is added to the dialysate.

CLINICAL APPLICATION:
Nursing Intervention Guidelines
Preventing Infection During Peritoneal Dialysis

- Maintain aseptic technique throughout dialysis procedure.
- Use sealed plastic dialysate bags.
- Change dialysis tubing regularly per protocol.
- Swab or soak tubing connections and injection ports with bactericidal solution before adding medications or breaking closed system.
- Assess patient continuously for signs and symptoms of peritonitis (pain, cloudy effluent, fever).
- Change exit site dressing daily using aseptic technique until healing occurs. Assess daily for increase in inflammation or drainage.
- If infection is suspected, obtain appropriate culture, and begin antibiotic according to protocol or physician's order.

Glucose

Supplemental insulin can be added to the dialysate to control hyperglycemia. Blood glucose levels should be monitored closely in patients with diabetes mellitus and hepatic disease.

Pain

Patients may experience mild abdominal discomfort at any time during the procedure. It is probably related to the constant distention or chemical irritation of the peritoneum. If a mild analgesic does not provide relief, inserting 5 mL of 2% lidocaine directly into the catheter may help. The patient may be more comfortable if nourishment is given in small amounts, when the fluid is draining out rather than when the abdominal cavity is distended.

Severe pain may indicate more serious problems of infection or paralytic ileus. Infection is not likely in the first 24 hours. Aseptic technique and prophylactic antibiotics minimize the risk of infection. Periodic cultures of the outflowing fluid will assist early detection of pathogenic organisms.

Immobility

Immobility may lead to hypostatic pneumonia, especially in the debilitated or older patient. Deep breathing, turning, and coughing should be encouraged during the procedure. Leg exercises and the use of elastic stockings may prevent the development of venous thrombi and emboli.

Discomfort

Because peritoneal dialysis results in slower clearance of waste products than hemodialysis, it rarely is associated with the disequilibrium seen with hemodialysis. Because the treatment is longer, however, boredom is a frequent problem. Nursing measures are directed toward making the patient as comfortable as possible. Diversions such as reading, watching television, and visitors should be encouraged. Educating the patient about peritoneal dialysis and involving the patient in the care may reduce some of the anxiety and discomfort.

■ PERITONEAL DIALYSIS AS A CHRONIC TREATMENT

Intermittent peritoneal dialysis (IPD) has been used for chronic therapy for some time, but it requires the patient to remain stationary for 10 to 14 hours three times per week. Because of this inconvenience to the patient and increased staff time needed if this therapy is performed in-center, IPD seldom is used and is not available in many dialysis centers.

Peritoneal dialysis has gained popularity as a chronic form of dialysis therapy, especially since *continuous ambulatory peritoneal dialysis* (CAPD) has become available. CAPD is taught easily to patients and does not limit ambu-

lation between dialysate fluid exchanges. It uses the dialysis fluid that is continuously present in the peritoneal cavity 24 hours a day 7 days a week. Dialysis fluid is drained by the patient and replaced with fresh solution three to five times per day. The number of solution exchanges needed per day depends on the patient's individual needs. Although the patient is required to perform dialysis techniques every day, CAPD is attractive to many end-stage renal disease patients because they can accomplish it easily and independently. It also may be the preferred therapy for patients who benefit from a slow, continuous removal of sodium and water, as in those with refractory congestive heart failure.

Another variation of chronic peritoneal dialysis therapy is continuous cyclic peritoneal dialysis (CCPD). Patients who choose this form of therapy perform IPD at night during sleep using a cycling machine and in the morning instill dialysis fluid, which remains in the abdomen during the whole day. This is most convenient for those who require the help of working family members to perform their exchanges.

As with acute peritoneal dialysis, peritonitis is the greatest potential problem with chronic forms of dialysis. Peritoneal catheters are permanent and inserted in the operating room. Such catheters have one or two Teflon cuffs that the surgeon sutures to the abdominal wall or subcutaneous tissue or both to anchor the catheter and provide a permanent seal against invading bacteria. Patients are taught how to recognize any potential problem associated with the catheter or treatment and to seek help from the CAPD team when needed.

Patients who perform IPD, CAPD, or CCPD at home generally visit the dialysis unit every 4 to 8 weeks. At this time, a nursing assessment is done, techniques are reviewed, and required blood studies are drawn. All health team members, including the physician, nurse, dietitian, and social worker, work together with the patient and family to ensure successful adaptation to the chosen mode of treatment.

Clinical Applicability Challenges

Self-Challenge: Critical Thinking

1. *Keeping track of fluid balance during a CVVH/D treatment is difficult unless you can organize the data so they are easily accessible. Start with an hourly fluid loss goal. Remember that you must account for hourly intake (including dialysate, any intravenous lines, any flushes, oral intake, blood products, and replacement fluid), hourly output (including ultrafiltrate and dialysate, any urine output, gastric drainage, and so forth) to calculate the next hour's replacement fluid. Devise a flow sheet that lets you keep track of fluid balance at a glance.*

2. *Your patient's renal function is not recovering, and he will need to continue dialysis after hospital discharge. He is diabetic but with good eyesight and dexterity and has a supportive family. There are plenty of outpatient dialysis units in the area. Explore with him the different forms of chronic dialysis to help him decide which one is best for him.*

3. *Your hospital is setting up a program to perform CVVH/D. You are asked to help develop a protocol in collaboration with the acute care dialysis nurses. To prepare for the meeting, outline responsibilities for equipment setup and patient teaching.*

Study Questions

1. *Which statement about hemodialysis is* not *true?*
   a. *It rapidly removes metabolic wastes and excess fluid.*
   b. *Heparin is always needed to keep the blood from clotting in the system.*
   c. *It removes excess body water by effecting a pressure differential between the blood and fluid compartments.*
   d. *It can restore a physiological level of electrolytes.*

2. *When a CVVH/D filter and lines begin to turn dark, ultrafiltration diminishes, and venous pressure rises, what would you do?*
   a. *Call the dialysis nurse immediately to change the circuit.*
   b. *Check the patient's blood pressure and oxygen saturation.*
   c. *Administer a saline bolus to inspect the circuit for clotting.*
   d. *Immediately give the patient more heparin because he is probably clotting.*

3. *You are doing a peritoneal dialysis exchange and notice that the drained fluid is cloudy. What do you do?*
   a. *Obtain a sample of the drained fluid, send it to the laboratory for culture and sensitivity and cell count, and obtain an order for an antibiotic.*
   b. *Wait until the next exchange to see if it clears up.*

   c. *Send a sample of the drained fluid for urea nitrogen, creatinine, and electrolytes.*
   d. *Do nothing because the fluid will usually clear up spontaneously.*

REFERENCES

1. Daugirdis J: Acute hemodialysis prescription. In Daugirdis J, Ing T (eds): Handbook of Dialysis (2nd Ed), pp 78–91. Boston, New York, Little Brown and Company, 1994
2. Nissenson A: Complications of chronic dialysis therapy. In Gutch L, Stoner M, Corea A (eds): Review of Hemodialysis for Nurses and Dialysis Personnel (5th Ed), pp 190–210, St. Louis, Mosby-Year Book, 1993
3. Martin R, Jurshak J: Nursing Management of Continuous Renal Replacement Therapy. Seminars in Dialysis 9(2):192–199, 1996

BIBLIOGRAPHY

Daugirdis J: Acute hemodialysis prescription. In Daugirdis J, Ing T (eds): Handbook of Dialysis (2nd Ed). Boston, New York, Little Brown and Company, 1994

Gokal R, Nolf K (eds): The Textbook of Peritoneal Dialysis. Boston, Kluwer Academic Publishers, 1994

Gutch L, Stoner M, Corea A (eds): Review of Hemodialysis for Nurses and Dialysis Personnel (5th Ed). St. Louis, Mosby-Year Book, 1993

Lancaster L (ed): Core Curriculum for Nephrology Nursing (3rd Ed). Pitman, NJ, AJ Jannetti, 1995

Mehta RL (guest ed): A symposium on practical issues in the use of continuous renal replacement therapies. Seminars in Dialysis 9(2):79–224, 1996

30

Common Renal Disorders

OBJECTIVES

Based on the content in this chapter, the reader should be able to:

- Describe the causes and treatment principles of volume imbalance.
- Explain the causes and treatment of imbalances of the major electrolytes of the body.
- Demonstrate knowledge of the causes of acute renal failure (ARF).
- Describe urine production during the nonoliguric, oliguric, and diuretic stages of ARF.
- Identify the clinical manifestations of hypoperfusion that can lead to ARF: decreased cardiac output, altered peripheral vascular resistance, and hypovolemia and hemorrhage.
- Identify the clinical manifestations of ARF according to their categories: prerenal, intrarenal, and postrenal.
- Discuss nursing assessment parameters used to identify the alteration in ARF.
- Develop a nursing care plan for managing the shock and postshock states of ARF.

*P*rognosis of acute renal failure (ARF) varies with the cause and severity of the disease. Although many patients recover completely, some patients may have residual renal insufficiency, requiring medication, dietary restriction, and continued monitoring. Some patients may not recover and may require long-term renal replacement therapy (dialysis and transplantation). Despite advances in dialysis and intensive care, the mortality rate for patients with severe, ischemic ARF remains in high, excess of 60%. Patients who have multisystem organ failure and require dialysis are at increased risk with mortality rates as high as 80%.[1,2]

It is necessary for the intensive care unit nurse to understand fluid and electrolyte balance and imbalance. Renal failure affects these balances. Because of this fact, this chapter begins with a brief discussion and summary tables on fluid and electrolyte imbalance.

Fluid and Electrolyte Imbalances

The nurse's role in the assessment and management of fluid and electrolyte disorders in the critically ill patient is vital. Careful monitoring of the patient's symptoms, general appearance, weight, and vital signs and interpretation of laboratory results can provide early clues to the diagnosis of disorders of fluid and electrolyte balance.

▓ BODY FLUIDS

Approximately 60% of the adult's body weight is fluid. This body fluid is either *intracellular*, inside the cell, or *extracellular*, outside the cell. Extracellular fluid (ECF) is further subdivided into *intravascular fluid* (plasma) and *interstitial fluid* (fluid lying between the cells). Also part of the ECF are transcellular fluids, such as secretions in the salivary glands, pancreas, liver, and biliary tract, and fluids in the gastrointestinal and respiratory tracts, sweat glands, cavities in the eye, cerebrospinal fluid, and kidneys.[3] In adults, two thirds of the body fluid exists in the intracellular space, and the remaining one third is found between the cells and in the plasma.[4]

Body fluid is composed primarily of water and electrolytes. Electrolytes are substances that develop an electrical charge when dissolved in water. Electrolytes that develop a positive charge are called cations, and examples of cations include sodium (Na), potassium (K), calcium (Ca), and magnesium (Mg). Electrolytes that develop negative charges are called anions, and they include chloride (Cl) and bicarbonate (HCO_3). In all body fluids, anions and cations are always present in equal amounts because positive and negative charges must be equal.

The electrolyte content of intracellular fluid (ICF) differs significantly from that of ECF. Table 30–1 shows the differences in the electrolyte content in the plasma or ECF and ICF. Because special techniques are required to measure electrolytes in the ICF; in the clinical setting, only the electrolyte content of ECF, namely plasma, is measured. Some tests are performed on serum (the portion of plasma left after clotting); however, for practical purposes, the terms serum electrolytes and plasma electrolytes are used interchangeably.

▓ PATHOPHYSIOLOGICAL PRINCIPLES

Alterations in Urinary Output and Solute Load

The normal kidney can maintain solute balance when urine volume is reduced to between 5 and 600 mL/d because the kidneys can increase the urine concentration from 1,000 to 1,200 mOsm/kg. In the average person producing 600 mOsm of metabolic solute from dietary intake and metabolic conversion, approximately 500 mL of urine is required to excrete this if solute urine-concentrating ability is normal. If, however, solute load is increased as a result of increased intake (eg, from high-protein diets, hyperalimentation, or hypercatabolism), a greater urine volume will be required to excrete the metabolic solute load.

Because the urine-concentrating ability normally decreases progressively after 40 years of age, older people require a greater urine volume to maintain homeostasis in the face of "normal" intakes. Even if urine-concentrating ability is reduced to 600 mOsm/kg, however, only 1,000 mL of urine would be required to excrete an "average" 600 mOsm solute load generated per day. Older people may eat considerably less and therefore a smaller urine volume is required to maintain homeostasis. The same sort of decreased urine-concentrating ability is noted in patients with chronic renal disease as their disease progresses. In addition to increased solute load from hyperalimentation, glycosuria associated with poorly controlled diabetes and radiological contrast agents can result in a solute diuresis, with a greater urine volume than normal.

In chronic renal disease, the kidneys have the ability to adapt significantly to maintain water and electrolyte levels that are equivalent to normal levels, until the glomerular filtration rate (GFR) drops below 15 to 20 mL/min. This adaptation is accomplished through increased solute and water excretion per nephron and is modulated in part by

---

TABLE 30-1

Differences in Electrolyte Content in Plasma and Intracellular Fluid

Electrolyte	Content	
	Plasma (in mEq/L)	Intracellular (in mEq/L)
Cations		
Sodium	142	12
Potassium	5	150
Calcium	5	<1
Magnesium	2	40
Total cations	154	200
Anions		
Chloride	103	Not typically measured
Bicarbonate	26	10
Phosphates	2	150
Sulfate	1	
Organic acids	5	0
Proteinate	17	40
Total anions	154	200

changes in systemic and local intrarenal hormone production, possibly by the so-called natriuretic factor.

When either too much or too little sodium and water are taken in, the kidney's ability to compensate may be restricted in chronic renal failure. For example, when sodium intake decreases abruptly, the kidneys may take longer than the normal 2 to 3 days to adapt, and a relative state of "salt wasting" may occur. Some patients may actually have true sodium wasting and require greater than normal sodium intake to maintain sodium balance. This condition is rare, however, and most patients with chronic renal failure can adapt if sodium restriction takes place slowly. In addition, unless acidosis is present, as with hyporeninemic hypoaldosteronism or with more severe decreases in GFR, serum potassium levels and the ability to excrete potassium also are maintained. When the GFR decreases to below 10 mL/min, patients with end-stage renal disease may require restriction of sodium, potassium, and water intake to maintain balance. This regimen usually requires major adjustments in the diet.

Chronic renal disease and ARF are quite different. Because patients with classic ARF have oliguria or anuria (<500 mL/d or <100 mL/d, respectively), they demand much more attention to electrolyte and water balance than patients with comparable degrees of chronic renal failure. Sodium, water, protein, and potassium restrictions become necessary because of the limited capacity of the kidneys to excrete these substances. In addition, the hypercatabolic state, with generation of excess metabolic water and with shifts of solutes between intracellular and extracellular compartments as a result of acidosis, adds to the effects of uremia in most patients with ARF.

Those at risk for decreased output include patients with the following:

- Increased solute intake (eg, hyperalimentation)
- Decreased ability to concentrate urine (eg, older adults)
- Chronic renal failure
- ARF

Disorders of Water Balance

Primary disorders of water balance, hyponatremia and hypernatremia, occur when water is retained or lost from the body in excess of sodium.

HYPONATREMIA

In a number of disease states, the serum sodium concentration may be reduced (hyponatremia) because of an inability of the kidneys to excrete free water. This is due to either a persistent release of antidiuretic hormone (ADH) in response to a decrease in the total or effective intravascular volume or to inappropriate stimulation of ADH release.

States of actual or effective intravascular volume depletion also contribute to the hyponatremia by decreasing distal delivery of fluid in the nephron, thereby limiting the amount of water that can be excreted.

Hyponatremia may be associated with an increased total body sodium and edema, a decreased total body sodium and hypovolemia, or a normal or slightly increased total body sodium and increased blood volume, depending on the clinical disorder that gives rise to the hyponatremia.

In patients with edema resulting from cirrhosis, congestive heart failure, or the nephrotic syndrome, hyponatremia occurs frequently and may be enhanced by the use of diuretics. In these conditions, although there is an overall increase in body sodium and water, ADH release is stimulated because the effective blood volume is decreased. As a result, the kidneys tend to reabsorb a greater percentage of filtered fluid in the proximal tubule. This reabsorption causes further fluid retention and hyponatremia, especially if the patient has unlimited access to water, because the little fluid reaching the distal tubule is reabsorbed more completely owing to the high plasma ADH level.

Treatment with thiazide diuretics, furosemide, or ethacrynic acid can produce or seriously compound the hyponatremia because these drugs may decrease further the effective blood volume and decrease sodium transport in the ascending loop of Henle, which is necessary for the kidneys' ability to excrete free water and maximally dilute the urine.

Patients with volume depletion as a result of loss of sodium or blood also may have hyponatremia when the volume depletion is great enough to stimulate ADH release. In this situation, body sodium and blood volume are reduced, and edema is not present. Diuretic administration, renal salt wasting, adrenal insufficiency, and hemorrhage are examples of this type of condition. ADH release occurs and stimulates water reabsorption in an attempt to restore intravascular volume, regardless of serum osmolality. If the patient ingests water without salt or if hypotonic fluids are administered intravenously, hyponatremia will result.

In addition, the following situations can cause hyponatremia: increased thirst, central nervous system disease, and decreased renal water excretion resulting from the use of drugs that stimulate vasopressin release (eg, cyclophosphamide and diazepam) or drugs that interfere with the action of vasopressin on the kidney (eg, chlorpropamide and nonsteroidal anti-inflammatory drugs). Table 30–2 summarizes causes and management of hyponatremia and hypernatremia.

HYPERVOLEMIA

Hypervolemia occurs when there is excess ECF. It may occur in the patient with heart failure, because decreased blood flow to the kidneys results in decreased excretion of urine. The patient with renal dysfunction also may have

TABLE 30-2
Sodium Electrolyte Abnormalities

Causes	Management
Sodium	
Hypernatremia	
Na > 145 mEq/L	
Deprivation of water (most common in those unable to perceive or respond to thirst) Increased insensible water loss (as in hyperventilation) Watery diarrhea Ingestion of salt in unusual amounts Excessive parenteral administration of sodium-containing solutions • Hypertonic saline (3% or 5% NaCl) • Sodium bicarbonate • Isotonic saline Near drowning in sea water Heatstroke Diabetes insipidus if water intake is inadequate	• Treat underlying cause. If water loss is the cause, water needs to be added. If sodium excess is the cause, sodium needs to be removed. • If patient is hypovolemic with hypernatremia, administer isotonic saline until volume is restored. Patients with pure free water losses should receive hypotonic fluid. Lower the sodium plasma level no faster than 2 mEq/L per hour (to prevent cerebral edema). • Monitor plasma electrolytes at frequent intervals. • Monitor intake and output, urine sodium, and daily weight • Monitor level of consciousness for signs of cerebral irritability
Hyponatremia Na < 135 mEq/L *Loss of sodium* • Use of diuretics • Loss of gastrointestinal fluids • Adrenal insufficiency • Osmotic diuresis • Salt-losing nephritis *Gains of water* • Excessive administration of D₅W • Psychogenic polydipsia • Excessive water administration with isotonic or hypotonic tube feedings *Disease states associated with SIADH* • Oat-cell carcinoma of lung • Carcinoma of duodenum or pancreas • Head trauma • Stroke • Pulmonary disorders (tuberculosis, pneumonia, asthma, respiratory failure) *Pharmacological agents that may impair renal water excretion* • Chlorpropamide (Diabenese) • Cyclophosphamide (Cytoxan) • Vincristine (Oncovin) • Thioridazine (Mellaril) • Fluphenazine (Prolixin) • Carbamazepine (Tegretol) • Oxytocin (Pitocin)	• Treat underlying cause. • Replace sodium orally, by gastrointestinal tube, or by the parenteral route. • If the plasma volume is below normal, administer lactated Ringer's solution of isotonic saline. • In the normovolemic patient, water restriction may be recommended, or increased water excretion may be implemented by loop diuretics in conjunction with increased sodium and potassium intake. • Monitor intake and output, daily weights, vital signs for evidence of fluid overload. • Monitor plasma electrolytes at frequent intervals.

D₅W, Dextrose 5% in water; SIADH, syndrome of inappropriate antidiuretic hormone secretion.

hypervolemia because of fluid and sodium retention. Liver disease may result in hypervolemia secondary to hypoproteinemia; the hypoproteinemia causes decreased production of albumin, which results in decreased serum colloid osmotic pressure. In turn, this causes leakage in interstitial fluid from capillaries.

HYPERNATREMIA

Hypernatremia occurs when the sodium level in the ECF is above normal. It almost always is associated with a loss of body fluids in excess of sodium. For example, it may occur as a result of inadequate fluid intake or profuse diarrhea. Aldosteronism, which causes increased sodium retention by the kidneys, is another cause of hypernatremia. Inhalation of salt water in a near-drowning incident can result in hypernatremia because of absorption of salt water from the alveoli into the pulmonary capillaries. Finally, therapies such as hypertonic tube feedings; drugs such as steroids, lithium, and doxycycline; and overzealous infusion of intravenous saline solution all may result in hypernatremia. These circumstances all interfere with the kidney's ability to conserve water by responding appropriately to vasopressin.

HYPOVOLEMIA

Hypovolemia is caused by a deficit in ECF that usually is accompanied by a loss of electrolytes. Hypovolemia also may be referred to as dehydration. When it is accompanied by a loss of electrolytes (often combined water and sodium deficits), it usually is referred to as volume depletion. Patients with the following clinical conditions are at risk for becoming hypovolemic:

- Decreased oral intake because of physical or mental debilitation or difficulty in swallowing
- Increased output from renal losses (eg, diuretics) gastrointestinal losses (diarrhea, vomiting, or suctioning), or skin losses (diaphoresis or draining wounds)
- Blood loss
- Impaired renal function
  - Kidneys unable to concentrate urine
  - Too much fluid removed during dialysis
- Diabetes insipidus (decreased secretion of ADH)
- Collection of third-space fluids (eg, effusions, decreased osmotic pressure that causes capillary leakage, ascites)

▆ MANAGEMENT OF VOLUME IMBALANCES

After patient evaluation and reviewing the intake and output records for the current and previous day, the nurse can make a decision about whether to increase or decrease fluid intake. In the absence of symptoms of fluid retention, when intravenous fluids are behind schedule and intake is inadequate for the patient's condition, missed fluids should be given. The nurse watches the patient's fluid status closely, especially the urine output, for the next few hours to evaluate whether or not the increase in fluid intake corrected the patient's fluid imbalance. If, however, urine output is zero or diminished in the presence of adequate fluid intake, no more fluids are given, and the physician is notified immediately. If a patient presents any of the symptoms of fluid overload, all fluid intake is restricted, and the physician is notified immediately.

Fluid replacement can be calculated for any period of time, depending on the severity of the situation. For example, a 24-hour calculation of intake for a patient who is oliguric with normal insensible losses could be as follows:

Previous 24-hour urine output: 100 mL
Insensible loss replacement: 500 mL
Total 24-hour fluid allowance: 600 mL

Although the physician will specify the total amount of fluid replacement, the details of fluid distribution often are decided by the nurse. Priority is given to fluid needed for administration of drugs, both intravenous and oral. Distribution of the remaining fluid is then made according to patient preference. The nurse helps the patient avoid using up the entire day's allowance early in the day by guiding the selection. Because sodium and potassium may be restricted in the patient with renal failure, fluids such as ginger ale, 7-Up, and Kool Aid, which are low in sodium and potassium, are given.

▆ MANAGEMENT OF IMBALANCES OF OTHER MAJOR ELECTROLYTES

Although water and sodium imbalances frequently are seen in critically ill patients, such patients are also at risk for imbalances of other major electrolytes, including potassium, calcium, magnesium, and phosphate. The diagnosis of these electrolyte abnormalities is based on careful assessment of the patient and specific laboratory tests for each electrolyte (see Chapter 28). There are multiple causes for abnormal levels of each of these electrolytes. Some of these electrolyte imbalances occur because of dysfunction of more than one body system. The nurse must be aware of the impact of these disorders on electrolyte balance and assess the patient accordingly.

The treatment for abnormally high or low electrolytes is based on similar principles. Namely, if the electrolyte level is too low, treatment focuses on the cause and replacement therapy. If the electrolyte level is too high, treatment focuses on the cause and decreasing the serum or tissue level of that electrolyte. Emergency or life-threatening situations resulting from electrolyte imbalances require invasive or special methods to correct the toxic effects rapidly. Table 30–3 gives a more detailed discussion of causes and treatment of each major electrolyte imbalance.

1

TABLE 30-3
Other Major Electrolyte Imbalances

Causes	Management
Potassium *Hyperkalemia* *K > 5.0 mEq/L* *Pseudohyperkalemia* • Prolonged tight application of tourniquet; fist clenching and unclenching immediately before or during blood drawing • Hemolysis of blood sample • Leukocytosis • Thrombocytosis *Decreased potassium excretion* • Oliguric renal failure • Potassium-conserving diuretics • Hypoaldosteronism *High potassium intake* • Improper use of oral potassium supplements • Excessive use of salt substitutes • Rapid intravenous potassium administration • Rapid transfusion of aged blood *Shift of potassium out of cells* • Acidosis • Tissue damage, as in crushing injuries • Malignant cell lysis after chemotherapy	• Treat underlying cause. • Restrict potassium intake and drugs potentiating hyperkalemia. • Administer drugs to promote potassium excretion, such as sodium polystyrene sulfonate (Kayexalate). • Administer dialysis when needed. • In emergencies, treat severe hyperkalemia by giving (1) calcium gluconate, (2) sodium bicarbonate, and (3) insulin and hypertonic dextrose. • Monitor electrocardiogram (ECG) for tall pointed T waves, which can occur in hyperkalemia. • Monitor plasma electrolytes. • Monitor intake and output and vital signs.
Hypokalemia *K < 3.5 mEq/L* *Gastrointestinal loss* • Diarrhea • Laxative abuse • Prolonged gastric suction • Villous adenoma *Renal loss* • Potassium-losing diuretics • Hyperaldosteronism • Sodium penicillin, carbenicillin, or amphotericin B • Steroid administration • Osmotic diuresis *Shift into cells* • Alkalosis • Excessive secretion or administration of insulin • Hyperalimentation *Poor intake* • Anorexia nervosa • Alcoholism • Debilitation	• Treat underlying cause. • Provide diet with potassium-rich foods, such as bananas, apricots, orange juice, and broccoli. • Administer potassium chloride orally or parentally (slowly). • Monitor plasma electrolytes at frequent intervals. • Monitor ECG for evidence of U waves (small upright waves following the T wave). • Monitor intake and output and vital signs. • Have emergency equipment if potassium level is <3 mEq/L.
Calcium *Hypercalcemia* *Ca > 10.5 mg/dL* Hyperparathyroidism Malignant neoplastic disease (lung tumors, breast tumors, and multiple myeloma account for more than 50% of the cases) *Drugs* • Thiazide diuretics • Excessive vitamin A or D • Overuse of calcium supplements • Overuse of calcium-containing antacids	• Treat underlying cause. • Eliminate drugs that contribute to hypercalcemia. • Administer isotonic saline to dilute the plasma calcium. • Monitor ECG for shortening of the QT interval. • Monitor plasma electrolytes at frequent intervals. • Monitor intake and output, daily weights, and vital signs.

(continued)

TABLE 30-3
Other Major Electrolyte Imbalances *(Continued)*

Causes	Management
• Lithium • Theophylline Prolonged immobilization	
Hypocalcemia *Ca < 8.5 mg/dL* Surgical hypoparathyroidism (may follow thyroid surgery or radical neck surgery for cancer) Primary hypoparathyroidism Malabsorption Acute pancreatitis Excessive administration of citrated blood Alkalotic states (causing decreased calcium ionization) Hyperphosphatemia Sepsis Hypomagnesemia Medullary carcinoma of thyroid Hypoalbuminemia (as in cirrhosis, nephrotic syndrome, and starvation)	• Treat underlying cause. • Give oral calcium supplements. Acute symptomatic hypocalcemia is an emergency requiring prompt administration of intravenous calcium. • Monitor ECG for lengthening of the QT interval. • Monitor intake and output, daily weights, and vital signs. • Monitor plasma electrolytes at frequent intervals.
Phosphate *Hyperphosphatemia* *P > 4.5 mg/dL* Renal failure Chemotherapy, particularly for acute lymphoblastic leukemia and lymphoma Large intake of milk, as in treatment of peptic ulcer Use of cow's milk in infants Overzealous administration of phosphorus supplements, orally or IV Excessive use of Fleet's phosphosoda as enema solution or laxative, particularly in children and individuals with slow bowel elimination Large vitamin D intake (increases phosphorus absorption)	• Treat underlying cause. • Restrict dietary intake of phosphate-containing foods, such as dietary products. • Administer phosphate-binding agents, such as aluminum hydroxide and aluminum carbonate. • If kidney function is normal, give isotonic saline to promote renal phosphate excretion. • Administer hypertonic dextrose with regular insulin to temporarily drive phosphorus into the cell. • Use dialysis for patients with compromised renal functions. • Monitor plasma electrolytes at frequent intervals.
Hypophosphatemia *P < 3 mg/dL* Glucose administration Refeeding after starvation Hyperalimentation Alcohol withdrawal Diabetic ketoacidosis Respiratory alkalosis Phosphate-binding antacids Recovery phase after severe burns	• Treat underlying cause. • Provide phosphate-rich foods, such as milk products. • Administer phosphorus-replacement therapy orally, and for severe hypophosphatemia, give intravenously. • Monitor for signs of infection because patients with severe hypophosphatemia are at greater risk for infection because of changes in white blood cell function. • Monitor plasma electrolytes at frequent intervals.
Magnesium *Hypermagnesemia* *Mg > 2.1 mEq/L* Acute and chronic renal failure (particularly when magnesium-containing medications are used) Excessive magnesium administration during treatment of eclampsia or to delay labor (affects both mother and fetus) Excessive doses of magnesium during treatment of hypomagnesemia Excessive use of magnesium-containing antacids or laxatives by older people (who have age-related decreased renal function) Adrenal insufficiency Hemodialysis with excessively hard water or with a dialysate high in magnesium content	• Treat underlying cause. • Eliminate any magnesium-replacement therapy. • In emergencies, administer intravenous calcium gluconate because it antagonizes the neuromuscular and cardiac toxicity of hypermagnesemia. Dialysis may be needed for hypermagnesemic renal failure in patient, and temporary cardiac pacemaker may be required to treat life-threatening bradydysrhythmias. • Monitor plasma electrolytes at frequent intervals.

(continued)

TABLE 30-3
Other Major Electrolyte Imbalances *(Continued)*

Causes	Management

Hypomagnesemia
  Mg < 1.4 mEq/L
Inadequate intake
Prolonged administration of magnesium-free fluids
Starvation
TPN without adequate magnesium supplementation
Chronic alcoholism
Increased gastrointestinal losses
Diarrhea
Laxative abuse
Fistulas
Prolonged nasogastric suction
Vomiting
Malabsorption syndromes
Increased renal losses
Drugs
  Loop and thiazide diuretics
  Mannitol
  Cisplatin
  Cyclosporine
  Aminoglycosides
  Carbenicillin
  Amphotericin B
  Digitalis
  Pentamidine
Diuresis
  Uncontrolled diabetes mellitus
  Hyperaldosteronism
SIADH
Changes in magnesium distribution
Pancreatitis
Thermal injury
Drugs causing shift into cells
  Insulin
  Glucose
  Catecholamines
Citrate chelation
  Citrated blood products
  Plasmapheresis
Hungry bone syndrome
	• Treat underlying cause.
	• Administer magnesium-replacement therapy, and monitor renal patients receiving magnesium replacement therapy carefully for signs of hypermagnesemia.
	• Provide magnesium-rich foods, such as dairy products, green vegetables, meat, seafood, and cereals.
	• Monitor vital signs of patients receiving rapid magnesium administration because it may cause respiratory or cardiac arrest.
	• Monitor plasma electrolytes at frequent intervals.

Metheny NM: Fluid and Electrolyte Balance: Nursing Considerations. Philadelphia, Lippincott-Raven, 1996

Acute Renal Failure

The sudden (hours to a few days) loss of renal function characterized by an increase in blood urea nitrogen (BUN) and serum creatinine is considered ARF. Although no exact criteria for BUN and creatinine can be set, an increase in BUN from 15 to 30 mg/dL and a rise in creatinine from 1 to 2 mg/dL suggest ARF in patients with preexisting normal renal function. In patients with preexisting renal disease, larger variations may be required to suggest the diagnosis because small changes in renal function, not related to ARF, may be magnified when nephron loss already is present.

CATEGORIES OF RENAL FAILURE

There are three general categories of ARF according to the precipitating factors and the symptoms manifested by the disease. These categories are prerenal, intrarenal, and postrenal. The ability to distinguish among patient conditions associated specifically with these ARF categories will enable the nurse to provide individualized care.

PRERENAL

Prerenal causes of ARF include physiological events that result in decreased circulation (ischemia) to the kidneys. Most commonly, these include hypovolemia and cardiovascular failure; however, any other event that leads to an acute decrease in the oxygenation of the kidneys can fall into this category, which sometimes is described as prerenal azotemia (see display).

INTRARENAL

The intrarenal category of ARF includes physiological events directly affecting kidney tissue structure and function. These often include events causing damage to the interstitium and the nephron tissue. The kidneys lose their ability to excrete nitrogen waste produced by protein metabolism. Tubule damage leads to an inability to concen-

trate the urine. Also, when conditions causing prerenal failure create kidney tissue destruction, the disease progresses to the intrarenal stage (see display). Acute tubular necrosis (ATN) is a common example of this category of ARF.

POSTRENAL

The postrenal category includes any obstruction in urine flow from the collection ducts in the kidney to the external urethral orifice or venous blood flow from the kidney. The obstructions may be from anatomical or functional causes. Anatomical causes usually are events such as strictures, tumors, or stones. Functional causes can include drugs, such as ganglionic blocking agents, that interrupt autonomic supply to the urinary system. Bilateral renal venous obstruction is rare; however, it also is categorized as a postrenal cause of ARF. It is seen most often secondary to intraabdominal neoplasms and iatrogenic causes (see display).

PATHOPHYSIOLOGICAL PRINCIPLES

Prerenal Azotemia

The adverse effect of reduced renal perfusion on renal function is distinct. Because of the large amount of renal blood flow required to maintain normal renal function, changes

---

General Categories of Acute Renal Failure Based on Precipitating Factors and Symptoms

Prerenal Failure	*Intrarenal Failure*	*Postrenal Failure*
Dehydration	Acute glomerulonephritis	Kidney stones
Sepsis/shock	Severe renal ischemia	Clots
Hypovolemic shock	Chemicals (eg, radiographic dyes, commercial chemicals)	Structure malformation
Vena cava obstruction		Tumors
Trauma with bleeding	Certain drugs (ie, anti-inflammatory drugs, antibiotics)	Prostatitism
Sequestration (burns, peritonitis)		Rupture of the bladder
Hypovolemia (ie, diuretics)	Neoplasms	Ureteral obstruction
Cardiovascular failure (ie, myocardial failure, tamponade, vascular pooling, congestive heart failure, dysrhythmia)	Malignant hypertension	Retroperitoneal fibrosis
	Systemic lupus erythematosus	Bilateral renal venous occlusion
	Diabetes mellitus	Neurogenic bladder
Hemorrhage	Complications of pregnancy (ie, eclampsia)	
Gastrointestinal losses (diarrhea, vomiting)	Streptococcal infections	
Extreme acidosis	Vasopressors	
Anaphylaxis/shock	Microangiopathy	
Renal artery stenosis or thrombosis	Hyperviscosity states	
	Hypercalcemia	
	Postrenal transplant	
	Myeloma	
	Interstitial nephritis	
	Transfusion reactions	
	HIV nephropathy	
	Heroin nephropathy	

in urinary composition occur early when renal perfusion is decreased.

When renal blood flow is severely compromised as a result of either reduction in effective blood volume, fall in cardiac output, or decrease in blood pressure below 80 mmHg, characteristic changes occur in renal function. The capacity for complete autoregulation is exceeded. The GFR falls. The amount of tubular fluid is reduced, and the fluid travels through the tubule more slowly. This results in increased sodium and water reabsorption. Because of the reduced renal circulation, the solutes reabsorbed from the tubular fluid are removed more slowly than normal from the interstitium of the renal medulla. This results in increased medullary tonicity, which in turn further augments water reabsorption from the distal tubular fluid. Therefore, the urinary changes are typical in the underperfused state. The urinary volume is reduced to less than 400 mL/d (17 mL/h), urine specific gravity is increased, and urinary sodium concentration is low (usually less than 5 mEq/L; Fig. 30–1).

In addition, substances such as creatinine and urea, which normally are filtered but poorly reabsorbed from the renal tubule, are present in high concentration in the urine as a result of the increased water reabsorption. Because of the characteristic changes associated with renal underperfusion, measurement of urinary volume and specific gravity is a simple method of determining the effect of management on renal perfusion.

An increase in systemic blood pressure does not necessarily imply improvement in renal perfusion. This may be especially evident when drugs such as norepinephrine are used to correct the hypotension associated with states of volume depletion. These drugs may be associated with further reduction in renal blood flow as a consequence of constriction of renal arteries. This is manifested by a further fall in urinary volume and rise in specific gravity.

In turn, if the hypoperfusion state is more appropriately and specifically treated by replacement of volume, improvement of cardiac output, and correction of dysrhythmias, the improved renal perfusion will be manifested as an increased urinary volume and a fall in specific gravity of the urine.

Intrarenal Acute Renal Failure

MECHANISMS OF INTRARENAL ACUTE RENAL FAILURE

Renal Underperfusion

When renal underperfusion persists for a sufficient period of time (the exact duration of which is unpredictable and varies with the clinical circumstances), the kidneys may become damaged so that restoration of renal perfusion no longer effects an improvement in glomerular filtration. In this situation, intrinsic renal failure (intrarenal category, such as ATN) occurs. This effect may be exaggerated by concomitant administration of nephrotoxic drugs or antibiotics such as the aminoglycosides. Alternatively, these agents and an increasing number of nephrotoxic substances may produce ARF, even in the absence of systemic hypotension and renal ischemia, as a direct result of their toxic effects on the kidney.

In both situations, the kidney may or may not reveal significant morphological changes associated with the inciting insult. For example, in postischemic ARF, the kidney may appear edematous and swollen but show only minor histological changes on microscopic examination. In nephrotoxic ARF, however, histological changes, most commonly in the late proximal convoluted tubule and pars recta, may be seen more frequently in association with distal tubular dilation and accumulation of cellular debris and intralumi-

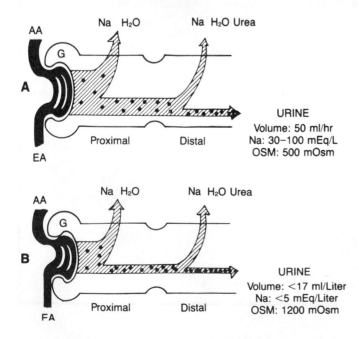

FIGURE 30-1

(**A**) Normal perfusion of the kidney compared with (**B**) underperfusion. Underperfusion of the kidney results in decreased renal blood flow and glomerular filtration; increase in the fraction of filtrate reabsorbed in the proximal tubule; and low urine flow with low sodium content and increased concentration. **B** characterizes the prerenal category of ARF.

nal casts. Despite severe reduction in renal function, pathological changes may be minimal and may not reflect the nature of the underlying process unless detailed evaluation of the fine renal architecture is made by electron microscopy. Regardless of the extent of histological damage, most patients recover complete renal function. Recovery time varies from days to weeks, depending on the severity and etiology of the process.

Glomerular Filtration Reduction

The exact mechanism that reduces glomerular filtration in any patient with ARF may be difficult to ascertain owing to the complexity of clinical circumstances. The mechanisms that are discussed represent those proposed for relatively pure circumstances of hypoperfusion-induced (prerenal) and nephrotoxin-induced (intrarenal) renal failure, as defined by human and laboratory animal studies. Despite years of investigation, there is no overwhelming evidence that supports one potential mechanism over another, and it is likely that several operate together.

Renal blood flow has been found to be reduced to approximately one third of normal in ATN, whereas the GFR is almost completely suppressed. This is in contrast to other states in which a similar reduction in renal blood flow is accompanied by much better maintenance of glomerular filtration and renal function.

Numerous animal studies have suggested that intratubular obstruction from casts and cellular debris may be involved in the suppression of glomerular filtration. If this obstruction is relieved, renal function returns. Other studies have suggested that there is disruption of the tubule epithelium with excessive back flow of the filtrate out of the tubule lumen, thus explaining the lack of urine formation in the face of continuing, although reduced, renal blood flow (Fig. 30–2).

Superficial Blood Flow Decrease

The mechanism responsible for the decreased superficial cortical blood flow in the kidney with ATN has not been defined. Earlier, discovery of converting enzyme in the kidney suggested that renin–angiotensin may play a role in this phenomenon. Subsequent studies, however, clearly have ruled out the renin–angiotensin system as the sole mediator of renal vasoconstriction and the decrease in GFR. Rather, the abnormalities are mediated by excesses or deficiencies of numerous vasoactive substances, both vasoconstrictors and vasodilators, and by lack of intrinsic myogenic tone in the renal vasculature. It is likely that no single factor, but rather an imbalance of vasoconstrictors and vasodilators acting in unison on the glomerular vasculature, is at fault in the observed renal ischemia (Fig. 30–3). In certain cases, increases of angiotensin II or vasopressin or decreases in prostaglandins or bradykinin may be the overriding phenomenon that disrupts the maintenance of renal blood flow and GFR. Prostaglandin inhibitors, for example, may decrease renal blood flow and GFR in states of stress, such as volume depletion, and further induce ARF.

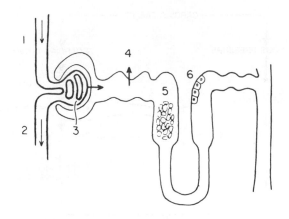

FIGURE 30-2
Potential mechanisms causing ARF include decreased filtration pressure because of constriction in the renal arterioles (*1* and *2*); decreased glomerular capillary permeability (*3*); increased permeability of the proximal tubules with back-leak of filtrate (*4*); obstruction of urine flow by necrotic tubular cells (*5*); increased sodium delivery to the macula densa (*6*); which causes an increase in renin–angiotensin production and vasoconstriction at the glomerular level.

Prostaglandin inhibitors also may enhance renal failure caused by gentamicin and myoglobin, at least in the experimental setting. More studies are needed to define these etiological associations.

Measurable Physiological Changes

Regardless of the mechanism, measurable physiological changes predictably occur. First, urine volume generally is reduced, in most cases produced by ischemic and nephrotoxic etiologies. Exceptions do occur, however, especially with nephrotoxic ARF caused by aminoglycosides, in which azotemia can occur without the urine flow rate ever being interrupted. The decreased GFR is accompanied by a rising serum creatinine and BUN and by characteristic urinary findings that differ from those seen in prerenal azotemia. First, urinary concentration (osmolality or specific gravity) falls to levels similar to plasma concentration, and the urine concentrations of urea and especially of creatinine are decreased, in contrast to findings made in the prerenal state of azotemia. Both reflect failure of distal tubules to concentrate the urine appropriately. The mechanism may be direct distal tubular toxicity or ischemia, or it may be disruption of the normal medullary solute concentration gradient necessary to produce a concentrated urine. Also, urinary sodium concentration no longer reflects systemic volume status and becomes disproportionately high (usually >30 mEq/L), indicating an inability to modulate sodium concentration appropriate for the clinical circumstance. This is assessed more accurately by the fractional sodium excretion (or by the renal failure index), which usually is greater than 1% and often greater than 3%, probably also reflecting decreased tubular function in residual filtering nephrons.

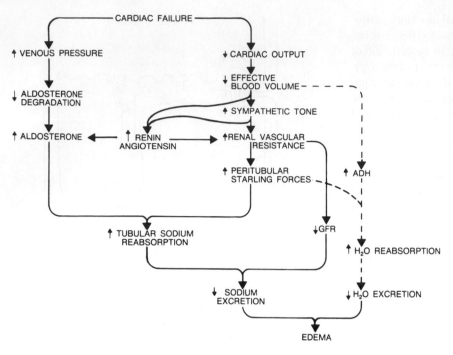

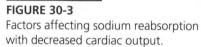

FIGURE 30-3
Factors affecting sodium reabsorption with decreased cardiac output.

MAIN CAUSES OF INTRARENAL ACUTE RENAL FAILURE

The causes of ARF are numerous but can be divided into two main groups: *ischemic* and *nephrotoxic*, as summarized in the accompanying display. If the history and clinical features are not consistent with an ischemic or nephrotoxic etiology, a kidney biopsy may be indicated to establish the diagnosis and to guide therapy.

Ischemic Acute Renal Failure

As indicated in the display, anything that reduces renal blood flow as a result of intravascular volume depletion can result in ARF. In traumatic shock, the duration and severity of hypotension play major roles in the development of ARF. The incidence and average duration of shock have been reduced because of prompt and effective therapy with blood products and volume expanders. ARF is more likely to

---

Common Causes of Intrarenal Acute Renal Failure

Ischemic (Prolonged)

Hemorrhagic hypotension
Severe volume depletion
Surgical aortic cross-clamping
Cardiac and biliary surgery
Defective cardiac output, including open heart
  surgery
Septic shock
Pregnancy
Pancreatitis
Immune suppression (cyclosporine, tacrolimus)
Nonsteroidal anti-inflammatory drugs

Nephrotoxic

Antibiotics: aminoglycosides, penicillins, tetra-
  cycline, amphotericin
Heavy metals: mercury, lead, *cis*-platinum,
  uranium, cadmium, bismuth, arsenic
Hemoglobinuria (from hemolysis)
Myoglobinuria (rhabdomyolysis, cocaine,
  ethanol)
Radiologic contrast agents
Drugs: phenytoin, phenylbutazone, cimetidine,
  cyclosporine
Organic solvents: carbon tetrachloride
Fungicides and pesticides
Uric acid
Ethylene glycol
Anesthetics (methoxyfluorane)
Disseminated intravascular coagulation
Plant and animal substances (mushrooms,
  snake venom)

occur *after* hospitalization as a result of septic complications or nephrotoxic antibiotic administration than as a result of the shock itself.

Nephrotoxic Acute Renal Failure

Many diverse chemicals and drugs have been implicated in the production of ARF (see display). In the hospitalized patient, the most common offending nephrotoxic agents are the antibiotics, especially the aminoglycosides. Examples of these agents are as follows, listed in decreasing order of the severity with which they produce dose-dependent damage to the proximal tubule: neomycin > tobramycin > kanamycin > gentamicin > amikacin > secomicin > netilmicin > streptomycin. Aminoglycoside nephrotoxicity accounts for up to 16% of all cases of ARF, usually is nonoliguric, and frequently improves after cessation of the antibiotic therapy. Because these agents accumulate preferentially in the renal cortex and are excreted slowly, however, they sometimes do not produce measurable toxicity until up to 1 week after cessation of administration. Routine monitoring of BUN and creatinine, therefore, are necessary when these agents are administered. Also, because these agents are eliminated from the body primarily by the kidneys, dosage must be adjusted in patients with preexisting renal function impairment. Peak and trough blood levels must be measured frequently so that drug dosage can be adjusted to the correct therapeutic range.

Nephrotoxicity associated with radiocontrast media administration also must be considered in the critical care setting. Patients at the greatest risk for development of renal failure after a load of contrast dye are those with diabetes, and especially diabetics with underlying renal failure.[1,5] This type of renal failure usually is mild, nonoliguric, and reversible. Serum creatinine rises within 48 hours after contrast administration, peaks in 3 to 5 days, and returns to baseline in 7 to 10 days. If the oliguric episode is more severe, it may take 5 to 10 days for the creatinine to reach peak levels, and baseline renal function may not be reached for 2 to 4 weeks. The need to provide temporary or permanent dialysis is rare except in patients with advanced underlying renal insufficiency.

The risk of contrast media–associated nephrotoxicity may be lowered by reducing the total dose of contrast media, by ensuring volume expansion before the injection, by infusing mannitol in conjunction with the dye, or by administering loop diuretics and calcium-channel blockers. Some authors now advocate the use of low-osmolality contrast media because of the reduced incidence of adverse effects.[6,7]

In addition to diabetes with underlying renal failure, other risk factors are recognized for the development of radiocontrast-associated nephrotoxicity. These are dehydration, large contrast loads, previous episodes of contrast media–associated nephrotoxicity, congestive heart failure, repeated contrast exposure, and multiple myeloma.

The nonsteroidal anti-inflammatory agents also may induce ARF in patients with diabetes, particularly in the presence of congestive heart failure due to coronary artery disease. Baseline renal function should be restored when the drug is discontinued.

Postrenal Acute Renal Failure

Obstruction can occur at any point in the urinary tract. When urine cannot get around the obstruction, resulting congestion will cause retrograde pressure through the collecting system and nephrons. This slows the rate of tubular fluid flow and lowers the GFR. As a result, the reabsorption of sodium, water, and urea is increased, leading to lowered urine sodium and increased urine osmolality and BUN. Serum creatinine also will rise. With prolonged pressure from urinary obstruction, the entire collecting system will dilate, compressing and damaging nephrons. This unfortunate circumstance can be avoided by prompt removal of the obstruction.[2] Because a well-functioning kidney is adequate to maintain homeostasis, the development of ARF from obstruction requires blockage of both kidneys (ie, urethral or bladder neck obstruction or bilateral ureteral obstruction) or unilateral ureteral obstruction in patients with a single kidney.

▊ ASSESSMENT

Clinical Manifestations

NONOLIGURIC ACUTE RENAL FAILURE

Classically, patients have oliguria in association with ATN; this is not always so, however. A group of patients presents with acute nonoliguric (partially reversible) renal failure. This state is especially common in patients receiving nephrotoxic antibiotics. If antibiotics are discontinued before renal function is reduced markedly, the patient frequently sustains moderate functional impairment for 7 to 10 days with gradual return to normal. In general, patients with nonoliguric ARF have few symptoms, and the disease is much less serious than the oliguric form of ATN.

 Considerations for the Older Patient
Physiological Changes Affecting the Renal System

As the body ages, many physiological changes occur in several body systems. Changes in the vascular and musculoskeletal system need to be addressed when assessing kidney function. Lipid-laden plaques can build up in the renal artery (like coronary arteries) and can cause significant damage. Changes in muscle mass and protein metabolism are commonly seen in individuals as they age. It is important to consider this when assessing renal function in older adults; underlying renal insufficiency can be inadvertently overlooked. The following calculation should be part of the assessment plan when evaluating older adults to obtain corrected values. This calculation takes into account age and muscle mass for individuals and gives more accurate information to provide treatment.

$$\text{Creatinine clearance} = \frac{(140 - \text{age}) \times \text{Weight in Kg}}{72 \times \text{Serum creatinine}}$$

OLIGURIC ACUTE RENAL FAILURE

The more classic or oliguric form of ATN begins with an acute precipitating event, immediately followed by oliguria (urine volume less than 400 mL/d). The mean duration of oliguria is approximately 12 days, although it may last only 2 to 3 days or as long as 30 days. This is accompanied by a usual rise in BUN of 25 to 30 mg/100 mL/d and an increase in creatinine of 1.5 to 2 mg/100 mL/d. The most common complication in this period is overhydration with resulting cardiac failure, pulmonary edema, and death. In addition, the patient may have acidosis, hyperkalemia, and symptoms of uremia.

DIURETIC STAGE

The oliguric phase is followed by gradual return of renal function as manifested by a stepwise increase in urine volume (the diuretic stage). The degree of diuresis is determined primarily by the state of hydration at the time the patient enters the diuretic stage. If the patient is markedly overloaded, urinary volume eventually may exceed 4 to 5 L/d. This could result in marked sodium wasting, with death resulting from electrolyte depletion in a few patients.

Because of the slow return of renal function during the diuretic phase, the degree of azotemia may increase during the early part of the diuretic period, with complications similar to those noted in the oliguric phase. Several months are required for full recovery of renal function after the end of the diuretic period.

Diagnostic Studies

Intrarenal ARF must be differentiated from prerenal azotemia, or decreased perfusion, and from obstruction. The latter can be distinguished by history and the appropriate use of ultrasonography and abdominal computed tomography scanning. In current practice, rarely will retrograde catheterization of the urinary tract be necessary to exclude this diagnosis.

Differentiation of intrarenal ARF from prerenal azotemia may be clinically difficult in many patients because both conditions frequently are accompanied by oliguria. A carefully collected urine sample, however, may provide significant clues in making the distinction. By itself, the routine urinalysis may be of little diagnostic aid because mild proteinuria may be present in both conditions, in association with a few cellular elements and granular casts on microscopic examination. The latter are much more numerous in ARF than in prerenal azotemia and tend to be pigmented; these are highly characteristic but not diagnostic.

Procurement of a urine specimen for diagnostic chemistries and indices as indicated in Table 30–4 is invaluable in establishing the diagnosis of ARF. This urine sample should be obtained *before* a diagnostic challenge of diuretics because these agents may alter the urine's chemical composition. Urinary chemistry determinations distinguish between underperfusion of the kidney, in which most solutes except sodium tend to be concentrated, and intrarenal ARF, in which solute concentration tends to be reduced, resulting from an inability of the injured tubules to alter the urine composition.

Differential Diagnosis of Acute Renal Failure

1. Prerenal azotemia
   a. Hypovolemia
   b. Cardiovascular failure
      1. Myocardial failure
      2. Vascular pooling
   c. Hepatorenal syndrome
2. Vascular obstruction
   a. Arterial obstruction
      1. Embolization
      2. Thrombosis
      3. Dissection
   b. Venous obstruction
3. Intrinsic renal disease
   a. Glomerulonephritis
   b. Vasculitis
   c. Microangiopathic disease
      1. Hemolytic uremic syndrome
      2. Thrombotic thrombocytopenic purpura
   d. Malignant nephrosclerosis
4. Postrenal azotemia
   a. Obstructive uropathy
   b. Bladder rupture
   c. Prostatic hypertrophy

Diagnostic Clues in Acute Renal Failure

Urine

- *Urate crystals:* Tumor lysis, especially lymphoma (urate nephropathy)
- *Oxalate crystals:* Ethylene glycol nephrotoxicity, methoxyflurane nephrotoxicity
- *Eosinophils:* Allergic interstitial nephritis, especially methicillin
- *Positive benzidene without RBCs:* Hemoglobinuria or myoglobinuria
- *Pigmented casts:* Hemoglobinuria or myoglobinuria
- *Massive proteinuria:* Acute interstitial nephritis, thiazide diuretics, hemorrhagic fevers (eg, Korean, Scandinavian)
- *Anuria:* Renal cortical necrosis, bilateral obstruction, hemolytic uremic syndrome, rapidly progressive glomerulonephritis

Plasma

- *Marked hyperkalemia:* Rhabdomyolysis, tissue necrosis, hemolysis
- *Marked hypocalcemia:* Rhabdomyolysis
- *Hypercalcemia:* Hypercalcemic nephropathy
- *Hyperuricemia:* Tumor lysis, rhabdomyolysis, toxin ingestion
- *Marked acidosis:* Ethylene glycol, methyl alcohol
- *Eosinophilia:* Allergic interstitial nephritis

TABLE 30-4

Use of Laboratory Values in Differentiating Acute Tubular Necrosis From Decreased Renal Perfusion

Test	Acute Tubular Necrosis	Reduced Renal Blood Flow
Urine		
Volume	< 400 mL/24 h	< 400 mL/24 h
Sodium	40–10 mEq/L	< 5 mEq/L
Specific gravity	1.010	Usually > 1.020
Osmolality	250–350 mOsm/L	Usually > 400 mOsm/L
Urea	200–300 mg/100 mL	Usually > 600 mg/100 mL
Creatinine	< 60 mg/100 mL	Usually > 150 mg/100 mL
Fe_{Na}	> 3.0%	< 1.0%
Blood		
BUN:Cr	10:1	Usually > 20:1
Responses To		
Mannitol	None	None or flow increases to > 40 mL/h
Furosemide	None	Flow increases to > 40 mL/h

FE_{Na}, fractional excretion of sodium; BUN:Cr, blood urea nitrogen–creatinine ratio.

Thus, in prerenal azotemia, the urinary sodium is low, as are the renal failure index and fractional excretion of sodium (Fe_{Na}), whereas the urine osmolality and concentration of nonreabsorbable solutes are high. In intrarenal ARF, urine sodium is greater than 30 mEq/L, the renal failure index and Fe_{Na} are greater than 1%, and the urine osmolality is close to that of plasma, reflecting the inability of the damaged kidney to reabsorb sodium and concentrate the urine.

Also, ATN must be distinguished from all other intrinsic renal diseases that can rapidly reduce renal function. Many of these can be differentiated by their clinical picture and urinalyses. In some circumstances, the diagnosis may be difficult, such as with rapidly progressive glomerulonephritis without significant urine sediment abnormalities. In this situation, urine chemistries look more like those seen in prerenal azotemia than those observed in ATN and should be a clue to the diagnosis. There frequently are subtle clues that will aid in the diagnosis of ARF, and these should be sought carefully (see display).

■ MANAGEMENT

Primary management of renal function impairment is directed at the adequate and specific management of the hypoperfused state. The three most common causes for reduced renal perfusion are decreased cardiac output, altered peripheral vascular resistance, and hypovolemia.

Improvement of Cardiac Function

Factors such as cardiac dysrhythmias, acute myocardial infarction, and acute pericardial tamponade, all of which decrease cardiac output, may be associated with a reduction in renal blood flow. The reversibility of the renal failure thus depends on the ability to improve cardiac function.

In these conditions, cardiac output usually is acutely and severely compromised. When cardiac output is impaired to a lesser extent over a longer period of time, however, features of congestive heart failure occur. Again, there is reduced renal perfusion, although to a lesser extent. The major feature of this state, from the renal aspect, is avid sodium reabsorption, which results in increased ECF volume, elevated central venous pressure, and edema.

Several mechanisms are responsible for the increased tubular reabsorption of sodium (see Fig. 30–3). First, there is a greater reduction in renal blood flow than in glomerular filtration, bringing into play the mechanisms discussed previously. Second, it has been suggested that blood flow to the superficial cortex is reduced, whereas blood flow to the inner cortical area is increased. In addition, it is thought that the nephrons in the inner cortical region reabsorb a greater percentage of the filtered sodium than the nephrons in the outer cortex of the kidney.

Other factors include increased proximal and distal tubule sodium reabsorption. The mechanisms responsible for the increased proximal tubule sodium reabsorption are dependent largely on increased postglomerular oncotic pressure; however, aldosterone mostly is responsible for the increased distal tubule sodium reabsorption. Numerous mechanisms are responsible for the increased tubular reabsorption of sodium in congestive heart failure.

Therapy is directed largely at increasing urinary sodium excretion. At times, this can be accomplished by improvement of cardiac output, which in turn increases renal perfusion. This is not always possible, however.

Diuretics are used frequently to increase sodium excretion. These agents directly inhibit sodium reabsorption in the renal tubule. The potency of a diuretic is determined primarily by the site in the renal tubule where sodium reabsorption is blocked.

Commonly used loop diuretics include furosemide (Lasix), bumetanide (Bumex), torsemide (Demadex), and ethacrynic acid (Edecrin). These agents block sodium reabsorption in the ascending limb of the loop of Henle and in the distal tubule. It still is unclear whether they have an effect in the proximal tubule as well. The thiazide diuretics have their major site of action in the distal tubule and are therefore somewhat less potent than the previously mentioned agents.

Another commonly used diuretic is spironolactone (Aldactone), which increases urinary sodium by blocking the renal tubular effect of aldosterone. Spironolactone should be used with caution in patients with severe decreases in cardiac output and renal underperfusion because it decreases potassium excretion and can produce life-threatening hyperkalemia in such patients. The same is true of triamterene, another potassium-sparing diuretic.

Management of Altered Peripheral Vascular Resistance

Renal perfusion is compromised in these states as a result of increased size of the intravascular compartment and redistribution of blood volume. This may be a consequence of gram-negative septicemia, certain drug overdoses, anaphylactic reactions, and electrolyte disturbances, such as acidosis.

Management is directed primarily at treating the basic disturbance with appropriate specific therapy plus fluid, electrolyte, and colloid replacement. The controversy over the use of steroids and various pressor agents in gram-negative sepsis is beyond the scope of this discussion.

Management of Hypovolemia and Hemorrhage

Restoration of ECF and blood volume is of major importance in the management of any hypoperfused state. Evidence for extracellular volume depletion usually is obtained from the history and physical examination.

Historically, the patient may give evidence of external sodium and water loss as a result of vomiting, diarrhea, excessive sweating, or surgical procedures. Blood volume also may be compromised as a result of fluid redistribution, as seen both with burns and with inflammatory processes in the abdomen, such as pancreatitis or peritonitis. The physical findings associated with extracellular volume depletion are sunken eyes, dry mouth, loss of skin turgor, and tachycardia. Postural hypotension also may be noted.

Therapy is directed at sodium and water replacement or blood when hemorrhage is the cause. Response to treatment can be judged by changes in urinary volume, specific gravity, central venous pressure, and the aforementioned physical findings.

Maintenance of Urinary Flow

At times, despite adequate treatment, urinary volume remains low. This may be a result of either continuing functional impairment in the post-hypoperfusion period or parenchymal renal damage resulting from the hypoperfusion. It is necessary to differentiate these two states from each other because prolonged oliguria, if allowed to persist, eventually may lead to ATN. Mannitol and furosemide have been used in this situation for diagnosis and maintenance of urinary function.

Mannitol is the reduced form of the six-carbon sugar, mannose. It is distributed in the ECF and essentially is not metabolized. It is freely filtered at the glomerulus and not reabsorbed by the tubule. Because of its small molecular size, it exerts a significant osmotic effect and, in turn, increases urinary flow.

Mannitol usually is infused rather rapidly. The more rapid the infusion, the higher the blood level and, in turn, the filtered load. Urinary flow depends on the amount of mannitol filtered, and if the infusion is too slow, changes in urinary flow rate will be delayed and less apparent.

The usual test is 0.2 g/kg given intravenously as a 25% solution over 3 to 5 minutes. If urine flow increases to greater than 40 mL/h, the patient is thought to have reversible renal failure, and urine volume is then maintained at 100 mL/h with additional mannitol and fluid replacement as indicated.

More recently, *furosemide* and other diuretics have largely replaced mannitol in the diagnosis of reversible renal failure. A number of patients who fail to have diuresis after infusion of mannitol will have an acceptable increase in urinary volume after administration of furosemide or ethacrynic acid.

After correction of volume depletion, furosemide in dosages of 200 to 600 mg may be given intravenously. The peak diuresis usually occurs within 2 hours of its administration. If furosemide is effective in increasing urinary volume, it may be repeated at 4- to 6-hour intervals to maintain the urinary flow rate as long as fluids are administered to maintain urine.

Tinnitus and hearing impairment (reversible and irreversible) have been reported following intravenous furosemide. Ototoxicity usually is associated with rapid injection, excessively high dosage, or concomitant therapy with other ototoxic drugs (ie, aminoglycosides). The manufacturer recommends controlled intravenous infusion (not to exceed 4 mg/min) for high-dose parenteral furosemide therapy.

In patients failing to respond to furosemide, a diagnosis of ATN must be considered. In patients who respond to furosemide and mannitol, it is important to replace sodium and water losses to avoid depletion. Usually, urine volume is replaced by half-strength normal saline. In addition, potassium replacement frequently is required.

Low-dose dopamine (Intropin) at 1 to 3 µg/kg/min has also been used in euvolemic patients with oliguric ARF. Dopamine increases renal blood flow and GFR and decreases systemic and renal vascular resistance. There is, however, ongoing controversy about the therapeutic benefit of this approach.

Management of Complications

PREVENTION OF ACUTE TUBULAR NECROSIS

Because ATN continues to be associated with a high mortality, the major objective is preventing this complication. ATN can be prevented in patients with major traumatic injuries by rapid replacement of blood loss and correction of fluid and electrolyte disturbances.

Similarly, patients receiving potentially nephrotoxic agents should undergo serial determinations to evaluate renal function during the course of the administration of these agents. This is accomplished most easily by measuring serum creatinine levels on an every-other-day schedule. If the serum creatinine begins to rise, the drug should be discontinued. In most patients, functional deterioration stabilizes, and the patient recovers without the development of severe impairment of renal function.

Considerable debate remains with regard to the effectiveness of mannitol, diuretics, and low-dose dopamine in the prevention of ARF. Some evidence suggests that furosemide actually may increase the toxicity of certain nephrotoxic agents. Most authors, however, agree that a trial of furosemide up to 500 mg intravenously should be used. Often, this may correct oliguric to nonoliguric ARF, which is easier to manage clinically.

MANAGEMENT OF ACUTE TUBULAR NECROSIS

Volume Replacement

After development of ATN, the primary consideration is maintenance of fluid and electrolyte balance. During the oliguric phase, urinary volume usually is less than 300 mL/d. Insensible losses average 800 to 1,000 mL/d and are virtually free of electrolytes.

In general, fluid replacement should be insensible losses plus output. Additional water will be obtained from the water present in foods plus the water of oxidation from metabolism. The *danger of fluid overload* with resulting congestive heart failure and pulmonary edema exists throughout the oliguric period. In contrast, during the diuretic phase of ATN, extensive *sodium wasting* may occur in association with the increased urinary volumes. It thus is necessary to keep accurate intake and output records and daily weights during both phases. This is especially important when there are other avenues of fluid and electrolyte losses, such as vomiting, diarrhea, nasogastric suction, and drainages from fistulas. In general, losses occurring as a result of these problems should be replaced in full.

Nutrition

Besides replacing fluids and electrolytes, intake is directed at supplying the patient with calories in the form of carbohydrates and fats to decrease the rate of breakdown of body protein. Because 1 g of urea is formed from every 6 g of protein metabolized, protein intake usually is restricted to prevent the BUN from rising too fast.

With the development of nutritional teams, there has been a growing tendency to provide more calories and protein in the form of parenteral or enteral hyperalimentation in attempts to improve the overall condition of the patient and hasten recovery of renal function. Diets containing 2,000 to 3,000 calories per day with 40 to 60 g of protein or essential amino acids have been used with increased frequency. These diets contain more than the 500 mL of fluid recommended previously. Therefore, hyperalimentation re-

> ### Considerations for Home Care
> ### Dialysis Therapy
>
> Individuals who suffer from acute renal failure secondary to hypoperfusion or tubular injury may have a delayed recovery time. Maintenance hemodialysis may be required until normal function returns. If damage is permanent, which is unknown at times, the individual will need permanent dialysis therapy. Chronic dialysis includes both hemodialysis and peritoneal dialysis and potential kidney transplantation (see Chapter 46). If there is a possibility of the kidney recovering, time is needed for tissue repair, and outpatient dialysis therapy may be required. Modification in diet and fluid consumption will be necessary until the kidney is recovered. This restriction must be reviewed, and psychosocial implications discussed with the patient and family. Temporary dialysis support is dependent on the renal injury and can last for several weeks to months.

quires more frequent dialysis, especially in the oliguric period, often in combination with hemofiltration.

Control of Acidosis

Metabolic acidosis of moderate severity usually is present in patients with renal failure. This results from the inability of the kidneys to excrete fixed acids (eg, H_2PO_4) produced from normal metabolic processes. Acidosis usually can be controlled easily by giving the patient 30 to 60 mEq of sodium bicarbonate daily but does not require treatment unless the HCO_3 falls below 15 to 18 mEq/L.

Control of Hyperkalemia

Hyperkalemia commonly occurs in patients with ATN. This is a consequence of the reduced ability of the kidneys to excrete potassium and the release of intracellular potassium because of acidosis and tissue breakdown. The acidosis results in movement of the hydrogen ion into the cell, thus displacing potassium into the ECF. This maintains electrical neutrality but increases the hyperkalemic state.

An additional mechanism for producing hyperkalemia, often overlooked in acutely ill patients, is caloric restriction, especially glucose restriction. Transport of glucose and amino acids into cells is accompanied by potassium. In acutely ill, catabolic patients, when dietary intake is restricted or intravenous fluid therapy inadvertently disrupted, failure of transport of potassium intracellularly may contribute to hyperkalemia. Because this process requires insulin, insulin deficiency may have the same consequences, and diabetics may therefore be more prone to acute disturbances in potassium balance when renal failure occurs.

Hyperkalemia is manifested clinically by cardiac and neuromuscular changes. Both cardiac conduction disturbances and acute flaccid quadriplegia are life-threatening complications. These hyperkalemic changes are reversed rapidly by administration of intravenous calcium gluconate, which has a direct antagonist effect on the action of potassium. Serum potassium can be reduced by intravenous administration of sodium bicarbonate for treatment of acidosis. In addition, administration of glucose and insulin frequently is used as an additional method of shifting extracellular potassium to intracellular pools.

Sodium polystyrene sulfonate resin (Kayexalate) given orally (25 g four times a day in 10 mL of 10% sorbitol) may reduce the body potassium burden more slowly and should be instituted when hyperkalemia begins to develop. In addition, when life-threatening hyperkalemia develops and these treatments fail or do not restore serum potassium to normal, emergency intervention, either hemodialysis or peritoneal dialysis, should be instituted. Although hemodialysis will reduce body burden of potassium to a greater degree than peritoneal dialysis, peritoneal dialysis generally can be instituted much more quickly. Because plasma potassium equilibrates rapidly with peritoneal fluid, serum potassium can be reduced promptly.

Hyperkalemia usually can be prevented by avoidance of potassium supplements, institution of chronic therapy for acidosis, and use of sodium polystyrene sulfonate resin when serum potassium is even slightly elevated.

Sodium and Water Diuresis

During the oliguric phase of ATN, sodium retention may occur. With the onset of the diuretic period, however, urinary volume and sodium excretion may increase markedly.

Urinary volume largely is determined by the state of hydration at the onset of the diuretic period. Because urinary sodium concentration is relatively fixed, sodium losses are determined mostly by urinary volume. Therefore, if the patient is markedly overhydrated at the onset of the diuretic phase, sodium losses may be severe. Clinically, sodium depletion is characterized by either extracellular volume depletion, as manifested by tachycardia and postural hypotension, or water intoxication when sodium losses exceed water losses. This latter syndrome is characterized by markedly reduced serum sodium concentrations in association with personality changes, convulsions, coma, and death if allowed to progress untreated.

Prevention of Uremic Syndrome

In addition to electrolyte disturbances, the patient may have symptoms of uremia. Early findings are nausea, anorexia, and vomiting. Later, stupor, convulsions, and coma develop. In addition, bleeding abnormalities, uremic pneumonitis, pericarditis, and pleuritis may occur.

Dialysis is indicated before the development of clinical symptoms of uremia. With the availability of hemodialysis or peritoneal dialysis, the clinical features of uremia do not usually occur in patients with ATN. Most patients with oliguria for more than 4 to 5 days will require dialysis sometime during the course of ATN. Dialysis has improved survival in patients with ATN. Continuous hemofiltration also has been used to treat ATN.

Prognosis is determined largely by the primary event that led to the development of ATN. Among patients with ATN due to medical causes (eg, transfusion reactions, myoglobinuria, nephrotoxic agents, and simple volume depletion), the mortality rate is approximately 25%, whereas cases resulting from trauma and severe surgical complications are associated with a 60% to 70% mortality rate. Death usually results as a complication of poor wound healing and sepsis or the underlying disease.

Precaution With Drugs

Certain drugs should be avoided or dosage reduced in any patient with markedly impaired renal function. Because of the possibility of magnesium intoxication, *antacids* containing magnesium should be avoided. Because of the reduced renal function, *digitalis* excretion may be reduced. Dosage should be altered to avoid excessively high blood levels. In addition, certain *antibiotics* should be given in much smaller dosages than usual. Modifications may be made based on the dosage interval or on alterations of the percentage of the normal dose given at standard dosage intervals. Table 30–5 lists antibiotics that may require supplemental doses because of their removal by hemodialysis.

Insights Into Clinical Research

Klang B, Bjorvell H, Clyne N: Perceived well-being in predialysis uremic patients. ANNA Journal 23(2):223–229, 260, 1996

This descriptive correlational study focused on patients with renal insufficiency prior to starting a dialytic therapy. The patients had sufficient renal impairment that toxins were interfering with other body systems, presenting a constellation of symptoms referred to as uremia. Questionnaires were used to assess individuals' perceived health, frequency of their symptoms, and sense of coherence. The instruments were Likert-type scales, which were mailed to the individuals home with proper instruction and a self-addressed envelope.

The goal of this study was to examine the individual's sense of well-being in the face of uremia. The study reinforced the impact of uremia on an individual's sense of well-being. The study demonstrated a significant relationship between sense of coherence and perceived health; individuals with a strong sense of coherence perceived their health as better than those with a weak sense of coherence. No major differences were found in age or length of disease, but gender and educational and marital status influenced the individual's perception of health and the presence of symptoms.

Many important clinical findings were discussed, and the focus of treating presenting symptoms may assist the individual's perception of health. Nurses could interpret the importance of significant others/social support in the perception of health. Individuals with poor social support systems need more intensive planning and referral to the appropriate support groups or services. Most importantly, nurses must remember that others are important to a patient's sense of health.

TABLE 30-5
Supplemental Antibiotic Dosages for Patients on Hemodialysis*

Drug	Dosage Modification
Antifungal Drugs	
Amphotericin B	None
Fluconazole	100 mg
Miconazole	None
Antitubercular Drugs	
Ethambutol	15 mg/kg
Isoniazid	5 mg/kg
Rifampin	None
Antiviral Drugs	
Acyclovir	5 mg/kg
Amantadine	None
Ganciclovir	2.5 mg/kg
Zidovudine	200 mg
Carbapenem	
Imipenem	0.5 g
Quinolones	
Ciprofloxacin	None
Norfloxacin	Avoid
Ofloxacin	100 mg
Miscellaneous	
Aztreonam	125 mg
Chloramphenicol	None
Clindamycin	None
Erythromycin	None
Metronidazole	250 mg

* Give all supplements after dialysis.
Modified from Cutler R, Forland S: Removal of drugs by hemodialysis and continuous ambulatory peritoneal dialysis: Suggested dosing modifications. Dialysis and Transplantation 20(12):759–761, 1991

Before administering a drug to a patient with renal failure, the following questions should be reviewed:

- Does the drug depend on the kidney for excretion?
- Does an excess blood level affect the kidney?
- Does the drug add chemically to the pool of urea nitrogen?
- Does the effect of the drug alter electrolyte balance?
- Is the patient more susceptible to the drug because of kidney disease?

As new drugs are introduced into the clinical setting, it is imperative that nurses working with renal patients review the need to modify drug dosages or frequencies to avoid toxicity or to provide necessary supplementation.

Because GFRs can change rapidly with certain physiological dysfunctions and multisystem involvement, the nurse should monitor laboratory data, assessment parameters, and patient response closely to anticipate needed adjustments in drug therapy. Likewise, in patients receiving dialysis, the same precaution should be taken to ensure that serum levels remain therapeutic.

CLINICAL APPLICATION: Patient Care Study

Mrs. Landry, an 85-year-old woman with calcific aortic stenosis, was admitted with mild congestive heart failure. She complained of weakness, fatigue, and loss of appetite. She stated that she lived alone and had great difficulty caring for herself. Admission examination revealed Mrs. Landry appeared chronically ill and was mildly dyspneic but not edematous. Her mucous membranes were very dry, her tongue was coated, and her skin was dry and flaky. She reported two-pillow orthopnea and had been spending most of her time in bed during the last 2 weeks. Her weight was 53.3 kg; blood pressure, 120/60; pulse, 98 beats/min; temperature, 97.8°F; and respirations, 24/min. BUN was 13.4 mg/dL, and serum creatinine was 0.4 mg/dL. Mrs. Landry was maintained on her normal dose of digoxin (0.125 mg/d) and placed on a 1,200-calorie, 2-g sodium diet and given hydrochlorothiazide, 50 mg two times a day.

Mrs. Landry's cardiovascular symptoms gradually improved, but 1 week later, she was slightly confused and complained of dizziness on sitting up. Her blood pressure was 150/60; pulse, 108 beats/min; and weight, 47.7 kg. She did not recall voiding in the past 24 hours. A Foley catheter was inserted, and 15 mL of dark yellow urine was obtained. The following laboratory values were obtained:

- Serum

Na: 149 mEq/L	BUN: 144 mg/dL
Cl: 112 mEq/L	Creatinine: 2.1 mg/dL
CO_2: 29 mEq/L	Osmolality: 303 mOsm/L
K: 3.5 mEq/L	

- Urine

Na: 11 mEq/dL	Osmolality: 482 mOsm/L
K: 33 mEq/dL	Creatinine: 89 mg/dL

Care Study Discussion

The hypernatremia suggested mild dehydration. BUN was alarmingly high, and the serum creatinine of 2.1 mg/dL, although seemingly low in relation to the BUN, was four times greater than the value recorded on admission, suggesting a loss of 75% of initial renal function. A diagnosis of ARF secondary to volume depletion was considered. When urine chemistries returned, however, the low urinary sodium, the urinary osmolality (which was 1.6 × that of plasma), and the U/P creatinine ratio of 42/1 suggested intact renal function. The fractional excretion of sodium (U:P Na/U:P creatinine × 100) was calculated as follows: $Fe_{Na} = 11:149/89:2.1 \times 100 = 0.17\%$. This also was consistent with volume depletion and prerenal azotemia.

Mrs. Landry could have had either (1) ARF resulting from excessive volume depletion or from emboli due to cardiac disease or (2) prerenal azotemia resulting from volume depletion.

A challenge with 500 mL normal saline (N/S) IV over 1 hour produced a urine flow of 40 mL in the next hour. A slow infusion of N/S, 2 L/d, was given over the next 4 days and followed by increasing urine volumes. Mrs. Landry's weight increased to 51.1 kg, and the BUN and creatinine dropped to 22.4 and 0.9 mg/dL, respectively, without increased signs of cardiac decompensation. This dramatic response confirmed the laboratory-supported diagnosis of prerenal azotemia.

An overview of the management of patients with ARF is provided in the accompanying Collaborative Care Guide.

COLLABORATIVE CARE GUIDE
for the Patient With Acute Renal Failure

OUTCOMES	INTERVENTIONS

Oxygenation/Ventilation

Arterial blood gas values are within normal limits with no evidence of atelectasis.

- Provide routine pulmonary toilet, including the following:
  - Airway suctioning
  - Chest percussion
  - Incentive spirometer
  - Turn frequently
- Mobilize out of bed to chair.
- Monitor arterial blood gases as necessary.
- Monitor pulse oximetry.

Circulation/Perfusion

Blood pressure, heart rate, and hemodynamic parameters are within normal limits.

Blood pressure remains within normal limits during dialysis.

- Monitor vital signs q1–2h.
- Monitor pulmonary artery pressures and right atrial pressure q1h and cardiac output, SVR, and PVR q6–12h if pulmonary artery catheter is in place.
- Assess vital signs continuously or q15min during dialysis.
- Administer intravascular volume or blood products as indicated.

Fluids/Electrolytes

Patient is euvolemic.

There are no signs of hypervolemia.

Urine output >30 mL/ h (or >0.5 mL/kg/h).

Dialysis results in normalization of fluid balance, electrolytes, BUN, and creatinine.

Dialysis access remains patent and no complications are evident.

- Monitor intake and output q1h.
- Weigh daily.
- Monitor for hypertension, pulmonary edema, peripheral edema, neck vein distension, elevated CVP, RAP, or PAWP.
- Administer diuretics as indicated.
- Make sure Foley catheter is in place.
- Administer fluids and diuretics to maintain intravascular volume and renal function, per order.
- Monitor electrolytes daily and PRN.
- Replace electrolytes as ordered.
- Monitor BUN, creatinine, serum osmolarity, and urine electrolytes q6–12h and predialysis and postdialysis as ordered.
- Monitor and maintain dialysis access for chosen dialysis and hemofiltration method:
  - *Continuous veno-veno or arterial-veno:*
    qh ultrafiltrate and fluid replacement measurement, protect vascular access from dislodgement, change filter and tubing per protocol, monitor vascular access for infection, monitor patient temperature.
  - *Peritoneal dialysis:*
    Slowly infuse warmed dialysate, drain after appropriate dwell time, assess drainage for volume and appearance, send cultures qd, and assess access for infection.
  - *Intermittent hemodialysis:*
    Assess shunt for thrill and buzzing sound q12h, avoid blood pressures and venipunctures in arm with shunt, and assess for infection.

Mobility/Safety

There is no evidence of complications related to bed rest and immobility.

- Initiate deep vein thrombosis prophylaxis.
- Reposition frequently.
- Mobilize to chair when possible.
- Consult physical therapist.

(continued)

COLLABORATIVE CARE GUIDE
for the Patient With Acute Renal Failure (Continued)

OUTCOMES	INTERVENTIONS
	• Conduct range-of-motion and strengthening exercises.
Skin Integrity Skin will remain intact.	• Assess skin q8h and each time patient is repositioned. • Turn q2h. • Consider pressure-relief-reduction mattress. • Use Braden Scale to assess risk of skin breakdown.
Nutrition Caloric and nutrient intake meet metabolic requirements per calculation (eg, basal energy expenditure).	• Provide parenteral or enteral feeding. • Consult dietitian or nutritional support service. • Observe sodium, potassium, protein, and fluid restriction as indicated. • Provide small, frequent feedings. • Monitor albumin, prealbumin, transferrin levels.
Comfort/Pain Control Patient will have minimal pain and discomfort.	• Assess pain and discomfort from dialysis and pruritus. • Administer analgesics cautiously, and monitor patient response. • Bathe with lanolin-based soap. • Lubricate skin with emollients PRN.
Psychosocial Patient demonstrates decreased anxiety.	• Assess vital signs during treatments, discussions. • Cautiously administer sedatives. • Consult social services, clergy as appropriate. • Provide for adequate rest and sleep. • Provide support during periods of stress or discomfort during dialysis.
Teaching/Discharge Planning Patient/significant others understand procedures and tests needed for treatment during the acute phase and maintenance of a patient with chronic disease. Significant others understand the severity of the illness, ask appropriate questions, and anticipate potential complications. In preparation for discharge to home, patient/family demonstrates understanding of renal replacement therapy, fluid, and dietary and medication restrictions.	• Prepare patient/significant others for procedures, such as insertion of dialysis access, dialysis therapy, or laboratory studies. • Explain the causes and effects of renal failure and the potential for complications, such as hypertension and fluid overload. • Encourage significant others to ask questions related to the pathophysiology, dialysis, monitoring, and dietary or fluid restrictions. • Make appropriate referrals and consults early during hospitalization. • Initiate family education regarding home care of dialysis patient, what to expect, maintenance of renal function, and when to seek medical attention.

Clinical Applicability Challenges

Self-Challenge: Critical Thinking

1. Develop a nursing plan of care for Mrs. Landry (see Patient Care Study).
2. Formulate a teaching plan for a patient on a low sodium diet.

Study Questions

1. Mr. O'Keefe has mild congestive heart failure. His serum sodium is 130 mEq/L. He has pitting edema of the ankles and moist rales are heard in bilateral lung bases. He would benefit most from:
   a. hypertonic saline infusion administered IV.
   b. 5% dextrose in water administered IV.

c. vasopressin.

d. furosemide.

2. In prerenal azotemia, the events that lead to a decline in function occur

a. between the bladder and the ureters.

b. in the renal cortex.

c. at the level of the glomeruli.

d. before circulation reaches the kidney.

3. Events that cause kidney tissue damage along with renal failure are categorized as

a. severe renal ischemia.

b. hyperviscosity states.

c. intrarenal ARF.

d. postrenal ARF.

4. The primary focus of treating prerenal azotemia is to

a. restore renal circulation.

b. control serum sodium and potassium.

c. remove the enlarged prostate.

d. inspect urine for hematuria and stones.

5. What is the most common complication of oliguric renal failure?

a. Respiratory acidosis

b. Overhydration

c. Metabolic acidosis

d. Hyperglycemia

6. The most important aspect of nursing care during the diuretic phase of ARF is

a. relieving symptoms of uremia.

b. measuring serial potassium levels.

c. monitoring oxygen saturation.

d. maintaining fluid and electrolyte balance.

7. The primary danger of not correcting prerenal ARF is

a. cardiovascular collapse.

b. progression to intrarenal ARF.

c. pulmonary edema.

d. cerebral hemorrhage.

REFERENCES

1. Glassock R, Adler S: Diabetic nephropathy. In Levine D (ed): Care of the Renal Patient (2nd Ed). Philadelphia, WB Saunders, 1991

2. Lancaster L: Manifestations of renal failure. In Lancaster L (ed): Core Curriculum for Nephrology Nursing (2nd Ed), pp 79–107. Pitman, NJ, AJ Jannetti, 1990

3. Narims R (ed): Maxwell & Kleeman's Clinical Disorders of Fluids and Electrolytes Metabolism, p 11. New York, McGraw-Hill, 1994

4. Metheny NM: Fluid and Electrolyte Balance: Nursing Considerations, p 4. Philadelphia, Lippincott-Raven, 1996

5. Weisberg L, Kurnik P, Kurnik B: Risk of radiocontrast nephropathy in patients with and without diabetes mellitus. Kidney International 45:259, 1994

6. Berns J, Rudnick M: Radiocontrast media associated nephropathy. The Kidney 24(4):1–5, 1992

7. Solomon R, Werner C, Mann D, et al: Effects of saline, mannitol, and furosemide on acute decreases in renal function induced by radiocontrast agents. The New England Journal of Medicine 331:1416, 1994

BIBLIOGRAPHY

Bennett W, Henrich W, Stoff J: The renal effects of nonsteroidal anti-inflammatory drugs: Summary and recommendations. American Journal of Kidney Disease 28(1 Supp):S56–S62, 1996

Daugirdas JT, Ing TS: Handbook of Dialysis 2nd ed., Boston, Little & Brown, 1994

Lancaster L: Manifestations of renal failure. In Lancaster L (ed): Core Curriculum for Nephrology Nursing, 3rd ed., Pitman, NJ, AJ Jannetti, 1995

Levy E, Viscoli C, Horwitz R: The effect of acute renal failure on mortality. JAMA 275(19):1489–1495, 1996

Myers B: Pathogenetic processes in human acute renal failure. Seminars in Dialysis 9(6):444–453, 1996

Nolde-Hurlbert B: Drug removal during dialysis. Dialysis and Transplantation 22(6)316–322, 1993

Pavao dos Santos O, Boim M, Schor N: Acute renal failure and sepsis: Pathophysiology. Kidney 4:59–62, 1995

Stark J: Acute renal failure in trauma: current perspectives. Critical Care Nursing Quarterly 16(4):49–60, 1994

Nervous System

Anatomy and Physiology of the Nervous System

OBJECTIVES

Based on the content in this chapter, the reader should be able to:

- List the cellular units of the nervous system.
- Briefly explain the physiology of a nerve impulse.
- List two functions of cerebrospinal fluid.
- Explain the functions of the thalamus.
- Define the reticular activating system.
- Briefly define the sensory system and the motor system.
- List and explain the three cord reflexes.
- Explain the physiology of pain and the gate theory of pain regulation.

*T*raditionally the nervous system is discussed in both anatomical and functional divisions. Anatomical components are the central nervous system (CNS), which comprises the brain and spinal cord, and the peripheral nervous system, comprising the spinal and cranial nerves. Functional divisions are the sensory, interpretive, and motor (somatic and autonomic) divisions. Content in this chapter is ordered according to both divisions. First, however, cell anatomy and physiology are discussed.

CELLS OF THE NERVOUS SYSTEM

The cellular units are the *neuron*—the basic functional unit—and its attendant cells, the *neuroglias* and *Schwann cells*. It may be easier to treat the attendant cells first and then proceed to neuronal functioning.

Neuroglial Cells

The neuroglial cells constitute the supportive tissue that lies within the CNS around the neurons. There are three types of glial cells: microglia, astrocytes, and oligodendroglia. These last cells are thought to produce the myelin that covers nerve fibers within the CNS.

Whereas neurons lose their ability to undergo mitosis early in the life of the individual, neuroglial cells seem to retain mitotic abilities throughout a person's life span. Because of this, nonmetastatic CNS lesions involve glial cells rather than neurons. As the glial tumor enlarges, however, it adversely affects adjacent neurons early by exerting pressure and later by promoting an inflammatory reaction along with the pressure. The counterpart of the myelin-producing oligodendroglial cell in the peripheral nervous system is the cell of Schwann.

Neurons

The basic functional unit of the nervous system is the *neuron,* and all information and activity, whether sensory, motor, or integrative, is processed by it.

The precise characteristic of individual neurons is determined by their specific function. Some neurons are extremely large and may give rise to extremely long nerve fibers. Transmission velocities in the long fibers may be as high as 100 m/s, whereas smaller neurons with very small fibers demonstrate velocities of 1 m/s. Some neurons connect to many different neurons in a "network," and still others have few connections to other cells of the nervous system.

It has been estimated that there are 12 billion neurons in the CNS. Three fourths of these neurons are located in the cerebral cortex, where information transmitted through the nervous system is processed. This processing, as already indicated, includes not only the determination of appropriate and effective responses, but also the storage of memory and the development of associative motor and thought patterns.

Neuron Structure and Function

The neuron is also termed a *nerve cell.* It consists of a nerve cell body that contains nuclear and cytoplasmic material and processes arising from this. These processes are functionally differentiated into axons and dendrites (Fig. 31–1). *Axons* normally carry nervous impulses away from the cell body, whereas *dendrites* conduct the impulse toward the cell body. Axons and dendrites may be merely microscopic knobs or areas on the cell body surface, or they may be cylindrical processes that can, in certain cases, extend to over 1 m (4 ft) in length.

Neurons do not connect to one another. There are spaces between the axon (or axons) of one neuron and the dendrite (or dendrites) of another. This space is termed the *synapse.* Axons and dendrites may branch, enabling the axon of one neuron to synapse with dendrites of more than one other neuron. Similarly, axons from several neurons may synapse with a single neuron. The former is an example of divergence; the latter exemplifies convergence.

NERVES AND GANGLIA

Axons and dendrites are referred to collectively as *nerve fibers.* A bundle of nerve fibers together with their coverings is termed a *nerve.* A *ganglion* is a group of cell bodies.

NERVE FIBER COVERINGS

Within the CNS, some fibers are covered with a lipid-protein sheath termed the *myelin sheath.* This appears to be formed by the action of oligodendrocytes. Other fibers remain unmyelinated. Peripheral nerve fibers all are covered by a *neurilemma.* This is a sheath formed by the cells of Schwann, which wrap themselves around the fiber. The Schwann cells around some fibers also secrete myelin; others do not (see Fig. 31–1). The neurilemma of myelinated fibers comes in contact with the fiber at periodic intervals. These periodic constrictions of the neurilemmal sheath are termed the *nodes of Ranvier.* Such nodes produce a faster impulse conduction.

NERVE FIBER REGENERATION

If a nerve fiber is severed, the portion distal to the cell body will die. The part still attached to the cell body will regenerate. In peripheral neurons, the neurilemma itself provides a channel that can be followed by a regenerating fiber so that it may become reattached to its original anatomical connection (Fig. 31–2). Regeneration also occurs in the absence of a neurilemma, as in the case of CNS neurons. Because there is no channel to ensure correct anatomical reconnection, most such regeneration does not produce recovered function. The regrowing stump may wind aimlessly among other structures or curl into a useless tangle. A bigger hindrance to functional regeneration within the CNS has been discovered, however—an overgrowth of neurological cells that occurs in response to injury. This produces a glial thicket that acts as a barrier to the reconnection of severed neuronal networks.

NEURONAL CONDUCTION

The essence of the nerve impulse is the action potential and its self-propagated conduction. The neuronal membrane contains sodium–potassium pumps that keep the inside of the neuron more negatively charged than the outside interstitial fluid. As in cardiac tissue, the cytoplasm of the neuron contains anions (negatively charged particles) that are too large to leave the cell. These electrochemically attract, in part, positively charged potassium ions and positively charged sodium ions. If this were all that happened, the influx of positively charged ions would counterbalance the negatively charged ones, electroneutrality would be established within the neuron, and nothing further could occur. The active transport enzyme system within the neuronal membrane, however, pumps sodium out of the cell almost as fast as it enters. Although potassium is pumped into the cell, this is insufficient to counterbalance the anions. Thus, the inside of the neuron remains negative with respect to the outside as long as the sodium–potassium pumps are operating. This internal relative negativity is the *resting polarity* of the neuron and typically measures 85 mV.

A stimulus acts locally to turn off the sodium pumps. This causes a local influx of sodium and a consequent local *depolarization.* If enough pumps are inactivated temporarily, the resulting depolarization is large enough to inactivate sodium pumps in adjacent areas. The depolarization can spread through the entire neuron.

A depolarization of such self-propagating magnitude is termed an *action potential,* which is the essence of a nerve impulse. An action potential is a discrete temporary event because the sodium pumps are inactivated only temporar-

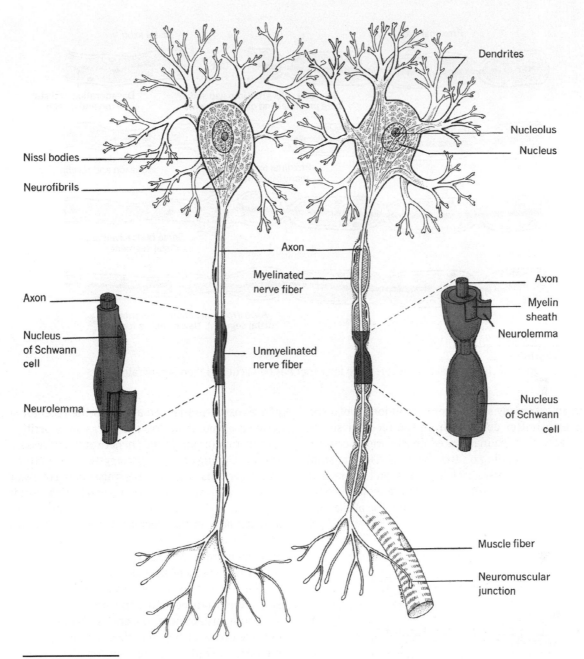

FIGURE 31-1
Typical efferent neurons (*left*, unmyelinated fiber; *right*, myelinated fiber).

ily. Once the pumps turn back on, the electrical events reverse, and the resting potential is restored (Fig. 31–3).

The electrical activity embodied in the action potential can be monitored in certain clinical situations. For example, the electroencephalogram depicts multiple action potentials from surface neurons of the brain.

SYNAPTIC TRANSMISSION

A synapse is made up of a presynaptic element, a postsynaptic element, and a small (150–1,000 A) space between elements called a synaptic cleft. A presynaptic element is any terminal portion of a neuron; a postsynaptic element is any part of another neuron in close proximity to the presynap-

tic element. One neuron stimulates or inhibits another by chemical transmission across the synapse. This involves the synthesis of the transmitter by the first neuron. Transmitter packets are then stored in the presynaptic element. As a nerve impulse passes down the axon, it triggers the release of a certain number of transmitter packets. These chemicals then diffuse across the synaptic cleft, where they attach temporarily to receptor binding sites on the dendrite surface of the postsynaptic element (Fig. 31–4).

While the transmitter is bound to the receptor site, the dendrite area is either stimulated (depolarized or hypopolarized) or inhibited (hyperpolarized). Most chemical transmitters are stimulators. Only one, gamma-aminobutyric acid (GABA), is known to hyperpolarize a neuron.

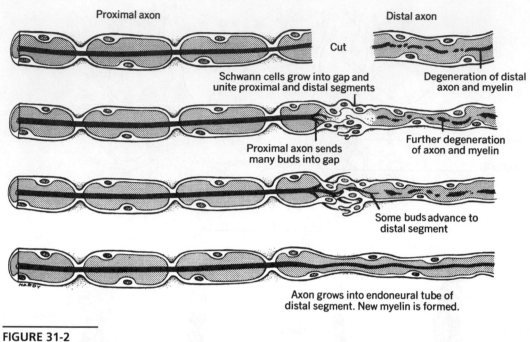

Proximal axon   Distal axon

Cut

Schwann cells grow into gap and   Degeneration of distal
unite proximal and distal segments   axon and myelin

Further degeneration
of axon and myelin

Proximal axon sends
many buds into gap

Some buds advance to
distal segment

Axon grows into endoneural tube of
distal segment. New myelin is formed.

FIGURE 31-2

Diagram of changes that occur in a nerve fiber that has been cut and then regenerates.

Within an extremely short interval (millionths of a second), the transmitter detaches from the receptor site. It may then reattach or be inactivated. Inactivation occurs in two basic ways, depending on the chemical. The transmitter norepinephrine diffuses back into the axon to be reused. The transmitter acetylcholine is destroyed by an enzyme present in the synaptic cleft. In either case, the availability

of a transmitter that can attach to the receptor sites is restricted temporarily. This enables rapid, repetitive, discrete stimulation (or inhibition) of neurons, a necessary factor in the functioning of the nervous system. From this picture, it can be seen that synaptic transmission is a one-way street—from the axon across the synaptic cleft to the dendrite of the next neuron. It cannot proceed in the opposite direction. It also can be seen that decreased destruction of transmitter can increase the effect of this transmitter on the postsynaptic membrane. Similarly, increased destruction of transmitter reduces its postsynaptic effects.

The best known synaptic transmitters are acetylcholine and norepinephrine. Other transmitters include dopamine, serotonin, histamine, endogenous opiates, and GABA. Most of these excite, or hypopolarize, the postsynaptic neuronal membrane; GABA and possibly some endogenous opiates inhibit, or hyperpolarize, the postsynaptic neuronal membrane.

It was not until the 1970s that it was known that peptides could act as neurotransmitters. Examples of these neuropeptides are the endorphins, enkephalins, and substance P, all of which appear to be involved in pain sensation. The endorphins and enkephalins, often described as the body's own morphine, contribute to a decrease in pain sensation. Substance P excites spinal neurons that respond to painful stimuli, so it is thought to be involved in transmission of pain information from the periphery to the CNS.

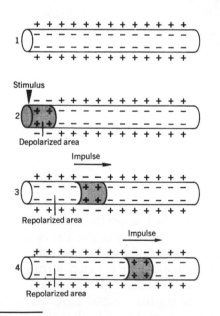

FIGURE 31-3

Propagation of impulses. (**1**) Resting membrane. (**2**) Action potential, first stage: stimulation of fiber results in depolarization. (**3**) Action potential, second stage: repolarization occurs as the resting potential is restored. (**4**) Propagation of impulses continues in direction of arrow.

NEURONAL THRESHOLDS

In the CNS (and sympathetic ganglia), the axons of several neurons may synapse with the dendrites or cell body of a single neuron. Some may release excitatory synaptic trans-

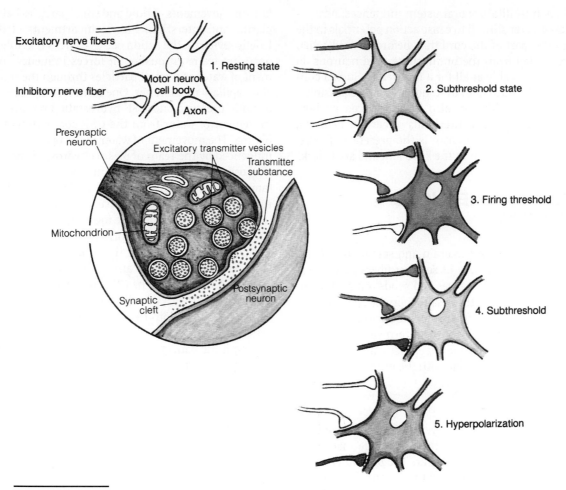

FIGURE 31-4

Conduction at synapses. *Left*, enlarged view of liberation chemical transmitter substance at a synapse; *right*, diagrams illustrating how a neuron may be excited or inhibited by transmitter substances liberated by presynaptic nerve fiber endings. Two excitatory and one inhibitory fiber are shown: (**1**) resting state; (**2**) subthreshold state; impulses from only one excitatory fiber cannot cause the postsynaptic neuron to fire; (**3**) firing threshold is reached by the addition of impulses from a second excitatory fiber; (**4**) subthreshold state is restored by impulses from an inhibitory fiber; (**5**) when the inhibitory fiber alone is carrying impulses, the postsynaptic neuron is in a state of hyperpolarization and is unable to fire.

mitters, whereas others may release an inhibitory transmitter. The excitatory transmitter released from a single axon often is insufficient to trigger an action potential in the postsynaptic neuron (ie, to excite the postsynaptic cell fully). Rather, it may be sufficient to depolarize, or excite, the postsynaptic membrane only partially. As such, it is termed a *subthreshold stimulus*. The partial depolarization, or hypopolarization, it produces renders the postsynaptic neuron more easily excitable by subsequent excitatory transmitter stimuli from other axons, provided such transmitters arrive while the postsynaptic membrane is hypopolarized. Thus, this initial subthreshold excitatory stimulus is said to "lower the threshold" of the postsynaptic neuron for stimulation by another presynaptic neuron. Full excitation of a postsynaptic membrane is a prerequisite to establishing an action potential and thus firing a nerve impulse along the postsynaptic neuron. It may require the near-

simultaneous depolarization produced by excitatory transmitters from two or more presynaptic neurons.

If the synaptic transmitter is an inhibitory one (eg, GABA), it will hyperpolarize, or "raise the threshold" of the postsynaptic neuron. This renders it more difficult to excite fully by excitatory transmitters. Figure 31–4 illustrates the action of three convergent presynaptic neurons on the threshold of a single postsynaptic neuron.

These principals underlie much of the normal functioning of cord neurons and spinal reflexes. For example, certain descending fibers from the brain stem deliver a low-level subthreshold stimulation to certain cord neurons. Although this stimulation is insufficient to activate cord neurons, it is enough of a background stimulus to make it easier for other input to excite these neurons fully. Such subthreshold stimuli would be said to be *facilitatory*. When the cord is severed, the distal portion also is separated from receipt of such facilitatory brain stem influences. As a result, it takes greater stimuli to cause action potentials in the neurons in this part of the cord than before. Indeed, when initially separated from the brain, these cord neurons do not function noticeably at all for a few weeks. Such a condition is termed *cord shock*. In it, no reflexes are possible.

Neuronal thresholds can also be influenced by hormones. *Thyroxine* lowers thresholds of certain neurons, and one sign of hyperthyroidism is the presence of exaggerated cord reflexes, such as the knee jerk and ankle jerk.

■ CENTRAL NERVOUS SYSTEM

The CNS is composed of the brain and spinal cord. It receives sensory input by way of sensory fibers (dendrites) within spinal and cranial nerves and sends out motor impulses by way of axons in these same nerves. The CNS also contains large numbers of neurons that are entirely contained within it. These neurons are termed *internuncial neurons*, or *interneurons*, and may exist within the brain and spinal cord or connect one with the other.

Meninges

The CNS is covered by three layers of tissue collectively called the *meninges* and consisting of the pia mater, the arachnoid layer, and the dura mater. The *pia mater* is the layer that lies next to the CNS. Next is the *arachnoid layer,* which contains a substantial vascular supply. Last is the *dura mater*, the thickest layer of all, lying next to the bones surrounding the CNS.

Cerebrospinal Fluid

Cerebrospinal fluid (CSF) functions as a fluid shock absorber, keeping the delicate CNS tissues from impacting against surrounding bony structures and being mechanically injured. It also functions in the exchange of nutrients between the plasma and cellular compartments. Cerebrospinal fluid is a plasma filtrate that is exuded by the capillaries in the roofs of each of the four ventricles of the brain. As such, it is similar to plasma minus the large plasma proteins, which stay behind in the bloodstream. Most of this fluid is made in the lateral ventricles, which are located in each cerebral hemisphere. It moves from there through the ducts and into the third ventricle of the diencephalon. From here it travels through the aqueduct of Sylvius of the midbrain and enters the fourth ventricle of the medulla. Then most of it passes through holes (foramina) in the roof of this ventricle and enters the subarachnoid space. (A small amount diffuses down into the spinal canal.) In the subarachnoid space, the CSF is reabsorbed into the bloodstream at certain points called the *subarachnoid plexes*.

The formation and reabsorption of CSF are governed by the same hydrostatic and colloid osmotic forces that regulate the movements of fluid and small particles between the plasma and interstitial fluid compartments of the body. Briefly reviewed, the action of these forces is as follows. Two opposing teams of push–pull forces influence the movement of water and small particles through the semipermeable capillary membranes. One team is composed of plasma osmotic pressure and CSF hydrostatic pressure. It favors movement of water from the CSF compartment into the plasma. The movement of water in the opposite direction is influenced by the team of plasma hydrostatic pressure and CSF osmotic pressure. Team influences are exerted simultaneously and continually. In the ventricles, the flow of CSF reduces CSF hydrostatic pressure. This tips the collective team influence in favor of the movement of water and small particles from plasma to ventricles. The low plasma hydrostatic pressure of blood in the venous sinuses next to the arachnoid villi tips the scales in favor of the movement of water and solute from the CSF compartment back into the bloodstream. Death of cells lining the CSF compartment will spill proteins into the CSF. This elevates CSF osmotic pressure and retards reabsorption (while also hastening formation if the damage is in ventricle walls). Increased CSF proteins from this or other causes can provoke or exacerbate a condition of excess CSF called *hydrocephalus*.

Brain

The basic anatomy of the brain is illustrated in Figure 31–5. The parts of the brain, in descending order, are the cerebral hemispheres, diencephalon, midbrain, pons, medulla, and cerebellum. The general appearance of the brain can be viewed as a stem extending upward from the spinal cord with an inferior small flowering overgrowth (cerebellum) covering the lower part of the stem and a large superior flowering overgrowth (cerebrum) covering most of the upper portion of the stem. The medulla, pons, and midbrain compose the brain stem. Some authors include the diencephalon.

CEREBRUM

Each of the two cerebral hemispheres (left and right) has a layer of cortex covering the surface. This cortical layer is made of several different types of unmyelinated neurons and glial cells arranged in six distinctive layers according to cell type and function. Underneath the cortex is white matter (myelinated nerve fibers). Deep within each hemisphere are several collections of nerve cell bodies, termed the *basal ganglia,* and a lateral ventricle containing CSF. The left and right hemispheres are connected and communicate with each other by a transverse band of nerve fibers termed the *corpus callosum*. Each hemisphere has four lobes named for and generally underlying each of the following skull bones: frontal, parietal, temporal, and occipital. For the most part, each hemisphere serves the contralateral side of the body (fibers cross over in the CNS).

One notable exception is Broca's speech area. This area of the cortex subserves all motor speech functions and is lo-

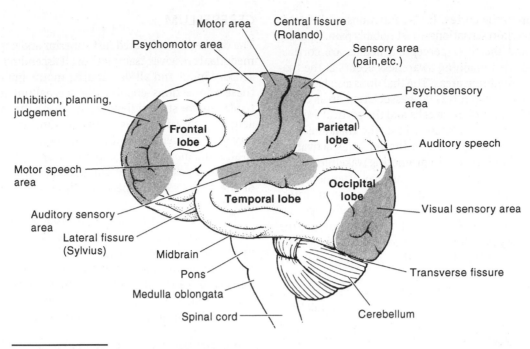

FIGURE 31-5
The human brain, showing the lobes and fissures of the cerebrum. Major functional areas are also indicated.

cated in a posterolateral area of the left frontal lobe for all right-handed and many left-handed people. Damage to this area in an adult produces motor dysphasia.

Cortex

The cortex is thought to operate in all higher mental functions, such as judgment, language, memory, creativity, and abstract thinking. It also functions in the perception, localization, and interpretation of all sensations and governs all voluntary and especially discrete motor activities (see Fig. 31–5). Various areas of the cortex have been identified as having different motor and sensory functions, but some of these areas are being implicated in other functions as well (eg, the occipital area is now known to function in some learning processes of blind people). Many areas of the cerebrum operate together to produce coordinated human function; the process of communication provides a good example of this.

Verbal communication depends on the ability to interpret speech and to translate thought into speech. Ideas usually are communicated between people by either spoken or written word. With the spoken word, the sensory input of information occurs through the primary auditory cortex. In auditory association areas, the sounds are interpreted as words and the words as sentences. These sentences are then interpreted by a common integrative area of the cerebral cortex as thoughts.

The common integrative area also develops thoughts to be communicated. Letters seen by the eyes are associated as words, thoughts, and sentences in the visual association areas and integrated into thought in this area as well.

Operating in conjunction with facial regions of the somesthetic sensory area, the common integrative area initiates a series of impulses, each representing a syllable or word, and transmits them to the secondary motor area controlling the larynx and mouth.

The speech center, in addition to controlling motor activity of the larynx and mouth, sends impulses to the respiratory center of the secondary motor cortex to provide appropriate breath patterns for the speech process.

Basal Ganglia

The basal ganglia function in cooperation with other lower brain parts in providing circuitry for basic and subconscious bodily movements. They provide the necessary background muscle tone for discrete voluntary movements, smoothness and coordination in functions of muscle antagonists, and the basic automatic subconscious rhythmic movements involved in walking and equilibrium maintenance. Lesions of these basal ganglia will produce various clinical abnormalities, such as chorea, hemiballismus, and Parkinson's disease.

DIENCEPHALON

Below the cerebrum lies the next brain area, the diencephalon. This area contains the third ventricle and the thalamus. Below is the hypothalamus, and above is the epithalamus or pineal gland (see Fig. 31-5). The diencephalon is the most superior portion of what most authors call the *brain stem* (diencephalon, midbrain, pons, and medulla).

The *thalamus* functions as a sensory and motor relay center. It relays sensory impulses, including those of sight and sound, up to the cortex. It also functions in the gross awareness of certain sensations, most notably pain. Discrete localization and the finer perceptual details are cortical functions, but the remaining awareness occurs at the thalamic and even midbrain areas. The thalamus also has other cells, the axons of which travel to association areas of the cortex. The functions of these cells and the cortical areas to which they attach are unknown. Last, the thalamus possesses some of the fiber tracts of the reticular activating systems (RAS) that function in promoting wakefulness and consciousness and possibly some aspects of attention.

The *hypothalamus* is the seat of neuroendocrine interaction. It is here that various neurosecretory substances are produced—hormones that previously were attributed to the posterior pituitary (antidiuretic hormone and oxytocin) and that stimulate or inhibit the secretion of anterior pituitary hormones.

This area of the brain also contains centers for coordinated parasympathetic and sympathetic stimulation, temperature regulation, appetite regulation, regulation of water balance by antidiuretic hormone, and regulation of certain rhythmic psychobiological activities (eg, sleep).

MIDBRAIN

The midbrain lies between the diencephalon and the pons of the brain stem. It contains the aqueduct of Sylvius, many ascending and descending nerve fiber tracts, and centers for auditory and visually stimulated nerve impulses. The *Edinger-Westphal nucleus* is located here. This nucleus contains the autonomic reflex centers for pupillary accommodations to light. It receives fibers from the retina by way of cranial nerve II and emits motor impulses by way of sympathetic and parasympathetic (cranial nerve III) fibers to the smooth muscles of the iris. Impaired pupillary accommodation signifies that at least one of these inputs or outputs is damaged or that the midbrain is suffering insult (often from tentorial herniation or stroke).

PONS

The *pons varolli* lies between the midbrain and the medulla oblongata of the brain stem and has cell bodies of fibers contained in cranial nerves V, VI, VII, and VIII. It contains pneumotaxic and apneustic respiratory centers and fiber tracts connecting higher and lower centers, including the cerebellum.

MEDULLA

The *medulla* lies between the pons and the cord. It contains autonomic centers that regulate such vital functions as breathing, cardiac rate, and vasomotor tone and centers for vomiting, gagging, coughing, and sneezing reflex behaviors. It also contains the fourth ventricle. Cranial nerves IX and XII have their cell bodies in this area. Impairment of any of these vital functions or reflexes suggests medullary damage.

CEREBELLUM

The cerebellum is located just superior and posterior to the medulla. It receives "samples" of all ascending somesthetic sensory input and all descending motor impulses. Use of these connections enables the cerebellum to match intended motor stimuli (before they reach the muscles) with actual sensory data. This ensures optimal match for voluntary motor "intention" with actual motor action, with time to alter the motor message in case of error. It sends its own messages up to the basal ganglia and cortex and to parts of the brain stem to perform three basic subconscious functions.

The cerebellum functions to produce smooth, steady, harmonious, and coordinated skeletal muscle actions; maintain equilibrium; and control posture without any jerky or uncompensated movements or swaying. Cerebellum disease can produce certain symptoms, the most prominent of which are disturbances of gait, equilibrium ataxia (overstability or understability of the walk), and tremors.

FUNCTIONALLY INTEGRATED BRAIN STEM SYSTEMS

Four networks within the brain stem should be mentioned. They are the integrated systems responsible for posture and equilibrium, consciousness, emotional reactions, and sleep.

Bulboreticular Formation

This is a network of neurons in the brain stem that functions in maintaining bodily support against gravity and equilibrium. Figure 31–6 illustrates the anatomical location of the bulboreticular formation. This area receives in-

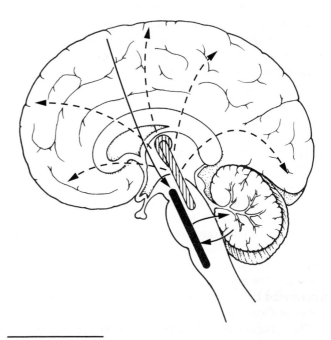

FIGURE 31-6
Bulboreticular and reticular activating systems. *Black area*, bulboreticular system; *striped area*, reticular activating system.

formation from a variety of sources, including all areas of the peripheral sensory receptors from the spinal cord, the cerebellum, the inner ear equilibrium apparatus, the motor cortex, and the basal ganglia. The bulboreticular formation, then, is an integrative area for sensory information, motor information from the cerebral cortex, equilibrium information from the vestibular apparatus, and proprioceptive information from the cerebellum. Output from the bulboreticular formation travels down descending fibers to internuncial neurons in the cord. This output alters the tonus of muscles maintaining equilibrium and positions of major body parts (trunk, appendages) necessary for the performance of discrete actions (eg, writing at a table, walking).

Reticular Activating System

The RAS is an ascending fiber system originating in the midbrain and thalamus (see Fig. 31–6). Branches extend up to the cortex. In this way, the RAS can stimulate the cortex. The RAS itself is stimulated by the arrival of a variety of sensory impulses and chemical stimuli from various sources. These include input from the optic and acoustic cranial nerves, somesthetic impulses from the dorsal column and spinothalamic pathways, and fibers from the cerebral cortex. In addition, it is stimulated by norepinephrine and epinephrine.

The stimulation of the cortex by the RAS seems to be the major physiological basis for consciousness, alertness, and attention to various environmental stimuli. Some of the aforementioned stimuli (eg, pain, noise), however, also can increase one's level of consciousness, at least temporarily. Decreased activity of the RAS produces decreased alertness or levels of consciousness, including stupor and coma. Inactivation of the RAS can result from anything that interrupts the entry of a critical amount of sensory input or by any damage that prevents the RAS fibers from sending impulses to the cortex. Normal inactivation of the cortex occurs during sleep.

Limbic System

The hypothalamus, cingulate, gyrus of the cortex, the amygdala and hippocampus within the temporal lobes, and the septum and interconnecting fiber tracts among these areas comprise a functional unit of the brain called the *limbic system*. This system provides a neural substrate for emotions (terror, intense pleasure, eroticism, and so forth). This region of the brain is involved in emotional experience and in the control of emotion-related behavior. Also, it is here that neural pathways provide a connection between higher brain functioning and endocrinological–autonomic activities.

Sleep Centers

The release of stored serotonin from the diencephalon, medulla, thalamus, and a small forebrain area (DMTF) results in inactivation of the RAS and activation of the DMTF. DMTF activity results in the first four stages of sleep, stages I, II, III, and IV. During stages III and IV, parasympathetic activity (with decreased heart rate, respiratory rate, and so forth) predominates and sleepwalking, sleep talking, and nocturnal enuresis occur.

Rhythmic discharges (about four to eight times per night, from 10–20 min/episode) from the pontine nuclei during sleep result in rapid eye movement sleep, during which about 80% of all dreaming occurs and sympathetic nervous system activity predominates. Based on circadian rhythmicity and decreasing cerebral serotonin levels, the RAS is reactivated in the morning, after 6 to 8 hours of sleep.

Spinal Cord

The spinal cord lies within the neural canal of the vertebral column, extending down and filling the neural canal to the level of the second lumbar vertebra. A pair of spinal nerves exists between adjacent vertebrae the entire length of the vertebral column. Below the point at which the cord terminates, the neural canal is filled with spinal nerves, extending to their point of exit (Fig. 31–7). Because neurons occupy less space in the canal at lower lumbar levels, it is here that spinal taps may be performed most safely. This anatom-

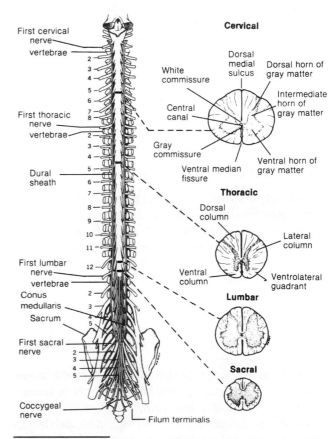

FIGURE 31-7

The spinal cord within the vertebral canal. The spinal canal and meninges have been opened. The spinal nerves and vertebrae are numbered on the left. Cross (transverse) sections with regional variations in gray matter and increasing proportions of white matter as the cord is ascended appear on the right.

ical fact also explains why injuries to lumbar and lower thoracic vertebrae can produce impairment at disproportionately lower body levels.

Within the cord lie interneurons, ascending sensory fibers, descending motor fibers, and the nerve cell bodies and dendrites of the second-order somatic (voluntary) and first-order autonomic motor neurons. The central area of the cord, the gray matter, contains nerve cell bodies and internuncial neurons (ie, nerve cells contained entirely within the cord). The gray matter has left and right dorsal and ventral projections, giving it an H-shaped appearance. Nerve cell bodies of motor neurons supplying skeletal muscles lie in the ventral horns. Left and right lateral projections or horns of gray matter exist in the thoracic, lumbar, and sacral cord. Within those lie the nerve cell bodies of autonomic neurons. Surrounding the gray matter is the white matter of the cord. It contains ascending and descending fiber tracts and fibers entering or leaving the cord. Its white color comes from the myelin that covers these fibers.

Spinal nerves contain both sensory and motor fibers. Each spinal nerve attaches to the cord by a dorsal and ventral root. The dorsal root houses the nerve cell bodies and fibers of sensory neurons. Motor fibers (whose nerve cell bodies lie within the gray matter) traverse the ventral root. Thus, damage to one root may impair sensory function without impairing motor function, or vice versa. A spinal nerve injury could damage both sensory and motor functioning.

Sensory Division

The sensory division of the nervous system is composed of sensory receptors, sensory neurons, sensory tracts, and perceptive areas of the brain.

SENSATIONS AND RECEPTORS

A wide variety of structures respond to diverse stimuli. They range in structure and function from light-sensitive retinal cells to stretch-sensitive structures in muscles and tendons. Stimulation of a sensory receptor initiates an electrical charge (generator potential), which stimulates the sensory neuron synapsing with the receptor. A series of nerve impulses travel along the sensory neuron to the CNS, where they in turn stimulate neurons in either brain or cord tracts to carry impulses to the appropriate centers in the brain (thalamus and cortex), where the sensation finally may be perceived consciously.

Sensations often are divided into those of the major senses (eg, vision, hearing, and smell) and those termed somesthetic sensations (eg, pain, touch, and stretch). Somesthetic sensations provide information on such things as body position and conditions of the immediate external and internal environment. These are called proprioceptive, exteroceptive, and visceral sensations, respectively. In this chapter, only somesthetic sensations are discussed.

Proprioceptive sensations describe the physical position state of the body, such as tension in muscle, flexion or extension of joints, tendon tension, and deep pressure in dependent parts like the feet while one is standing or the buttocks while one is seated. *Exteroceptive sensations* monitor the conditions on the body surface. These include temperature and pain. *Visceral sensations* are like exteroceptive sensations except that they originate from within and monitor pain, pressure, and fullness from internal organs.

The sensory receptors for somesthetic sensations include both free nerve endings and specialized end-organs. Free nerve endings are nothing more than small, filamentous branches of the dendrite fibers. They detect crude sensations of touch, pain, heat, and cold. The precision is crude because there are many interconnections between the free endings of different neurons. They are the most profusely distributed and perform the general discriminatory functions, whereas the more specialized receptors discriminate between very slight differences in degrees of touch, heat, and cold.

Structurally, the special exteroceptive end-organs for detection of cold, warmth, and light touch differ from one another and are specific in their function. The physiological basis for this specific function has not been determined but is presumed to be based on some specific physical effect on the organ itself.

There are three proprioceptive receptors. Joint kinesthetic receptors are found in the joint capsules and provide data on the angulation of a joint and the rate at which it is changing. Information from muscles concerning the degree of stretch is transmitted to the nervous system from the muscle spindle apparatus, whereas the Golgi tendon determines the overall tension applied to the tendons.

When a sensory receptor is stimulated, it responds with an increased frequency of firing (generator potential). At first there is a burst of impulses; if the stimulus persists, the frequency of impulses transmitted begins to decrease. All sensory receptors show this phenomenon of *adaptation* to varying degrees and at different rates. Adaptations to light tough and pressure occur in a few seconds, whereas pain and proprioceptive sensation adapt very little, if at all, and at a very slow rate. The determination of the intensity of sensation is made on a relative rather than an absolute basis and follows a logarithmic response. Therefore, the intensity of a sensation increases logarithmically, whereas the frequency of response in the nerve ending increases linearly.

Although there are structurally different receptors for detecting each type of sensation, the area of the brain to which the information is transmitted determines the *modality,* or type of sensation, a person feels. The thalamus and somesthetic areas of the cortex operate together to attribute various sensory qualities and intensities to nerve impulse information they receive.

SENSORY NEURONS

Stimulation of sensory receptors creates nerve impulses (action potentials) in sensory neurons. These neurons conduct such impulses to the CNS.

SENSORY PATHWAYS

Depending on the type of somesthetic receptor involved, fibers of sensory neurons may, on entering the cord, do one of three things. They may travel the white matter of the cord on the same side of the body as the sensory receptor. There they will synapse with a second set of neurons that then cross over to the opposite side of the brain and travel to the thalamus. This pathway is termed the *dorsal column* or *posterior column pathway* (Fig. 31–8) and is used for the conduction of impulses originating from stimulation of muscle, tendon, and joint proprioceptors; vibration-sensitive receptors; and receptors in the skin involved in precise localization of touch.

Alternatively, the sensory neuron may synapse immediately on entering the cord with a second neuron that then immediately crosses over to the opposite side of the cord. Fibers from this second neuron then travel up the white matter of the cord to the thalamus. This is called the *spinothalamic pathway* (see Fig. 31–8). It conducts impulses concerned with pain, temperature, poorly localized touch, and sex organ sensations. In the thalamus, neurons of both the spinothalamic pathway and the dorsal column pathway synapse with other neurons that transmit impulses to the appropriate area of the somesthetic cortex. Because of this, impulses from either pathway give rise to consciously perceived sensations.

Last, certain sensory neurons may synapse with a neuron belonging to the *spinocerebellar* pathway. Spinocerebellar neurons do not cross over, and they carry impulses only as far as the cerebellum (and possibly lower brain stem). This pathway carries impulses originating from stimulation of muscle, tendon, and joint proprioceptors. Because this pathway ends at the cerebellum, it transmits sensory information that never is perceived consciously. These data are used in reflex postural adjustments.

Motor System

The motor system technically comprises the areas of the brain, descending fiber tracts, and the motor neurons involved in producing or altering movement or adjusting tonus of skeletal, cardiac, and smooth muscles and in regulating the secretions of the various exocrine and certain endocrine gland cells of the body. In practical terms, the heart usually is excluded from this system. Muscle and glandular tissues are referred to as the *effector organs* of this system.

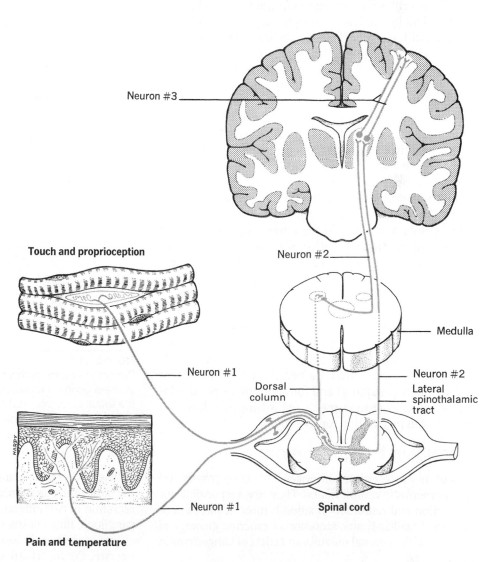

FIGURE 31-8
Diagrammatic representation of the decussation (crossing) of ascending tracts. First-order neurons for touch and proprioception ascend in the dorsal columns to the medulla; here they synapse with second-order neurons that cross to the opposite side before ascending to the thalamus. First-order neurons for pain and temperature enter the dorsal gray matter of the cord; here they synapse with second-order neurons that cross to the opposite side and ascend in the lateral spinothalamic tract to the thalamus. Third-order neurons connect the thalamus with the cerebral cortex.

The motor system can be divided on the basis of motor neurons and effector organs into *somatic* and *autonomic* subdivisions. The former involve skeletal muscles and motor neurons innervating them. The autonomic subdivision is composed of smooth muscle and gland cells plus the sympathetic and parasympathetic fibers innervating them.

SOMATIC MOTOR DIVISION

Figure 31–9 depicts the major descending fiber tracts from motor areas of the cerebral cortex. Some of these fibers cross over to the opposite side of the body in the brain. Many cross in the medulla. A few cross over in the cord centers. Descending fibers from motor areas of the cortex ultimately stimulate somatic motor neurons, the nerve cell bodies of which lie in the anterior (ventral) horn of the gray matter in the cord. The axons of these motor neurons travel within spinal nerves and terminate adjacent to the membranes of skeletal cells. The space between the somatic motor neuron axon and the muscle cell is termed the *myoneural junction*. When stimulated, somatic motor neurons conduct impulses to the ends of their axons. As the impulse arrives there, it triggers the release of a certain number of acetylcholine molecules that are stored in the terminal bouton. The acetylcholine diffuses across the myoneural junction and binds with receptor sites on a skeletal muscle cell. This triggers a chain of events leading to contraction. Thus, willed intentional motor movements are enacted.

Not shown in Figure 31–9 are descending fiber tracts that stimulate motor neurons responsible for the movement of skeletal muscles of the head (eg, tongue, face, jaw). The general pattern and myoneural transmitter are the same, except the somatic motor neuron nerve cell bodies lie within certain areas of the brain.

Also not shown in Figure 31–9 are several extrapyramidal tracts arising from the brain stem centers (eg, bulboreticular formation, midbrain). Some of these cross over, and others do not. Fibers in these tracts descend the cord and ultimately stimulate either somatic motor neurons, which stimulate skeletal muscle cells, or other motor neurons (gamma efferent) that alter the tensions of stretch receptor organelles (spindles) within the skeletal muscles. Alteration of spindle tension provokes a spinal reflex arc that efficiently and indirectly alters skeletal muscle tonus. These extrapyramidal pathways conduct impulses that produce the automatic coordinated alterations in skeletal muscle tonus and movement that are necessary for gross motor movements (eg, walking) and for appropriate posture for conduction of finer movements (eg, sitting at a desk with arm flexed in preparation for writing).

AUTONOMIC MOTOR DIVISION

The autonomic division comprises both *sympathetic* and *parasympathetic motor fibers.* They are responsible for contraction and relaxation of smooth muscle, rate of contraction of cardiac tissue, secretion of exocrine glands, and secretion of the adrenal medulla and islets of Langerhans in the pancreas.

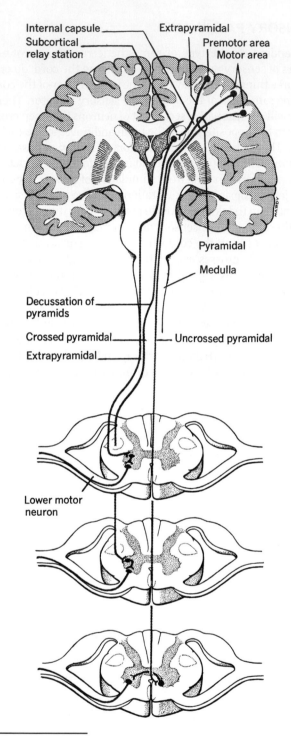

FIGURE 31-9

Diagram of motor pathways between the cerebral cortex, one of the subcortical relay centers, and lower motor neurons in the spinal cord. Decussation (crossing) of fibers means that each side of the brain controls skeletal muscles on the opposite side of the body.

The sympathetic and parasympathetic sections differ on the basis of the anatomical distribution of nerve fibers, the secretion of two different neural transmitters by the postganglionic fibers of the two divisions, and the antagonistic effects of the two divisions on some of the organs they innervate. Figure 31–10 shows the anatomy of the sympa-

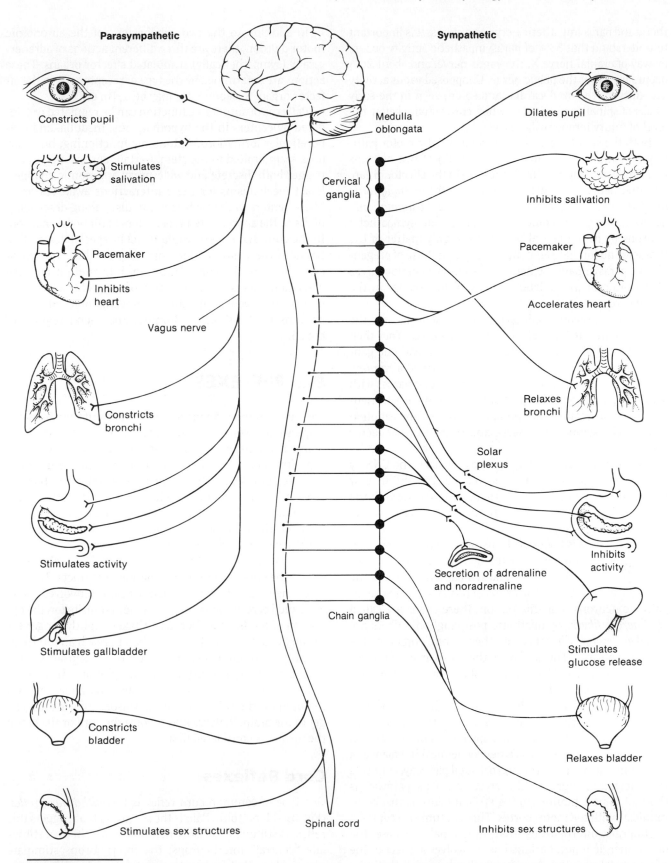

Parasympathetic

Constricts pupil

Stimulates salivation

Pacemaker

Inhibits heart

Vagus nerve

Constricts bronchi

Stimulates activity

Stimulates gallbladder

Constricts bladder

Stimulates sex structures

Sympathetic

Medulla oblongata

Cervical ganglia

Pacemaker

Vagus nerve

Solar plexus

Secretion of adrenaline and noradrenaline

Chain ganglia

Spinal cord

Dilates pupil

Inhibits salivation

Accelerates heart

Relaxes bronchi

Inhibits activity

Stimulates glucose release

Relaxes bladder

Inhibits sex structures

FIGURE 31-10

The autonomic nervous system and the organs it affects. The left side illustrates the actions of the sympathetic nervous system, which stimulates actions. The right side illustrates the parasympathetic nervous system, which inhibits actions.

thetic and parasympathetic nervous systems. It is important to understand that 80% of parasympathetic activity occurs by way of cranial nerve X, the vagus nerve, and about 20% occurs by way of the pelvic nerve. Unopposed vagus activity accounts for the bradycardia (and so on) seen in the early weeks of spinal cord injuries, when cord activity below the level of injury temporarily ceases.

Both the sympathetic and parasympathetic motor pathways essentially are composed of a chain of two neurons carrying nerve impulses from the CNS to the effector organ. The first neuron in the chain is termed the *preganglionic neuron*, and the second is termed the *postganglionic neuron*. Nerve cell bodies of preganglionic sympathetic neurons lie in the lateral horns of the gray matter of the thoracic and lumbar segments of the cord; those of preganglionic parasympathetic neurons lie either in certain areas of the brain or in the lateral horns of gray matter in the sacral cord.

Axons of preganglionic sympathetic neurons exit the cord and enter the ventral roots of spinal nerves. They then leave the spinal nerve to enter a nearby sympathetic ganglion (by way of a connecting pathway termed a *ramus*). Within a ganglion, the preganglionic neuron synapses with a postganglionic one. The postganglionic sympathetic neuron then may reenter the spinal nerve or exit the ganglion by a special sympathetic nerve and travel to the effector organ.

Parasympathetic preganglionic axons leave the CNS by certain cranial or spinal nerves and travel to the effector organ. At or near the effector organ, they synapse with the postganglionic neuron, which in turn innervates the effector organ.

Acetylcholine is the neurotransmitter at *all* synapses between preganglionic and postganglionic autonomic neurons—both parasympathetic and sympathetic. It also is the transmitter secreted by the axons of postsynaptic parasympathetic neurons. For this reason, these axons are called *cholinergic fibers*. Sympathetic postganglionic fibers are called *adrenergic fibers* because they secrete noradrenaline (norepinephrine). The actions of these two arms of the autonomic division and their chemical transmitters are summarized in Table 31–1.

The neurotransmitters balance each other. When there is a disruption in the production or destruction of one, clinical manifestations may become apparent. For example, in Parkinson's disease, there is a neurochemical imbalance. A dopaminergic pathway, the nigrostriatal pathway, connects the substantia nigra to the striatum. This pathway is thought to be inhibitory to the striatal neurons that communicate with the motor cortex. The striatum also contains cholinergic interneurons that functionally oppose the dopaminergic input. Parkinsonism involves a defect in the nigrostriatal pathway. As a result, the dopamine that normally is secreted in the striatum no longer is present. The neurons that secrete acetylcholine remain functional and in the absence of dopamine, become overactive, contributing to the motor symptoms of parkinsonism.

In addition to the two subdivisions of the autonomic motor division, there are three different actions of adrenergically (sympathetically) stimulated effector organs. These actions are determined by the type of receptor site in the effector organ. Receptor sites may be α, β_1, or β_2.

Patterns of autonomic function can be regulated or triggered by centers in the hypothalamus, medulla, and bulboreticular formations. Autonomic functioning, however, does seem limited to the stem. Certain cortical nerves can trigger both discrete and widespread autonomic changes. Exact mechanisms for these interactions await research. These centers in the CNS send impulses along descending fibers to the appropriate preganglionic autonomic neuron. In the cord, such fibers would travel by special descending tracts in the white matter until they reached the appropriate level of the cord. Thus, any interruption of these descending fibers (eg, transection of cervical tracts) would impede or prevent stimulation of preganglionic autonomic neurons in the thoracic, lumbar, and sacral regions of the cord.

◼ REFLEXES

Basically, a reflex is an instantaneous and autonomic motor response to a sensory input. It arises from a special autonomic relationship among sensory receptors, sensory neurons, interneurons, somatic or autonomic motor neurons, and effector organs. The effector is the end-organ that receives the motor impulse, such as skeletal, smooth, or cardiac muscles or an exocrine or endocrine gland.

Somesthetic sensory neurons involved in a reflex arc usually have branching axons. One branch participates in the arc, whereas the other travels up to the cerebrum by way of the dorsal column or spinothalamic tracts. This enables the person to perceive the sensation involved; however, such perception is not part of, nor requisite for, the operation of a reflex arc. Because it takes slightly longer for sensory data to reach the cortex than to reach an interneuron, a person often becomes aware of the sensation only during or after the occurrence of the reflex arc. Also, a cord reflex can occur even if the cord is transected above the level required for the reflex so that no sensory information can get to the brain. Reflexes may involve the cord or the brain; the former is considered first.

Cord Reflexes

One type of common cord reflex is the *withdrawal reflex* (Fig. 31–11, bottom). Pain is the sensation that triggers this reflex. It stimulates sensory neurons, which in turn stimulate "central" interneurons; the interneurons stimulate motor fibers that innervate skeletal muscles. When contracted, the skeletal muscles will produce withdrawal of the body part (here, a hand) from the painful stimulus. Its occurrence depends on the appropriate anatomical connections, or "wiring," along sensory and motor neurons within

TABLE 31-1

Responses of Effector Organs to Autonomic Nerve Impulses and Circulating Catecholamines

Effector Organs	Cholinergic Impulses Response	Noradrenergic Impulses	
		Receptor Type	Response
Eye			
Radial muscle of iris	—	α	Contraction (mydriasis)
Sphincter muscle of iris	Contraction (miosis)		
Ciliary muscle	Contraction for near vision	β	Relaxation for far vision
Heart			
SA node	Decrease in heart rate; vagal arrest	β_1	Increase in heart rate
Atria	Decrease in contractility and (usually) increase in conduction velocity	β_1	Increase in contractility and conduction velocity
AV node and conduction system	Decrease in conduction velocity; AV block	β_1	Increase in conduction velocity
Ventricles	—	β_1	Increase in contractility and conduction velocity
Arterioles			
Coronary, skeletal muscle, pulmonary, abdominal viscera, renal	Dilation	α β_2	Constriction Dilation
Skin and mucosa, cerebral, salivary glands	—	α	Constriction
Systemic Veins	—	α β_2	Constriction Dilation
Lung			
Bronchial muscle	Contraction	β_2	Relaxation
Bronchial glands	Stimulation	?	Inhibition (?)
Stomach			
Motility and tone	Increase	α, β_2	Decrease (usually)
Sphincters	Relaxation (usually)	α	Contraction (usually)
Secretion	Stimulation		Inhibition (?)
Intestine			
Motility and tone	Increase	α, β_2	Decrease
Sphincters	Relaxation (usually)	α	Contraction (usually)
Secretion	Stimulation		Inhibition (?)
Gallbladder and Ducts	Contraction		Relaxation
Urinary Bladder			
Detrusor	Contraction	β	Relaxation (usually)
Trigone and sphincter	Relaxation	α	Contraction
Ureter			
Motility and tone	Increase (?)	α	Increase (usually)
Uterus	Variable*	α, β_2	Variable*
Male Sex Organs	Erection	α	Ejaculation
Skin			
Pilomotor muscles	—	α	Contraction
Sweat glands	Generalized secretion	α	Slight, localized secretion†
Spleen Capsule	—	α β_2	Contraction Relaxation
Adrenal Medulla	Secretion of epinephrine and norepinephrine		—
Liver	—	α, β_2	Glycogenolysis

(continued)

TABLE 31-1

Responses of Effector Organs to Autonomic Nerve Impulses and Circulating Catecholamines (Continued)

Effector Organs	Cholinergic Impulses Response	Noradrenergic Impulses	
		Receptor Type	*Response*
Pancreas			
Acini	Secretion	α	Decreased secretion
Islets	Insulin and glucagon secretion	α	Inhibition of insulin and glucagon secretion
		β_2	Insulin and glucagon secretion
Salivary Glands	Profuse, watery secretion	α	Thick, viscous secretion
		β_2	Amylase secretion
Lacrimal Glands	Secretion		—
Nasopharyngeal Glands	Secretion		—
Adipose Tissue	—	β_1	Lipolysis
Juxtaglomerular Cells	—	$\beta(\beta_1?)$	Renin secretion
Pineal Gland	—	β	Melatonin synthesis and secretion

* *Depends on stage of menstrual cycle, amount of circulating estrogen and progesterone, pregnancy, and other factors.*
† *On palms of hands and in some other locations ("adrenergic sweating").*
(From Ganong WF: Review of Medical Physiology, Los Altos, Lange Medical Publications)

the cord. If these become nonfunctional (eg, cord shock or physical trauma), the reflex will not be possible.

Reflex withdrawal of one foot is associated with another reflex, the *crossed extensor reflex* (see Fig. 31–11, top). This reflex involves stimulation of various extensor muscles in the opposite leg so that the person's weight is fully supported while one lower extremity is withdrawn from a painful stimulus. Such a reflex is very complex and involves many levels of the cord. Any imbalance, however slight, during the operation of this reflex in a normal person will trigger the occurrence of additional reflexes involving the bulboreticular formation, cerebellum, and various muscles of arms and trunk to maintain balance and posture.

Another cord reflex is the *stretch reflex,* most commonly illustrated by the clinical test of the knee–jerk reflex (Fig 31–11, middle). Because of the anatomical connections within the cord, the stimulation of stretch receptors in a muscle or a tendon automatically triggers an immediate contraction of the muscle. In the knee–jerk reflex, the hammer blow stretches the tendon of the quadriceps. This reflexively causes contraction of the quadriceps, which causes the lower leg to kick forward. Other stretch reflexes of clinical importance are the ankle jerk and the biceps and triceps reflexes. All involve stretching the muscle by a hammer tap of its tendon.

An important feature of all cord reflexes involving skeletal muscles is *reciprocal inhibition,* which occurs in the antagonist muscle of the one stimulated. For example, when a flexor reflex stimulates the biceps, it also inhibits its an-

tagonist, the triceps, and provides for more efficient performance of motor activities in the upper arm.

Spinal cord activities also include reflex circuits, which aid in the *control of visceral functions* of the body. Sensory input arises from visceral sensory receptors and is transmitted to the spinal cord, where reflex patterns appropriate to the sensory input are determined. The signals are then transmitted to autonomic motor neurons in the gray matter of the spinal cord, which send impulses to the sympathetic nerves innervating visceral motor end-organs. A most important autonomic reflex is the *peritoneal reflex.* Tissue damage in any portion of the peritoneum results in the response of this reflex, which slows or stops all motor activity in nearby viscera. Other autonomic cord reflexes are capable of *modifying local blood flow* in response to cold, pain, and heat. This vascular control by autonomic reflexes in the spinal cord can operate as a backup mechanism for the usual brain stem control patterns in patients with transectional injuries at the brain stem.

Also included in the autonomic reflexes of the spinal cord are those causing the *emptying of the urinary bladder and the rectum.* When the bowel or bladder becomes distended, sensory signals from stretch receptors in the bowel or bladder wall are transmitted by sensory neurons to the internuncial neurons of the upper sacral and lower lumbar segments of the cord. These neurons in turn stimulate parasympathetic motor neurons innervating the wall of the bowel or bladder, and its internal sphincter muscles also are reflexively stimulated by the internuncials. The result of

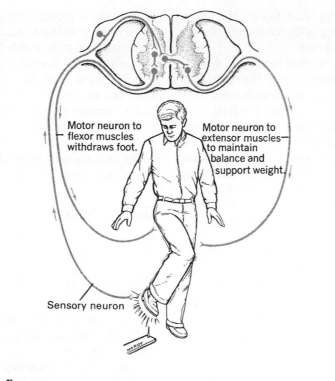

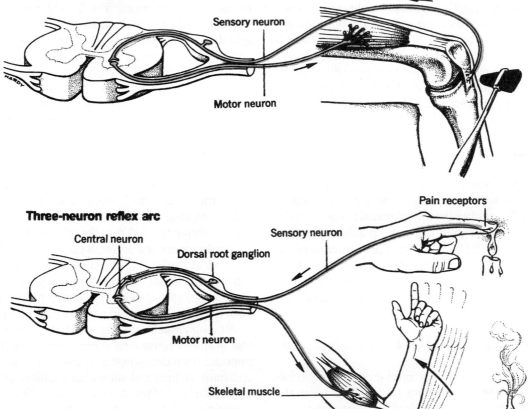

FIGURE 31-11

Reflex arcs showing pathways of impulses in response to a stimulus. *Bottom*, withdrawal reflex involves a three-neuron reflex arc: sensory, central, and motor neurons. *Top*, flexor and crossed extensor reflexes. *Middle*, example of a stretch reflex, involving only a two-neuron reflex arc: sensory and motor neurons.

such motor neuron stimulation is a reflex contraction of bowel or bladder and an opening of the sphincters, thereby permitting defecation or micturition.

Descending fibers from the cerebral cortex also synapse with the internuncials. These fibers inhibit the reflex emptying of bowel or bladder at times or places deemed inappropriate by the person. Toilet training of infants must await the functional maturation of these descending fibers. Cord transection or other damage above the level of the cord housing the neurons for the bowel or bladder evacuation reflexes will interrupt some or all of these descending fibers. This produces a condition wherein the patient cannot consciously control (ie, prevent) the emptying of the bowel or bladder or both. Damage to or interrupted function of that level of the cord housing the anatomical neuronal connections for these reflexes (eg, spina bifida, cord shock, severe injuries to the lower sacral or lumbar cord) will prevent reflex evacuation of bowel or bladder or both. Such a patient may exhibit retention with overflow but will not possess any effective mechanism for emptying the bowel or bladder or both.

Brain Reflexes

Brain reflexes operate in the same way as do cord reflexes, except that the brain houses the connection, not the cord. Brain reflexes include those involving the *cardioregulatory and vasomotor centers* of the medulla, plus the pupillary adjustment center, which involves the midbrain. Because the sensory and motor arms of the heart and vasopressure reflexes are commonly known, only the pupillary reflex is discussed.

Light in the retina causes stimulation of the optic nerve. Fibers in this nerve travel to the Edinger-Westphal nucleus in the midbrain. Here the sensory fibers synapse with interneurons. The result is outgoing autonomic motor impulses to the smooth muscles of the iris. Increases in parasympathetic impulses (by way of cranial nerve III) or decreases in sympathetic impulses cause pupillary constriction in response to the light. As the light stimulus of the retina decreases, this reflex causes pupillary dilation. Lack of this reflex signifies damage to the midbrain–optic fiber connection or to the oculomotor nerve (cranial nerve III).

■ PAIN SENSATION

The sensation of pain warrants special consideration because it plays such an important protective role for the body. Whenever there is tissue damage, nerve endings are stimulated and the sensation of pain is felt. This sensation usually is felt during the time that tissue is undergoing damage and ceases when the damage ends. This condition is due to the release of chemicals and metabolites, such as histamine and kinin, from damaged cells. Typical damage stimuli are physical trauma (cutting, crushing, tearing), ischemia, and intense heat and cold. In addition to these stimuli, acidity of the tissue fluid at the nerve fiber ending

is known to stimulate pain sensations, which can be eliminated by making this fluid alkaline.

Variation in pain thresholds among different people and within the same person at different times has been long known. This is in addition to the wide variation in people's reactions to pain. The exact mechanism for transmission and perception of pain is not clear. Neurophysiological, psychological, and sociological research has contributed to formulation of pain theories. Some theories developed in the 1880s and are still being developed because there is so much yet to learn about pain.

Gate Theory

More recent evidence points to the existence of gating mechanisms in the substantia gelatinosa at all levels of the spinal cord, which are capable of regulating the amount of pain impulses that can enter the spinothalamic tract and travel to the brain. This cord level of pain regulation opens new avenues to the treatment of pain.

Briefly, two types of fibers are involved. One is a small-diameter (S) fiber that carries impulses responsible for the sensation of pain (pain impulses). The other is a large-diameter (L) fiber that carries impulses responsible for cutaneous tactile sensations. The S and L fibers each synapse with two other cells—a gate cell and a T cell of the spinothalamic tract. The gate also synapses with the T cell and *inhibits* it (by hyperpolarization). L-fiber impulses stimulate the gate cell, thereby hyperpolarizing the T cell to a certain degree. S-fiber impulses inhibit the gate cell and stimulate the T cell. When the gate cell is inhibited, the T cell is stimulated. Thus, by itself, the S-fiber impulse readily gains access to the spinothalamic tract.

In theory, if tactile skin receptors *in the same dermatome* are stimulated simultaneously with S fibers, the action of the L fibers will (by way of the gate cell) hyperpolarize the T cell and thereby make it more difficult for S-fiber impulses to stimulate the T cell (gain access to the spinothalamic tract). Thus, the relative S- to L-fiber activity can determine the degree of pain impulses that can enter the CNS at the level of the cord (Fig. 31–12). Rubbing or other tactile sensation, such as provided by transcutaneous nerve (skin) stimulation, applied to a painful area may reduce the sensation of pain perceived by the patient.

Although much more remains to be learned, it is known that primitive sensations of pain occur once the ascending impulses from the spinothalamic tract reach the midbrain, and more refined and somewhat localized perception occurs at the level of the thalamus. Most refined and localized sensations and their significance to the person occur at the level of the cortex.

Referred Pain

Referred pain is perceived as arising from a site that is different from its true point of origin. Well known examples include the referring of pain from severe cardiac ischemia to the left arm or the referring of diaphragmatic pain to the

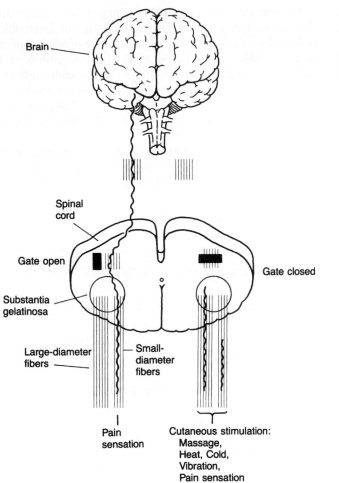

FIGURE 31-12
Gate control theory of pain.

tures, the referred locale is used preferentially over the more unfamiliar but true point of origin (Fig. 31–13).

Endogenous Opiates

These are substances that in terms of molecular structure and action resemble opiate drugs. Several types are known, including enkephalins, endorphins, and dynorphins. Enkephalins are pentapeptides synthesized by certain CNS neurons. They appear to function as inhibitory neurotransmitters in pathways conducting impulses concerning pain (nociception). Stimulation of "enkephalinergic neurons" produces analgesia similar to that produced by opiate drugs. Enkephalins bind to opiate receptors in the postsynaptic membrane. In most cases, this inhibits (hyperpolarizes) the postsynaptic neuron by decreasing its sodium influx.

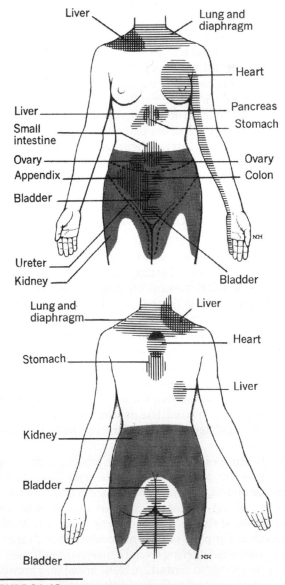

FIGURE 31-13
Areas of referred pain. *Top*, anterior view. *Bottom*, posterior view.

neck and shoulder. The "true point of origin" for this type of pain usually is some visceral organ or deep somatic structure, and the "point of reference" is some area of the body surface. A knowledge of the embryological development of various parts of the body provides an understanding of the physiological basis of referred pain. The true point of origin and its common referred areas were, at one time, embryologically close together and are innervated by sensory neurons that enter the same segment of the spinal cord. Although the two areas move farther apart in the normal growth and development of a person, their innervation persists. Thus, sensory impulses originating from painful stimuli in either the true or referred body areas will enter the same level of the cord and synapse with the same neurons of the spinothalamic pathway at this level. There is no way for the cerebral cortex to know whether a given spinothalamic neuron was stimulated originally by pain from the true point of origin or the referred area. In localizing the source of the pain stimulus, the cortex relies on prior experience regarding the person's geographical knowledge of his or her own body. Because surface areas are more familiar to a person than the locations of the visceral or deep somatic struc-

Opiate receptors and enkephalins have been discovered in various locations within the CNS. These locations function in the conduction of pain impulses up the cord and brain stem to the cortex, in areas associated with emotional effects produced by opiates, or in analgesic centers within the brain stem. One location is the part of the dorsal horn of gray matter housing the spinal gate. Here, enkephalinergic neurons, which receive impulses from descending fibers of the nucleus raphe magnus in the medulla, act on sensory neurons to inhibit the stimulation of T cells by small fibers. This inhibits the entry of pain impulses into the spinothalamic tract. Enkephalins and opiate receptors exist in the medullary respiratory center. The latter perhaps explains the potent action of opiate drugs on respiration. They also are found in certain limbic system structures (eg, amygdala). This may explain the emotional effects produced by natural and synthetic opiate drugs. It also suggests that endogenous opiates may function in naturally evoked feelings of pleasure or well-being. The role of enkephalins and opiate receptors found in other brain centers, such as the basal ganglia and neocortex, is unclear at this time.

Enkephalins and opiate receptors also are richly distributed in three central analgesic areas of the brain stem: the raphe magnus, the periaqueductal gray matter of the midbrain, and areas bordering the third ventricle in the thalamus. Electrical stimulation of these areas is known to produce varying but strong, widespread analgesic effects. Electrical stimulation of the first two areas produces a systemic analgesia that lasts for hours after the stimulation is stopped. It is one current modality for the treatment of intractable pain; however, its effects are limited because patients develop tolerance to therapy as they do to narcotics and there is cross-tolerance between such electrical stimulation-produced analgesia and narcotic drugs. The exact manner by which these areas produce analgesia is unknown, but enkephalins clearly are involved as mediators because opiate-blocking drugs, such as naloxone, will inhibit such electrical stimulation–produced analgesia.

The raphe magnus (in the medulla) functions in regulating the spinal gates. Descending fibers from the raphe synapse at all levels of the cord with enkephalinergic internuncial neurons that regulate the ability of pain-stimulated sensory neurons to stimulate spinothalamic neurons. Thus, the raphe magnus controls the entry of pain impulses into the pain conduction system in the first place. What cannot enter cannot be perceived. It is not clear whether this raphe is, in turn, regulated by either of the two higher analgesic centers.

Opiate drugs exert their effects by binding with the opiate receptors in many or all of these areas depending on dosage. Acupuncture and various placebo analgesics seem to act by causing a release of endogenous opiates because, in double-blind studies, their analgesic effects are blocked by naloxone. The parts of the CNS involved in such analgesia are unknown. Differing levels of enkephalinergic neuron activity (especially in central analgesic areas) may provide a physiological basis for individual differences in pain reports and tolerances.

Endorphins are part of the pro-opiomelanocortin (POMC) molecule that is secreted by the corticotrophic cells of the anterior pituitary. They consist of any segment of this POMC that also contains the five amino acid enkephalin sequence (represented by amino acids numbers 61–65). They bind to various opiate receptors in the brain, especially the basal ganglia and the limbic system, and seem to function in endogenously produced analgesia. Their exact role or roles are unknown.

Dynorphins are another opiate-like neuropeptide that bind to opiate receptors in the brain and produce analgesia. These substances are distributed widely and considered extremely potent.

Clinical Applicability Challenges

Self-Challenge: Critical Thinking

1. Compare and contrast the functions of the sympathetic and parasympathetic divisions of the autonomic nervous system.

2. Explain the process of synaptic transmission.

Study Questions

1. Which statement is true regarding the structure of neurons?
   a. Axons carry impulses toward the cell body.
   b. Dendrites carry impulses toward the cell body.
   c. Neurons connect one to the other.
   d. The synapse is the space between two axons.

2. Which is an example of a cord reflex?
   a. Withdrawal reflex
   b. Pupillary reflex
   c. Corneal reflex
   d. Action potential depolarization

3. Cholinergic responses would include
   a. an increase in heart rate.
   b. pupillary dilation.
   c. decreased stomach motility.
   d. arteriole dilation.

4. A major function of the brain stem is to
   a. provide a neural pathway for emotions.
   b. control posture and balance.
   c. stimulate sensory neurons, which in turn stimulate interneurons, which stimulate motor fibers that innervate skeletal muscles.
   d. control respiration, cardiac rate, and blood vessel diameter.

BIBLIOGRAPHY

Bullock B, Rosendahl P: Pathophysiology: Adaptations and Alterations in Function (4th Ed). Philadelphia, JB Lippincott, 1996

Guyton A, Hall J: Textbook of Medical Physiology (9th Ed). Philadelphia, WB Saunders, 1996

Hole J Jr: Human Anatomy and Physiology. Dubuque, IA, William C. Brown, 1992

Smeltzer S, Bare B (eds): Brunner and Suddarth's Textbook of Medical-Surgical Nursing (8th Ed). Philadelphia, JB Lippincott, 1996

32

Patient Assessment: Nervous System

OBJECTIVES

Based on the content in this chapter, the reader should be able to:

- Discuss the value of gathering neurological data in an orderly and objective manner.
- Correlate such data over time.
- Recognize patterns of assessment findings that imply a significant change in pathological condition for the patient.
- Evaluate the effect of neurological dysfunction on the patient's living patterns.
- Define brain death.
- Relate the procedure of selected neurodiagnostic tests to nursing implications for patient care.

*A*ssessment and care of a patient with a neurological problem constitute one of the biggest challenges for many critical care nurses. In basic nursing education and even in many critical care courses, an assessment of the functioning of the nervous system is frequently covered last. The curriculum may not address the nervous system to the depth or complexity of other body systems. It is not uncommon, then, for even the experienced caregiver to feel uncertain when gathering data about the nervous system.

There are three major objectives in the nursing assessment of a patient with a real or potential neurological problem. The first objective is to gather data about the functioning of the nervous system in an objective and orderly manner. Data can be considered objective if several examiners, seeing the same phenomenon or behavior, would give similar descriptions. (This is called inter-rater reliability.) A standard neurological check sheet should be used by all the nursing staff, with clearly defined grading scales or terms listed. This avoids potential inconsistency (eg, "stuporous" to one person may mean "lethargic" to another).

The second objective of neurological assessment is to correlate and trend the data over time. For such a correlation to be of value, the results of history, physical assessment, and diagnostic tests must be interrelated. Consideration of the information in a patterned format will help to establish medical and nursing diagnoses and guide the nurse in choosing and evaluating therapy. It is critical that

613

examination results be recorded clearly so changes in findings can be easily identified.

The third objective of the neurological nursing assessment is to determine the effect of dysfunction on the patient's daily living and ability to care for self. To this point, the goals of physicians and nurses in the care of a patient with a neurological problem are similar. Each discipline uses many of the same questions and techniques to determine normal and abnormal nervous system functioning. In contrast to medicine, the focus of nursing is to assist patients in coping with real or potential changes in daily living and self-care.

HISTORY

Neurological assessment begins at the first encounter with the patient. Conversation with the patient and family is a vital source of data needed to evaluate overall functioning. The focus of such an interview is twofold:

- Analysis of the current problem bringing the patient to the health care facility
- General survey of other systems to determine if other problem areas are evident in addition to those identified by the patient

When gathering this information, the nurse should ask questions geared to the detection of specific neurological problems and their effect on the patient. It may be helpful to have a family member or friend present who can confirm and clarify the patient's responses. The following list contains significant information the nurse should learn from the history questions:

- Recent trauma that could affect the nervous system (eg, a fall or an automobile crash)
- Recent infections, including sinusitis and ear or tooth infections
- Recent headaches or problems with concentration and memory
- Feelings of dizziness, loss of balance, "black-out" spells, tinnitus, and hearing problems
- Clumsiness or weakness of the extremities and difficulty walking
- Sensory distortions (eg, numbness, tingling, hypersensitivity, pain) or sensory loss in face, trunk, or extremities
- Impotence or difficulty with urination
- Recent difficulties in performing everyday activities
- Effects of problem on usual pattern of living, job performance, social interactions
- Tobacco, alcohol, and drug use
- Prescription and over-the-counter medication use, including dose, schedule, and therapeutic and adverse effects

---

Considerations for the Pediatric Patient
Neuroassessment

The principles (or objectives) of neuroassessment are the same for all patients: gather data, correlate and trend the data over time, and determine the effect of dysfunction on the patient and family. All aspects of this process can be difficult when the patient is a child.

- History may be difficult to obtain.
- Language skills may be limited so that degree of confusion is difficult to assess.
- If the nurse is unfamiliar with normal child behavior, deviation from the norm may not be apparent.
- Variations in physical capability and limitations in motor, social, and language skills can add to the difficulty of assessing the injured pediatric patient.
- When a child's level of consciousness is assessed, special attention should be given to the comments of the family caregiver. A child may seem calm to the nurse, but if the caregiver insists the child is "not acting right," further evaluation is warranted.
- Children who allow the nurse to examine them or perform painful diagnostic tests without protest are cause for special concern.
- A modified Glasgow Coma Scale can be used for assessing infants and toddlers (see scale at right).
- Pupil checks can most easily be accomplished by allowing

the child, if condition allows, to play with the flashlight; changes in pupils can be noted with the change in level of light.

Modified Glasgow Coma Scale for Infants, Toddlers, and Children

Best Eye-Opening Response	Score
Spontaneous	4
To verbal stimulus	3
To pain stimulus	2
None	1
Best Motor Response	
Normal spontaneous movement	6
Localizes pain	5
Withdraws to pain	4
Abnormal flexion	3
Abnormal extension	2
None	1
Best Verbal Response	
Smiles, interacts	5
Consolable	4
Cries to pain	3
Moans to pain	2
None	1

With permission from HealthONE EMS and Trauma Services, Columbia Swedish Medical Center, Englewood, CO

PHYSICAL EXAMINATION

Level of Consciousness

The quality of a patient's level of consciousness is the most basic and most critical parameter requiring assessment. The level of a patient's awareness of, response to, and interaction with the environment is the most sensitive indicator of nervous system dysfunction. Several systems are used for grading alterations in arousal and awareness. Terms such as *lethargic*, *stuporous*, and *semicomatose* are in common use in many areas (see terminology display).

In acute care settings where time for gathering data is limited, using the Glasgow Coma Scale (see Scale). can provide a useful shortcut. Such a scale allows the examiner to record objectively the patient's response to the environment in three major areas: eye opening, verbalization, and movement. In each category, the best response is scored. Maximum total score for a fully awake and alert person is 15. A minimum score of 3 indicates a completely unresponsive patient. An overall score of 8 or below is associated with coma; if maintained over time, it may be one predictor of a poor functional recovery. This scoring system was designed as a guide for rapid evaluation of the acutely ill or severely injured patient whose status may change quickly. It is not useful as a guide for evaluation of patients in long-standing comas or during prolonged recovery from severe brain injury.

An alternative to grading scales is to describe what stimulus is used and what the patient's response is. A suggested order of stimuli follows:

1. Call patient by name.
2. Call name louder.
3. Combine calling name with light touch.
4. Combine calling name with vigorous touch ("shake and shout").
5. Create pain.

A stimulus–reaction level scale is given in the accompanying display.

The Glasgow Coma Scale

Best Eye-Opening Response	Score
Spontaneously	4
To speech	3
To pain	2
No response	1

Best Verbal Response	Score
Oriented	5
Confused conversation	4
Inappropriate words	3
Garbled sounds	2
No response	1

Best Motor Response	Score
Obeys commands	6
Localizes stimuli	5
Withdrawal from stimulus	4
Abnormal flexion (decorticate)	3
Abnormal extension (decerebrate)	2
No response	1

When noxious stimuli are needed to evoke a response, the nurse should pay careful attention to where the painful stimulus is applied. It is not unknown for a misplaced examiner's hand to cause serious skin or tissue injury. Areas to avoid include the skin of the nipples and genital area. Instead, one should apply pain to the big toenail, the knuckles or nails of the fingers, the sternum, or the supraorbital ridge. When stimulating the last area, one should take care not to damage the eye itself.

More complex information about nervous system functioning may be obtained by gathering data about the pa-

---

Clinical Terminology

Grading Responsiveness

Alert: normal

Awake: may sleep more than usual or be somewhat confused on first awakening, but fully oriented when aroused

Lethargic: drowsy but follows simple commands when stimulated

Stuporous: very hard to arouse; inconsistently may follow simple commands or speak single words or short phrases

Semicomatose: movements are purposeful when stimulated; does not follow commands or speak coherently

Comatose: may respond with reflexive posturing when stimulated or may have no response to any stimulus

---

A Stimulus–Reaction Level Scale

Level	Description
1	Alert; no delay in response
2	Drowsy but responsive to gentle stimulation; confused about either name, place, or time
3	Very drowsy; responds to strong stimulation with orienting eye movements, obeying commands or localizing, and actively attempting to remove stimulus
4	Unconscious; localizes but not successful in removing stimulus
5	Unconscious; withdrawal movements to any stimulation
6	Unconscious; stereotypical flexion movements to pain
7	Unconscious; stereotypical extension movements to pain
8	Unconscious; no response to pain stimulation

CLINICAL APPLICATION: Assessment Parameters
Format for Mental Status Examination

Attention
Digit span forward and backward

Remembering
Short-term: recall of three items after 5 min
Long-term: recall of mother's maiden name, recall of break-fast menu, events of previous day, etc.

Feeling (Affective)
Facial, body expression of mood
Verbal description of affect
Congruence of verbal, body indicators of mood

Language
Content and quantity of spontaneous speech
Naming common objects, parts of objects
Repetition of phrases
Ability to read and explain short passage in newspaper, magazine
Ability to write to dictation, spontaneously

Thinking
Fund of information (example: current president, preceding three)
Knowledge of current events
Orientation to person, place, time (tested as part of arousal, see consciousness)
Calculation: add two numbers, subtract 7 from 100
Problem-solving: What would you do if you found a stamped envelope on the street? What would you do if you smelled smoke in a theater?

Spatial Perception
Copy drawings: square, cross, three-dimensional cube
Draw clock face, map of room
Point out right and left side of self
Demonstrate: putting on a coat, blowing out match, using a toothbrush

---

tient's ability to integrate attention, memory, and thought processes (see display). Such a mental status examination also may uncover clues about the presence of additional problems affecting the patient's lifestyle.

When gathering such a wealth of data, assessment of the patient's ability to communicate becomes paramount. Use of language requires comprehension of verbal and nonverbal symbols and the ability to use those symbols to communicate with others. Evaluation of the patient's understanding normally is accomplished through the spoken word (Table 32–1). Speech dysfunctions may make such evaluations exceedingly difficult.

TABLE 32-1
Patterns of Speech Deficits

Type	Deficit Location	Speech Patterns
Fluent dysphasia	Left parietal–temporal lobes (Wernicke's area)	• Fluent speech that lacks coherent content • Impaired understanding of spoken word in spite of normal hearing • May have normal-sounding speech rhythm but no intelligible words • May use invented, meaningless words (neologism), word substitution (paraphasia), or repetition of words (perseveration, echolalia)
Nonfluent dysphasia	Left frontal area (Broca's area)	• Slow speech with poor articulation • Inability to initiate sounds • Comprehension usually intact • Usually associated with impaired writing skills
Global dysphasia	Diffuse involvement of frontal, parietal, and occipital areas	• Nonfluent speech • Inability to understand spoken or written words
Dysarthria	Corticobulbar tracts; cerebellum	• Loss of articulation, phonation • Loss of control of muscles of lips, tongue, palate • Slurred, jerky, or irregular speech but with appropriate content

Movement, Strength, and Coordination

Muscle weakness is a cardinal sign of dysfunction in many neurological disorders. The nurse can test strength of extremities by offering resistance to various muscle groups, using the nurse's own muscles, or using gravity. As a quick test to detect weakness of the upper extremities, the nurse can have the patient hold the arms straight out with palms upward and eyes closed. Observe for any downward drift or pronation of the forearms. A similar test for the lower extremities includes having the patient raise the legs, one leg at a time, straight off the bed against the examiner's resistance. Weakness noted in any of these tests may indicate damage to the motor neuron pathways of the pyramidal system, which transmits commands for voluntary movement. A grading scale for muscle strength is given in the display.

Hemiparesis (weakness) and hemiplegia (paralysis) are unilateral dysfunctions resulting from a lesion contralateral to the corticospinal tract. Paraplegia may result from bilateral spinal cord or peripheral nerve dysfunctions. Quadriplegia is associated with bilateral spinal cord lesions, brain stem dysfunction, and large bilateral lesions in the cerebrum.

Each extremity should also be assessed for size, muscle tone, and smoothness of passive movement. Dysfunctions noted here may indicate problems in the basal ganglia (also called the extrapyramidal system). These pathways normally suppress involuntary movements through controlled inhibition. Assessment findings may include the "clasp-knife" phenomenon, in which initially strong resistance to passive movement suddenly decreases. Alternatively, "lead-pipe" rigidity may be present, which is steady, continuous resistance to passive movement and is characteristic of diffuse hemispheric damage. "Cog wheel" rigidity is characteristic of Parkinson's disease.

The nurse also should be alert for the presence of involuntary movements, from mild fasciculation to the violent, flailing movement of an extremity. This terminology is described in the display.

The cerebellum is responsible for smooth synchronization, balance, and ordering of movements. It does *not* initiate any movements, so a patient with cerebellar dysfunction is not paralyzed. Instead, ataxia, dysmetria, and lack of synchronization of movement are common manifestations.

A Grading Scale for Muscle Strength

0 = No muscle contraction
1 = Flicker or trace of contraction
2 = Moves but cannot overcome gravity
3 = Moves against gravity but cannot overcome resistance of examiner's muscles
4 = Moves with some weakness against resistance of examiner's muscles
5 = Normal power and strength

Clinical Terminology: Types of Involuntary Movements

Tremor	Purposeless movement
Resting	Lesion in basal ganglia
Intention	Lesion in cerebellum
Asterixis	Metabolic derangement
Physiological	Due to fatigue or stress
Fasciculation	Twitching of resting muscles; due to peripheral nerve or spinal cord lesion or to metabolic influences such as cold or anesthetic agents
Clonus	Repetitive movement; elicited with stretch reflex and implies lesion of the corticospinal tracts
Myoclonus	Nonrhythmic movement; single jerk-like movements, symmetrical, unknown etiology
Hemiballismus	Flailing movement of extremity; violent movement; not present during sleep; lesion in subthalamic nuclei of basal ganglia
Chorea	Irregular movements; involves limbs and facial muscles; asymmetrical movements at rest; involuntary movements may increase when purposeful movement attempted
Athetosis	Slow, writhing movements

Some of the more common tests for cerebellar synchronization of movement with balance include the following:

- *Romberg test*—performed by having the patient stand with feet together, first with eyes open, then with eyes closed. Observe for sway or direction of falling, and be prepared to catch the patient if necessary.
- *Finger to nose test*—performed by having the patient touch one finger to the examiner's finger, then touch own nose. Overshooting or past-pointing the mark is called *dysmetria*. Both sides are tested individually.
- *Rapidly alternating movement (RAM)*—checked on each side by having the patient oppose each finger and thumb in rapid succession or by performing rapid pronation and supination of the hand on the leg. Inability to perform RAM is termed *adiadochokinesia*; performing RAM poorly or clumsily is termed *dysdiadochokinesia*.

Assessment of movement and strength in a patient who cannot follow commands or is unresponsive can be difficult. For such a patient, it is important to note what, if any, stimuli initiate a response and to describe or grade the type of response obtained.

Motor response in the comatose person may be appropriate, inappropriate, or absent (Fig. 32–1). Appropriate responses, such as localization or withdrawal, mean that the sensory pathways and corticospinal pathways are functioning (see Fig. 32–1A, B). There may be monoplegia or hemiplegia, indicating that the corticospinal pathways are interrupted on one side.

Inappropriate responses include decorticate rigidity and decerebrate rigidity. *Decorticate* rigidity results from lesions of the internal capsule, basal ganglia, thalamus, or cerebral hemisphere, which interrupt corticospinal pathways. It is characterized by flexion of the arms, wrists, and fingers; adduction of the upper extremities; and extension, internal rotation, and plantar flexion of the lower extremities (see Fig. 32–1C).

Decerebrate rigidity consists of extension, adduction, and hyperpronation of the upper extremities and extension of the lower extremities, with plantar flexion of the feet (see Fig. 32–1D). Many times, the person also is opisthotonic and has clenched teeth. Injury to the midbrain and pons results in decerebration. At times, the inappropriate responses of decortication and decerebration may switch back and forth. If there is no response to noxious stimuli or only very weak flexor responses, the person probably has extensive brain stem dysfunction (see Fig. 32–1E).

Reflexes

A reflex occurs when a sensory stimulus evokes a motor response. Cerebral control and consciousness are not required for a reflex to occur. Superficial and deep reflexes are

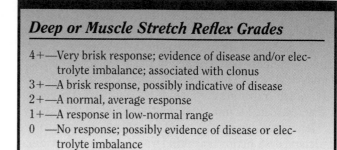

Deep or Muscle Stretch Reflex Grades

4+—Very brisk response; evidence of disease and/or electrolyte imbalance; associated with clonus
3+—A brisk response, possibly indicative of disease
2+—A normal, average response
1+—A response in low-normal range
0 —No response; possibly evidence of disease or electrolyte imbalance

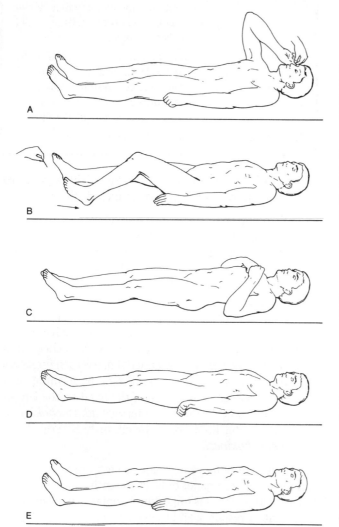

(A) Localizing pain. An appropriate response is to reach up above shoulder level toward the stimulus. Remember, a focal motor deficit such as hemiplegia may prevent a bilateral response.

(B) Withdrawal. An appropriate response is to pull the extremity or body away from the stimulus. As brain stem involvement increases, your patient may respond by assuming one of the following postures. Each one shows more advanced deterioration.

(C) Decorticate posturing. One or both arms in full flexion on the chest. Legs may be stiffly extended.

(D) Decerebrate posturing. One or both arms stiffly extended. Possible extension of the legs.

(E) Flaccid. No motor response in any extremity. An extremely ominous sign.

FIGURE 32-1
Motor responses to pain. When a painful stimulus is applied to an unconscious patient's supraorbital notch, the patient will respond in one of these ways.

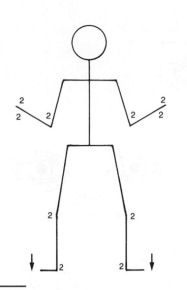

FIGURE 32-2
Documentation of selected deep and cutaneous reflexes. Reflexes shown here at major muscle stretch reflex sites are normal and symmetrical.

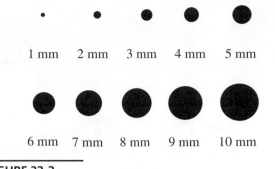

FIGURE 32-3
Pupil size chart.

tested on symmetrical sides of the body and compared by reference to the strength of contraction elicited.

Muscle stretch reflexes, also called deep tendon reflexes, are elicited by a brisk tap with a reflex hammer. The target for this sensory stimulus is a stretched tendon of a muscle group. The desired motor response is contraction of the muscle group that was stimulated. Deep tendon reflexes commonly are graded on a scale of 0 to 4; grade 2 indicates normal response (see scale).

Cutaneous or superficial reflexes occur when certain areas of skin are lightly stroked or tapped, causing contraction of the muscle groups beneath. Such reflexes are graded simply as normal, abnormal (pathological), or absent. An example is the plantar reflex. The sensory stimulus is applied by briskly stroking the outer edge of the sole and across the ball of the foot with a dull object, such as a tongue blade or key. The normal motor response is downward or plantar flexion of the toes. An abnormal response (Babinski's sign) is upward or dorsiflexion of the big toe, with or without fanning of the other toes. A positive Babinski's sign may indicate a lesion in the pyramidal tract.

A "shorthand" method of documenting reflex responses is to draw a stick figure with grades or direction of responses indicated (Fig. 32–2).

Pupillary Changes

Pupils should be examined for their size (best specified in millimeters) and shape (Fig. 32–3). The patient focuses on a distant point in the room. The examiner places the edge of one hand along the patient's nose. A bright light is directed into one eye, and the briskness of pupillary constriction (direct response) is noted. The other pupil also should constrict (consensual response). The procedure is repeated with the other eye. *Anisocoria* (unequal pupils) may be normal in a small percentage of the population or may be an indication of neural dysfunction. If it is a normal variant, the difference in pupil size should be less than 1 mm.

To test accommodation, an object is held 8 to 12 inches in front of the patient's face. The patient focuses on the object as the examiner moves it in toward the patient's nose. The pupils should constrict as the object gets closer, and the eyes turn inward to maintain a clear image. The normal response to testing may be documented as PERRLA, or pupils equal, round, reactive to light, and accommodation.

Some important pupillary abnormalities are shown in Figure 32–4. Causes of small, reactive pupils include metabolic abnormalities and bilateral dysfunction in the diencephalon. Large, fixed pupils 5–6 mm) that may show slight rhythmic constriction and dilation when stimulated may indicate midbrain damage. Midposition-fixed pupils (4–5 mm) also may indicate midbrain dysfunction, with sympathetic and parasympathetic pathways interrupted. Pinpoint, nonreactive pupils are seen after damage to the pons area of the brain stem (remember the phrase "pontine pupils are pinpoint"), with selected eye medications, and with opiate administration. A unilaterally dilated, nonreactive ("blown") pupils will be seen with third cranial (oculomotor) nerve damage when the uncal portion of the temporal

---

CLINICAL APPLICATION:
Assessment Parameters
Quick Guide to Causes of Pupil Size Changes

Pinpoint pupils
- Drugs: opiates
- Drops: medications for glaucoma
- "Nearly dead": damage in the pons area of the brain stem

Dilated pupils
- Fear: panic attack, extreme anxiety
- "Fits": seizures
- "Fast living": cocaine, crack, phencyclidine (PCP) use

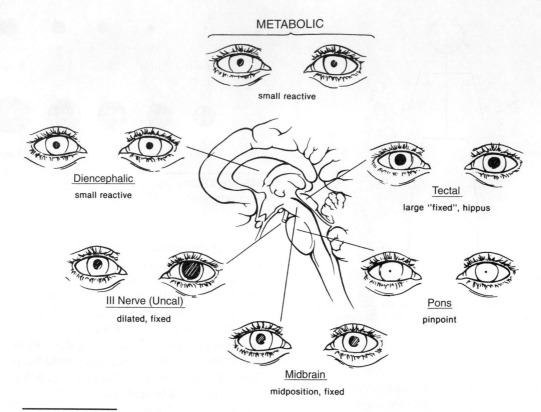

FIGURE 32-4

Abnormal pupils. (Adapted from Plum F, Poser J: The Diagnosis of Stupor and Coma [3rd Ed]. Philadelphia, FA Davis).

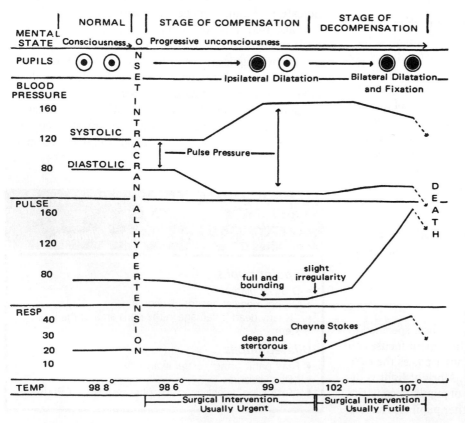

FIGURE 32-5

Vital sign changes during elevated ICP. Chart showing changes in mental state, pupils, blood pressure, pulse rate, respiratory rate, and temperature before and after the onset of fatal increased ICP.

lobe herniates through the small opening in the tentorium. When structures are compressed around the opening in the tentorium or fold of dura that separates the cerebrum from the cerebellum and brain stem, loss of functioning of the parasympathetic nerves to the pupil on that side results in an ipsilaterally dilated pupils. A quick guide to changes in pupil size is given in the display (p. 7).

Vital Signs

Classic signs of *increased intracranial pressure* include an elevated systolic pressure in conjunction with a widening pulse pressure, slow bounding pulse, and respiratory irregularities. This combination is termed Cushing's response.

After any emergency treatment that may be indicated (eg, maintenance of the airway for adequate ventilation), vital signs should be taken immediately and checked frequently. Any indication of shock should alert the nurse to search for signs of thoracic and intra-abdominal injuries. Vital signs are only signs and are not infallible in determining the patient's neurological status (Fig. 32–5).

Hypoventilation after cerebral trauma can lead to respiratory acidosis. As the blood carbon dioxide increases and blood oxygen decreases, cerebral hypoxia and edema can result in secondary brain trauma. *Hyperventilation* after cerebral trauma produces respiratory alkalosis with increased blood oxygen and decreased blood carbon dioxide levels. This causes vasoconstriction of cerebral vessels and decreases oxygen consumption, resulting in cerebral hypoxia.

Because temperature elevation increases cellular metabolism, measures should be implemented to maintain temperature in the normal range. Hypothermia may be induced if indicated, but care must be taken to avoid shivering.

Cranial Nerves

I. OLFACTORY

The first cranial nerve contains sensory fibers for the sense of smell. This test usually is deferred unless the patient complains of an inability to smell. One tests the nerve, with the patient's eyes closed, by placing aromatic substances near the nose for identification. Fragrances that have a distinct smell (eg, soap, coffee, or cinnamon) should be used. Ammonia should not be used because the patient will respond to irritation of the nasal mucosa rather than to the odor. Each nostril is checked separately. Loss of smell may be caused by a fracture of the cribriform plate or a fracture in the ethmoid area.

The patient also may have anosmia (loss of sense of smell) from a shearing injury to the olfactory bulb after a basilar skull fracture or from cerebrospinal fluid (CSF) rhinorrhea.

II. OPTIC

Gross visual acuity is checked by having the patient read ordinary newsprint. The patient's preinjury need for glasses should be noted. Visual field can be tested by having the patient look straight ahead with one eye covered. The examiner will move a finger from the periphery of each quadrant of vision toward the patient's center of vision. The patient should indicate when the examiner's finger is seen. This is done for both eyes, and the results are compared to the examiner's visual fields, which are assumed to be normal (Fig. 32–6). Damage to the retina will produce a blind spot. An optic nerve lesion will produce partial or complete blindness on the same side. Damage to the optic chiasm results in bitemporal hemianopsia, blindness in both lateral visual fields. Pressure on the optic tract can cause homonymous hemianopsia, half-blindness on the opposite side of the lesion in both eyes. A lesion in the parietal or temporal lobe may produce contralateral blindness in the upper or lower quadrant of vision, respectively, in both eyes (this is known as *quadrant deficit*). Damage in the occipital lobe may cause homonymous hemianopsia with central vision sparing (Fig. 32–7).

III. OCULOMOTOR; IV. TROCHLEAR; VI. ABDUCENS

These cranial nerves are checked together because they all innervate extraocular muscles. The parasympathetic fibers of the oculomotor nerve are responsible for lens accommodation and pupil size through control of the ciliary muscles. The motor fibers of the oculomotor nerve innervate the muscles that elevate the eyelid and those that move the eyes up, down, and medially. These include the superior rectus, inferior oblique, inferior rectus, and medial rectus muscles. The trochlear nerve innervates the superior oblique muscle to move the eyes down and in. The lateral rectus muscle

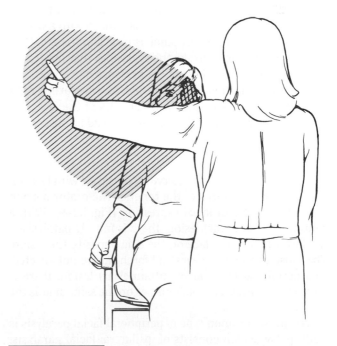

FIGURE 32-6
Confrontational method of testing visual fields.

VISUAL FIELD DEFECTS

DESCRIPTION

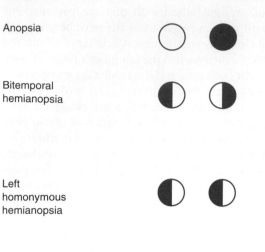

Anopsia

Blindness in one eye;
due to complete lesion of the right
optic nerve, as in trauma.

Bitemporal
hemianopsia

Also called central vision; due to lesions around the optic chiasm such as pituitary tumors or aneurysms of the anterior communicating artery. Affected fibers originate in the nasal half of each retina.

Left
homonymous
hemianopsia

Half-vision involving both eyes with loss of visual field on the same side of each eye; due to lesion of right temporal or occipital lobes with damage to the right optic tract or optic radiations.

Left eye   Right eye

FIGURE 32-7
Visual field defects associated with lesions of the visual system.

moves the eyes laterally and is innervated by the abducens nerve. Diplopia, nystagmus, conjugate deviation, and ptosis may indicate dysfunction of these cranial nerves. These nerves are tested by having the patient follow the examiner's finger as it is moved in all directions of gaze (Fig. 32–8).

V. TRIGEMINAL

The trigeminal nerve has three divisions: ophthalmic, maxillary, and mandibular. The sensory portion of this nerve controls sensation to the face and cornea. The motor portion controls the muscles of mastication. This nerve is partially tested by checking the corneal reflex; if it is intact, the patient will blink when the cornea is stroked with a wisp of cotton or a drop of normal saline is placed in the eye. Care must be taken not to stroke the eyelash as that may cause the eye to blink regardless of the presence of a corneal reflex. Facial sensation can be tested by comparing light touch and pinprick on symmetrical sides of the face. The ability to chew or clench the jaw also should be observed.

VII. FACIAL

The sensory portion of this nerve is concerned with taste on the anterior two thirds of the tongue. The motor portion controls muscles of facial expression (Fig. 32–9). With a central (supranuclear) lesion, there is muscle paralysis of the lower half of the face on the side opposite the lesion. The muscles about the eyes and forehead are not affected. In a peripheral (nuclear or infranuclear) lesion, there is complete paralysis of facial muscles on the same side as the lesion.

The most common type of peripheral facial paralysis is Bell's palsy, which consists of ipsilateral facial paralysis. There is drooping of the upper lid with the lower lid slightly everted. Facial lines on the same side are obliter-

ated with the mouth drawn toward the normal side. Artificial tears or ophthalmic ointment and taping the eye closed may be indicated to prevent corneal abrasion and irritation.

VIII. ACOUSTIC

This nerve is divided into the cochlear and vestibular branches, which control hearing and equilibrium, respectively.

The cochlear nerve is tested by air and bone conduction. A vibrating tuning fork is placed on the mastoid process; after the patient can no longer hear the fork, he or she should be able to hear it for a few seconds longer when it is placed in front of the ear (Rinne test). The patient may complain of tinnitus or decreased hearing if this nerve is damaged.

The vestibular nerve may not be evaluated routinely. The nurse should be alert, however, to complaints of dizziness or vertigo from the patient.

IX. GLOSSOPHARYNGEAL; X. VAGUS

These cranial nerves usually are tested together. The glossopharyngeal nerve supplies sensory fibers to the posterior third of the tongue and the uvula and soft palate. The vagus innervates the larynx, pharynx, and soft palate and conveys autonomic responses to the heart, stomach, lungs, and small intestines. Autonomic vagal functions usually are not tested because they are checked during the general physical examination. These nerves can be tested by eliciting a gag reflex, observing the uvula for symmetrical movement when the patient says "ah," or observing midline elevation of the uvula when both sides are stroked. Inability to cough forcefully, difficulty with swallowing, and hoarseness may be signs of dysfunction.

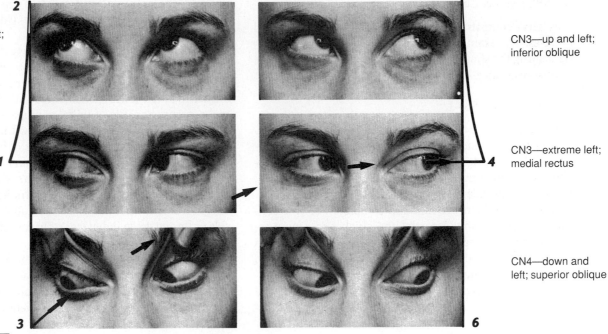

CN3—up and right; superior rectus inferior oblique

CN3—up and left; inferior oblique

CN6—extreme right; lateral rectus

CN3—extreme left; medial rectus

CN3—down and right; inferior rectus

CN4—down and left; superior oblique

FIGURE 32-8
Muscles used in conjugate eye movements in the six cardinal directions of gaze. Lead the patient's gaze in the sequence numbered 1 through 6. (Adapted from Bates B: A Guide to Physical Examination and History Taking. Phildelphia, JB Lippincott,1995).

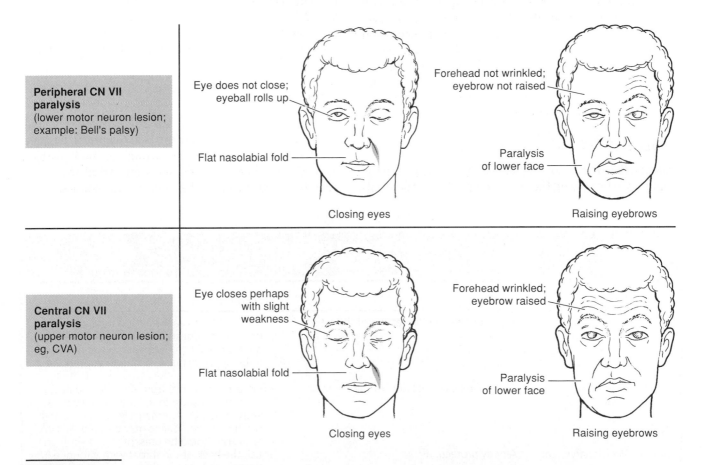

Peripheral CN VII paralysis
(lower motor neuron lesion; example: Bell's palsy)

Eye does not close; eyeball rolls up

Flat nasolabial fold

Closing eyes

Forehead not wrinkled; eyebrow not raised

Paralysis of lower face

Raising eyebrows

Central CN VII paralysis
(upper motor neuron lesion; eg, CVA)

Eye closes perhaps with slight weakness

Flat nasolabial fold

Closing eyes

Forehead wrinkled; eyebrow raised

Paralysis of lower face

Raising eyebrows

FIGURE 32-9
Facial movements with upper and lower motor neuron facial paralysis. (Adapted from Bates B: A Guide to Physical Examination [5th Ed], pp 550–551. Philadelphia, JB Lippincott, 1991)

XI. SPINAL ACCESSORY

This nerve controls the trapezius and sternocleidomastoid muscles. The examiner tests this nerve by having the patient shrug the shoulders or turn the head from side to side against resistance.

XII. HYPOGLOSSAL

This nerve controls tongue movement. It can be checked by having the patient protrude the tongue. The examiner should check for deviation from midline, tremor, and atrophy. If deviation is noted secondary to damage of the nerve, it will be to the side of the lesion.

Testing cranial nerve function completely is time consuming and exacting. A partial and quicker screening assessment may be performed, focusing on nerves in which dysfunction may indicate serious problems or interfere with activities of daily living. The cranial nerves of primary importance in a screening examination are the optic (II) and oculomotor (III), trigeminal (V) and facial (VII), and glossopharyngeal (IX) and vagus (X; Table 32–2).

Ocular Signs in the Unconscious Patient

Ocular position and movement are among the most useful guides to the site of brain dysfunction in the comatose person. When observing the eyes at rest, it is not uncommon to note a slight divergence of gaze. If both eyes are conjugately deviated to one side, there is possible dysfunction either in the frontal lobe on that side or in the contralateral pontine area of the brain stem. Downward deviation suggests a dysfunction in the midbrain.

"DOLL'S EYES" AND CALORIC REFLEX

Although the unconscious patient cannot participate in the examination by moving the eyes through fields of gaze voluntarily, the examiner still can test the range of ocular movement using the oculocephalic ("doll's eyes") and oculovestibular (caloric) reflexes.

The oculocephalic reflex can be assessed by quickly rotating the patient's head to one side and observing the position of the eyes (Fig. 32–10). This maneuver must *never* be performed in a person with possible cervical spine injury. A normal response consists of initial conjugate deviation of the eyes in the opposite direction, then, within a few seconds, smooth and simultaneous movement of both eyes back to midline position. This is indicative of an intact brain stem.

An abnormal reflex response occurs when one eye does not follow the normal response pattern. Absence of any ocular movement when the head is rotated briskly to either side or up and down indicates an absent reflex and portends severe brain stem dysfunction.

The examiner tests oculovestibular reflex (caloric test) by elevating the patient's head 30 degrees and irrigating each ear separately with 30 to 50 mL of iced water (Fig. 32–11). This test never should be performed in a patient who does not have an intact eardrum or who has blood or fluid collected behind it. The external ear canal should be unobstructed by cerumen or debris. In an unconscious patient with an intact brain stem, the eyes will exhibit horizontal nystagmus with slow, conjugate movement toward the irrigated ear followed by rapid movement away from the stimulus. When the reflex is absent, both eyes remain fixed in midline position, indicating midbrain and pons dysfunction. The oculovestibular reflex can usually be elicited later than the oculocephalic reflex.

Sensation

The primary forms of sensation are tested first. These include perception of touch (cotton wisp), pain (pinprick), temperature (hot, cold), and proprioception (limb position). With the patient's eyes closed, multiple and symmetrical areas of the body are tested, including the trunk and extremities.

TABLE 32-2   CLINICAL APPLICATION: Assessment Parameters
A Quick Screening Test for Cranial Nerve Function

	Nerve	Reflex	Procedure
II III	Optic Oculomotor	Pupil constriction (protection of the retina)	Shine a light into each eye and note if the pupil on that side constricts (direct response). Next, shine a light into each eye and note if the opposite pupil constricts (consensual response).
V VII	Trigeminal Facial	Corneal reflex (protection of the cornea)	Approaching the eye from the side and avoiding the eyelashes, touch the cornea with a wisp of cotton. Alternatively, a drop of sterile water or normal saline may be used. A blink response should be present.
IX X	Glossopharyngeal Vagus	Airway protection	Touch the back of the throat with a tongue depressor. A gag or cough response should be present.

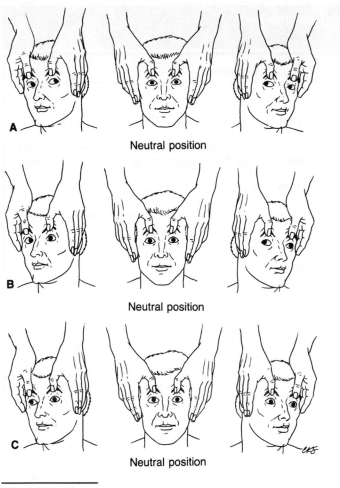

FIGURE 32-10
Test for oculocephalic reflex response (doll's eyes phenomenon). (**A**) Normal response—when the head is rotated, the eyes turn together to the side opposite to the head movement. (**B**) Abnormal response—when the head is rotated, the eyes do not turn in a conjugate manner. (**C**) Absent response—as head position is changed, eyes do not move in the sockets.

The patient's ability to perceive the sensation should be noted, with distal areas compared to proximal areas and right and left sides compared at corresponding areas. The nurse should determine whether sensory change involves one entire side of the body. Abnormal results may indicate damage somewhere along the pathways of the receptors in the skin, muscles, joints and tendons, spinothalamic tracts, or sensory area of the cortex (Table 32–3).

Cortical forms of sensation also should be tested. Disturbances of these forms when the primary forms of sensation are intact indicate damage to the parietal lobe.

The inability to recognize objects by sight, touch, or sound is termed *agnosia*. The ability to recognize and identify objects by touch is called *stereognosis* and is a function of the parietal lobe. Identification of an object by the sense of sight is a function of the parieto-occipital junction. The temporal lobe is responsible for identification of objects by sound. Each of these senses should be tested separately. For example, a patient may not be able to identify a whistle by its sound but may recognize it immediately if he or she holds it or looks at it.

Other cortical forms of sensation include the following:

- *Graphesthesia*—the ability to recognize numbers or letters traced lightly on the skin. Bilateral sides are compared.
- *Point localization*—the ability to locate the precise spot on the body touched by the examiner. One version of dysfunction in this area is called *extinction phenomenon*, the inability to recognize bilateral sensations when the examiner simultaneously touches two symmetrical areas on opposite sides of the body.
- *Two-point discrimination*—tested by using two sharp objects and determining the smallest area in which two points can be perceived.
- *Texture discrimination*—the ability to recognize materials, such as cotton, burlap, and wool, by feeling them.

Other Observations

- *Battle's sign*—bruising over the mastoid areas suggests basal skull fracture.
- *Raccoon's eye*—periorbital edema and bruising suggests frontobasilar fracture.
- *Rhinorrhea*—drainage of CSF from the nose suggests fracture of the cribriform plate with herniation of a fragment of the dura and arachnoid through the fracture.
- *Otorrhea*—drainage of CSF from the ear usually is associated with fracture of the petrous portion of the temporal bone.

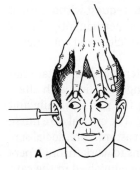
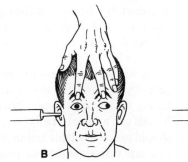
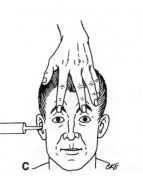

FIGURE 32-11
Test for oculovestibular reflex response (caloric ice-water test). (**A**) Normal response—ice water infusion in the ear produces conjugate eye movements. (**B**) Abnormal response—infusion produces dysconjugate or asymmetrical eye movements. (**C**) Absent response—infusion produces no eye movements.

TABLE 32-3   CLINICAL APPLICATION: Assessment Parameters
Testing Superficial and Deep Sensations

Sensation	Stimuli	Dysfunction
Spinothalamic Tracts Carry Impulses for		
Pain	Alternate sharp and dull ends of a pin, asking patient to discriminate between the two (superficial pain). Squeeze nail beds; apply pressure on the orbital rim; rub sternum (deep pain).	• Ipsilateral sensory loss implies a peripheral nerve lesion. • Contralateral sensory loss is seen with lesions of the spinothalamic tract or in the thalamus.
Light touch	Use a wisp of cotton on skin and ask patient to identify when it touches.	• Bilateral sensory loss may indicate a spinal cord lesion. • Paresthesia is an abnormal sensation, such as itching or tingling.
Temperature	Use test tubes filled with hot and cold water or use small metal plates of varying temperatures. (Test only if pain and light touch sensations are abnormal.)	• Causalgia is a burning sensation that can be caused by peripheral nerve irritation.
Posterior Columns Carry Impulses for		
Vibration	Apply a vibrating tuning fork on bony prominences, and note patient's ability to sense and locate vibrations bilaterally.	• Ipsilateral sensory loss may be due to spinal cord injury or to peripheral neuropathy.
Proprioception	Move the patient's finger or toe up and down and ask patient to identify final resting position.	• Contralateral loss may occur from lesions of the thalamus or of the parietal lobes.

• *Meningeal irritation*—this can be detected by the presence of nuchal rigidity in conjunction with fever, headache, and photophobia. A positive Kernig's sign, pain in the neck when the thigh is flexed on the abdomen and the leg is extended at the knee, also may be present. Brudzinski's sign, involuntary flexion of the hips when the neck is flexed toward the chest, is another indication of meningeal inflammation (Fig. 32–12).

Evaluation of Dysfunction in Patient's Living Patterns

Neurological nursing assessment would be incomplete if the process consisted solely of gathering data and identifying abnormal functions. Nursing expertise should expand the scope to include an evaluation of the impact of dysfunction on the patient's living patterns and ability to care for self. For example, diplopia (double vision) is an abnormal finding and may be an indicator of problems with the ocular muscles or with the nervous system; however, it also may be a clue suggesting difficulty in carrying out daily activities.

▆▆▆ PERSISTENT VEGETATIVE STATE

Vegetative state is a term used to describe a chronic condition that sometimes is the consequence of severe brain injury. It is characterized by a period of sleep-like coma followed by a return to the awake state but with a total lack of apparent cognition.[1] In persistent vegetative state, the higher cortical functions of the cerebral hemispheres have been damaged permanently, but the lower functions of the brain stem remain intact. The patient's eyes may open spontaneously, or they may open seemingly in response to verbal stimuli. Sleep–wake cycles exist. The patient maintains normal blood pressure and respiratory control. Also seen are involuntary lip smacking, chewing, and roving eye movements.

The issue of "chronic comatose-like" states first came to national attention in the early 1970s with the case of Karen Ann Quinlan, whose parents finally won a protracted legal battle to remove ventilatory support from their daughter. Even after the removal, Ms. Quinlan survived for several more years in a persistent vegetative state. More recently, the case of Nancy Cruzan was the first "right-to-die" case to be decided by the United States Supreme Court. In that landmark decision, the Court ruled that Ms. Cruzan's legal guardian, her father, had the right to request withdrawal of nutrition and hydration from his permanently brain-injured daughter in accordance with "clear and convincing evidence" of her wishes.[2]

Caring for the patient in a persistent vegetative state can be a physical and emotional challenge. Dealing with alternating cycles of hope and grief on the part of family and friends can be emotionally battering. The critical care nurse should use all available resources of pastoral care, social service, and various assistance programs to work through personal thoughts and feelings. Everyone involved in the care

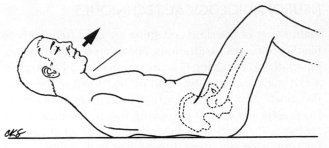

Brudzinksi's sign

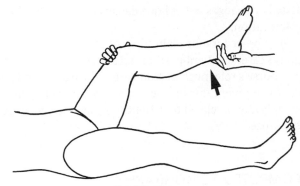

Kernig's sign

FIGURE 32-12
Two signs of meningeal irritation.

of such patients should have a realistic understanding of the prognosis of persistent vegetative state. Supporting the family in the process of gathering information and making decisions is difficult but essential.

■ BRAIN DEATH

The patient's condition may be so severe that brain death is the final outcome. The accompanying display summarizes clinical criteria for determining brain death. The critical care nurse provides essential nursing care to such a patient as treatment is continued or as life-support measures are withdrawn. The nurse may be involved in determining whether the patient has suffered brain death, although a physician legally must make the final determination.

Many years ago, the common acceptable understanding of death was "total stoppage of the circulation of the blood and a cessation of vital functions such as respiration, pulsation, etc." In the 1960s, the advent of cardiopulmonary resuscitation measures made this criterion of death obsolete. In 1968, a landmark report was published by the Ad Hoc Committee of the Harvard Medical School to Examine the Definition of Death. This committee established the first widely accepted criteria to determine brain death. Finally, in 1979, the American Medical Association House of Delegates passed a model bill on the following definition of death:

> **NURSING PERSPECTIVE**
> *Summary of Clinical Criteria for Determining Brain Death*

Nature of the Comatose State Must Be Determined

- Drugs must be excluded as a possible cause of the coma.
- The patient may not be hypothermic (ie, body temperature must exceed 33°C, or 91.4°F).
- There must be an appropriate period of observation of patient in comatose state for adequate assessment.

Absence of All Cortical/Brain Stem Function Must Be Established

- Absence of all cerebral responses to light, noise, motion, and pain
- Absence of all reflexes or muscle activity unless the reflex activity is determined to be of spinal cord origin
- Absence of spontaneous respirations with respirator disconnected for at least 3 min, with a PCO$_2$ of at least 55 mmHg to stimulate respiratory response. Some institutions do not advocate arterial blood gases and do not recommend complete apnea for 3 min for fear of causing more neuronal death if viable brain function remains. In such institutions, high levels of oxygen are administered passively through endotracheal or tracheostomy tubes for rather prolonged periods without respiration for confirmation of apnea.
- Absence of cranial nerve reflexes: fixed pupils that do not react to light and absence of oculovestibular reflex (caloric ice test response)

In addition, other tests may be required, for example:

- Isoelectric electroencephalogram (EEG). Some institutions require only one isoelectric EEG; others require two, 12 h apart.
- Absence of intracranial blood flow, as demonstrated by angiography, radioisotope techniques, echo pulsation, or computed tomography scan after administration of contrast medium

An individual who has sustained either (a) irreversible cessation of circulatory and respiratory functions, or (b) irreversible cessation of all functions of the entire brain, should be considered dead. A determination of death shall be made in accordance with accepted medical standards.[3]

The first legal statute recognizing the concept of brain death was enacted in Kansas in the early 1970s. Since then, all states have passed similar statutes. The adoption of clinical criteria to determine brain death has been facilitated by larger medical centers and by institutions actively involved in organ transplant surgery. The National Organ Transplant Act of 1984 requires every hospital receiving Medicare reimbursement to offer the opportunity for organ and tissue donation to the family of every patient who dies; this has effectively mandated that every hospital have a policy on declaration of brain death.

The role of the nurse who is caring for a potentially brain-dead patient is fourfold:

- Question the possibility of brain death.
- Assist in gathering data necessary to determine brain death.
- Provide support, understanding, and empathy for the patient's family.
- Maintain the optimal functioning of organs for potential transplantation.

These tasks may be difficult for the critical care nurse. It often is very hard to "switch gears" from fighting for a person's life one day to accepting death the next day.

◼ NEURODIAGNOSTIC STUDIES

Many diagnostic tests are available to assist in the diagnosis of neurological and neurosurgical problems. Such neurodiagnostic testing is performed in conjunction with a thorough neurological examination. The ease of availability and the diagnostic accuracy of current technology benefit the patient in an acute setting by shortening the time required to arrive at a diagnosis and institute therapy. The choice of which investigative test to perform should be based on the examiner's ability to integrate the findings with neurological assessment and locate the cause of the abnormality.

The nurse's role in neurodiagnostic testing involves patient and family preparation and monitoring the critically ill patient during and after the procedure for potential complications. Although there has been a definite increase in the number of tests that can be performed at the bedside, many still require the patient to be transported to the imaging department or even out of the institution, further expanding the role of the critical care nurse. Table 32–4 summarizes some of the diagnostic tests and outlines nursing implications.

NEURORADIOLOGICAL TECHNIQUES

Plain x-rays of the skull and spine are used frequently to identify fractures, dislocations, and other bony anomalies, especially in the setting of acute trauma. In addition, plain x-rays may be diagnostic when displacement of the calcified pineal gland is visible, which is an immediate clue to the presence of a space-occupying lesion. The presence of air inside the skull also allows diagnosis of an open skull fracture, such as a frontal or basilar skull fracture, that may not be readily apparent externally. Plain x-rays of the skull also may demonstrate infection or neoplasm manifested by changes in the bone density or other intracranial calcification.

The procedure for plain films of the skull and spine requires careful patient positioning and is relatively painless. The nurse's role involves monitoring the patient and attendant equipment during the procedure and being alert for complications related to patient position and the length of the procedure.

COMPUTED TOMOGRAPHY

Computed tomographic (CT) scanning has been in use in the United States since 1973. It permits more refined measurement of the density of tissues, blood, and bone within the body. The value of this technique is illustrated best in the trauma setting, where the ability to image rapidly and accurately the intracranial contents and position of vertebrae and spinal cord has dramatically changed the treatment of neurological patients. CT scanning can reliably detect such conditions as skull fractures, tissue swelling, hematomas, tumors, and abscesses. The use of radiographic contrast material allows better visualization of vascular areas and enhances lesions previously seen on noncontrast films. Sometimes two technologies are used in combination, such as myelography with CT scanning, to provide a more refined image of anatomical structures of the spinal cord and vertebral column. With current technology, a routine scan now takes less than 5 minutes to survey the patient, analyze the data, and display a finished image.

MAGNETIC RESONANCE IMAGING

Magnetic resonance imaging (MRI), known in the past as nuclear magnetic resonance imaging, has become widely available in medium and large medical centers. This modality uses nonionizing forms of radiation to produce computerized cross-sectional images in much the same fashion as a CT scan. It provides much more finely detailed images, however, that look remarkably like anatomical slices of the body. The MRI is superior to in the early diagnosis of cerebral infarction and the detection of demyelinating disorders, such as multiple

TABLE 32-4 *CLINICAL APPLICATION: Diagnostic Studies*
Neurodiagnostic Tests

Diagnostic Test	Description	Information Obtained	Nursing Considerations and Interventions
Computed tomography, or CT scan (invasive and noninvasive)	A scanner takes a series of radiographic images all around the same axial plane. A computer then creates a composite picture of various tissue densities visualized. The images may be enhanced with the use of IV contrast dye.	CT scans give detailed outlines of bone, tissue, and fluid structures of the body. They can indicate shift of structures due to tumors, hematomas, or hydrocephalus. A CT scan is limited in that it gives information only about structure of tissues, not about functional status.	Instruct the patient to lie flat on a table with the machine surrounding, but not touching, the area to be scanned. Patient also must remain as immobile as possible; sedation may be required. The scan may not be of the best quality if the patient moves during the test or if the x-ray beams were deflected by any metal object (ie, traction tongs, ICP monitoring devices).
Magnetic resonance imaging (MRI)	A selected area of the patient's body is placed inside a powerful magnetic field. The hydrogen atoms inside the patient are temporarily "excited" and caused to oscillate by a sequence of radiofrequency pulsations. The sensitive scanner measures these minute oscillations, and a computer-enhanced image is created.	An MRI scan creates a graphic image of bone, fluid, and soft-tissue structures. It gives a more defined image of anatomical details and may help one diagnose small tumors or early infarction syndromes.	Risk factors for this new technique are not well identified. This test is contraindicated in patients with previous surgeries where hemostatic or aneurysm clips were implanted. The powerful magnetic field can cause such clips to move out of position, placing the patient at risk for bleeding or hemorrhage. Inform patient the procedure is very noisy. Use caution if patient is claustrophobic. Other contraindications include patients with cardiac pacemakers, valve prosthesis, bullet fragments, orthopedic pins. The patient (and caregivers) must remove all metal objects with magnetic characteristics (eg, scissors, stethoscope).
Positron emission tomography (PET); single-photon emission computer tomography (SPECT)	The patient either inhales or receives by injection radioactively tagged substances, such as oxygen or glucose. A gamma scanner measures the radioactive uptake of these substances, and a computer produces a composite image, indicating where the radioactive material is located, corresponding to areas of cellular metabolism.	These diagnostic tests are the only ones to measure physiological and biochemical processes in the nervous system. Specific areas can be identified as to functioning and nonfunctioning. Cerebral metabolism and cerebral blood flow can be measured regionally. PET and SPECT scans help diagnose abnormalities (tumors, vascular disease) and behavioral disturbances, such as dementia and schizophrenia, that may have a physiological basis.	The patient receives only minimal radiation exposure because the half-life of the radionuclides used is from a few minutes to 2 h. Testing may take a few hours. The patient must remain very still and immobile. Procedure is very expensive.

(continued)

TABLE 32-4   CLINICAL APPLICATION: Diagnostic Studies
Neurodiagnostic Tests (Continued)

Diagnostic Test	Description	Information Obtained	Nursing Considerations and Interventions
Cerebral angiography (invasive)	This is a radiographic contrast study in which radiopaque dye is injected by a catheter into the patient's cerebral arterial circulation. The contrast medium is directed into each common carotid artery and each vertebral artery, and serial radiographs are then taken.	The contrast dye illuminates the structure of the cerebral circulation. The vessel pathways are examined for patency, narrowing, and occlusion, as well as structural abnormalities (aneurysms), vessel displacement (tumors, edema), and alterations in blood flow (tumors, AV malformations).	In preparation for this test, inform the patient as to the location of the catheter insertion (femoral artery is a common site) and that a local anesthetic will be used. Also warn that a warm, flushed feeling will occur when the dye is injected. After this procedure, assess the puncture site for swelling, redness, and bleeding. Also check the skin color, temperature, and peripheral pulses of the extremity distal to the site for signs of arterial insufficiency due to vasospasm or clotting. A large amount of contrast medium may be needed during this test, with resulting increased osmotic diuresis and risk of dehydration and renal tubular occlusion. Other complications include temporary or permanent neurological deficit, anaphylaxis, bleeding or hematoma at insertion site, and impaired circulation to the extremity used for injection.
Digital subtraction angiography (invasive)	In this test, a plain radiograph is taken of the patient's cranium. Then, radiopaque dye is injected into a large vein, and serial radiographs are taken. A computer converts the images into digital form and "subtracts" the plain radiograph from the ones with the dye. The result is an enhanced radiographic image of contrast medium in the arterial vessels.	Extracranial circulation (arterial, capillary, and venous) can be examined. Vessel size, patency, narrowing, and degree of stenosis or displacement can be determined.	There is less risk to the patient for bleeding or vascular insufficiency because the injection of dye is intravenous rather than intraarterial. The patient must remain absolutely motionless during the examination (even swallowing will interfere with the results).
Radioisotope brain scan (noninvasive)	In this test, radioactive isotope is usually injected intravenously. The scanning device produces films of areas of concentration of the isotope within the patient's head.	Because damaged brain tissue absorbs more isotope, the presence of an intracranial lesion can be diagnosed, as well as cerebral infarction or contusion. Lack of uptake of the isotope may indicate cerebral brain death.	Minimal patient preparation is required. The isotope may not be readily available within the institution. Movement will make the test difficult to interpret. Test is less commonly used than CT scan or MRI.

(continued)

TABLE 32-4   CLINICAL APPLICATION: Diagnostic Studies
Neurodiagnostic Tests (Continued)

Diagnostic Test	Description	Information Obtained	Nursing Considerations and Interventions
Myelography (invasive)	A myelogram is a radiographic study in which a contrast substance (either air or dye) is injected into the lumbar subarachnoid space. Fluoroscopy, conventional radiographs, or CT scans are used to visualize selected areas.	The spinal subarachnoid space is examined for partial or complete obstructions due to bone displacements, spinal cord compression, or herniated intervertebral disks.	Instruct the patient as for a lumbar puncture. In addition, advise that a special table will tilt up or down during the procedure. Postprocedure care is determined by the type of contrast material used. Oil-based contrast dye: • flat in bed for 24 h • force fluids • observe for headache, fever, back spasms, nausea and vomiting Water-based contrast dye: • head of bed elevated for 8 h • keep patient quiet for first few hours • do not administer phenothiazines • observe for headache, fever, back spasms, nausea and vomiting, seizures
Electroencephalogram, or EEG (noninvasive)	An EEG is a recording of electrical impulses generated by the brain cortex that are sensed by electrodes on the surface of the scalp.	Analysis of the resulting tracings helps detect and localize abnormal electrical activity occurring in the cerebral cortex. It aids in seizure focus detection, localization of a source of irritation such as a tumor or abscess, and diagnosis of metabolic disturbances and sleep disorders.	Reassure the patient that he or she will not feel an electrical shock or pain during this test. The nurse also may need to clarify for the patient that the machine cannot "read minds" or indicate the presence of mental illness. The patient's scalp and hair should be free of oil, dirt, creams, and sprays because they can cause electrical interference and thus an inaccurate recording. Inform the EEG technician of electrical devices around the patient that may cause interference during the procedure (eg, cardiac monitor, ventilator).
Cortical evoked potentials (noninvasive) Somatosensory-evoked potentials (SSEP) Brain stem auditory-evoked response (BAER) Visual-evoked potentials (VEP)	In this test, a specialized device senses central or cortical cerebral electrical activity by skin electrodes in response to peripheral stimulation of specific sensory receptors. The sensory receptors stimulated can be those for vision, hearing, or tactile sensation. The signals are graphically	Cortical evoked potentials provide a detailed assessment of neuron transmission along particular pathways. It has value in determining the integrity of visual auditory and tactile pathways in patients with multiple sclerosis and spinal cord injury. This test also may be used in the as-	This test may be used in conscious as well as unconscious patients and can be performed at the bedside. The patient must be as motionless as possible during some phases of this test to minimize musculoskeletal interference. Depending on the sensory pathway being tested, the

(continued)

TABLE 32-4 CLINICAL APPLICATION: Diagnostic Studies
Neurodiagnostic Tests (Continued)

Diagnostic Test	Description	Information Obtained	Nursing Considerations and Interventions
	displayed by a computer, and characteristic peaks, and the intervals between them, are measured.	sessment of a sensory pathway before, during, and after surgery.	patient may be instructed to watch a series of geometric designs or listen to a series of clicking noises.
Transcranial Doppler sonography (TCD)	This is a test in which high-frequency ultrasonic waves are directed from a probe toward specific cerebral vessels. The ultrasonic energy is aimed through cranial "windows," areas in the skull where the bony table is thin (temporal zygoma) or where there are small gaps in the bone (orbit or foramen magnum). The reflected sound waves are analyzed for shifts in frequency, indicating flow velocity.	The speed or velocity at which blood travels through cerebral vessels is an indicator of the size of the vascular channel and the resistance to blood flow. An approximation of cerebral blood flow may be determined. Cerebral autoregulation can be monitored by observing the response of intracranial vessels to changes in arterial carbon dioxide and to the partial occlusion of the proximal vessels, as may occur in vasospasm.	The test is noninvasive and may be performed at the bedside by the physician or ultrasound technician in 30–60 min. There are no known adverse effects, and the procedure may be repeated as often as necessary. The testing is accomplished with the patient initially supine, and later on his or her side, with the head flexed forward.
Lumbar puncture (invasive)	A hollow needle is positioned in the subarachnoid space at L3–4 or L4–5 level, and CSF is sampled. The pressure of the CSF also is measured. Normal pressure varies with age from 45 mm H_2O in full-term newborns to 120 mm H_2O in adults.	The CSF is examined for blood and for alterations in appearance, cell count, protein, and glucose. The opening pressure is roughly equivalent to the ICP for most patients, if done recumbent and no block is present.	This test is contraindicated in patients with suspected increased ICP because a sudden reduction in pressure from below may cause brain structures to herniate, leading to death. In preparation for this test, position the patient on side with knees and head flexed. Explain to the patient that some pressure may be felt as the needle is inserted and not to move suddenly or cough. After this procedure, keep the patient flat for 8 to 10 hours to prevent headache. Encourage liberal fluid intake.

sclerosis. Traditional CT scanning is superior for scanning for bony abnormalities, which visualize poorly on MRI.

Although superior in many ways to CT scanning, MRI has its limitations. The powerful magnetic fields interfere with the functioning of devices such as cardiac pacemakers. Patients with surgical clips and prosthetic implants made of ferrous metal cannot be scanned. It also is difficult to study patients on life-support equipment because most ventilators and monitors are constructed in part of ferrous metal. If emergency therapy is needed, the patient must be removed from the scanning chamber and the imaging suite before resuscitation can begin.

POSITRON EMISSION TOMOGRAPHY AND SINGLE-PHOTON EMISSION COMPUTED TOMOGRAPHY

Positron emission tomography is a process by which molecules labeled with radioactive isotopes are located within the brain and recorded by radiation-sensitive detectors outside the head. It has the capacity to measure cerebral blood flow and cerebral metabolism as the isotope-labeled glucose or oxygen is used within the body. It is superior to previous technologies that could image structure only and not function. However, the complexity of the testing, the comparatively high cost per scan, and the need to have a cyclotron nearby to produce the short-lived radioactive isotopes make this modality impractical and unwieldy in the clinical setting.

Single-photon emission computed tomography (SPECT) combines the imaging ability of conventional nuclear medicine scanners with the technology of transaxial CT scanning to overcome some limitations. Using more stable radioisotopes, SPECT scanning has been able to detect diminished perfusion in an area of stroke before conventional CT evidence of infarction and alterations in regional blood flow in patients with Alzheimer's disease.

ANGIOGRAPHY AND DIGITAL SUBTRACTION ANGIOGRAPHY

Cerebral angiography remains the study of choice for evaluating cerebrovascular problems. It is the only test that can reveal large and small aneurysms and arteriovenous malformations and their relationship to adjacent structures and vessels. It involves the passage of a radiographic catheter through a large artery (usually femoral) to each of the arterial vessels bringing blood to the brain and spinal cord. Radiopaque contrast dye is then injected into each vessel. A rapid sequence of films is taken after the dye has passed through small arterial branches and capillaries and into the venous circulation.

Digital subtraction angiography makes use of radiographic contrast to illuminate the cerebral circulation but in considerably smaller quantities than required for conventional angiography. The dye may be injected into the arterial or the venous systems. Films are taken before and after the dye injection and converted into digital information in the accompanying computer. The images are "subtracted" from each other, removing all images in common. The resultant image displays only the enhanced circulatory system, free of other anatomical distortion.

CEREBRAL BLOOD FLOW STUDIES

Cerebral blood flow in the diagnostic setting is evaluated most commonly by a radioisotope brain scan. A radioactive isotope, such as technetium 99m, is injected intravenously. In unusual circumstances, the isotope can also be administered orally or intra-arterially. The brain is then scanned to determine which areas show an accumulation of the radioactive substance. If there is blood flow to the brain, damaged areas absorb more of the isotope. The test may be used to determine brain death, which is evidenced if there is no flow to the cerebral hemispheres. In certain disorders, such as carbon monoxide poisoning, there may be increased blood flow to the brain, yet anoxic brain death may still occur.

MYELOGRAPHY

Myelography is a contrast study of the spinal cord and surrounding structures. It involves the introduction of water-soluble material (metrizamide) into the CSF by way of a lumbar or cisternal puncture, performed under fluoroscopy. Because metrizamide is lighter than CSF, it allows for better visualization of nerve roots and surrounding structures. However, because of its rapid dispersal into the subarachnoid space, the patient's position cannot be adjusted. At times, a heavier, oil-based preparation is used (iophendylate [Pantopaque]) that must be removed at the end of the procedure. Because metrizamide does not require removal, the patient should be kept well hydrated to facilitate dye excretion. It also is potentially toxic to cerebral tissue, as evidenced by grand mal seizures, so the patient must be maintained with the head up at least 30 to 45 degrees, and phenothiazine medications, which increase the toxic symptoms, must be avoided.

ELECTROPHYSIOLOGICAL STUDIES

Electroencephalogram

Using electroencephalographs (EEGs), a record is made of the brain's electrical activity. Small plate electrodes are placed in specific locations over the patient's scalp, and 16 to 21 channels transcribe the electrical potentials generated by the brain. Waveforms are classified in terms of voltage and amplitude. It is most valuable in the diagnosis and treatment of patients with seizures. In addition, it may help in the localization of structural abnormalities, such as tumors and abscesses, and aid in the differentiation of structural from metabolic abnormalities. It also may provide confirmatory criteria in the diagnosis of brain death. In recent years, a modified form of EEG is being used at the bedside in critical care to monitor the effects of pharmacological agents that reduce cerebral blood flow and hence reduce electrical activity.

A computerized technique that dramatically compresses standard EEG data and converts them into a more easily interpreted and colorized form is called *compressed spectral array*. This technique also is seen at the bedside in neurological intensive care units to monitor patients with severe head injuries.

Evoked Potentials

An evoked potential is an electrical manifestation of the brain's response to an external stimulus: auditory, visual, somatic, or a combination of these. The measurement of the response evoked by a certain sensory stimulus provides an assessment of the function of neuropathways from the periphery through the spinal cord and brain stem and finally to cortical structures (Fig. 32–13). This technique has been most helpful in the diagnosis of multiple sclerosis and Guillain–Barré syndrome and in the prognosis of the reversibility of coma in the brain stem–injured patient.[4] It also may be used during surgery to monitor potential injury during manipulations of spinal nerves and structures. The three most frequently used techniques in head trauma evaluation are somatosensory-evoked potentials (SSEP), brain stem auditory-evoked response, and visual-evoked potentials. Somatosensory-evoked potentials assess neurological function in specific neural pathways postinjury and detect further central nervous system insults from secondary processes, such as hypoxia and hypertension.

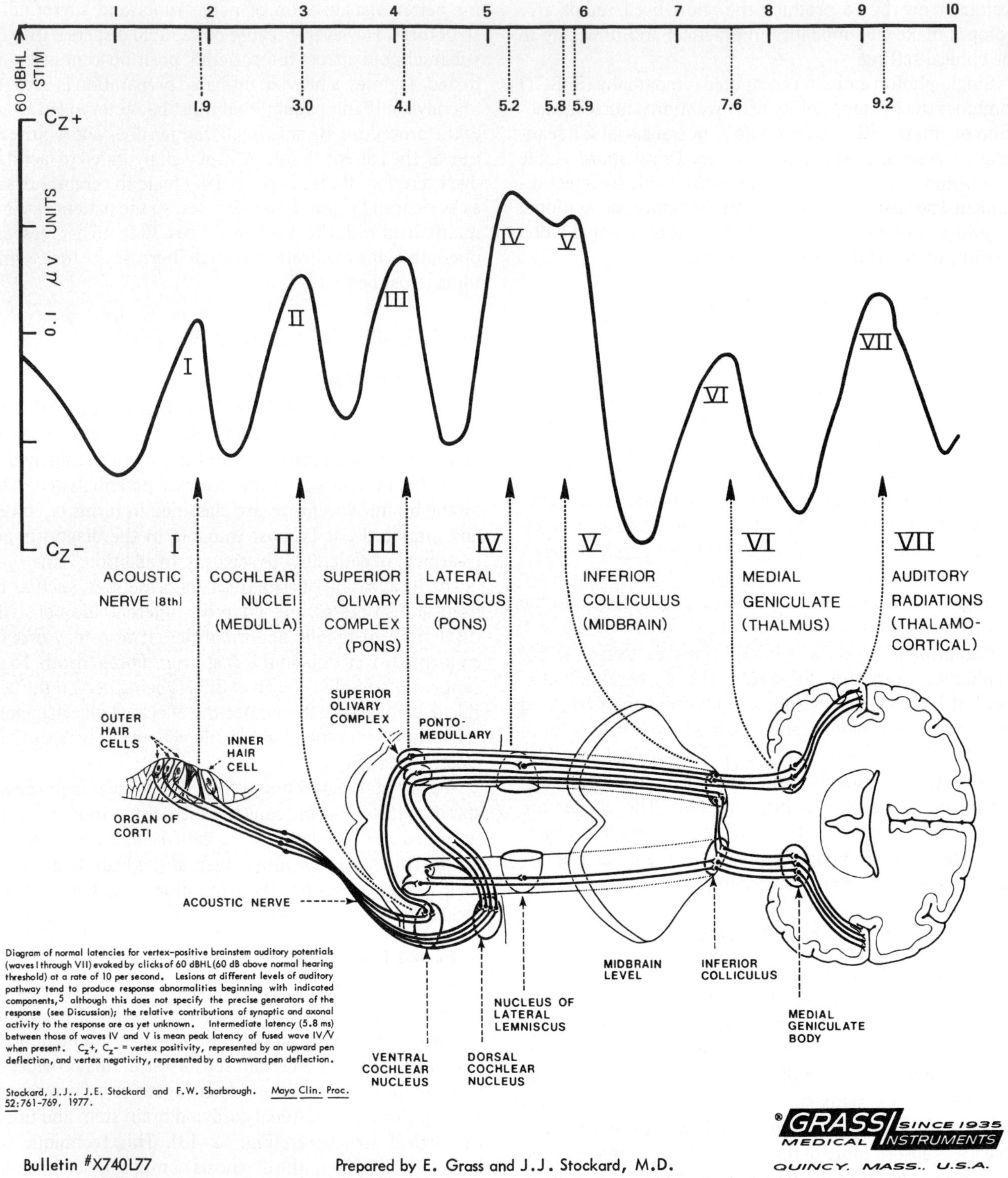

1 2 3 4 5 6 7 8 9 10
60 dBHL STIM
1.9 3.0 4.1 5.2 5.8 5.9 7.6 9.2
Cz+
0.1 μV UNITS
Cz−
I II III IV V VI VII
I ACOUSTIC NERVE (8th)
II COCHLEAR NUCLEI (MEDULLA)
III SUPERIOR OLIVARY COMPLEX (PONS)
IV LATERAL LEMNISCUS (PONS)
V INFERIOR COLLICULUS (MIDBRAIN)
VI MEDIAL GENICULATE (THALMUS)
VII AUDITORY RADIATIONS (THALAMO-CORTICAL)
OUTER HAIR CELLS
INNER HAIR CELL
ORGAN OF CORTI
SUPERIOR OLIVARY COMPLEX
PONTO-MEDULLARY
ACOUSTIC NERVE
MIDBRAIN LEVEL
INFERIOR COLLICULUS
MEDIAL GENICULATE BODY
NUCLEUS OF LATERAL LEMNISCUS
VENTRAL COCHLEAR NUCLEUS
DORSAL COCHLEAR NUCLEUS
Diagram of normal latencies for vertex-positive brainstem auditory potentials (waves I through VII) evoked by clicks of 60 dBHL (60 dB above normal hearing threshold) at a rate of 10 per second. Lesions at different levels of auditory pathway tend to produce response abnormalities beginning with indicated components,5 although this does not specify the precise generators of the response (see Discussion); the relative contributions of synaptic and axonal activity to the response are as yet unknown. Intermediate latency (5.8 ms) between those of waves IV and V is mean peak latency of fused wave IV/V when present. Cz+, Cz− = vertex positivity, represented by an upward pen deflection, and vertex negativity, represented by a downward pen deflection.
Stockard, J.J., J.E. Stockard and F.W. Sharbrough. Mayo Clin. Proc. 52:761-769, 1977.
GRASS SINCE 1935 MEDICAL INSTRUMENTS
QUINCY. MASS., U.S.A.
Bulletin #X740L77
Prepared by E. Grass and J.J. Stockard, M.D.

FIGURE 32-13
The waveform of a normal brain-stem auditory-evoked response. (Courtesy of Grass Instrument Company, Quincy, MA)

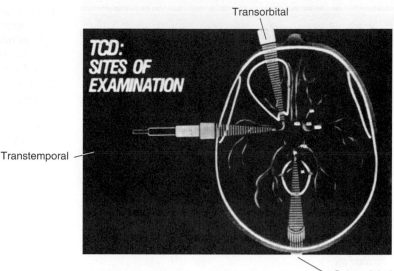

FIGURE 32-14

Transcranial Doppler: sites of examination via transcranial windows. (Adapted from March K: Transcranial Doppler sonography: Non-invasive monitoring of intracranial vasculature. Journal of Neuroscience Nursing 22:113, 1990)

TRANSCRANIAL DOPPLER SONOGRAPHY

Transcranial Doppler ultrasound studies provide a noninvasive means for monitoring intracranial hemodynamics at the bedside. The examination is performed through cranial "windows," areas in the skull where the bone is relatively thin, such as the temporal area, or where there are small spaces between bones, such as the orbit (Fig. 32–14). The ultrasonic probe transmits sound waves at certain frequencies to a specified depth. The resultant reflected signal from blood traveling through cerebral vessels is interpreted for speed or velocity. As resistance or vascular size changes, it is reflected as a change in blood flow velocities. The data may be used to monitor therapy, aid in determining prognosis, and provide early recognition of cerebral vasospasm in patients after subarachnoid hemorrhage or severe head injury.

LUMBAR PUNCTURE FOR CEREBROSPINAL FLUID EXAMINATION

A lumbar puncture for CSF analysis may be performed to aid in the diagnosis of autoimmune disorders or infections. Occasionally, it is performed to verify subarachnoid hemorrhage, although the CT scan is the procedure of choice and is safer for such a patient. CSF is obtained by the insertion of a long, 18- to 22-gauge needle between the vertebrae at the L3-4 or L4-5 levels. The fluid is sent for content analysis and for culture, sensitivity, and other serological tests (Table 32–5).

TABLE 32-5 CLINICAL APPLICATION: Diagnostic Studies
Normal and Abnormal Values for Cerebrospinal Fluid

Characteristic	Normal	Abnormal
Color	Clear, colorless	Cloudy often due to presence of WBC or bacteria Xanthochromic due to presence of RBC
WBC	0–5/mm³, all mononuclear	Elevated count accompanies many conditions (tumor, meningitis, subarachnoid hemorrhage, infarct, abscess)
RBC	None	Presence may be due to traumatic tap or subarachnoid hemorrhage
Chloride	120–130 mEq/L	Low concentration associated with meningeal infection and tuberculous meningitis Elevated level not neurologically significant
Glucose	50–75 mg/100 mL	Decreased level associated with presence of bacteria in CSF Elevated level not neurologically significant
Pressure	70–180 mm H₂O	Low pressure associated with inaccurate placement of needle, dehydration, or block along subarachnoid space or at foramen magnum Elevated pressure associated with benign intracranial hypertension; cerebral edema; CNS tumor, abscess, or cyst; hydrocephalus; muscle tension or abdominal compression; subdural hematoma
Protein	14–45 mg/100 mL	Decreased level not neurologically significant Increased level associated with demyelinating or degenerative disease, Guillain-Barré syndrome, hemorrhage, infection, spinal block, tumor

(From Cammermeyer M, Appeldorn C [eds]: Core Curriculum for Neuroscience Nursing. 4th ed. Chicago, American Association of Neuroscience Nurses, 1996)

Clinical Applicability Challenges

Self-Challenge: Critical Thinking

1. You have just been assigned to the care of a newly admitted patient with a leaking cerebral aneurysm. Develop a plan for your initial assessment of this patient.

2. Compare and contrast the advantages and disadvantages of a CT scan versus an MRI scan on a critically ill, ventilated patient.

Study Questions

1. A patient whose movements are purposeful when stimulated but who does not follow commands would be described as
   a. semicomatose.
   b. stuporous.
   c. comatose.
   d. lethargic.

2. All of the following may cause dilated pupils except
   a. fear.
   b. seizure.
   c. morphine.
   d. cocaine.

3. Approaching the eye from the side and touching the cornea to elicit a blink reflex tests which of the cranial nerves?
   a. Optic
   b. Facial
   c. Oculomotor
   d. Trigeminal

4. The most common cause for bitemporal hemianopsia is
   a. pyramidal tract damage.
   b. pituitary tumor pressing on the optic chiasm.
   c. lesion in the medulla.
   d. bilateral dysfunction in the diencephalon.

5. Tremor and deviation of the tongue indicate damage to cranial nerve
   a. X.
   b. XI.
   c. XII.
   d. IX.

REFERENCES

1. Daley BJ: Withholding nutrition and hydration revisited. Nursing Management 26(5):30–38, 1995
2. Hall JK: Caring for corpses or killing patients? Nursing Management 25(10):81–89, 1994
3. American Medical Association: Model Bill. Chicago, American Medical Association, 1979
4. Sloan TB: Electrophysiologic monitoring in head injury. New Horizons 3(3):431–438, 1995

BIBLIOGRAPHY

Bates B: A Guide to Physical Examination and History Taking (6th Ed). Philadelphia, JB Lippincott, 1996
Cammermeyer M, Appledorn C (eds): Core Curriculum for Neuroscience Nursing (4th Ed). Chicago, American Association of Neuroscience Nurses, 1996
Cardona VD, Hurn PD, et al (eds): Trauma Nursing From Resuscitation to Rehabilitation (2nd Ed). Philadelphia, WB Saunders, 1994
Day L: Practical limits to the uniform determination of death act. J Neurosci Nurs 27(5):319–322, 1995
Way C, Segatore M: Development and preliminary testing of the Neurological Assessment Instrument. J Neurosci Nurs 26(5):278–287, 1994

33

Patient Management: Nervous System

OBJECTIVES

Based on the content in this chapter, the reader should be able to:

- Discuss indications for intracranial pressure (ICP) monitoring.
- Identify five techniques for obtaining ICP measurements.
- Describe cerebral perfusion pressure.
- Explain three interventions used to promote adequate cerebral blood flow in the presence of increased ICP.
- List three possible nursing diagnoses for the patient with intracranial hypertension, and describe the nursing interventions for each diagnosis.
- Explain the rationale for using induced hypothermia in a clinical situation.
- List and explain two methods for inducing hypothermia in the clinical setting.
- Identify three causes of unintentional (accidental) hypothermia.
- Describe three nursing diagnoses and their appropriate nursing interventions for the hypothermic patient.

Intracranial Pressure Monitoring

Intracranial pressure (ICP) is the pressure exerted by the combined volume of three intracranial components: brain tissue, cerebrospinal fluid (CSF), and blood. *Intracranial hypertension* (also called *increased ICP*) is a serious complication of severe head injury, coma-producing subarachnoid hemorrhage, hydrocephalus, space-occupying mass lesions, intracranial infections, and hypoxic or ischemic insults to the brain; it may cause cerebral herniation with respiratory and cardiac arrest.

The management of patients with intracranial hypertension has changed greatly in the last 5 years. In today's environment of managed care and cost control, it is important for the clinician to be aware of indications for ICP monitoring, the various monitoring devices and methods available, and assessment, management, and interpretation skills. This chapter includes a review of physiological principles and the various types of ICP monitoring equipment and methods available, indications for ICP monitoring, waveform interpretation, and management of intracranial hypertension.

◼ PHYSIOLOGICAL PRINCIPLES

Intracranial Dynamics

The management of intracranial hypertension is based on the Monro-Kellie Doctrine of a fixed intracranial volume, which states that the volume of the intracranium is equal to the volume of the cerebral blood (3%–10%) plus the volume of the CSF (8%–12%). Any alterations in the volume of any of these components of the cranial vault or a lesion may lead to an increase in ICP. A normal ICP measurement varies between 0 and 15 mmHg. An ICP measurement greater than 15 mmHg is considered intracranial hypertension.

The normal brain has the ability to autoregulate cerebral blood flow (CBF). Normal CBF is provided by a cerebral perfusion pressure in the range of 60 to 100 mmHg. Normally, autoregulation ensures a constant blood flow through the cerebral vessels over this range of perfusion pressures by changing the diameter of vessels in response to changes in cerebral perfusion pressure (CPP). The measurement of CPP provides an estimate of the adequacy of the cerebral circulation in delivering oxygen to brain tissue.

Factors that alter the ability of the cerebral vessels to constrict or dilate, such as ischemia, hypoxia, hypercapnia, and brain trauma, interfere with autoregulation. Carbon dioxide is the most potent vasodilator of cerebral vessels, causing increased CBF that can result in an increased volume within the cranium, leading to intracranial hyperten-

sion. For autoregulation to be functional, carbon dioxide levels must be in an acceptable range and pressures must be within the following ranges: CPP over 60 mmHg, mean arterial pressure (MAP) under 160 mmHg and systolic pressure between 60 to 140 mmHg, and ICP under 30 mmHg. Brain injury also may impair autoregulation. When autoregulation is impaired, the CBF fluctuates in correlation with the systemic blood pressure (BP). In patients with impaired autoregulation, any activity that causes an increase in BP, such as coughing, suctioning, and anxiety, can cause an increase in CBF that could increase ICP.

The brain can accommodate or compensate for minimal changes in volume by partial collapse of the cisterns, ventricles, and vascular systems and by decreasing production and increasing reabsorption of CSF. The following are ICP compensatory mechanisms:

- Shunting of CSF into the spinal subarachnoid space
- Increased CSF absorption
- Decreased CSF production
- Shunting of venous blood out of the skull

During this compensatory period, the ICP remains fairly constant. When these compensatory mechanisms have been used fully, pressure increases rapidly until herniation occurs, and the blood supply to the medulla is cut off (Fig. 33–1). (Herniation is the displacement of brain tissue to another area of the brain or outside the cranial vault.) The ability of the intracranial contents to compensate depends on the location of the lesion, the rate of expansion, and the compliance or volume-buffering capacity of the system.

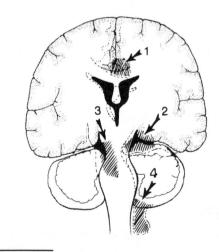

FIGURE 33-1

Major types of brain herniation: (**1**) herniation of cingulate gyrus under the falx; (**2**) herniation of the uncus of the temporal lobe beneath the free edge of the tentorium; (**3**) herniation of the central or transtentorial portion of the brain; (**4**) downward displacement of the midbrain through the tentorial arch.

The classic syndrome of intracranial hypertension, which includes increased pulse pressure, decreased pulse, and decreased respirations with pupillary changes, usually occurs only in association with posterior fossa lesions and seldom with the more commonly observed supratentorial mass lesions, such as subdural hematoma. When these classic Kocher-Cushing signs do accompany a supratentorial lesion, they are associated with a sudden pressure increase and usually herald a state of decompensation. Brain damage usually is irreversible at this point, and death is imminent.

In the stage between the onset of intracranial hypertension and herniation, many treatments are available to reduce ICP. Therapies used to normalize ICP and maintain adequate cerebral perfusion include hyperventilation to reduce intracerebral blood volume; CSF drainage to reduce intracerebral CSF volume; various pharmacological agents to induce diuresis, sedation, or paralysis; and surgery.

Volume–Pressure Curve

The intracranial volume–pressure curve, also called a pressure–volume index, demonstrates the relationship between changes in volume and changes in ICP. The rate at which the ICP rises in response to a change in intracranial volume depends on the compliance of the brain. The term *compliance* may be defined as a change in volume resulting from a change in pressure. The term *elastance* refers to a change in pressure resulting from a change in volume. The term compliance, however, is frequently used in place of the term elastance, as in the following explanation of the volume–pressure curve. When the intracranial compartment has low compliance (stiffness), a small volume change will cause a large increase in ICP. In Figure 33–2A, the initial portion of the curve illustrates compliance, as the compensatory mechanisms maintain ICP in the normal range during increases in intracranial volume. Little change occurs in the ICP during the initial increase in volume, because the increase in volume added to the cranium is compensated for by volume displacement. As the compensatory mechanisms become exhausted, the volume added becomes greater than the volume displaced, and there is a larger increase in ICP with a smaller volume increase. This is illustrated by the steeper portion of the curve in Figure 33–2B. This disproportionate rise in pressure represents elastance. The cranial contents become stiffer, and free communication of CSF between the lateral ventricles and infratentorium is lost.

Knowledge of the patient's position on the volume–pressure curve is useful in managing interventions, such as minimizing stimuli and volume increases that could lead to impaired cerebral perfusion. Usually a physician determines the volume–pressure curve by injecting fluid, usually 1 mL, into the ventricles to create a pressure response change. Because the procedure puts the patient at risk for an increase in ICP and for infection, measures should be taken to reduce complications. Drastic increases in ICP may result from hypercarbia, hypoxia, rapid eye movement sleep, pyrexia, or the administration of certain anesthetics. A

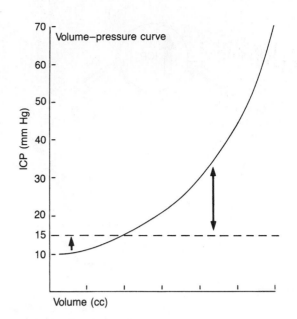

FIGURE 33-2

Volume–pressure curve. Volume–pressure response (VPR), also referred to as the pressure–volume index (PVI), provides a method of estimating the compensatory capacity of the intracranial cavity. Note that the intracranial pressure (ICP) remains within the normal limit of 0–15 mmHg as long as compliance is normal and fluid can be displaced by the additional volume (**A**). Once the compensatory system is exhausted, a small additional volume causes a greater increase in pressure (**B**). Acute changes can cause serious and sometimes fatal neurological deterioration.

major reason for controlling and decreasing ICP is the maintenance of cerebral oxygenation by adequate CBF, which is estimated clinically by the measurement of CPP.

Cerebral Perfusion Pressure

Normal CBF is provided by a CPP in the range of 60 to 100 mmHg. When the CPP is greater than 100 mmHg, there is a potential for hyperperfusion and increased ICP. When the CPP is less than 60 mmHg, blood supply to the brain is inadequate, and neuronal hypoxia and cell death may occur. Hypotensive patients, such as postcardiac resuscitation or trauma patients, with normal ICPs (0–15 mmHg) may have impaired CPP. Because an acutely injured brain requires higher CPPs than a normal brain, a minimum CPP of 70 mmHg or higher is required for maintenance of adequate cerebral perfusion and potentially improved patient outcome in head-injured patients.[1] When perfusion pressure decreases, the cardiovascular response is a rise in systemic pressure. The autoregulation system for maintenance of constant blood flow does not function at pressures less than 40 mmHg. A severe reduction in CPP is accompanied by an absence of brain stem auditory evoked potentials, indicating changes in brain stem function. Increased ICP leads to ischemia, brain shifts, and possible herniation (Fig. 33–3).

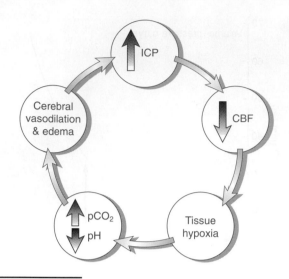

FIGURE 33-3

Cycle for malignant progressive brain swelling. As the intracranial pressure (ICP) increases, cerebral blood flow (CBF) decreases, leading to tissue hypoxia, a decrease in pH, an increase in PCO_2, cerebral vasodilation, and edema, thus leading to further pressure increases. This malignant cycle continues until herniation occurs.

When brain damage is severe, as with widespread brain edema or when blood flow has been arrested in the brain, CBF may be reduced at relatively normal levels of CPP. This is due to impedance to the flow of blood across the cerebrovascular bed. CBF may not increase despite increases in CPP if autoregulation is impaired. This condition is referred to as *pressure–flow dissociation* or *vasomotor paralysis*.

CPP is determined by substracting the mean ICP from the mean systemic arterial pressure (MAP):

$$CPP = MAP - ICP$$

When the CPP is zero, there is no CBF. In other words, when ICP equals MAP, CPP equals zero, and CBF is zero. CBF may cease totally at pressures somewhat above zero. A variety of bedside hemodynamic monitors calculate and continuously display ICP and CPP.

EQUIPMENT FEATURES

The proven value of ICP monitoring and the need for an accurate, reliable, low-risk, and cost-effective method of measurement have resulted in the development of numerous methods of monitoring ICP and a variety of devices to facilitate each method or technique. ICP monitoring equipment may be categorized as internal or external measurement systems. The initial ICP monitoring systems consisted of an external pressure transducer (the same type used for systemic arterial BP measurement) attached by a fluid-filled system of tubing and stopcocks to an intraventricular catheter, subarachnoid bolt, and subdural or epidural catheter device; it had ICP waveforms and pressure displayed on a standard bedside monitor. These fluid-coupled external systems continue to be used widely. A variety of disposable ICP kits are available for placement of various ICP monitoring devices.

Internal measurement systems now are available that measure ICP directly from the site. Fiberoptic transducer-tipped catheters are inserted directly into the brain tissue, ventricles, or subdural-subarachnoid spaces, with the ICP waveforms and pressure displayed on a dedicated amplifier system. They eliminate the need for a fluid-filled system between the patient and the transducer. There is considerable variation in the average cost of the intracranial, extracranial, and disposable components for ICP monitoring systems (Table 33–1). Although the actual purchase cost of fluid-coupled ICP systems tends to be less than other systems, the benefits of fiberoptic and catheter tip pressure transducers include ICP measurements that are independent of the patient's head position, the ability to measure ICP during transport, and the reduction of damping errors related to fluid coupling. Both external and internal measurement systems are discussed in more detail in the discussion of ICP procedures that follows.

American National Standard for ICP Monitoring Devices*

ICP monitoring device should have:

- Pressure range from 0–100 mmHg
- Accuracy $\pm$ 2 mmHg in range of 0–20 mmHg
- Maximum error 10% in range of 20–100 mmHg

*Established by the Association for the Advancement of Medical Instrumentation in association with a Neurosurgical Committee [2]

INDICATIONS FOR INTRACRANIAL PRESSURE MONITORING

Monitoring ICP provides information that facilitates interventions to prevent cerebral ischemia and brain stem distortion. There are no reliable clinical signs of increasing ICP in a comatose patient prior to cerebral herniation. For ICP monitoring to be safe, effective, and within cost-containment guidelines, the indications, methods, and ethical considerations for patient care and nursing practice must be taken into account for each patient. In addition to diagnosis, factors that affect patient selection include the patient's prognosis and likelihood of developing impaired perfusion; the alteration of therapy if the ICP value is known; knowledge of insertion, maintenance, and data interpretation; availability of medical and nursing personnel; and availability of monitoring equipment and other assessment techniques, such as computed tomography (CT) scans. In addition to its usefulness in improving patient outcome by providing information on the likelihood of cerebral herniation and facilitating calculation of CPP, ICP

> ### NURSING PERSPECTIVE TABLE 33-1
> #### Summary of Intracranial Pressure Monitoring Technologies

Technique	Rank*	Cost of Disposable Components† (1994)
Intraventricular (72%)	1	$235–$672
Parenchymal (47%)	2	$270–$285
Subarachnoid (25%)	3	$132–$325
Epidural (15%)	4 or 5	N/A
Subdural (5%)	4 or 5	$41–$1,705**

*Ranking based on frequency of use.[2] (%) Percentage of use.[2]

†Includes combined cost of disposable pressure transducer and components, such as ventricular catheters, CSF drainage bags, bolts, and kits.

**Intracranial catheter tip transducer for 6 to 10 uses.[2]

Note: Some studies rank epidural as the least used technique, others list subdural.

monitoring is helpful in guiding the use of potentially harmful treatments, such as hyperventilation, mannitol, and barbiturates. In a study on the use of ICP monitoring, 81% of the 279 patients monitored had interventions based on ICP monitoring: mannitol (81%), emergency CT (22%), surgical decompression (3%), or barbiturate coma (2%).[3]

Diagnostic conditions that may be indications for ICP measurement include head injury (patients with an abnormal CT scan and selected patients with normal scans, because the CT scan looks only at anatomy and its disruption, not brain function), subarachnoid hemorrhage, brain tumors, cardiac arrest, strokes, and surgery. The decision to use ICP monitoring should be based on clinical and radiographic evaluation and the CT diagnosis. Because severe head injury usually involves intracranial hypertension, for

illustration, various aspects of ICP management are related to head injury in this discussion. Most of these management techniques are also used for patients with other diagnoses who are at risk for or develop intracranial hypertension.

CT scanning and ICP monitoring are major diagnostic tools in managing severely head-injured patients. The CT scan identifies intracranial pathology and is therefore of value in evaluating severity, prognosis, and the need for surgery. The ICP monitor is useful for diagnosis and prognosis and provides direct feedback for management of intracranial hypertension and manipulating cerebral perfusion.[1]

HEAD INJURY

Intracranial hypertension occurs almost universally in patients in whom intracranial mass lesions develop after head injury. Uncontrollable elevation of ICP is the cause of death in approximately half of fatally injured patients. Ischemic brain damage has been documented in more than 90% of patients with fatal head injuries. Increased morbidity is associated with patients exhibiting moderate elevations of ICP. Brain electrical dysfunction and disturbances of CBF frequently are associated with ICPs greater than 40 mmHg.

Monitoring of ICP may be indicated when head injury is associated with the following:

- Inability to obey commands or utter recognizable words despite cardiopulmonary stabilization
- Abnormal CT scan
- Abnormal multimodality-evoked potentials
- A Glasgow Coma Scale (GCS) score ≤ 8 or a GSC motor scale score ≤ 5 (ie, not following commands)

It is recommended that ICP monitoring be used on severely head-injured patients with normal CT scans and two or more of the following factors on admission: systolic BP ≤ 90 mmHg, age ≥ 40 years, or unilateral or bilateral motor posturing. Extreme vigilance should be maintained during transport to CT scanning and during the scan to avoid secondary brain insult, such as hypoxia or hypotension.

> ### CLINICAL APPLICATION:
> #### Assessment Parameters
> #### Indications for ICP Monitoring
>
> **Increased Volume of Brain**
> Cerebral edema
> Trauma
> Surgery
> Stroke
> Tumor
>
> **Increased Volume of Blood**
> Hematomas
> AV malformations
> Aneurysm
> Stroke
> Increase in PCO_2
>
> **Increased Volume of Cerebrospinal Fluid (CSF)**
> Decreased CSF reabsorption
> Congenital hydrocephalus
>
> **Lesions**
> Tumors
> Abscesses

Continued monitoring is also recommended for all patients with burr holes, who fail to regain consciousness within 48 hours after injury, and whose level of consciousness deteriorates, unless the patient has meningitis or a brain abscess.

Patients with intracranial mass lesions after head injury often have early, severe intracranial hypertension; patients with acute subdural hematomas seem to be most prone to elevations in ICP; and patients who maintain ICPs of 45 to 60 mmHg the first 48 hours after injury, despite all therapeutic intervention, have a mortality rate approaching 100%.

In patients with diffuse brain injury, any elevation above 10 mmHg on admission results in a progressively worsening prognosis. The initial level of ICP is to some degree an indication of the extent of diffuse brain damage. Recurrent or persistent intracranial hypertension is more frequently a problem with intracerebral lesions, contusion, hematoma, and brain swelling than with discrete extracerebral hematomas, whether epidural or subdural. Recurrent or persistent intracranial hypertension is associated with a poorer outcome.

SUBARACHNOID HEMORRHAGE

The level of ICP correlates well with the clinical grade of the hemorrhage. The ICP is of value in determining the best time for surgery, predicting and detecting rebleeding, and determining the etiology of neurological deterioration. When the subarachnoid hemorrhage is from ruptured intracranial aneurysms, cerebral vasospasm is an important cause of neurological deterioration. ICP monitoring facilitates the use of various drugs and other management techniques, such as hyperventilation and continuous ventricular fluid drainage or a permanent shunt to compensate for CSF absorption impairment.

BRAIN TUMORS

In patients with brain tumors, ICP tends to remain normal, with episodic increases seen particularly at night. Elevations in ICP tend to occur when the mass has enlarged to the point at which the patient is demonstrating neurological deterioration with papilledema, headache, and vomiting. Metastatic tumors can cause massive edema. Patients may be monitored before surgery to determine their response to the preoperative therapeutic regimen and to assist in determining the optimal time for surgery. After surgery, they may be monitored to assist with the diagnosis and treatment of diffuse generalized cerebral edema secondary to extensive manipulation of the brain during surgery.

CARDIAC ARREST

Of long-term cardiac arrest survivors, 10% to 20% suffer permanent severe brain damage ranging from intellectual changes to vegetative states after global ischemic–anoxic insults. ICP measurement has been of value in the development of new, specific neuron-saving therapies for "postresuscitation disease" to assist in the restoration of mentation.

STROKE

Increases in ICP are common with spontaneous intracerebral hemorrhage and routinely occur in comatose patients. In ischemic stroke, high ICP is likely after cerebral infarction has progressed to coma with midline brain shift. ICP monitoring has been effective in the initiation and maintenance of therapeutic intervention. It also has provided valuable information for research on the mechanisms and amelioration of focal brain ischemia.

SURGERY

During surgery, ICP monitoring assists in determining the optimal position for the patient and the responses to various anesthetic agents and ventilatory support. ICP can be increased by adverse responses to surgery, such as hypertension, tachycardia, coughing, straining, airway manipulation, and anesthetic agents, which can exacerbate hemodynamic instability and increase cerebral blood volume.[4]

◼ CONTRAINDICATIONS TO INTRACRANIAL PRESSURE MONITORING

Coagulopathy (an early complication of severe head injury), systemic infection, or a localized infection at the site of insertion of the ICP monitoring device may be considered contraindications to ICP monitoring.

◼ PROCEDURES

Techniques

There are five basic techniques, as shown in Figure 33–4, for measuring ICP in the critical care setting: intraventricular, subarachnoid, subdural, parenchymal, and epidural (extradural). All of these methods require strict aseptic technique during insertion and maintenance. Despite many years of research, ICP telemetry systems for long-term monitoring of selected patients, such as those with hydrocephalus, metabolic encephalopathies, and brain tumors, are seldom used at this time. The patient's pathophysiology may influence the type of ICP monitoring selected. For example, a patient with collapsed ventricles secondary to cerebral edema will probably require absorption other than intraventricular, whereas a patient with subarachnoid hemorrhage will benefit from the drainage of CSF as a means of controlling and reducing intracranial hypertension. The usual duration for any ICP monitoring is 3 to 5 days. Advantages and disadvantages of each technique are shown in Table 33–2.

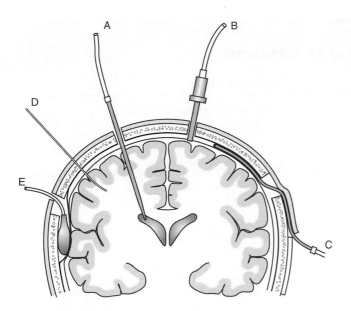

FIGURE 33-4

Intracranial pressure (ICP) monitoring systems. (**A**) intraventricular; (**B**) subarachnoid; (**C**) subdural; (**D**) parenchymal; (**E**) epidural.

INTRAVENTRICULAR TECHNIQUE

The intraventricular technique of ICP measurement remains the most frequently used because it is considered the most accurate and reliable method of monitoring ICP, facilitates CSF drainage, and is cost-effective. It consists of placement of a catheter into the lateral ventricle. A twist drill hole or small burr hole is placed lateral to the midline at the level of the coronal suture, usually on the nondominant side. A ventriculostomy catheter is placed through the cerebrum into the anterior horn of the lateral ventricle. On occasion, the occipital horn is used. Connected to the ventricular catheter by a stopcock or pressure tubing is a pressure transducer. Sterile saline or Ringer's lactate solution is used to provide the fluid column between the CSF and diaphragm of the transducer. A continuous-flush device is not used for ICP measurement.

The miniature transducer may be positioned directly on the patient's head. A standard-size transducer is mounted at the bedside, with the venting port positioned at the level of the foramen of Monro. External landmarks for this position are the edge of the brow or the tragus of the ear. For every 1 inch of discrepancy between the level of the transducer and the pressure source, there is an error of approximately 2 mmHg.

A disposable fiberoptic transducer-tipped catheter may be used instead of an external transducer. This eliminates the need for the fluid-filled system required with external transducers. A Y-connector at the proximal end of the catheter facilitates attachment to the monitor and a CSF drainage system. The advantages and disadvantages of the intraventricular technique are listed in Table 33–2.

SUBARACHNOID TECHNIQUE

The measurement of ICP by means of a subarachnoid screw is accomplished by inserting the screw device through a twist drill hole and extending it into the subdural or subarachnoid space. Although the cerebrum is not penetrated, pressures, as with the intraventricular technique, are measured directly from the CSF. A transducer filled with saline or Ringer's lactate solution may be fastened directly to a stopcock on the screw or connected by pressure tubing. As with any technique for monitoring ICP, a continuous-flush device is contraindicated.

An alternate technique for monitoring subarachnoid pressure is the fiberoptic subarachnoid tipped catheter. The disposable fiberoptic transducer tipped catheter is introduced through a small subarachnoid-subdural bolt, with the catheter extending just beyond the tip of the bolt. Volume–pressure responses have been determined with these techniques. Subarachnoid pressures usually correlate well with intraventricular pressures. The advantages and disadvantages of the subarachnoid technique are listed in Table 33–2.

SUBDURAL TECHNIQUE

For subdural monitoring, fluid-filled catheters connected to external transducers or fiberoptic systems are placed between the dura and subarachnoid space. Subdural monitors are most commonly placed during surgery and facilitate postoperative clot evacuation. Advantages and disadvantages are listed in Table 33–2.

PARENCHYMAL TECHNIQUE

A disposable fiberoptic transducer tipped catheter is placed directly into brain tissue, usually 1 cm below the subarachnoid space, using a small subarachnoid bolt device. The parenchymal technique provides a means of obtaining ICP recordings in patients with compressed and dislocated ventricles, with pressures that correlate well with ventricular pressure and waveforms distinct enough for analysis, though not as good as with intraventricular monitoring.

It is not necessary to balance the transducer after insertion. The mean ICP is displayed continuously on a portable monitor that interfaces with a standard monitoring system for oscilloscopic display and printout of ICP waveforms and values. The advantages and disadvantages of the intraparenchymal technique are listed in Table 33–2.

EPIDURAL TECHNIQUE

This technique involves placement of an epidural device, such as a balloon with radionuclides, a radio transmitter, or a fiberoptic or pneumatic transducer, between the skull and the dura. Some researchers believe that dural compression, surface tension, and thickening of the dura during prolonged monitoring cause inaccuracies in the pressure readings. Although subarachnoid, parenchymal, and intraventricular pressures correlate well with each other, there have

TABLE 33-2
Advantages and Disadvantages of Techniques of ICP Monitoring

Technique	Advantages	Disadvantages
Intraventricular	• Direct measurement of pressure from the cerebrospinal fluid (CSF) • Access for CSF drainage or sampling • Access for determining volume–pressure responses (VPRs) • Access for instillation of drugs	• Need to puncture the brain • Difficulty in locating the lateral ventricle after midline shifting of the ventricle or collapse of the ventricle as a normal compensatory mechanism for increases in pressure • Blockage of the catheter by fluid components or the ventricle wall • Risks of intracranial hemorrhage and infection
Subarachnoid	• Direct pressure measurement for CSF • No need to penetrate cerebrum to locate ventricle • Access for determining VPRs • Access for CSF drainage and sampling • Ease of insertion	• Risk of complications comparable to those associated with intraventricular technique • Need for closed skull • Greater difficulty in VPR studies and with CSF drainage than with ventricular catheters • Possible blockage of the measuring devices from high intracranial pressure (ICP) • Possible underestimation of ICP when it is elevated
Subdural	• Clot evacuation • Allows for trending	• Inaccurate • Damping as brain resumes normal shape
Parenchymal	• Accurate—correlates well with ventricular pressures • Ease of insertion • No fluid- or air-filled system • Eliminates effect of hydrostatic pressure on readings • Minimizes artifact, leaks, drift, and infection • No need to balance after insertion • No calibration required • No problem with transducer position • Adequate waveform	• Catheter breakage with bending, tension, or rough manipulation • No route for CSF drainage and sampling • Inability to zero or calibrate after insertion • Requires dedicated equipment • Cost • Risks of hemorrhage, infection, and CSF leakage
Epidural	• Less invasive • Usefulness of selected transducers for anterior fontanelle monitoring	• Questionable reflection of CSF pressure. With high ICPs, epidural pressures may overread ventricular pressures considerably. • Slow response time. Many systems are unable to pick up transient peaks caused by Valsalva maneuvers and respiratory changes. • No route for CSF drainage and sampling • Infeasible VPRs • Inability to zero and calibrate some systems after measurement is initiated • Transducer placement. Transducer must touch but not indent the dura and must be parallel to, or coplanar with, the dura. If the dura is stretched, the pressure recording will be affected by dural compliance.

been inconsistent correlations between direct CSF pressure and pressure measurement using various epidural techniques. A study comparing extradural ICP measurements to intraparenchymatous pressures obtained with a fiberoptic system showed extradural pressures reading higher than intraparenchymatous pressures. The authors concluded that the lack of agreement was probably due to the unreliability of extradural pressure for the measurement of ICP.[5] The advantages and disadvantages of the epidural technique are listed in Table 33–2.

Interpretation of Results

RANGE OF NORMAL VALUES

Normal measurements of ICP range between 0 and 10 mmHg, with an upper limit of 15 mmHg. During coughing or straining, a normal ICP may increase to 100 mmHg. In acute situations, patients often become symptomatic at pressures ranging from 20 to 25 mmHg.

The patient's tolerance of a change in ICP varies with the acuteness of its onset. Patients with a slower buildup of ICP, as occurs with certain brain tumors, are more tolerant of elevations in the ICP than patients in whom pressure changes rapidly, as seen in those with acute subdural hematoma. Uncontrolled ICP between 20 and 25 mmHg is considered the "kiss of death" for the head-injured patient. Sustained intracranial hypertension greater than 60 mmHg usually is fatal.

The ICP may rise to the level of the MAP. The greater the variations in the mean ICP, the more nearly exhausted are the compensatory mechanisms for intracranial volume increases.

Although protocols vary, measures to reduce ICP usually are initiated if the patient shows neurological deterioration, such as a score of 7 or less on the GCS or an ICP of 15 mmHg or greater.

Although ICP is monitored routinely as a mean pressure, systolic and diastolic pressures should be noted. Because there is a linear relationship between pulse pressure and ICP, pulse pressure may be used to estimate intracranial elastance, particularly in the patient with cerebral vasoparalysis.

For patients with head injury, the mortality rate is between 22% and 57%. Remaining comatose with an elevation of ICP within 72 hours of injury combined with a GCS score of less than 9 and older age appear to be associated with a poor outcome.

INTRACRANIAL PRESSURE WAVEFORMS

Waveforms of ICP provide an index of ICP dynamics, such as changes in intracerebral compliance. The appearance of ICP waveforms varies according to the technique of measurement being used, the patient's pathological status and activities, interventions, or environmental changes. Hemodynamic and respiratory oscillations can be observed in ICP traces. Sometimes, the waveforms closely resemble arterial pressure waveforms; at other times, they resemble central venous pressure waveforms. To varying degrees, oscillations corresponding to intracranial arterial pulsations with retrograde venous pulsations are seen with each heartbeat (Fig. 33–5, top).

At times, a small "a" wave is superimposed on diastole, reflecting right atrial pressure.

Alterations in arterial driving force, disturbance of venous outflow, and cerebral vasodilation have been correlated with changes in waveform appearances.

In patients with ICP less than 20 mmHg, a slower waveform, synchronous with respiration and caused by changes in intrathoracic pressure, can be seen (see Fig. 33–5, middle).

Some patients exhibit waveform variation, most commonly A, B, and C waves. *A waves*, also known as *plateau waves*, are spontaneous, rapid increases of pressure between 50 and 200 mmHg, occurring at variable intervals (see Fig. 33–5, bottom). They tend to occur in patients with moderate elevations of ICP, last 5 to 20 minutes, and fall spontaneously. The plateau waves usually are accompanied by a

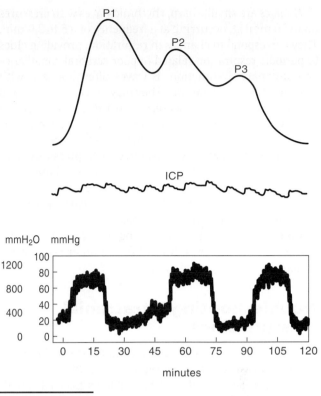

FIGURE 33-5

Intracranial pressure (ICP) waveforms. *Top,* A normal ICP pulse waveform may demonstrate three or more descending peaks. P1, the pressure wave, originates from choroid plexus pulsations. P2, the tidal wave, is more variable in shape and amplitude and ends on the dicrotic notch. P3, the dicrotic wave, follows the dicrotic notch and tapers down to the diastolic position unless retrograde venous pulsations cause a few more peaks. The P2 portion of the waveform most directly reflects the state of intracerebral compliance. As mean ICP rises, P2 progressively elevates, causing the pulse wave to appear more rounded. When a state of decreased compliance exists, the P2 component is equal to or higher than P1. *Middle,* An ICP waveform demonstrating hemodynamic and respiratory oscillations. Note the vascular pressure-type notches in the waveforms and the baseline variations that reflect respirations. *Bottom,* "A" or plateau waves, associated with decreased intracranial compliance, may be secondary to an increase in blood volume with a simultaneous decrease in blood flow.

temporary increase in neurological deficit. Although the mechanism of A waves has not been established firmly, it is thought that they indicate decreased intracranial compliance, and measures should be used to prevent their occurrence. They may result from an increase in blood volume with a simultaneous decrease in blood flow. The sudden reversal of high pressure may be caused by increased CSF absorption with reduction of CSF pressure. Falls in CPP with intact autoregulation and low intracranial compliance have been correlated with the initiating plateau waves. Plateau waves may be set off by a stimulus to vasodilation or by nonspecific stimuli, such as hypoventilation or hyperventilation, pain, and aroused mental activities.

B waves are small, sharp, rhythmic waves with pressures up to 50 mmHg, occurring at a frequency of 0.5 to 2.0/min. They correspond to changes in respiration, providing clues to periodic respiration related to poor cerebral compliance or pulmonary dysfunction. B waves often are seen with Cheyne-Stokes respirations. They may precede A waves and increase as compliance decreases. At times, they occur in patients with normal ICP and no papilledema. They may be secondary to oscillations of cerebral blood volume.

C waves are small, rhythmic waves with pressures up to 20 mmHg, occurring at a rate of approximately 6/min. They are related to BP. Like A waves, they indicate severe intracranial compression, with limited remaining volume residual within the intracranial space.

Computerized systems are being developed to analyze waveforms and integrate ICP, CPP, and other relevant parameters.

Troubleshooting Intracranial Pressure Lines

Each type of system has potential complications. To ensure accurate measurements and reduce morbidity, it is necessary to be aware of and alert to problems associated with fluid-coupled ICP monitoring systems that could cause incorrect ICP measurements and complications, such as infection.

When the monitor indicates a change in ICP, the nurse must determine first whether the reading is accurate. If the reading is accurate, an attempt is then made to determine the reason for the pressure change. Table 33–3 provides a guide to troubleshooting ICP lines.

■ MANAGEMENT OF INCREASED INTRACRANIAL PRESSURE

Monitoring of ICP is used in conjunction with clinical assessment and other invasive and noninvasive assessment techniques, such as intracranial CT scanning, magnetic-resonance imaging, cerebral oximetry, and bedside CBF measurements, either direct or more commonly indirect by transcranial Doppler (TCD) ultrasonography, jugular venous O_2 saturation measurements, and multimodality-evoked potentials (somatosensory evoked potentials [SSEP], visual evoked potentials [VEP], brain stem auditory evoked responses [BAER]). When used this way, ICP monitoring frequently reduces the time required for accurate diagnosis, increases the time available for treatment, provides continual feedback on responses to selected patient care activities and therapies, and assists with determination of prognosis for patients at risk for developing or with actual intracranial hypertension.

There are many methods of treating intracranial hypertension. No single management routine is appropriate for all patients. In addition to clinical pathways and nursing care protocols, algorithms for incremental application and weaning of ICP management have been developed. Figure 33–6 provides an algorithm for first-tier (conventional) and second-tier (refractory) treatments of intracranial hypertension. First-tier therapy includes ventricular CSF drainage, mannitol hyperventilation, and sedation. Second-tier therapy includes hypothermia, barbiturate coma, optimized hyperventilation, hypertensive CPP therapy, and decompressive craniectomy.

Most management techniques for ICP are oriented toward control of cerebral blood volume and CSF circulation, the two major mechanisms responsible for the regulation of ICP. Although protocols vary, measures to reduce ICP are usually initiated when the patient's ICP increases to approximately 15 mmHg.

Although no one therapeutic regimen has been accepted universally, the goals of treatment for the patient with intracranial hypertension are as follows:

- Reduce ICP
- Improve CPP
- Reduce brain shift and distortion and the systemic effects that they induce

Remember that nursing care activity can compound primary and secondary intracranial insults, contributing to rapid deterioration in the unstable patient who has lost intracranial compliance, autoregulation, and vasomotor tone. It is important to assess the patient for extracranial causes (see display) and potential causes of intracranial hypertension and provide appropriate interventions to prevent elevations in ICP or to decrease ICP. For example, it has been shown that in comatose patients with GCS scores of > 6, emotionally related conversation tended to increase ICP, probably due to increasing anxiety and stress. Conversations unrelated to the patient tended to decrease ICP.

The following discussion includes measures used in the management of intracranial hypertension.

Position

The head is elevated 15 to 30 degrees unless contraindicated by limb fractures or hepatorenal failure. In patients with grade 4 hepatic coma, head elevation of less than 20 degrees has been associated with lowering ICP, whereas a greater than 20-degree elevation is associated with an increase in ICP and a decrease in CPP. Decerebrate or decorticate posturing may increase ICP.

Flexion of the knees is contraindicated, and patients at risk for a pathological increase in ICP should not be positioned with the neck in flexion or the head turned to either side. These positions restrict venous drainage from the head through the internal jugular system and the vertebral venous plexus, increasing the total intracranial content. Rotation of the head to the right causes the greatest increase in ICP.

TABLE 33-3
Troubleshooting ICP Lines

Problem	Cause	Nursing Considerations and Interventions
No ICP waveform	Air between the transducer diaphragm and pressure source	Eliminate air bubbles with sterile saline.
	Occlusion of intracranial measurement device with blood or debris	Flush intracranial catheter or screw as directed by physician: 0.25-mL sterile saline is often used.
	Transducer connected incorrectly	Check connection, and be sure the appropriate connector for amplifier is in use.
	Fiberoptic catheter bent, broken	Replace fiberoptic catheter.
	Incorrect gain setting for pressure or patient having plateau waves	Adjust gain setting for higher pressure range.
	Trace turned off	Turn power on to trace.
False high-pressure reading	Transducer too low	Place the venting port of the transducer at the level of the foramen of Monro. For every 2.54 cm (1 in) the transducer is below the pressure source, there is an error of approximately 2 mmHg.
	Transducer incorrectly balanced	With transducer correctly positioned, rebalance. Transducer should be balanced every 2 to 4 h and before the initiation of treatment based on a pressure change.
	Monitoring system incorrectly calibrated	Repeat calibration procedures.
	Air in system: air may attenuate or amplify pressure signal	Remove air from monitoring line.
High-pressure reading	Airway not patent: an increase in intrathoracic pressure may increase PCO_2	Suction patient. Position. Initiate chest physiotherapy.
	Ventilator setting incorrect	Check ventilator settings.
	PEEP	Draw arterial blood gases, because hypoxia and hypercarbia cause increases in ICP.
	Posture	Head should be elevated 15 to 30 degrees unless contraindicated by other problems, such as fractures.
	Head and neck	The head should be positioned to facilitate venous drainage.
	Legs	Limit knee flexion.
	Excessive muscle activity during decerebrate posturing in patients with upper brain stem injury may increase ICP.	Muscle relaxants or paralyzing agents sometimes are indicated.
	Hyperthermia	Initiate measures to control muscle movement, infection, and pyrexia.
	Excessive muscle activity	
	Increased susceptibility to infection	
	Fluid and electrolyte imbalance secondary to fluid restrictions and diuretics	Draw blood for serum electrolytes, serum osmolality. Note pulmonary artery pressure. Evaluate input and output with specific gravity.
	Blood pressure: vasopressor responses occur in some patients with elevating ICP.	Use measures to maintain adequate CPP.
	Low BP associated with hypovolemia, shock, and barbiturate coma may increase cerebral ischemia.	
False low-pressure reading	Air bubbles between transducer and CSF	Eliminate air bubbles with sterile saline.
	Transducer level too high	Place the venting port of the transducer at the level of the foramen of Monro. For every 2.54 cm (1 in) the transducer is above the level of the pressure source, there will be an error of approximately 2 mm Hg.

(continued)

TABLE 33-3
Troubleshooting ICP Lines (Continued)

Problem	Cause	Nursing Considerations and Interventions
False low-pressure reading	Zero or calibration incorrect Collapse of ventricles around catheter	Rezero and calibrate monitoring system. If ventriculostomy is being used, there may be inadequate positive pressure. Check to make sure a positive pressure of 15 to 20 mm Hg exists. Drain CSF slowly.
	Otorrhea or rhinorrhea	These conditions cause a false low-pressure reading secondary to decompression. Document the correlation between drainage and pressure changes.
	Leakage of fluid from connections Dislodgement of catheter from ventricle into brain	Eliminate all fluid leakage. Contact physician regarding appropriate diagnostic studies and intervention. Use soft catheter designed for intraventricular measurement.
	Occlusion of the end of a subarachnoid screw by the necrotic brain	In most cases, remove screw.

Steroids

Recent research with severely head-injured patients has demonstrated that high-dose glucocorticoid therapy is ineffective in altering the course of intracranial hypertension or improving long-term neurological outcome. High-dose glucocorticoid therapy, such as dexamethasone, is effective in reducing vasogenic edema associated with primary and metastatic brain tumors, brain abscesses, and spinal cord tumors.[6]

Antihypertensive Therapy

The regulation of BP is an important aspect of managing the patient with intracranial hypertension. BP is directly related to cerebral blood volume, cerebroperfusion pressure, cerebral ischemia, and cerebral compliance.

The normal intact brain has the ability to maintain a stable CBF (40–50 mL/g/min) over a wide range of perfusion pressures (50–150 mmHg) by varying the degree of vasoconstriction or vasodilation. This autoregulation may be abnormal in injured brains. Patients with ischemic or traumatic injury may require pharmacological therapy to treat life-threatening hypertension despite the risks associated with the use of antihypertensive therapies in the presence of intracranial ischemia or space-occupying pathology. For these patients, the principal goal is to reduce systemic hypertension while maintaining adequate CPP, thereby avoiding secondary ischemic brain damage. For patients with acute brain injury, the optimal method and agents of choice for reduction of arterial BP remain controversial. Several treatment options are available for the acute treatment of hypertensive crisis in patients with intracranial ischemic or space-occupying pathology (Table 33–4).

Because calcium-channel blockers have a direct effect on cerebral vasodilation, patients receiving them require frequent neurological assessment. The use of calcium-channel blockers may be contraindicated in patients with cerebral edema or space-occupying intracranial lesions.[7] Calcium-channel antagonists cause cerebral vasodilation with associated increased ICP and should be used only with great caution in head-injured patients.

Significant drops in BP have been documented with nimodipine. One approach that has been used to prevent abrupt decreases in BP is to divide the dose and give it more frequently. For example, if 60 mg is being given every 4 hours, the dose is changed to 30 mg every 2 hours, which seems to eliminate hypotensive episodes in most patients.

Hemodynamic Monitoring

For brain-injured patients, the preservation of CPP (MAP – ICP) and maintenance of systemic oxygen availability (cardiac index × arterial oxygen content) are the two most important goals. Most head-injured patients have increased metabolic oxygen consumption, mild hypertension, and increased cardiac indices.[8]

Because brain-injured patients are at risk for secondary injury caused by hypotension and hypoxia, *invasive BP monitoring* is routinely used to provide continuous and accurate BP measurements and CPPs during the acute management phase. MAP, the driving force for peripheral blood flow, is the preferred BP measurement in unstable patients. The MAP is essential for the calculation of CPP.

For head-injured patients, the overall hemodynamic goals are as follows:

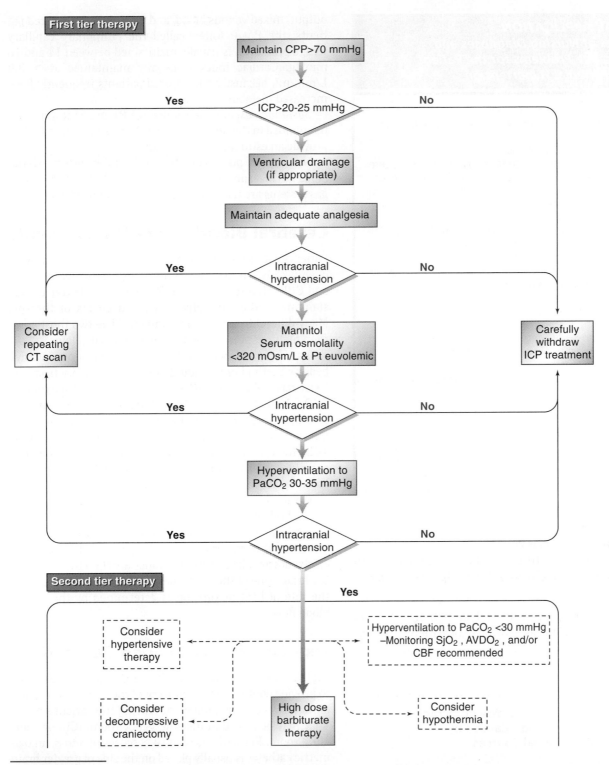

First tier therapy

Maintain CPP>70 mmHg

ICP>20-25 mmHg — Yes / No

Ventricular drainage (if appropriate)

Maintain adequate analgesia

Intracranial hypertension — Yes / No

Consider repeating CT scan

Mannitol
Serum osmolality
<320 mOsm/L & Pt euvolemic

Carefully withdraw ICP treatment

Intracranial hypertension — Yes / No

Hyperventilation to PaCO₂ 30-35 mmHg

Intracranial hypertension — Yes / No

Second tier therapy

Yes

Consider hypertensive therapy

Hyperventilation to PaCO₂ <30 mmHg
–Monitoring SjO₂ , AVDO₂ , and/or CBF recommended

Consider decompressive craniectomy

High dose barbiturate therapy

Consider hypothermia

FIGURE 33-6

Algorithm for management of intracranial hypertension. Increased intracranial pressure (ICP), cerebral perfusion pressure (CPP), computed tomography (CT), jugular venous saturation (SjO₂), cerebral blood flow (CBF), cerebral oxygen consumption, arteriovenous difference (AVDO₂). Intracranial hypertension is usually defined as an ICP greater than 20 to 25 mmHg. The first tier indicates conventional treatment. The second tier indicates treatments for refractory intracranial hypertension. (From Randall M: Chestnut: Medical management of severe head injury: Present and future. New Horizons: The Science and Practice of Acute Medicine 3(3):585, 1995 with permission)

Decreased Intracranial Adaptive Capacity
  Related to cerebral edema or space-occupying lesion (hemorrhage or tumor)
Altered Cerebral Tissue Perfusion
  Related to decreased space for cerebral perfusion, cerebral tissue edema, decreased systemic perfusion, or absent cerebral perfusion due to embolus or cerebral vascular flow interruption
Fluid Volume Deficit
  Related to diabetes insipidus (DI), diuretic therapy, high metabolic needs, diaphoresis, renal failure
Ineffective Breathing Pattern
  Related to subdued level of consciousness, brain tissue injury near medulla or pons, inability to maintain adequate airway, lack of control over respiratory muscles, severe hypoventilation, or pulmonary complications
Risk for Altered Body Temperature
  Related to brain tissue injury or infection
Risk for Infection
  Related to invasive lines, decreased level of consciousness, and immobility
Risk for Injury
  Related to decreased level of consciousness, agitation, restlessness, or seizure activity
Risk for Altered Nutrition: Less Than Body Requirements
  Related to decreased level of consciousness, mechanical ventilation, or increased metabolic needs

- A normal or slightly increased CPP
- Normal intravascular volume
- MAP < 140 mmHg (the upper limit of autoregulation) usually between 115 to 120 mmHg, even if ICP is elevated

Pulmonary artery pressures and *pulmonary artery occlusive pressure* (PAOP) can provide information on cardiac and pulmonary problems, intravascular volume, cardiac

- Position of neck, head, and hips
- Cardiovascular instability
- Increased intrathoracic pressure
- Increased abdominal distention
- Decerebrate posturing and agitation
- Metabolic abnormalities
- Nontherapeutic touch and painful procedures
- Extraneous sounds
- Suctioning
- Hygienic measures
- Emotionally charged conversations

output, mixed venous blood, and SvO_2. In head-injured patients, the PAOP (often called the pulmonary capillary wedge pressure), is usually maintained between 14 and 16 mmHg. Cardiac index is usually maintained at > 3.0 L/min/m², because brain-injured patients frequently have increased metabolic rates.

Systemic vascular resistance (SVR) and SVR index are maintained in the normal range. BP, cardiac index, and SVR provide an estimation of perfusion.

Noninvasive pulse oximetry (SpO_2), intermittent arterial blood gas measurements, and invasive bedside arterial blood gas systems are used to determine arterial oxygen content.

Cerebral Blood Flow Measurements

Patients with severe head injury are at risk of secondary ischemia caused by derangements of the cerebral vasculature and CBF. Monitoring of CBF is useful for a better understanding of the pathophysiology and effects of therapy. Many different methods are available. The two most common methods seen in the ICU are discussed below.

Transcranial Doppler ultrasonography is a noninvasive bedside method of recording blood flow velocity from the basal cerebral arteries. (See Chapter 32 for a discussion of TCD.) Applications for TCD include detection of vascular spasm, intracranial arterial emboli, and increases in resistance of the cerebral circulation. High ICP is indicated by TCD. Relative change in CBF in response to various circumstances in the intensive care unit (ICU) can be measured by monitoring the middle cerebral artery.[9]

For direct measurement of CBF, CBF probes are placed on the brain's cortical surface for measurement of cerebral flow during and after a craniectomy procedure. They may be removed postoperatively at the patient's bedside. Two electrodes are placed a fixed distance apart on the surface of the brain. One of the electrodes is very slightly heated, and the rate of heat dissipation is determined by the rate of blood flow.

Jugular Venous Oxygen Saturation

Jugular venous oxygen saturation (SjO_2) catheters are used to provide continuous monitoring of the oxygen saturation of mixed venous cerebral blood leaving the patient's brain. They may be placed in the emergency room, ICU, or operating room. For patients with GCS scores of 3 to 8, an oximetric catheter is usually placed on the side of greater brain injury with a technique similar to placing an internal jugular central venous line. The major difference is that the SjO_2 catheter is directed toward the patient's head. Continuous jugular venous oxygen saturation measurements provide information on cerebral metabolism, optimal timing of neurosurgical interventions, and general information on prognosis. The average mixed jugular venous oxygen saturation in normal subjects is 62% (range 55%–71%). In head-injured patients, a sustained saturation of 50% to 55% requires investigation of the cause of desaturation.

TABLE 33-4   CLINICAL APPLICATION: Drug Therapy
Major Classes of Pharmacological Agents Used in Acute Antihypertensive Intervention for Patients With Intracranial Pathology

Class	Mechanisms	Drugs	Comments
Direct vasodilators (smooth muscle relaxants)	Directly dilate the peripheral vasculature and lower vascular resistance	• Sodium nitroprusside • Nitroglycerin • Hydralazine • Adenosine • Diazoxide	Dilate the cerebral vascular bed, ↑CBV and ↑ICP while ↓MAP and ↓CPP
Ganglionic blockers	Halt neuronal transmission through nicotinic receptors of both parasympathetic and sympathetic automatic ganglia Reduce BP by decreasing CO and SVR Do not cross the blood–brain barrier	• Trimethaphan (Arfonad)	Prevent reliable examination of pupillary muscle Few CNS side effects Little or no effect on CBF or ICP May cause transient increase in ICP during induction of hypotension Most likely to increase ICP when administered rapidly in patients with reduced intracranial compliance 1:1 mixture of nitroprusside and trimethaphan effective in decreasing dosage and dose-related side effects of both drugs
α-Adrenergic antagonists	Pharmacological blockade to vascular smooth muscle causing vasodilation, decreased peripheral vascular resistance, and reduction of MAP	• Phentolamine (reversible)	The relatively long duration of action after IV dose (10–15 min) may be a problem in patients with labile pressure-dependent cerebral perfusion, because overdosage may cause profound hypotension with the potential for additional brain injury. If CPP is decreased, CBF may be reduced with no known effect on CBF or ICP within the normal autoregulation range.
β-Adrenergic antagonists	β-adrenergic receptor antagonism	• Propranolol • Esmolol	Do not affect CBF Have been used during intracranial hemorrhage after adverse effect on ICP Use caution when Cushing's response present (bradycardia, hypertension and increased ICP) because β-adrenergic receptor antagonists can potentiate bradycardia Minimal effect on cerebral circulation Duration of action half-life of 9 min Frequently administered by continuous IV
Mixed α- and β-adrenergic antagonists	Selective α-, and nonselective β-, and β$_2$-adrenergic receptor antagonist Cause a reduction in SVR	• Labetalol	Improve CPP and do not increase ICP. Use with caution in patients with Cushing's response because it slows heart rate.
Calcium-channel antagonists	Prevent inward transport of calcium ions in vascular smooth muscle by inhibiting voltage-dependent calcium-channels, resulting in vasodilation, decreased myocardial contractility, decreased heart rate, and decreased rate of conduction at the atrioventricular node	• Nifedipine • Verapamil • Diltiazem • Nicardipine	Cause cerebral vasodilation with increased ICP Use with caution in patients with brain injury May be contraindicated in patients with space-occupying lesions or cerebral edema Frequent neurological examinations required on patients receiving these drugs

(continued)

TABLE 33-4   CLINICAL APPLICATION: Drug Therapy (Continued)
Major Classes of Pharmacological Agents Used in Acute Antihypertensive Intervention for Patients With Intracranial Pathology

Class	Mechanisms	Drugs	Comments
Angiotensin converting enzyme (ACE) inhibitors	Shift the upper and lower limits of autoregulation Influence CBF autoregulation by inhibiting angiotensin II-mediated vascular tone in large cerebral arteries while small resistance vessels constrict	• Captopril • Enalaprilat	Preserve CBF after single dose and increase CBF with chronic treatment Have the potential to increase ICP in patients with intracranial hypertension by increased CBF
Barbiturates	Decrease CBF through an effect on cerebral metabolism and direct vasoconstriction effect on cerebral blood vessels Have systemic cardiovascular effect with arterial BP decreasing as a consequence of peripheral venodilation and pooling of blood	• Pentobarbital (long-acting) • Thiopental (short-acting)	Used for treatment of intracranial hypertension and may be the preferred class of drug for treatment of hypertension in brain-injured patients Used for treatment of hypertension in patients with space-occupying pathology; neurological monitoring required (eg, ICP, SSEPs, EEG, TCD) Barbiturates decrease both CBF and oxygen metabolism; potential for secondary ischemic injury decreased, despite reduction of CBF Do not interfere with CBF autoregulation; possible alteration of cerebral vasodilatory responses to hypoxia and hypercapnia by drug-induced metabolic depression

For patients with intracranial ischemia or space-occupying pathology, the treatment of acute hypertensive crisis requires consideration of both cerebrovascular and cardiovascular effects. Most antihypertensive drugs have an adverse affect on CBF and ICP. Nitroprusside is now the drug of choice for most hypertensive emergencies in patients with intracranial pathology, due to its immediate onset and ease of titration.

Contraindications to this catheter include cervical spine injuries, bleeding diathesis, local infection, and impairments of cerebral venous drainage. Because of the increased potential for infection, the presence of a tracheostomy is considered a relative contraindication.[10]

Ventricular Cerebrospinal Fluid Drainage (Ventriculostomy, Shunt)

Ventriculostomy catheters are used for ICP monitoring and treatment of intracranial hypertension. In situations involving impaired absorption of CSF, such as after a subarachnoid hemorrhage; impaired circulation of CSF, as with hydrocephalus and certain brain tumors; or elevation of ICP without total collapse of the ventricles, controlled CSF drainage may facilitate a reduction in ICP (Fig. 33–7). Ventriculostomy catheters may be placed during surgery, in the ICU or in the emergency room. In patients with midline shift of the ventricles, ultrasonography may be useful for locating the ventricles. Ventricular drainage always should be against a positive pressure of 15 to 20 mmHg to prevent ventricular collapse. Best results are obtained when there is bilateral dilation of the ventricles. Decompression should be gradual, particularly in children.

Although CSF drainage is done routinely by intraventricular catheter (ventriculostomy), in selected patients, CSF can be drained by a subarachnoid screw or bolt. It is recommended that external ventricular drainage (ventriculostomy) systems be changed every 3 to 5 days, when three-quarters filled, or if the drainage becomes excessively bloody. Strict sterile technique is required during catheter insertion, dressing changes, and drainage bag changes to reduce the risk of infection. Disruption of the drainage system must be minimized.

The amount and appearance of CSF drainage and the condition of the catheter site after surgery should be documented.

Mannitol

Mannitol, a hypertonic crystalloid solution that decreases brain water content, is the only pharmacological agent used as routine therapy for reducing ICP. It is now the first choice for reducing ICP after brain injury, replacing other

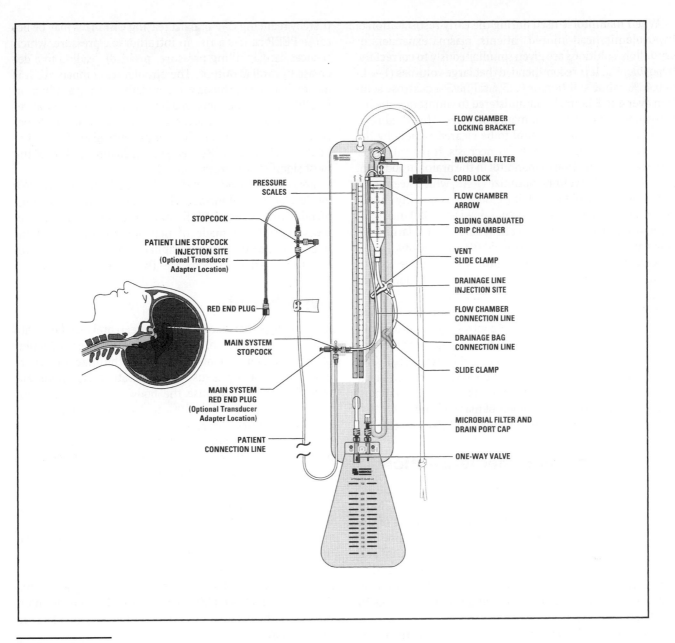

FLOW CHAMBER
LOCKING BRACKET

MICROBIAL FILTER

CORD LOCK

PRESSURE
SCALES

FLOW CHAMBER
ARROW

STOPCOCK

SLIDING GRADUATED
DRIP CHAMBER

PATIENT LINE STOPCOCK
INJECTION SITE
(Optional Transducer
Adapter Location)

VENT
SLIDE CLAMP

DRAINAGE LINE
INJECTION SITE

RED END PLUG

FLOW CHAMBER
CONNECTION LINE

DRAINAGE BAG
CONNECTION LINE

MAIN SYSTEM
STOPCOCK

SLIDE CLAMP

MAIN SYSTEM
RED END PLUG
(Optional Transducer
Adapter Location)

MICROBIAL FILTER AND
DRAIN PORT CAP

PATIENT
CONNECTION LINE

ONE-WAY VALVE

FIGURE 33-7

Becker external drainage and monitoring system for intracranial pressure monitoring and intermittent cerebrospinal fluid drainage. A pressure transducer is attached to the intraventricular catheter or main system stopcock. Physician orders should specify the desired level of ICP or the volume of CSF to be drained. (Courtesy of Medtronic PS Medical, Goleta, CA)

osmotic diuretics, such as urea. Mannitol may be used when high ICP is suspected, with neurological deterioration, prior to CT scanning, preoperatively or intraoperatively in patients with intracranial hematomas, and with demonstrated intracranial hypertension. When mannitol is used, the bladder must be catheterized (Foley catheter) as soon as possible. To reduce potential side effects and optimize the risk–benefit ratio, mannitol administration should be based directly on ICP measurements.

Mannitol is safer and more effective when administered as a bolus intravenous infusion over 10 to 30 minutes in doses ranging from 0.25 to 1.0 g/kg body weight. Studies have demonstrated mannitol's beneficial effects on ICP,

CPP, CBF, and brain metabolism and have shown a beneficial effect on neurological outcome. CBF and cerebral oxygen metabolism are increased by the immediate plasma-expanding effect of mannitol, which reduces the hematocrit level and blood viscosity, permitting cerebral arterioles to decrease in diameter; this lowers cerebral blood volume and ICP while maintaining constant CBF. When mannitol is given as a continuous infusion, it accumulates in the brain, which leads to a reverse osmotic shift that increases brain swelling and ICP. Because mannitol is excreted entirely by the urine, if it is administered in large doses and serum osmolality is > 320 mOsm, there is a significant risk of acute renal failure (acute tubular necrosis).

When mannitol is used during the early resuscitation of hypovolemic head-injured patients, plasma expanders or crystalloid solutions are given simultaneously to correct the hypovolemia. It is recommended that large volumes (1–2 L) of 0.45% saline solution or 0.45% saline/5% dextrose solution over 4 to 8 hours be administered to counteract the hyperosmolar effect of serial mannitol doses. This fluid regimen may allow the mannitol to be cleared rapidly by the kidney, preventing renal tubular necrosis. It may also prevent the accumulation of mannitol in the brain. In addition, the intravascular volume optimizes MAP, which keeps CPP levels high. To avoid renal failure, serum osmolality should be measured frequently and maintained at < 320 mOsm. It is important to monitor the patient carefully for large fluid shifts and osmotic diuresis to avoid BP fluctuations.

Recent studies indicate mannitol is an effective "small-volume resuscitation fluid," for acute resuscitation of patients with hypertension and concomitant brain injury.[11]

Although a small study has reported that tromethamine base (THAM) is as effective in ICP control as mannitol, mannitol is the standard of practice in the management of head-injured patients with suspected or actual increased ICP. The practice of using loop diuretics, such as furosemide (Lasix) in conjunction with mannitol administration is no longer recommended due to the danger of massive diuresis, causing depletion of intravascular volume and electrolytes.

Ventilation and Hyperventilation

Maintaining adequate oxygenation and hypocapnea are essential in the patient with intracranial hypertension. Neuronal damage or death may occur within 5 minutes of the onset of hypoxemia. Uncorrected hypercapnia causes vasodilation of cerebral blood vessels with increased CBF and increased ICP, leading to cerebral ischemia. Hyperventilation with hypocapnia usually to a $PaCO_2$ of 30 to 35 mmHg, may cause ICP to decrease by causing cerebral arteries to constrict, reducing cerebral blood volume.

Endotracheal intubation usually is used with a tracheostomy performed by the third day if ventilation still is required. Intermittent positive pressure ventilation is indicated in patients with a head injury and in a coma, ICPs greater than 30 mmHg after cranial surgery, chest injuries, or decerebrate spasms or uncontrolled seizures secondary to brain damage.

Ventilation usually is done at a slow rate (approximately 10–12 cycles/min) with a high tidal volume (15 mL/kg body weight) to moderate hypocapnia (30–35 mmHg). The use of sedatives, analgesics, and paralytics may be indicated for some patients. Reduction of PCO_2 below 20 mmHg causes no further vasoconstriction. Lowering PCO_2 below 25 mmHg may increase lactic acid and dysrhythmias. Arterial PO_2 is maintained at more than 70 mmHg.

Positive end-expiratory pressure (PEEP) is used at levels up to 20 cm of water to improve oxygenation in patients with pulmonary dysfunction and requires ICP monitoring. The use of PEEP can increase ICP or reduce arterial BP, thereby reducing CPP and decreasing CBF. This may be because PEEP causes a rise in intrathoracic pressure, which reduces cardiac filling pressure (preload), leading to a decrease in cardiac output. The circulatory compensation is incomplete and the blood pressure falls, causing a reduction in CPP. ICP may be increased by impedance to cerebral venous outflow. In one study, significant increases in ICP occurred in approximately 50% of patients given PEEP. Patients with baseline ICPs greater than 25 mmHg showed the most significant increases in ICP.

For optimal titration of PEEP in the patient who is at risk for development of intracranial hypertension, it is recommended that ICP and BP be monitored continuously and measurements be made of neurological status and intracranial and pulmonary compliance. Volume pressure responses and arterial blood gases therefore are indicated.

Hypothermia

Although hypothermia decreases the cerebral metabolic rate of oxygen consumption, used alone it may cause a reduction of CBF. Except in patients in induced barbiturate coma, normothermia usually is used. Temperature elevations are treated promptly, because the body's metabolic rate increases by approximately 10% to 13% per °C increase in body temperature. There is a significant relationship between fever and a poor neurological outcome. Rectal temperatures alone may significantly underestimate brain tissue temperature.[10] A catheter that measures both ICP and the temperature within the brain is currently in development.

Hypothermia has been used successfully in conjunction with induced barbiturate coma. The combination may offer synergistic protection, acting through different mechanisms to control increased ICP. The National Acute Brain Injury Study: Hypothermia, a 4-year multicenter protocol, is testing the effect of moderate systemic hypothermia (32°–33°C [89.6°–91.4°F]) in patients with severe brain injury.[12] See the detailed discussion of hypothermia later in this chapter.

Sedation, Analgesia, and Neuromuscular Blockade

Patients with severe head injury frequently require sedation, analgesia, and neuromuscular blockade (NMB) to facilitate mechanical ventilation or therapy for intracranial hypertension. Prior to the initiation or increase of sedation, analgesia, or neuromuscular blocking (paralysis), every effort should be made to manage causes of agitation and confusion, such as hypoxia, drug or alcohol withdrawal, pain, meningitis, or other systemic infections and cerebrovascular events. At this time, there are many concerns and questions about the use of these drugs to control or limit intracranial hypertension, including the time between discontinuing the drugs and awakening, incidences of prolonged weakness after NMB, and the effect of those drugs on patient outcome.

Because NMB drugs do not have sedative, amnestic, or analgesic activity, they must be accompanied by sedative and analgesic drugs. Although patients receiving these drugs have the external appearance of being quiet, calm, and comfortable, patients may still be able to hear and process tactile stimuli. Every effort should be made to verbally reassure and orient patients.

SEDATIVES

Sedatives, such as propofol, are used to decrease anxiety and diminish awareness of noxious stimuli. When possible, the administration of sedation should be periodically discontinued to facilitate evaluation of mental status and neurological responsiveness. Patients in pain who receive sedation without analgesia may become agitated and combative. Sedatives and analgesia may potentiate each other, allowing patients to be more calm and comfortable at lower doses. In severely head-injured patients (GCS score < 8), sedatives and analgesia are used to reduce agitation, discomfort, and pain; facilitate mechanical ventilation; suppress coughing; limit responses to stimuli, such as suctioning; and limit ICP increases. Various sedative, analgesic, and NMB drugs may compromise the immune system and be factors in the development of nosocomial infections. Benzodiazepines, the most commonly used sedatives in the ICU, include midazolam (Versed), diazepam (Valium), lorazepam (Ativan), and propofol (Diprivan). Diazepam, lorazepam, and midazolam are anticonvulsants and cause little or no change in CBF, ICP, or the cerebral metabolic rate for oxygen ($CMRO_2$). Propofol decreases CBF, ICP, CPP, and $CMRO_2$. An additional reason for its extensive use in the ICU is that patients awaken promptly and with clear mental functions. Bolus propofol may cause hypotension. Because of the risk of bacterial or fungal infection associated with the use of propofol, the propofol infusion should be changed every 6 hours. A side effect of this drug is the development of green hair and urine.

Because ketamine increases BP, CBF, and ICP, it is not used as a sedative in head-injured patients. Etomidate is not recommended because continuous infusion increases mortality secondary to adrenal suppression.

ANALGESICS

Fentanyl or morphine are frequently used to limit pain, facilitate mechanical ventilation, and potentiate the effect of sedation. They do not increase $CMRO_2$, CBF, or ICP.

NEUROMUSCULAR BLOCKADES

Drugs that are NMBs, such as vecuronium, can effectively counteract increases in ICP associated with the reflex motor response to suctioning and facilitate mechanical ventilation. The use of NMB drugs with head trauma patients is controversial and usually is a last resort. Because the primary effect of NMB drugs is muscle paralysis, patients must have a secured, patent, artificial airway; adequate ventila-

tion; appropriate inspired oxygen concentration; concurrent sedation and analgesia; prophylaxis for deep venous thrombosis (intermittent compression stockings); and be protected from pressure points around the eyes, peripheral nerves, and skin.

Hand-held peripheral nerve stimulators or neuromuscular transmission monitors are routinely used to monitor the depth of NMB in patients receiving prolonged paralytic therapy. The use of peripheral nerve stimulation monitoring every 4 hours or when the drug dosage is changed may prevent the complications of persistent paralysis following drug withdrawal. Usually the train-of-four technique is used, with visual observation of thumb movement following four 2-Hz stimuli of 0.2 msec duration delivered at intervals of 0.5 second to the ulnar nerve at the wrist. If four thumb twitches occur, paralysis is insufficient. If no twitches occur, paralysis is excessive, and a reduction is required in the paralytic dose. Two to three twitches generally indicate an adequate degree of NMB.

For a conscious patient, the inability to move and communicate following administration of a paralytic agent can be frightening. All patients receiving paralytics must be treated with a sedative and usually with an analgesic to reduce pain and anxiety, relieve discomfort due to positioning and the ICU environment, and promote rest and comfort. The two most commonly used intermediate-acting paralytics are atracurium (Tracrium) and vecuronium (Norcuron). A bolus of 0.1 mg/kg of vecuronium induces paralysis for 35 to 45 minutes. The usual vecuronium dosage by infusion is 1 to 2 µg/kg/min. Vecuronium does not cause hypotension, and recovery from paralysis occurs approximately 45 to 60 minutes after the drug is discontinued. Rocuronium (Zemuron) is a newer intermediate acting paralytic that induces paralysis within 60 to 90 seconds, has no cardiovascular effects, and does not accumulate in patients with renal failure.

Long-acting paralytics include the newer drugs pipercuronium (Arduan) and doxacurium (Nuromax), which have a longer duration of action than pancuronium (Pavulon) without the cardiovascular side effects.

Avoiding interactions between paralytics and other drugs being used for the patient is necessary because some drugs, such as cardiovascular agents, including certain antiarrhythmics and diuretics, calcium blockers, and beta blockers, and antibiotics, such as aminoglycosides, polymyxin B, clindamycin, and tetracycline, can potentiate the action of paralytics. Phenytoin, carbamazepine, theophylline, and corticosteroids are included in medications with the potential for antagonizing the action of paralytics.

Alterations in body temperature or acid–base balance or electrolyte disturbances can potentiate or antagonize the actions of paralytics.[1,13-16]

Barbiturate Coma

Although controversial, induced barbiturate coma has been documented as increasing survival and decreasing morbidity, particularly in patients with refractory or intractable elevation in ICP. Barbiturates suppress seizure activity and reduce cerebral metabolic activity and cerebral oxygen demand.

MECHANISM OF ACTION

The mechanism by which ICP is reduced in barbiturate coma has not been established firmly. Barbiturates affect CBF, $CMRO_2$, electroencephalogram (EEG), and systemic hemodynamics. Reductions of approximately 50% have been documented in CBF and $CMRO_2$. The reduction in CBF requirements decreases cerebral blood volume, decreasing ICP. The barbiturate appears to have a direct, restrictive effect on cerebral vasculature, diverting small amounts of the blood from well perfused areas to ischemic areas, thereby improving cerebral pressure and collateral circulation. Vascular spasms are reduced, improving CBF. It lowers the systemic BP, thereby decreasing blood–brain barrier disruption. Effects of noxious stimuli, such as ICU noise, are blunted, and patients are more tolerant of positioning and suctioning. The total muscle relaxation and immobilization reduce cerebral venous pressure. Both BP and ICP become less labile.

INDICATIONS

Criteria vary extensively. Barbiturate coma may be initiated in head-injured patients with a GCS score of 7 or less and in whom the ICP reaches 25 mmHg for longer than 10 minutes with the patient at rest while being treated with hyperventilation, steroids, mannitol, and CSF drainage.

PROCEDURE

Before administration of the barbiturate (usually pentobarbital [Nembutal]) or thiopental [Pentothal]), ICP, BP, pulmonary artery pressure, and electrocardiogram monitoring with assisted ventilation are initiated. Baseline EEG and BAER recordings are taken. An EEG is taken before initiation of barbiturate coma so that spontaneous electrocortical activity can be documented, and BAERs are recorded so that brain stem integrity can be assessed. Many ICUs are now using continuous electroencephalogram neurological monitors, or neuromuscular transmission monitors. The loading dose of pentobarbital is 5 to 10 mg/kg over 30 minutes, followed by 5 mg/kg IV for 3 hours, followed by a maintenance dose of 1 mg/kg/h IV until EEG burst suppression is documented.[17] The EEG pattern of burst suppression is the most commonly used method to establish barbiturate dosing. The initial loading dose may be supplemented with 200 mg IV for burst suppression. The EEG is used to titrate the barbiturates. Although high serum barbiturate levels will suppress electrocortical activity totally, BAER will remain as long as there is brain stem function. Because barbiturates are metabolized in the liver and excreted by the kidneys, impaired liver or kidney function will affect serum barbiturate levels.

Barbiturate serum levels are poor guides to therapeutic efficacy and systemic toxicity.

NURSING MANAGEMENT

The patient in barbiturate coma becomes dependent. Clinical neurological evaluation is almost impossible, making extensive, accurate monitoring of physiological responses to therapy mandatory. Artificial ventilation is required, and all vital functions must be maintained by the critical care team. Hypotension secondary to vasodilation is frequently seen, and a reduction in cardiac output may occur. Vasopressors should be available when barbiturates are administered for ICP control. One study indicated that vasopressor support was required in 95% of barbiturate-treated patients.[18] The patient is at risk for deep venous thrombosis, pulmonary embolism, hypostatic pneumonia, and infectious complications secondary to suppressed leukocyte and lymphocyte activity. Treatment of elevated ICP with high-dose barbiturates and mild hypothermia make it difficult to assess the patient for the complication of sepsis. Septic shock may be the first sign of sepsis recognized in the patient in barbiturate coma, adding the complication of hypotension to the morbidity associated with this intervention.

INDICATIONS FOR DISCONTINUING BARBITURATE COMA

Barbiturate coma should be discontinued if any of the factors listed in the accompanying display exist. The barbiturates are tapered gradually over 24 hours to several days. Arousal is gradual and prolonged, even after blood levels have been zero for several days. Patients must be weaned slowly and carefully from the respirator because of muscle weakness resulting from the therapy. The average length of treatment with pentobarbital coma is 72 hours.

Patients have vacuous facial expressions for several days despite normal blood barbiturate levels. Occasionally, during the first 24 hours, they have slow, abnormal movements that appear athetotic. Dysarthria is common. Anticonvulsants are used for control of withdrawal seizures. Status epilepticus has been reported.

CLINICAL APPLICATION:
Assessment Parameters
Indications for Discontinuing Barbiturate Coma

- Intracranial pressure (ICP) less than 15 mmHg for 24 to 72 hours
- Normal volume–pressure response (<3 mmHg/mL)
- Systolic blood pressure less than 90 mmHg despite the use of vasopressors, such as dopamine
- Lack of ICP response
- Progressive neurological impairment, such as deterioration of brain stem auditory evoked responses
- Abolition of the need for vasodilator therapy to reduce systolic blood pressure below 160 mmHg
- Cardiac arrest

Complications of Intracranial Pressure Devices Hemorrhage

- Intraventricular — 1.1%
- Subarachnoid bolts — 0
- Subdural catheters — 0
- Parenchymal — 2.8%
- Overall — 1.4%
- Hematomas* — 0.5%

*Significant hematomas requiring surgical evacuation.

Table 33-5 Bacterial Colonization by Intracranial Pressure Monitoring Site

Technique	Average	Range
Intraventricular	5%	0%–9.5%
Subarachnoid	5%	0%–10%
Subdural	4%	1%–10%
Parenchymal	14%	11.7%–16.6%

Surgical Decompression

Neurosurgical procedures are used for the management of subdural, epidural, and intracerebral hematomas; cerebral contusions; and injuries from penetrating objects. Intracranial mass lesions are evacuated as early as possible, usually with replacement of the bone flap, although for patients with cerebral edema, craniectomy may be used.[19]

COMPLICATIONS IN INTRACRANIAL PRESSURE MONITORING

The monitoring and management of ICP are not without risks. Complications of ICP monitoring include infections, hemorrhage, device misplacement, and inaccurate readings secondary to position or damping (see accompanying display and Table 33–5). There have been no reports of clinically significant intracranial infections in large prospective studies. Bacterial colonization of ICP devices increases significantly after 5 days of implantation and is treated by removal of the device. Irrigation of fluid-coupled ICP devices significantly increases bacterial colonization, with one study reporting an increased incidence from 6% to 19%.[2,3] Infection is the most common complication associated with ICP monitoring. Infections may increase patient discomfort, prolong hospitalization, and increase the cost of care. A central nervous system infection, such as meningitis, brain abscess, or ventriculitis, may cause permanent disability or death. Factors that affect infection rates include the type of device used, differences in patient population, definitions of infection, methods of data analysis, and duration of monitoring. Patients monitored for 5 days or less have a negligible incidence of infection.

It appears that intracranial complications do not significantly alter outcome in patients with severe head injury, whereas extracranial complications are often associated with an unfavorable outcome.

CONCLUSION

There is considerable variation in the management of ICP pressure. The measurement of ICP is useful in determining ischemia, cerebral herniation, and CPP. ICP monitoring is essential to the safe and effective management of intracranial hypertension, as demonstrated by the following:

- Successful ICP management and lower rates of morbidity and mortality
- Reduction of risks associated with the administration of drugs and therapies, such as hyperventilation
- Early warning signs of intracranial hypertension of herniation
- Accurate management of CPP

Hypothermia

CLASSIFICATIONS OF HYPOTHERMIA

Hypothermia (lowered body temperature) occurs when the core temperature is less than 35°C (95°F). Hypothermia may be classified as induced (therapeutic, protective–preserva-tive, prearrest, and intra-arrest), unintentional (accidental, inadvertent), or resuscitative (postinsult, postarrest). Severe unintentional or prolonged hypothermia is life threatening with death rates as high as 80% when body temperature falls below 34°C (93.2°F).[20,21] Conversely, hypothermia has the potential to be protective and resuscitative to the ischemic or traumatic brain and other vital organs.

Clinical Terminology: Hypothermia
(core temperatures)

Mild hypothermia	32°–35°C
	89.6°–95°F
Mild therapeutic hypothermia	34°–36°C
	93.2°–96.8°F
Moderate hypothermia	28°–32°C
	82.4°–89.6°F
Severe hypothermia	< 28°C
	< 82.4°F

Induced Hypothermia

Induced therapeutic hypothermia is the intentional lowering of a patient's body temperature, usually by heat exchange through a heart–lung machine or by surface cooling. Induced hypothermia is a well established method of preventing postischemic brain damage after total circulatory arrest for cardiothoracic surgery.[22,23] During the last 5 years there has been considerable research on the use of therapeutic mild or moderate hypothermia for the treatment of cerebral ischemia and traumatic brain injury to preserve central nervous system tissue and improve functional outcome.

Unintentional Hypothermia

Accidental hypothermia is a spontaneous decrease in core temperature to 35°C (95°F) or below in a cold environment. It is an acute problem most commonly seen with neonates; older adults; unconscious, immobile, or drugged people; and people who become exhausted in a cold environment, such as snowmobile riders, hikers, mountain climbers, and skiers.[24] Primary accidental hypothermia occurs in people with normal thermoregulation, overwhelming exposure to cold, and often in the presence of traumatic injury. In trauma patients, hypothermia is frequently associated with exposure to the environment, heat loss during initial clinical assessment, multiple transfusions of refrigerated blood products, and visceral exposure during prolonged surgical procedures.

Inadvertent hypothermia occurs to some degree in more than 90% of patients undergoing surgery.[25] When muscle relaxants, central nervous system depressants, and general anesthesia are used, the patient loses the natural ability to produce internal body heat. In addition, some anesthetic agents are potent vasodilators that may cause the body to lose heat through radiation and conduction, leading to hypothermia. One study also demonstrated that during standard external CPR of 5 to 60 minutes, 50% of the patients developed spontaneous mild hypothermia with tympanic membrane temperatures of ≤ 35°C (95°F). Tympanic and esophageal temperatures were similar.[22]

Resuscitative Hypothermia

The third type of hypothermia is resuscitative (postinsult) therapeutic hypothermia used to reduce secondary brain injury after cardiac arrest. A method for inducing rapid cerebral hypothermia for cardiac arrest victims is peritoneal cold lavage and head and neck surface cooling with ice bags.

▬ PHYSIOLOGICAL PRINCIPLES

Compensatory Mechanisms

The hypothalamus uses a complex feedback system in an attempt to maintain the body's core temperature between 36.8°C and 37.9°C (98.2°F–100.2°F), adjusting for environmental and physiological temperature changes. Imbalances between heat dissipation and heat production can lead to hypothermia. Heat loss may be secondary to conduction, convection, radiation, respiration, and evaporation.

When the body senses heat loss, muscles become tense, and vasoconstriction and shivering result. Shivering starts when the hypothalamic temperature reaches 36.5°C (97.7°F) and can cause the metabolic demand for oxygen to increase 400% above normal. The aerobic muscle activity associated with shivering can raise the body's metabolic rate fivefold.[25] Shivering increases myocardial workload, oxygen consumption, and carbon dioxide production, while decreasing glycogen stores, arterial oxygen saturation, and mixed venous saturation. Shivering can result in decreased cardiac output and oxygen transport to tissues.

Liver and pancreatic function are impeded with hypothermia, causing decreased insulin levels in the tissue and increased serum glucose levels. Renal blood flow decreases, which impairs glomerular filtration and leads to a rise in blood urea nitrogen and creatinine levels. Hypothermia causes physiological changes in all organ systems, with progressive depression of metabolic processes and nerve conduction, which may lead to death.

In a normal brain, hypothermia reduces the cerebral metabolic rate 7% with every 1°C (33.8°F) reduction in brain temperature.[22] At 30°C (86°F), a patient who is not shivering has a 54% reduction in brain metabolism, a 30% decrease in CBF, and a 20% decrease in brain volume.

Hematological Effects

Hematological effects of hypothermia include cold-induced diuresis, edema, and splenic contracture that can cause hemoconcentration with increased hemoglobin–hematocrit. Platelet counts drop as temperature decreases. Bleeding from a hypocoagulable state (hypothermic coagulopathy, disseminated intravascular coagulation) is a life-threatening complication of hypothermia.

Hypothermia-induced reversible platelet dysfunction, significantly prolonged activated coagulation time, and prolongation of activated partial thromboplastin time, prothrombin time, and thrombin time have been associated with temperature reductions, with a 15% decrease in thromboxane B_2 production for each 1°C (33.8°F) decrease in temperature.[26] Restoration of normothermia results in normal bleeding time and concentration of thromboxane B_2, the metabolite that constricts blood vessels and aggregates platelets at the bleeding site.[21,26]

Physiological Manifestations of Hypothermia

Because the critical care nurse usually is responsible for monitoring the hypothermic patient, the clinician must be aware of the physiological manifestations of the various phases of body cooling. The body's initial reaction to cold exposure is an attempt to conserve body heat and increase heat production. *Skin pallor* that occurs is due to a vasoconstrictor response that limits superficial blood flow and thus loss of body heat. Intense activity in the form of *shivering* occurs to maintain body heat. The effects of these compensatory responses will be reflected in the vital signs, and the nurse must understand these transient variations and consider them in evaluating the patient.

During the first 15 to 20 minutes of hypothermia induction, all *vital signs* increase, as shown in the display. Pulse and BP rise in response to the increased venous return produced by vasoconstriction. Respiratory rate increases to meet the added oxygen requirements of increased metabolic activity produced by shivering and to eliminate the additional carbon dioxide produced. If the patient hyperventilates with shivering, respiratory alkalosis can develop. The initial rise in temperature is a reflection of this increased cellular activity.

Because the patient requiring hypothermia usually has an existing cellular oxygenation problem, the increased oxygen consumption induced by shivering is undesirable. For this reason, chlorpromazine (Thorazine) may be given at the beginning of induction to reduce hypothalamic response. *Hypoglycemia* is a potential occurrence during vig-

orous shivering because increased glucose is required for the increased metabolic activity.

After approximately 15 minutes, the vasoconstrictor effect is broken by means of a negative feedback loop, and warm blood flow to the body surface is reestablished. This accounts for the reddened skin color after initial skin pallor. (This same phenomenon can be seen by holding an ice cube in the hand for a short period of time.)

As superficial warm blood flow is reestablished, body heat is lost, and body temperature begins to drop. Because blood cooled at the body surface continues to circulate through the body core, downward drift of the temperature usually continues for approximately 17.2°C (1°F) after the cooling blanket is turned off.

When the desired level of induced hypothermia is achieved, usually around 32°C (89.6°F), other physiological changes become apparent (Table 33–6). All the vital signs at this stage are diminished. The development of respiratory acidosis is a real possibility because at deeper levels of hypothermia, ventilation falls off more rapidly than does reduced carbon dioxide production. Also, with increasing hypothermia, the oxygen dissociation curve shifts to the left, and at lower tensions, oxygen is not released readily by hemoglobin to the tissues. Because of the developing circulatory insufficiency and increased metabolic activity due to shivering, metabolic acidosis also is a possibility.

Secretion of antidiuretic hormone is inhibited, and an increase in urine output may be noted with a drop in the specific gravity. During hypothermia, water shifts from the intravascular spaces to the interstitial and intracellular spaces. This results from movement of sodium into the cell

---

CLINICAL APPLICATION: Assessment Parameters
Physiological Reactions During the First 15 to 20 Minutes of Hypothermia Induction

Skin: Pallor
Motor activity: Shivering
Pulse: Increased
Blood pressure: Increased
Respiratory rate: Increased
Temperature: May increase initially due to increased cellular activity

---

RED FLAG

Table 33-6 Possible Complications of the Hypothermic State

Response	Possible Complications
Skin	
Decreased circulation, leading to crystal formation in cells	Fat necrosis
Vital signs	
Diminished	Respiratory acidosis Metabolic acidosis
Urinary output	
Increased	
Fluid volume	
Hemoconcentration	Embolization; hypothermic coagulopathies
Sensorium	
Fades at 34°–33°C (93°–91.4°F)	Increased difficulty in determining mental status
Hearing	
Fades at 34°–33°C (93°–91.4°F)	
Cardiac rhythm	
Myocardial irritability below 30°C (86°F)	Dysrhythmias

in exchange for potassium and movement of water with it. This fluid shift produces hemoconcentration.

Because all cellular activity diminishes with hypothermia, cerebral activity decreases, and hearing fades at approximately 34° to 33°C (93°–91.4°F) due to reduced cochlear response. At 18° to 30°C (82°–86°F), there is no corneal or gag reflex, and pulse irregularities may be noted as the result of myocardial irritability, which probably occurs because of the movement of potassium into the cell. Asystole usually occurs at 22° to 24°C (71.6°–75.2°F). Ventricular fibrillation is a common occurrence at 28° to 30°C (82°–86°F). Defibrillation of patients with temperatures below 28° to 30°C (82.4°–86°F) usually is unsuccessful. Many dysrhythmic, hypothermic patients will convert automatically to a sinus rhythm at a core temperature above 30°C (86°F).

EQUIPMENT FEATURES

WARMING AND COOLING SYSTEMS

A variety of microprocessor-controlled systems are available for cooling and heating patients. In addition to the hyperthermia–hypothermia blanket systems, convective air-warming systems with an inflated warming tube and alarm system are available. Most commonly used with postoperative hypothermia, they provide a continuous flow of heated air to peripheral areas of the body. Convective warming therapy reduces the incidence of shivering.

TEMPERATURE DEVICES

For patients with hypothermia, the temperature of the blood circulating in the body "core" provides the best determination of the thermal state of the body. The continuous measurement of core body temperature is done with an esophageal temperature probe (most commonly in the operating room), pulmonary artery thermistor catheter, or urinary bladder thermistor catheter (temperature-sensing Foley catheter). Ear (tympanic, aural) thermometers set in the core mode are used for noninvasive measurements of intermittent core temperatures[27-29] (Fig. 33–8).

INDICATIONS FOR INDUCED HYPOTHERMIA

Induced hypothermia, lowering a patient's core temperature below 30°C (86°F), reduces metabolic and oxygen demands and protects the brain, heart, and other vital organs during low blood flow periods. This is the rationale for using hypothermia during open heart and neurosurgical procedures, in the presence of major organ ischemia, and following cardiac arrest.

After traumatic brain injury, rapid triage, early tracheal intubation, ICP monitoring, and in selected patients, the

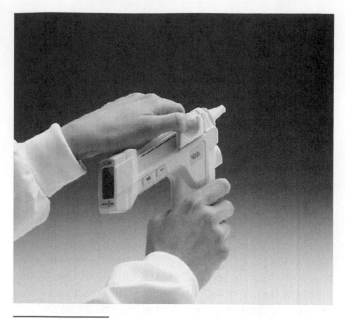

FIGURE 33-8
An infrared aural (ear, typanic) thermometer can be used to obtain intermittent core temperatures from the auditory canal. The ear thermometer offers a safe, fast, noninvasive method of measuring infrared emissions from the tympanic membrane, providing reflected core temperature readings within 1 second. (Welch Allyn Model 9000 Infared Aural Thermometer, courtesy of Diatek A Welch Allyn Company, San Diego, CA)

use of mild or moderate hypothermia and other techniques, such as combination treatments, including CBF promotion (hypertension, hemodilution, and normocapnia), have improved outcome. Prolonged moderate hypothermia can prevent or delay increases in ICP, reduce the cerebral metabolic rate for oxygen, and reduce the volume of the traumatic brain injury lesion. Complete functional recovery of the brain after cardiac arrest has been demonstrated with mild resuscitative (early postarrest) hypothermia 34°C (93.2°F).[30] Hypothermia has also proven beneficial with focal brain ischemia (stroke). Because hypothermia reduces the basal cerebral metabolic rate for oxygen, some feel it is more efficacious than barbiturates in ameliorating ischemic brain damage.[22]

PROCEDURES

Inducing Hypothermia

Although the method of inducing hypothermia will depend on the situation and the equipment available, essentially the three ways to proceed are surface cooling, the more direct method of bloodstream cooling, and peritoneal cold lavage.

Surface cooling, which involves the use of blankets that circulate a refrigerant, is the method usually used in ICUs. The cooling blanket, with a disposable cover, may be placed directly against the patient. The important point here is to avoid placing any degree of thickness between the patient and the blanket, because this will insulate and impede the cooling process.

When cooling is initiated, one blanket may be placed under the patient and another placed on top to hasten the cooling process. If a top blanket is used, exercise care in observing the patient's respiratory status because the weight of the cooling blanket may limit chest excursion. Keeping the blanket in contact with areas of superficial blood flow, such as the axilla and groin, also will expedite cooling. In the event that a cooling device is not available, apply ice bags to initiate the cooling process, using these same principles. In anesthetized patients, body surface cooling with refrigerated blankets or fanning requires 30 to 60 minutes to achieve an esophageal temperature of 32°C (89.6°F).

Bloodstream (core) *cooling* is the method used during open heart surgical procedures when the blood passes through the cooling coils in the cardiopulmonary bypass machine. Immediate cardiac arrest and flaccidity of the heart muscle is produced by injection of a pharmacological cardioplegic solution at 4°C (39.2°F).

Peritoneal cold lavage has recently been suggested for resuscitative (postinsult) hypothermia. It provides a rapid way to induce mild cerebral hyupothermia of 34°C (93.2°F) within 15 minutes when combined with surface cooling of the head and neck with icebags. The beneficial effects of this treatment have been confirmed in recent clinical studies. Peritoneal lavage is now carried out in approximately 80% of severely head-injured patients to rule out abdominal hemorrhage.[22]

Rewarming

Patients are rewarmed gradually to allow their bodies to adjust to shifts in temperatures. For patients who have undergone cardiac surgical procedures, the problems of obtaining postoperative normothermic temperatures may be compounded by compromised cardiac functions.

Rewarming techniques can be classified as external and core rewarming. External rewarming is recommended for patients with core temperatures of 30°C (86°F) or above whose cardiovascular function is adequate. Passive external rewarming includes warm (nonelectric) blankets and room temperature normal saline administered intravenously. Active core rewarming is recommended for patients with core temperatures below 30°C (86°F) or severe cardiovascular abnormalities. Following completion of a cardiac surgical procedure, the heat exchange in the cardiopulmonary bypass pump gradually rewarms the patient's blood. In addition, the temperature regulating blanket is usually set to 40°C (104°F) and the operating room temperature increased to 26.7°C (80°F).

In hypothermic cardiopulmonary bypass patients and trauma surgical patients, bleeding time and blood loss are reduced by rewarming. Maintaining the temperature of platelets and fresh-frozen plasma at 37°C (99°C) with a blood warmer during transfusion helps facilitate optimum function of blood products. Normal hemostasis requires the optimum platelet and clotting protein function that occurs during normothermia.

The patient with accidental hypothermia requires general supportive measures and specific rewarming techniques, including peritoneal dialysis; hemodialysis; warm air ventilation; irrigation of stomach, bladder, bowel, or mediastinum with warmed fluids; closed thoracic cavity lavage; and cardiopulmonary bypass with extracorporeal circulation. Peritoneal dialysis and cardiopulmonary bypass are recommended for severely hypothermic patients. Although hemodialysis can increase temperature more rapidly, peritoneal dialysis has the advantages of not requiring vascular access or the use of heparin for anticoagulation. Cardiopulmonary bypass is the most rapid method of rewarming but does not correct electrolyte and acid–base disturbances or remove drugs or toxins.[24] Rewarming facilitates optimum function of platelets and clotting proteins. For hypothermic patients in hemorrhagic shock, rewarming effectively restores both core and peripheral temperatures to normal and helps prevent the bleeding diathesis associated with ambient temperature-induced hypothermia.

▬ ASSESSMENT AND MANAGEMENT

The treatment and outcome of hypothermia are affected by length or type of exposure, nutritional status, infection, injury, age, state of health, and medication or intoxicant ingestion.

Cooling Phase

Reduction of body temperature is at best an unpleasant experience for the conscious patient. Adequate explanation and support for the patient and family are integral parts of nursing care.

In management of the patient undergoing hypothermia, a core temperature reading is required to determine the degree of hypothermia. Normal core temperature is 36.8° to 37.9°C (98.2°–100.2°F). SpO_2, SvO_2, or both are monitored using a pulmonary artery catheter to monitor arterial oxygen saturation and oxygen consumption.

Cardiac patients with low oxygen reserves may not be able to tolerate the decreased cardiac output and oxygen transport associated with shivering and may require measures to compensate for the increase in oxygen demands. Meperidine provides pharmacological treatment of shivering with minimal hemodynamic effects.

In the obese patient, a greater degree of downward drift may be experienced after removal of a cooling device. For this reason, the cooling device should be turned off before the desired hypothermic level actually is attained. Temperature must be monitored closely to determine whether the trend remains downward or whether an increase in temperature occurs, requiring use of the blanket again.

Skin care becomes particularly crucial due to the presence of cold and its circulatory effects. The clinician can change the patient's position to eliminate pressure points, taking care to move the blanket with the patient so that body contact is maintained with the cooling device. To prevent embolization secondary to hemoconcentration, nursing measures, such as passive range-of-motion exercises and frequent change of position, are initiated.

For the neurological patient who already has a depressed sensorium, other measures for evaluation of changes in the patient's level of response must be used, such as assessment of purposeful or nonpurposeful movements in response to painful stimuli and the degree of painful stimulus necessary to elicit a response.

Hypothermic Phase

The patient with mild hypothermia (32°–35°C, 89.6°–95°F) is intensely cold to the touch and is usually conscious but may be stuporous or confused. At temperatures below 32°C (89°F) consciousness levels deteriorate rapidly, and coma usually occurs below 30°C (86°F). BP becomes difficult to detect with noninvasive instruments, shivering ceases, and muscles and joints become rigid. Below 28°C (82.4°F), brain stem and deep tendon reflexes are not seen, and cardiac dysrhythmias begin, with a slowing of the heart rate and respirations. On arrival at the hospital, the patient with severe accidental hypothermia may have combinations of muscle stiffness, absence of pupillary reflexes, and minimal pulse and respirations. Because the brain and other organs are temporarily protected by cold hypometabolism, the development of asystole does not preclude survival. At this time, the myocardium can be extremely sensitive to mechanical irritation, and resuscitation methods may trigger ventricular fibrillation.[20] Noncardiogenic pulmonary edema caused by increased lung microvascular permeability has been associated with accidental hypothermia. Rising CSF pressure during rewarming has been associated with neurogenic pulmonary edema.[31]

When the patient with induced hypothermia has reached the desired therapeutic level, vital signs will level out at reduced values. Changes in vital signs therefore must be evaluated in light of the patient's hypothermic state. For example, if the nurse is caring for a neurosurgical patient cooled to 32°C (89.6°F) and if the vital signs have decreased (as would be expected), an increase in pulse, respirations, or BP to "normal" levels must be interpreted in view of the hypothermic state. Is an infectious process present? Are changes occurring in the patient's neurological status? Is ICP increasing?

Nursing measures should be performed gently, with a minimal degree of activity on the patient's part to prevent an increase in body heat, such as when providing passive range-of-motion exercises. The patient should be bathed with tepid or cool water to avoid increasing temperature in this manner.

Prevention of pulmonary problems in the hypothermic patient is dependent almost entirely on nursing care. Change of position allowing for postural drainage, measures to promote adequate ventilation, and suctioning to remove accumulated secretions all are extremely important in this patient.

Rewarming Phase

During the rewarming phase, the patient must be monitored closely for indications necessitating recooling. With the patient's normothermic status used as a baseline, these indications would include a fading sensorium, greater increase in pulse and respirations than normally would be expected with the warming process, and a drop in BP. Another important facet to be monitored is the cumulative effect of drugs given previously.

One of the hazards of artificially induced external rewarming is that the skin and muscles may be warmed before the heart. The heart remains in a cooled state and is unable to maintain sufficient cardiac output to meet the oxygen demands of the superficial areas. Further warming increases the dilation of peripheral vessels and blood pools, resulting in decreased circulating volume, decreased venous return, decreased cardiac output, hypotension, and a drop in core temperature (afterdrop). Core temperature may continue to drop up to 20 minutes after removal of the cold stimuli. Acidosis occurs as a result of the increase in metabolic activity in those areas already warmed and an insufficient circulation to meet the metabolic requirements of this increased activity. Oliguria also may result, probably because of antidiuretic hormone secretion.

With active core rewarming, warmed arterial blood from the central organs travels to the cold peripheral vessels and then returns to the heart and lungs significantly colder; thus, the core temperature drops. Combination methods of rewarming are used with some patients, such as cardiac surgery patients or patients with profound accidental hypothermia, to eliminate or minimize the problem of afterdrop.

Afterdrop is more prevalent in patients who undergo cardiopulmonary bypass procedures, older and young patients, obese patients, and victims of cold water immersion. This sequence of events can be avoided if the heart is warmed first, as in the bloodstream method, in conjunction with external rewarming or if the body is allowed to rewarm naturally.

■ COMPLICATIONS

Many possible complications are associated with induced and unintentional hypothermia. The surgical patient's risk of wound infection and prolonged surgical recovery are increased by the loss of nitrogen and protein associated with hypothermia. Hypothermia-related hypokalemia leads to cardiac and respiratory complications. Increased blood viscosity, decreased perfusion of vital organs, deep vein thrombosis, and pulmonary emboli are also associated with hypothermia.

Cumulative Drug Effects

Drugs tend to have a cumulative effect in the hypothermic patient. Decreased perfusion at the injection site and decreased enzyme activity result in slower chemical reactions. Therefore, the intravenous route is preferred, and intramuscular or subcutaneous injections should be avoided. If a drug must be given hypodermically, it should be given deeply intramuscularly, and vigilance must be maintained during the rewarming phase for cumulative effects. Prior to the administration of insulin, a patient should be rewarmed to a normothermic state to prevent rewarming hypoglycemia as insulin is ineffective at hypothermic temperatures.

Fat Necrosis

Another potential occurrence during hypothermia is that of fat necrosis. This results from prolonged exposure to cold and decreased circulation, which allows crystals to form in the fluid elements of the cells, leading to necrosis and cellular death. Nursing measures that can minimize fat necrosis include turning the patient frequently, massaging the skin to increase circulation, and avoiding prolonged application of cold to any one area.

■■■ TROUBLESHOOTING RELATED TO TEMPERATURE INACCURACIES

Temperature inaccuracies can be a problem in hypothermia management. In devices that use temperature as a control input, such as warming and cooling blanket units, the thermometer probe specified by the device's manufacturer should be used to ensure accuracy.

The tympanic membrane shares a common blood supply with the hypothalamus, making it possible to obtain accurate, intermittent, noninvasive core temperature readings with medical grade ear thermometers.

When using an ear (tympanic, infrared aural) thermometer for the measurement of intermittent core temperatures, the nurse must remember that within the ear canal, the temperature between the opening of the ear canal and the area of the tympanic membrane can vary by as much as 15°C (5°F). To eliminate false low readings caused

by ambient air at the opening of the ear canal, the thermometer probe should be positioned snugly to close off the ear canal (Fig. 33–9).

Urinary bladder temperatures reflect the temperature of arterial and venous blood in the periureteral tissues. Because the temperature of the urine is partially a function of urine flow, urine output should be measured when urinary bladder temperatures are used to monitor core temperature. Urinary bladder temperatures usually are slightly higher than pulmonary artery temperatures.

Pulmonary artery temperatures reflect the temperature of mixed venous blood and are considered true core temperatures. They are affected by inspired gases and are higher when the patient is shivering. Because shivering does not affect the temperature of urine, there is an increase in the temperature gradient between the pulmonary artery temperature and urinary temperature during shivering.

■■■ CONCLUSION

Induced hypothermia can be a life-saving therapy. Unintentional hypothermia, however, becomes a life-threatening condition requiring swift and knowledgeable interventions. A major challenge for the nurse is to interpret clinical changes in the hypothermic patient on the basis of the physiological effects brought about by hypothermia and during the rewarming phase.

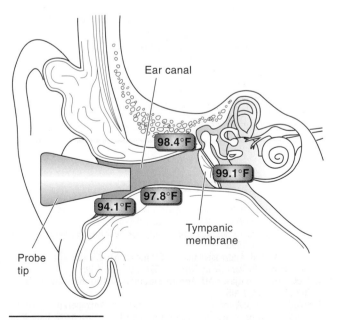

FIGURE 33-9

There is a temperature gradient of up to 5°F within the ear canal, with temperature lowest at the external opening of the ear canal and highest at the deepest portion of the ear canal near the tympanic membrane. (Courtesy of Diatek A Welch Allyn Company, San Diego, CA)

Clinical Applicability Challenges

Self-Challenge: Critical Thinking

1. *Identify ethical considerations related to safety, effectiveness, and cost containment in patient care and nursing practice for ICP monitoring.*

2. *Discuss the importance of accurate temperature readings in various classifications of hypothermia.*

Study Questions

1. *Initial treatment for increased intracranial pressure usually includes which of following?*
   a. *Craniectomy*
   b. *Induced barbiturate coma*
   c. *Pancuronium or curare*
   d. *Ventricular CSF drainage, mannitol, and hyperventilation*

2. *Nursing measures that may prevent or reduce intracranial hypertension include which of the following?*
   a. *Frequent suctioning with aggressive hyperventilation*
   b. *Flushing ICP lines q1h and PRN*
   c. *Elimination of extracranial causes of elevated ICP*
   d. *Frequent turning and repositioning*

3. *Continuous-flush devices are not used for ICP monitoring because*
   a. *a small increase in the volume of fluid in the cranial vault of a decompensated patient may initiate herniation.*
   b. *the infused flush solution is under too much pressure.*
   c. *ICP may be greater than 300 mmHg.*
   d. *of high infection risk.*

4. *A definition of shivering includes which of the following (more than one may be used):*
   1. *Is a compensatory response to maintain body heat*
   2. *Increases oxygen consumption*
   3. *Increases carbon dioxide production*
   4. *Can result in hypoglycemia*
      a. *1 & 2 only*
      b. *2 only*
      c. *2, 3 & 4*
      d. *all of the above*

REFERENCES

1. Chesnut RM: Medical management of severe head injury: Present and future. New Horizons 3(3):581–593, 1995
2. Ghajar J: Intracranial pressure monitoring techniques. New Horizons 3(3):395–399, 1995
3. Eddy VA, et al: Aggressive use of ICP monitoring is safe and alters patient care. The American Surgeon 61(1):24–29, 1995
4. McGrath BJ, Matjasko MJ: Anesthesia and head trauma. New Horizons 3(3):523–533, 1995
5. Bruder N, et al: A comparison of extradural and intraparenchymatous intracranial pressures in head injured patients. Intensive Care Med 21:850–852, 1995
6. Kelly DF: Steroids in head injury. New Horizons 3(3):453–455, 1995
7. Tietjen CS, et al: Treatment modalities for hypertensive patients with intracranial pathology: Options and risks. Critical Care Medicine 24(2):311–322, 1996
8. Tonnesen AS: Hemodynamic management of brain-injured patients. New Horizons 3(3):499–505, 1995
9. Newell DW: Transcranial Doppler measurements. New Horizons 3(3):423–430, 1995
10. Robertson CS, Cormio M: Cerebral metabolic management. New Horizons 3(3):410–422, 1995
11. Bullock R: Mannitol and other diuretics in severe neurotrauma. New Horizons 3(3):448–452, 1995
12. Clifton GL: Hypothermia and hyperbaric oxygen as treatment modalities for severe head injury. New Horizons 3(3):474–478, 1995
13. Lang EW, Chesnut RM: Intracranial pressure and cerebral perfusion pressure in severe head injury. New Horizons 3(3):400–409, 1995
14. Zellinger M: Paralytics and Sedatives in the ICU. Current Issues in Critical Care Nursing: 17–20, 1995
15. Prielipp RC, Coursin DB: Sedative and neuromuscular blocking drug use in critically ill patients with head injuries. New Horizons 3(3):456–468, 1995
16. Mirski MA, et al: Sedation for the critically ill neurologic patient. Critical Care Medicine 23(12):2038–2053, 1995
17. Wilberger JE, Cantella D: High-dose barbiturates for intracranial pressure control. New Horizons 3(3):469–473, 1995
18. Lee ML, et al: The efficacy of barbiturate coma in the management of uncontrolled hypertension following neurosurgical trauma. Journal Neurotrauma 11:325–331, 1994
19. Pieper DR, et al: Surgical management of patients with severe head injuries. AORN Journal 63(5):854–867, 1996
20. Wake D: Accidental hypothermia: A guide to treatment in the field. Nursing Times 92(3):32–33, 1996
21. Staab DB, et al: Coagulation defects resulting from ambient temperature-induced hypothermia. Journal of Trauma 36(5):634–638, 1994
22. Marion DW, et al: Resuscitative hypothermia. Critical Care Medicine 24(2):S81–S89, 1996
23. Kern FH, Greeley WJ: Cerebral perfusion and hypothermia. Can J Anaesth 42(11):959–963, 1995
24. Hernandez E, et al: Hemodialysis for treatment of accidental hypothermia. Nephron 63:214–216, 1993
25. Dennison D: Thermal regulation of patients during the perioperative period. AORN Journal 61(5):827–832, 1995
26. Valeri CR, et al: Effects of temperature on bleeding time and clotting time in normal male and female volunteers. Critical Care Medicine 23(4):698–704, 1995
27. Smith RN, et al: Comparison of temperature readings from infrared ear thermometers, electronic oral thermometers and core temperature techniques. Critical Care Medicine 23(1):838, 1995
28. Erickson RS, Meyer LT: Accuracy of infrared ear thermometry and other temperature methods in adults. American Journal of Critical Care 3(1):40–54, 1994
29. Erickson RS, Kirklin SK: Comparison of ear-based, bladder, oral, and axillary methods for core temperature measurements. Critical Care Medicine 21(10):1528–1534, 1993
30. Gisvold SE, et al: Cerebral resuscitation from cardiac arrest: Treatment potentials. Critical Care Medicine 24(2):S69–S80, 1996
31. Morales CF, Strollo PJ: Noncardiogenic pulmonary edema associated with accidental hypothermia. Chest 103(3):971–973, 1993

BIBLIOGRAPHY

Cruz J, et al: Cerebral blood flow, vascular resistance, and oxygen metabolism in acute brain trauma: Redefining the role of cerebral perfusion pressure? Critical Care Medicine 23(8):1412–1417, 1995

Marion DW, et al: Hyperventilation therapy for severe traumatic brain injury. New Horizons 3(3):439–447, 1995

McArthur CJ, et al: Gastric emptying following brain injury: Effects of choice of sedation and intracranial pressure. Intensive Care Med 21:573–576, 1995

Nurse S, Corbett D: Neuroprotection after several days of mild, drug-induced hypothermia. Journal of Cerebral Blood Flow and Metabolism 16:474–480, 1996

Walder AD, et al: The abbreviated injury scale as a predictor of outcome of severe head injury. Intensive Care Med 21:606–609, 1995

Ward JD: Pediatric issues in head trauma. New Horizons 3(3):539–545, 1995

Zhuang J, et al: Colloid infusion after brain injury: Effect on intracranial pressure, cerebral blood flow, and oxygen delivery. Critical Care Medicine 23(1):140–148, 1993

34

Head Injury

OBJECTIVES

Based on the content in this chapter, the reader should be able to:

- Identify possible mechanisms of head injury associated with trauma.
- Describe various types of head injuries and their associated symptomatology.
- Explain the pathophysiological process of potential patient problems resulting from head injuries.
- Discuss the rationale for medical and nursing management in the therapy of the head-injured patient.

*H*ead injuries (or brain injuries) are among the most devastating and lethal catastrophes in humans. In the United States, head injury is the leading cause of death and disability among children and young adults [1], occurring most often in the 15- to 24-year-old age group and occurring twice as often in men as in women. Approximately 2 million people in the United States receive head injuries each year. Of the 500,000 patients hospitalized each year with brain damage secondary to traumatic head injury, 75,000 to 100,000 die, and an additional 70,000 to 90,000 have lifelong disabling neurological dysfunction. Approximately 5,000 people develop epilepsy and 2,000 people remain in a persistent vegetative state.[2] The majority of head injuries are caused by motor vehicle crashes, followed by falls and assaults.[3]

The critical care nurse must understand the psychological and physiological changes that head-injured patients undergo in the acute care setting so that he or she can collaborate with the physician and other health care team members to focus on specific therapies based on the consequences of the patient's pathological condition.

Descriptive Terms

Multiple terms are used to describe or classify patients with head injuries. In earlier years, the terms "open" and "closed" and "coup" and "contra coup" were used. These terms are misleading if used to describe the degree of injury severity. An open head injury could be a scalp laceration or a bullet through the brain. A closed head injury could apply equally to a patient with a mild concussion or to one with diffuse cerebral edema. The terms coup and contra coup describe the location of most of the internal damage in relation to the site of impact. A coup injury causes most of the damage relatively close to the impact site, whereas in a contra coup injury, the damage is opposite to the site of impacting forces (Fig. 34–1).

The Traumatic Coma Data Bank is a multinational effort begun in 1979 to gather data about the frequency of head injuries, their classification, and the role of therapy on outcome. The severity of head injury now is defined by the Traumatic Coma Data Bank on the basis of the Glasgow Coma Scale score (Table 34–1). The terms minor, moderate, and severe head injury are useful in relating assessment parameters to therapy and outcome along a continuum of care. However, the reader should not be misled into think-

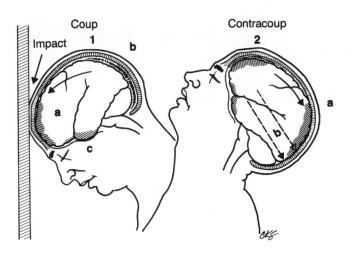

Mechanics of coup, contracoup

Coup _ _ _ _ _

Countracoup ----------

Impact point ◄

FIGURE 34-1
Coup and contrecoup head injury after blunt trauma. *1,* Coup injury: impact against object. *a,* Site of impact and direct trauma to brain; *b,* Shearing of subdural veins; *c,* Trauma to base of brain. *2,* Contrecoup injury: impact within skull. *a,* Site of impact from brain hitting opposite side of skull; *b,* Shearing forces throughout brain. These injuries occur in one continuous motion—the head strikes the wall (coup), then rebounds (contrecoup).

Severity	Description	Frequency
Minor	GCS 13–15 May have loss of consciousness or amnesia but for less than 30 min No skull fracture, cerebral contusion, hematoma	55%
Moderate	GCS 9–12 Loss of consciousness or amnesia for more than 30 min but less than 24 h May have a skull fracture	24%
Severe	GCS 3–8 Loss of consciousness or amnesia for more than 24 h Also includes those with a cerebral contusion, laceration, or intracranial hematoma	21%

TABLE 34-1   CLINICAL APPLICATION: Assessment Parameters
Categories Defining Head Injury Severity Based on Glasgow Coma Scale (GCS) Score

ing a minor head injury will result in minor or no problems for the patient. Such a patient may experience posttraumatic amnesia as well as memory problems that may significantly alter the patient's postinjury lifestyle.

PATHOPHYSIOLOGICAL PRINCIPLES

Mechanisms of Injury

The mechanisms of injury play a large part in determining the pathophysiological consequences of head trauma. An acceleration injury occurs when a moving object strikes the stationary head, such as in a missile injury or one from a blunt object. A deceleration injury is one in which the head strikes a relatively immobile object, such as an automobile frame or the ground. Both of these forces may occur together when there is sudden head movement without direct contact, such as that produced when torso position is altered violently and rapidly. These forces may be combined with rotational displacement of the head, causing stretching and shearing injury to the white matter and the brain stem.

A primary injury, occurring at the time of impact, may be due to bruising on the brain surface, laceration of brain matter, or shearing injuries or hemorrhage. As a result, secondary injury may occur as cerebral autoregulatory ability is diminished or absent in the injured areas. The consequences include hyperemia (increased blood volume) in areas of increased capillary permeability and arterial vasodilation, both leading to increased intracranial content and eventually to increased intracranial pressure (ICP). Some conditions, such as hypoxia, hypercarbia, and hypotension, may cause secondary brain injury. Hypotension is particularly detrimental, being associated with up to a 150% increase in mortality.[4]

Gennarelli and colleagues introduced the terms "focal" and "diffuse" injuries as categories of severe head injuries in an attempt to trace outcome more specifically.[5] *Focal* brain injuries result from localized damage, including cerebral contusions and intracerebral hematomas, and from secondary damage caused by expanding mass lesions, brain shifts, and herniation. *Diffuse* brain injuries are associated with more widespread damage and occur in four forms: diffuse axonal injury, hypoxic brain damage, diffuse brain swelling, and multiple small hemorrhages throughout the brain. These types of injury cause coma not by compression of the brain stem, but by diffuse injury to the cerebral hemispheres, the brain stem, or both.

Specific Head–Brain Injuries

SKULL FRACTURE

The arrangement of the layers of the skull along with the scalp help to dissipate energy from a head impact so that less force is transmitted to the brain surface. Nevertheless, skull fractures are common in severely head-injured patients, although the incidence varies from 12% to 80%, depending on the study reported. In general, children seem less susceptible than adults. Skull fractures occur in various patterns. *Linear fractures* are the most common, occurring in 70% of patients with skull fractures, and are caused by the application of forces over a relatively wide area of the skull.[6]

Basilar skull fractures may be limited to the floor of the skull or occur in association with fractures of the cranial vault, such as parts of the frontal or temporal bones. Fractures of the base of the skull are serious in that they may lead to contact between the cerebrospinal fluid (CSF) in the subarachnoid space and the air-containing sinuses of the face or skull. This communication may allow CSF to leak out through the sinus passages to the nose (rhinorrhea) or ears (otorrhea) and allow bacteria contained within the sinus drainage to contaminate the spinal fluid.

Depressed skull fractures are caused by forces driving bone fragments downward toward the brain deeper than the thickness of the skull itself. These fractures may be associated with scalp lacerations or with lacerations of the dura or brain.

CEREBRAL CONCUSSION

A concussion is a syndrome involving a mild form of diffuse brain injury resulting in temporary and reversible neurological dysfunction. There is usually loss of consciousness ranging from a few seconds or minutes to several hours. The classic presentation of mild concussion includes a brief period of disorientation and confusion, and the patient often exhibits retrograde amnesia (inability to recall events just preceding the precipitating event) or posttraumatic amnesia. Most patients recover completely and quickly, but a few develop postconcussive syndrome and may have continued symptoms, such as headache, inability to concentrate, memory problems, dizziness, and irritability. These symptoms may persist for up to 1 year.[6]

CEREBRAL CONTUSION

Cerebral contusion describes an area of the brain that is "bruised" without being punctured or lacerated. The bruise generally is on the surface and is composed of an area of small hemorrhage that is diffused throughout the brain substance in that area, rather than being in one discrete location. Cerebral contusion is the most frequently seen lesion after a head injury. The signs and symptoms of contusions vary, depending on the location and degree. There may be small, localized contusions resulting in focal neurological deficits, or larger areas may be involved. These larger areas may expand over 2 to 3 days after the injury and create widespread dysfunctions as a result of increasing cerebral edema. This larger contused area produces a mass effect seen on computed tomography scanning and may cause profound changes in ICP, raising the mortality rate to as high as 45%.

EPIDURAL HEMATOMA

Epidural hematoma is an accumulation of blood in the space between the inner table of the skull and the outermost layer of meninges, the dura (Fig. 34–2). Such hematomas

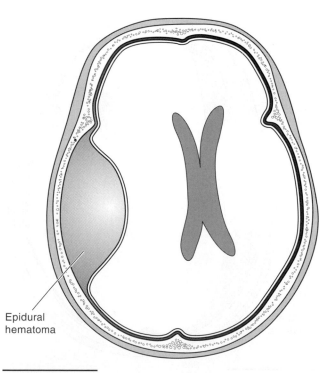

FIGURE 34-2
A large epidural hematoma showing the typical lenticular (lens) shape.

Epidural
hematoma

occur because of tearing of small branches of the middle meningeal artery or the frontal meningeal artery. Approximately 85% are associated with a linear skull fracture, usually of the temporal bone just in front of and above the ear, which disturbs the artery embedded in shallow depressions of the inner skull table. The incidence varies from 2% to 3% up to 9% in severely injured patients.[6] Approximately 33% of patients with epidural hematoma fall into what Lobato and associates described as the "talk and die" category.[7] The classic signs and symptoms include a brief loss of consciousness at the time of impact, followed by a relatively lucid period of minutes to hours. This "talk" period is then followed by rapid neurological deterioration from confusion to coma, from purposeful movement to decorticate or decerebrate posturing, and from equal pupils to anisocoria. These all are signs of rapid herniation and must be treated quickly to prevent the patient's death. Although the lucid interval is classic, it is important to remember that not all patients will exhibit the classic symptoms.

SUBDURAL HEMATOMA

A subdural hematoma is an accumulation of blood below the dural meningeal layer and above the arachnoid covering of the brain (Fig. 34–3). The cause usually is tearing of surface veins or dislodgment of pools of venous blood (called sinuses) that are found in this area. It often is associated with an underlying cerebral contusion from acceleration–deceleration or rotational forces of impact. Two adult patient groups in which this injury is seen more frequently are older adults and alcoholics. Both groups have in com-

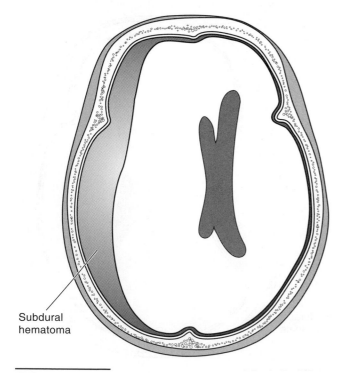

FIGURE 34-3
A large acute subdural hematoma covering the entire hemisphere and compressing the ipsilateral ventricle.

Subdural hematoma

mon frequent falls and some degree of cortical atrophy that puts the bridging vein structure leading from the brain surface under more tension. Although blood in the subdural space is common to all types, subdural hematomas are classified as acute, subacute, and chronic based on the time from injury to onset of symptoms.

Patients with acute subdural hematoma manifest symptoms within 24 to 48 hours after injury. The manifestations are those of an expanding mass lesion and rapidly increasing ICP and require immediate intervention. Patients with subacute subdural hematomas exhibit clinical symptoms from 2 days to 2 weeks after injury. The onset of symptoms is slower and often more innocuous than in acute hematoma. The patients usually do not deteriorate to the point of herniation or brain stem compression.

Chronic subdural hematomas occur from 2 weeks to 3 to 4 months after the initial injury. The initial hemorrhage may be quite small. Within 1 week or so after the hemorrhage, the clot develops a fibrous membrane that encapsulates it. Further expansion of the mass occurs with slow capillary leaking, causing symptoms once it becomes large enough to put pressure on surrounding structures. Common symptoms include headache, lethargy, confusion, seizures, and occasionally dysphasia. If surgical intervention is required in the case of hematoma expansion and worsening symptoms, a craniotomy usually is required to remove both the fibrous capsule and the "currant jelly–like" hematoma within. Drains may be placed in the bed of the hematoma, and after surgery, the head of the patient's bed may be ordered to be *flat* for the first 24 hours. This facilitates reexpansion of the brain, which may have been compressed for several weeks.

INTRACEREBRAL HEMATOMA

An intracerebral hematoma is a collection of 25 mL or more of blood within the brain parenchyma. It is difficult to distinguish radiographically from a brain contusion with bleeding deep within the brain substance itself. Traumatic causes include depressed skull fractures, penetrating missile injuries, and sudden acceleration–deceleration movements. Treatment of patients with intracerebral hematomas is controversial as to whether surgery is indicated or medical management is the best course. In general, surgical intervention is used only if the lesion is continuing to expand and causing further neurological deterioration.

Impairments

BREATHING PATTERNS

Because the neurophysiology of respiration is so complex, a neurological insult can produce problems at any number of levels. Numerous locations in both cerebral hemispheres regulate voluntary control over the muscles used in breathing, with the cerebellum synchronizing and coordinating the muscular effort. The cerebrum also has some control over the rate and rhythm of respiration. Nuclei in the pons and midbrain areas of the brain stem regulate the automaticity of respiration. Cells in these areas are responsive to small changes in pH and oxygen content of surrounding blood and tissues.

These centers can be injured by elevated ICP, hypoxia, interruption of blood supply, or direct trauma. Cerebral trauma that alters the level of consciousness usually results in alveolar hypoventilation due to shallow respirations. These factors ultimately can lead to respiratory failure, which accounts for a high mortality rate among head-injured patients. Different respiratory patterns can be identified when there is a dysfunction in a correlating intracranial area (Fig. 34–4).

Cheyne-Stokes breathing is periodic breathing in which the depth of each breath increases to a peak and then decreases to a state of apnea. The hyperpneic phase usually lasts longer than the apneic phase. Cheyne-Stokes breathing patterns may be a normal result of aging when they occur in an older person during sleep. The pattern also may be seen with bilateral lesions located deep in the cerebral hemispheres. With traumatic brain injury, the onset of Cheyne-Stokes breathing might be due to herniation of the cerebral hemispheres through the tentorium, indicating a deteriorating neurological condition. This herniation also can cause compression of the midbrain, and *central neurogenic hyperventilation* will be observed. This hyperventilation is sustained, regular, rapid, and fairly deep. It usually is caused by a lesion above the midbrain.

Apneustic breathing is characterized by respiration with a long pause at full inspiration or full expiration. The etiology of this pattern is loss of all cerebral and cerebellar control of breathing, with respiratory function at a brain stem level only.

Cluster breathing may be seen when the lesion is high in the medulla or low in the pons. This pattern of respiration is seen as gasping breaths with irregular pauses.

The critical centers of inspiration and expiration are located in the medulla oblongata. Any rapidly expanding intracranial lesion, such as cerebellar hemorrhage, can compress the medulla, and *ataxic breathing* will result. This is totally irregular breathing consisting of both deep and shallow breaths associated with irregular pauses. When this pattern of respiration occurs, a ventilator should be available because neither adequate respiratory rhythm nor continuation of respiratory effort can be predicted.

Interference with some cranial nerves also can influence respiration. The brain stem centers receive information from chemoreceptors in the carotid artery and aorta and from stretch receptors in the lungs by way of the glossopharyngeal (IX) and the vagus (X) nerves. Outgoing information from the brain stem then travels by way of the phrenic nerve, which leaves the spinal cord with the third cervical nerve and activates the diaphragm. The intercostal muscles that expand the chest wall are activated by the intracostal nerves of the thoracic spinal cord.

PHYSICAL MOBILITY

A major result of severe brain injury can be its effect on body movement. Hemiparesis or hemiplegia may occur as a result of damage to the motor areas of the brain. In addition, the patient may have voluntary control over movements yet encounter difficulties in self-care and daily living related to abnormal posturing, spasticity, or contractures. Nursing interventions should be based on an assessment of the patient's motor functioning and impact on living patterns.

Voluntary movement occurs as a result of the synapsing of two large groups of neurons. Nerve cells in the first group originate in the posterior portion of each frontal lobe, called the precentral gyrus, or motor strip. Axons from these

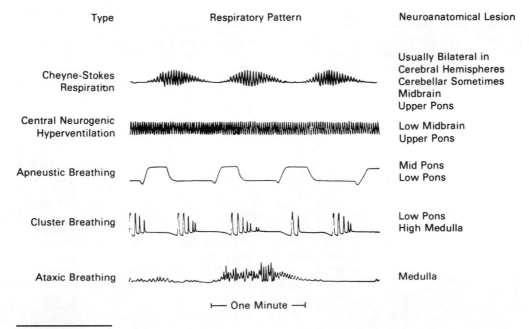

FIGURE 34-4
Respiratory patterns in neurological dysfunctions.

"upper" motor neurons terminate either in the brain stem or in the anterior gray horns at various levels in the spinal cord. Here they synapse with "lower" motor neurons, which travel from the brain stem or spinal cord to specific muscles. Each of these neuron groups transmits particular information on movement. Thus, the patient will exhibit specific symptoms if either of these two neuron pathways is injured (Table 34–2).

With bilateral hemispheric dysfunction or with dysfunction at the brain stem level, there is loss of cerebral inhibition of involuntary movements. There are disorders of muscle tone and the appearance of abnormal postures, which, in time, can create complications such as increased spasticity and contractures.

HYDRATION BALANCE

Nearly all severely head-injured patients have a problem with maintenance of a balanced hydration state. For some, it is a self-limiting response to the stress of trauma. In a physiological stress state, more antidiuretic hormone (ADH) and more aldosterone are produced, resulting in fluid and sodium retention. The process usually reverses itself within a day or two when diuresis occurs.

In some patients with neurological trauma—especially those with skull fractures, damage to the pituitary or hypothalamus, or elevated ICP—the clinical picture may be complicated by *diabetes insipidus*. In this condition, there is a dysfunction in the production and storage of ADH, with a subsequent decrease in the amount of ADH present in the blood. Without ADH, the kidneys excrete too much water, leading to dehydration. The same cerebral pathological condition sometimes leads to an opposite problem of ADH being produced in excess of the body's needs. This *syndrome of inappropriate ADH* (*SIADH*) is characterized by fluid retention and consequent hemodilution (Table 34–3). See Chapter 43 for a discussion of SIADH and diabetes insipidus.

SWALLOWING

Adequate nutrition plays a primary role in recovery from illness and often is neglected. A state of catabolism and negative nitrogen balance is a common finding in head-injured patients. Standard intravenous solutions generally are inadequate to prevent this problem. In addition, the body's demand for energy and substrates for repair and growth can cause breakdown of body proteins at an accelerated rate.

The acts of chewing and swallowing are integrated at the brain stem level through a complex feedback system involving multiple motor and sensory branches of several cranial nerves. For the most part, this is a reflex response to the presence of something in the mouth and pharynx. Higher centers in the cerebral cortex, cerebellum, and basal ganglia participate in the speed and coordination of this reflex.

Swallowing is a three-stage process that begins with placement of food in the mouth. Solids are masticated and mixed with saliva to a softer consistency. In the oral stage, the tongue controls a bolus of food or liquid by pressing it against the soft palate and forming a seal around it

---

TABLE 34-2

A Comparison of Upper and Lower Motor Neuron Function

Neuron	Pathway/Names	Functions	Signs of Dysfunction
Neuron group 1, or "upper" motor neurons	From motor area of cerebral cortex to brain stem (corticobulbar tracts) or to spinal cord (corticospinal tracts)	Carries commands for voluntary movement of specific body parts Carries inhibition commands to control the response of the next neuron pathway	Loss of voluntary muscle control Loss of inhibition of lower motor neurons, resulting in: 　Preservation of reflex arcs 　Pathological reflex responses 　Spastic muscles 　Increased muscle tone 　Little or no muscle atrophy
Neuron group 2, or "lower" motor neurons	From brain stem or spinal cord to specific muscle groups; names end in the word "nerve" (eg, femoral nerve, radial nerve)	Relays commands from the upper motor neurons to effect voluntary muscle movement Forms the effector response branch of the reflex arc	Loss of voluntary muscle movement No reflex arc activity, resulting in: 　Flaccid muscles 　No pathological reflex responses 　Decreased muscle tone 　Significant muscle atrophy

TABLE 34-3
Comparison of Diabetes Insipidus (DI) and the Syndrome of Inappropriate Antidiuretic Hormone (SIADH)

	DI	SIADH
Clinical manifestations	Increased thirst drive in the awake patient Polyuria, usually more than 5 L/d Urine specific gravity 1.001 to 1.005 Volume depletion, as evidenced by slightly elevated hematocrit and serum sodium levels	Lethargy and confusion, leading to coma and seizures Decreased urine output, usually less than 500 mL/d Urine specific gravity usually greater than 1.025 Hemodilution, as evidenced by decreased hematocrit and hyponatremia
Medical therapy	Appropriate oral or intravenous fluid replacement or both Supplemental ADH therapy using injectable vasopressin (Pitressin) or nasal spray solutions of desmopressin (DDAVP)	Fluid restriction Furosemide diuretics Drug therapy with demeclocycline hydrochloride (Declomycin), which blocks the effect of ADH on the kidney

(Fig. 34–5A). There is a respiratory pause on inspiration as the larynx moves up and forward to close and protect the airway. The seal around the bolus is broken as the soft palate elevates and closes the nasopharynx to prevent nasal regurgitation.

In the pharyngeal stage, with the soft palate elevated and the airway occluded, the tongue propels the bolus back against the posterior pharyngeal wall (Fig. 34–5B). The muscles of the pharynx contract sequentially to move the bolus downward, forcing the epiglottis closed over the tra-

cheal opening (Fig. 34–5C). The cricopharyngeal sphincter relaxes and opens in the esophageal stage as the bolus of food enters the esophagus (Fig. 34–5D). Waves of peristalsis carry the bolus downward toward the stomach.

Disorders of the motor and sensory areas of the cerebral hemispheres impair the ability to detect the presence of food in the affected side of the mouth and to manipulate it by cheek and tongue movements. In addition, the brain stem reflexes of swallowing may be either hyperactive or di-

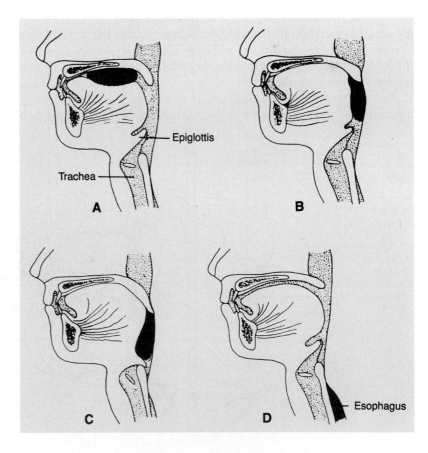

FIGURE 34-5
Stages of normal swallowing or deglutition: (**A**) oral; (**B** and **C**) pharyngeal; and (**D**) esophageal. (Mitchell PH, Cammermyer M, et al: Neurological Assessment for Nursing Practice. Reston VA, Reston Publishing)

minished to absent. The functional result is choking, ineffective or absent coughing, and aspiration of food or fluid.

COMMUNICATION

It is not unusual for the patient with cerebral trauma to present with a breakdown in the ability to communicate. This dysfunction is the most frequently occurring handicap in head-injured people. Such an impairment results from the combined effects of disorganized and confused language processing and specific aphasic disorders, if present.

Patients who have sustained injury to certain areas of the dominant cerebral hemisphere may evidence dysphasia, the loss of the ability to use language in some or all of its forms (Fig. 34–6). Language is the entire system of symbols that we learn as children to communicate efficiently with one another. This language system consists of the ability to interpret sounds as words, letters and numbers used to read and write to communicate without drawing detailed pictures, and the ability to produce certain sounds to convey thoughts to other people. Speech is merely the sounds made with the mouth to convey language.

▨ ASSESSMENT AND MANAGEMENT

Prehospital Treatment

In 1995, evidence-based guidelines for treating the severely head-injured patient were developed by a group of neurosurgeons supported by the Brain Trauma Foundation, the American Association of Neurological Surgeons, and the Congress of Neurologic Surgeons.[8] Figure 34–7 illustrates the decision making process in the prehospital treatment of the severely head-injured person.

The primary goals of resuscitation in the multiple-injured patient include treatments, such as massive fluid infusion, that can be in direct conflict with the traditional treatment of elevated ICP. Particularly in the prehospital setting where ICP monitoring is not available, there should be reasonable assurance that intracranial hypertension exists prior to initiating treatment to reduce ICP. Data supporting the detrimental effects of systemic hypotension far outweigh data supporting the efficacy of prehospital treatment of intracranial hypertension. Thus, there must be reasonable confidence that systemic hypotension will *not* result from any treatment modalities initiated to address *potential* intracranial hypertension.

Respiratory Care

The patient should be positioned on the side or in the coma position (Fig. 34–8). Care must be taken to avoid extreme neck flexion because both the airway and ICP may be compromised. An oral airway may be used to prevent obstruction of the upper airway by the tongue, although care must be taken not to stimulate the gag reflex. Frequent position changes or use of a rotokinetic bed will help prevent pooled secretions in dependent lung fields.

The nurse should assess the patient's respiratory rate and effort, skin color, breath sounds, and chest expansion. If an abnormality is encountered, arterial blood gases (ABGs) should be measured to evaluate the effectiveness of ventilation. When suctioning is required, the patient should be hyperoxygenated before, during, and after the procedure so that secondary brain injury due to hypoxia and elevated ICP is minimized. Care, however, should be taken not to excessively hyperventilate the patient during the process. Recent studies indicate that aggressive hyperventilation, particularly in the early stages of head injury, may be linked with ischemia and hypoxic secondary brain injury. Further studies are needed to differentiate between the effects of transient hyperventilation using bag-valve-mask and therapeutic hyperventilation using ventilator settings.[9,10] In ad-

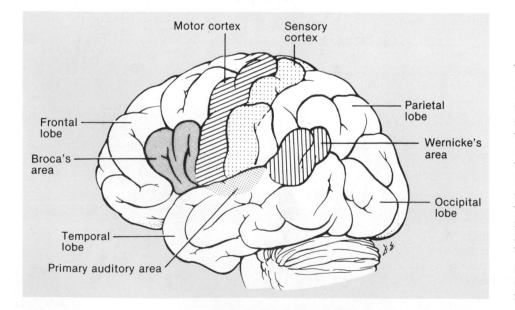

FIGURE 34-6

Cerebrocortical areas involved in communication. The frontal lobe contains the motor cortex, which controls voluntary movement, and the Broca's area, which controls the output of language. The primary auditory cortex and Wernicke's area, which control comprehension of spoken and written language, are located in the temporal lobe. The occipital lobe contains the primary visual area, which interprets written language and visual input.

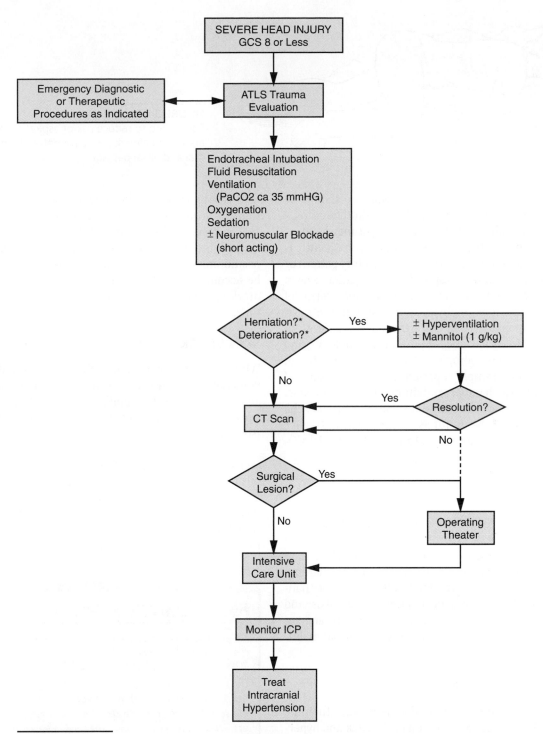

FIGURE 34-7

Flowchart for resuscitation of the severe head injured patient prior to ICP monitoring. *Presence of signs of herniation (pupillary dilation or motor posturing) or progressive neurological deterioration not attributable to extracranial factors. GCS, Glasgow Coma Scale; ATLS, advanced trauma life support; CT, computed tomography; ICP, intracranial pressure.

(Chestnut RM: Medical Management of Severe Head Injury: Present and Future. New Horizon 3[3]:583, 1995, with permission)

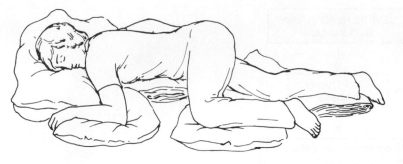

FIGURE 34-8
Positioning to reduce risk of aspiration. Shoulders are turned almost prone for better drainage of the oral and nasal passages.

dition, suctioning through the nasopharynx should be avoided in a patient with suspected basilar skull fracture.

The very critically ill head-injured patient may be managed initially on a ventilator. In such cases, it frequently is not possible to determine a particular respiratory pattern or a definite rhythm or rate of respiration of the patient's own. One technology that is useful in the ongoing monitoring of such patients is capnography. Capnography is the measurement and graphic display of the carbon dioxide level appearing at the airway entrance. A portable technology using infrared spectroscopy compares the amount of infrared light absorbed by a sample of patient gas to the amount of light absorbed in a chamber containing no carbon dioxide. This technology allows a continuous approximation of the alveolar CO_2 and can be useful as an early warning device that ABGs need to be monitored to maintain arterial CO_2 levels within the desired range.

Mobility

It is easier to "mold" a patient's posture and muscle tone early postinjury. Initial critical care management of the brain-injured patient is focused on life-saving rather than function-sparing activities. Attention to proper positioning, however, helps inhibit abnormal tone, allows for easier handling by the physical and occupational therapists and nurses who are helping the patient maintain full range of motion, and offers the best opportunity for normal mobility postrecovery.

ABNORMAL POSTURING

Most common in the brain-injured patient is opisthotonic posturing. This is a forward arching of the back and hyperextension of the head with all extremities rigid and straight or hyperextended. This posturing is exaggerated when the patient is supine. Trunk rotation and flexion of the lower extremities, such as that shown in Figure 34-9, will help break up this posturing. If the patient is left flat on the back with legs out straight, an increase in extensor muscle tone will be seen. Turning the hips to a side-lying position and flexing the knees will relax the tone.

Head positioning is important because of an asymmetrical tonic neck reflex. This reflex is demonstrated when the extremities on the same side to which the head is turned extend and the opposite extremities flex. Therefore, the nurse

who is attempting to do range-of-motion exercises on a tightly drawn-up arm should try turning the head to that side and see whether the muscle tone decreases.

Each brain-injured patient will have different reflexive positioning, and the nurse must evaluate what positions can be accomplished. The goal of effective positioning is to break up reflexive patterns and decrease abnormal muscle tone.

SKIN BREAKDOWN

With loss of motor function, the brain-injured patient is vulnerable to skin breakdown. The unconscious patient, and anyone who is immobilized, is prone to skin problems because of pressure, moisture, shearing forces, and diminished sensation.

One major rule must be followed to maintain skin integrity: prevent pressure. With current technology, numerous tools can help achieve this goal. Specialty beds distribute the patient's body weight evenly over the skin while giving support on a cushion of air, keep the patient in continual motion from side to side, or facilitate turning while maintaining body alignment. A variety of items may be

---

Insights into Clinical Research

Geraci EB, Geraci T: A look at recent hyperventilation studies: Outcomes and recommendations for early use in the head-injured patient. J Neurosci Nurs 28(4):222–233, 1996

During the past decade, mounting controversy surrounding the use of hyperventilation for the treatment of head injury has raised concerns about its safety and therapeutic benefits. A recent investigation of the medical literature was conducted to determine if outcomes for the head-injured patient continued to support the use of indiscriminate, and often unmonitored, hyperventilation in the prehospital and early hospital phases of care. Another goal was to determine if current investigators are recommending the use of hyperventilation for the initial treatment of all unconscious head-injured patients. Findings suggest that early head-injured patients in the prehospital and early phases of care are at increased risk for suffering hyperventilation-induced secondary brain injury. Researchers are now recommending a highly monitored, cautious, and selective approach to care; this investigation calls the current practice into question.

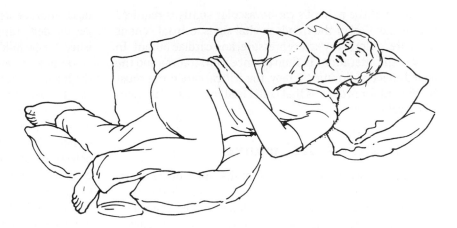

FIGURE 34-9
Positioning to relax extensor muscle tone in brain-injured patients. This position uses trunk rotation and lower extremity flexion to relax abnormal muscle tone.

placed on the bed to make pressure less of a problem. These items include alternating pressure air mattresses, water mattresses, gel pads, and sheepskin. The fact remains, however, that pressure sores can develop over time in any immobile patient who is not turned regularly. Each patient must be evaluated individually as to skin tolerance (how fast the skin turns red without the patient being turned). The average skin-pressure tolerance time for an acutely ill patient is less than 2 hours.

Padding above and below prominent bony processes also helps prevent pressure problems. For example, when the patient is on the side, the nurse can place a rectangular foam pad or small pillow above and below the hip trochanter, above the lateral malleolus of the ankle, and between bony pressure points, such as the knees (Fig. 34–10A). The nurse should place a hand under the bony processes to confirm that pressure has been relieved. When the patient is on his or her back, the nurse should place a pad above and below the sacrum and above the heels, as shown in Figure 34–10B. Circular pads called "doughnuts" actually may impair circulation by causing circular pressure around the protected area. Use of rectangular pads al-

lows for collateral circulation while relieving pressure. The pads should be made of firm, open-cell foam rather than rolled towels or blankets. They should be soft enough to redistribute the patient's weight evenly over a large area. Rolled towels or blankets apply pressure to a narrow section of skin only and are not recommended.

Skin massage with lotion is helpful in stimulating circulation to a pressure area, but the skin should be dried carefully because moisture can lead to irritation.

Another prime cause of breakdown in skin integrity is the shearing effect of linen against skin. A lift sheet (folded draw-sheet or bath blanket) should be used to maneuver the patient in the bed. To shield the patient's elbows and heels, soft foam or sheepskin protectors should be used.

Hydration

Accurate measurement of intake and output and evaluations of changes in weight from day to day are essential to the assessment of fluid balance. The nurse also should assess the patient's skin and mucous membranes for drying and cracking, which predispose to further injury. Close ob-

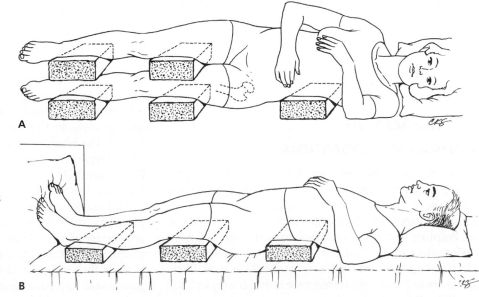

FIGURE 34-10
Positioning the patient in bed. (**A**) Side-lying position. Pads are used above and below the trochanter and lateral malleolus to relieve pressure. (**B**) Supine position. Pads are used above and below the sacrum and above the heels to relieve pressure. A pad above the knees prevents hyperextension of the knees and relieves pressure on the popliteal space.

servation of the patient's cardiovascular status is required with evaluation of the trends in vital signs, central venous pressure, pulmonary artery pressure, and cardiac output. In view of the alterations in fluid balance from trauma and the added effect of diuretic therapy, the critical care nurse must be vigilant for problems that could lead to a secondary neurological injury.

Initiation of Oral Intake

Nursing literature supports the fact that inadequate nutrition is a risk for the head-injured patient. A 12% loss in body weight is not uncommon and is related to the hypermetabolic and catabolic state. Not all physicians, however, begin early feeding of head-injured patients. Some feel that early implementation of enteral or parenteral feeding may make it more difficult to control elevated ICP.[6]

Factors to consider before initiating oral feedings include the patient's ability to swallow, respiratory status and method of airway management, and the strength of cough. After oral feedings resume, the nurse continually evaluates the possible need to discontinue the feedings. Indications for discontinuation include signs and symptoms of aspiration pneumonia (including right lower lobe infiltration, increased right lower lobe sounds after feeding, or sudden temperature spike) or other complications that require priority treatment.

Elimination

Monitoring the acute head-injured patient for bowel or bladder problems may seem of low priority in the intensive care unit (ICU). It is the nurse at the bedside, however, who may first become aware of changes in frequency, amount, or characteristics of urine or stool. Such changes may be an indication of hydration problems, medication intolerance, or even previously undetected physical injury. The urinary catheter may have been inserted in the emergency department during resuscitation in less than sterile conditions, and the Foley catheter should not be forgotten as a potential source of infection.

Bowel and bladder retraining are seldom initiated in the ICU, but it is an important part of the patient's rehabilitation process.

Communication

DYSPHASIA AND DYSARTHRIA

Many brain-injured patients have difficulty using or understanding language (dysphasia) as a result of their injury. When communicating with a dysphasic patient, it is best to use simple language with clear gestures and environmental cues. Pointing to the desired object, tone of voice, facial expression, time of day, and hospital routine contributes to understanding. A normal tone of voice should be used. Such patients are not deaf (unless they were before the injury) but have difficulty understanding the meaning of what they

hear. Short sentences should be used; the patient may forget the beginning of a long sentence by the time it is finished. "Baby talk" is not appropriate.

Dysphasic patients quickly become adept at "filling in the blanks" when they do not understand completely. It is easy to overestimate their level of auditory comprehension and to assume that the patient understands everything being said. It is important to check this level of understanding fairly. The nurse should ask the patient to point to objects in the room, being careful not to nod or point in the correct direction. This often is difficult to do, because we all use gestures naturally. The questions that are asked of patients should be modified because the patient will learn quickly what responses are expected. Not only is getting a clear picture of the level of understanding important clinically, but it also will decrease frustration and confusion for the staff. Patients may be labeled as uncooperative, cross, or irrational when staff members believe patients understand but the patients behave as if they do not.

Other brain-injured patients may develop dysarthria, a group of speech disorders resulting from disturbances in muscular control of the speech mechanism (weakness, slowness, poor coordination, or altered muscle tone) due to damage to the central or peripheral nervous system. Motor processes of speech that may be affected include respiration, phonation, resonance, and articulation. These patients are also likely to have swallowing difficulties because of muscle weakness or poor coordination.

Patients who are difficult to understand because of slurred, dysarthric speech should be encouraged to reduce their rate of speaking and to "overemphasize" speech movements. They may need to use an alphabet board, a simple communication board, or a felt pen on a white board to communicate. The nurse may need to try several communication methods to allow the patient to communicate his or her needs successfully.

INAPPROPRIATE BEHAVIOR RESPONSES

Neurological damage does not occur without effecting some change in a person's behavior response. The personality and entire characteristic behavior pattern will undergo some changes, either temporary or permanent, depending on the locus and severity of the injury.

Cognition involves the ability to perceive, integrate, and interpret both internal and external environmental stimuli appropriately. In this way, behavior is regulated and controlled. The brain-injured patient will perceive, integrate, and interpret the surroundings in a disorganized fashion. Consequently, behavioral response can seem inappropriate, confused, hostile, or apathetic. Nursing assessment of the patient's cognitive abilities will aid in formulating the best way to approach a brain-injured patient at various stages during recovery (Table 34–4). During the early stages of recovery, patients may be unable to respond to any stimulation. As they progress, they may eventually respond in a generalized way. An example is when the nurse moves the patient's arm to position the blood pressure cuff, and the pa-

TABLE 34-4   CLINICAL APPLICATION: Nursing Intervention Guidelines
Cognitive Behavior Levels of Brain-Injured Patients and Nursing Considerations

Cognitive Behavior Level	Nursing Considerations and Interventions
1. *No response* to any stimuli occurs. 2. *Generalized response:* Stimulus response is inconsistent, limited, nonpurposeful with random movements or incomprehensible sounds. 3. *Localized response:* Responses to stimuli are specific but inconsistent. Patient may withdraw or push away, may make sounds, follow some simple commands, or respond to certain family members.	Levels 1, 2, and 3 • Assume that patient can understand all that is said. Converse *with* not *about* the patient. • Do not overwhelm the patient with talking. Leave some moments of silence between verbal stimuli. • Manage the environment to provide only one source of stimulation at a time. If talking is taking place, the radio or TV should be off. • Encourage the family to provide short, random periods of sensory input that is meaningful to the patient. A favorite TV program, or tape recording or 30 min of music from the patient's favorite radio station will provide more meaningful stimulation than constant radio accompaniment, which becomes as meaningless as the continual bleep of the cardiac monitor.
4. *Confused–agitated:* Response is primarily to internal confusion with increased state of activity; behavior may be bizarre or aggressive; patient may attempt to remove tubes or restraints or crawl out of bed; verbalization is incoherent or inappropriate; patient shows minimal awareness of environment and absent short-term memory.	Level 4 • Be calm and soothing when handling the patient. Approach with gentle touch to decrease the occurrence of defensive emotional and motor reflexes. • Watch for early signs that the patient is becoming agitated (eg, increased movement, vocal loudness, resistance to activity). • When the patient becomes upset, do not try to reason with him or "talk him out of it." Talking will be an additional external stimulus that the patient cannot handle. • If the patient remains upset, either remove him from the situation or remove the situation from him.
5. *Confused, inappropriate, nonagitated:* Patient is alert and responds consistently to simple commands; has short attention span and easily distracted memory impaired with confusion of past and present events; can perform previously learned tasks with maximal structure but is unable to learn new information; may wander off with vague intention of "going home." 6. *Confused–appropriate:* Patient shows goal-directed behavior but still needs external direction; can understand simple directions and reasoning; follows simple directions consistently and requires less supervision for previously learned tasks; has improved past memory depth and detail and basic awareness of self and surroundings.	Levels 5 and 6 • Present the patient with only one task at a time. Allow time to complete it before giving further instructions. • Make sure that you have the patient's attention by placing yourself in view and touching the patient before talking. • If the patient becomes confused or resistant, stop talking. Wait until he appears relaxed before continuing with instruction or activity. • Use gestures, demonstrations, and only the most necessary words when giving instructions. • Maintain the same sequence in routine activities and tasks. Describe these routines to the patient and relate them to time of day.
7. *Automatic–appropriate:* Patient is able to complete daily routines in structured environment; has increased awareness of self and surroundings but lacks insight, judgment, and problem-solving ability.	Level 7 • Supervision is still necessary for continued learning and safety. • Reinforce the patient's memory of routines and schedules with clocks, calendars, and a written log of activities.
8. *Purposeful–appropriate:* Patient is alert, oriented, able to recall and integrate past and recent events; responds appropriately to environment; still has decreased ability in abstract reasoning, stress tolerance, and judgment in emergencies or unusual situations.	Level 8 • The patient should be able to function without supervision. • Consideration should be given to job retraining or return to school.

tient's entire body moves in response to the stimulation (see Table 34–4, cognitive levels 1 and 2). The therapy goal during these early phases of recovery is to help increase the brain-injured patient's awareness of self and the surroundings. *Coma stimulation* or *sensory stimulation* describe the approaches used to accomplish this goal.

One of the most common results of brain injury is an inability to screen incoming sensations to concentrate only on certain ones. For this reason, a planned approach of sensory stimulation will assist the patient in learning to attend selectively to the environment. Such an approach begins with selective stimulation of the basic senses of sound, sight, touch, and smell. The senses of taste and movement also may be included. Nursing interventions related to sensory stimulation are listed in the accompanying display.

DIAGNOSTIC STUDIES

Although head or brain injury may be suspected in any patient with an abnormal neurological examination, more definitive tests are required in many cases to verify and quantitate an injury. The diagnostic test most commonly performed on a patient with suspected head injury is a computed axial tomography scan of the head. This test is particularly useful when the patient exhibits behaviors that might also be attributed to the effects of drugs or alcohol. Magnetic resonance imaging (MRI) is being used increasingly as more facilities have such equipment available. Although an MRI can detect more subtle injuries, there are limitations in performing this test on a critically injured patient. Diagnostic cerebral angiography is more often used in the nontrauma patient. (See Chapter 32 for a thorough discussion of neurological diagnostic tests.)

COMPLICATIONS

Increased Intracranial Pressure

Potentially the most lethal complication of a brain injury is increased ICP. If not successfully treated, sustained ICP elevations may lead to brain stem compression or herniation and death. Traditional methods of treatment have included keeping the head of the bed elevated, limiting nursing interventions and treatments, decreasing stimulation, hyperventilation, steroids, sedation, mannitol or other diuretics, and the use of paralytics and barbiturate coma. Chapter 33 discusses these management modalities in depth for the treatment of elevated ICP.

Pulmonary Edema

A serious pulmonary complication of head-injured patients is pulmonary edema. It may be primarily neurogenic in origin or may occur with adult respiratory distress syndrome. Neurogenic pulmonary edema may result from an injury to the brain that causes the Cushing's reflex. An increase in systemic arterial pressure occurs as a sympathetic nervous system response to increasing ICP. This increase in vasoconstriction throughout the body causes more blood to be shunted to the lungs. Altered permeability of the pulmonary blood vessels contributes to the process by allowing fluid to move into the alveoli. The impaired diffusion of oxygen and carbon dioxide from the blood can lead to further increases in ICP (Fig. 34–11).

Seizures

Seizures occur in approximately 10% of head-injured patients during the acute stage. The risk of late seizures exceeds 30% for patients with penetrating head injury, intracerebral hematoma, subdural hematoma, depressed skull fracture or seizure within the first week of injury.[11]

The nurse should make preparations for the possibility of seizures by having a padded tongue blade or oral airway at the bedside and suction equipment close at hand. The bed side rails should be kept up. Padding the rails with pillows or foam cushions may minimize the risk of secondary injury from a seizure. During a seizure, the nurse should focus attention on maintaining a patent airway while observing the progression of seizure events and preventing further injury to the patient. If there is enough time before

---

CLINICAL APPLICATION: Nursing Intervention Guidelines
Sensory Stimulation

Sound

- Explain to the patient what you are going to do.
- Play the patient's favorite television or radio program for 10–15 min. Alternatively, play a tape recording of a familiar voice of a friend or family member.
- Another approach is to clap your hands or ring a bell. Do this for 5–10 sec at a time, moving the sound to different locations around the bed.
- During the program, do not converse with others in the room or perform other activities of patient care. The goal is to minimize distractions so the patient may learn to attend to the stimulus selectively.

Sight

- Place a brightly colored object in the patient's view. Present only one object at a time.
- Alternatively, use an object that is familiar, such as a family photo or favorite poster.

Touch

- Stroke the patient's arm or leg with fabrics of various textures. Alternatively, the back of a spoon can simulate smooth texture and a towel rough texture.
- Rubbing lotion over the patient's skin will also stimulate this sense. For some, firm pressure may be better tolerated than very light touch.

Smell

- Hold a container of a pleasing fragrance under the patient's nose. Use a familiar scent, such as perfume, aftershave, cinnamon, or coffee.
- Present this stimulation for very short periods (1–3 min maximum).
- If a cuffed tracheostomy or endotracheal tube is in place, the patient will not be able to appreciate this stimulation fully.

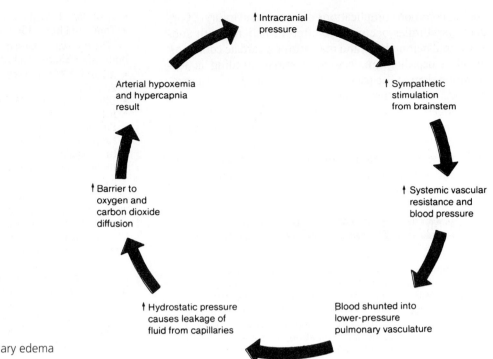

FIGURE 34-11
Mechanism of neurogenic pulmonary edema in brain-injured patients.

muscle spasticity begins and the jaws clench, a padded tongue blade, an oral airway, or a plastic bite stick should be inserted between the patient's teeth. This will prevent the patient from biting his or her tongue and will keep the airway clear. Nothing should be forced between the teeth, nor should the jaws be pried open. The patient should be turned to the side to allow secretions to drain or to be suctioned more easily. The person's movements should be restrained only enough to prevent hitting objects, causing bruising or injury.

The only medical treatment for seizures is drug therapy. Diazepam is the most widely used drug and is slowly given intravenously. Because the drug depresses respirations, the patient's respiratory rate and rhythm should be monitored carefully. Once the seizure has been terminated, the physician may order phenobarbital or phenytoin (Dilantin) to maintain seizure control. Because phenytoin is a cardiac depressant, the nurse should pay careful attention to the patient's cardiac rate and rhythm. This intravenous drug should be given no faster than 50 mg/min. Phenytoin may not be effective in preventing late seizures.[11] (See Chapter 35 for a full discussion of seizure disorders.)

Cerebrospinal Fluid Leak

It is not uncommon for some head-injured patients with a skull fracture to leak CSF from the ears or nose. This may result from a fracture in the anterior fossa near the frontal sinuses or from a basilar skull fracture of the petrous portion of the temporal bone. In either case, the fractured bone causes damage to the thin meningeal tissues that lie adjacent, allowing CSF to escape. Any clear drainage from the nose or ears of the trauma patient should be considered CSF

until proven otherwise. The presence of CSF can be detected by testing the clear, watery drainage for sugar using blood glucose test strips. Reagent strips designed to detect sugar in urine should not be used because the results may be misleading. CSF will be positive for sugar; mucus will not. Blood-tinged drainage should be collected on a sterile gauze pad and observed for the "halo" sign of blood surrounded by a clear or yellow-colored ring of spinal fluid. The presence of blood will make the results from blood glucose test strips inaccurate.

When CSF rhinorrhea or otorrhea has been detected, the drainage areas should not be cleaned, irrigated, or suctioned. A sterile pad may be placed under the nose or over the ear and should be changed when damp. The nurse must instruct the awake patient not to blow the nose or sniff and not to put a finger in the nose or ear. Drainage usually slows down quickly, and the dural tear closes without any problem.

Medical Complications

In addition to the preceding neurological complications, the recovery of a patient with severe head injury is adversely influenced by medical complications. The most frequent medical complications include disturbances of serum electrolytes, particularly serum sodium, which occurs in as many as 60% of patients, and pneumonia, which occurs in as many as 40% of patients, with aspiration pneumonia being the most frequently occurring. Endotracheal intubation protects the airway best against large particles entering the bronchial tree; gastric fluids still pose a risk to the patient. Hypotension occurs commonly in both the prehospital and inpatient setting (22%) and may cause secondary brain injury. Coagulopathies (18%) and septicemia (10%)

are less common complications of severe head injury.[12] Cardiac dysrythmias occur more often in patients with subarachnoid hemorrhage and may mimic a cardiac contusion on electrocardiogram. Gastrointestinal bleeding is less common than in the past, in part due to heightened awareness and vigorous prophylactic treatment.

Septicemia, nosocomial pneumonia, coagulopathy, and hypotension are associated with increased morbidity and mortality. Prevention or effective treatment of these major and frequent extracranial complications following severe head injury could reduce morbidity and mortality in this group of patients.[12]

CLINICAL APPLICATION: Patient Care Study

Sharon, a 17-year-old girl, was admitted to the intensive care unit (ICU) after a head-on automobile crash. She was a non–seatbelted passenger in the car driven by her boyfriend and was thrown about 40 ft from the car. The driver, who was wearing his seat belt, was uninjured. After skull and spine radiographs, computer tomography scan of the head and abdomen, and medical evaluation, Sharon's medical diagnoses were severe closed head injury with moderate cerebral edema, no intracranial bleeding, and probable basilar skull fracture.

The following medical orders were written:

- ICP monitor
- 25% mannitol, 1–3 g/kg IV PRN for ICP > 20 mm
- Notify MD if sustained ICP > 25 mm
- VS and neurological checks q30min
- Foley catheter to straight drainage
- NGT to suction
- HOB elevated 34 degrees
- Diphenylhydantoin 100 mg IV q8h
- Acetaminophen 650 mg suppository prn for temperature greater than 38°C (100.4°F)
- Hypothermia blanket prn for temperature greater than 38°C (101.3°F)
- Ventilator with settings of $FIO_2 = 0.5$; $V_T = 1200$ mL; IMV = 18; CPAP = 0
- End-tidal CO_2 monitor; maintain CO_2 26–34 mmHg

- IV of D5/0.2 NS at 50 mL/h
- Total fluid limit: 1500 mL/24 h

The following assessment data were obtained a few hours after Sharon's admission:

- ABGs: pH 7.32, CO_2 42 mmHg, PaO_2 60 mmHg, HCO_3 20 mEq/L
- BP: 180/68; P: 60; RR: 26; T: 39.2°C (102.5°F)
- ICP: 32 mmHg
- Pupils equal, 4 mm, sluggishly reactive
- No response to commands; assumes decerebrate posture to pain
- Breath sounds: rhonchi in upper lung fields; rales in both bases

An evaluation of the above data by the critical care nurse demonstrated several areas in which the patient needed immediate intervention. Sharon had impaired gas exchange related to neurogenic pulmonary edema, despite a respiratory rate suggestive of hyperventilation. This contributed to CO_2 retention, which, in turn, increased her ICP. The cerebral perfusion pressure is normal for now, because of systemic hypertension. Adding to the potential for secondary brain injury and increased cerebral edema is the elevated temperature and resultant increased cerebral metabolic rate.

Sharon was treated for about 1 week in the ICU, and then she was transferred to a progressive care setting specializing in the care of brain-injured patients. Approximately 3 months after injury, she was in a rehabilitation setting. Sharon was alert and able to respond to simple commands. Her speech was slow and slurred, but she was able to state her needs in single words and short phrases. She recognized her immediate family but had no memory of the accident or of events several weeks before it. Sharon progressed slowly on oral feedings because aspiration was still a risk, and the old tracheostomy site had not completely healed.

HOB, head of bed; V_T, tidal volume; IMV, intermittent mandatory ventilation; CPAP, continuous positive airway pressure

It is obvious that the care of the head-injured patient is both complex and demanding. The accompanying Collaborative Care Guide outlines the expected outcomes and nursing interventions associated with this clinical problem.

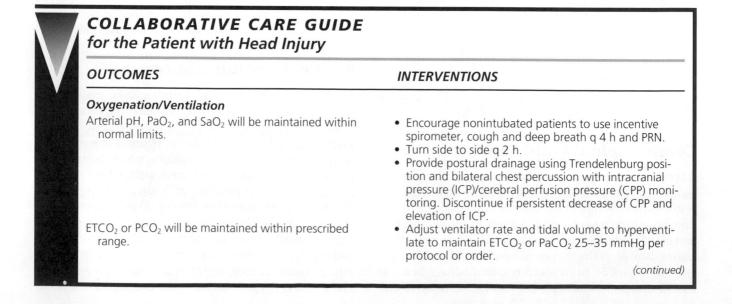

COLLABORATIVE CARE GUIDE
for the Patient with Head Injury

OUTCOMES	INTERVENTIONS
Oxygenation/Ventilation	
Arterial pH, PaO_2, and SaO_2 will be maintained within normal limits.	• Encourage nonintubated patients to use incentive spirometer, cough and deep breath q 4 h and PRN. • Turn side to side q 2 h. • Provide postural drainage using Trendelenburg position and bilateral chest percussion with intracranial pressure (ICP)/cerebral perfusion pressure (CPP) monitoring. Discontinue if persistent decrease of CPP and elevation of ICP.
$ETCO_2$ or PCO_2 will be maintained within prescribed range.	• Adjust ventilator rate and tidal volume to hyperventilate to maintain $ETCO_2$ or $PaCO_2$ 25–35 mmHg per protocol or order.

(continued)

COLLABORATIVE CARE GUIDE
for the Patient with Head Injury (Continued)

OUTCOMES	INTERVENTIONS
Patient will maintain a patent airway. Lungs will be clear on auscultation. There will be no evidence of atelectasis or pneumonia.	• Auscultate breath sounds q 2–4 h and PRN. • Suction only when rhonchi are present or secretions visible in endotracheal tube. • Hyperoxygenate and hyperventilate before and after each suction pass. • Avoid suction passes > 10 sec. • Monitor ICP and CPP during suctioning and chest physiotherapy. • Provide meticulous oral hygiene. • Monitor for signs of aspiration.
Circulation/Perfusion Cerebral perfusion pressure will be > 60 mmHg. Intracerebral pressure will be < 15 mmHg. Serum lactate will be < 2.2 mmol/L within 36 h of injury.	• Monitor blood pressure continuously. • If device is in place, monitor ICP and CPP continuously. • Elevate head of bed 30°–45°, increase to 90° for ICP control. • Administer sedatives, barbiturates, paralytics, diuretics (mannitol) per order/or protocol. • Monitor oxygen delivery (hemoglobin SaO_2, cardiac output). • Administer red blood cells, inotropes, intravascular volume as indicated.
Fluids/Electrolytes Serum electrolytes will be within normal limits. Serum osmolality will remain within prescribed range.	• Monitor intake and output. • Monitor laboratory tests minimally q 24 h for serum osmolarity, electrolytes, and glucose. • Administer mannitol as ordered or per protocol. • Observe fluid restriction and administration per protocol.
Mobility/Safety There will be minimal and transient changes in ICP/CPP during treatments or patient care activities. ICP/CPP will return to baseline within 5 min. There will be no evidence of complications related to prolonged immobilization (eg, deep vein thrombosis [DVT], pneumonia, ankylosis). There will be no evidence of seizure activity. Patient will not harm self.	• Make neurological checks q 1–2 h. • Plan care activity or treatments around patient's vital signs and ICP/CPP response. • Administer medications as indicated prior to activity. • Avoid extreme hip flexion. • Maintain head and neck alignment. • Reposition q 2–4 h. • Consider kinetic therapy bed. • Institute DVT prophylaxis. • Provide range of motion exercises q 4–6 h. • Apply and remove therapeutic extremity splints per schedule. • Consult with occupational and/or physical therapy service. • Monitor and facilitate clearance of cervical spine injury before removing cervical collar and/or mobilizing out of bed. • Monitor for seizure activity. • Assess anticonvulsant levels q day. • Maintain calm, quiet environment. • Institute seizure precautions. • Institute falls precautions. • Utilize patient protective device as indicated and per hospital policy. • Closely monitor patients with Ranchos Los Amigos Scale level III to VI for intentional self-harm.

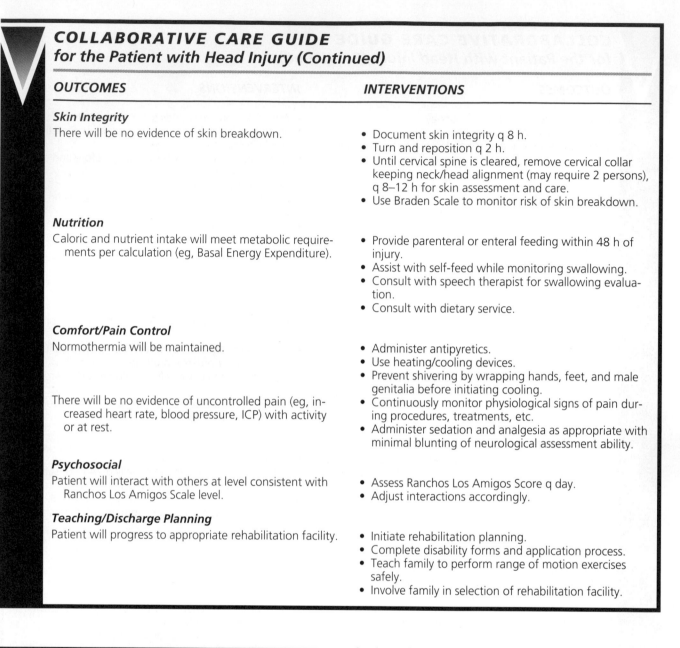

COLLABORATIVE CARE GUIDE
for the Patient with Head Injury (Continued)

OUTCOMES	INTERVENTIONS
Skin Integrity There will be no evidence of skin breakdown.	• Document skin integrity q 8 h. • Turn and reposition q 2 h. • Until cervical spine is cleared, remove cervical collar keeping neck/head alignment (may require 2 persons), q 8–12 h for skin assessment and care. • Use Braden Scale to monitor risk of skin breakdown.
Nutrition Caloric and nutrient intake will meet metabolic requirements per calculation (eg, Basal Energy Expenditure).	• Provide parenteral or enteral feeding within 48 h of injury. • Assist with self-feed while monitoring swallowing. • Consult with speech therapist for swallowing evaluation. • Consult with dietary service.
Comfort/Pain Control Normothermia will be maintained. There will be no evidence of uncontrolled pain (eg, increased heart rate, blood pressure, ICP) with activity or at rest.	• Administer antipyretics. • Use heating/cooling devices. • Prevent shivering by wrapping hands, feet, and male genitalia before initiating cooling. • Continuously monitor physiological signs of pain during procedures, treatments, etc. • Administer sedation and analgesia as appropriate with minimal blunting of neurological assessment ability.
Psychosocial Patient will interact with others at level consistent with Ranchos Los Amigos Scale level.	• Assess Ranchos Los Amigos Score q day. • Adjust interactions accordingly.
Teaching/Discharge Planning Patient will progress to appropriate rehabilitation facility.	• Initiate rehabilitation planning. • Complete disability forms and application process. • Teach family to perform range of motion exercises safely. • Involve family in selection of rehabilitation facility.

Clinical Applicability Challenges

Self-Challenge: Critical Thinking

1. Based on Sharon's care study, defend the need to suction the patient in light of the fact that suctioning will increase ICP.

2. Anticipate the most likely change in Sharon's neurological examination if the ICP continues to rise.

Study Questions

1. A concussion
   a. always is associated with loss of consciousness.
   b. never is associated with loss of consciousness.
   c. produces irreversible neurological dysfunction.
   d. produces reversible neurological dysfunction.

2. The neurophysiology of respiration includes all the following except
   a. the motor strip of the cerebral cortex.
   b. the medulla oblongata in the brain stem.
   c. the cranial nerves IX and X.
   d. the cervical and thoracic spinal nerves.

3. Cheyne-Stokes breathing is characterized by
   a. respiration with a long pause at full inspiration or full expiration.
   b. the depth of each breath increasing to a peak and then decreasing to a period of apnea.
   c. gasping breaths with irregular pauses.
   d. totally irregular breathing with both deep and shallow breaths with irregular pauses.

4. When communicating with a dysphasic patient, all of the following techniques are recommended except
   a. using simple language punctuated with gestures.
   b. not using baby talk.
   c. using longer sentences to force the patient to concentrate.
   d. speaking in a normal tone of voice.

REFERENCES

1. Ghajar J, et al: Survey of critical care management of comatose, head-injured patients in the United States. Critical Care Medicine 23(3): 560–567, 1995
2. Pieper DR, et al: Surgical management of patients with severe head injuries. AORN Journal 63(5):854–867, 1996
3. American Trauma Society: Trauma Quiz 1994.
4. Chestnut RM, Marshall LF, Klauber MR, Blunt BA, Baldwin N, Eisenberg HM, Jane JA, Marmarou A, Foulkes MA: The role of secondary brain injury in determining outcome from severe head injury. J Trauma 34(2):216–222, 1993
5. Gennarelli TA, Spielman GM, Langfitt TW: Influence of the type of intracranial lesion on outcome from severe head injury. J Neurosurg 56:26–36, 1982
6. Mitchell PH: Central nervous system I: Closed head injuries. In Cardona VD (ed): Trauma Nursing From Resuscitation Through Rehabilitation, pp 383–434. Philadelphia, WB Saunders, 1994
7. Lobato R, Rivas J, Gomez P, et al: Head-injured patients who talk and deteriorate into coma. J Neurosurg 75:256–261, 1991
8. Chesnut RM: Medical management of severe head injury. New Horizons 3(3):581–591, 1995
9. Geraci EB, Geraci T: A look at recent hyperventilation studies: Outcomes and recommendations for early use in the head-injured patient. J Neurosci Nurs 28(4):222–244, 1996
10. Marion DW, Firlik A, McLaughlin MR: Hyperventilation therapy for severe traumatic brain injury. New Horizons 3(3):439–445, 1995
11. Temkin NR, Haglund MM, Winn HR: Causes, prevention, and treatment of post-traumatic epilepsy. New Horizons 3(3):518–522, 1995
12. Piek J: Medical complications in severe head injury. New Horizons 3(3):534–538, 1995

BIBLIOGRAPHY

Cammermeyer M, Appledorn C (eds): Core Curriculum For Neuroscience Nurses (4th Ed). Chicago, American Association of Neuroscience Nurses, 1996
Cardona VD, Hurn PD, et al (eds): Trauma nursing from resuscitation to rehabilitation (2nd Ed). Philadelphia, WB Saunders, 1994
Chudley S: The effect of nursing activities on intracranial pressure. British Journal of Nursing 3(9):454–459, 1994
Eisenhart K: New perspectives in the management of adults with severe head injury. Critical Care Nursing Quarterly 17(2):1–12, 1994
Hsiang JK, Chesnut RM, et al: Early routine paralysis for intracranial pressure control in severe head injury: Is it necessary? Critical Care Medicine 22(9):1471–1476, 1994
Wald SL: Advances in early management of patients with head injury. Surg Clin North Am 75(2):225–242, 1995

35

Common Neurological Disorders

OBJECTIVES

Based on the content in this chapter, the reader should be able to:

- Name three common clinical manifestations of a right hemispheric stroke; a left hemispheric stroke.
- Discuss two treatment modalities available for the patient with an arteriovenous malformation; a cerebral aneurysm.
- Describe three appropriate nursing interventions for a patient with a cerebral aneurysm before surgery.
- Discuss three important facts a patient taking phenytoin should be taught.
- Differentiate between partial and generalized seizures.
- Explain the pathophysiology of Guillain-Barré syndrome.
- Formulate a teaching plan for a patient with myasthenia gravis.
- Describe several signs and symptoms that might prompt a person with a brain tumor to seek medical attention.

Nurses in the intensive care unit (ICU) caring for patients who have the neurological disorders discussed in this chapter serve as the patient's first line of defense. To ensure superior care, a multitude of routine supportive acts must be performed in repetition. Concomitantly, the nurse must carry out frequent neurological and (in cases of multiple systems injuries) other evaluations with constant vigil for subtle changes in blood pressure, pulse rate and regularity, respiratory activity, sensorial status (level of consciousness [LOC]), and motor and sensory function. When alterations occur, they may be the initial indication of impending deterioration, leading to rapid death unless immediate action is taken.

Experience helps the nurse to recognize slight changes that may be the precursors of the full constellation of signs associated with life-threatening conditions. Experience also strengthens the nurse's confidence.

Cerebrovascular Disease

Cerebrovascular disease (CVD) is the most frequent neurological disorder of adults. It is the third leading cause of morbidity and mortality in the United States after heart disease and cancer.[1] Cerebrovascular disease includes any pathological process that involves the blood vessels of the brain. Most CVD is due to thrombosis, embolism, or hemorrhage (Fig. 35–1). The mechanism of each of these etiologies is different, but the result is the same—ultimate ischemia or hypoxia to a focal area of the brain. Ischemia may lead to brain necrosis (infarction).

Brain Vasculature

The brain is supplied with blood from two major sets of vessels: the carotid or anterior circulation and the vertebral or posterior circulation (Fig. 35–2). Each system comes off the aortic arch as a pair of vessels: the left and right common carotids and the left and right vertebrals. Each carotid bifurcates to form the internal and external carotid artery. The vertebral arteries arise from the subclavian arteries. The vertebrals join to form the basilar artery, that in turn divides to form the two posterior cerebral arteries, which supply the medial and inferior surfaces of the brain and the lateral portions of the temporal and occipital lobe (Fig. 35–3).

The circle of Willis is the area in which the branches of the basilar and internal carotid arteries unite. The circle of Willis is composed of the two anterior cerebral arteries, the anterior communicating artery, the two posterior cerebral arteries, and the two posterior communicating arteries (Fig. 35–4). This circular network permits blood to circulate from one hemisphere to the other and from the anterior into the posterior areas of the brain. This system allows for collateral circulation if one vessel is occluded. It is not unusual, however, for some vessel within the circle of Willis to be atrophic or even absent. This accounts for different clinical presentations among patients with the same lesion. For example, a person with an occluded carotid artery and a fully patent circle of Willis may be totally asymptomatic, but a patient in whom the circle of Willis is incomplete may demonstrate a massive cerebral infarction.

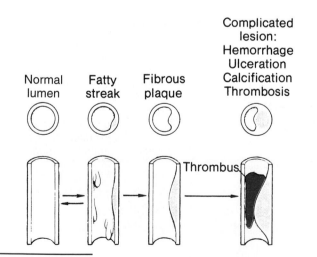

FIGURE 35-1
Atherosclerotic vascular changes preventing blood flow. (Brunner LS, Suddarth DS: Textbook of Medical-Surgical Nursing, [8th ed.] Philadelphia, Lippincott-Raven, 1996).

STROKE ("BRAIN ATTACK")

Stroke is now referred to as "brain attack" to encourage professionals and the public to think about stroke as a medical emergency.[1] This term resembles heart attack, which is viewed by most as a medical condition requiring immediate attention. To reverse cerebral ischemia, patients must be seen early. Ischemic brain injury occurs when arterial occlusion lasts longer than 2 to 3 hours. Delay in seeking

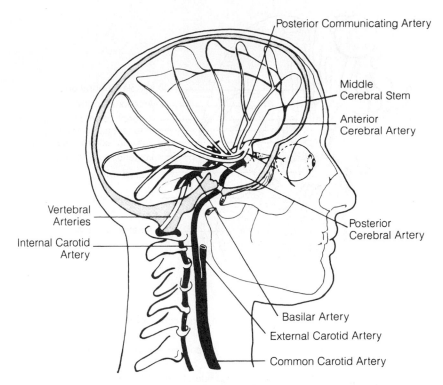

FIGURE 35-2
The major vessels to the brain. The internal carotid, anterior, and middle cerebral arteries constitute the anterior circulation. The vertebral, basilar, and posterior cerebral arteries and branches comprise the posterior circulation.

medical care may eliminate the potential for tissue-saving therapy with thrombolytic agents.

A stroke may be defined as a neurological deficit that has a sudden onset, lasts more than 24 hours, and results from CVD. Approximately three fourths of strokes are due to vascular obstruction (thrombi or emboli), resulting in ischemia and infarction. About one fourth of strokes are hemorrhagic, resulting from hypertensive vascular disease (which causes an intracerebral hemorrhage), a ruptured aneurysm, or an arteriovenous malformation (AVM).

Each of the three types of stroke has a fairly typical time course. Thrombotic strokes may be subdivided into transient ischemic attacks (TIAs), stroke in evolution, or completed stroke. Thrombotic strokes may occur suddenly and be complete early, or they may progress over time, depending on how much blood is able to get through the vascular lumen. Both embolic and hemorrhagic strokes typically present suddenly and progress rapidly over minutes or hours. There usually is little or no warning.

Sixty percent of thrombotic strokes occur during sleep. If the stroke is not complete at the time of the initial attack, symptoms may evolve over several hours or days. There may be some temporary improvement in clinical deficits, but then there follows a rapid progression of permanent deficits. This symptom development is referred to as stroke-in-evolution.

Stroke is the third most common cause of death in North America. Approximately 550,000 strokes occur per year in the United States, and about 150,000 of these individuals do not survive.[1] According to the National Stroke Association, stroke is one of the leading causes of permanent disability in adults. Of long-term stroke survivors, 15% require insti-

tutional care, 30% are dependent in activities of daily living, and 60% have decreased socialization outside the home.[2] The American Heart Association estimates that $15 to $20 billion are spent annually on stroke and stroke-related disorders.[3]

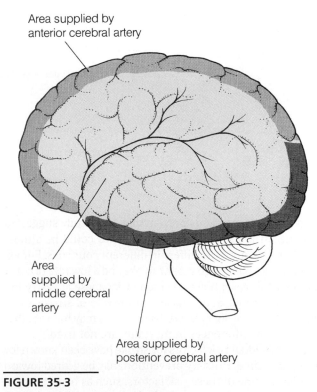

Area supplied by anterior cerebral artery

Area supplied by middle cerebral artery

Area supplied by posterior cerebral artery

FIGURE 35-3
Arterial supply to areas in the brain.

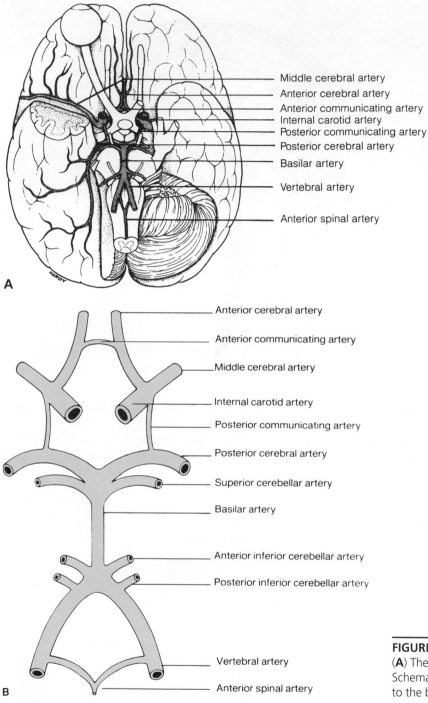

Middle cerebral artery
Anterior cerebral artery
Anterior communicating artery
Internal carotid artery
Posterior communicating artery
Posterior cerebral artery
Basilar artery
Vertebral artery
Anterior spinal artery

A

Anterior cerebral artery
Anterior communicating artery
Middle cerebral artery
Internal carotid artery
Posterior communicating artery
Posterior cerebral artery
Superior cerebellar artery
Basilar artery
Anterior inferior cerebellar artery
Posterior inferior cerebellar artery
Vertebral artery
Anterior spinal artery

B

FIGURE 35-4
(**A**) The circle of Willis seen from below the brain. (**B**) Schematic of the circle of Willis (arterial blood supply to the brain).

In principle, stroke is preventable. One study suggested that the estimate of preventable strokes could be almost 80%.[4] Stroke mortality differs in different countries. For example, Japan has a high rate of stroke and a low rate of coronary heart disease; however, men of Japanese ancestry living in the United States have a lower rate of stroke and a higher rate of coronary heart disease. This may indicate that international differences in mortality are not fixed.

The individual risk factors for stroke have been known for quite some time. Primary prevention may be geared toward modifying some of these risk factors, such as hypertension, serum cholesterol, smoking, obesity, impaired glucose tol-

erance, alcohol abuse, use of oral contraceptives in people at risk, and diet. Additionally, the appropriate use of warfarin or aspirin in patients at risk for cardiac sources of emboli (eg, atrial fibrillation) constitutes primary prevention.[5]

Pathophysiological Principles

When blood flow to any part of the brain is impeded as a result of a thrombus or embolus, oxygen deprivation of the cerebral tissue begins. Deprivation for 1 minute can lead to reversible symptoms, such as loss of consciousness. Oxygen deprivation for longer periods can produce microscopic necrosis of the neurons. The necrotic area is then said to be infarcted.

The initial oxygen deprivation may be due to general ischemia (from cardiac arrest or hypotension) or hypoxia from an anemic process or high altitude. If the neurons are only ischemic and have not yet necrosed, there is a chance to save them. This situation is analogous to the focal injury caused by a myocardial infarction. An occluded coronary artery can produce an area of infarcted (dead) tissue. Surrounding the infarcted zone is an area of ischemic tissue, which has been marginally deprived of oxygen. This ischemic tissue, as in the brain, may either be salvaged with appropriate treatment or killed by secondary events.

Strokes due to embolus may be a result of blood clots, fragments of atheromatous plaques, lipids, or air. Emboli to the brain most often come from the heart, secondary to myocardial infarction or atrial fibrillation.

If hemorrhage is the etiology of a stroke, hypertension often is a precipitating factor. Vascular abnormalities, such as AVMs and cerebral aneurysms, are more prone to rupture and cause hemorrhage in the presence of hypertension.

The most frequent neurovascular syndrome seen in thrombotic and embolic strokes is due to involvement of the middle cerebral artery. This artery mainly supplies the lateral aspects of the cerebral hemisphere. Infarction to that area of the brain may cause contralateral motor and sensory deficits. If the infarcted hemisphere is dominant, speech problems result, and dysphasia may be present.

With a thrombotic or embolic stroke, the amount of brain ischemia and infarction that might occur is difficult to predict. There is a chance that the stroke will extend after the initial insult. There can be massive cerebral edema and an increase in intracranial pressure (ICP) to the point of herniation and death after a huge thrombotic stroke. The prognosis is influenced by the area of the brain involved and the extent of the insult. Because thrombotic strokes often are due to atherosclerosis, there is risk of a future stroke in a patient who already has had one. With embolic strokes, patients also may have subsequent episodes of stroke if the underlying cause is not treated. If the extent of brain tissue destroyed from a hemorrhagic stroke is not excessive and is in a nonvital area, the patient may recover with minimal deficits. If the hemorrhage is large or in a vital area of the brain, the patient may not recover. About 30% of intracerebral hemorrhages are less massive, making survival possible.

Assessment

HISTORY AND PHYSICAL EXAMINATION

Diagnosis of a stroke is based on physical examination and history. The age of the patient is useful to know because strokes are more likely to occur in older people. It is helpful to know about the onset of symptoms. If the symptoms began suddenly and were severe within an hour, the most likely diagnosis is embolic ischemic brain infarction or intracranial hemorrhage. Nonvascular diseases, such as tu-

mors, abscesses, subdural hematomas, and encephalitis, rarely progress that quickly.

The history will be helpful in determining what has happened to the patient. It is important to obtain a description of the neurological event, how long it lasted, whether the symptoms are resolving, completely gone, or the same as at the time of onset. Knowing the type of symptoms may help determine and locate a possible vascular etiology. Determination of risk factors for stroke, such as hypertension, chronic atrial fibrillation, elevated serum cholesterol, smoking, oral contraceptive use, or a familial history of stroke, also will help in diagnosis.

If atrial fibrillation or a carotid bruit is found on physical examination, it may suggest the diagnosis of stroke. It is important to note the LOC when the patient presents. Ischemic CVD usually does not cause a depression in the LOC. Nonvascular processes and intracranial hemorrhage must be considered if the person has a depressed LOC.

CLINICAL MANIFESTATIONS

A patient with CVD may present with a TIA. This is a neurological deficit that totally resolves within 24 hours. Its average duration is 10 minutes, after which the symptoms completely disappear. A patient also may present with a reversible ischemic neurological deficit. This event may persist beyond the 24-hour duration of a TIA, but it eventually will clear completely. The third possible clinical presentation is a completed stroke, which leaves the person with a permanent deficit.

Of those who have TIAs, one third will have a major stroke, one third will continue to have TIAs but will not have a major stroke, and one third will have a resolution of their TIAs.

Symptoms seen with TIAs depend a great deal on the vessels involved. When the carotid and cerebral arteries are involved, the patient may have blindness in one eye, hemiplegia, hemianesthesia, speech disturbances, and confusion. When the vertebrobasilar artery is involved, dizziness, diplopia, numbness, visual defects in one or both fields, and dysarthria can be seen. Table 35–1 lists common deficits seen with a brain attack and suggested nursing interventions.

Some generalizations can be made about the probable disabilities of a patient if one knows both the side of the brain in which the stroke occurred and the "handedness" of the patient. Ninety-three percent of people are right handed. This means that their left hemisphere is dominant. Of the 7% of the population who are left handed, about 60% have their dominant speech center in the left hemisphere, as do right-handed people. The display on p. xxx lists probable disabilities associated with stroke.

DIAGNOSTIC STUDIES

A computed tomography (CT) scan may be useful in differentiating between cerebrovascular lesions and nonvascular lesions. For example, a subdural hemorrhage, brain abscess, tumor, or intracerebral hemorrhage will be visible on the

TABLE 35-1 CLINICAL APPLICATION: Nursing Intervention Guidelines
Common Deficits and Emotional Reactions to Stroke

Common Motor Deficits	Nursing Interventions
1. Hemiparesis or hemiplegia (side of the body opposite the cerebral episode)	1. Position the patient in proper body alignment; use a hand roll to keep the hand in a functional position. • Provide frequent passive range-of-motion exercises. • Reposition the patient every 2 h. • Keep heel on affected leg elevated off bed to prevent pressure sores.
2. Dysarthria (muscles of speech impaired)	2. Provide for an alternative method of communication.
3. Dysphagia (muscles of swallowing impaired)	3. Test the patient's palatal and pharyngeal reflexes before offering nourishment. • Elevate and turn the patient's head to the unaffected side. • If the patient is able to manage oral intake, place food on the unaffected side of the patient's mouth.

Common Sensory Deficits	Nursing Interventions

1. Visual deficits (common because the visual pathways cut through much of the cerebral hemispheres)
  a. Homonymous hemianopsia (loss of vision in half of the visual field on the same side)
 	
  b. Double vision (diplopia)
  c. Decreased visual acuity
	1. Be aware that variations of visual deficits may exist and compensate for them.
	  a. Approach the patient from the unaffected side; remind the patient to turn the head to compensate for visual deficits.
	  b. Alternate an eye patch to reduce double vision.
	  c. Provide assistance as necessary. Keep frequently used items within reach.

2. Absent or diminished response to superficial sensation (touch, pain, pressure, heat, cold)	2. Increase the amount of touch when administering patient care. • Protect the involved areas from injury. • Protect the involved areas from burns. • Examine the involved areas for signs of skin irritation and injury. • Provide the patient with an opportunity to handle various objects of different weight, texture, and size. • If pain is present, assess its location, type, and duration.
3. Absent or diminished response to proprioception (knowledge of position of body parts)	3. Teach the patient to check the position of body parts visually.

4. Perceptual deficits (disturbance in correctly perceiving and interpreting self or environment)
  a. Body scheme disturbance (amnesia or denial for paralyzed extremities; unilateral neglect)
 	
  b. Disorientation (to time, place, and person)
 	
  c. Apraxia (loss of ability to use objects correctly)
  d. Agnosia (inability to identify the environment by means of the senses)
  e. Defects in localizing objects in space, estimating their size, and judging distance
  f. Impaired memory for recall of spatial location of objects or places
 	
  g. Right–left disorientation
	4. Compensate for the patient's perceptual–sensory deficits.
	
	  a. Protect the involved area.
	    • Accept the patient's self-perception.
	    • Position the patient to face the involved area.
	  b. Control the amount of change in the patient's schedule.
	    • Reorient the patient as necessary.
	    • Talk to the patient; tell him or her about the immediate environment.
	    • Provide a calendar, clock, pictures of family, and so forth.
	  c. Correct misuse of objects, and demonstrate proper use.
	  d. Correct misinformation.
	
	  e. Reduce any stimuli that will distract the patient.
	
	  f. Place necessary equipment where the patient will see it, rather than telling the patient, "It is in the closet" and so forth.
	  g. Phrase requests carefully, like "Lift this leg." (Point to the leg.)

(continued)

TABLE 35-1   CLINICAL APPLICATION: Nursing Intervention Guidelines
Common Deficits and Emotional Reactions to Stroke (Continued)

Language Deficits	Nursing Interventions
1. Expressive dysphasia (difficulty in transforming sound into patterns of understandable speech)—can speak using single-word responses	1. Ask the patient to repeat the individual sounds of the alphabet as a start at retraining.
2. Receptive dysphasia (impairment of comprehension of the spoken word)—able to speak, but uses words incorrectly and is unaware of these errors	2. Speak clearly and in simple sentences; use gestures as necessary.
3. Global dysphasia (combination of expressive and receptive dysphasia)—unable to communicate at any level	3. Evaluate what language skills are intact; speak in very simple sentences, ask the patient to repeat individual sounds, and use gestures or any other means to communicate.
4. Alexia (inability to understand the written word)	4. Point to the written names of objects, and have the patient repeat the name of the object.
5. Agraphia (inability to express ideas in writing)	5. Have the patient write words and simple sentences.

Intellectual Deficits	Nursing Interventions
1. Loss of memory	1. Provide information as necessary.
2. Short attention span	2. Divide activities into short steps.
3. Increased distractibility	3. Control any excessive environmental distractions.
4. Poor judgment	4. Protect the patient from injury.
5. Inability to transfer learning from one situation to another	5. Repeat instructions as necessary.
6. Inability to calculate, reason, or think abstractly	6. Do not set unrealistic expectations for the patient. Be concrete with requests/instructions.

Emotional Deficits	Nursing Interventions
1. Emotional lability (exhibits reactions easily or inappropriately)	1. Disregard bursts of emotions; explain to the patient that emotional lability is part of the illness.
2. Loss of self-control and social inhibitions	2. Protect the patient as necessary so that his or her dignity is preserved.
3. Reduced tolerance to stress	3. Control the amount of stress experienced by the patient.
4. Fear, hostility, frustration, anger	4. Be accepting of the patient; be supportive. Set limits.
5. Confusion and despair	5. Clarify any misconceptions; allow the patient to verbalize.
6. Withdrawal, isolation	6. Provide stimulation and a safe, comfortable environment.
7. Depression	7. Provide a supportive environment.

Bowel and Bladder Dysfunction	Nursing Interventions
Bladder: Incomplete Upper Motor Neuron Lesion	*Do not suggest insertion of an indwelling catheter immediately after the stroke.*
1. The unilateral lesion from the stroke results in partial sensation and control of the bladder, so that the patient experiences frequency, urgency, and incontinence. (Cognitive deficits affect control.)	1. Observe the patient to identify characteristics of the voiding pattern (eg, frequency, amount, forcefulness of stream, constant dribbling).
2. If the stroke lesion is in the brain stem, there will be bilateral damage, resulting in an upper motor neuron bladder with loss of all control of micturition.	2. Maintain an accurate intake and output record.
	Nursing note: Incontinence after regaining consciousness is usually attributable to urinary tract infection caused by use of an indwelling urinary catheter.
3. Possibility of establishing normal bladder function is excellent.	3. Try to allow the patient to stay catheter-free: • Offer the bedside commode or urinal frequently. • Take the patient to the commode frequently. • Assess the patient's ability to make his or her need for help with voiding known.
	If a catheter is necessary, remove it as soon as possible and follow a bladder training program.

(continued)

TABLE 35-1   CLINICAL APPLICATION: Nursing Intervention Guidelines
Common Deficits and Emotional Reactions to Stroke (Continued)

Bowel and Bladder Dysfunction	Nursing Interventions
Bowel	
1. Impairment of bowel function in a stroke patient is attributable to: • Deterioration in the level of consciousness • Dehydration • Immobility 2. Constipation is the most common problem, along with potential impaction.	1. Develop a bowel training program: • Give foods known to stimulate defecation (prune juice, roughage). • Initiate a suppository and stool softener regimen. Initiate laxatives if suppository and softener are ineffective. 2. Institute a bowel program. Enemas are avoided in the presence of increased intracranial pressure.

Adapted from Hickey JV: The Clinical Practice of Neurological and Neurosurgical Nursing (4th Ed), pp 529–530. Philadelphia, Lippincott-Raven, 1996

CT scan. An area of infarction may not show on the CT scan for 48 hours.

A brain scan has limited value in the acute setting but may be helpful if it is positive. A brain scan will show major infarcted areas, but not as early as the CT scan.

Angiography was done more often before the CT scan was available to distinguish cerebrovascular lesions from nonvascular ones. Early angiography in a patient with a stroke often is performed if an intracranial hemorrhage is suspected, if the patient is rapidly deteriorating neurologically, or if the patient has a suspected acute carotid occlusion.

A lumbar puncture may be performed to look for blood in the cerebrospinal fluid (CSF). The CT scan may not show low concentrations of blood in the CSF. It is important to know whether hemorrhage is present because this information will help the physician decide whether or not to anticoagulate the patient.

Magnetic resonance imaging (MRI) also may help in the differential diagnosis of stroke. Ultrasound or Doppler studies are noninvasive procedures that are useful in diagnosing blocked arteries. An electrocardiogram will help determine if a dysrhythmia is present, which may have caused the stroke. Other electrocardiogram changes that might be found are an inverted T wave, ST depression, and QT elevation and prolongation.

No laboratory tests are definitive in confirming a diagnosis of stroke; however, commonly drawn blood tests include hematocrit and hemoglobin, which, when elevated, indicate a more severe occlusion; prothrombin time and partial thromboplastin time, which provide a baseline should anticoagulation therapy be initiated; and a white blood cell count, which may indicate an infection, such as subacute bacterial endocarditis.

In many cases, the etiology of the stroke remains undetermined, and a significant proportion of patients will have evidence of more than one potential mechanism.

Management

REDUCTION OF ISCHEMIC DAMAGE

With a cerebral infarction, there is a central core of brain tissue that is irreversibly lost. Around this dead zone is an area of tissue that may be salvageable. It should be the focus of initial treatment to save as much of the ischemic area as possible. Three ingredients necessary to that area are oxygen, glucose, and adequate blood flow. The oxygen level can be monitored through arterial blood gases, and oxygen can be given to the patient if indicated. Hypoglycemia can be evaluated with serial checks on blood glucose.

Cerebral perfusion pressure is a reflection of the systemic blood pressure, the ICP, the autoregulation still functioning in the brain, and the heart rate and rhythm. The parameters most easily controlled externally are the cardiac rhythm, rate, and blood pressure. Dysrhythmias usually can be corrected. Causes of tachycardia, such as fever, pain, and dehydration, can be treated.

Probable Disabilities Associated With Stroke

Left Hemispheric Stroke
• Right-sided hemiparesis or hemiplegia
• Slow and cautious behavior
• Right visual field defect
• Expressive, receptive, or global dysphasia
• High frustration

Right Hemispheric Stroke
• Left-sided hemiparesis or hemiplegia
• Spatial–perceptual deficits
• Poor judgment
• Distractibility
• Impulsive behavior
• Apparent unawareness of deficits of affected side and therefore susceptibility to falls or other injuries
• Left visual field defect

Not widely used as yet is monitoring with a retrograde jugular catheter. Such a catheter allows for sampling of the venous blood leaving the cerebral hemispheres, permitting calculation of venous oxygen saturation. The calculated SjO_2 (saturation of jugular oxygen) reflects what is happening at the cellular level better than ICP or cerebral perfusion pressure. Monitoring the arteriovenous difference of oxygen ($AVDO_2$) and the SjO_2 allows the physician to determine if therapies are harming or improving oxygen delivery. Normal SjO_2 is 60% to 80%.

THROMBOLYSIS

Thrombolytic agents are exogenous drugs that dissolve clots. Several drugs currently approved by the Food and Drug Administration are listed in the display.

Some centers have a cerebrovascular team that evaluates patients in the emergency department, facilitates the diagnostic process to rule out intracerebral hemorrhage, and initiates intra-arterial thrombolytic therapy. Local thrombolytic therapy should be initiated within 3 hours or less of the onset of neurological symptoms.[6] The accompanying display outlines contraindications for this treatment.

Thrombolytic therapy for acute stroke was briefly attempted in the late 1950s prior to the widespread use of CT. Patients with hemorrhagic rather than thrombotic strokes were difficult to distinguish in that era, so early outcomes were not very good because of complications from hemorrhage. Recent technological advances have allowed this approach to be revisited with better outcomes. Intracranial vasculature can now be accessed by use of microcatheters and steerable microguide wires, making localized intra-arterial infusion of thrombolytic agents possible. Thus, an occluded cerebral artery can be reopened. State-of-the-art brain imaging and neuronal protection agents have also aided this approach.

For intra-arterial therapy, a femoral arterial sheath is usually inserted, through which a microcatheter can be threaded under fluoroscopy. The catheter tip is positioned into the clot and advanced as the clot dissolves. The femoral sheath usually remains in place for 24 hours in case of recurrent vessel occlusion. The accompanying display discusses nursing management of the patient undergoing thrombolytic therapy.

Reperfusion injury is a risk of thrombolytic therapy, as is bleeding. There is also reason to believe that restoring blood flow to the infarcted area may increase edema and cause neurological deterioration.[7]

Currently there is no agreement on the optimal fibrinolytic agent, the optimal dose, or the rate of administration. The critical time after which thrombolytic therapy is no longer beneficial has not been firmly established. Other areas of controversy involve the choice of catheter (end hole versus multiple hole), the best catheter position (prethrombus, intrathrombus, or post-thrombus), and even the advisability of mechanical thrombus disruption. More data are needed before intra-arterial fibrinolysis can be adequately assessed and made available on a wider basis.

CLINICAL APPLICATION: Drug Therapy
Thrombolytic Agents Approved by the Food and Drug Administration

Streptokinase
- Oldest and best known thrombolytic agent
- Not clot specific, so causes a systemic lytic state characterized by fibrinogen depletion
- Half-life of approximately 20 minutes
- Bacterial product, so may produce allergic response characterized by rash and fever
- Hypotension (infusion-rate dependent) and bronchospasm possible
- Steroids and diphenhydramine to treat symptoms or prophylactically
- May form antibodies to streptokinase, preventing future thrombolysis with this drug

Urokinase
- Human enzyme, so does not cause allergic or anaphylactic responses; may be given repeatedly because no antibody formation
- Half-life of 10–16 minutes
- Systemic lytic state up to 24 hours
- May be given as IV bolus without causing hypotension

Tissue-Type Plasminogen Activator (t-PA)
- Clot specific, so risk of systemic lytic state reduced compared with streptokinase and urokinase if given in doses under 100 mg
- Half-life of 5–7 minutes

Anisoylated Plasminogen Streptokinase Activator (APSAC)
- Decreased risk of systemic lytic state
- Not fibrin selective
- Half-life of 70–120 minutes
- Acts as a sustained-release form of streptokinase
- Same allergic potential as streptokinase

RED FLAG — Contraindications to Thrombolytic Therapy

Absolute Contraindications
- Active internal bleeding
- Intracranial aneurysm, arteriovenous malformation or neoplasm
- Recent (within 2 months) stroke or intracranial or intraspinal surgery or trauma

Major Relative Contraindications
- Recent (within 10 days) major surgery, serious gastrointestinal bleeding, organ biopsy, obstetrical delivery, or previous puncture of noncompressible vessel
- Severe uncontrolled hypertension (systolic blood pressure >180–200 mmHg, diastolic blood pressure >110 mmHg)
- Recent serious trauma

CLINICAL APPLICATION: Nursing Intervention Guidelines
Thrombolytic Therapy

Prior to Thrombolysis

- Complete all invasive procedures, including establishment of two peripheral intravenous (IV) lines, one for administration of the thrombolytic agent and the second for blood administration if needed. Subclavian and jugular sites are avoided because they are noncompressible, and blood could be lost into the chest or neck. Some type of blood sampling device is established to prevent numerous venipunctures to monitor laboratory studies. Arterial access is obtained, usually using a femoral sheath.
- Obtain baseline blood samples. Usually these include a complete blood count, platelet count, partial thromboplastin time, prothrombin time, fibrinogen level, and chemical panel.
- Document baseline vital signs and neurological assessments.
- Give the patient a thorough explanation of what to expect.

Following Thrombolysis

- Protect femoral arterial sheath until removed, which is usually after coagulation studies return to normal. The patient's leg should remain straight while on bed rest. Popliteal, dorsalis pedis, and posterior tibialis pulses should be checked in the leg with the sheath. Changes in color, sensation, and temperature in the leg should also be noted. Observations are made for oozing or hematoma formation at the femoral cannulation site.
- Monitor vital signs and neurological status.
- Evaluate patient for signs of internal bleeding, such as tachycardia, hypotension, or confusion. Changes in level of consciousness may reflect intracranial bleeding. Complaints of low back pain, leg numbness, or muscle weakness may indicate retroperitoneal bleeding. Watch for hematuria and heme-positive stools. Decline in hemoglobin,

hematocrit, and mean corpuscular volume may also indicate bleeding.
- Prevent administration of contraindicated medications for 24 hours after the thrombolysis, such as heparin, aspirin and aspirin-containing drugs, and warfarin.
- Watch for signs of increased intracranial pressure, such as a change in level of consciousness and later, hypertension, bradycardia, and widened pulse pressure. Changes in level of consciousness, pupillary reflexes, or other neurological changes are more likely attributable to hemorrhage from the thrombolytic agent than from changes caused by the ischemic stroke. Neurological deterioration is usually an indication for an immediate computed tomography scan.
- Prevent hypotensive episodes to maintain adequate cerebral perfusion. A drop of 10 to 15 mmHg in blood pressure may result in reduced cerebral perfusion pressure, which can extend the area of cerebral infarction. If treating hypotension with intravenous fluids, dextrose in water should be avoided, because dextrose metabolism facilitates production of lactic acid and contributes to ischemia and edema in the brain. If hypotension does not respond to fluid challenges, vasopressors may be indicated.
- Avoid use of sedatives and hypnotics because they make neurological assessment difficult, and they impede neuronal recovery.
- Initiate deep vein thrombosis prevention while the patient is on bed rest. Subcutaneous heparin can be administered 24 hours after receiving thrombolysis. Patients can also use support stockings or sequential air compression stockings.
- Monitor laboratory studies including coagulation tests and glucose and electrolytes. Hyperglycemia two to three times normal can change minor ischemic areas to areas of infarction.

CONTROL OF HYPERTENSION AND INCREASED INTRACRANIAL PRESSURE

Control of hypertension, ICP, and cerebral perfusion pressure may take the efforts of both the nurse and the physician. The nurse must assess for these problems, recognize them and their significance, and ensure that medical interventions are initiated.

Patients with moderate hypertension usually are not treated acutely. If their blood pressure is lowered after the brain is accustomed to the hypertension for adequate perfusion, the brain's perfusion pressure will fall along with the blood pressure. If the diastolic blood pressure is above about 105 mmHg, it may need to be lowered gradually. This may be accomplished effectively with nitroprusside.

If ICP is elevated in a stroke patient, it usually occurs after the first day. Although this is a natural response of the brain to some cerebrovascular lesions, it is destructive to the brain. The destructive response, such as edema or arterial vasopasm, sometimes can be treated or prevented. The usual methods of controlling increased ICP may be insti-

tuted, such as hyperventilation; fluid restriction; head elevation; avoidance of neck flexion or severe head rotation that would impede venous outflow from the head; use of osmotic diuretics, such as mannitol; and perhaps administration of dexamethasone, although its use remains controversial. Refer to Chapter 33 for a detailed discussion of the management of elevated ICP.

PHARMACOLOGICAL THERAPY

Anticoagulation may be initiated if the stroke was not hemorrhage, although heparinization of patients with an acute ischemic stroke has the potential for causing hemorrhagic complications. Low-molecular-weight heparinoids (LMWH) offer an alternative to heparin, and there is a decrease in bleeding tendency with their use. Low-molecular-weight heparinoids interact differently from standard heparin within the coagulation system and with platelets. They have no significant effect on platelet function and aggregation, and on partial thromboplastin and prothrombin times.

Heparinoids should be initiated soon after symptom onset, preferably within 24 hours. Baseline laboratory studies prior to drug initiation may include a complete blood count (CBC) with differential and coagulation studies, including platelet count. Another CBC with platelet count may be recommended on day 3 of the protocol. When administering LMWH subcutaneously, as with heparin, an air bubble should be left at the end of the syringe for injection after the medication is injected. This ensures that all the heparinoid solution has been injected and prevents escape of the drug from the injection site.

If the patient has not had a stroke but a TIA, antiplatelet drugs may be indicated. Such drugs include dipyridamole (Persantine), sulfinpyrazone (Anturane), and aspirin. They reduce the platelet adhesiveness and are given in the hope of preventing a future thrombotic or embolic event. Antiplatelet drugs are contraindicated in the presence of a hemorrhagic stroke, as is heparin.

Calcium-channel blockers, such as nimodipine, may be used to treat cerebral vasospasm. These drugs relax the smooth muscle of the vessel walls. Vasospasm is most common after rupture of a cerebral aneurysm. (See "Vasospasm" under the discussion of aneurysms.)

SURGICAL INTERVENTION

Transient ischemic episodes often are viewed as a warning of impending stroke due to occlusion of a vessel. Some patients with atherosclerotic disease of extracranial or intracranial vessels may be good surgical candidates. Carotid endarterectomy may be beneficial to a patient with narrowing of the vessels. See Chapter 21 for a discussion of this procedure.

Cranial bypass surgery involves anastomosing an extracranial artery that perfuses the scalp to an intracranial artery distal to the occluded site. The procedure often used when there is intracranial involvement is the superior temporal artery anastomosis to the middle cerebral artery (STA-MCA). Collateral circulation thus is provided to areas of the brain supplied by the middle cerebral artery. Many STA-MCA anastomoses are performed with the hope of preventing a future stroke in people with unilateral focal cerebral ischemia who present with TIAs.

PREVENTION OF COMPLICATIONS

The nurse will play a significant role in preventing the complications associated with immobility, hemiparesis, or any neurological deficit produced by stroke. Preventive measures are particularly important in the area of urinary tract infections, aspiration pneumonia, pressure sores, contractures, thrombophlebitis, and corneal abrasions.

EMOTIONAL AND BEHAVIORAL MODIFICATION

Victims of stroke may display emotional problems, and their behavior may be different from the prestroke baseline. Emotions may be labile; for example, the patient may cry one moment and laugh the next, without explanation or control. Tolerance to stress may be reduced. A minor stress in the prestroke state may be perceived as a major problem

after the stroke. Families may not understand the behavior. Stroke victims may use loud profanity with the nursing staff or with their family members, yet the family cannot understand it because the patient may never have used any profanity before the stroke. It is the nurse's role to help the family understand these behavioral changes. There is much that the nurse can do to modify the patient's behavior, such as controlling stimuli in the environment, providing rest periods throughout the day to prevent the patient from becoming overtired, giving positive feedback for acceptable behavior or positive accomplishments, and providing repetition when the patient is trying to relearn a skill.

COMMUNICATION

Stroke victims may demonstrate much frustration with their deficits. Probably no deficit produces more frustration for the patient and those trying to communicate with him or her than the one involving the production and understanding of language. Dysphasia can involve motor abilities or sensory function, or both. If the area of brain injury is in or near the left Broca's area, the memory of motor patterns of speech are affected (see Fig. 34-6). This results in an expressive dysphasia, in which the patient understands language but is unable to use it appropriately.

Receptive dysphasia usually is a result of injury to the left Wernicke's area, which is the control center for recognition of spoken language. The patient thus is unable to understand the significance of the spoken word. Presence of both expressive dysphasia and receptive dysphasia is referred to as global dysphasia. The accompanying display summarizes differences between expressive and receptive problems.

It is important for the nursing staff to tell families that having dysphasia does not mean that a person is intellectually impaired. Communication at some level should be attempted, whether it is by writing, pointing at alphabet charts, or using gestures.

Complications in Stroke

Three primary complications of subarachnoid hemorrhage (SAH) may result from a stroke, AVM, or aneurysm. They are vasospasm, hydrocephalus, and dysrhythmias.

In addition, patients with stroke who are on anticoagulation therapy are at risk for bleeding from other sites, and vigilance and early intervention are required to prevent serious complications. The Collaborative Care Guide defines the specific outcomes and interventions for the patient who has had a stroke.

■ ARTERIOVENOUS MALFORMATIONS

Most AVMs occur in patients younger than 30 years. Each AVM is a tangled mass of arterial and venous blood vessels that shunt blood directly from the arterial system into the venous system, bypassing the capillary system.

Comparison of Expressive and Receptive Dysphasia

Expressive Dysphasia	Receptive Dysphasia
Hemiparesis is present because motor cortex is near Broca's area.	Hemiparesis is mild or absent because lesion is not near motor cortex.
	Hemianopsia or quadrantanopsia may be present.
Speech is slow, nonfluent; articulation is poor; speaking requires much effort. Total speech is reduced in quantity. Patient may use telegraphic speech, omitting small words.	Speech is fluent; articulation and rhythm are normal. Content of speech is impaired; wrong words are used.
Patient understands written and verbal speech.	Patient does not understand written and verbal speech.
Patient writes dysphasically.	Content of writing is abnormal. Penmanship may be good.
Patient may be able to repeat single words with effort. Phrase repetition is poor.	Repetition is poor.
Object naming is often poor, but it may be better than attempts to use spontaneous speech.	Object naming is poor.
Patient is aware of deficit, often experiencing frustration and depression.	Patient is often unaware of deficit.
Curses or other ejaculatory speech may be well articulated and automatic. Patient may be able to hum normally.	Patient may use wrong words and sounds.

These congenital developmental defects in the capillaries may occur at any site in the central nervous system (CNS) but frequently are found in the area of the middle cerebral artery. The capillaries in an AVM have failed to develop normally between the arterial and venous blood supplies, so the channels of the two blood supplies are connected by abnormally thin vessels.

Arteriovenous malformations are not confined to the cerebral circulation. They may be seen in the spinal cord, the gastrointestinal tract, under the skin, or in the renal system. Small, superfical AVMs may be detected by port wine stains of the skin.

Pathophysiological Principles

There is degeneration of the brain parenchyma around and within the malformation. Blood is shunted directly from the arterial to the venous system. This pathway offers less resistance to blood flow than the normal capillary bed, so the AVM consequently receives a large blood flow. Arteries dilate to handle the increased perfusion of the AVM, and veins enlarge to drain the additional blood away. Collateral vessels may dilate in an attempt to carry the additional load, adding to the mass of the lesion.

Large AVMs may cause an "intracerebral steal" situation whereby arterial blood is diverted away from one area of the brain because of lowered vascular resistance in another. It is thought that AVMs can steal enough blood from adjacent areas of the brain to cause ischemic damage in the otherwise normal area. The neurological signs and symptoms seen in the patient correlate with the area of the brain that is deprived of blood flow. The size, shape, and location of the AVM also determine the deficits seen.

Assessment

HISTORY

Initial assessment of the patient depends on the presenting symptoms. The patient may or may not be able to provide a history. A history of headache or seizures may cause the patient to seek medical attention but may not be very helpful in pinpointing the diagnosis of AVM.

CLINICAL MANIFESTATIONS

Onset of symptoms may occur in childhood or early adult life. The chief complaint in many patients is headache, which often is unilateral. Another initial symptom may be seizures: first focal, then developing to generalized. Hemorrhage occurs in about 50% of patients before they are admitted to the hospital. An AVM that has bled once has a one in four chance of bleeding again within 4 years. An AVM that has bled more than once has a one in four chance of bleeding again within 1 year. Hemorrhage associated with an AVM can be intracerebral, subdural, or subarachnoid.

Alteration of brain tissue within the AVM and depletion of blood perfusion to adjacent areas may cause the patient to exhibit paresis or mental deterioration. Transient episodes of dizziness, syncope, sensory deficits or tingling, visual deficits (usually hemianopsia), and confusion may occur. If the bleeding is severe, there may be elevation of ICP with brain stem compression and unconsciousness.

A few patients report a constant swishing sound in the head with each heartbeat, representing a bruit, which may be auscultated occasionally by placing a stethoscope over the skull.

COLLABORATIVE CARE GUIDE
for the Patient Who Has Had a Stroke

OUTCOMES	INTERVENTIONS
Oxygenation/Ventilation	
Arterial pH, PO$_2$, and SaO$_2$ will be maintained within normal limits.	• Provide chest physiotherapy, turn, deep breath, cough, incentive spirometer q 4 h and PRN.
	• Provide postural drainage using Trendelenburg position per ICP protocol (see head injury care guide)
ETCO$_2$ or PCO$_2$ will be maintained within prescribed range.	• Adjust ventilator rate and tidal volume to hyperventilate to maintain ETCO$_2$ or PaCO$_2$ per protocol or order.
Patent airway will be maintained.	• Auscultate breath sounds q 2–4 h and PRN.
Lungs clear on auscultation.	• Suction only when rhonchi are present or secretions visible in endotracheal tube.
There will be no evidence of atelectasis or pneumonia.	• Hyperoxygenate and hyperventilate before and after each suction pass.
	• Monitor ICP and cerebral perfusion pressure (CPP) during suctioning and chest physiotherapy.
	• Provide meticulous oral hygiene.
	• Monitor for signs of aspiration.
Circulation/Perfusion	
Cerebral perfusion pressure will be > 60 mmHg.	• Monitor blood pressure continuously.
Intracerebral pressure will be < 15 mmHg.	• If device is in place, monitor ICP continuously.
	• Administer medications to reduce blood pressure (post initial hemorrhage).
	• Administer medications, intravenous fluids to raise blood pressure (post vasospasm).
	• Elevate head of bed 30–45 degrees.
	• Maintain calm, quiet environment.
	• Administer sedatives, barbiturates, paralytics, diuretics (mannitol) per order or protocol.
Fluids/Electrolytes	
Serum electrolytes will be within normal limits.	• Monitor intake and output.
Serum osmolality will remain within prescribed range.	• Monitor laboratory tests minimally q 24 h for serum osmolality, electrolytes, and glucose.
	• Administer mannitol as ordered or per protocol.
	• Observe fluid restriction and administer per protocol.
	• Take daily weights.
Mobility/Safety	
Changes in ICP/CPP during treatments or patient care activities will be minimal and transient.	• Plan care activity or treatments around patient's vital signs and ICP/CPP response.
ICP/CPP will return to baseline within 5 minutes.	• Administer medications as indicated prior to activity.
There will be no evidence of complications related to prolonged immobilization (eg, deep vein thrombosis [DVT], pneumonia, ankylosis).	• Avoid extreme hip flexion.
	• Maintain head and neck alignment.
	• Reposition q 2–4 h.
	• Consider kinetic therapy bed.
	• Institute DVT prophylaxis.
	• Provide range of motion exercises q 4–6 h.
	• Apply therapeutic extremity splints.
	• Utilize space boots or high-top tennis shoes, 2 h on, 2 h off, and monitor skin closely.
	• Consult with occupational and/or physical therapy service.
There will be no evidence of seizure activity.	• Monitor closely for seizure activity.
	• Maintain calm, quiet environment.
Patient will not harm self.	• Institute seizure precautions.
	• Administer medications per protocol to manage seizures.

(continued)

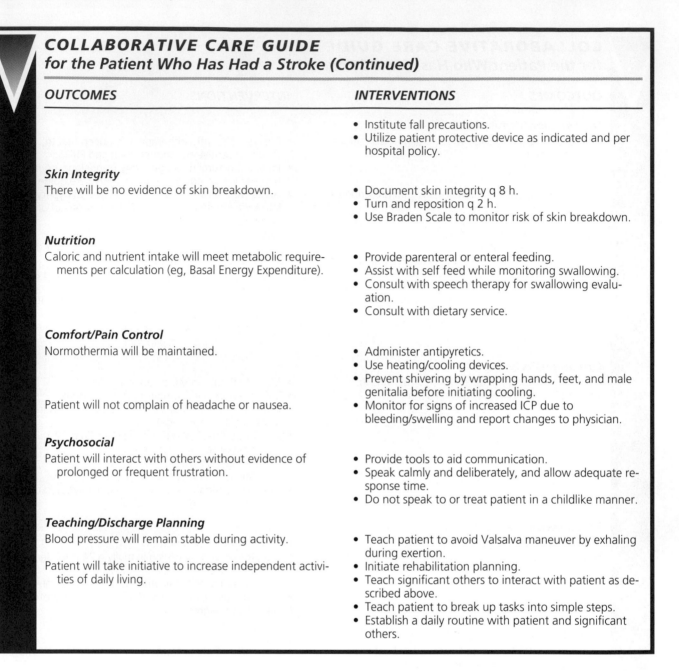

COLLABORATIVE CARE GUIDE
for the Patient Who Has Had a Stroke (Continued)

OUTCOMES	INTERVENTIONS
	• Institute fall precautions. • Utilize patient protective device as indicated and per hospital policy.
Skin Integrity There will be no evidence of skin breakdown.	• Document skin integrity q 8 h. • Turn and reposition q 2 h. • Use Braden Scale to monitor risk of skin breakdown.
Nutrition Caloric and nutrient intake will meet metabolic requirements per calculation (eg, Basal Energy Expenditure).	• Provide parenteral or enteral feeding. • Assist with self feed while monitoring swallowing. • Consult with speech therapy for swallowing evaluation. • Consult with dietary service.
Comfort/Pain Control Normothermia will be maintained. Patient will not complain of headache or nausea.	• Administer antipyretics. • Use heating/cooling devices. • Prevent shivering by wrapping hands, feet, and male genitalia before initiating cooling. • Monitor for signs of increased ICP due to bleeding/swelling and report changes to physician.
Psychosocial Patient will interact with others without evidence of prolonged or frequent frustration.	• Provide tools to aid communication. • Speak calmly and deliberately, and allow adequate response time. • Do not speak to or treat patient in a childlike manner.
Teaching/Discharge Planning Blood pressure will remain stable during activity. Patient will take initiative to increase independent activities of daily living.	• Teach patient to avoid Valsalva maneuver by exhaling during exertion. • Initiate rehabilitation planning. • Teach significant others to interact with patient as described above. • Teach patient to break up tasks into simple steps. • Establish a daily routine with patient and significant others.

DIAGNOSTIC STUDIES

If an AVM is suspected from the clinical manifestations or from a noncontrast scan, a CT with contrast usually is done to better visualize the cerebral vasculature. An electroencephalogram (EEG) may be done to localize the focus of any seizure activity or to demonstrate areas of cerebral ischemia or atrophy. For confirmation of the diagnosis, an angiogram is performed to identify the arteries feeding the AVM and the veins that are draining it.

Management

Available management techniques for AVMs include embolization, surgical excision, balloon occlusion, adjunctive pharmacological therapy, and proton beam irradiation. In some cases, conservative management may be the treatment of choice.

EMBOLIZATION AND SURGERY

In past years, embolization of an AVM was accomplished by the introduction of small Silastic beads into the internal carotid artery, where they subsequently entered the AVM. This resulted in thrombosis and destruction of the lesion (Fig. 35–5). This technique was effective for AVMs supplied by the middle cerebral artery because the Silastic beads tended to follow the flow pattern of the middle cerebral artery. Sometimes the AVM might appear occluded after the procedure, but collateral circulation redeveloped, providing a new vascular supply to the area, and the AVM reactivated.

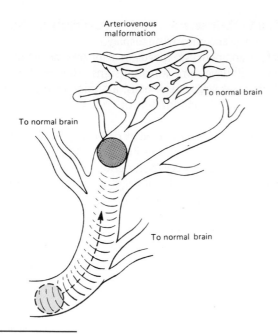

Arteriovenous malformation

To normal brain

To normal brain

To normal brain

FIGURE 35-5
Small Silastic beads or spheres are introduced into the artery to block blood flow to the arteriovenous malformation.

In recent years, tremendous improvements have been made in imaging equipment, microcatheter techniques, and embolotherapy materials. These components, in conjunction with digital subtraction angiography, have enabled very selective catheterization of distal vessels as well as the nucleus of the AVM.

Newer embolic materials include polyvinyl alcohol (PVA) and Gelfoam particles, which are fairly easy to use, but which are not permanent substances. N-butyl-cyanoacrylate (NBCA) is a liquid polymerizing agent that is short acting, permanent, but not yet readily available.

Complete surgical excision eliminates the possibility of recurrent bleeding. Protection from hemorrhage is not provided by ligation of the feeder vessels. Surgery is usually performed after the patient has stabilized from the hemorrhage—about 2 to 3 weeks. Sometimes an embolization procedure is performed first, followed by surgical excision 4 weeks later.

BALLOON OCCLUSION

A third treatment modality involves use of an intravascular detachable balloon. Carotid–cavernous sinus fistulas and vertebrovertebral fistulas have had the best results. Specific vascular anatomy with large feeding vessels deep to the nidus or aneurysms within feeding arteries favor the use of the detachable balloon over other embolic agents. Preoperative use of balloon occlusion may reduce the difficulty of surgical resection of the malformation. There usually is marked reduction of flow into the AVM by occlusion of major arterial fistula feeders. This procedure is used most often as an adjunct surgical intervention.

PHARMACOLOGICAL THERAPY

Propranolol hydrochloride (Inderal) may be prescribed before and after surgery to reduce the risk of postoperative hemorrhage. Because an AVM can cause an increase of blood flow by 50% to 100% above normal, cerebral autoregulation may be disrupted. After excision of the AVM, the increased blood flow gets rerouted into the brain's normal circulation, which was accustomed to minimal flow. Hyperperfusion is the result, and a hemorrahge may develop in adjacent parts of the brain. Propranolol will reduce cerebral blood flow and cardiac output.

IRRADIATION

A noninvasive treatment for AVM available in only a few centers in this country is the proton beam, which uses radiation energy given off by protons in a cyclotron. This shrinks the AVM and is very useful in treating deep-seated intraparenchymal AVMs that are not accessible to surgical management.

The nursing care of patients with an AVM or a cerebral aneurysm is similar. See the discussion under "Management" for cerebral aneurysm in the next section.

Complications in Arteriovenous Malformation

Complications for patients with an AVM and subsequent subarachnoid bleed are similar to those seen in the setting of an aneurysm.

CEREBRAL ANEURYSMS

An aneurysm is a round, saccular dilation of the arterial wall that develops as a result of weakness of the wall. Concern arises if the outpouching in the vessel wall ruptures or becomes large enough to exert pressure on surrounding brain structures.

Between 20% and 40% of the victims die at the time of the initial bleed of their aneurysms. Rebleeding is the leading cause of death in patients with a history of ruptured aneurysm. Of those who survive the first hemorrhage, 35% to 40% bleed again, with a mortality rate of about 42% at that time. Rebleeding most often occurs around the seventh day after the original bleed. Predictors of good recovery by 1 month after the bleed include a high score on the admission Glasgow Coma Scale, youth, and absence of blood on the first CT.[8,9]

Pathophysiological Principles

Arterial vessels are composed of three layers: endothelial lining, smooth muscle, and connective tissue. A defect in the smooth muscle layer allows the endothelial lining to bulge through, creating an aneurysm.

Some aneurysms are called "berry aneurysms" because they look like a berry, having a stem and neck. Saccular aneurysms do not have a neck but resemble a ballooning of the vessel (Fig. 35–6).

Most aneurysms arise from larger arteries around the anterior section of the circle of Willis. The most frequent site of occurrence is the juncture of the posterior communicating artery and the internal carotid artery. Other common aneurysm sites include the basilar artery, anterior cerebral artery, anterior communicating artery, and middle cerebral artery. Only about 15% of aneurysms occur within the vertebrobasilar system. Aneurysms most often form at the bifurcation of arteries.

Because aneurysm-forming vessels usually lie in the space between the arachnoid and the brain, hemorrhage from an aneurysm usually occurs in the subarachnoid space. Sometimes, however, the force of the rupturing vessel can be so great that it pushes blood through the pia mater and into the brain substance, causing an intracerebral hemorrhage, or through the arachnoid into the subdural space, causing a subdural hemorrhage.

Assessment

HISTORY

The nursing history should include identification of risk factors, such as familial predisposition, hypertension, cigarette smoking, or use of over-the-counter medications (eg, nasal sprays or antihistamines that have vasoconstrictive properties). Occupational history may be relevant, because if the patient has an occupation involving strenuous activity, there may be a significant delay in going back to work or the need to change occupations entirely.

CLINICAL MANIFESTATIONS

Many aneurysms are silent and never cause a problem but may be discovered on postmortem examination. If an aneurysm does cause problems, they usually will occur in the 35- to 60-year age group. Aneurysms are graded ac-

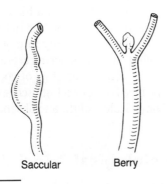

Saccular   Berry

FIGURE 35-6
Saccular and berry aneurysms. (Hickey J: Clinical Practice of Neurological and Neurosurgical Nursing, [4th ed]. Philadelphia, Lippincott-Raven, 1996).

cording to their severity. Such a classification system is shown in the accompanying display.

Before an aneurysm bleeds or ruptures, about half the patients will have some warning signs. These may include headaches, lethargy, neck pain, a "noise in the head" (a bruit), and optic, oculomotor, or trigeminal cranial nerve dysfunction.

After an aneurysm has bled or ruptured, the patient usually complains of an explosive headache. There is a decrease in the LOC, cranial nerve dysfunction, visual disturbances, perhaps hemiparesis or hemiplegia, and often vomiting. All these signs are related to an increase in ICP. With an SAH, there will be signs of meningeal irritation, such as a stiff and painful neck, photophobia, blurred vision, irritability, fever, and positive Kernig's and Brudzinski's signs. Exactly which deficits are present depends on the location of the aneurysm, the subsequent hemorrhage, and the severity of the bleeding.

The actual amount of blood loss through an aneurysm usually is quite small because of the severe vasoconstriction of vessels in the area of the aneurysm. This vasospasm may help stop the bleeding, but it also can cause ischemia to parts of the brain, resulting in localized neurological deficits.

When there is blood in the subarachnoid space, it irritates the brain stem, causing abnormal activity in the autonomic nervous system centers, often with cardiac dysrhythmias and hypertension. Another complication of blood in the subarachnoid space is hydrocephalus. This may occur as the result of obstruction of the narrow channels through which the CSF flows (eg, the aqueduct of Sylvius) by red cells in the CSF. The blood in the subarachnoid space also may impede reabsorption of the CSF from the arachnoid villi. Both these situations will cause hydrocephalus, with enlargement of the lateral and third ventricles.

DIAGNOSTIC STUDIES

The diagnosis of a cerebral aneurysm usually is made on the basis of the history, physical examination, lumbar puncture, cerebral arteriogram, and often a CT scan.

Transcranial Doppler ultrasonography may be used in patients to diagnose and help treat vasospasm, a common complication of SAH.[10] Daily serial correlations can be made to the patient's neurological status, as measured by the National Institutes of Health Stroke Scale. Trends can be established over time, and it also is a predictor of impending vasospasm (see discussion under "Stroke" and Table 32–4).

Management

GENERAL MEASURES

Management of a patient with a ruptured or leaking aneurysm before surgical repair includes a quiet environment and minimal stimulation. Sedation may be used. The number of visitors may need to be limited. Hot or cold beverages and caffeine products may be prohibited. Constipa-

Botterell Classification of Aneurysms	
Grade	*Criteria*
Grade I (minimal bleed)	Patient is alert, with no focal neurological signs and no signs of meningeal irritation.
Grade II (mild bleed)	Patient is alert with minimal deficits and usually signs of meningeal irritation.
Grade III (moderate bleed)	Patient is lethargic, confused, with or without neurological deficits and signs of meningeal irritation.
Grade IV (moderate to severe bleed)	Patient is stuporous or comatose with some purposeful movements. Major neurological deficits may or may not be evident.
Grade V (severe bleed)	Patient is comatose and often decerebrate. Patient appears moribund.

tion should be prevented, as should straining or vigorous coughing.

PHARMACOLOGICAL THERAPY

Some physicians use aminocaproic acid (Amicar) in their management of a patient with an aneurysm. This is an antifibrinolytic agent that delays the lysis of blood clots. At the time of hemorrhage from an aneurysm, about 10 to 20 mL of blood escapes from the vessel. Loss of 30 to 50 mL of blood would be a massive hemorrhage, and the person probably would not survive. A blood clot normally forms over the bleeding vessel, then dissolves several days later. Aminocaproic acid may be used to prevent the breakdown of the clot over the aneurysm.

A calcium antagonist, such as nimodipine, may be used to reduce cerebral ischemia and vasospasm. Plasma volume should not be allowed to fall. Hyponatremia must be anticipated, which may result from hemodilution as a result of inappropriate secretion of antidiuretic hormone.

Stool softeners often are used in the management of patients with an aneurysm to prevent straining. Mild analgesics may be used for relief of headache; acetaminophen or codeine can be used without masking neurological signs. If hypertension is present, a drug such as hydralazine hydrochloride (Apresoline) or methyldopa (Aldomet) can control it.

Blood in the subarachnoid space will cause an elevated temperature. An antipyretic, usually acetaminophen, and hypothermia blankets are used if necessary. Steroids are controversial, but if used, dexamethasone (Decadron) is the steroid of choice. Fluids often are restricted to prevent cerebral edema.

SURGICAL INTERVENTION

Surgical excision or clipping may be considered if the aneurysm is in an accessible area. Aneurysms of the vertebrobasilar system often present a problem of surgical inaccessibility. Some aneurysms may be wrapped in a gauze-like material and coated with an acrylic substance that gives the aneurysm support. There is some controversy about when to intervene surgically in an aneurysm. Some physicians believe in stabilizing the patient after the hemorrhage for 7 to 10 days. Others believe that surgery should be performed immediately after the hemorrhage. The current trend is to operate sooner rather than later.

After AVM excision or aneurysm clipping, the patient may be intubated and on mechanical ventilation to minimize postoperative cerebral swelling. The hyperventilation will keep the PCO_2 low, causing vasoconstriction of cerebral vasculature, reducing the volume of blood flow to the head, and thus reducing the ICP. Maintenance of an adequate airway is vital. If suctioning is necessary, it is important that the suction catheter go in and out quickly so that a PCO_2 buildup is avoided and sustained coughing is prevented.

Signs of vasospasm, such as hemiparesis, visual disturbance, seizures, or a decreasing LOC, should be noted and reported so that rapid medical interventions can be initiated (see discussion under "Complications").

Control of increased ICP is a collaborative effort. Nurses should keep the patient's head elevated without neck flexion or severe head rotation. Osmotics may be used as necessary.

Control of temperature is important, because fever increases the metabolic demands in the brain. Whenever blood gets into the subarachnoid space, whether from a leaking AVM or a ruptured aneurysm, the patient will be febrile. Control usually is by acetaminophen suppositories and a cooling blanket.

NURSING INTERVENTION

Severity and duration of any postoperative disability will depend largely on the location and extent of the vascular lesion and the resultant ischemia. Immediately after surgery, the patient should be watched for a change in neurological status, especially a change in LOC. The nurse must be alert for the development of new deficits or for a worsening of those present before surgery. Cerebral edema may develop after surgery, causing a change in neurological status.

A patent airway is required, and mechanical hyperventilation may be necessary to reduce ICP. Management of fluids and electrolytes includes a careful watch for hyponatremia, which can cause an increase in cerebral edema. Accurate intake and output records are important.

Monitoring of vital signs is crucial. The goal is to avoid any significant change, especially in blood pressure. Hypotension must be treated immediately to prevent a drop in cerebral perfusion. Cardiac dysrhythmias may be present, especially if there was bleeding into the subarachnoid space. Many dysrhythmias cause a drop in cardiac output, and consequently the cerebral perfusion falls. For this reason, dysrhythmias should be treated.

The critical care nurse may help awaken an unconscious patient by talking directly to the person. Research, however, indicates that even in an unconscious person, talking *about* that person around the bed causes a rise in ICP. Conversation over the unconscious person's bed should be limited to what would be said if the patient were fully awake. One can never be sure when the patient's brain stem is intact and conversation is being perceived, regardless of whether there is motor response to demonstrate this. The critical care nurse should talk to the patient about what is going to be done, even if the LOC is impaired.

Preoperative education of patient and family will make the postoperative period less stressful. Rehabilitation for specific deficits should begin early, and family participation in the rehabilitation program should be encouraged.

Nurses caring for a patient with an SAH should be aware of the person's baseline neurological status and be alert to changes. Patients are sometimes difficult to assess clinically when they are receiving sedation. A change in LOC is probably the first clinical sign that will be seen if the patient is deteriorating, unless an ICP monitoring device is in place, in which case increased ICP may be recognized immediately. Size and reactivity of the patient's pupils are important to document, along with changes in motor and sensory function. Sudden appearance of a cranial nerve defect or increasing severity of headache should be reported immediately. Blurred vision and dysphasia also may be present, along with other neurological deficits.

Complications in Cerebral Aneurysms

VASOSPASM

Vasospasm can occur after as well as before surgery in the person with an aneurysm. In fact, 30% to 50% of patients have preoperative vasospasm, whereas 65% have postoperative vasospasm. The aneurysm may have been clipped successfully, but because of this complication, the patient may end up with a large area of ischemic or infarcted brain and severe deficits.

Vasospasm usually occurs from 3 to 12 days after SAH. The peak incidence is between days 7 through 10, although there is some variation.[11] Vasospasm is of clinical significance because it decreases cerebral blood flow, depriving

---

Insights Into Clinical Research

Solenski N, Haley E, Kassell N et al: Medical complications of aneurysmal subarachnoid hemorrhage: A report of the multicenter, cooperative aneurysm study. Critical Care Medicine 23(6): 1007–1017, 1995

The purpose of this study was to describe the nonneurological complications following subarachnoid hemorrhage. Data from 457 patients over 18 years old who were seen at a neurosurgical center within 7 days of their aneurysm rupture were analyzed. Although 100% of the patients had at least one medical complication, 40% experienced at least one life-threatening complication. A low Glasgow Coma Score was predictive of at least one severe complication.

Anemia (37%), hypertension (37%), and cardiac dysrhythmias (35%) were the most frequent medical complications. Dysrhythmias tended to occur in the first 7 hospital days, appearing most often on the day of or after aneurysm surgery. Pulmonary edema (23%) appeared most frequently on the third hospital day.

These nonneurological complications are potentially preventable. This study demonstrates that mortality from medical complications approximates mortality from the more obvious complications, such as vasospasm and rebleeding, and illustrates the importance of the critical care nurse's vigilance and timely intervention.

---

brain tissue of oxygen and promoting accumulation of metabolic waste products, such as lactic acid.

The exact etiology of vasospasm is not clear. There does seem to be a positive correlation between the size of the hemorrhage seen on CT scan and subsequent development of spasm. There is a release of calcium ions from lysed red blood cells, and it is believed that calcium ions are mediators for spasm. There has been some success with use of nimodipine after SAH, improving patient outcomes after the bleed. There may be an inflammatory response to SAH, and this may stimulate release of vasoactive mediators. Some neuroprotective drugs are being tested that protect the cell membrane from this reaction.

Neuroprotective agents used to suppress development of secondary cerebral injury by interrupting the progression of delayed injury are still experimental. Delayed injury occurs as a result of the process of reperfusion to a part of the brain that previously was ischemic. When perfusion is reestablished, there is swelling of the capillary lumen and a drop in adenosine triphosphate (ATP) production. Because ATP powers the sodium pump in the cells, cellular metabolism slows and blood flow slows. This results in a secondary round of ischemia and cellular death and extension of the primary insult. Oxygen free radicals, lipid peroxidation, and excitatory amino acids are being studied as potential mediators of this reperfusion injury. Figure 35–7 demonstrates the role and interaction of these mediators.

"Triple-H" therapy is the standard for prevention and treatment of vasospasm. This consists of hypervolemic expansion, hemodilution, and induced hypertension in post-

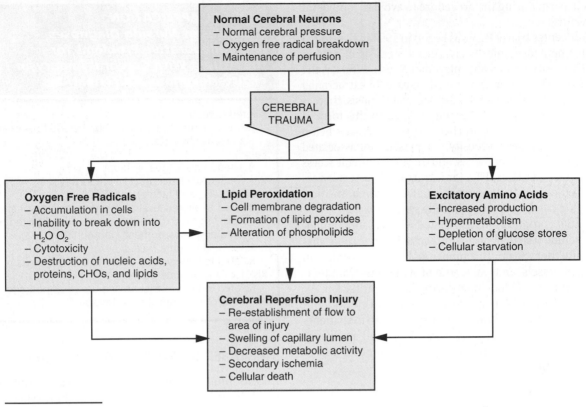

FIGURE 35-7
Influence of three key mediators on reperfusion injury.
(From Hilton G: Experimental neuroprotective agents: Nursing challenge. Dimensions of Critical Care 14[4]: 182, 1995)

operative patients. Along with this therapy, the calcium-channel blocker nimodipine is used. These measures reduce smooth muscle spasm and maximize perfusion when spasm occurs. Outcome is improved up to 21% by these therapies.[11]

Hypervolemia is accomplished by volume expansion, using both colloid and crystalloid solutions. Objectives of hypervolemia are to have a pulmonary capillary wedge pressure of approximately 14 mmHg (usual baseline is 6–8 mmHg) and a cardiac output of 6.5 to 8 L/min (4.5–5.0 L/min is normal). Hemodilution decreases blood viscosity, increases regional cerebral blood flow, and may decrease infarction size and increase oxygen transport. The goal for hemodilution is to reduce the hematocrit by 15% to 20%. Pressor agents are used to induce hypertension; the combination of dobutamine and dopamine is used frequently. The objective is to maintain systolic blood pressure at greater than 20 mmHg over normal.

For this therapy to be effective against vasospasm, the nurse must monitor hemodynamic parameters closely and assess frequently for signs of acute pulmonary edema. Recent attempts to prevent the spasmogenic effect of SAH have had some success. Erythrocytes that get trapped in the subarachnoid cisterns slowly hemolyze, and as they do, they release potent spasmogens, such as oxyhemoglobin. This causes the arterial vessel smooth muscle to spasm. Oxyhemoglobin also contributes to free radical release and lipid peroxidation.[12]

Thrombolytic agents, such as tissue plasminogen activator (t-PA), have been tried in SAH. This is a naturally occurring enzyme that activates plasmin, the fibrin-splitting enzyme, and dissolves fibrin clots. Blood from SAH is probably cleared by several mechanisms: thrombolysis, hemolysis, and phagocytosis. Instillation of t-PA into the basal cisterns after an aneurysm has been clipped, followed by irrigation, improves the natural process of clot clearance and most of the red blood cell destruction is eliminated.[13]

There appear to be no systemic effects from the local use of t-PA in the basal cisterns. There is, however, a potential complication of remote cerebral hemorrhage and bleeding from the craniotomy site. For this reason, it is recommended that postoperative dressings be checked at least hourly for evidence of bleeding during the first 24 hours, and CSF be examined for red blood cells if the patient has an external ventricular or lumbar drain.

When conventional medical therapy has not been effective, acute arterial vasospasm secondary to SAH is being managed in some centers by balloon angioplasty. Recent advances in microballoon technology now allow access to the cerebral vasculature with soft, flexible angioplasty balloons that mechanically dilate and improve cerebral blood flow through the major arterial segments affected by vasospasm.

Patients undergoing percutaneous transluminal angioplasty (PTA) are systemically anticoagulated with intravenous heparin during the procedure to avoid thromboembolic events.

A multicenter trial of PTA was begun in 1995 in the United States for hemodynamically significant stenosis of greater than 70% in extracranial and intracranial vessels. So far, the results from PTA appear favorable when used for extracranial vascular stenosis. However, for intracranial stenosis, there is significant morbidity and mortality related to this form of therapy, likely due to the smaller size of the vessels being treated, the increased tortuosity, the presence of associated small perforating side branches, and the more difficult access to these vessels.[14] Thus, PTA for intracranial vessels is recommended only if the patient has failed maximal medical therapy and continues to be clinically symptomatic.

Potential complications associated with cerebral angioplasty include vascular occlusion, vessel perforation, dissection, further spasm, thromboemboli, stroke, occlusion of adjacent vessels, and worsening of symptoms from temporary occlusion of blood flow during balloon inflation.

In the future, PTA may prove to be useful not only in treatment of some cerebral vasospasm, but also for patients with atherosclerosis, vasculitis, vessel dissection, radiation-induced vasculopathy, and postoperative stenosis due to intimal hyperplasia.

HYDROCEPHALUS

Hydrocephalus indicates an imbalance between the production and absorption of the CSF. It occurs in 15% to 20% of patients with SAH. When there is blood in the subarachnoid space, the red blood cells can occlude the very small channels leading from one ventricle to another. If that occurs, an obstructive hydrocephalus develops in the patient; that is, there is an obstruction to the normal flow of CSF, very often between the third and fourth ventricles or at the exits from the fourth ventricle. There also is potential for a reabsorption problem when there is blood in the subarachnoid space. The red blood cells occlude the arachnoid villi, impeding reabsorption and resulting in a communicating hydrocephalus. A shunt may be placed, often between one of the lateral ventricles and the peritoneal cavity (a V-P shunt) to drain the CSF and relieve the hydrocephalus.

DYSRHYTHMIAS

Dysrhythmias of any type may occur in patients with SAH, perhaps because blood in the CSF that bathes the brain stem is irritating to that area. The brain stem influences heart rate, so the presence of a chemical irritation can result in irregular rhythms.

REBLEEDING

Another complication in patients with an SAH can be a rebleed if the AVM or aneurysm is not repaired. At least 10% of all patients with SAH have another bleed within hours of the initial hemorrhage. Without intervention, the risk of rebleeding in the remaining patients is at least 30% during the subsequent 4 weeks. The immediate mortality of rebleeding is about 70%.[11]

CLINICAL APPLICATION:
Examples of Nursing Diagnoses and Collaborative Problems for the Patient With Cerebral Aneurysm or Arteriovenous Malformations

Altered Cerebral Tissue Perfusion
 Related to interruption in cerebral blood flow or intracranial hypertension
Pain
 Related to meningeal irritation
Risk for Sensory/Perceptual Alterations (visual, auditory, kinesthetic, and tactile)
 Related to altered level of consciousness, disorientation, impaired communication skills, restricted or unfamiliar environment, photophobia
Risk for Fluid Volume Excess
 Related to hypervolemia used to treat vasospasm
Risk for Fluid Volume Deficit
 Related to fluid restriction and use of osmotics to control intracranial hypertension

INCREASED INTRACRANIAL PRESSURE

In CNS injury, elevated ICP is a potential complication. It may be the result of ischemia after a stroke or a hemorrhagic stroke where the blood causes a mass lesion effect. It may result from a leaking AVM or aneurysm or may be postoperative after manipulation of the brain during a craniotomy.

Many nursing interventions can minimize this potentially fatal complication. Early medical interventions, such as hyperventilation, use of osmotics, steroids, barbiturate coma, hypothermia, and fluid restriction, also are valuable in treating this complication. (Osmotics are not used when there is an active cerebral hemorrhage, however, because they may increase the bleeding by shrinking the brain and releasing the tamponade effect of the leaking vessel.)

CLINICAL APPLICATION: Patient Care Study

Mrs. B was a 50-year-old woman who, while playing with her dog, collapsed, grabbing her head. She was rushed to the hospital where she was diagnosed as having a small ruptured cerebral aneurysm. She was awake on entering the intensive care unit but complained of a severe headache and a stiff neck. She was taken to surgery within 4 hours, where the aneurysm was clipped successfully. Postoperative angiogram demonstrated no evidence of vasospasm. On day 5, Mrs. B became confused, disoriented, weak in one arm, and wanted to sleep more than usual. She was sent to radiology for an emergent CT scan, where hydrocephalus and rebleeding were ruled out. Transcranial Doppler ultrasonography confirmed vasospasm.

"Triple-H" therapy (hypervolemia, hemodilution, and induced hypertension) and nimodipine were initiated, and follow-up transcranial Doppler ultrasonography showed normal lumen diameter of the vessels. By the next day, Mrs. B was oriented and following commands, had normal strength in all extremities, and was neurologically intact. She was discharged home 2 weeks later, doing well.

Seizure Disorders

A seizure is the sudden discharge of a group of neurons, resulting in a transient impairment of consciousness, movement, sensation, or memory. The term *seizure disorder* may refer to one isolated occurrence or to a recurrent situation. The term *epilepsy* usually is reserved for a chronic disorder involving recurrent seizures. There seems to be less social stigma associated with the term *seizure disorder* than with *epilepsy*.

Seizures may be caused by a variety of pathological conditions, including brain tumors, trauma, blood clots, meningitis, encephalitis, electrolyte disorders, alcohol and drug overdose and withdrawal, metabolic disorders, uremia, overhydration, toxic substances, and cerebral anoxia. Some seizures are idiopathic.

Between 5% and 50% of patients with head trauma have post-traumatic seizures. When trauma is the cause, the seizures occur within 2 years of the injury in 90% of the cases. Craniotomies may leave scar tissue, which can be a future site of seizure activity.

Seizures develop in 10% to 20% of patients with strokes. CNS infections result in 17% to 34% of those people having seizures. Lesions of the brain can be produced by degenerative CNS disease, such as multiple sclerosis, Alzheimer's disease, and Huntington's chorea, and these can be a site for seizure activity. Seizures usually are a symptom of some cerebral pathological condition and not a disease entity in themselves.

Pathophysiological Principles

The exact mechanism that causes seizure activity in the brain is not fully understood. Some trigger causes a sudden abnormal burst of electrical stimulation, disrupting the brain's normal nerve conduction. In a non–seizure-prone brain, there is a balance between excitatory and inhibitory synaptic influences on postsynaptic neurons. In a seizure-prone brain, this balance somehow is disrupted, causing imbalanced patterns of electrical conduction called paroxysmal depolarization shifts. These shifts may be seen either when there is excessive excitatory influence or insufficient inhibitory influence.

The pathophysiological process is different with different types of seizures, leading to a variety of clinical manifestations (see "Clinical Manifestations," under "Assessment").

Classification of Seizures

Seizures are classified according to clinical and EEG criteria established by the Commission of Classification and Terminology of the International League Against Epilepsy (see display). The two main categories are generalized and focal, or partial, seizures. Generalized seizures show synchronous involvement of all regions of the brain in both hemispheres.

Partial seizures show clinical or EEG evidence of a focal onset, involving one particular part of the brain.

PARTIAL SEIZURES

There are two types of seizures: simple and complex. Partial seizures of either type may progress to a generalized seizure if the abnormal electrical discharges spread from the initial focus to involve the remainder of the brain. Differentiation of the two types of partial seizures is based on whether consciousness is retained or impaired. When there is no impairment of consciousness, the attack is termed a simple partial seizure, which may be motor, sensory, autonomic, or psychic in nature, depending on the seizure focus. If the focus is in the posterior frontal lobe near the cortex, there will be motor involvement of the contralateral side of the body.

The old term, "jacksonian seizure," is an example of a simple partial seizure with motor involvement. Clinically, there are repetitive, usually unilateral involuntary contractions of a specific muscle group, such as thumb flexors. Adjacent muscle groups are affected progressively, often until one entire side of the body is involved. In the individual patient, the seizure almost always begins in the same area and migrates in the same pattern, called the jacksonian march.

If the focus is in the anterior parietal lobe, which is involved with the sensory cortex, no clinical evidence of seizures may appear. The patient may describe sensory phe-

---

International Classification of Epileptic Seizures

I. Partial seizures
  A. Simple partial (consciousness retained)
    1. Motor
    2. Sensory
    3. Autonomic
    4. Psychic
  B. Complex partial (consciousness impaired)
    1. Simple partial, followed by impaired consciousness
    2. Consciousness impaired at onset
  C. Partial seizures with secondary generalization
II. Generalized seizures
  A. Absences
    1. Typical
    2. Atypical
  B. Generalized tonic–clonic
  C. Tonic
  D. Clonic
  E. Myoclonic
  F. Atonic
III. Unclassified seizures

nomena related to the focus in the contralateral side of the brain. Partial seizures with psychic symptoms are rare.

Complex partial seizures (also known as temporal lobe, psychomotor seizures, or automatisms) often have their focus in or near the temporal lobe, although sometimes the focus is in the frontal lobe. There always is an impairment in the LOC. Clinical manifestations with this type of seizure are varied, and the behavior exhibited may be quite bizarre. There may be visual, auditory, or olfactory hallucinations. A visceral sensation, such as nausea, vomiting, or profuse sweating, may precede the seizure.

The patient may demonstrate automatisms, or automatic behaviors, such as playing with buttons on clothing or becoming preoccupied with some other motor activity. During the seizure, the person usually is not combative, but if provoked or if someone attempts restraint, the person may become agitated and asocial. After the seizure episode, the patient has no recall of behavior displayed. Such a person may be misdiagnosed as having a psychiatric problem because behaviors often are similar.

GENERALIZED SEIZURES

In a generalized seizure, the entire brain is activated at once, synchronously, without a focal onset. There is no aura or prodromal warning unless it is a partial seizure that has generalized.

Typical absence seizures are diagnosed by 3-second spike wave activity on EEG (ie, 3 cycles/second [Hz]). These seizures usually occur in children and often are outgrown by puberty. After puberty, the person may not have any further seizure activity, or the type of seizure may change to a generalized type of activity.

Clinically, a typical absence seizure does not involve any violent involuntary movements or incontinence. There may be minor manifestations, such as blinking. There is a transient, often unnoticed loss of consciousness or contact with the environment. The behavior, with vacant staring, may resemble daydreaming and is over within a few seconds.

Atypical absence seizures clinically resemble typical absence seizures. The primary difference is demonstrated on EEG; only the typical absence seizure demonstrates 3-second spike wave activity. Atypical absence seizures may be seen in both children and adults. There may be minor automatisms. The patient usually has other types of seizures as well, which often are refractory to medical therapy. Atypical absence seizures frequently are associated with mental retardation.

In the old classification, generalized tonic-clonic seizures were called grand mal, or major motor, seizures. These seizures involve a bilateral tonic extension of the extremities followed by synchronous bilateral jerking movements. There may be a cry, incontinence of stool or urine or both, tongue-biting, and foaming at the mouth. There is a sudden loss of consciousness. The seizure is followed by a postictal period, during which the patient is exhausted and extremely difficult to arouse. As the person awakens, diffuse muscle soreness and initial confusion may be experienced.

Tonic or clonic generalized seizures exhibit only one phase of the previously described tonic–clonic activity.

Myoclonic seizures are typified by synchronous asymmetrical rapid jerking of one or more extremity, the trunk, or a specific muscle group. They may be seen with metabolic encephalopathies, such as hepatic failure; with infectious processes; and with degenerative processes. There is no loss of consciousness associated with myoclonic seizures.

Atonic seizures, previously classified as "drop attacks" or akinetic seizures, are another type of generalized seizure. There usually is loss of consciousness, but the episode may be so brief that the patient is unaware of the blackout. The patient is aware of the sudden loss of muscle tone as he or she falls to the ground.

UNCLASSIFIED SEIZURES

Some seizures do not fit any of the aforementioned classifications, perhaps because clinically or electrographically they do not meet the criteria of the established categories. Sometimes the diagnosis of a seizure disorder needs to be confirmed with observation and in-hospital monitoring, rather than on an outpatient basis.

STATUS EPILEPTICUS

Status epilepticus is a medical emergency characterized by a series of seizures without recovery of the baseline neurological status between the seizures. Most authorities agree that clinical, or EEG, seizure activity that lasts 30 minutes or more constitutes status epilepticus. Classification of status epilepticus is shown in the display.

PSEUDOSEIZURES

Pseudoseizures are psychologically based. They have no associated abnormal discharges from the brain. They may resemble epileptic seizures closely, thus making the diagnosis difficult. Some patients may have both pseudoseizures and a real seizure disorder.

Pseudoseizures are frequent in children and adolescents (the mean age range is 18.5–27.5 years), and the incidence is twice as high in women as in men. The onset of a pseudoseizure may be gradual or sudden, and it usually is no longer than an epileptic seizure. Pseudoseizures occur more often around witnesses. Environmental influences can affect the course of a pseudoseizure and may precipitate

---

Classification of Status Epilepticus

I. Convulsive status
   A. Generalized tonic–clonic status
   B. Partial motor status ("epilepsia partialis continua")
II. Nonconvulsive status
   A. Absence status (petit mal status)
   B. Complex partial status (psychomotor status)
   C. Partial sensory status

it. Patients may follow commands and focus their eye contact on a witness.

Abnormal motor activity occurs with pseudoseizures. One unusual type is opisthotonus, in which the head and legs are bent backward and the trunk arches forward. Protective mechanisms, such as breaking a fall with the arms and protecting the head from hitting the ground, are present in patients who have pseudoseizures but not in those who have real seizures.

With pseudoseizures, there is no tongue biting, incontinence, or dilated pupils; the corneal reflex is present; and there is response to painful stimulation. Confusion after the pseudoseizure usually is absent. Table 35–2 distinguishes epileptic seizures from pseudoseizures.

Assessment

HISTORY AND PHYSICAL EXAMINATION

A complete neurological examination should be performed in a seizure workup because a focal finding may help determine the origin of some seizure activity. Along with the neurological examination, a history should be elicited. Often the history will reveal precipitating factors that may have provoked the seizure, even in usually well controlled patients. Some common precipitating factors may be fever, injury, menses, sleep deprivation, drug use, physical exhaustion, and hyperventilation. Emotional stress from the home or work environment also is a possible precipitating factor.

An often invaluable piece of information in the assessment of seizure disorders is a description of the attack by an eyewitness. The patient also may be able to help in the description of the event, especially if an aura was felt before the attack.

The critical care nurse who witnesses an actual seizure can help the physician diagnose the type of seizure and localize the focus. A specific description of the seizure should include the factors listed in the assessment display.

DIAGNOSTIC STUDIES

A CT scan usually is part of the seizure diagnostic workup. Such pathological conditions as tumor, edema, infarct, congenital lesion, hemorrhage, AVM, or ventricular enlargement can be seen on CT scan.

Skull x-rays usually are not of much help in the diagnostic workup of seizures, except perhaps to rule out a fracture. The CT scan is more inclusive. An MRI also may be done to determine the presence of pathological CNS changes.

A metabolic workup may be useful. Tests for blood glucose, electrolytes, calcium, and hepatic and renal function often are obtained. The presence of infection may be investigated. Platelet count, sedimentation rate, and serological or immunological tests also may be ordered. A lumbar puncture may help determine presence of an infection, such as meningitis. The CSF also is examined for cells, protein, glucose, and cultures. In the presence of a CNS infection, white blood cells and protein may be elevated and glucose level decreased compared with the serum values. Normally, the CSF glucose is one-half to two-thirds the serum value.

An EEG often is beneficial in confirming the seizure diagnosis and localizing a lesion if one exists. Electroencephalograms show neurological function, whereas CT scans demonstrate anatomy. Most EEGs are done during a time when the patient is not actively seizing. The EEG may not be very helpful, unless the patient happened to be seizing during the EEG recording. Sometimes, photic stimulation and hyperventilation can provoke a generalized seizure of the absence type. These stimuli usually are included during the routine EEG recording. If a patient appears to be clinically seizing and the concurrent EEG is normal, the possibility of hysterical seizures or pseudoseizures should be considered.

TABLE 35-2
Criteria for Distinguishing Epileptic Seizures From Pseudoseizures

	Epileptic	Pseudoseizure
Apparent cause	Absent	Emotional disturbance
Warning	Varies, but more commonly unilateral or epigastric aura	Palpitation, malaise, choking, bilateral foot aura
Onset	Commonly sudden	Often gradual
Scream	At onset	During course
Convulsion	Rigidity followed by "jerking"; rarely rigidity alone	Rigidity or "struggling"; throwing limbs and head about
Biting	Tongue	Lips, hands, or more often other people and things
Micturition	Frequent	Never
Defecation	Occasional	Never
Duration	A few minutes	Often half an hour or several hours
Restraint needed	To prevent self-injury	To control violence
Termination	Spontaneous	Spontaneous or artificially induced (eg, water)

- *Onset.* Determine whether the seizure had a sudden onset or whether it was preceded by a warning aura.
- *Duration.* Timing of the seizure from onset to end is important. What was the frequency of seizures?
- *Motor activity.* Note the parts of the body involved and determine whether both left and right sides were involved. In what part of the body did the seizure begin, and how did it progress? Was rigidity, jerking, or twitching observed?
- *Eyes and tongue.* Notice whether there was any deviation of the eyes or tongue to one side or the other.
- *State of consciousness.* Arousability is important. Was the patient arousable during the seizure or immediately after it? If there was unconsciousness, the duration of that period should be timed. Was there confusion or awareness and clear memory of the event after the seizure?
- *Distractibility.* Determine whether the patient responds to the environment during the seizure, such as when his or her name is called. Some patients, often drug abusers, may try to feign seizures, which will be revealed when they respond to their names.
- *Pupils.* Note any change in size, shape, or equality of the pupils and their reaction to light or any deviation to one side.
- *Teeth.* Observe whether the teeth were clenched or open.
- *Respirations.* Observe the rate, quality, or absence of respiration and the presence of cyanosis.
- *Body activities.* Report incontinence, vomiting, salivation, and bleeding from the mouth or tongue.
- *After the seizure.* After a seizure there can be a transient paralysis, weakness, numbness, tingling, dysphasia, other injuries, a postictal period, or amnesia regarding the seizure and events before and after it.
- *Precipitating factors.* By talking to the patient, the nurse may uncover a precipitating factor. Fever, emotional or physical stress, and anticonvulsant noncompliance all may precipitate a seizure.

Management

PHARMACOLOGICAL THERAPY

Drug management of *any* seizure activity should be systematic. The accompanying display lists principles of treatment. Different types of seizures respond better to specific drugs. Partial seizures (simple or complex) and generalized seizures of the tonic–clonic type respond to carbamazepine, phenytoin, primidone, and phenobarbital. Some studies suggest that valproate, chlorazepate, clonazepam, and methsuximide are useful in some refractory cases of complex partial seizures.

Ethosuximide is the drug of choice for simple absences, and phenobarbital usually is the second choice. Valproate or clonazepam is useful in atypical absences, atonic seizures, and myoclonic seizures. Myoclonic seizures may be treated with adrenocorticotropic hormone or a ketogenic diet or both.

Therapeutic blood levels should be checked periodically. Drug screens can identify patients who are not compliant with their treatment, those who may metabolize the drugs at different rates, or those who are not absorbing it. Most anticonvulsive drugs may be taken once or twice daily and still maintain therapeutic levels because of the long half-life of these drugs.

Baclofen recently has had some success as an adjunct to conventional anticonvulsant therapy to control complex partial seizures. Animal studies indicate that baclofen increases the threshold for induced seizures.

Treatment of status epilepticus usually involves the use of diazepam, phenytoin, phenobarbital, or any combination of these drugs. Diazepam, a rapid-acting drug with short duration, may stop all types of status epilepticus activity immediately. Because of the rapid onset of action, it can be dose regulated according to the effects it has. The dosage of diazepam is 5 to 20 mg, injected intravenously at a rate of 5 mg or less per minute, while the nurse watches for respiratory depression. Because the duration of action of diazepam is short, 10% to 50% of patients treated with this drug alone experience recurrent seizure activity.

Diazepam should be accompanied by another drug, such as phenytoin. Phenytoin provides long-term control in about 80% of cases of status epilepticus. The dose of phenytoin is 12 to 18 mg/kg. A loading dose of 1 to 1.5 is given to most adults. The drug should be administered at a rate of 40 to 50 mg/min while the patient is on a cardiac monitor. If the drug is given too rapidly, there may be a widening of the

---

Principles of Treatment of Seizures

1. Establish the diagnosis and rule out underlying cerebral pathological condition.
2. Classify seizure type, using clinical and electroencephalogram criteria.
3. Select drug of first choice for seizure type.
4. Increase dose slowly until end point is reached:
   - Complete seizure control
   - Optimum plasma drug level
   - Toxic side effects
5. If poor seizure control, gradually withdraw first drug while replacing with second drug of choice for seizure type: monotherapy is preferable to polypharmacy.
6. If improvement is only partial, other drugs may be necessary.
7. Adjust dose gradually according to plasma levels, keeping in mind:
   - Pharmacokinetics of each drug
   - Potential drug interactions
8. If best medical therapy is unsuccessful, refer to specialized epilepsy center for intensive monitoring and possible surgical therapy.

QRS complexes, cardiac conduction disturbances, bradycardia, hypotension, and cardiac arrest.

Phenytoin is highly alkaline and will precipitate easily in any intravenous solution that contains dextrose. It should be given in normal saline or lactated Ringer's solution. The onset of action is 10 to 20 minutes. When given with diazepam, which acts immediately, the phenytoin will be effective by the time the diazepam is beginning to wear off. Phenytoin usually is not effective against typical absence seizures.

Phenobarbital may be given intravenously to stop status epilepticus, or the drug may be administered to treat seizures on a long-term basis. The dose is 5 to 8 mg/kg, and the effects are seen in 5 to 25 minutes. The rate of injection is 40 to 60 mg/min. When phenobarbital is given along with diazepam, the respiratory depression effect of each may be compounded, so respirations should be monitored carefully.

Once the status epilepticus is under control, the etiology should be determined because seizures often are a sign of an underlying pathological process and not a disease entity in themselves.

SURGICAL INTERVENTION

Recent advances in diagnostic and microsurgical techniques have made surgical intervention more possible for selected patients who are resistant to drug therapy. Technology now exists to map electrical activity from deep within the brain. Stereotactic surgical techniques are also available.

Studies on vagal nerve stimulation are underway. This treatment involves an implantable neurocybernetic prosthesis (NCP), which is similar in construction to a cardiac pacemaker. The NCP stimulates the vagus nerve with intermittent electrical impulses to prevent or reduce some complex partial seizures. An electronic device is implanted under the skin between the clavicle and the nipple. It is programmable from outside the skin, so changes can be made in its initial setup. The NCP delivers a stimulation every 5 to 20 minutes, with a duration of 30 to 90 seconds. It is hypothesized that stimulation of the vagus nerve desynchronizes cerebral electrical activity, giving an antiepileptic effect. Preliminary reports on the effectiveness of NCP are favorable.

PATIENT EDUCATION

Teaching the patient and family about the importance of anticonvulsant medications is a vital part of the nurse's role. Side effects and toxic effects should be taught. Information on what to do if a seizure occurs may help alleviate some anxiety in the patient and family as well. This information empowers the patient and family to control the unpredictability of seizure activity to some extent. A battle plan of sorts can be established and put into use if a seizure occurs.

If one particular trigger, such as flashing lights, is identified as the precipitating event to a seizure, this trigger can be avoided. When the stimulus is not clear, general advice may include avoidance of becoming overtired, tackling too many stressful activities at once, and consuming alcohol and excessive caffeine. Patients should be advised to wear a medical alert bracelet or necklace and stay hydrated.

NURSING INTERVENTION

If a nurse encounters a person who is seizing, he or she should stay with the patient to offer protection from the environment. A seizing patient never should be restrained. Any tight or restrictive clothing can be loosened. If the patient already has the teeth clenched, the nurse should not attempt to insert an oral airway or tongue blade because such action may break off teeth, which the patient might aspirate. A patent airway should be maintained during the seizure. It may help to turn the patient on the side to prevent aspiration. The nurse should reassure and reorient the patient if the seizure has caused fright and disorientation.

Complications in Seizures

PHYSICAL AND DENTAL INJURY

Some common complications after seizures are physical injury and broken teeth if someone tries to insert a tongue blade or oral airway after the teeth already are clenched tight. Teeth can also be aspirated into the lungs.

RHABDOMYOLYSIS AND MYOGLOBINURIA

Another complication of seizure activity may be rhabdomyolysis and myoglobinuria. Myoglobin is an iron-containing pigment found in skeletal muscle, especially in those specialized for sustained contraction. There is muscle damage with seizure activity, as with many other activities. Severe exercise, such as jogging, performing military calisthenics, marathon running, and riding mechanical bulls, can cause the same type of muscle breakdown. Patients who are found after lying unconscious for a period of time, those who present with amphetamine or heroin overdoses (with the accompanying shaking chills), and those who demonstrate phencyclidine (PCP, angel dust) abuse may have profound rhabdomyolysis when there is unusual muscular hyperactivity.

The protein from the destroyed tissue turns the patient's urine red or cola colored. The muscle cell breakdown releases myoglobin into the bloodstream, which is rapidly filtered by the kidneys, producing the dark red or brown urine. The myoglobin can occlude the kidneys, and renal failure may result. The critical care nurse may be the first to recognize the signs of this serious complication.

Treatment of rhabdomyolysis involves flushing the kidneys. Extensive skeletal muscle necrosis may be associated with massive loss of arterial volume into necrotic muscle and subsequent shock. The large volume replacement necessary for these patients approximates that seen in extensively burned patients. Furosemide, mannitol, or both are used sometimes for diuresis, along with volume replacement. Hyperkalemia due to the cellular breakdown and renal dysfunction also may require treatment.

PSYCHOLOGICAL ABERRATIONS

The psychological reaction of a patient with a known seizure disorder is varied. One response to the feelings of dependency and loss of self-esteem that seizures may precipitate is social withdrawal. This may seem to the patient to be an adequate coping mechanism, but it can foster feelings of depression.

People with long histories of seizures may have personality disorders. They may be manipulative, hostile, and aggressive. Children may demonstrate personality disorders through temper tantrums, hyperactivity, or antisocial behavior. The reaction of others to people with seizure disorders must be one of acceptance and support. Therapeutic interaction can help the patient achieve resocialization.

Denial is another psychological coping mechanism that may be displayed by patient or family. If the interval between seizures is long, this mechanism is easier to use. When a patient uses denial, there may be concurrent noncompliance with medical therapy.

Guillain-Barré Syndrome

Guillain-Barré syndrome (GBS) is most commonly thought to be an inflammatory peripheral neuropathy in which lymphocytes and macrophages strip myelin from axons. The diffuse inflammatory reaction may be seen in the peripheral nervous system, cranial nerves, and the ventral and dorsal spinal nerve roots. The etiology is uncertain, but an autoimmune response is strongly suspected. Some researchers believe the syndrome has a viral origin, but no virus has been isolated thus far.

Guillain-Barré occurs with equal frequency in both sexes and in all races. A slight peak seems to occur in the 16- to 25-year age group, but it may develop at any age. About half the victims have a mild febrile illness 2 to 3 weeks before onset of symptoms. The febrile infection usually is of respiratory or gastrointestinal origin. The annual incidence in 0.75 to 2.0 cases per 100,000 population.[15]

Pathophysiological Principles

In GBS, the myelin sheath surrounding the axon is lost. The myelin sheath is quite susceptible to injury by many agents and conditions, including physical trauma, hypoxemia, toxic chemicals, vascular insufficiency, and immunological reactions. Demyelination is a common response of neural tissue to any of these adverse conditions.

Myelinated axons conduct nerve impulses more rapidly than nonmyelinated axons. Along the course of a myelinated fiber are interruptions in the sheath (nodes of Ranvier) where there is direct contact between the cell membrane of the axon and the extracellular fluid. The membrane is highly permeable at these nodes, thus making conduction good. The movement of ions into and out of the axon can occur rapidly only at the nodes of Ranvier (Fig. 35–8); thus, a nerve impulse along a myelinated fiber may jump from node to node (saltatory conduction) quite rapidly. Loss of the myelin sheath in GBS makes saltatory conduction impossible, and nerve impulse transmission is aborted.

A current theory regarding the disease process of GBS speculates that a primary lymphocytic T-cell mechanism is the cause of the inflammation. Cells migrate through the vessel walls to the peripheral nerve; the result is edema and perivascular inflammation. Macrophages then break down the myelin.

Another causal theory holds that the process of demyelination is initiated by an antibody attack on the myelin early in the course of the disease. Demyelination causes axon atrophy, which causes slowed or blocked nerve conduction.

Assessment

HISTORY

The history often is one of an upper respiratory or gastrointestinal disorder occurring 1 to 4 weeks before onset of neurological manifestations. The history of the onset of symptoms may be revealing, because those of GBS usually begin with weakness or paresthesias (numbness and tingling) of the lower extremities and ascend in a symmetrical pattern.

Significant interest has developed in the preceding infections and the development of autoantibodies. Some studies show a relationship between clinical findings and *Campylobacter jejuni* infection and also between clinical findings and cytomegalovirus infections. In the first group, patients tend to have a pure motor GBS with predominantly distal motor involvement and a rapid onset of weakness. In the second group, there is more involvement of the sensory system; cranial nerves are more often involved as are more proximal muscles, resulting in a high incidence of mechanical ventilation.

CLINICAL MANIFESTATIONS

A flaccid, symmetrical, ascending paralysis quickly develops. The trunk and cranial nerves may become involved. Respiratory muscles may become affected, resulting in respiratory insufficiency.

Autonomic disturbances, such as urinary retention and postural hypotension, sometimes occur. Superficial and deep tendon reflexes may be lost. Usually no muscle wasting is noted because the flaccid paralysis develops so rapidly. Some patients experience tenderness and pain on deep pressure or movement of some muscles.

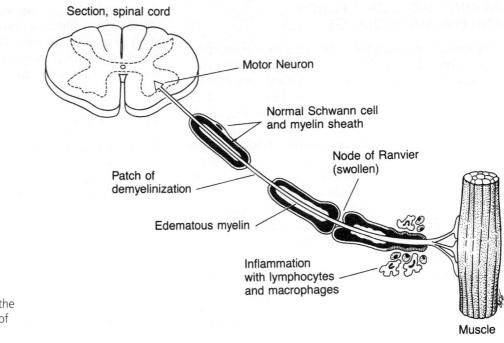

Section, spinal cord

Motor Neuron

Normal Schwann cell
and myelin sheath

Node of Ranvier
(swollen)

Patch of
demyelinization

Edematous myelin

Inflammation
with lymphocytes
and macrophages

Muscle

FIGURE 35-8
Pathological changes with
Guillain-Barré syndrome. Note the
patchy demyelination and loss of
the Schwann cell.

Sensory symptoms of paresthesias, including tingling "pins and needles" and numbness, may occur transiently. If cranial nerves are involved, the facial (VII) nerve is affected most often. GBS does not affect LOC, pupillary signs, or cerebral function.

Symptoms usually peak within 1 week, but may progress for several weeks. The level of paralysis may stop at any point. Motor function returns in a descending fashion. Demyelination occurs rapidly, but the rate of remyelination is only about 1 to 2 mm/d.

DIAGNOSTIC STUDIES

Diagnosis of GBS depends a great deal on the history and the clinical progression of symptoms. No one test will confirm the diagnosis of GBS; it is a "rule out" disorder. Lumbar puncture may reveal a normal protein level initially, with an elevation in the fourth and sixth week.

Nerve conduction studies record impulse transmission along the nerve fiber, and in a patient with GBS, the velocity of conduction will be reduced.

About 25% of people with this disease have antibodies to either cytomegalovirus or Epstein-Barr virus. It has been suggested that an altered immune response to peripheral nerve antigens may contribute to development of the disorder.

Pulmonary function tests may be done when GBS is suspected, so that a baseline is established for comparison as the disease progresses. Declining pulmonary function capacity may indicate the need for mechanical ventilation.

Management

The major goals in caring for a patient with GBS are to provide functional maintenance of the body systems, to treat life-threatening crises promptly, to prevent infections and complications of immobility, and to provide psychological support for the patient and family.

RESPIRATORY AND CARDIOVASCULAR SUPPORT

If the respiratory musculature is involved, mechanical ventilation will be necessary. Tracheostomy may be needed if the patient cannot be weaned from the ventilator in a couple of weeks. Respiratory failure should be anticipated until the progress of the disorder plateaus because it never is clear how far the paralysis will ascend.

If there is autonomic nervous system involvement, drastic changes in blood pressure (hypotension or hypertension) and heart rate can occur, and the patient should be monitored closely. Cardiac monitoring will allow dysrhythmias to be identified and treated quickly. An autonomic nervous system disturbance may be triggered by the Valsalva maneuver, coughing, suctioning, and position changes, so these activities should be performed very carefully.

PLASMAPHERESIS

Plasmapheresis may be used both for GBS or myasthenia gravis to remove the offending antibodies from plasma. The patient's plasma is separated selectively from whole blood, and its abnormal constituents are washed out, or the plasma is exchanged with normal plasma or a colloidal substitute. Many centers begin this plasma exchange (PE) if it appears the patient is worsening and will be unable to return home within about 2 weeks, approximately the time it would take to complete a course of PEs. If plasmapheresis is started 3 weeks or longer after the onset of symptoms, it does not appear to be very effective.

IMMUNE GLOBULIN INFUSION AND PLASMA EXCHANGE

Intravenous immunoglobulin (IVIG) is a blood product that contains pooled plasma from many people. The major component is immunoglobulin G, with a trace amount of immunoglobulin A. IVIG has been used in the past to treat disorders such as idiopathic thrombocytopenic purpura, an autoimmune process in which antibodies attack the patient's platelets. It has been suggested that IVIG may also be effective in treating other autoimmune disorders, such as GBS, myasthenia gravis, multiple sclerosis, chronic inflammatory demyelinating polyneuropathy, polymyositis, dermatomyositis and intractable childhood seizures.[16]

Trials are still underway to evaluate the effects of immune globulin therapy versus PE versus a combination of PE followed by immune globulin therapy. The effects of immune globulin therapy alone or in combination with corticosteroids (methylprednisolone and immune globulin therapy may have a synergistic effect) are also being evaluated. Initial research indicates that immunoglobulins have a specific effect in certain subgroups, such as patients with *C. jejuni* infection or cytomegalovirus infection.

Immune globulins can be infused easily, even in the home setting, without expensive equipment. The optimal dosages and frequency of administration are yet to be determined. This therapy is less invasive than PE.

Plasma exchange removes circulating antibodies and immunoglobulins, both those that are beneficial and those that are harmful to the patient. This immunosuppression must be closely monitored, because it places the patient at significant risk for infection. Positive clinical responses to PE may include shortened duration of muscle weakness, prevention or reduction of the need for mechanical ventilation, and reduced long-term disability. Thus, PE may shorten the duration and severity of the syndrome.

It is believed that PE removes 65% to 70% of circulating antibodies, but that the antibodies reenter the plasma continuously, reaching previous levels in 7 to 20 days. Likewise, immune globulin, which binds to receptors on T cells or to receptors on nerves, would be expected to induce only a temporary improvement because of the turnover of T cells or the loss of antibodies from the receptors. Daily treatments of IVIG or PE may be most beneficial with acute GBS in which the patient is deteriorating rapidly.

Medications are usually not administered before or during PE to avoid their immediate removal along with the plasma. Blood levels must be monitored, with supplemental dosing to ensure that therapeutic drug levels are maintained.

Some studies suggest that both immune globulin therapy and PE are efficacious. There are specific situations, however, in which immune globulin therapy would be the treatment of choice: in patients in whom venous access for PE is a problem and when apheresis equipment is not readily available.

Improvement demonstrated in patients who receive either therapy might be due to axonal regeneration, remyelination, or decrease of conduction block. Dyck and associates believe that only a decrease of conduction block is fast enough to explain the rapid improvement seen with these therapies.[17]

PAIN MANAGEMENT

Pain management may be of concern in a patient with GBS. Severe muscle pain usually subsides as muscle strength improves. Transcutaneous electrical stimulation units are helpful for some. Later, pain commonly is hyperesthetic. Some drugs may provide temporary relief. Pain usually is worse between 10 PM and 4 AM, preventing sleep, and narcotics may be used liberally at night if the patient is not so marginally compensated that narcotics will cause respiratory failure. In that case, the patient usually is intubated and then given narcotics.

Pain may persist several years after the acute phase of GBS. In this situation, it is a challenge to determine if the persisting discomfort is actually a residual effect of the GBS or if it represents a new problem. Arthritic problems, diabetic neuropathy, carpal tunnel syndrome, and pinched low back nerves should be ruled out, because these may mimic some of the abnormal sensations seen with GBS. Nerve blocks may be considered for intractable pain.

COMFORT AND SLEEP

Sleep deprivation can become a serious problem for a patient with this disorder, especially because the pain seems to accelerate at night. Comfort measures, analgesics, and careful control of the environment (eg, turning out the lights and providing a quiet room) may help to promote sleep and rest. A patient who is paralyzed and perhaps on

Insights Into Clinical Research

Dyck P, Litchy W, Kratz K, Suarez G, Low P, Pineda A, Windebank A, Karnes J, O'Brien P: A plasma exchange versus immune globulin infusion trial in chronic inflammatory demyelinating polyradiculoneuropathy. Annals of Neurology 36(6):838–844, 1994

The purpose of this study was to evaluate two treatment regimens in patients with chronic inflammatory demyelinating polyradiculoneuropathy. Thirteen patients received both plasma exchange and immune globulin infusion, four patients received only plasma exchange, and two patients received only immune globulin infusion. When the effectiveness of the two treatments was compared, statistically significant differences between the two were not found. There was statistically significant improvement shown with both therapies as measured by the neurological disability score. It is felt that with use of these modalities, improvement or maintenance of good neuromuscular ability is now achievable, and the high cost of medical treatment can be offset, at least in part, by the patient's ability to return to work.

mechanical ventilation may be very frightened to be alone at night for fear of being unable to summon help if he or she gets into trouble. A call light or some mechanism should be available so the patient knows he or she can call for help. Setting up a routine schedule of checking on the patient may help overcome the fear.

NUTRITION

Adequate nutrition must be maintained. If the patient is unable to take oral feedings, tube feedings may be initiated. Tube feedings, however, may cause diarrhea and a resultant electrolyte imbalance, so careful monitoring by physician and nurse is required (see Chapter 39).

EMOTIONAL SUPPORT

Fright, hopelessness, and helplessness all may be seen in patients and families during the often long course of this disorder. Frequent explanations of the interventions and the progress will be very useful. The patient should be allowed to make as many decisions as possible over the course of recovery.

Sometimes these patients are very difficult to care for because they require much nursing time. They may use the call light excessively if insecure about being alone. The nurse should consider allowing the family to spend more time with the patient. Having a primary nurse may give the patient and family more security, knowing there is one person from whom they can get consistent information. Team conferences with the patient and family should be held on a routine basis to discuss progress and plans.

Complications in Guillain-Barré Syndrome

RESPIRATORY FAILURE

The most severe complication of GBS is respiratory failure. Weakened respiratory muscles put the patient with this disorder at great risk for hypoventilation and repeated pulmonary infections. Fifty percent of patients with GBS have some respiratory compromise, resulting in reduced tidal volume and vital capacity, or possibly, complete respiratory arrest. Dysphagia also may be present, leading to aspiration. There may be the same complications of immobility as seen in the stroke patient.

CARDIOVASCULAR ABERRATIONS

There may be a disturbance of the autonomic nervous system with GBS that could result in a fatal cardiac dysrhythmia or drastic life-threatening changes in vital signs.

PLASMA EXCHANGE COMPLICATIONS

A patient with GBS or myasthenia gravis receiving PE is at risk for some complications with that procedure. An infection may develop at the site of vascular access. Hypovolemia may result in hypotension, tachycardia, dizziness, and diaphoresis. Hypokalemia and hypocalcemia may lead to cardiac dysrhythmias. The patient may experience temporary circumoral and distal extremity paresthesias, muscle twitching, and nausea and vomiting related to administration of citrated plasma. Careful observation and assessment are necessary to prevent these problems.

CLINICAL APPLICATION: Patient Care Study

Mr. A was a 32-year-old businessman who presented in the physician's office with a chief complaint of weakness and numbness in both feet that had been developing over the past 4 days. At first, only the bottom of his feet were involved. Now the numbness was up to his ankles. Two weeks before this, he stated he had had a "mild case of the stomach flu."

The physician admitted him to the hospital and ruled out many disorders with extensive laboratory tests. Over the next 6 days, the patient lost his ability to walk. His feet and legs felt like "pins and needles" up to groin level, and he had no motor ability in his legs. The symptoms were ascending in a symmetrical pattern. The symptom progression and history made the physician highly suspicious that this was Guillain-Barré syndrome.

Mr. A's symptoms plateaued after 6 days and did not ascend further than his hips. He went to a rehabilitation center, where over the next 4 months he gradually regained the strength in his lower extremities. The symptom onset was rapid, but the recovery was much slower. After the disease was explained to him, Mr. A considered himself extremely lucky the disease plateaued where it did and did not involve his upper extremities or his respiratory muscles.

Myasthenia Gravis

Myasthenia gravis is a neuromuscular transmission disorder caused by an autoimmune response. Myasthenia gravis means "grave muscle weakness," which is the primary clinical feature, along with abnormal fatigability. It is seen more often in women than men. Symptoms most commonly show up in the third decade of life, although any age group may be affected. The annual incidence of myasthenia gravis is 9 to 10 per million, up from previous figures of 2 to 4 per million.[18]

Pathophysiological Principles

Most researchers believe that the autoimmune response in myasthenia gravis occurs at the neuromuscular junction, specifically on the postsynaptic membrane of the muscles, where antibodies destroy acetylcholine receptor sites. By reducing the number of functioning acetylcholine receptor sites, complete depolarization of the muscle is difficult or impossible. This causes striated voluntary muscle weakness, which characteristically is greater after activity and improves after rest.

There are several other theories about the exact nature of the transmission deficit at the neuromuscular junction. Some researchers think there is a deficient amount of acetylcholine released from the presynaptic membranes into the synapse. This deficiency may be in the synthesis of the enzyme choline acetylase, impaired transport of the acetylcholine into the synapse, or other possible defects.

Abnormalities in the thymus gland are frequent in patients with myasthenia gravis. The thymus is involved intimately in the immune responses of the body. Eighty percent of victims of myasthenia gravis have structural changes of the thymus, such as thymic hyperplasia. These data support the pathogenic role of the immune system in myasthenia gravis.

Assessment

HISTORY

Diagnosis of myasthenia gravis is based on the history and clinical presentation. A history of muscle weakness after activity and partial strength restoration after rest is highly suspect for myasthenia gravis. The patient may complain of weakness after simple physical tasks. A history of drooping eyelids on upward gaze also may be significant, as is evidence of other cranial muscle weakness.

CLINICAL MANIFESTATIONS

There may be extraocular muscle weakness causing ocular palsy, drooping eyelid, or intermittent diplopia. Facial expression may be masklike when facial muscles are affected. The patient may have dysphagia and difficulty chewing. Speech may be dysarthric.

If muscular involvement of the trunk and extremities is present, the proximal muscles usually are affected more severely than the distal ones. This disorder may produce mild ocular involvement to severe muscular involvement of the diaphragm, intercostal muscles, and abdominal and external sphincters. Dyspnea and dysphagia are two life-threatening symptoms that may result in aspiration and acute respiratory failure. If the patient's vital capacity falls below 1.2 L or if the patient is unable to cough, intubation should be done. Delivery of oxygen alone will not relieve respiratory symptoms, because the problem is one of impaired muscle strength and not gas exchange.

Pupillary signs and cerebral function remain intact. There may be remissions and relapses.

DIAGNOSTIC STUDIES

The edrophonium chloride (Tensilon) test is the classic diagnostic tool for this disorder. Edrophonium chloride is a short-acting anticholinesterase, and when injected, it transiently inhibits the breakdown of acetylcholine at the neuromuscular junction. The patient shows marked improvement of muscle strength within 30 seconds that lasts up to 5 minutes.

Electromyography also may help confirm the diagnosis. This involves repetitive nerve stimulation at a slow rate, which in a normal person produces very little decrease in muscle action potential. In the patient with myasthenia gravis, this repetitive slow stimulation produces a rapid decline in muscle action potential because of the deficient number of acetylcholine receptors available.

Because myasthenia gravis often is seen along with other conditions, other studies that might be performed are a CT scan of the thymus, thyroid studies, serum creatine phosphokinase, sedimentation rate, antinuclear antibody levels, and immunological studies. The presence of serum antibodies to the muscle acetylcholine receptors also helps confirm a diagnosis of myasthenia gravis.

Management

MEDICAL THERAPY

Medical management includes medication therapy with anticholinesterases and steroids. Drugs such as neostigmine (Prostigmin) inactivate or destroy cholinesterase so the acetylcholine is not immediately destroyed. Steroids, by reducing the amount of antibodies produced through the immune response, block the immune mechanism and restore chemical reaction at the myoneural junction. Azathioprine (Imuran) or other immunosuppressive drugs may be useful.

Patients should receive a list of medications that may impair neuromuscular function and exacerbate myasthenia gravis. While no medications are absolutely contraindicated, with the exception of D-penicillamine, some drugs increase myasthenic weakness (see the display).

Thymectomy may be indicated because it is thought that this procedure removes a source of antigen and reduces the immune response. Plasmapheresis or PE may be initiated to remove circulating antiacetylcholine receptor antibodies from the plasma, resulting in some clinical improvement. As with GBS, respiratory failure may occur, and mechanical ventilatory support may be necessary.

CLINICAL APPLICATION: Drug Therapy
Drugs to Be Used Cautiously in the Patient With Myasthenia Gravis

Contraindicated: D-penicillamine
Drugs that increase myasthenic weakness:
Muscle relaxants: curare, succinylcholine
Psychotropics: lithium carbonate, phenothiazines
Anticonvulsants: phenytoin, mephenytoin, trimethadione
Cardiac drugs: quinidine, beta-blockers, procainamide
Antibiotics: tetracycline, aminoglycosides, "mycins," polymyxin B and E, colistin

EMOTIONAL SUPPORT

Like GBS, myasthenia gravis can be a very frightening disease. Unlike GBS, it is a chronic disorder in that once an exacerbation is treated, it does not reverse itself and go away. Chronic management is indicated for myasthenia gravis. Keeping the patient and family informed and giving honest information will help them make decisions about options for care.

Complications in Myasthenia Gravis

A patient may experience two types of crises: myasthenic crisis and cholinergic crisis. *Myasthenic crisis* is a condition in which the symptoms of myasthenia gravis are exaggerated, and the patient requires more anticholinesterase drugs. This crisis usually is precipitated by stress, such as infection, emotional turmoil, pregnancy, alcohol ingestion, or cold, but in some cases, the cause cannot be identified readily. Myasthenic crisis is not distinguished easily from *cholinergic crisis,* in which the patient has received too much anticholinesterase drug. Cholinergic crisis often involves nausea, vomiting, pallor, diarrhea, diaphoresis, bradycardia, and salivation.

To determine the type of crisis, edrophonium chloride may be used. With its administration, there will be marked improvement of symptoms in myasthenic crisis. There will be a transient exacerbation of symptoms if the patient is having a cholinergic crisis. Atropine, a cholinergic reactivator, may be given for cholinergic crisis. Neostigmine may be given for myasthenic crisis, because the edrophonium chloride quickly wears off. Because there often is a narrow range of therapeutic control, the patient must understand the importance of taking the correct amount of medication and not skipping doses or doubling up on a dose if a previous dose was missed.

Some of the complications experienced by the patient with GBS are similar to those experienced by the patient with myasthenia gravis. Refer to the section on complications of GBS for further information.

Brain Tumors

Pathophysiological Principles

Tumors of the CNS may be classified as benign or malignant; however, the location, invasiveness, size, and rate of growth of these tumors are often more significant than the degree of malignancy. Tumors inside the head produce a mass effect, causing pressure on surrounding tissues and causing increased ICP at some point in their development. A benign tumor in an inaccessible area of the brain may be just as damaging as one designated malignant.

Primary brain tumors are those that arise from the brain tissue itself or surrounding structures. Ninety percent of brain tumors are primary, meaning that they develop from CNS tissue. Metastatic brain tumors have their origin or primary site elsewhere in the body, but cells have migrated to the brain. Seventy-five percent of tumors in adults are supratentorial and of the primary type. Ten percent of all primary tumors occur in children, and 70% are infratentorial.[19]

Brain tumors are classified or named based on the type of cells present at the tumor site (eg, astrocytomas arise from astrocyte cells), on anatomical location, on cellular differentiation or grading (see display), or according to intra-axial versus extra-axial location.

Table 35–3 outlines common brain tumors and their characteristics.

Assessment and Diagnosis

Diagnosis of a CNS tumor starts with a detailed history and a careful neurological examination. The history should include questions about headache and seizures; these are often early symptoms of tumor presence. Pain may be described as dull, nonlocalized, and most severe on awakening, tending to improve throughout the day. The headache pain is usually aggravated by any activity that increases intra-abdominal or intrathoracic pressure, such as coughing, stooping over, or straining. Inquiry should also be made regarding visual disturbances. Vomiting may be experienced, especially in patients with posterior fossa tumors. Nausea often does not precede the vomiting nor is vomiting related to intake of food.

The presence of memory loss, altered judgment or social skills, impaired LOC, hemiparesis, hemiplegia, and ataxia should also be determined. Family members may be more aware than the patient of subtle cognitive changes. A history of depression or labile emotions may be significant.

Cranial nerve testing is very important. During physical assessment, a visual field and funduscopic examination will reveal any visual field deficits or papilledema. Abnormal audiometric tests and caloric testing (oculovestibular reflex) suggest acoustic neuroma. Dysphagia, apraxia, ataxia, or incoordination should be noted.

Cellular Differentiation (Grading) of Brain Tumors

Tumors are graded according to the amount of cellular differentiation. The better the differentiation, the better the prognosis:

- Grade I—well-differentiated cells
- Grade II—moderately differentiated cells
- Grade III—poorly differentiated cells
- Grade IV—very poorly differentiated cells

Grade III and IV tumors are typically malignant.

TABLE 35-3
Characteristics of Common Brain Tumors

Tumor Type	Etiology	Characteristics
Glioma (subclassified into five tumor types according to predominant glial cell type):	Originates from neuroglial cells	Most common adult primary intracranial tumor Rapidly growing and infiltrative
Astrocytoma	Originates from astrocytes	Infiltrative, making surgical removal difficult
Glioblastoma multiforme	Composed of various cell types (multiforme)	Highly vascular Extremely malignant Rapidly growing; invasive Resistant to combinations of surgery, radiotherapy, and chemotherapy Average survival in treated patients is 12 to 18 mo from onset of clinical symptoms
Medulloblastoma	Type of primitive, undifferentiated, neural ectodermal tumor	Rapidly growing, invasive, highly malignant Often invades fourth ventricle and metastasizes to subarachnoid spaces of hemisphere and spinal cord; produces obstructive hydrocephalus Occurs frequently in children
Ependymoma	Originates from cells within the ventricular system, most often in fourth ventricle	Tends to form small canals (rosettes) within the tumor, and tumor cells align themselves around blood vessels (pseudorosettes) Causes obstructive hydrocephalus Most benign but may become malignant Response to radiation poor for grades I and II; but may be beneficial for grades III and IV Slow growing; often in inaccessible areas
Oligodendroglioma	Originates from oligodendroglial cells that form myelin in the CNS	Frontal lobe most common site for 40%–70% cases May be slow growing and produce long-term focal problems or may grow rapidly and be associated with hemorrhage Tend to form focal calcifications, which may be seen on skull x-rays; however, tumor possibly diffusely infiltrated Recurrence frequent Radical surgery often followed by radiation
Meningioma	Primary tumor arising from meninges	Vascular; well-circumscribed; encapsulated; may penetrate adjacent bone Most benign and slow growing If not completely excised, may recur Prognosis largely dependent on location
Pituitary adenoma (subdivided into three types):	Originate from cells of pituitary gland	Encapsulated Benign Initial symptoms—hormonal disturbances or visual field defects
Adrenocorticotropic hormone (ACTH)-producing pituitary adenoma	Primarily composed of basophil cells	Usually small, so adjacent tissue not compressed Hypersecretion of ACTH—Cushing's syndrome
Pituitary adenoma inducing gigantism and acromegaly	Primarily composed of acidophilic cells	Usually small, slow growing Cause an increase in growth hormone resulting in gigantism if the tumor occurs before the bone epiphyses have fused; in adults, results in acromegaly Combination of surgical debulking and radiation for treatment of large tumors

(continued)

TABLE 35-3

Characteristics of Common Brain Tumors (Continued)

Tumor Type	Etiology	Characteristics
Nonsecreting pituitary adenoma	Primarily composed of chromophobe cells	Most common pituitary tumor Usually large May cause hypopituitarism by compressing anterior region of pituitary gland, resulting in amenorrhea, loss of libido, loss of body hair, sterility in women, and impotence in men due to decreased gonadotropin secretion, hypoglycemia, hypotension, and electrolyte imbalance Surgical removal beneficial using transsphenoidal microsurgery
Hemangioblastoma	Originates from capillary vessel-forming endothelial cells and stromal cells	Tumor of blood vessels Slow growing; vascular Occurs most often in cerebellum Symptoms: cerebellar signs and polycythemia (because they secrete erythropoietin) Surgery followed by radiation possibly useful for recurrences Tends to run in families
Acoustic neuroma (schwannoma and neurofibroma)	Originates from the sheath of Schwann cells in vestibular portion of eighth cranial nerve	Benign; slow growing; encapsulated Often located at cerebellopontine angle, causing unilateral cranial nerve symptoms Other symptoms: impaired hearing, weakness, vertigo, ataxia, deafness, hydrocephalus (causing increased ICP), tinnitus, loss of extraocular eye movements, drooling, difficulty swallowing, and loss of corneal reflex Complete excision of small tumors—excellent outcome; incomplete excision—30% mortality in 3–4 y; 50% of patients with incomplete removal—recurrence
Developmental tumor	Originates from cells that develop abnormally and persist throughout prenatal growth	Congenital
Dermoid and teratoma	Common origin: ventricular system, causing obstruction to CSF flow, and thus hydrocephalus and increased ICP	Infiltrating; difficult to treat Often impairs endocrine function and may result in early puberty
Cholesteatoma (epidermoid tumor)	Composed of encapsulated epithelial debris	Simulates acoustic neuromas when located in cerebellopontine angle Benign but may enlarge and cause erosion of adjacent bone Complete excision difficult Slow growing
Chordoma	Usually originates at base of brain	Malignant, slow growing Locally invasive; causes bone erosion and invasion of dura Highly invasive Complete excision probably impossible
Craniopharyngioma	Develops over the sella turcica from epithelium developed from Rathke's pouch	Solid or cystic tumor (encapsulated) Rupture of cystic fluid within tumor or cyst—bouts of "sterile" meningitis or sometimes bacterial meningitis

(continued)

TABLE 35-3
Characteristics of Common Brain Tumors (Continued)

Tumor Type	Etiology	Characteristics
		Pressure on pituitary gland, optic chiasm, and base of brain, producing symptoms of pituitary hypofunction, visual disturbances, diabetes insipidus, and hydrocephalus
		May be resected if in accessible area; radiation sensitive after surgery
Metatastic tumor	Most common primary sites: lungs (45%) and breast (20%)	Most common in children
	May result from a primary site in gastrointestinal tract, kidney, bone, ovary, or from melanoma	Usually solid circumscribed mass surrounded by vasogenic edema, but multiple small masses throughout CNS
		Usually spread by way of arterial system and lodge at junction of white and gray matter where there is rapid spread beneath cortical surface.
		Extensive white matter edema; mass effect, which may cause increased ICP and death
		Surgery palliative
		Poor prognosis even with surgery, radiotherapy, and chemotherapy
Lymphoma	Originates from lymphatic system	Tumors of the immune system
	Most in CNS classified as large B-cell lymphomas (B cells mediate antibody responses)	Increasing incidence of primary lymphomas, which may be due to greater numbers of immunosuppressed individuals from drugs given after organ transplantation or altered immune system from HIV
		May be localized or infiltrative

DIAGNOSTIC STUDIES

Based on neurological deficits identified, radiological tests may be indicated. Refer to Table 32-4 for an explanation of specific procedures.

Skull x-rays show deviation of a calcified pineal body by a brain mass, erosion of bone, and calcified parts of a tumor. CT scan will demonstrate the presence of hydrocephalus and the size and location of the tumor. Injected isotopes may be used to outline the blood supply to the tumor. An abnormal amount of radioactive isotope will accumulate in the area of the tumor; vascular or small tumors may be missed by this test. Angiography will outline the vascularity in the brain and in the tumor. Positron emission tomography illustrates the metabolism of the tumor and the surrounding brain tissue.

An MRI will give a more detailed picture of successive layers of the brain. An EEG may help to localize a lesion. Seventy-five percent of patients with brain tumors have abnormal EEG tracings. Somatosensory-evoked potentials (SEEPs) may localize sensory deficits. Sensory pathway conduction may be slowed from the tumor compressing normal brain tissue and from abnormal vascularization. SEEPs look at the efficiency of the sensory pathway from a peripheral nerve to the sensory cortex by electrically stimulating the appropriate nerve and documenting afferent activity during the conduction.

If there is no obvious evidence of increased ICP, a lumbar puncture may be done. CSF protein will be elevated in one third of patients with intracranial neoplasms. Cytology studies may show cancerous cells, and chest x-ray and other routine studies may be done to find the primary site. Cisternal myelogram with tomography may be needed to visualize the cerebellopontine angle if acoustic neuroma is suspected.

Pituitary tumors are detected with endocrine, ophthalmological, and radiological studies. Radioimmunoassays reveal the amount of circulating pituitary hormones. Endocrine tests may be especially abnormal with pituitary adenomas and craniopharyngiomas. Tumor markers are substances made by tumor cells that are sometimes unique to a particular type of tumor. If the tumor is accessible, biopsy will give a definitive diagnosis of tumor type.

Management

SURGICAL INTERVENTION

Surgery may be an option in the management of a brain tumor. A biopsy, if obtainable, helps determine the medical management. If the tumor is not totally accessible, only partial removal may be possible. This will decompress the brain and reduce the ICP. Often only partial removal is possible with large infiltrating or very vascular tumors, such as glioblastoma multiforme and hemangioblastomas. Complete surgical excision is usually possible with small, well-circumscribed tumors located in an accessible area. Surgery is the preferred treatment when possible. Meningiomas, pituitary tumors, and acoustic neuromas usually meet the criteria for surgical excision.

Stereotactic localization for resection of the tumor is a method of precisely locating areas in the brain with use of three-dimensional coordinates. The advantage of stereotaxis is that manipulation and exposure of neural tissue are minimized, which reduces the risk for increased ICP and herniation. Because of minimized cerebral edema, the blood supply in the microcirculation is not impeded. Exacted localization provides the surgeon with more precise feedback on tumor margin than may be visually possible during open craniotomy. Stereotaxis has many current uses in addition to surgical tumor resection, as detailed in the display.

Image-guided surgery involves an interplay between computers and surgical instruments that pinpoints the location of a tumor during surgery. Laser and ultrasound technology, including ultrasonic aspiration and intraoperative ultrasonography, permit aggressive resection of large tumor volumes from the brain with little manipulation of adjacent healthy tissue.

RADIATION THERAPY

Radiation therapy may be used in addition to surgical intervention, by itself, in combination with chemotherapy, or for palliation in metastatic tumors. The goal is to destroy tumor cells while minimizing side effects and effects on surrounding normal brain tissue.

Stereotactic radiosurgery, accomplished using the gamma knife, is another method of tumor management. The gamma knife, not really a knife at all, is a curved steel helmet that fits over the patient's head. Along the curved half-circle of the helmet are 201 small portals that emit beams of ionizing radiation from cobalt-60 sources that are focused to a single point on the intracranial lesion. The patient is positioned using a specially designed frame so that the tumor lies at the focal point of the machine where the highest radiation dose is delivered, thus sparing the surrounding tissue from high doses of radiation. Basically, images from the CT and MRI are fed into the gamma knife computer, and a plan is developed to deliver a single or multiple doses of radiation to cover the entire tumor. The advantages of the gamma knife include its rapid, noninvasive, and painless application to the patient.

Interstitial radiation therapy is accomplished by surgically implanting radioactive seeds directly into the tumor. This is a local therapy and does not address undetected cancer cells elsewhere in the brain.

> ### *Applications for Stereotaxis*
>
> - Surgical tumor resection
> - Localization of seizure foci
> - Brain or tumor biopsy
> - Implantation of radioactive sources for interstitial irradiation
> - Implantation of pellets containing chemotherapeutic agents
> - Removal of thrombosed arteriovenous malformations
> - Ventriculostomy of third ventricle
> - Thalamotomy for intractable cancer pain or tremor
> - Implantation of heat sources for interstitial hyperthermia
> - Target localization for stereotactic radiosurgery

HYPERTHERMIA

Hyperthermia treatment of brain tumors is used occasionally as an adjuvant therapy for certain recurrent intracranial malignancies. Interstitial hyperthermia involves application of relatively low levels of heat ($40°–43°C$ [$104°–109.4°F$]) for a period of time sufficient to damage and destroy neoplastic cells.

The rationale for this therapy is that some evidence suggests that cancer cells may be more heat sensitive and thus incur damage at temperatures not cytotoxic to normal cells. Heat may alter the cell membrane permeability, making the cancer cell more sensitive to chemotherapeutic drugs. Hypoxia, hypometabolism, decreased vascularity, and hyperacidity, all common features in the inner regions of brain tumors, enhance sensitivity to hyperthermia. So the effects of hyperthermia are more profound in regions of the tumor with these characteristics.

Hyperthermia may be used not only in conjunction with chemotherapy, but also with radiation therapy. Heat seems to inhibit the cell's ability to repair radiation damage. This enhancement of lethality seems to be greatest when the time interval between application of hyperthermia and radiation is no more than 1 to 2 hours. There is a maximum synergistic effect when the two are administered simultaneously.

There are still many unanswered questions about the use of hyperthermia. Controversies exist regarding thermotolerance, correct thermal dosing, methods of generating the heat (eg, microwaves, conductive heat), and the most effective combination of modalities. Research continues for treatments that will improve the expected life span of patients without producing significant neurological deficits.

PHARMACOLOGICAL THERAPY

Chemotherapy

Generally, chemotherapy that does not cross the blood–brain barrier is of no value in the treatment of metastatic brain tumors. Research involving manipulation of the blood–brain barrier so that drugs can enter the brain is ongoing. Some forms of chemotherapy can be effective against metastatic brain tumors resulting from breast cancer, including cyclophosphamide, 5-FU, and methotrexate. Tamoxifen may also be effective.

Intra-arterial chemotherapy is being investigated for treatment of lung cancer metastases to the brain. Also, application has been made to the FDA for use of the Gliadel wafer in the treatment of malignant brain cancer. The wafer is implanted into the surgical cavities created when a brain tumor is resected. As the wafer dissolves, it releases the chemotherapeutic agent carmustine in high concentrations for an extended period directly into the tumor site.

Hormone Therapy

Hormones are another class of drugs that may be used to treat brain tumors. If the primary tumor is hormone dependent, hormones or hormone-blocking agents may be useful. For example, breast cancers that are estrogen receptor positive are treated with tamoxifen, which may also shrink coexisting metastatic tumors. Steroids may act as hormones in patients with lymphoma.

Tamoxifen is considered an antiestrogen drug and has been used to treat breast cancer for some time. New research demonstrates its promise in treating brain tumors. The basis for its use is the enzyme protein kinase C (PKC), which seems to regulate the growth of malignant gliomas. Tamoxifen is thought to inhibit the production of PKC, thus interrupting the signals that prompt cancer cells to proliferate. Early studies indicate that doses of tamoxifen five times the dosage given to breast cancer patients are required.[20]

Immunotherapy

Immunotherapy is another approach to the management of brain tumors. Tumors produce an antigen that normally stimulates production of an antibody. Patients with intracranial tumors have a depressed immune system, and this normal response does not take place. Immunotherapy involves giving a patient drugs to enhance the body's immune system or to help develop an active immunity to the tumor cells. Immunotherapy uses immune cells or biological response modifiers, which either kill the tumor cells directly or stimulate the immune system to produce substances on its own to restrict tumor growth.

Other Drugs

Steroids are thought to slow tumor growth and reduce cerebral swelling from the tumor itself or from radiation edema. Phenytoin is often given prophylactically to patients with tumors or who have had a brain tumor surgically resected. The tumor or scar tissue in the brain may become a focus for abnormal electrical discharges. Analgesics for headache may be given to a patient who has a brain tumor or following treatment of a tumor. Stool softeners may be indicated to prevent straining, which can cause increased ICP.

CLINICAL APPLICATION: Patient Care Study

Jane was a 30-year-old woman who saw her physician because of a chief complaint of generalized headache, worse on awakening in the morning. She demonstrated no neurological deficits, and her vital signs were normal. Papilledema was seen on funduscopic examination.

Jane was referred to a neurologist for further workup. A computed tomography scan showed a well-circumscribed mass in the anterior left frontal lobe. She was considered a candidate for stereotactic resection of the tumor mass.

The stereotactic head frame was fixed to Jane's skull, and she was transported to magnetic resonance imaging and then to radiology. When the stereotactic imaging was completed, the target coordinates were determined, and she was taken to the operating room. With the specific coordinates to localize the mass, minimal surrounding tissue was disturbed. The tumor was dissected free from the dura and removed.

Her postoperative course was uneventful, and she demonstrated no neurological deficits. She was placed on prophylactic phenytoin and was weaned off steroids. There was no indication for radiation or chemotherapy. On follow-up, she reported no further headaches.

NURSING INTERVENTION

The nursing care of the patient following surgery for a brain tumor is similar to that for the patient with an aneurysm or stroke. Close monitoring for signs of increased ICP and neurological deficits is extremely important. Generally, these patients spend limited time in the ICU. Nonetheless, even for an abbreviated stay, it is important to remember that these patients and their families are usually under extreme emotional stress related to the diagnosis and potential sequelae. A supportive and caring approach can ameliorate some of this stress.

Complications in Brain Tumors

The primary complication seen with brain tumor is increased ICP. As the mass grows, it takes up space inside the skull and causes compression of healthy tissue. All clinical signs of increased ICP may be present or only some subtle signs until the tumor enlarges enough to create increased ICP. Chapter 33 discusses increased ICP in depth.

Side effects of chemotherapy or radiation, such as fatigue and hair loss, may be observed during treatment of the tumor. With some types of tumor, recurrence is possible after initial treatment.

Clinical Applicability Challenges

Self-Challenge: Critical Thinking

1. *Compare and contrast myasthenic crisis and cholinergic crisis in a patient with myasthenia gravis.*

2. *Construct factors in a critical path for a patient with a stroke about to have thrombolytic therapy.*

3. Examine the pathophysiological reasons "triple-H" therapy is useful in treating vasospasm in a patient following aneurysm clipping.

Study Questions

1. Which cerebrovascular problem may present with a chief complaint of unilateral headache?

    a. Stroke

    b. Arteriovenous malformation

    c. Hydrocephalus

    d. Guillain-Barré syndrome

2. Hemorrhage from an aneurysm most often occurs in which space in the brain?

    a. Subdural space

    b. Epidural space

    c. Subarachnoid space

    d. Intracerebral space

3. The most serious and most common type of status epilepticus is

    a. absence status.

    b. partial motor seizures.

    c. generalized tonic–clonic status.

    d. complex partial status.

4. How can a myasthenic crisis be distinguished from a cholinergic crisis?

    a. The clinical manifestations are different.

    b. Atropine will cause improved muscle strength in myasthenic crisis.

    c. Neostigmine will cause improved muscle strength in cholinergic crisis.

    d. Edrophonium chloride will cause improved muscle strength in myasthenic crisis.

5. Which statement is true of brain tumors?

    a. They may cause increased ICP.

    b. Most are malignant.

    c. Most have metastasized from another site.

    d. They are invasive of adjacent tissue.

REFERENCES

1. National Stroke Association Fact Sheet: Brain Attack Statistics. Englewood, CO, National Stroke Association, 1996
2. Goldstein LB, Matchar DB: Clinical assessment of stroke. JAMA 271(14):1114–1119, 1994
3. American Heart Association: Heart and Stroke A-Z Guide: Stroke (Brain Attack Statistics). Dallas, American Heart Association, 1996
4. Gorelick PB: Stroke prevention. Arch Neurol 52(4):347–355, 1995
5. Raps EC, Galetta SL: Stroke prevention therapies and management of patient subgroups. Neurology 45(2 Suppl 1):S19–S24, 1995
6. National Institute of Neurological Disorders and Stroke rt-PA Stroke Study Group: Tissue Plasminogen Activator for Acute Ischemic Stroke. N Engl J Med 333(24):1581–1587, 1995
7. Hilton G: Experimental neuroprotective agents: Nursing challenge. Dimensions of Critical Care Nursing 14(4):181–188, 1995
8. Longstreth WT Jr, Nelson LM, et al: Clinical course of spontaneous subarachnoid hemorrhage: A population-based study in King County, Washington. Neurology 43(4):712–78, 1993
9. Schievink WI, Wijdicks EF, et al: Sudden death from aneurysmal subarachnoid hemorrhage. Neurology 45(5):871–874, 1995
10. Fearon, M, Rusy K: Transcranial Doppler: Advanced technology for assessing cerebral hemodynamics. Dimensions of Critical Care Nursing 13(5):241–248, 1994
11. Mayberg MR, Batjer HH, et al: Guidelines for the management of aneurysmal subarachnoid hemorrhage. Stroke 25(11):2315–2328, 1994
12. Vollrath B, Weir B, MacDonald R, Cook D: Intracellular mechanisms involved in the responses of cerebrovascular smooth-muscle cells to hemoglobin. J Neurosurg 80:261–268, 1994
13. Bell T, Kongable G: Innovations in aneurysmal subarachnoid hemorrhage, Intracisternal t-PA for the prevention of vasospasm. J Neurosci Nurs 28(2):107–113, 1996
14. Higashida R, Tsal F, Halbach V, Barnwell S, Dowd C, Hieshima G: Interventional neurovascular techniques in the treatment of stroke-state-of-the-art therapy. J Int Med 237:105–115, 1995
15. Jiang GX, de Pedro-Cuesta J, et al: Guillain-Barré syndrome in southwest Stockholm, 1973–1991, 1. Quality of registered hospital diagnoses and incidence. Acta Neurologica Scandinavica 91(2):109–117, 1995
16. Chipps E, Skinner C: Intravenous immunoglobulin: Implications for use in the neurological patient. J Neurosci Nurs 26(1):8–17, 1994
17. Dyke P, Litchy W, Dratz K, Suarez G, Low P, Pineda A, Windebank A, Karnes J, O'Brien P: A plasma exchange versus immune globulin infusion trial in chronic inflammatory demyelinating polyradiculoneuropathy. Ann Neurol 36(6):838–845, 1994
18. Schon F, Drayson M, Thompson RA: Myasthenia gravis and elderly people. Age Ageing 25(1):56–58, 1996
19. Central Brain Tumor Registry of the United States: 1995 First Annual Report. Chicago, Central Brain Tumor Registry of the United States (CBTRUS), 1996
20. Couldwell W, Weiss M, DeGiorgio C, Weiner L, Hinton D, Ehresmann G, Conti P, Apuzzo M: Clinical and radiographic response in a minority of patients with recurrent malignant gliomas treated with high-dose Tamoxifen. Neurosurgery 32(3):485–489, 1993

BIBLIOGRAPHY

Benbadis S, Stagno S, Kosalko J, Friedman A: Psychogenic seizures: A guide for patients and families. J Neurosci Nurs 26(5):306–308, 1994

Bronstein K: Epidemiology and classification of brain tumors. Critical Care Nursing Clinics of North America 7(1):79–89, 1995

Buzea C: Understanding computerized EEG monitoring in the intensive care unit. J Neurosci Nurs 27(5):292–297, 1995

Donohoe K: Nursing care of the patient with myasthenia gravis. Neurol Clin 12:369–385, 1994

Ferguson R, Ferguson J: Cerebral intraarterial fibrinolysis at the crossroads: Is a phase III trial advisable at this time? Am J Neuroradiol 15:1201–1216, 1994

Hilton G: Secondary brain injury and the role of neuroprotective agents. J Neurosci Nurs 26(4):251–255, 1994

Kernick C, Kaminski H: Myasthenia gravis: Pathophysiology, diagnosis and collaborative care. J Neurosci Nurs 27(4):207–215, 1995

Lucke K, Derr M, Chovanes G: Continuous bedside cerebral blood flow monitoring. J Neurosci Nurs 27(3):164–173, 1995

Macabasco A, Hickman J: Thrombolytic therapy for brain attack. J Neurosci Nurs 27(3):138–149, 1995

Price C, McCarley P: Physical assessment for patients receiving therapeutic plasma exchange. American Nephrology Nurses Association 21(4):149–154, 1994

Welsh D: Hyperthermia treatment of malignant brain tumor. Critical Care Nursing Clinics of North America 7(1):115–124, 1995

36

Spinal Cord Injury

OBJECTIVES

Based on the content in this chapter, the reader should be able to:

- Differentiate between a complete and an incomplete spinal cord injury.
- Explain the pathophysiological processes involved with Brown-Séquard syndrome, central cord syndrome, anterior cord syndrome, and posterior cord syndrome.
- Describe three clinical features of spinal shock.
- Describe two immediate nursing actions to take after autonomic dysreflexia is recognized.
- Develop a holistic plan of care for a patient with an acute spinal cord injury.

Every year there are 8,000 to 10,000 new spinal cord injuries in the United States. Spinal cord injury (SCI) is most common in young adults ages 16 to 30, and most are men (82% men versus 18% women). Approximately 35% of SCIs result from vehicle accidents; falls account for approximately 20%, acts of violence 30%, and sports 8%. Etiology varies in different groups depending on age of onset, sex, and racial or ethnic background. Motor vehicle accidents occur most in 15 to 30 year olds, but those older than 60 years have more spinal injuries due to falls. Violence as a cause of SCI is increasing in the 16- to 30-year-old group and primarily in nonwhite people. Motor vehicle accidents account for most SCIs among Caucasians.

Slightly more than one half of all new injuries involve the cervical spine. Thoracic vertebral injuries account for more than one third of all new injuries, and lumbar and sacral injuries account for the remainder. Motor vehicle accidents cause an equal number of tetraplegias and paraplegias. Tetraplegia results mostly from sports injuries, especially diving accidents and contact sports. Paraplegia results mostly from penetrating wounds, such as from a knife or bullet.

Statistics compiled on SCI during the last several decades by the National Spinal Cord Injury Database located in Birmingham, Alabama, have helped to develop profiles that describe the demographics of spinal injury. The typical profile is a young, single male between 16 and 30 years old with a high school education, whose injury occurs in July.

The combination of early onset of spinal injury that results in severe disability, coupled with advances in health care that allow almost a full life expectancy, can result in catastrophe in terms of human disability and social economics. Economic consequences of this type of injury, especially if there are repeated hospitalizations, may be staggering.

■ PATHOPHYSIOLOGICAL PRINCIPLES

Complete Versus Incomplete Injuries

The level of SCI is defined by the number of the most distal uninvolved segment of the cord. Functional abilities at the different levels of SCI are not completely determined for every patient. Functional performance may vary among patients depending on whether the lesion is complete or incomplete. An incomplete lesion implies preservation of motor or sensory fibers (or both) below the level of the lesion, whereas a complete lesion implies total loss of voluntary muscle control and sensation below the injury. When an SCI is incomplete, segments distal to the lesion still may be intact, although the orthopedic level of injury is higher. For instance, the orthopedic level of injury may be a C5 fracture, but the patient may be neurologically intact to C6. Because it is important to know what level of performance a patient can achieve, the neurological level to which he or she can perform is more significant than knowledge of the location of orthopedic injury.

With a complete cord injury, the orthopedic level of injury also can be the same as the neurological level of injury. No segments distal to the injury are preserved. A person with complete cord injury will closely follow the dermatome pathways for the level of sensory loss shown in Figure 36–1. Table 36–1 discusses the motor and sensory

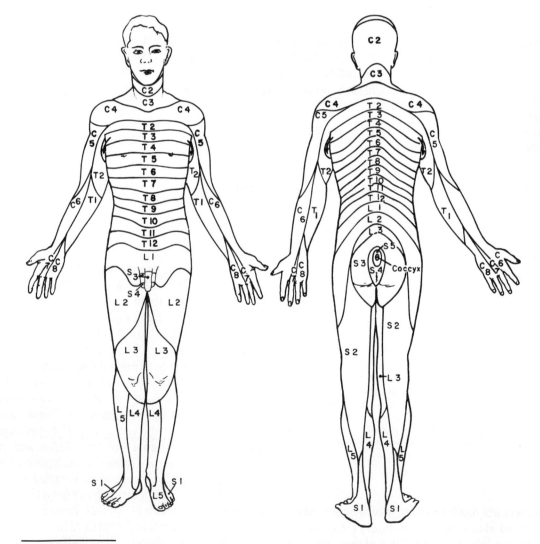

FIGURE 36-1
Sensory dermatomes illustrating the area of skin supplied by a single dorsal root ganglion. (Barr M: The Human Nervous System, p 85. New York, Harper & Row, 1993)

TABLE 36-1
Effects of Spinal Cord Injury on Patient Functioning

Level of Injury	Physical Deficits	Daily Functioning
Cervical Injuries		
C1–C4	With a C1–C4 lesion, the trapezius, sternomastoid, and platysma muscles remain functional. Intercostal muscles and the diaphragm are paralyzed, and there is no voluntary movement (physiological or functional) below the spinal injury. Sensory loss for levels C1 through C3 includes the occipital region, the ears, and some regions of the face. Sensory loss is illustrated by a diagram of the dermatomes of the body (see Fig. 36–1).	A patient with a C1, C2, or C3 tetraplegia requires full-time attendance because of dependency on a mechanical ventilator. This person also is dependent in all daily living skills, such as feeding, bathing, and dressing. A person with this level of injury is able to operate an electric wheelchair (which should have a high back for head support) with chin or breath control. A mouthstick can be used to operate a typewriter or a telephone. A C4 tetraplegic usually also needs a mechanical ventilator, but may be removed from it intermittently. The patient usually is dependent on others in daily living skills, although he or she may be able to self-feed with the aid of feeding devices. This patient still needs an electric wheelchair, although because of better head control, a high-backed chair is not essential.
C5	When the C5 segment of the cord is damaged, the function of the diaphragm is impaired secondary to post-traumatic edema in the acute phase. Intestinal paralysis and gastric dilation may compound the respiratory distress. The upper extremities are rotated outwardly from impairment of the supraspinous and infraspinous muscles. The shoulders may be elevated markedly due to uninhibited action of the levator scapulae and trapezius muscles. After the acute phase, reflexes below the level of the lesion are exaggerated. Sensation is present in the neck and the triangular area of the anterior aspect of the upper arms.	A C5 tetraplegic usually is dependent in activities such as bathing, shaving, and combing of hair, but the patient has better hand-to-mouth coordination, allowing self-feeding with the aid of a feeder or brace. These aids permit the patient to brush teeth and to dress upper extremities. With the use of mechanical aids, this patient usually can write. Assistance is needed, as with higher-level tetraplegia, in transfers from wheelchair to bed or vice versa. An electric wheelchair still is preferable with a C5 tetraplegic, although a manual wheelchair may be managed if it has quad pegs (projections on the hand rim that allow for greater ease of movement of the wheelchair). A person with this level of injury may find that manual manipulation of a wheelchair is very tiring.
C6	In a C6 segment injury, respiratory distress may occur because of intestinal paralysis and ascending edema of the spinal cord. The shoulders usually are elevated, with arms abducted and forearms flexed. This is due to the uninhibited action of the deltoid, biceps, and brachioradialis muscles. Functional recovery of the triceps depends on correct positioning of the arms (forearm in extension, arm in adduction). Sensation remains over the lateral aspect of the arms and dorsolateral aspect of the forearms.	A C6 tetraplegic is independent in most hygiene requirements and sometimes is successful in lower extremity dressing and undressing. This patient is independent in feeding with or without mechanical aids. Light housework can be accomplished, and the person is able to drive a car with hand controls.
C7	Cord injuries at the level of C7 allow the diaphragm and accessory muscles to compensate for the affected abdominal and intercostal muscles. The upper extremities assume the same position as in C6 lesions. Finger flexion usually is exaggerated when the reflex action returns.	A C7 tetraplegic has the potential for independent living without the care of an attendant. Transfers are independent, as are upper and lower extremity dressing and undressing, feeding, bathing, light housework, and cooking.

(continued)

TABLE 36-1

Effects of Spinal Cord Injury on Patient Functioning (Continued)

Level of Injury	Physical Deficits	Daily Functioning
C8	The abnormal position of the upper extremities is not present in C8 injuries because the adductors and internal rotators are able to counteract the antagonists. The latissimus dorsi and trapezius muscles are strong enough to support a sitting position. Postural hypotension may occur when the patient is raised to the sitting position owing to the loss of vasomotor control. This postural hypotension can be minimized by having the patient make a gradual change from the lying to the sitting position. The patient's fingers usually assume a claw position.	A C8 tetraplegic should be able to live independently. This person is independent in dressing, undressing, driving a car, homemaking, and self-care.
Thoracic Injuries **T1–T5**	Injuries in the T1–T5 region may cause diaphragmatic breathing. The inspiratory function of the lungs increases as the level of the thoracic damage descends. Postural hypotension usually is present. A partial paralysis of the adductor pollicis, interosseous, and lumbrical mucles of the hands is present, as is sensory loss for touch, pain, and temperature.	Patients with damage at a thoracic level should be functionally independent.
T6–T12	Injuries at the T6 level abolish all abdominal reflexes. From the level of T6 down, individual segments are functioning, and at the level of T12, all abdominal reflexes are present. There is spastic paralysis of the lower limbs. The upper limits of sensory loss in thoracic lesions are T2 Entire body to inner side of the upper arm T3 Axilla T5 Nipple T6 Xiphoid process T7, T8 Lower costal margin T10 Umbilicus T12 Groin	Bowel and bladder function may return with the reflex automatism.
Lumbar Injuries **L1–L5**	The sensory loss involved in L1–L5 injuries is as follows: L1 All areas of the lower limbs, extending to the groin and back of the buttocks L2 Lower limbs, except the upper third of the anterior aspect of the thigh L3 Lower limbs and saddle area L4 Same as in L3 lesions, except the anterior aspect of the thigh L5 Outer aspects of the legs and ankles and the lower limbs and saddle area	Patients should attain total independence.
Sacral Injuries **S1–S6**	With injuries involving S1–S5, there may be some displacement of the foot. From S3 through S5, there is no paralysis of the leg muscles. The loss of sensation involves the saddle area, scrotum, glans penis, perineum, anal area, and the upper third of the posterior aspect of the thigh.	Patients should attain total independence.

changes associated with injury at various levels of the spinal cord and the degree of patient functioning that can be expected.

Spinal Cord Syndromes

Incomplete cord injuries often fit into recognizable neurological syndromes that are classified according to the area damaged.

CENTRAL CORD SYNDROME

Damage to the spinal cord in this syndrome is centrally located. Hyperextension of the cervical spine often is the mechanism of injury, and the damage is greatest to the cervical tracts supplying the arms. Clinically, the patient may present with paralyzed arms but with no deficit in the legs or bladder (Fig. 36–2A).

BROWN-SÉQUARD SYNDROME

The damage in this syndrome is located on one side of the spinal cord, such as a hemisection from a stab wound. The clinical presentation is one in which the patient has either increased or decreased cutaneous sensation of pain, temperature, and touch on the same side at the level of the lesion. Below the level of the lesion on the same side, there is complete motor paralysis. On the patient's opposite side, below the level of the lesion, there is loss of pain, temperature, and touch because the spinothalamic tracts cross soon after entering the cord. The posterior columns will be interrupted ipsilaterally, but this does not cause a major deficit because some fibers cross instead of running ipsilaterally. Clinically, the patient's limb with the best motor strength has the poorest sensation. Conversely, the limb with the best sensation has the poorest motor strength (see Fig. 36–2B).

ANTERIOR CORD SYNDROME

The area of damage in this syndrome is, as the name suggests, the anterior aspect of the spinal cord. Clinically, the patient usually has complete motor paralysis below the level of injury (corticospinal tracts) and loss of pain, temperature, and touch sensation (spinothalamic tracts), with preservation of light touch, proprioception, and position sense (posterior columns; see Fig. 36–2C).

POSTERIOR CORD SYNDROME

Posterior cord syndrome is usually the result of a hyperextension injury at the cervical level and is not commonly seen. Position sense, light touch, and vibratory sense are lost below the level of the injury.

Spinal Shock

Spinal shock (or posttransectional areflexia) is a condition that occurs very quickly after SCI and is characterized by the loss of motor, sensory, reflexic, and autonomic function

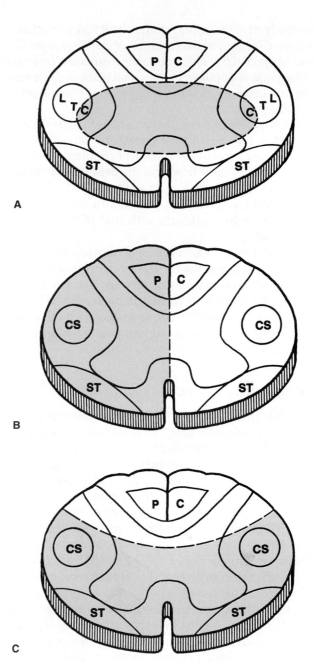

FIGURE 36-2
(**A**) Cross-section of the spinal cord to show the area involved in the **central cord syndrome**. Sensory loss typically is slight, and weakness is greater in the arms and hands than in the legs because of the distribution of nerve fibers in the corticospinal tracts. *L*, descending lumbar nerve fibers; *T*, thoracic nerve fibers; *C*, cervical nerve fibers. (**B**) Cross-section of the spinal cord to show the area involved in the **Brown-Séquard syndrome**. There are hemiparesis and loss of position and vibratory sense on the side of the lesion, with contralateral loss of pain and temperature. *PC*, posterior columns; *CS*, corticospinal tract; *ST*, anterolateral spinothalamic tract. (**C**) Cross-section of the spinal cord to show the area involved in the **anterior cord syndrome**. There are motor paralysis and loss of pain and temperature to the level of the lesion (or just below it), but position and vibratory sense are relatively spared.

below the level of the injury with resultant flaccid paralysis. It is caused by the sudden cessation of impulses from the higher brain centers, which normally maintain a continuous discharge of impulses to the spinal neurons. This cessation may occur because of the disruption of neural pathways at the injury site.

Clinically, loss of sympathetic pathway transmissions manifests as unopposed parasympathetic activity. There is vasodilation, subsequent pooling of circulating volume in the periphery, and hypotension. Bradycardia occurs from reflex vagal stimulation. In addition, the body's ability to control temperature is lost, and the patient's temperature tends to equilibrate with that of the external environment.

If the SCI produces an incomplete transection, the suppression of function below the level of injury is temporary, lasting a few days, to weeks or months. The duration of spinal shock is variable depending on the severity of the insult. Reflex activity usually returns gradually with those reflexes associated with the area surrounding the injured cord returning last.

Neurogenic Shock

Neurogenic shock (vasomotor shock) is a condition caused by the loss of vasomotor tone. The constriction and dilation of blood vessels are controlled by the vasomotor center in the medulla and by the sympathetic nerve fibers exiting the spinal cord and innervating the peripheral vessels. Any condition that interferes with the function or integrity of these structures can precipitate neurogenic shock. For example, SCI disrupts the sympathetic pathways at the level of the injury and can cause neurogenic shock. The medullary vasomotor center may be directly affected by a higher level cord injury (cervical or upper thoracic) or may also be directly depressed by high doses of certain drugs, such as anesthetic agents, opiates, and barbiturates. The vasomotor center may be indirectly affected by way of a condition, such as head injury, which produces cerebral edema and resultant pressure on the medulla and the vasomotor center contained therein, causing loss of vasomotor function.

The same clinical findings pertaining to disruption of the sympathetic transmissions in spinal shock will pertain in neurogenic shock (ie, hypotension, bradycardia, and loss of temperature control). Isolated syncopal episodes are often an example of neurogenic shock.

▦ ASSESSMENT

Initial Evaluation

Because elapsed time from injury significantly affects prognosis, the patient with SCI should be transported as rapidly as possible to a specialized unit or a hospital with adequate

diagnostic and treatment facilities to handle such trauma. A primary survey done at the scene of an accident includes a rapid assessment of airway, breathing, and circulation (ABCs). Along with checking for airway patency, the cervical spine and spinal cord are immobilized. Unfortunately, a significant number of neurological injuries occur or are aggravated during emergency extrication, transport, and evaluation of the patient.[1]

The patient is assessed for presence of spontaneous respirations, and breath sounds are auscultated. Circulation is checked by presence or absence of a pulse. The patient also is assessed for external hemorrhage or signs of shock. The primary survey also includes a brief neurological assessment to see if the patient is alert, responds to verbal or

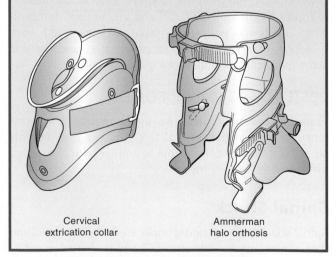

painful stimuli, or is unresponsive. Clothing is removed to assess for hidden injuries.

Secondary Assessment

Secondary survey includes obtaining a history of what happened; taking vital signs; noting any odors, such as alcohol, fuel, urine, or feces; and performing a more thorough neurological examination, including pupil check and head-to-toe survey. (Chapter 32 discusses a complete neurological assessment.)

From 25% to 65% of patients with SCI have other injuries associated with the spinal cord trauma. Head injuries are the most common and usually accompany a cervical cord injury. Chest injury often accompanies thoracic spinal cord trauma. The chest, head, and abdomen should be examined for evidence of concomitant injuries. Appropriate radiographs of the chest, skull, abdomen, and long bones may be indicated. Placement of a nasogastric tube and urinary catheter also can help to evaluate the patient for other injuries. During the early assessment of the SCI patient, a digital rectal examination is important in determining whether the injury is incomplete or complete. The lesion is incomplete if the patient can feel the palpating finger or can contract the perianal muscles around the finger voluntarily. Sensation may be present in the absence of voluntary motor activity. Sensation seldom is absent when voluntary perianal muscle contraction is present. In either case, the prognosis for further motor and sensory return is good. Preservation of sacral function might be the only finding that indicates an incomplete lesion, and significant neurological recovery may occur in the patient with an incomplete cord injury.

Rectal tone by itself, without the presence of voluntary perianal muscle contraction or rectal sensation, is not evidence of an incomplete cord injury. Some rectal tone may be accounted for by local reflexes.

Clinical Manifestations

RESPIRATORY SYMPTOMS

Clinical manifestations other than those associated with concomitant injuries may include hypoventilation or respiratory failure, particularly with high cervical injuries. Hypoventilation from inadequate innervation of respiratory muscles is a common problem after SCI. It is important to assess whether the intercostal muscles are functioning or whether the patient has only diaphragmatic breathing. The diaphragm, the major respiratory muscle, is innervated by the phrenic nerve, which travels through the third, fourth, and fifth cervical segments of the cord.

Anytime a person has a cervical cord injury, respiratory failure should be anticipated. Although the patient initially may have what appears to be adequate diaphragmatic breathing (the intercostals would not be functioning because they are innervated from the thoracic region of the cord), cord edema can act like an ascending lesion and may compromise function of the diaphragm. Frequent checks of tidal volume and vital capacity and frequent auscultation of breath sounds should be routine.

The SCI patient may have further respiratory compromise because of preexisting pulmonary disease or coexistent chest injuries. Alveolar ventilation may be affected directly by the pulmonary collapse or by consolidation from retained secretions or aspiration of vomitus. Pulmonary edema also may result from incorrect management of intravenous fluids. Paralytic ileus and gastric dilation may increase the pressure on the diaphragm and cause further respiratory embarrassment. Interference with the cough reflex and fluid imbalance may combine to obstruct the airways.

SPINAL SHOCK

During the spinal shock phase, vasomotor tone is lost, and blood pools in the periphery, lowering blood pressure because of the decreased circulating volume. Orthostatic hypotension also may occur because the patient is unable to compensate for changes in position. The vasoconstricting message from the medulla cannot reach the blood vessels because of the cord injury. Thus, hypotension is a common manifestation following SCI. Frequently, bradycardia is present owing to reflex vagal activity. The effects of the vagus nerve (parasympathetic innervation to the heart) are unopposed by sympathetic response. Figure 36–3 outlines the mechanisms involved in spinal shock.

There also may be flaccid paralysis and loss of reflex activity below the level of the injury, along with loss of sensation. Hypothermia often results from vasodilation and excessive loss of body heat. The patient tends to take on the temperature of the environment.

Incontinence of urine and possibly feces may have occurred at the scene of the accident. Urine incontinence or retention may result from injury to the spinal cord. There may be an imbalance between parasympathetic and sympathetic innervation to the bowel and thus a loss of voluntary control.

Spinal shock may last from weeks to months. The vasodilation usually resolves within a few days, but it may be months before deep tendon reflexes reappear.

METABOLIC DERANGEMENT

The patient with SCI demonstrates a surprisingly florid metabolic response to an injury that usually is associated with little tissue damage. If the injury is uncomplicated, the metabolic derangement reaches a peak within 48 to 72 hours postinjury. A return to normal may be anticipated between 10 and 14 days postinjury.

When the spinal injury is complicated by other factors, such as surgical intervention or other medical problems, the metabolic response is greater and more prolonged. This

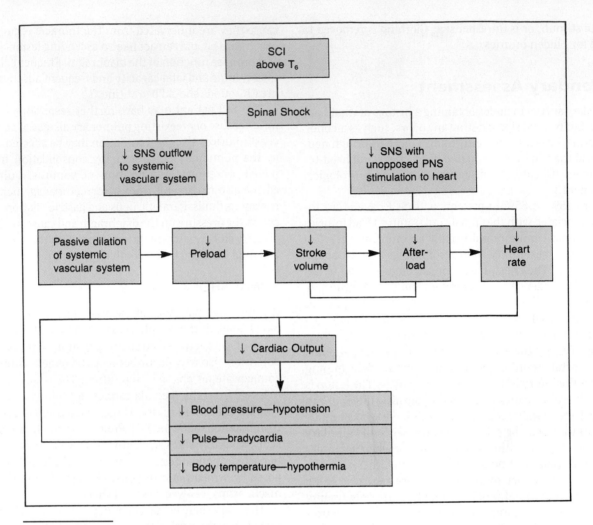

FIGURE 36-3

Mechanisms involved in spinal shock: *SNS*, sympathetic nervous system; *PNS*, parasympathetic nervous system. (Zejdlik C: Management of Spinal Cord Injury. Boston, Jones and Bartlett Publishers, 1992. Reprinted by permission. Based on L. Belange, SCI Unit, Shaughnessy Site, Vancouver, BC, unpublished material)

metabolic response is characterized by a marked retention of sodium and water, increased potassium excretion, breakdown of body protein, and an oliguric period followed by diuresis. A reduced glomerular filtration rate secondary to hypotension compounds the sodium and water retention.

Starvation also is a factor in the metabolic disturbance because most cord-injured patients are unable to tolerate oral food or fluid for at least 1 week after the injury. This can lead to negative nitrogen balance. Cord-injured patients also have a decrease in testosterone levels that is significant enough to contribute to the negative nitrogen balance.

Research on metabolic and endocrine changes in patients with SCI has provided some interesting data. Apparently, body areas that have become insensitive as a result of the cord injury do not secrete anti-inflammatory steroids in adequate amounts. This lack of secretion may play a role in the genesis of pressure sores in the patient with SCI. This attenuation of the normally expected rise in corticosteroid

levels also is seen during surgical procedures. Because excessive inflammation of the surgical site may occur as a result of the minimal cortisol release, this must be kept in mind if the patient undergoes surgery.

Diagnostic Studies

Diagnostic tests common for patients with SCI include radiographic evaluation of spine fractures and possible cord compression. Magnetic resonance imaging also may be used to assess the amount of cord compression and the type of injury (ie, either hemorrhage or edema). Computed tomography (CT) scanning will outline the spine and perispinal structures.

Tomography or polytomography is being replaced by CT scanning in many areas but still may be useful to assess the extent of bony injury. Somatosensory evoked potentials whereby a peripheral nerve below the level of injury is stimulated and the neurological response (evoked potential) is recorded from the cerebral cortex through scalp electrodes may be recorded to clarify the prognosis. See Chapter 32 for a detailed discussion of these procedures.

MEDICAL MANAGEMENT

Restoration of Hemodynamic Stability

During the initial postinjury period, medical management often focuses on regulation of blood pressure and heart rate. Adequate tissue perfusion to the spinal cord and other vital organs, such as the kidneys, needs to be addressed. Careful intravenous fluid replacement will provide hydration without fluid overload. Vasopressors may not be needed to maintain blood pressure during spinal shock, but when the blood pressure is not high enough to sustain vital organ perfusion, usually low-dose dopamine is used. The bradycardia during spinal shock also may not need treatment, but if necessary, atropine may be used to speed up the heart rate.

Cord Decompression and Immobilization

Decompression of the cord by realignment of the spinal canal is of initial concern. Closed reduction of a cervical fracture often may be accomplished with skeletal traction. Cervical traction is used when the fracture is unstable or if subluxation has occurred. Once the fracture or subluxation is reduced, a halo device is often applied to allow mobilization of the patient. Gardner-Wells tongs or Crutchfield tongs are common forms of cervical traction; however, because of all the complications that accompany prolonged immobility, long-term traction with tongs is seldom used since the advent of the halo vest.

Surgical reduction may be indicated for other spinal fractures. Surgical stabilization is accomplished by placement of Harrington rods, laminectomy and fusion, or by anterior fusion. Bone for fusion usually is taken from the iliac crest, tibia, or ribs.

Pharmacological Management

Animal studies suggest that preservation of a relatively small number of spinal axons can support neurological recovery from SCI. The focus of the second National Acute

Spinal Cord Injury Study (NASCIS2) was on enhancing tissue preservation by inhibiting posttraumatic spinal cord lipid peroxidation (which causes the injury-induced degenerative cascade) through the use of methylprednisolone. NASCIS2 demonstrated that use of methylprednisolone in large doses, given within 8 hours of injury, results in improved neurological function.[2] The accompanying display gives administration protocol. Methylprednisolone also helps reverse the intracellular calcium accumulation, which causes cord degeneration and ischemia after SCI, retards secondary neuronal degeneration, maintains spinal cord blood flow, and improves the functioning of the cellular sodium–calcium pump.

Several experimental drugs are being developed. They include a number of opioid antagonists that are more specific than naloxone, which has not proven to be beneficial. Research is focusing on the *N*-methyl-D-aspartate receptors and glutamate antagonists. Benzamil is an experimental sodium–calcium exchange blocking agent that limits the amount of intracellular calcium and ischemia at the injury site.

Nutrition

Nutrition is of significant concern even during the acute phase of injury and must not be overlooked while hemodynamic stability is being addressed. Optimal nutrition is necessary for this stability to be achieved. Once the patient is in negative nitrogen balance, this contributes to skin breakdown, poor wound healing, and lack of energy for rehabili-

---

CLINICAL APPLICATION: Drug Therapy
Methylprednisolone Administration Protocol for Spinal Cord Injury*

Dosage:
- Loading dose—30 mg/kg IV over 15 minutes
- Maintenance dose—5.4 mg/kg/h IV for 23 hours

Administration:
- Loading dose must be given within 8 hours of injury.
- Maintenance dose must begin within 1 hour of loading dose.

Indications:
- Evidence of cord injury, including penetrating injuries
- Injury < 8 hours old

Relative contraindications:
- Pregnancy
- Uncontrolled diabetes mellitus
- Medication allergy
- Severe comorbidity
- Injury > 8 hours old

---

*Based on NASCIS 2 study.
From Nolan S: Current trends in the management of acute spinal cord injury. Critical Care Nursing Quarterly 17(1):71, 1994

---

tative efforts. Caloric requirements should be calculated to ensure adequate, but not excessive, nutritional support. Some studies have demonstrated that human growth hormone has no effect on nitrogen balance in highly stressed, immobilized patients after head or spinal injury, but it does significantly enhance constitutive serum protein concentrations and other indices of nutritional repletion.[3]

Treatment of Paralytic Ileus

Early medical management includes NPO status, particularly for cervical-injured patients, and usually nasogastric tube placement with intermittent suction for the paralytic ileus that frequently accompanies SCI. Peristalsis should be stimulated as soon as bowel sounds are present. This may be done safely with stool softeners, mild laxatives, or suppositories. Enemas, other than the oil-retention type, should be avoided because the risk of intestinal perforation is high.

Urinary Management

Acute tubular necrosis may occur during the first 48 hours postinjury as a result of hypotension. An indwelling urinary catheter is necessary to allow for hourly measurement of urinary output during this phase, with a goal of keeping it at least 30 mL/h. Fluid and electrolyte balance must be monitored closely. Removal of the indwelling catheter as soon as spinal shock has resolved will reduce the risk of infection.

The long-range objective of bladder management, regardless of the level of the injury, is to achieve a means whereby the bladder consistently empties, the urine is sterile, and the patient remains continent. The ultimate goal is to have the patient catheter free, with consistent low residual urine checks, no urinary tract infection, and no evidence of damage to the upper urinary tract structures.

One method of bladder management is accomplished by intermittent catheterization, and it may begin in the early recovery phase after spinal shock is resolved. The purpose of this program is to exercise the detrusor muscle, again with the goal of keeping the patient catheter free. The advantage of this method is that no irritant remains in the bladder; consequently, the risk of urinary tract infection, periurethral abscess, and epididymitis is reduced.

▬ NURSING MANAGEMENT

Respiratory Care

Although a patient with an injury below C4 will have an intact diaphragm, during the initial period after a cervical SCI, there may be ascending cord edema that will temporarily impair functioning of the diaphragm. During the duration of the edema, the patient may require mechanical ventilation. Anyone with a cervical cord injury should have respiratory parameters, such as tidal volume and vital capacity, measured frequently, along with frequent auscultation of breath sounds. Respiratory failure should be anticipated.

Normally, ventilation is accomplished through a complex interaction between muscles of the chest, the abdominal wall, and the diaphragm. An SCI results in paralysis of inspiratory and expiratory muscles. Dysfunction of intercostal and accessory muscles decreases ventilation and predisposes the patient to atelectasis. Dysfunction of abdominal muscles and expiratory intercostal muscles diminishes the patient's ability to generate a cough to clear secretions. The intercostal muscles also normally provide support to the lateral chest wall. When the intercostals are impaired, this part of the chest wall collapses during inspiration as the abdomen expands. This breathing pattern is easily discernible and results in ineffective ventilation.

The degree of respiratory compromise is determined primarily by the level of the injury, although not entirely. For example, a 28-year-old C5 tetraplegic with no lung disease may have better ventilation than a 65-year-old C8 quadriplegic with a long history of smoking and chronic obstructive pulmonary disease.

Respiratory complications are the leading cause of death in the acute and chronic phases of SCI, especially among tetraplegics. Therefore, careful respiratory assessment and early intervention are important.

Assisting the patient with the quad coughing technique may help clear airways more effectively despite weakness or loss of the respiratory muscles that produce the automatic cough reflex. With this quad coughing technique, the sides of the patient's chest (if patient is on side or abdomen) or the diaphragm (if supine) are compressed during exhalation. This technique often is most helpful after postural drainage or vibration of the chest.

Suctioning may be necessary if the patient's airway cannot be cleared effectively with other techniques. Nurses should remember that suctioning (or nasogastric tube insertion) may trigger an abnormal vasovagal response, resulting in bradycardia.

When turning a patient to the prone position on a Stryker frame, the nurse needs to remain at the bedside for the first few turns to evaluate the patient's respiratory tolerance of the turn. High-level tetraplegics can experience respiratory arrest in the prone position because movement of the diaphragm is compromised. Bradycardia in the prone position also is common.

Temperature Control

An SCI above the thoracolumbar outflow of the sympathetic nervous system disconnects the thalamic thermoregulatory mechanisms. As a result, the patient fails to sweat to get rid of body heat, and there is an absence of vasoconstriction, resulting in the patient's inability to shiver to increase body heat. The degree of thermal control and dysfunction is directly proportional to the extent of body area with loss of thermal regulation. Hence, a tetraplegic has a more difficult time with thermoregulation than a paraplegic.

Hypothermia usually is managed using warmed blankets. Electric heating blankets or hot water bottles may present a danger for body parts with no sensation. An attempt is made to stabilize the patient's temperature above 96.5°F (35.8°C). Over the long term, thermal control can be facilitated by use of clothing appropriate for the weather conditions.

Prevention of Deep Venous Thrombosis

Measures to prevent deep venous thrombosis (DVT) may include low-dose heparin or low-molecular-weight heparin and antiembolic stockings. During the acute phase, devices that sequentially compress the lower extremities may be used. Many SCI centers use prophylactic anticoagulation or low-molecular-weight heparin; others rely on passive range-of-motion exercises and early mobilization. The RotoRest bed also is available for use in preventing this complication by keeping the patient in continuous motion. Functional electrical stimulation, with the help of computers, provides electrical neuromuscular stimulation that causes muscle contractions and movement and functional activities of paralyzed extremities. It is still considered an experimental therapy and requires a great deal of patient energy to use, but it may have some future application in helping prevent DVT formation.

Leg veins should not be used as sites from which to draw blood lest the trauma to the vessel wall enhance platelet aggregation and clot formation. Smokers should be encouraged to quit because nicotine causes vasoconstriction, thus slowing blood flow through the periphery.

There is some controversy about the effectiveness of serial leg measurements in monitoring for DVT. If leg measurements are used, a standard measurement protocol should be established and followed by all staff. For example, use a special measuring tape rather than sewing tape, take independent measurements by two nurses, and use running averages.[4]

Mobilization and Skin Care

Pressure is a common cause of structural damage to a muscle and its peripheral nerve supply. There is a definite time–pressure relationship in the development of pressure sores. Skin can tolerate minute pressure indefinitely, but great pressure for a short time is disruptive. Microscopic tissue changes secondary to local ischemia occur in less than

30 minutes. Pressure interferes with arteriolar and capillary blood flow.

When the pressure is prolonged, there is definite damage to superficial circulation and tissue. The damage may be associated with congestion and induration of the area or blistering and loss of superficial epidermal layers of skin. As the pressure continues, the deeper skin layers are lost, leading to necrosis and ulceration. Serous drainage from such an ulceration can constitute a continuous protein loss of as much as 50 g/d. Prolongation of the pressure results in deep penetrating necrosis of the skin, subcutaneous tissue, fascia, and muscle. The destruction may progress to gangrene of the underlying bony structure. Pressure necrosis can begin from within the tissue over a bony prominence, where the body weight is greatest per square inch.

A turn schedule for the patient is important. Turning should be carried out at least every 2 hours. Use of an air or egg-crate mattress does not preclude the need to turn. The condition of the skin should be checked before and after the position change.

Numerous kinetic beds that are in continuous motion are available. They slowly turn from side to side, but may be stopped in any position. They are helpful for mobilizing pulmonary secretions, improving gas exchange, and preventing skin breakdown. These beds are useful for preventing and treating complications of immobility.

Medication Administration

Nurses administering medications to patients with SCI should recognize several special considerations. Subcutaneous and intramuscular injections are not absorbed well because of the lack of muscle tone. Sterile abscesses may result, causing autonomic dysreflexia or an increase in spasms. Injection sites are the deltoid area, the anterior thigh, and the abdominal area. These sites should be rotated, and the volume injected should not exceed 1 mL at any one site.

As a rule, sensation in the cord-injured patient is limited. Intractable pain may be present after spinal shock and is due to nerve root damage. Abnormal sensation may occur at the level of the lesion in injuries causing diverse nerve root damage, such as occurs with gunshot or knife wounds. Narcotics are not favored because of the high probability of addiction. Attention to position and other comfort measures, along with the use of mild analgesics, such as aspirin or acetaminophen, is a more acceptable approach.

Nurses often start peripheral intravenous lines, but the intravenous site of choice is the subclavian vein. In this area of high blood flow, there is less chance of thrombosis secondary to vasomotor paralysis, especially during spinal shock. For this reason, the veins of the lower extremities never should be used for intravenous administration.

Psychological Support

Psychological adjustment to the loss of previous physical abilities is unique to each person. The rate at which a person works through this process varies, and none of the stages is static. A person can move back and forth between stages. The emotions felt and displayed by someone with a cord injury are no different from the emotions felt by everyone one time or another, and recognition of that fact may help promote empathy with the patient.

Whatever names are given to the stages of grief, certain emotions are felt after a cord injury.

- *Stage I—shock and disbelief.* During this phase, the patient does not request an explanation of what has happened. The patient is overwhelmed by the injury. There may be more concern with whether he or she will live than with whether he or she will walk again. This period may result in extreme dependence on the staff members. Staff members at the same time may feel that the patient does not understand the ramifications of the injury. The staff may identify with the feelings of being overwhelmed because they are often overwhelmed with the acute medical management of this catastrophic illness.
- *Stage II—denial.* The process of denial is an escape mechanism. Generally, the whole disability is not denied, but particular aspects of it are. For instance, the patient may say he or she cannot walk now but will be able to in 6 months. Bargaining, instead of being a separate stage, can be considered a form of denial. Bargains with God may be in the form of offering Him the legs if He will just return function of the arms. Staff often find it difficult to deal with patients in this stage.

A helpful approach is to focus on the present problems. This is not the stage to discuss long-term

---

Sample Stages of Grief in the Person With a Spinal Cord Injury

Stage I: Shock and disbelief
  Patient is overwhelmed by injury and does not ask for explanation of cause of injury.
Stage II: Denial
  Patient uses escape mechanism and denies certain aspects of disability.
Stage III: Reaction
  Patient expresses and verbalizes impact of injury.
Stage IV: Mobilization
  Patient looks to the future and desires to develop self-care.
Stage V: Coping
  Patient no longer holds injury as center of life.

changes, such as ordering a wheelchair or making modifications to the home. More appropriate matters to deal with would be skin care and range-of-motion exercises.

- *Stage III—reaction*. During this stage, instead of denying the impact of the injury, the patient expresses this impact. There may be severe depression and loss of motivation and involvement. Previous hobbies or interests lose their meaning. There is great helplessness during this period, and there may be suicidal statements.

   Staff members can help at this stage by listening to the patient as feelings are verbalized. The staff should avoid setting up failure situations, which could happen if they push the patient too fast.

   It is important to note that both the sudden absence of muscular activity and sensations in the patient with SCI and the mental state of helplessness appear to alter central nervous system metabolism. Depression coincides with a fall in a brain metabolite excreted in the urine as tryptamine. Thus, it is important for the nurse to understand that depression in some SCI patients might have a metabolic basis and that a trial of pharmacological therapy might be beneficial.

- *Stage IV—mobilization*. Problem-solving behavior can be seen during this stage. The patient is looking toward the future and wants to learn about self-care. In fact, the patient may become very possessive of the therapist or nurse and resent the time spent with other patients. This is a time of sharing and planning between patient and staff.

- *Stage V—coping*. Some authorities think that patients do not accept the disability *per se* but instead learn to cope with it. Disability still is an inconvenience, but it is no longer the center of their lives. Life is again meaningful to the person, and the patient is again involved with others.

All staff should have an understanding of the types of feelings and reactions the patient with an SCI may exhibit. This process of recovery can be shared with family members in helping them to support the injured person and participate in recovery. Psychological support should be provided for family members as well. They no doubt have many concerns, such as finances, role changes, long-term outcomes, and more. It is important to be supportive of them and help them and the patient with coping strategies.

Sexual Concerns

After a cord injury, patients are concerned about their ability to function sexually, although they may not verbalize this concern immediately. It is essential that nurses address this area of concern. While nurses in the intensive care unit probably will not deal with this problem specifically, it is important for them to have some knowledge of the functional potential of the patient in order to begin to deal with the patient's fears and concerns in this area early on. By avoiding discussion of this important issue, professionals validate the patient's fear that there can be no sex after SCI, which is certainly not true.

Most cord-injured men believe that their total sexuality is tied to erection and ejaculation. There are three general types of erection in men: psychogenic, reflexogenic, and spontaneous.

A psychogenic erection can result from sexual thoughts. The area of the cord responsible for this type of erection is between T11 and L2. Therefore, if the lesion is above this level, the message from the brain cannot get through the damaged area.

Reflexogenic erections are a direct result of stimulation to the penis. Some patients may get this type of erection when changing their catheter or pulling the pubic hairs. The length of time the erection can be maintained is variable; thus, its usefulness for sexual activity is variable. Reflexogenic erections are better with higher cervical and thoracic lesions. Damage to lumbar and sacral regions may destroy the reflex arc.

The third type of erection is spontaneous. This may occur when the bladder is full, and it comes from some internal stimulation. How long the spontaneous erection lasts will determine its usefulness for sexual activity. The ability to achieve a reflexogenic or spontaneous erection comes from nerves in the S2, S3, and S4 segments of the cord.

In 50% of cord-injured women, the menstrual pattern is interrupted for approximately 6 months after injury but then is reestablished. Women with SCI are able to become pregnant and seem to have no increase in rate of miscarriage. There are potential complications for the pregnant spinal cord-injured woman, such as urinary tract infection, pressure sores, and anemia, but with careful medical attention, complications usually can be avoided or minimized.

Labor may be painless, or the woman may experience other signs that indicate labor is occurring (eg, abdominal or leg spasms, back pain, difficulty breathing). Autonomic dysreflexia is a complication of labor in women with injuries above T4 to T6 and should be anticipated so it can be controlled. Women with SCI can breast-feed their infant if desired.

▬ COMPLICATIONS

Autonomic Dysreflexia

Autonomic dysreflexia, or hyperreflexia, is a syndrome that sometimes occurs after the acute phase in patients with a spinal cord lesion at T7 or above and constitutes a medical emergency. The syndrome presents quickly and can precipitate a seizure or stroke. Death can occur if the cause is not relieved.

The syndrome can be triggered by bladder or intestinal distention, spasticity, decubitus ulcers, or stimulation of the skin below the level of the injury. Ejaculation in the man can initiate the reflex, as can strong uterine contractions in the pregnant woman. Potential precipitating factors are listed in the accompanying display.

These stimuli produce a sympathetic discharge that causes a reflex vasoconstriction of the blood vessels in the skin and splanchnic bed below the level of the injury. The vasoconstriction produces extreme hypertension and a throbbing headache.

Vasoconstriction of the splanchnic bed distends the baroreceptors in the carotid sinus and aortic arch. They in turn stimulate the vagus nerve, producing a bradycardia, in an attempt to lower the blood pressure. The body also attempts to reduce the hypertension by superficial vasodilation of vessels above the SCI. As a result, there is flushing, blurred vision, and nasal congestion. Because the SCI interrupts transmission of the vasodilation message below the level of the injury, the vasoconstriction continues below the level of the injury until the stimulus is identified and interrupted. The vasoconstriction results in pallor below the injury, whereas flushing occurs above the injury. Other signs and symptoms of autonomic dysreflexia are listed in the display.

When autonomic dysreflexia is recognized, there are several things the alert nurse can do quickly and can teach the patient to do (see Procedure display). The head of the bed should be elevated and frequent checks of blood pressure made. The bladder drainage system should be checked

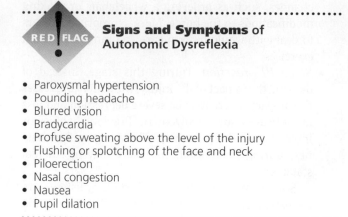

Signs and Symptoms of
Autonomic Dysreflexia

- Paroxysmal hypertension
- Pounding headache
- Blurred vision
- Bradycardia
- Profuse sweating above the level of the injury
- Flushing or splotching of the face and neck
- Piloerection
- Nasal congestion
- Nausea
- Pupil dilation

quickly for kinks in the tubing, and the urine collection bag should not be overly full. Some protocols for checking the patency of the urinary drainage system include irrigation of the catheter with 10 to 30 mL of irrigating solution. The nurse should make sure that absolutely no more than that amount is used because the addition of the fluid may aggravate the massive sympathetic outflow already present. If the symptoms persist after these checks are made, the catheter should be changed so that the bladder can empty. If the patient did not have a catheter in place when the hyperreflexia began, one should be inserted.

If the urinary system does not seem to be the cause of the stimulus, the patient should be checked for bowel impaction. The impaction should not be removed until the symptoms subside. Dibucaine or lidocaine ointment can be applied to the rectum to anesthetize the area until symptoms subside.

If the patient's blood pressure does not return to normal, sublingual nifedipine (Procardia) may be very effective. Use of a sympathetic ganglionic blocking agent such as atropine sulfate, guanethidine sulfate (Ismelin), reserpine (Reserfia), or methyldopa (Aldomet) may be used. Hydralazine (Apresoline) and diazoxide (Hyperstat) also may be used.

Pulmonary Problems

Pulmonary complications are most commonly associated with death in people with SCI, both in the acute and chronic phases. These pulmonary complications are especially prevalent in people injured above T10. If there is concomitant chest trauma or preexisting pulmonary disease, a history of smoking, or older age, there is higher risk for these complications.

Atelectasis is possible in any immobilized patient. Early mobilization, ensuring the airways are clear of secretions, and bronchial hygiene may be useful in minimizing or preventing atelectasis. Pneumonia also may result from hypoventilation and inability to keep airways clear. Adequate

CLINICAL APPLICATION:
Assessment Parameters
Precipitating Factors in Autonomic Dysreflexia

- Bladder distention or urinary tract infection
- Bladder/kidney stones
- Distended bowel
- Pressure areas or decubiti
- Thrombophlebitis
- Acute abdominal problems, such as ulcers, gastritis
- Pulmonary emboli
- Menstruation
- Second stage of labor
- Constrictive clothing
- Heterotopic bone
- Pain
- Sexual activity; ejaculation by a man
- Manipulation/instrumentation of bladder or bowel
- Spasticity
- Exposure to hot or cold stimuli

CLINICAL APPLICATION:
Nursing Intervention Guidelines
Procedure for Managing Autonomic Dysreflexia

1. Elevate the head of bed.
2. Apply blood pressure cuff, and check blood pressure every 1 to 2 minutes.
   - If BP is above 180/90, proceed to step 5.
   - If BP is below 180/90, proceed as follows.
3. Quickly insert bladder catheter or check bladder drainage system in place to detect possible obstruction.
   - Check to make sure plug or clamp is not in catheter or on tubing.
   - Check for kinks in catheter or drainage tubing.
   - Check inlet to leg bag to make sure it is not corroded.
   - Check to make sure leg bag is not overfull.
   - If none of these are evident, proceed to step 4.
4. Determine if catheter is plugged by irrigating the bladder slowly with no more than 30 mL of irrigation solution. Use of more solution may increase the massive sympathetic outflow already present. If symptoms have not subsided, proceed to step 5.
5. Change the catheter and empty the bladder.
6. When you are sure the bladder is empty and if BP is:
   - Above 180/90, call physician immediately.
   - Below 180/90, proceed as follows:
     Give sublingual nifedipine (Procardia) if protocol calls for it. Give atropine according to physician's order. If BP rises or fails to subside, call physician immediately. Guanethidine monosulfate (Ismelin), hydralazine (Apresoline), or inhaled amyl nitrate may then be ordered by the physician. Dibenzylene may be used for chronic dysreflexia.
7. Ideally, this procedure requires three people: one to check the BP, one to check the drainage system, and one to notify the physician.

If bladder overdistention does not seem to be the cause of the dysreflexia,

- Check for bowel impaction. Do not attempt to remove it, if present. Apply Nupercainal ointment or Xylocaine jelly to the rectum and anal area. As the area is anesthetized, the BP should fall. After the BP is again stable, using a generous amount of anesthetizing ointment or jelly, manually remove impaction.
- Change the patient's position. Pressure areas may be the source of dysreflexia.

hydration helps keep secretions liquefied for ease of removal, and bronchoscopy may be necessary to remove mucous plugs. Supplemental oxygen administration is used to treat hypoxia. Ventilator-dependent patients need exquisite pulmonary care (see Chapter 24). Especially during the acute phase of SCI, pulmonary embolus is a potential problem. Many emboli break off a DVT and lodge in the lung. Patients particularly at risk for a fat embolus are those with long bone fractures. Signs of chest or neck petechiae and low-grade fever may be early indications.

CLINICAL APPLICATION: Patient Care Study

Adam Davis is a 19-year-old college student who fell 30 feet to the ground while rock climbing. He was picked up at the scene of the accident by paramedics who found him lying in a supine position, unable to move any extremities and complaining of some neck pain. He appeared awake, alert, and oriented to his current location, the date and day of the week, and details of the fall. His pupils were equal and reactive to light. He showed no other signs of injury except for several scrapes on his arms. Vital signs were BP 110/72, pulse 86, respirations 18, unlabored and regular. The paramedics applied a cervical collar, placed him on a backboard, and he was transported to the medical center by helicopter.

On initial examination, his vital signs were BP 100/60, pulse 68, respirations 24 and somewhat shallow, temperature 99.8°F (37.7°C). His color was dusky, skin warm and dry, and his arm veins were quite distended. He had no motor function or sensation past a couple of inches below midaxillary level. He could tighten his biceps but could not overcome gravity to raise his arms. There were no deep tendon reflexes.

Full spine, skull, and chest radiographs were done. Intravenous lactated Ringer's solution was started, and a Foley catheter was inserted into his bladder. A nasogastric tube was inserted and connected to low intermittent suction.

The radiographs revealed that Adam had a dislocated fracture of C5 and C6. The chest film showed a lack of full lung field expansion. Blood work was normal with the exception of arterial blood gases, which showed respiratory acidosis (pH 7.30).

The treatment plan for his spinal shock included careful intravenous fluid replacement to avoid overhydration, the use of dopamine or a similar drug if his hypotension compromised adequate perfusion of vital organs, atropine to correct the bradycardia if he became symptomatic, and careful monitoring of his respiratory function. Although an injury at C5 to C6 would spare his diaphragm, mechanical ventilation might become necessary owing to ascending edema around the cord. The respiratory acidosis probably reflected hypoventilation with resultant CO_2 retention.

During the spinal shock phase, it is important to measure urine output to ensure adequate renal perfusion. Because he probably had an atonic bladder, to ensure emptying with no retention and to monitor output accurately, an indwelling catheter was inserted. The nasogastric tube will decompress a possible distended stomach and prevent aspiration, and if an ileus is present, nasogastric drainage will facilitate its resolution.

Neurosurgeons stabilized Adam's neck by using traction to reduce the fracture. Once the spine was in proper alignment, a halo vest was applied that he would wear for 13 weeks to allow healing to occur. (See earlier display on nursing management of a patient in a halo vest.) Once past the acute phase of his injury, Adam was transferred to a rehabilitation facility for further recovery and adaptation to his injury.

The following Collaborative Care Guide details care of the patient with a spinal cord injury.

COLLABORATIVE CARE GUIDE
for the Patient with Spinal Cord Injury

OUTCOMES	INTERVENTIONS
Oxygenation/Ventilation	

Arterial blood gas values will be within normal limits. No evidence of atelectasis is demonstrated.	• Provide routine pulmonary toilet including
	  –airway suctioning
	  –chest percussion
	  –incentive spirometer.
	• Turn frequently.
	• Mobilize out of bed to chair.
	• Apply abdominal binder when out of bed.

Circulation/Perfusion	
There will be no evidence of neurogenic (spinal) shock (T10 injuries and higher). Blood pressure will be adequate to maintain vital organ function. There will be no development of deep vein thrombosis. There will be no evidence of orthostatic hypotension.	• Monitor for bradycardia, vasodilation, and hypotension. • Prepare to administer intravascular volume, vasopressors, and positive chronotropic agents. • Begin DVT prophylaxis on admission (eg, external compression device, low dose heparin). • Measure calf and thigh circumference daily and at same location; report increase. • Apply Ace wraps to lower extremities before mobilizing out of bed.
Fluids/Electrolytes	
Serum electrolytes will be within normal limits. Fluid balance will be maintained as evidenced by stable weight, absence of edema, normal skin turgor.	• Monitor laboratory studies as indicated by patient condition. • Administer mineral/electrolyte replacement as ordered. • Monitor gastrointestinal and insensible fluid loss. • Make accurate daily fluid intake and output measurements. • Weigh daily.
Mobility/Safety	
Joint range of motion will be maintained and contractures prevented. Skin integrity will be maintained under or around stabilization devices (cervical collar, Yale brace, halo vest, etc.).	• Begin range of motion exercises early after admission. • Use high top tennis shoes, moon boots, extremity splints routinely. • Consult with physical and occupational therapist. • Monitor skin and/or pin sites of stabilization devices. • Use meticulous skin care/pin care under or around stabilization devices.
Skin Integrity	
Skin will remain intact.	• Reposition at least every 2 hours while in bed. • Position to prevent pressure on bony prominences. • Use upright, straight-backed chair when out of bed (not a reclining chair). • Reposition/shift weight every hour when sitting upright. • Use Braden Scale to monitor risk of skin breakdown.
Nutrition	
Protein, carbohydrate, fat, and calorie intake will meet minimum daily requirements.	• Consult dietitian. • Encourage fluids, high fiber diet. • Monitor fluid intake and output, calorie count. • Administer parenteral and enteral nutrition as appropriate. • Assist with feeding/feed as needed.

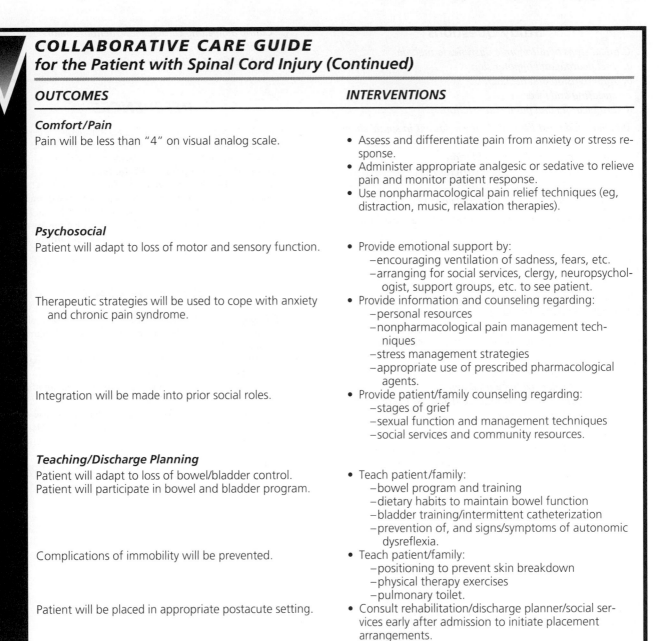

COLLABORATIVE CARE GUIDE
for the Patient with Spinal Cord Injury (Continued)

OUTCOMES	INTERVENTIONS
Comfort/Pain	
Pain will be less than "4" on visual analog scale.	• Assess and differentiate pain from anxiety or stress response.
	• Administer appropriate analgesic or sedative to relieve pain and monitor patient response.
	• Use nonpharmacological pain relief techniques (eg, distraction, music, relaxation therapies).
Psychosocial	

Patient will adapt to loss of motor and sensory function.	• Provide emotional support by:
	  –encouraging ventilation of sadness, fears, etc.
	  –arranging for social services, clergy, neuropsychologist, support groups, etc. to see patient.

Therapeutic strategies will be used to cope with anxiety and chronic pain syndrome.	• Provide information and counseling regarding:
	  –personal resources
	  –nonpharmacological pain management techniques
	  –stress management strategies
	  –appropriate use of prescribed pharmacological agents.

Integration will be made into prior social roles.	• Provide patient/family counseling regarding:
	  –stages of grief
	  –sexual function and management techniques
	  –social services and community resources.

Teaching/Discharge Planning	

Patient will adapt to loss of bowel/bladder control.
Patient will participate in bowel and bladder program.
	• Teach patient/family:
	  –bowel program and training
	  –dietary habits to maintain bowel function
	  –bladder training/intermittent catheterization
	  –prevention of, and signs/symptoms of autonomic dysreflexia.

Complications of immobility will be prevented.	• Teach patient/family:
	  –positioning to prevent skin breakdown
	  –physical therapy exercises
	  –pulmonary toilet.

Patient will be placed in appropriate postacute setting.	• Consult rehabilitation/discharge planner/social services early after admission to initiate placement arrangements.

CONCLUSION

Acute SCI can result in devastating physical and emotional consequences for the patient. Care of these patients requires a thorough knowledge of the pathophysiological principles underlying various levels of injury and the syndromes associated with specific injuries.

Nursing assessment and intervention require constant vigilance and skill and present an ongoing challenge for the critical care nurse. The nurse must deal with many physical and emotional needs of the patient and often with personal emotions precipitated by this catastrophic injury.

Clinical Applicability Challenges

Self-Challenge: Critical Thinking

1. *Develop a checklist of the possible complications of spinal shock during the first week postinjury and the usual management of each.*

2. *Formulate a teaching plan that will discuss autonomic dysreflexia with a patient with a new C5 to C6 SCI. Include causes, prevention, and treatment.*

Study Questions

1. Clinical signs of autonomic dysreflexia include
   a. tachycardia and hypotension.
   b. hypertension and headache.
   c. sweating and fever.
   d. bradycardia and pupil constriction.

2. Which would most likely describe a patient in spinal shock as he or she would present initially?
   a. Pink, warm, dry skin; vasodilation
   b. Pale, cool, wet skin; vasoconstriction
   c. Bradycardia and hypertension
   d. Pounding headache and blurred vision

3. At what level of quadriplegia is a patient usually ventilator independent?
   a. C3
   b. C4
   c. C5
   d. C7

4. In teaching a patient about a bowel program, which statement is true?
   a. The bowel program should begin as soon as spinal shock is resolved.
   b. A bowel program is necessary only for tetraplegics.
   c. Laxatives will need to be used daily.
   d. Autonomic dysreflexia may be triggered in some patients with each bowel program.

5. Which statement holds true for bladder training?
   a. Force fluids with an intermittent catheterization program.
   b. Restrict fluids with an intermittent catheterization program.
   c. Clamp indwelling catheter several hours before discontinuing it.
   d. Restrict fluids with a suprapubic catheter.

REFERENCES

1. Chandler D, Nemejc C, Adkins R, Waters R: Emergency cervical-spine immobilization. Ann Emerg Med 21(10):1185–1188, 1992
2. Nolan S: Current trends in the management of acute spinal cord injury. Crit Care Nursing Q 17(1):64–78, 1994
3. Behrman S, Kudsk K, Brown R et al: The effects of growth hormone on nutritional markers in enterally fed immobilized trauma patients. Journal of Parenteral and Enteral Nutrition 19(1):41–45, 1995
4. Swarczinski C, Dijkers M: The value of serial leg measurements for monitoring deep vein thrombosis in spinal cord injury. J Neurosci Nurs 23:306–317, 1991

BIBLIOGRAPHY

Chai T, Chung A, Belville W, Faerber G: Compliance and complications of clean intermittent catheterization in the spinal cord injured patient. Paraplegia 33:161–163, 1995

Hickey J: The Clinical Practice of Neurosurgical and Neurologic Nursing (4th Ed). Philadelphia, JB Lippincott, 1996

Hudson L (Issue ed): Topics in Spinal Cord Injury Rehabilitation: Sexuality. 1(2). Gaithersburg, MD, Aspen Publishers, 1995

Nayduch D, Lee A, Butler D: High-dose methylprednisolone after acute spinal cord injury. Critical Care Nurse August:69–78, 1994

Tippett J: Spinal immobilization of the multiply injured patient. Accident and Emergency Nursing 1:25–33, 1993

Young W: Secondary injury mechanisms in acute spinal cord injury. J Emerg Med 11:13–23, 1993

Gastrointestinal System

Anatomy and Physiology of the Gastrointestinal System

OBJECTIVES

Based on the content in this chapter, the reader should be able to:

- Describe the functions of the major structures of the gastrointestinal system.
- Examine the processes of ingestion, digestion, absorption, and elimination.
- Explain digestion and absorption of carbohydrates, proteins, fats, vitamins, and minerals.
- Compare and contrast the processes involved in emesis and defecation.
- Describe bile production, secretion, and excretion.

*A*ll cells require nutrients to sustain function and grow. The primary function of the gastrointestinal (GI) system is to provide those nutrients through the processes of ingestion (taking in food), digestion (breaking down food), and absorption (movement of food particles into the bloodstream). Nutrients are then carried to body cells through the bloodstream. Elimination is the process by which waste is eliminated from the body.

The organs of the GI system include the alimentary canal (oropharyngeal cavity, esophagus, stomach, small intestine, colon, rectum). Associated organs include the liver, pancreas, and gallbladder. Gastrointestinal function is influenced by the autonomic nervous system and a variety of hormones, including those of stress.

STRUCTURE OF THE GASTROINTESTINAL TRACT

Macrostructure

The structure of the digestive system is shown in Figure 37–1. It is composed of the alimentary canal, a tube about 8 m (25 ft) long that begins at the oral cavity and ends at the anus. The accessory glands (eg, salivary glands) and organs (eg, liver and pancreas) empty products into this tube.

The oral cavity opens into the pharynx, a structure that allows the passage of nutrients and air. The anterior pharynx is divided into an oropharynx and nasopharynx, connecting to the oral and nasal cavities, respectively. The posteroinferior end of the pharynx (at about the level of the sixth cervical vertebra) connects to the esophagus and larynx. A thin cartilaginous flap covered by soft tissue, the epiglottis, reflexively covers the larynx during swallowing. Thus, food and water pass into the esophagus, not the trachea.

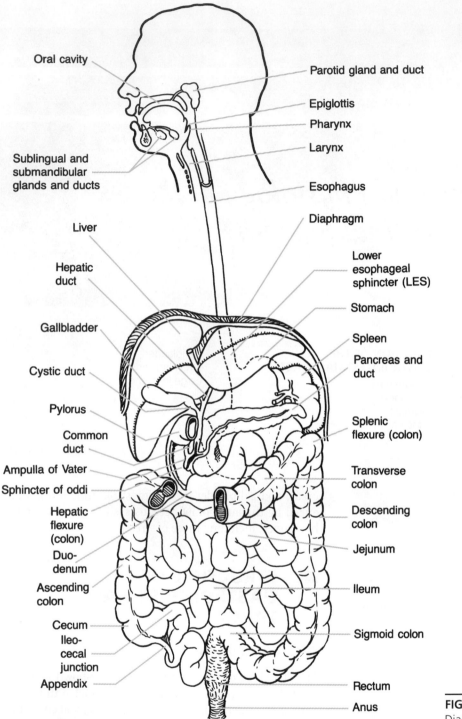

FIGURE 37-1
Diagram of the digestive tract.

The esophagus is a 25-cm (10-in) tube leading to the stomach. The walls of the upper one third of this tube are composed of skeletal muscle, as are the walls of the mouth and pharynx. The remaining esophageal walls contain smooth muscle, as does the remainder of the alimentary canal until the external anal sphincter, which again is composed of skeletal muscle. The lower esophageal sphincter (LES) is the muscular ring between the stomach and esophagus. It is thicker with more tone than other esophageal muscle. It prevents reflux of gastric contents into the esophagus. The other end of the stomach opens into the small intestine. This opening is surrounded by the pyloric sphincter, a structure that minimizes intestinal reflux.

The first 25 to 30 cm (10–12 in) of the intestine is the duodenum. The next 2.6 m (8.5 ft) is the jejunum and ileum and the last 1.1 m (3.6 ft), the colon. The opening of the ileum into the colon (cecum) is guarded by the ileocecal valve, which prevents reflux of colonic contents into the ileum. Protruding inferiorly from the cecum is a blind-ended 2.5- to 20-cm (1–8 in) tube called the vermiform appendix. The ascending colon extends superiorly from the cecum to the inferior border of the liver. The colon then flexes transversely and crosses to the left side of the abdominal cavity to a point just inferior to the stomach, where it curves again to become the descending colon. This part of the colon passes down on the left side of the abdomen to the level of the iliac crest, where it becomes the sigmoid colon. The S-shaped portion of colon bends first toward the right side of the abdomen, but almost immediately, it sharply bends posteriorly and upward toward the sacrum. It then curves anteriorly again, completing its S shape, and then continues downward to the pelvic floor as the rectum. The last 2.5 cm (1 in) or so of the rectum, the anal canal, passes between the levator and muscles of the pelvic floor and opens to the exterior body surface as the anal orifice. Two sphincters guard this orifice: an internal one composed of smooth muscle and an external one composed of skeletal muscle.

Innervation

The GI tract is innervated by the peripheral and autonomic nervous systems. Autonomic components include parasympathetic and sympathetic elements and the enteric nervous system, located within the GI tract. Peripheral fibers innervate the voluntary muscles of chewing, swallowing, and defecating. Parasympathetic fibers promote motility, relax sphincters, and promote secretion. Sympathetic innervation tends to slow or inhibit motility and secretion and increase sphincter tone. The enteric nervous system coordinates function. Figure 37–2 illustrates innervation of the gut.

Parasympathetic Nervous System

Parasympathetic efferents (motor control) to the GI system are preganglionic fibers carried in the vagus and pelvic nerves. Vagal parasympathetic efferent preganglionic fibers richly innervate the GI tract, including the esophagus, stomach, and small intestine. It is generally accepted that in humans, vagal efferents innervate the colon, but the distribution and function are controversial. Cell bodies for the vagal efferents are located primarily in the dorsal motor nucleus of the vagus. Vagal efferents synapse onto neurons in Auerbach's myenteric plexus. Postganglionic fibers then synapse with secretory and smooth muscle cells.

Vagal afferent (sensory) fibers originate in the esophagus, stomach, small intestine, and possibly the large intestine. The cell bodies are located in the nodose ganglion, lo-

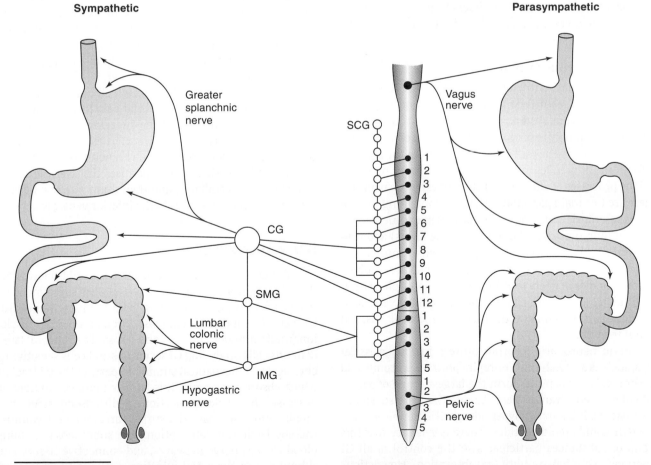

FIGURE 37-2
Extrinsic efferent innervation of the gut. (From Johnson LR (ed): Physiology of the Gastrointestinal Tract, p.508. New York, Raven Press, 1987) SCG, superior cervical ganglion; CG, celiac ganglion; SMG, superior mesenteric ganglion; IMG, inferior mesenteric ganglion

cated in the neck, then join the vagus high in the neck. Afferent fibers relay information about pain and distention to the brain and spinal cord.

In humans, the pelvic nerve, issuing from spinal routes S_2 to S_4 carries parasympathetic afferent and efferent fibers to innervate the rectum and descending colon. For sacral efferents, the cell bodies are located in the spinal cord. Afferent cell bodies are in the corresponding dorsal root ganglia.

Sympathetic Nervous System

Sympathetic efferent fibers exit the spinal cord and synapse on ganglia near the spinal cord. Then long postganglionic fibers travel to the gut and synapse on blood vessels, myenteric plexus ganglia, and secretory cells. The esophagus receives rich sympathetic innervation, but origin and course of the fibers are not clear. Interestingly, although the muscle of the upper esophagus is primarily striated (ie, skeletal voluntary muscle) the area receives dense sympathetic innervation. Stress-related impaired swallowing may be elicited by these fibers. Sympathetic fibers to the stomach and duodenum exit T_6 to T_9, synapse in the celiac ganglion, then travel along the celiac artery. Sympathetic fibers exiting at T_9 and T_{10} synapse in the superior mesenteric ganglion and then travel with the celiac artery to the large and small intestine. Fibers terminate on enteric neurons, blood vessels; a few fibers innervate the muscle layers.

Enteric Nervous System

The GI tract has an intrinsic nervous system, the enteric nervous system, coordinating GI motility and secretion. The enteric nervous system is considered the third component of the autonomic nervous system. It is a complex network embedded in the wall of the GI tract from the pharynx to the anus. It includes intrinsic neurons (enteric neurons) and the processes of afferent and efferent extrinsic neurons. There are two main ganglionic plexuses containing the cell bodies of enteric neurons: myenteric plexus (Auerbach's; between longitudinal and circular muscle layers) and submucosal plexus (Meissner's; between circular muscle and the mucosa). From these two ganglionic plexuses emerge smaller bundles of fibers forming nonganglionic plexuses in longitudinal and circular muscle, around blood vessels, in the muscularis mucosae, at the base of mucosal glands, and within the villi.

Enteric neuronal neurotransmitters include classical ones, such as acetylcholine, norepinephrine, serotonin, and dopamine. Neuropeptides form the largest group of potential enteric neurotransmitters. Among these are substance P, vasoactive intestinal polypeptide, gastric inhibitory peptide (GIP), and opioid peptides. There is evidence that this group of substances participates in the control of all GI functions (secretion, motility, and absorption). How actions of these substances integrate with those of more classic neurotransmitters is an important aspect of current investigative work.

Circulation

The GI system receives about one fourth of the resting cardiac output, more than any other organ system. Supply to the abdominal GI organs and spleen is called the splanchnic circulation. When circulation is impaired (as in shock), perfusion is shifted from the splanchnic bed to the systemic circulation. Because splanchnic organs normally extract only about 20% of the oxygen in the perfusing blood, splanchnic perfusion can be reduced without compromising splanchnic organs. However, severe reduction in splanchnic perfusion can damage the gut mucosal lining.

The esophageal artery, branching from the thoracic aorta, perfuses the esophagus. Three abdominal aortic branches perfuse GI organs: celiac (perfusing lower esophagus, stomach, duodenum, gallbladder, liver), superior mesenteric (perfusing small intestine to transverse colon), and inferior mesenteric (perfusing descending colon, sigmoid colon, rectum). Areas of perfusion overlap, providing some protection against ischemia.

Venous drainage of the stomach and small and large intestine is primarily through the portal vein, which leads to the liver and then the hepatic vein. Blood from the lower rectum and the lower esophagus bypasses the portal system. Blood from the rectum drains into the inferior vena cava through the rectal veins and then the external iliac vein. Blood from the esophagus drains through the hemizygous and azygous veins into the inferior vena cava.

The liver is unique in receiving its blood supply from both venous and arterial sources (Fig. 37–3). The venous supply is by way of the portal vein, which drains most of the blood from the GI tract. The portal vein forms behind the spleen at the confluence of the superior mesenteric and splenic veins and leads to the liver. The arterial supply is by the common hepatic artery, which branches from the celiac trunk near the aorta and then perfuses the liver. Both sets of vessels form capillaries and then drain into the hepatic vein, which in turn feeds into the inferior vena cava.

Microstructure

The alimentary tract is composed of a central hollow tube, the lumen, through which food passes. It is surrounded by five layers of tissue. Proceeding from the lumen outward, they are the mucosa, submucosa, circular smooth muscle, longitudinal smooth muscle, and serosa. The mucosal layer contains cells producing GI secretions and cells sensitive to chemical and mechanical stimuli. In parts of the GI tract in which absorption occurs, this layer is more convoluted or possesses fingerlike projections (villi). Such structural modifications increase the surface area per unit volume, thereby facilitating absorption. The submucosa contains blood vessels, nerve networks, and connective tissue. The submucosa of the small intestine contains aggregates of lymphatic tissue (Peyer's patches), which are especially numerous within the ileum. Viral and bacterial antigens are absorbed by specialized mucosal cells that lie above the

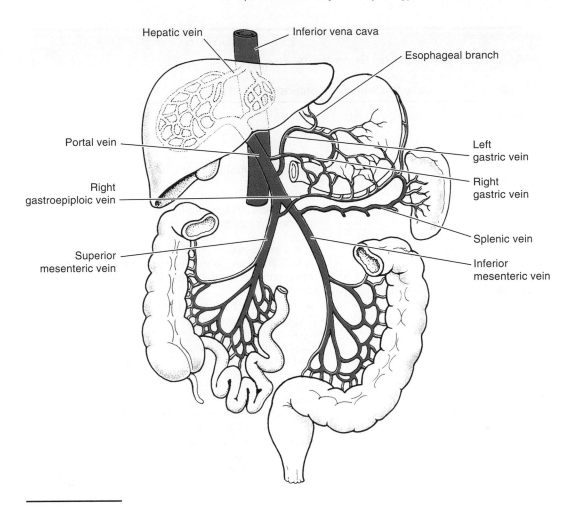

FIGURE 37-3
Portal circulation. Blood from the gastrointestinal tract, spleen, and pancreas travels to the liver by way of the portal vein before moving into the inferior vena cava for return to the heart.

patches of lymphatic tissue in the small intestine. These specialized cells pass on the antigens together with a chemical that sensitizes the lymphatic cells to manufacture and secrete antibodies of immunoglobulin class A (IgA) against this particular antigen the next time (or times) this antigen enters the small intestine.

The two smooth muscle layers function in the two major types of GI motility: propulsive motion and mixing movements. The stomach has an additional layer of smooth muscle to facilitate its food-mixing movements. The outer serosa layer is continuous with the mesentery and forms part of the visceral peritoneum.

Two nerve networks extend the length of the GI tract: the submucosal plexus and the myenteric plexus. The submucosal network consists of sensory neurons that receive stimulation from the sensory cells in the mucosal layer. The myenteric plexus, located between the two smooth muscle layers, is a network of motor neurons that stimulate the smooth muscle of the GI tract. The myenteric plexus receives sensory input from the submucosal plexus. Together, these two plexuses function in locally coordinated regulation of GI motility (eg, peristalsis) and secretion (eg, certain gastric secretions).

FUNCTION OF THE GASTROINTESTINAL TRACT

Oropharynx

SECRETION

Saliva is produced by three pairs of salivary glands: submaxillary, sublingual, and parotid. Saliva (Table 37–1) is composed of mucus, a lubricant to facilitate swallowing, lingual lipase (a fat-digesting enzyme secreted by tongue glands), salivary amylase (a starch-digesting enzyme), class A antibodies (IgA) that provide a first line of defense against bacteria and viruses, and bacteriostatic and anticariogenic chemicals. Lingual lipase is estimated to digest about 30% of the dietary fat in the stomach. About one half of digestive amylase is secreted by the salivary glands; the rest is from the pancreas.

Stimuli eliciting salivation include sight, smell, and thought of food and a pleasant taste and smooth texture of food in the mouth. Rough, bad-tasting, unpleasant-smelling foods reduce salivary gland secretions. Stimuli are received by the two salivary centers in the medulla of the

TABLE 37-1
Major Gastrointestinal Secretions

Location	Daily Volume	Composition and (Action)
Mouth	1,000–2,000 mL	Amylase (carbohydrate digestion) Lipase (fat digestion) Immunoglobulins Mucus Water, electrolytes
Esophagus	300–800 mL	Mucus
Stomach	2,000 mL	Intrinsic factor (vitamin B_{12} absorption) Hydrochloric acid (activates pepsinogen) Pepsinogen (protein digestion) Mucus Water, electrolytes Gastrin (stimulates hydrochloric acid release; trophic effects on mucosa, especially in stomach)
Pancreas	1,200–1,800 mL	Enzymes • Amylase (carbohydrate digestion) • Trypsinogen (protein digestion) • Chymotrypsin (protein digestion) • Elastase (protein digestion) • Carboxypeptidase (protein digestion) • Lipase (fat digestion) • Colipase (fat digestion) • Esterase (cholesterol digestion) • Phospholipase (phospholipid digestion) • Nucleases (RNA and DNA digestion) Bicarbonate (protects lumenal wall by neutralizing acid) Water, electrolytes
Liver	500–1,000 mL	Bile salts (emulsifies fats) Bilirubin (excretory end-product of hemoglobin breakdown) Water, electrolytes
Small intestine	3,000–4,000 mL	Enzymes • Enterokinase (activates trypsinogen) • Lipase (fat digestion) • Enteropeptidase (protein digestion) • Peptidase (protein digestion) • Nucleases (RNA and DNA digestion) • Maltase (carbohydrate digestion) • Lactase (carbohydrate digestion) • Sucrase (carbohydrate digestion) Mucus Bicarbonate Water, electrolytes Cholecystokinin into blood (stimulates pancreatic secretion and gallbladder contraction) Glucose-dependent insulinotropic peptide into blood (stimulates insulin release and gastric motility, secretion) Gastrin (stimulates gastric acid secretion)
Large intestine	Variable	Mucus

brain stem. These centers then send impulses to the salivary glands through the seventh and ninth cranial nerves (parasympathetic fibers) and the first and second thoracic nerves (sympathetic fibers). Parasympathetic stimulation, or the administration of drugs that mimic such stimulation (cholinergics) or enhance it (neostigmine), promotes copious secretion of watery saliva. Sympathetic stimulation or sympathomimetic drug administration produces a scanty output of thick saliva. Cholinergic blockers (eg, atropine) also produce scanty salivation.

MOTILITY

Food is mechanically broken down in the mouth by chewing. This produces a bolus of food held together and lubricated by saliva that then can be swallowed. Swallowing has two phases: an initial voluntary phase, described here, involving the first third of the esophagus, and an involuntary phase, described below.

Swallowing is triggered by the presence of food or fluid in the pharynx. This presence mechanically stimulates pharyngeal sensory receptors that initiate impulses through the fifth cranial nerve to the swallowing center in the medulla. Sensory impulses reflexively trigger the outflow of impulses down motor fibers in the ninth and tenth cranial nerves to pharyngeal and laryngeal structures. This causes the following coordinated events, which propel the solid or fluid substance into the esophagus:

1. The soft palate pulls upward, sealing off the nasopharynx.
2. The epiglottis closes over the larynx.
3. The muscles of the upper esophagus relax.
4. The pharyngeal muscles contract, moving food or fluid into the opened esophagus.

Damage to sensory or motor fibers (in cranial nerves V, IX, or X) or to the swallowing center in the brain stem can weaken or eliminate the ability to swallow or can cause poorly coordinated swallowing, wherein food or fluid enters the nasopharynx or larynx or both.

Esophagus

SECRETIONS

Esophageal mucosal cells secrete mucus (see Table 37–1). This protects the esophageal lining from damage by gastric secretions or food and acts as a lubricant to facilitate the passage of food.

MOTILITY

Once food or fluid enters the esophagus, it is propelled through the first third of the lumen by reflexes from the swallowing center from the ninth and tenth cranial nerves. Food or fluid stimulates receptors in the wall of the esophagus, in turn initiating impulses to the swallowing center. Reflex output from the swallowing center to the muscle (by way of the ninth and tenth cranial nerves) produces a pattern of esophageal relaxation ahead of the food or fluid and esophageal muscle contraction behind it, thereby propelling the matter being swallowed through this part of the esophagus.

In contrast, food or fluid is propelled along the remainder of the esophagus by local reflexes involving sensory receptors and the two nerve plexuses in the wall of the esophagus. This process, peristalsis, occurs as food or fluid distends the esophageal area. The distention stimulates stretch receptors that reflexively (by the two plexuses) promote both relaxation of the esophageal muscles ahead of the area of distention and contraction of the esophageal muscles in and behind it. This squeezes the food or fluid ahead into the newly relaxed area, which then becomes the distended one. The peristalsis reflex repeatedly recurs until the

food or fluid arrives at the LES. The LES is the last centimeter (0.5 in) or so of the esophagus, in which smooth muscles generally remain contracted, preventing gastric reflux and damage to the esophagus caused by gastric acid. The wave of peristalsis causes the LES to relax, thereby allowing food to enter the stomach. Tonus of the LES can be altered by a variety of agents (Table 37–2). Some people suffer from a hypertrophic LES, which impedes esophageal emptying (and can lead to overdistention of the lower esophagus), whereas others have an incompetent LES, which results in repeated episodes of gastric reflux (which can lead to lower esophageal strictures).

Stomach

SECRETION

In addition to mucus-secreting cells, three types of secretory cells are contained in the gastric mucosa: parietal cells, which secrete hydrochloric acid (HCl) and intrinsic factor; chief cells, which secrete digestive enzymes; and G cells (in antrum only), which secrete the hormone gastrin (see Table 37–1). The luminal surface membrane of the gastric mucosal cell and the tight fit against one another provide a protective barrier against damage caused by the HCl. This barrier can be disrupted by a variety of agents, including bile salts, alcohol, and aspirin.

The digestive enzyme pepsinogen is secreted as an inactive precursor, which is activated by HCl in the gastric lumen to provide three pepsins that digest proteins. The chemical action of HCl also breaks down food molecules. Intrinsic factor is necessary for the intestinal absorption of vitamin B_{12}. Gastrin stimulates secretion by the chief and parietal cells and promotes the growth of the gastric mucosa (Table 37–3).

Stomach secretions are regulated in three phases: cephalic, gastric, and intestinal, as outlined in Table 37–4. These phases are controlled by neural and hormonal mechanisms.

TABLE 37-2
Factors Influencing Lower Esophageal Sphincter Tone

Increased Tone	Decreased Tone
Food substances:	Food substances:
protein	Fats
Drugs:	Coffee
metoclopramide	Chocolate
Some prostaglandins (F_2)	Alcohol
	Cholecystokinin
	Progesterone (as in pregnancy)
	Somatostatin
	Dopamine
	Some prostaglandins (E_2, A_2)
	Cigarette smoking

TABLE 37-3
Major Hormones Controlling Secretion and Motility

Hormone	Source	Stimulation of Release	Major Function
Gastrin	Stomach, small intestine	Gastric distention, presence of partially digested protein near pylorus	Stimulates • Gastric acid secretion • Gastric intrinsic factor secretion • Gastric motility • Intestinal motility • Mucosal growth • Pancreatic growth • Pancreatic insulin release • Lower esophageal tone
Secretin	Small intestine	Acid entering small intestine	Stimulates • Pancreatic bicarbonate secretion • Pancreatic enzyme secretion • Pancreatic growth • Gastric pepsin secretion • Bile bicarbonate secretion • Gallbladder contraction Inhibits • Gastric emptying • Gastric motility • Intestinal motility
Cholecystokinin (CCK)	Small intestine	Fatty acid and amino acids in small intestine	Stimulates • Gastric acid secretion • Gastric motility • Intestinal motility • Colonic motility • Gallbladder contraction and sphincter of Oddi relaxation (thus increasing bile flow into small intestine) • Pancreatic bicarbonate secretion • Pancreatic enzyme release • Pancreatic growth Inhibits • Lower esophageal tone • Gastric emptying
Gastric inhibitory peptide (GIP)	Small intestine	Fatty acids and lipids in small intestine	Inhibits • Gastric acid secretion • Gastric emptying • Gastric motility Stimulates • Insulin release • Intestinal motility

In the cephalic phase, sight, smell, taste, or thought of food acts on brain stem centers, reflexively prompting parasympathetic (vagal) stimulation of salivation, pancreatic secretion, bile release, and gastric secretions by the chief (pepsinogen) and parietal (HCl) cells. Sympathetic stimulation can alter cephalic phase response, providing a mechanism by which emotions can influence GI secretions. Fear, anger, and depression decrease secretions.

The gastric phase refers to the stimulation of gastric secretions by the presence of food (chyme) in the stomach. Distention of the stomach by food stimulates stretch receptors in the stomach wall. Chemicals, mainly proteins, stimulate chemoreceptors in the mucosa. The stretch receptors and chemoreceptors in turn activate neurons in the submucosal plexus, which then stimulate neurons in the myenteric plexus, which in turn stimulate secretion by the parietal and chief cells. Proteins in the chyme also directly promote gastrin secretion by G cells; the gastrin provides an additional stimulus for parietal and chief cell secretion. The gastric phase is eventually halted by a combination of events. The stretch receptors and chemoreceptors in the wall of the stomach become refractory to stimulation, the acidity of the chyme inhibits further gastrin secretion, and GIP decreases HCl secretions and gastric motility.

TABLE 37-4
Phases of Gastric Digestion

Phase	Stimulus to Secretion	Effect

Cephalic (neuronal)	Sight, smell, taste of food initiates central nervous system impulse mediated by vagus	Gastric effects:
		  Hydrochloric acid (from parietal cells)
		  Pepsinogen (from chief cells)
		  Mucus secretion
		Other effects:
		  Salivation
		  Pancreatic secretion
		  Bile release

Gastric (neuronal and hormonal)	Food in antrum initiates central nervous system impulse mediated by vagus	Gastrin release Hydrochloric acid release Pepsinogen release
Intestinal (hormonal)	Chyme in small intestine	pH of chyme <2: release of secretin, gastric inhibitory polypeptide, cholecystokinin (decreases gastric acid secretion) pH of chyme >3: release of gastrin (increases gastric acid secretion)

The intestinal phase begins after chyme reaches the duodenum. The acidity of this mixture stimulates duodenal mucosal cells to release secretin into the bloodstream, proteins trigger the release of cholecystokinin (CCK) into the blood from similar cells, and glucose and fat stimulate the secretion of GIP. Secretin and CCK cause pancreatic secretion and release of gallbladder contents into the duodenum. GIP stimulates the release of insulin from the islets of Langerhans and decreases gastric motility and secretions (see Table 37–3). Stretch receptors in the duodenum trigger peristalsis so that chyme is degraded, mixed with enzymes and diluents, and moved past the highly absorbent small intestinal lumen. If the chyme is less acidic, gastrin is released.

Gastric parietal cells contain receptors for acetylcholine, histamine, and gastrin. Stimulation of these receptors prompts the parietal cell to secrete HCl. Acid secretion is inhibited by chemicals that block the histamine receptor (eg, H_2 antagonists, such as cimetidine [Tagamet] and ranitidine [Zantac]) of the acetylcholine receptor (eg, atropine). Excess HCl secretion can damage tissue. Some prostaglandins inhibit HCl secretion. Another drug, omeprazole (Prilosec), inhibits an intracellular step in the HCl secretion process in parietal cells. Other factors that stimulate gastric secretions are alcohol, caffeine, and hypoglycemia. The first two factors act directly by way of gastric chemoreceptors and the intramural nerve plexuses in the stomach wall. Hypoglycemia acts by way of the brain stem and vagal fibers.

MOTILITY

The passage of food from the esophagus into the stomach reflexively initiates receptive relaxation. After the stomach has filled with food, peristaltic contractions mix the food and squirt small amounts into the duodenum. The pyloric sphincter plays a minor role in gastric emptying. Its main function is to prevent duodenal reflux. The bile acids in the chyme that reenters the stomach through duodenal reflux damage the chemical barrier that coats the surfaces of gastric mucosal cells. Mild peristaltic contractions that persist after the stomach has completely emptied are called hunger contractions. They play no obligatory role in appetite regulation. Gastric emptying can be retarded by vagotomy; by the presence of fats, proteins, or HCl in the duodenal chyme; by duodenal distention; and by intestinal hormones.

Emesis

Vomiting results from the relaxation of the LES and the rest of the esophagus combined with simultaneous strong contractions of abdominal muscles and diaphragm and closure of the epiglottis over the airway. The contractions squeeze the stomach and force its contents into the esophagus and out the mouth. In addition, irritation of the small intestine (by materials in the chyme, by inflammation, or by disease process) can cause movements that reverse peristalsis. These movements move chyme toward the pyloric valve. They can be sufficiently strong to force open the pylorus and enter the stomach. This is how intestinal contents are vomited. If golden yellow bile from the duodenum spends any appreciable time in the stomach, acids turn it green. Occasionally, vomiting of intestinal contents can be so rapid that the vomitus contains golden yellow bile. If blood is allowed time in the stomach, acids turn it brownish black (coffee-ground color). If vomiting does not allow sufficient time for this acid action to occur; blood in the vomitus has its normal red color.

Pancreas

This organ contains both exocrine tissue and endocrine tissue. The latter constitutes the islets of Langerhans, discussed in Chapter 41, Anatomy and Physiology of the Endocrine

System. The exocrine (acinar) cells are arranged in lobules and empty secretions into an internal pancreatic ductal system (see Fig. 37–1). These internal ducts drain into an external pancreatic duct (duct of Wirsung) that joins the common bile duct to form a shared short duct called the ampulla of Vater. This ampulla, carrying bile and pancreatic secretions, opens into the duodenum. It is encircled by a smooth muscle ring, the sphincter of Oddi. Because of the anatomical arrangements between the common bile duct and the duct of Wirsung, a gallstone that obstructs the ampulla of Vater can obstruct the normal flow of bile and pancreatic secretions. (Such obstruction, although rare, can lead to a stasis of pancreatic secretion, resulting in acute pancreatitis.) Some people have a second external pancreatic duct (duct of Santorini) that opens into the duodenum near the pylorus.

SECRETIONS

The large amount of water secreted by the pancreas is instrumental in diluting chyme before absorption. The exocrine acinar cells secrete both a watery alkaline bicarbonate solution and digestive enzymes (see Table 37–1). The bicarbonate neutralizes the highly acidic chyme from the

stomach. The pancreatic enzymes digest proteins (trypsin, chymotrypsin, elastase, and carboxypeptidase), fats (lipase, calipase, and esterase), phospholipase and nucleic acids (nucleases), and starch (amylase). These are secreted from the pancreas in inactive forms. Once the pancreatic secretions arrive in the duodenum, inactive trypsin (trypsinogen) is activated by an intestinal mucosal enzyme, enterokinase. Active trypsin then activates the other pancreatic enzymes. Regulation of pancreatic secretion occurs by neural and hormonal means. Vagal stimulation results in the secretion of pancreatic enzymes. Hormonal regulation occurs as a result of duodenal mucosal responses to chyme and is discussed later.

Gallbladder

In the duodenum, chyme mixed with pancreatic secretions is watery. The fat in chyme is not water soluble and requires a solvent–enzyme mixture from the liver to render it absorbable by intestinal human cells.

Hepatocytes, among many other metabolic functions, also make bile (Table 37–5). Bile is a mixture of bile salts, cholesterol, bilirubin, and acids suspended in water. This so-

---

TABLE 37-5
Hepatic Function

General Category	Specific Description
Carbohydrate metabolism	Glycogenesis (conversion of glucose to glycogen)
	Glycogenolysis (breakdown of glycogen to glucose)
	Gluconeogenesis (formation of glucose from amino acids or fatty acids)
Protein metabolism	Synthesis of nonessential amino acids
	Synthesis of plasma proteins (albumin, prealbumin, transferrin, clotting factors, complement factors; not gamma globulin or immunoglobulins)
	Urea formation from NH_3 (NH_3 formed by deamination of amino acids in liver and by action of colonic bacteria on proteins)
Lipid and lipoprotein metabolism	Synthesis of lipoproteins
	Breakdown of triglycerides into fatty acids and glycerol
	Formation of ketone bodies
	Synthesis of fatty acids from amino acids and glucose
	Synthesis and breakdown of cholesterol
Bile acid synthesis and excretion	Bile formation (containing bile salts, bile pigments [bilirubin, biliverdin]), cholesterol
	Bile excretion (about 1 L/d)
Storage	Glucose (as glycogen)
	Vitamins (A, D, E, K, B_1, B_2, B_{12}, folic acid)
	Fatty acids
	Minerals (Fe, Cu)
	Amino acids (as albumin, beta globulins)
Biotransformation, detoxification, excretion of endogenous and exogenous compounds	Inactivation of drugs and excretion of the breakdown products
	Clearance of procoagulants, activated clotting factors, byproducts of coagulation
Removal of pathogens	Clearance of microorganisms by macrophages
Steroid catabolism	Conjugation and excretion of gonadal steroids
	Conjugation and excretion of adrenal steroids (cortisol, aldosterone)

lution emulsifies the fat in chyme, breaking the fat into small globules that can be absorbed across the intestinal lumen. Fat-soluble vitamins are ionized into absorbable forms by the action of bile. Bile also suspends cholesterol, triglycerides, and multiple-density lipoproteins in the bloodstream, preventing precipitation and deposition of these molecules in the vasculature, until they can be catabolized.

Bile is stored and concentrated in the gallbladder. Under the influence of vagal activity, or CCK, the gallbladder contracts, emptying bile into the duodenum to mix with chyme.

Small Intestine

SECRETION

Chyme in the duodenum is mixed with digestive enzymes, alkaline substances, water, mucus, and bile from the stomach, pancreas, and gallbladder. Intestinal enzymes are added to this mixture.

Secretin, CCK, and enterokinase, which converts trypsinogen from the pancreas into trypsin, have already been discussed. The small intestine secretes mucus, and Brunner's glands in the duodenal mucosa secrete more bicarbonate and water in response to acid, secretin, and gastrin.

MOTILITY

The small intestine has two types of movement: mixing and peristaltic contraction. The intramural plexuses initiate and coordinate these movements, but they can be enhanced or retarded by extrinsic autonomic stimulation, as discussed previously. Peristalsis propels food. During mixing movement, intestinal distention provokes (by the intramural reflex arcs) constrictions at intervals along its length. This makes the distended area resemble links of sausage. These constrictions then relax, and new areas become constricted. Repetition of this process continually kneads the chyme, thereby eventually exposing all molecules of this material to the absorptive surfaces of the intestinal mucosa.

Emptying of the small intestine into the colon occurs in the same way as gastric emptying. Peristaltic waves build up pressure in the ileum behind the ileocecal valve and push the chyme through the valve into the colon. The valve then prevents backflow. Ileal emptying can be retarded by intramural reflexes, which are initiated by a full (distended) colon.

ABSORPTION

The mucosal layer of the small intestine has many folds covered with numerous finger-like projections (villi). The luminal surface of each villus is covered with microvilli, increasing the absorptive area of the small intestine.

Carbohydrates

Breakdown of carbohydrates (CHO) begins in the mouth, through the action of salivary amylase, and continues in the duodenum. Conversion to simple sugars continues in the small intestine by intestinal enzymes. Both active and pas-

sive transport are used to absorb sugars across the intestinal lumen into the bloodstream.

Proteins

Protein degradation begins in the stomach by HCl and pepsin. Polypeptides in the small intestine are degraded into peptide fragments and amino acids by trypsin, chymotrypsin, and carboxypeptidase. Amino acids are absorbed into the blood by active and passive diffusion.

Fats

Triglycerides, lipids, and phospholipids are first degraded in the small intestine. Bile salts, in a process called emulsification, facilitate the creation of small droplets of fats from larger globules. Pancreatic enzymes then degrade the fats into fatty acid chains and monoglycerides. These smaller molecules form into even smaller globules, called micelles. Fatty acids and monosaccharides are transported across the intestinal mucosa from a micelle passively, leaving bile behind.

In the submucosa, free fatty acids are passed into the blood directly, if small enough. If too large for direct passive diffusion, the free fatty acid is reorganized into a triglyceride, coupled with lipoproteins and cholesterol, and passed into the lymph fluid as chylomicron.

The bile left behind in the intestine after absorption of fats from a micelle is reabsorbed in the ileum. If bile salts enter the colon, they decrease the reabsorption of sodium and water, thereby increasing the liquidity of the undigested food residues in the colon. Most fat is absorbed by the time chyme reaches the middle of the jejunum.

Vitamins, Minerals, and Water

Most vitamins, whether they are fat or water soluble, diffuse across the intestinal mucosa and submucosa into the blood. Fat-soluble vitamin B_{12} couples with intrinsic factor, forming a larger molecule. In this form, B_{12} is absorbed.

Minerals and electrolytes vary in their absorption. Sodium and iron require active transport, whereas other minerals and electrolytes diffuse passively.

Water is absorbed passively throughout the stomach and small and large intestines. The GI tract is highly permeable, in *both* directions, to water. Should a hypertonic solution enter the duodenum, osmosis occurs in the lumen. The converse is true: A hypotonic chyme in the stomach and duodenum causes an extremely rapid movement of water into the bloodstream.

Large Intestine

SECRETION

The mucosal cells of the colon secrete mucus, which lubricates the passage of chyme (see Table 37–1).

MOTILITY

Colonic movements include mixing and peristaltic movements. These operate as described for the small intestine. A third movement, unique to the colon, is mass movement.

This consists of simultaneous contractions of colonic smooth muscle over large portions of the descending and sigmoid portions of the colon. Mass movement rapidly moves the undigested food residue (feces) from these areas into the rectum.

Humans cannot digest the cellulose, hemicellulose, or lignin in plant tissues. These plant materials form a large portion of the undigested food residue. They are usually termed "vegetable fiber" or "dietary bulk." These fibers attract and hold water, causing a larger, softer stool. Low quantities of bulk result in a relatively inactive colon, leading to bowel movements that are relatively infrequent and feces that are relatively small, dry, and difficult to pass. Epidemiological reports suggest that high-fiber diets are associated with a decreased incidence of diverticulitis and colon cancer.

Defecation

Filling of the rectum triggers the defecation reflex by stimulating stretch receptors in the rectal wall. Stimulation of the stretch receptors causes sensory (afferent) nerve fibers to transmit impulses to the lower spinal cord. Because of anatomical arrangements of neurons in this part of the cord, these afferent impulses reflexively cause nerve impulses to travel out of the cord along parasympathetic motor fibers that innervate the smooth muscles of the descending and sigmoid colon, the rectum, and the internal anal sphincter. The afferent impulses also reflexively cause nerve impulses to be sent out of the cord along somatic motor neurons that innervate the skeletal muscle of the external anal sphincter. The total effect of these events is to produce coordinated expulsive contractions of the colon and rectum, relaxation (opening) of the sphincters, and output of feces from the anus.

The urge to defecate begins after the pressure within the rectum reaches 18 torr. After intrarectal pressure reaches 55 torr, reflex bowel evacuation occurs. This defecation reflex is inhibited in a continent person by descending neuronal impulses from higher brain centers to inhibit the actions of the somatic motor neurons that innervate the external sphincter. Such inhibition keeps the external anal sphincter closed, thereby averting inappropriate defecation. After a few minutes, the defecation reflex subsides, but it usually becomes active again a few hours later. Defecation is a spinal cord reflex that does not require intact pathways between the sacral cord and the brain. In the early post-traumatic phase of spinal shock, the reflex does not work. After cord shock is ended, reflex defecation occurs once again, but voluntary inhibition is not possible (neurogenic bowel).

ABSORPTION

In the large intestine, most of the water and potassium are absorbed from the chyme. This produces a semisolid residue of undigested food (feces) that can be eliminated from the body. Diarrhea can reduce the transit time for chyme, thereby limiting such potassium and water reabsorption. This can result in hypokalemia and dehydration. Diarrhea also can be caused by materials that hold water in the chyme (eg, $MgSO_4$), resulting in semiliquid stool.

COLONIC BACTERIA

At birth, the colon is sterile, but large colonic bacterial populations become established soon afterward. Some of these organisms produce vitamin K and a number of B vitamins. Other bacteria produce ammonia, which is absorbed. Normally, this is removed from the blood once it reaches the liver. However, in people with seriously impaired liver function or with collateral circulatory routes that bypass the liver (usually the result of portal hypertension), such ammonia can remain in the circulation and lead to encephalopathy.

Liver

STRUCTURE

This organ has two lobes (right and left) and lies just below the diaphragm, with its greatest portion located to the right side of the body. Its superior (rounded) surface fits into the curve of the diaphragm and is in contact with the anterior wall of the abdominal cavity. The inferior surface is molded over the stomach, the duodenum, the pancreas, the hepatic flexure of the colon, the right kidney, and the right adrenal gland.

The liver is covered with a thin layer of peritoneum and under that, a thin fibrous coat called Glisson's capsule. This fibrous capsule encases and partitions the liver, sending inward fibrous sheets that divide the liver into functional units called lobules. Each lobule consists of sheets of hepatocytes organized around a core cluster of vessels called the portal triad. The portal triad includes the two sets of afferent vessels (portal vein and hepatic artery) and small bile ducts. The afferent vessels lead to the liver sinusoids, which drain into the efferent hepatic vein, lying at the periphery of each lobule. These structures are illustrated in Figure 37–4.

The lobule measures approximately 1.5 mm in diameter and 8 mm in length. Each lobe of the liver contains between 50,000 and 100,000 lobules. Rows of hepatocytes radiate from a central venule like spokes of a wheel. Branches of the hepatic artery and the hepatic portal vein lie at the periphery of the wheel. Blood from these branches is poured into open channels (hepatic sinuses) that run between alternate rows of hepatocytes. Kupffer's cells, specialized white cells of the reticuloendothelial system, phagocytize bacteria, debris, and other foreign matter in the sinus blood. The sinuses drain into the central venule, which in turn carries blood to the hepatic vein. Approximately 400 mL of blood, held within the venous sinuses, can be made available in emergencies to compensate for hypovolemia. Blind-ended bile canaliculi arise between the other rows of hepatocytes. They carry newly secreted bile to larger ducts located at the periphery. These smaller ducts eventually drain into the common bile duct. Bile that is leaving the liver is concentrated and stored in the gallbladder. Fluid and electrolyte reabsorption in the gallbladder can increase the concentration of bile salts, cholesterol, and bilirubin twelve-fold.

Cross section of liver lobule

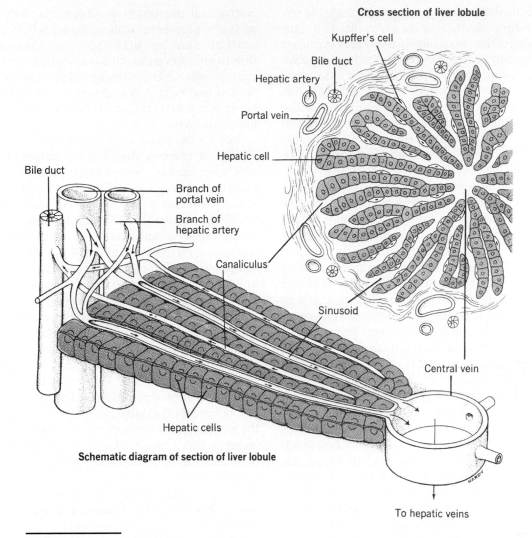

FIGURE 37-4

A section of liver lobule showing the location of the hepatic veins, hepatic cells, liver sinusoids, and branches of the portal vein and hepatic artery.

Thus, the gallbladder, with a maximum capacity of 50 mL, can hold a 24-hour output of bile (600 mL) from the liver. The intestinal hormone CCK and vagus nerve activity stimulate gallbladder contraction. CCK and local reflexes initiated by duodenal peristalsis open the sphincter of Oddi. These events permit an outflow of bile down the common bile duct into the duodenum.

The common bile duct and the main duct from the pancreas usually unite just before the duct enters the lumen of the duodenum. There is often a dilation of the tube after this junction (the ampulla of Vater). The opening of the common bile duct in the duodenum is about 8 to 10 cm from the pylorus.

FUNCTION

The liver cells perform many functions (see Table 37–5). They degrade steroid hormones, thereby preventing excess serum levels of estrogen, testosterone, progesterone, aldosterone, and glucocorticosteroids.

Another hepatic function concerns protein metabolism. Hepatocytes deaminate proteins and synthesize nitrogenous wastes (eg, uric acid). They also convert ammonia into urea and synthesize plasma proteins (eg, albumins and globulins). The albumins maintain normal plasma oncotic pressure. A fall in this pressure leads to edema (both systemic and pulmonary) and contributes to ascites. The globulins bind thyroid and adrenal hormones. Bound, the hormones are inactive. Decreased hepatic protein levels can lead to a clinical excess of these hormones.

Hepatocytes also make bile, which contains water, bile salts, cholesterol, bilirubin, gluconate, and inorganic acids. Bile salts aid digestion by emulsifying dietary fats and fostering their absorption and the absorption of fat-soluble vitamins through the intestinal mucosa. They also prevent the cholesterol in the bile from precipitating out of solution and forming calculi. More than 90% of the daily output of bile is reabsorbed for recycling by an active transport process of the ileal mucosa.

The liver contributes to adipose stores through the metabolism of triglycerides, fatty acids, and cholesterol. During fasting, triglycerides from adipose tissue are catabolized by the liver into fatty acids and glycerols. The free fatty acids in prolonged fasting are further catabolized into acetyl coenzyme-A and then into ketone bodies. Ketone bodies provide an energy source for some (non-neuronal) tissues.

Fat-soluble vitamins and many minerals are stored in the liver. These vitamins and minerals are released under the influence of hormones and serum concentrations of inorganic elements.

Another hepatic function is elimination of bilirubin from the body. Old or defective erythrocytes are phagocytosed by large reticuloendothelial cells lining the large veins and the sinuses of the liver and spleen. These phagocytes degrade the hemoglobin of these cells into biliverdin, iron, and globulin molecules. The last two components are recycled by the body in future erythropoiesis. The biliverdin is almost immediately converted to free bilirubin. Because this is an insoluble compound, it is transported bound to plasma albumin molecules. The hepatocytes convert this insoluble bilirubin into a soluble (and thus excretable) form by conjugating it with glucuronic acid to form bilirubin gluconate. This soluble form of bilirubin is then added to the bile and is eliminated from the body by the feces. Bilirubin gluconate gives the bile its normal golden yellow color. Organisms in the intestine convert most of the bilirubin gluconate into a darker brown compound, urobilinogen, which gives the feces its natural brown color. Because it is soluble in water, urobilinogen can also be absorbed from the colon back into the bloodstream and be excreted by way of the kidneys. Excess plasma levels of either the conjugated (direct) or unconjugated (indirect) bilirubin produce jaundice. Excess unconjugated bilirubin can cross the immature or damaged blood–brain barrier and bind with the basal ganglia, resulting in kernicterus.

The liver participates in carbohydrate metabolism. Serum glucose levels are maintained by *hepatic glucostatic function*, involving two mechanisms. If plasma glucose levels are high, hepatocytes remove glucose from the plasma. This glucose is stored in polymer form as glycogen. As plasma glucose levels decline, the hepatocytes convert the glycogen back into glucose molecules (glycogenolysis) and release them into the bloodstream. Although many body tissues have the requisite cellular enzymes for glycogenolysis, hepatocytes are one of the few cell types that can release this intracellular glucose into the bloodstream. Hepatocytes do not simply respond directly to plasma glucose. These glucostatic functions are mediated by several hormones; some (eg, insulin) promote hepatic glucose uptake, and others (eg, glucagon, growth hormone, and epinephrine) stimulate glycogenolysis and the release of glucose from liver cells.

The liver does not contain enough glycogen reserves to be able to buffer plasma glucose during prolonged fasting or severe exercise. During these times, low plasma glucose levels stimulate the secretion of one or more hormones (glucagon, glucocorticoids, or thyroxine) that trigger the biochemical conversion of intracellular fatty and amino acids into glucose (gluconeogenesis), which the liver cell can then release into the bloodstream or store as glycogen. Only hepatocytes possess the enzyme that is critical for gluconeogenesis. Glycogen storage is important for other functions of liver cells. A glycogen-rich hepatocyte conjugates bilirubin at a faster rate and is more resistant to toxins and infectious agents.

Hepatocytes possess a *mixed-function–oxidase system* (MFOS) of enzymes that degrade certain drugs, among which are alcohol, benzodiazepines, tranquilizers, phenobarbital, phenytoin (Dilantin), and sodium warfarin (Coumadin). This system operates in addition to other intracellular systems that also degrade some of these drugs. Its clinical significance lies in the nature of the drugs that this system catabolizes and in the fact that MFOS activity can be either inhibited or augmented (induced) by these same drugs, depending on *when* they are taken. Administration of two MFOS-catabolized drugs within a few hours of one another or together causes each agent to act competitively, slowing down the degradation of the other. For example, simultaneous ingestion of diazepam (Valium) and alcohol can result in slower degradation of each drug. The outcome is higher blood levels of both chemicals for a longer time after administration. The repeated administration of one MFOS-catabolized drug for several days causes the MFOS system to enlarge physically and to possess more enzymes. This is called induction. Once induced, the MFOS degrades drugs more rapidly (including the drug that initiated the induction). If administration of a second MFOS-catabolized drug is begun after MFOS induction, a larger dose of this drug will be required to produce a given effect. For example, induction of the MFOS by diazepam increases the dosage of warfarin needed to produce a given therapeutic effect. Other drugs are degraded by various hepatic systems.

Many elements that constitute the coagulation cascade are synthesized in the liver. Fibrinogen, prothrombin, proaccelerin, proconvertin, plasma, thromboplastin component, and Stuart factor are all made in the liver. Coagulation is delayed in patients with deficient liver function. Also, several complement proteins are synthesized there.

Clinical Applicability Challenges

Self-Challenge: Critical Thinking

1. *Explore mechanisms by which stress can impair swallowing.*

2. *Compare and contrast the effects of vagotomy and vagal stimulation on swallowing and gastric emptying.*

3. *Jaundice can be caused by prehepatic (hemolytic), hepatic, and posthepatic (obstructive) conditions. Contrast laboratory findings in each type of condition with respect to serum bilirubin elevations.*

Study Questions

1. The pancreas secretes
   1. amylase.
   2. bicarbonate.
   3. hydrochloric acid.
   4. secretin.
      a. 1 and 2
      b. 3 and 4
      c. 1 and 3
      d. 2 and 4

2. The colon is a major site for
   a. digestion.
   b. absorption of digested foodstuffs.
   c. reabsorption of water and electrolytes.
   d. secretion of secretin and gastrin.

3. Which of the following is not a liver function?
   a. Manufacture of clotting factors
   b. Lipid digestion
   c. Synthesis of nitrogenous wastes
   d. Synthesis of immunoglobulins

4. Defecation
   1. is initiated by pressure of feces on the internal anal sphincter.
   2. is initiated by stretching of the rectal wall.
   3. cannot occur after recovery from a complete transection of the spinal cord in the lumbar region.
   4. is a cord reflex that can be voluntarily inhibited if central nervous system pathways between the cerebral cortex and the sacral cord are intact.
      a. 1 and 2
      b. 3 and 4
      c. 1 and 3
      d. 2 and 4

BIBLIOGRAPHY

Johnson LR (ed): Physiology of the Gastrointestinal Tract (3rd Ed). New York, Raven Press, 1994

Ganong WF: Review of Medical Physiology (17th Ed). Norwalk, Ct, Appleton & Lange, 1995

38

Patient Assessment: Gastrointestinal System

HISTORY

PHYSICAL EXAMINATION
Oral Cavity
Abdomen
Rectal Area

DIAGNOSTIC STUDIES
Laboratory Tests
Diagnostic Tests
   X-rays
   Gastrointestinal Endoscopy
   Colonoscopy
   Barium Contrast Studies

Ultrasonography
Computed Tomography and
   Magnetic Resonance Imaging
Biopsy
Arteriography
Paracentesis

OBJECTIVES

Based on the content in this chapter, the reader should be able to:

- Explore the major concepts involved in performing a history and physical examination of the gastrointestinal system.
- Discuss six tests used to diagnose common gastrointestinal disorders.
- Explain the nursing role in assessing the patient with gastrointestinal compromise.

*W*hen a patient is critically ill, assessment of the gastrointestinal (GI) system helps determine whether assessment findings relate to the current clinical problem or herald a new complication. For example, is a pulmonary disorder causing the comatose patient's respiratory distress or is a mucous plug lodged in the nasopharynx? Is the bright red blood in the stool a result of GI bleeding or from external bleeding hemorrhoids? Is the abdominal pain due to recent bowel surgery or to a distended stomach?

Assessing the GI system helps determine the cause of nutritional issues, acid–base imbalance, bleeding episodes, and GI-related pain. It also helps identify nursing diagnoses and the need for health teaching.

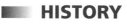 HISTORY

Unless emergency conditions require immediate action to preserve life, an assessment of the GI system begins with the history. The nurse asks the patient about past or current problems with anorexia, indigestion, dysphagia, nausea, vomiting, pain, jaundice, constipation, gas, diarrhea, bleeding, or hemorrhoids. A nutritional history is important and includes dietary intake, changes in appetite, food allergies, food intolerances, special diets, taste sensations, difficulty swallowing, heartburn, and indigestion. A history about cigarette smoking and alcohol and coffee intake is also obtained. Recent weight gain or loss, bowel habits, recent surgeries (including dental work), and any family history of ulcers, colitis, or cancer are recorded. The nurse inquires about recent emotional upsets, depression, and anxiety. A thorough medication history is also necessary. Additional questions describe each symptom: when it appeared, the severity and frequency, what precipitated the symptom, what relieved it, what made it worse, and its course. Pain should also be described by type, location, quality, duration, and associated signs and symptoms (eg, hyperventilation, guarding, and tachycardia). The accompanying display lists some conditions that produce abdominal pain.

CLINICAL APPLICATION:
Assessment Parameters
Factors in Intra-abdominal Pain and Tenderness

- Perforated peptic ulcer
- Dissecting or ruptured aneurysm
- Pancreatitis
- Cholecystitis
- Regional enteritis
- Ulcerative colitis
- Diverticulitis
- Appendicitis
- Occlusion of mesenteric artery
- Ruptured ectopic pregnancy
- Acute renal infections
- Pelvic inflammatory disease
- Hepatitis
- Extra-abdominal causes
    Myocardial disease
    Respiratory disease
    Diabetic or thyroid crisis
    Spinal cord lesion
    Acute intermittent porphyria
    Pneumonia
    Acute glaucoma

■ PHYSICAL EXAMINATION

Physical examination begins with general observations that include overall appearance, motor activity, body position, gait, hair, skin color (jaundice, cyanosis, pallor), edema, facial expression, level of consciousness, and signs of depression, anxiety, confusion, or irritability.

Oral Cavity

The oral cavity is examined by inspection and palpation using a good light source, a tongue depressor, an examining glove, and a mask. The nurse explains the procedure. The patient assumes a comfortable position that facilitates examination. Sitting upright is the best position for this part of the examination.

The lips and jaw are inspected for abnormal color, texture, lesions, symmetry, and swellings. The temporomandibular joints are palpated for mobility, tenderness, and crepitus. The nurse retracts the lips to allow adequate visualization. Dentures are inspected for fit, and they are removed for the oral examination. A good light source is used to inspect all structures inside the mouth and the buccal mucosa. Missing, broken, loose, and decayed teeth are identified, while the nurse notes redness, pallor, white patches, plaques, ulcers, petechiae, bleeding, and masses. A pool of saliva under the tongue helps assess hydration. The parotid and submaxillary ducts are palpated.

The nurse palpates suspicious areas with a gloved finger to determine tenderness or induration. The patient sticks out his or her tongue, while the nurse checks for symmetry of movement, swellings, lesions, and an abnormal coating. While the nurse depresses the tongue with a tongue blade, he or she observes the movement of the soft palate and uvula as the patient says *ahhhh*. These structures should rise symmetrically. This is a good time to inspect the hard and soft palates, the uvula, the tonsils, the pillars, and the posterior pharynx. Unusual breath odors are characteristic of GI disease, such as peptic ulcer disease, severe bowel obstruction, hepatic failure, and neoplasms of the esophagus.

Abdomen

The patient's comfort is kept in mind as the nurse performs the abdominal examination. The patient empties his or her bladder just prior to the examination. A supine position with arms down and knees slightly bent is used. This position relieves tension on the abdominal wall. Draping exposes the abdomen but protects the patient's modesty. If the patient is experiencing pain, the need for an examination is evaluated. Likewise, if the procedure increases discomfort or intensity of pain, the examination is stopped. An abdominal examination is not conducted if the patient has appendicitis, dissecting abdominal aortic aneurysm, polycystic kidneys, or an organ transplantation.

The order of the abdominal examination is inspection, auscultation, percussion, and palpation. Auscultation precedes percussion and palpation because the latter can alter the frequency and quality of bowel sounds. The abdomen is divided into four quadrants: right upper quadrant (RUQ), left upper quadrant (LUQ), left lower quadrant (LLQ), and right lower quadrant (RLQ). The underlying structures are shown in Figure 38–l.

Observation

The examination begins with the nurse standing at the foot of the patient and inspecting for symmetry of the ab-

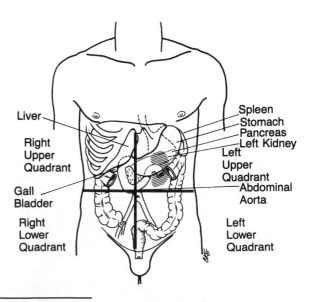

FIGURE 38-1
A map of abdominal organs

domen, visible masses, and pulsations. He or she also observes for tense, shiny skin; rashes; striae; ecchymoses; lesions; scars; and prominent or dilated veins. A blue-tinged umbilicus, known as Cullen's sign, can indicate intra-abdominal bleeding. A hernia will become visible with a cough. The nurse moves to the patient's side and assumes a position to obtain an eye-level view across the abdomen. Size, shape, asymmetry, eversion of the umbilicus, and movements from respirations, peristalsis, vascular pulsations, and exaggerated movement are inspected. Pulsation of the aorta is normally seen in the epigastric area. In a thin person, the femoral pulses may be visible. When ascites or abdominal bleeding is suspected, the abdominal girth is measured.

Auscultation

Light pressure on the diaphragm of the stethoscope is used when auscultating the four quadrants of the abdomen. To prevent contraction of the abdominal muscles, which can obscure sounds, the stethoscope must be lifted completely off the abdominal wall when changing its location. It may be necessary to listen for 2 minutes or longer to confirm hypoactive or absent bowel sounds. Frequency and character of sounds are noted. Normal bowel sounds are irregular gurgles that occur every 5 to 15 seconds. High-pitched, tinkling sounds indicate that fluid and air are under tension in the intestine and may signal a partial obstruction.

Edema of the abdominal wall can be detected when an imprint of the diaphragm remains after light auscultation. The nurse uses the bell of the stethoscope to listen for bruits (continuous purring, blowing, or humming sounds) over the abdominal aorta and the renal and femoral arteries. If a bruit is heard, percussion and palpation are not performed. If a bruit is a new finding, the physician is notified.

Percussion

Following auscultation, percussion of all four quadrants will identify air, gas, and fluid in the abdomen and help to determine organ size. The percussion sound depends on the density of the underlying structure. A dull sound is heard over solid organs, such as the liver, a stool-filled colon, abdominal masses, or pleural effusions. A tympanic sound is heard over air, as in the gastric bubble. The size of the liver is determined by percussing along the right midclavicular line. One method is to begin at the iliac crest and work upward. The point at which the sound becomes dull is marked. Percussion is performed down from the clavicle. The dull sound of a rib should not be mistaken for the superior edge of the liver. After the superior edge is marked, the nurse measures the distance between the marks in centimeters. The normal liver measures 6 to 12 centimeters in height at the midclavicular line (Fig. 38–2).

Palpation

Light palpation should be performed first to identify muscular resistance and areas of tenderness. The appre-

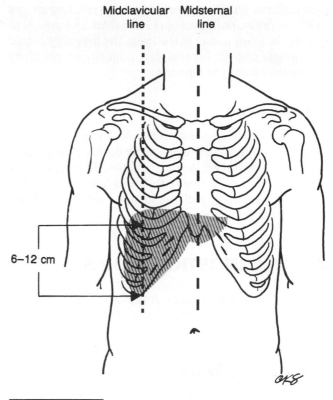

FIGURE 38-2
Location of the liver for percussion.

hensive patient will relax if he or she participates in performing palpation. The examiner places his or her hand over the patient's hand during early palpation. As the patient becomes more relaxed, palpation continues without problems. This method also helps with a ticklish patient.

One or two fingers are used to depress the abdominal wall 1 cm (0.5 in). Skin temperature, muscle resistance, tender areas, and masses are recorded. The femoral artery is palpated bilaterally. A symptomatic area is always palpated last to ensure patient cooperation and relaxed muscles.

When disease is present, palpation may result in somatic or organ pain. Somatic pain is localized and reflects inflammation of the skin, fascia, or abdominal surfaces. It is accompanied by guarding of the abdominal muscles. Organ pain is visceral in nature and is usually dull, diffuse, and generalized.

Deep palpation is used to locate organs (enlarged spleen, liver edge, poles of right and left kidney) and large masses. The tips of the fingers are used to depress the abdominal wall firmly to a depth of 7.5 cm (3 in). Palpation is performed in the epigastric area for the pulse of the aorta. If an area of tenderness is found with light palpation, rebound tenderness should be checked by quickly withdrawing the fingertips following depression. Rebound tenderness usually indicates an inflammation of the peritoneum.

The liver is best palpated by placing one hand under the patient at the level of the 11th rib, while the other hand is placed on the abdomen at the level of the percussed liver edge dullness. With the abdominal fingers pointing upward to lift the organ, push the upper hand down and upward to palpate the lower border of the liver. The liver edge should be firm and smooth. An enlarged, nodular, or irregularly shaped liver should be reported.

Rectal Area

The rectum is assessed by inspection and palpation. The skin around the rectum is normally darker than the surrounding area. Inspect for inflammation, lesions, fissures, and hemorrhoids. Palpate with a well-lubricated rubber-gloved finger for outpouching, nodules, tenderness, irregularities, and fecal impaction.

■■■ DIAGNOSTIC STUDIES

A variety of diagnostic studies can be used to help in the diagnosis of GI and abdominal disorders in the critical care setting.

Laboratory Tests

Laboratory tests used to diagnose common GI disorders include electrolytes, end products of metabolism, enzymes, proteins, and hematology. They are described in Table 38–1. However, laboratory values may vary among laboratories. Their significance in specific GI disease is discussed in Chapter 40, Common Gastrointestinal Disorders. Serology tests for hepatitis are also discussed in Chapter 40.

Diagnostic Tests

X-RAYS

The abdominal series, or three-way view of the abdomen, consists of films of the flat abdomen, films of the upper abdomen and upper chest with the patient erect, and films obtained with the patient lying on one side (decubitus). Radiographs help delineate free air in the abdomen caused by problems such as a perforated viscus or a ruptured abscess. They also show organ size, position, and intactness. Bowel obstructions, as indicated by dilated loops of bowel with air fluid levels or intestinal volvulus, can be seen on these films. Decubitus films help determine the presence and mobility of ascites.

Gastric Lavage

Gastric lavage may be used for diagnosis of upper GI bleeding and to prepare for further testing. Bloody gastric aspirate from a nasogastric tube indicates bleeding proximal to the jejunum. While false-negatives are uncommon, they may occur if the tube is coiled in the fundus, bleeding is intermittent, or blood is not refluxing back from the duodenum. Lavage with room temperature water or saline can clear the stomach of clots prior to endoscopy. It can also help assess the amount of bleeding occurring in the patient with bright red blood after nasogastric tube placement.

GASTROINTESTINAL ENDOSCOPY

This procedure is an important adjunct to the barium studies because it allows direct observation of portions of the intestinal tract (Fig. 38–3). A flexible fiberoptic endoscope is used. Designed with a movable tip, it can be manipulated through the intestinal tract by the operator. It also includes an instrument channel that allows for biopsy of lesions, such as tumors, ulcers, or inflammation. Fluids can be aspirated from the lumen of the intestinal tract, and air can be insufflated to distend the intestinal tract for better observation. Cytology brushes and electrocautery snares can also be passed through the scope. The basic upper intestinal endoscope and the colonoscope are designed in a similar fashion and differ only in their diameters and lengths. A side-viewing upper intestinal endoscope has also been designed for special studies of the common bile duct and the pancreatic duct. This is called endoscopic retrograde cholangiopancreatography (ERCP).

The indications for upper intestinal endoscopy are multiple. In the critical care setting the most common indication is acute GI hemorrhage, which can be caused by ulcers, gastritis, or esophageal varices. Endoscopy is helpful in diagnosing neoplasms of the upper intestinal tract. Biopsies or brushings of these abnormal areas can be done to obtain diagnostic material.

Endoscopic studies require an empty stomach for good visualization. It may be necessary to lavage the stomach with a wide-bore gastric tube before beginning these tests. Because of the size of these tubes, they are passed into the stomach orally and left in place only as long as necessary to empty the stomach of food or blood clots. Before passage of the endoscope, the patient is placed on the left side, three-fourths prone. This position provides easy access to the pylorus and improves viewing of the greater curvature of the stomach. A local anesthetic is applied to the throat, and a sedative such as diazepam (Valium) or midazolam hydrochloride (Versed) is administered intravenously.

During the procedure, the patient is observed closely for changes in condition and untoward reactions to the test. A thorough history assists in anticipating reactions, and nursing intervention can prevent unfavorable responses, such as a drug reaction or pain and discomfort due to positional limitations.

COLONOSCOPY

Colonoscopy is used to evaluate for the presence of tumors, inflammation, or polyps within the colon. It is also used to evaluate a surgical anastomotic site from a previous surgery and to assess the degree of stricture from their previous surgeries or inflammation.

The colonoscope can be passed from the rectum through the full length of the colon into the cecum. From here the ileocecal valve can be assessed, as well as other abnormalities, such as early carcinomas or polyps of the right side of the colon. These polyps can be removed through the endoscope, or they can be fulgurated and cauterized. Specific

TABLE 38-1
Laboratory Tests Used for Gastrointestinal Disorders

Tests	Normal Values	Comments
Electrolyte/Chemistry		
Calcium	8.9–10.3 mg/dL (total)	These electrolytes are absorbed by the
	4.6–5.1 mg/dL (free)	small intestine and may be lost, de-
Chloride	97–110 mmol/L	pleted, or increased with gastrointesti-
Magnesium	1.3–2.2 mEq/L	nal disorders. Ammonia increases as
Potassium	3.3–4.9 mmol/L	breakdown of proteins or urea sur-
Sodium	135–145 mmol/L	passes the clearance ability of the hepa-
Ammonia	19–43 μmol/L	tobiliary system.
Bilirubin		
Total	0.2–1.3 mg/100 mL	These values measure the ability of the
Conjugated (direct)	0.0–0.2 mg/100 mL	liver to conjugate and excrete bilirubin.
Unconjugated (indirect)	0.2–0.7 mg/100 mL	
Enzymatic		
Lipase	2.3–20 IU/dL	Lipase and amylase are increased with
Amylase	35–118 IU/dL	pancreatic disease. AST/ALT are hepato-
AST/SGOT	11–17 IU/L	cellular enzymes that are released with
ALT/SGPT	7–53 IU/L	hepatic disruption or destruction. ALT is
Alkaline Phosphatase	30–120 IU/L	found primarily in the liver, while AST
GGT	0–30 IU/100 mL	may be found in the heart, skeletal
LDH	165–300 units/100 mL	muscle, kidney, and brain. Alkaline
5'-nucleotidase	2–16 IU/L	phosphatase is found in bone, intestine,
		liver, and placental tissue and is re-
		leased with destruction of these tissues.
		GGT is found primarily in the liver and if
		elevated along with alkaline phospha-
		tase, usually indicates biliary disease.
		Increased 5'-nucleotidase and alkaline
		phosphatase reflects hepatobiliary
		sources of enzyme elevation.
Proteins		
Total (serum)	6.5–8 g/100 mL	Proteins are responsible for maintaining
Albumin	3.6–5.0 g/100 mL	osmotic pressures between blood and
Globulins	2–3 g/100 mL	tissue and transporting hormones and
Haptoglobins	44–303 mg/dL	drugs.
Fibrinogen	150–360 mg/dL	Some have primary clotting and transport
		functions or assist in antibody produc-
		tion.
Hematologic		
Prothrombin time	11.0–14.0 s	Reflects the abnormality of clotting fac-
Partial thromboplastin time	25.0–36.0 s	tors and intestinal uptake of vitamin K
Hematocrit	male: 40.7%–50.3%	(required for some clotting factor func-
	female: 36.1%–44.3%	tion). Partial thromboplastin time may
		be prolonged in severe liver disease.

AST, aspartate transaminase; also called SGOT, serum glutamic–oxaloacetic transaminase
ALT, alanine transaminase; also called SGPT, serum glutamic–pyruvic transaminase
GGT, gamma-glutamyltransferase
LDH, lactate dehydrogenase

sites of bleeding, such as occurs in colitis, polyps, tumors, or angiodysplasia (a collection of abnormal blood vessels that can bleed extensively), can be observed.

Because patients are usually sedated for endoscopic procedures, it is important to guard their airways to prevent respiratory depression or aspiration and to monitor vital signs.

BARIUM CONTRAST STUDIES

These studies are extremely important to define abnormalities within the intestinal tract. The upper GI x-ray or barium swallow is performed by having the patient drink radiopaque barium while the radiologist observes the coating of this material within the esophagus, stomach, and small

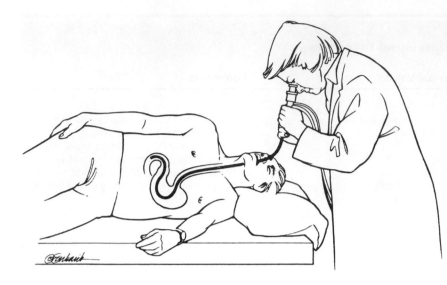

FIGURE 38-3
Patient undergoing gastrointestinal endoscopy. (From Smeltzer S, Bare B: Brunner and Suddarth's Textbook of Medical Surgical Nursing [8th Ed]. Philadelphia, Lippincott-Raven, 1996)

intestine. The barium outlines structural defects, such as tumors or ulcers and can define inflammation or strictures. The barium enema is performed by instilling barium through the rectum in a retrograde fashion into the entire colon. A thin coat of barium helps to outline tumors, polyps, diverticula, or inflammation such as Crohn's disease or ulcerative colitis. This test should be performed *after* any tests that require visualization of the intestinal mucosa. Studies of the upper GI tract require withholding all oral intake (food, liquids, oral medications) for 8 to 10 hours before the test is performed. The patient may be given an oral contrast substance to take just before testing. Studies of the lower intestinal tract require a low-residue diet and the administration of a potent laxative the evening before the test. Enemas can be given the morning of the test to make certain the rectum and colon are completely empty. No more than three enemas should be necessary.

After a barium study, stools should be observed to be sure barium is expelled. The protocol may call for administration of a laxative to promote barium excretion. Following an endoscopic procedure, the patient must be observed for signs of bleeding (hematemesis, melena, tachycardia, hypotension), perforation (pain on swallowing, epigastric substernal pain increased with breathing and movement, shoulder pain, abdominal pain, back pain, dyspnea, tachycardia, hypotension), and adverse drug reactions (anxiety, erythema, fever, angioedema, wheezing, dyspnea, cyanosis, palpitations, hypotension, vomiting, diarrhea). If an ERCP has been performed, watch for signs of cholangitis (fever, chills, hyperbilirubinemia) or pancreatitis.

ULTRASONOGRAPHY

This noninvasive test uses echowaves to detect abnormalities in the abdominal cavity. Dilation of the common bile duct, distended gallbladder with gallstones, and pancreatic abnormalities, such as tumors, pseudocysts, or abscesses, can be defined. Abdominal aortic aneurysms can be quantitated to help decide if surgical excision is required. Thickening of the descending colon and sigmoid colon

with pericolonic abscesses caused by such conditions as diverticulosis can be identified. When used in conjunction with Doppler flow studies, the degree of portal hypertension and retrograde or forward flow may be determined. This procedure is usually performed in the radiology department of a hospital but can be performed in the critical care setting.

COMPUTED TOMOGRAPHY AND MAGNETIC RESONANCE IMAGING

Tumors of the liver, pancreas, esophagus, stomach, and colon can be identified using these scans. Retroperitoneal tumors or lymph nodes can be seen as well.

Nuclear medicine techniques are often used to help diagnose abnormalities of the hepatogastrointestinal systems. Radionuclide liver scans can help determine hepatic cell dysfunction. Computed axial tomography, also called computed tomography (CT) scanning, can be used to define tumors or abscesses within the liver or upper abdomen.

Cholescintograms can be performed to determine the functional capacity of the biliary system and the patency of the bile ducts and the cystic duct. In recurrent intestinal bleeding, if the source has not been found, technetium scans can be helpful. In this technique, the blood is labeled with technetium, and if the patient is actively bleeding, a "hot spot" can show up on the scan of the abdomen. It is a nonspecific test for locating the exact site of the bleeding but can help in directing the surgeon to the general site. Angiodysplasia and a bleeding Meckel's diverticulum can be diagnosed with this procedure.

BIOPSY

Biopsy of intestinal structures may be necessary to determine the source and extent of disease processes and for tissue cytology and culture studies. Liver biopsy is a valuable method for diagnosing the extent and source of liver disease, while pancreatic cysts and growths may be biopsied or drained using a similar technique. Biopsy samples may be obtained percutaneously, without the use of concurrent imaging studies to guide the needle, or they may be performed in conjunction with CT or ultrasound to facilitate exact placement of the probe. Transjugular liver biopsy sampling allows the physician to obtain a sample under fluoroscopy with a catheter and biopsy needle threaded through the vasculature into the liver.

ARTERIOGRAPHY

This procedure is useful in defining the sites of bleeding that are otherwise difficult to determine. The catheter is placed in either the superior or inferior mesenteric artery, and contrast is injected to highlight areas of bleeding. Arteriography is also extremely helpful in defining aneurysms of the aorta.

PARACENTESIS

Peritoneal tap with lavage of the peritoneal cavity can be most useful in trauma cases in which intra-abdominal hemorrhage must be defined. Testing the peritoneal fluid for amylase and lipase can help diagnose pancreatitis, while cytology studies on peritoneal fluid help detect tumors. Paracentesis can be a comfort measure by alleviating the accumulation of ascitic fluid and a diagnostic measure when protein and albumin tests aid in determining the source and speed of fluid accumulation. Local anesthetic and strict sterile technique are used for paracentesis. The patient's bladder must be empty at the time of the tap to prevent accidental puncture of the bladder. The patient is positioned according to the physician's preference. Emotional support is provided during the procedure, and condition changes are monitored. Following paracentesis, the patient must be observed for signs and symptoms of internal bleeding due to laceration of a blood vessel or peritonitis due to perforated viscus. Because of sedation, respiratory rate, depth, and effort must be carefully monitored, and the health care team must be ready to respond to respiratory compromise. Pulse oximeters may also be used to monitor oxygen levels.

Clinical Applicability Challenges

Self-Challenge: Critical Thinking

1. Review the patient care studies in Chapter 40 about Mr. Lane who has GI bleeding and Mr. Jackson who has acute pancreatitis. Analyze the risk factors in each history. Compare and contrast their examination and diagnostic findings.

Study Questions

1. During percussion of the abdomen, a dull sound is heard over
   a. solid organs.
   b. hollow organs.
   c. a gastric air bubble.
   d. an empty colon.

2. The diagnostic study that allows for direct visual observation of the intestinal tract is the
   a. abdominal x-ray.
   b. endoscopy.
   c. ultrasonography.
   d. computed tomography.

3. If a patient is to receive each of the following four tests, which one should be done last?
   a. Arteriography
   b. Barium swallow
   c. Colonoscopy
   d. Endoscopy

BIBLIOGRAPHY

Bates B: A Guide to Physical Examination and History Taking (6th Ed). Philadelphia, JB Lippincott, 1995

Beachley M, Farrar J: Abdominal trauma: Putting the pieces together. Am J Nurs 93(11):26–34, 1993

Fuller J, Schaller-Ayers J: Health Assessment, A Nursing Approach (2nd Ed). Philadelphia, JB Lippincott, 1994

Kirton CA: Physical assessment: Assessing for ascites. Nursing 26(4):53, 1996

Walsh S: Oh no, the patient is six, not sixty!: The pediatric endoscopy patient. Gastroenterol Nurs 18(2):57–61, 1995

Patient Management: Gastrointestinal System

OBJECTIVES

Based on the content in this chapter, the reader should be able to:

- Explain how physiological stresses of illness and injury alter the body's need for energy.
- Explore assessment findings that help determine nutritional status.
- Compare and contrast the indications, procedures, management, and complications for patients receiving enteral and parenteral feedings.

*H*ealth and nutrition go hand in hand. Physiological stressors such as illness and injury increase the body's metabolic and energy demands. When energy expenditures exceed supply, malnutrition can rapidly develop. Early nutritional intervention can lessen these risks in the critically ill patient. This chapter presents an overview of energy requirements for patients under physiological stress, nutri-

tional assessment, and methods, management, and complications of nutritional support.

PHYSIOLOGICAL PRINCIPLES

The total energy expended by the body is the sum of physical activity, growth, and basal metabolic rate (BMR). The BMR is the energy a person requires to perform essential physiological processes at rest. There must be a balance between energy supply and energy expenditure to maintain homeostasis.

The body must also maintain nitrogen balance. This is crucial because nitrogen is a major component of amino acids, which represent the building blocks of protein. One gram of nitrogen equals 6.25 g of protein, which is equal to about 30 g of lean mass.

Nitrogen balance is a very important measure of protein synthesis and metabolism. This balance is calculated from the amount of nitrogen intake versus that excreted in the urine as urea. If the body is building protein, a state of anabolism exists, and nitrogen balance is positive. If the body is breaking down protein, a state of catabolism exists, and the nitrogen balance is negative. Catabolism represents 8the breakdown of protein for energy purposes. The loss of protein influences many body functions because it is necessary for enzymes, cell membranes, contractile protein in muscle, and maintaining cellular osmotic pressure. Catabolism often occurs in trauma, sepsis, and many diseases.

Metabolic Response to Injury

A traumatic event, regardless of its cause, triggers a complex series of hormonal responses that significantly alter the body's metabolism. The major effect is an increase in protein and fat catabolism, with a retention of water and sodium and a loss of potassium. Antidiuretic hormone (ADH) is released from the pituitary in response to such factors as hypovolemia, pain, stress, and drugs. By acting on the collecting ducts of the kidney, ADH reduces free water excretion, thus correcting the hypovolemic state. Corticotropin (ACTH) also is released from the pituitary and stimulates the adrenal gland to secrete mineralocorticoids and glucocorticoids. The mineralocorticoid aldosterone causes sodium retention and potassium excretion by its action on the kidney. This function, along with the action of ADH, is the major volume regulatory system in which the body maintains blood pressure in the face of trauma.

The glucocorticoids, of which cortisol is the most important, act in several ways to produce energy for the body during stress. They act on the liver to stimulate gluconeogenesis but also are catabolic in that they cause muscle protein breakdown to amino acids and decreased protein synthesis. They also release free fatty acids from lipid stores. Fatty acids meet the requirements of all organs with the exception of those that specifically require glucose (eg, the brain and nervous system).

The catecholamines, epinephrine and norepinephrine, are released from the adrenal medulla during stress. They also set into motion a series of reactions aimed at increasing energy for the body.

Lipolysis results from increased catecholamine secretion. Free fatty acids are then available for use as an energy source by the liver, kidney, lung, heart, and skeletal muscle. Ketone bodies are formed from fatty acids by the liver. These also are used as an energy source.

Catecholamines cause hyperglycemia to develop during stress; this is called "stress diabetes." This clinical state arises through a variety of mechanisms. Liver glycogen and muscle glycogen are converted to glucose. Insulin released from the pancreas is suppressed, and glucagon is released. Uptake of glucose in the peripheral tissues also is reduced.

Both ACTH and catecholamines act to release glucagon. Glucagon then acts on the liver to promote gluconeogenesis. It also helps break down skeletal muscle glycogen to glucose and acids in oxidation of fat.

Corticotropin, catecholamines, glucagon, insulin, and growth hormone act in synergism to supply the body with energy substrate and to control blood volume to help ensure survival during stress. This stress can be either starvation or trauma. However, in starvation, the levels of cortisol and catecholamines are not elevated to the magnitude seen in severe trauma. This can account for the fact that there is a rise in metabolic rate in the post-traumatic state rather than the fall that occurs in starvation. In starvation, the body tends to preserve lean body mass and protein, but in trauma, protein becomes the major source of calories. The mechanisms for this are not well understood.

During the initial phase of stress, the body uses carbohydrates in the form of glycogen. These stores can last as long as 8 to 12 hours. After this, the body uses amino acids from protein and to some degree, fatty acids for energy.

Although drastic losses of lean body mass cannot be avoided, they can be offset by an adequate supply of calories and amino acids. If nutrition is supplied and other factors of support, such as blood pressure and respiratory status, are maintained, the body enters a phase of "available opportunity." During this time, the levels of catecholamines, cortisol, and glucagon drop, and the insulin level rises. Protein breakdown is curtailed, and protein resynthesis is favored.

If catabolism is allowed to continue without the support of calories and amino acids, wound healing, immune function, and muscular strength are compromised. At this point, there is direct competition for these substances by the rest of the body. If this situation continues, malnutrition can occur.

TYPES OF MALNUTRITION

There are two major classifications of malnutrition: protein and protein-calorie. Either can occur in critically ill patients. Protein malnutrition is characterized by general apathy, decreased visceral protein synthesis as indicated by decreased plasma albumin and transferrin, edema, muscular wasting, and a decreased total lymphocyte count.

Protein-calorie malnutrition is accompanied by a recent unplanned loss of 10% or more of body weight, decreased subcutaneous fat stores, muscle mass atrophy, diarrhea, and anorexia.

■ NUTRITIONAL ASSESSMENT

Assessing for malnutrition and identifying high-risk patients are important because there is a significant difference in morbidity and mortality rates between groups of malnourished and well-nourished patients. High-risk patients include those with chronic disease, severe catabolism, inability to use the gastrointestinal tract, intravenous support for more than 5 days, and beginning signs or symptoms of malnutrition.

Assessing the patient who may need nutritional assistance includes a health history, anthropometric measurements, and tests for visceral proteins, immunological response, and nitrogen balance.

NUTRITIONAL HISTORY

The nutritional history includes a description of the patient's usual diet; food preferences, including cultural influences; changes in weight; appetite; or difficulty eating. Because many illnesses and injuries influence nutrition, the patient's history helps assess nutritional needs. For example, does the patient have problems associated with chewing, swallowing, digestion, absorption, and elimination? Is there a history of liver disease, gastrointestinal disease, diabetes, or alcoholism? Ask about current medications because they can interfere with appetite and absorption of nutrients. Age can help determine metabolic needs and absorption of nutrients. Obtain the history as soon as possible. If the patient is unable to provide this information, family members can often assist. (See Chapter 38, Patient Assessment: Gastrointestinal System.)

ANTHROPOMETRIC MEASUREMENTS

Anthropometric measurements are physical measures of the body that provide an estimate of fat content and muscle mass. They include height, weight, midarm circumference, and the thickness of skin folds. Additional measures, such as frame size and body mass index, can be extrapolated. Charts of normal ranges help interpret the data. Weight is the most common measure used during critical illness.

The patient's admission height and weight are compared with ideal body weight. The 1983 Metropolitan Life Weight-Height Chart is an accepted standard for ideal body weight. A general rule is that weight 10% below the ideal suggests mild malnutrition. Although dehydration or fluid retention can alter weight, acute weight loss is an important assessment parameter. Therefore, critically ill patients should be weighed daily to determine the loss of lean body mass.

Approximately 50% of the body's total fat stores are subcutaneous, while muscles contain approximately 60% of the body's total protein. When energy expenditure exceeds the amount provided by nutritional intake, the muscles become the major site of protein breakdown. Measuring skinfold thickness and midarm circumference help estimate fat stores and skeletal muscle mass. Skinfold thicknesses are measured using a set of specially designed calipers. The tricep arm area is the primary measure; however, subscapular and thigh skinfolds can also be measured to improve accuracy. The midarm circumference is measured with a tape. These measures are less accurate in older people because of loss of muscle mass and sagging tissues. They can also be altered by edema, gender, and clinician technique.

PROTEIN MEASUREMENTS

Serum protein concentrations reflect the protein mass of the internal organs (visceral proteins). The proteins most often measured to determine malnutrition are albumin, transferrin, and prealbumin (Table 39–1). Many factors alter protein levels, such as metabolic response to injury, amount of amino acids available for plasma synthesis in the liver, fluid volume, administration of blood and blood products, and liver and kidney disease. Therefore, serial protein levels are more useful than a single level in evaluating the patient's response to nutritional interventions.

Albumin is stored in large concentrations in the body and has a long half-life of 20 days. As a result, it is a poor marker of early nutritional deficiencies and is best at predicting complications associated with malnutrition. Serum transferrin is stored in smaller quantities and has a half-life of 8 to 10 days, making it a more sensitive indicator of protein depletion. Prealbumin has the shortest half-life, 24 to 48 hours, and may therefore be the most sensitive indicator of acute protein depletion. Any sudden stress to the body will rapidly depress serum prealbumin levels.

IMMUNOLOGICAL MEASURES

Skin tests containing antigens to tuberculosis, mumps, and *Candida* are used to measure cellular immunity. If cutaneous reactions do not occur, it may indicate altered immunocompetence. Absent or delayed reactions can be caused by malnutrition. Reduced total lymphocyte counts may also be found. A total lymphocyte count of less than 1,500/mm^3 may indicate impaired immune function.

URINARY UREA NITROGEN MEASURE

The urea nitrogen in a 24-hour urine sample is measured, and the following formula is used to calculate nitrogen balance. Nitrogen balance = protein intake (g) divided by 6.25 g minus the urinary urea nitrogen + 4 g. The 4 g added to the equation is the amount of nitrogen lost in the stool. Additional protein loses occur through wounds and diaphoresis. Zero indicates nitrogen balance; a higher number means that protein intake exceeded output, and protein is available for tissue building; a deficit means the amount needed by the body exceeded intake.

The amino acid and nitrogen needs of the patient can be calculated by this measurement. Maintaining a state of positive nitrogen balance allows for wound healing. A 4- to 6-g positive balance is ideal, although this is difficult to achieve in the critically ill patient. The focus is then to decrease the negative nitrogen balance.

DETERMINING NUTRITIONAL REQUIREMENTS

Determining an individual's nutritional requirements is the next step in a nutritional assessment. This involves calculating calorie, protein, carbohydrate, fat, vitamin, and mineral requirements.

Energy requirements are estimated using the Harris-Benedict equation, *Basal Energy Equivalents* at rest. This formula has been adapted to include correction factors that

TABLE 39-1 CLINICAL APPLICATION: Diagnostic Studies — Determining Nutritional Status		
Proteins	**Half-life**	**Normal Value**
Albumin	20 d	>3.5 g/dL
Transferrin	8 d	>200 mg/dL
Prealbumin	2 d	>15 mg/dL

Basal Energy Expenditure (BEE)

Females:

BEE = 655 + (9.6 × weight in kg) + (1.7 × height in cm) − (4.7 × age [y])

Males:

BEE = 66 + (13.75 × weight in kg) + (5 × height in cm) − (6.76 × age [y])

Stress Factors:

Hypermetabolism:

Mild (uncomplicated postoperative state):	1.2
Moderate (multiple trauma)	1.2–1.5
Severe (severe burns and multiple organ dysfunction)	1.5–2.0

Activity Factors:

Bed rest = 1.2
Ambulatory = 1.3

Calorie needs for 24 hours = BEE × stress factor × activity factor

References: Young ME: Malnutrition and wound healing. Heart Lung 17:1, 60–69, 1988; Kimbrell JD: "Alterations in Metabolism" In Huddleston VB (ed): Multisystem Organ Failure: Pathophysiology and Clinical Implications, pp 11, 125–139. St Louis, MO, Mosby-Year Book, 1992; Mainous MR, Deitch EA: Nutrition in infection. Surg Clin North Am 74(3):659–676, 1994

---

assess stress and activity (see display). The goal is to provide enough calories to meet energy requirements without overfeeding or underfeeding. This equation may overestimate a patient's calorie need and result in overfeeding. Another method is to provide 25 to 30 kcal/kg for ideal body weight. All calculations should be done using ideal body weight.

Optimal therapy provides a ratio of nonprotein calories (glucose) to nitrogen (amino acids) of 150:1. This ratio preserves the nitrogen balance of the body by allowing glucose to be used for calories and amino acids to be used for protein synthesis. If this ratio is not preserved, excess amino acids are lost in the urine when adequate glucose is present, or amino acids are used for calories if adequate glucose is not present.

The critically ill patient requires 1.5 g/kg/d of protein. Some patients, such as those with thermal injuries who lose larger amounts of protein through their wounds, should receive 2 g/kg/d. Carbohydrates should be supplied at a rate of 4 to 7 g/kg/d, or 50% to 60% of total calories. Carbohydrates improve nitrogen retention and assist in restoring nitrogen balance, provided adequate protein is supplied. Fat should be supplied approximately at a rate of 1 g/kg/d, or 25% to 40% of total calories. In addition, critically ill patients may need increased amounts of vitamins and minerals due to the illness, the risk of malabsorption, and some medications that increase requirements.

METHODS OF NUTRITIONAL SUPPORT

After determining nutritional needs, an administration route is selected. Administration routes for providing nutrition are enteral feeding and parenteral nutrition. Parenteral nutrition can be administered through a peripheral intravenous line or through a central venous catheter. If enteral feedings alone do not meet nutritional needs, they can be supplemented with peripheral parenteral nutrition. If the patient's intestinal tract cannot be used for feeding, parenteral nutrition is given through a centrally placed catheter. Figure 39–1 provides an explanation of routes to deliver nutritional support in adults.

Enteral Feeding

INDICATIONS

Patients who have functioning gastrointestinal tracts can receive enteral feedings. This is the least dangerous route for these patients. It is also the least complicated and the least costly way of providing nutritional support. Furthermore, the intestinal mucosa has important functions and contains the normal flora that aids digestion of nutrients. On the other hand, nonuse and hypoxia of the intestines cause atrophy of gut mucosa that predisposes the patient to ulceration and the escape of enteric bacteria.

Considerations for the Older Patient
Determination of Nutritional Requirements

- The risk for malnutrition increases as functional abilities decrease.
- Protein requirements remain the same.
- There is decreased ability to tolerate glucose loads.
- There is a greater chance of having a higher gastric pH (achlorhydria).

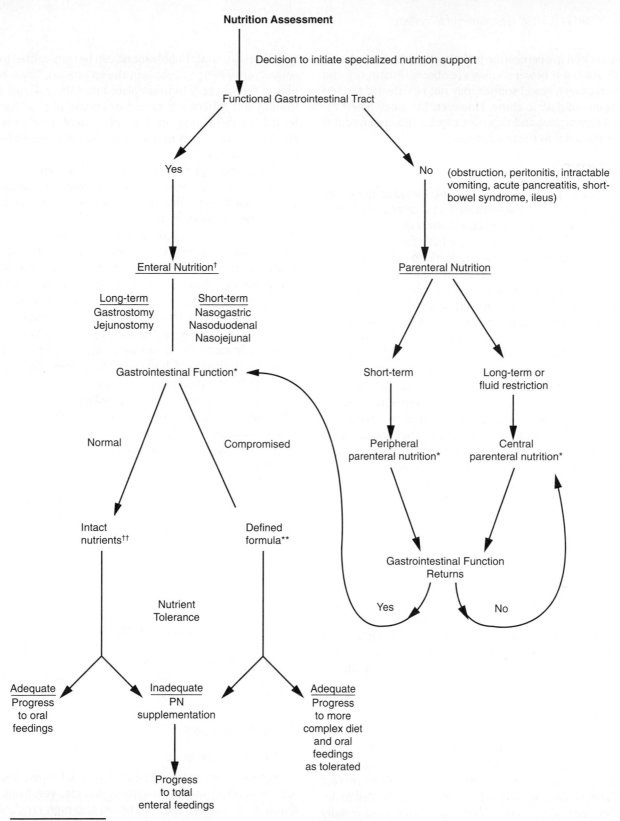

Nutrition Assessment

Decision to initiate specialized nutrition support

Functional Gastrointestinal Tract

Yes

No (obstruction, peritonitis, intractable vomiting, acute pancreatitis, short-bowel syndrome, ileus)

Enteral Nutrition†

Long-term
Gastrostomy
Jejunostomy

Short-term
Nasogastric
Nasoduodenal
Nasojejunal

Parenteral Nutrition

Gastrointestinal Function*

Short-term

Long-term or fluid restriction

Normal

Compromised

Peripheral parenteral nutrition*

Central parenteral nutrition*

Intact nutrients††

Defined formula**

Gastrointestinal Function Returns

Yes

No

Nutrient Tolerance

Adequate
Progress to oral feedings

Inadequate
PN supplementation

Adequate
Progress to more complex diet and oral feedings as tolerated

Progress to total enteral feedings

FIGURE 39-1
Algorithm for clinical decision making concerning the route of nutrition support. (Reference: ASPEN Board of Directors: Guidelines for the use of parenteral and enteral nutrition in adults and pediatric patients. J Paren Ent Nutr 17(4 suppl), 1993)
*Formulation of enteral and parenteral solutions should be made considering organ function (eg, cardiac, renal, respiratory, hepatic).
†Feeding may be more appropriate distal to the pylorus if the patient is at increased aspiration risk.
**Elemental low/high fat content, lactose-free, fiber-rich, and modular formulas should be provided according to patient's gastrointestinal tolerance.
††Polymeric, complete formulas, or pureed diets are appropriate.

A common misperception is that enteral feedings should not be started if bowel sounds are absent. Postinjury and postoperatively, bowel sounds may not be detected for 3 to 5 days due to gastric atony. However, the small bowel retains its absorptive and digestive capabilities, and feedings can be started into the duodenum.

SOLUTIONS

Commercially prepared elemental nutritional solutions are usually used because they deliver 1 to 2 calories per milliliter and contain carbohydrate, fat, protein, and vitamins. However, various formulas are available for enteral nutrition: polymeric, peptide, elemental, and modular. All of the solutions contain proteins, carbohydrates, fats, vitamins, and minerals. The difference lies in how they are structured and provided. The dietary formula selected is based on the patient's ability to digest and absorb major nutrients, the total nutrient requirements, and fluid and electrolyte restrictions. Polymeric solutions contain proteins that require normal pancreatic enzymes for digestion. Peptide and elemental solutions require a minimal amount of digestion and are virtually residue free. They are recommended for patients with compromised gastrointestinal function.

Modular formulas are also available. They contain individual protein carbohydrates and fats and can be used to create specific formulas. Dietitians assist with these formulas because improper mixing can result in metabolic abnormalities. Special formulas have been developed for specific patient populations, such as patients with pulmonary disease, hepatic or renal failure, and hypermetabolism due to sepsis, burns, and trauma.

PROCEDURE

Enteral feedings are delivered by several methods. A tube can be inserted through the nose and placed in the stomach (nasogastric), duodenum, or jejunum (nasoenteric). A tube can be surgically or percutaneously inserted through the abdomen into the stomach (gastrostomy) or jejunum (jejunostomy).

Nasogastric tubes are used for short-term feeding. They are less comfortable for patients because they are larger in diameter and made of stiffer material than nasoenteric tubes. Patients with nasogastric tubes are also at greatest risk for aspiration, especially when they are unconscious, mechanically ventilated, or otherwise less able to protect their airway. Gastric contents can be easily aspirated to determine feeding residuals. Nasoenteric tubes are usually more comfortable for patients because they have a smaller diameter and are more flexible. There is less likelihood of aspiration because the tube is placed past the pylorus. It is more difficult to check feeding residual, however, because the lumen is smaller and tends to collapse when aspirated.

Proper tube placement is confirmed by abdominal x-ray before beginning feedings. Gastric tube placement can be verified every 4 hours by aspirating gastric contents from the tube. Injecting air into the tube and auscultating the gastric bubble is not an accurate method for verifying placement because an air bubble sound can be transmitted to the epigastrum when the tube is in the esophagus. These techniques do not apply to tubes placed past the pylorus. Suctioning and patient movement or coughing have the potential for dislodging the tube placement. Any time the exact tube location is in question, the tube should be removed and reinserted.

The patient's tolerance to enteral feeding depends on the rate of flow and the osmolality of the formula. Feedings can be administered by bolus, intermittent infusion, on continuous infusion. Bolus feedings are considered the most natural method physiologically and they allow the bowel to rest between feedings. However, they are generally not well tolerated. They are often accompanied by nausea, bloating, cramping, diarrhea, or aspiration. Intermittent slow-gravity drip feedings are administered four to six times a day over a period of 30 to 60 minutes. Continuous infusions are administered with the aid of a feeding pump to ensure a constant flow rate. The continuous method is best suited to the critically ill patient, because it allows more time for nutrients to be absorbed in the intestine.

Continuous infusions are required when the patient has a feeding tube placed past the pylorus, because the small bowel cannot handle large amounts, such as those delivered by bolus feedings. The maximum recommended rate is 125 mL/h.

A full-strength solution is started at a slow rate (20 mL/h) and increased by 10 mL every 4 hours until the goal rate is achieved. The goal of nutritional therapy is to achieve full-strength feedings in the shortest possible time. Diluting feedings is not recommended because it may contribute to osmotic diarrhea and increase the time needed to meet the nutritional requirements.

The ultimate goal is for patients to return to oral eating. As their condition improves, enteral feedings can be changed from continuous to nighttime only. Discontinuing daytime feedings allows the appetite to return. Enteral feeding can be discontinued when patients can drink enough liquid to maintain hydration and can eat two thirds of their nutritional requirements.

COMPLICATIONS

Gastric Intolerance

Signs and symptoms of gastrointestinal intolerance to enteral feeding include diarrhea, nausea, vomiting, abdominal discomfort and distention, and high residual returns. Diarrhea is the most frequent problem and can be caused by an infusion rate that is too rapid or by intolerance of lactose, fat, or osmolality. Reducing the infusion rate, changing to a peptide-based formula that is easier to digest, and giving an absorbing product, such as Metamucil, may help. Liquid medications may also cause diarrhea because they have a hypertonic, sorbitol base. Antidiarrhea medication should not be given until *Clostridium difficile* infection has been ruled out. Diarrhea can also be due to hypoalbuminemia.

Diarrhea can also be caused by bacterial contamination of the solution or administration set. To prevent this, hang no more than 4 hours of feeding solution in the container at one time, and use open solution within 24 hours. Change administration sets daily, rinse them between bolus feedings, and use good handwashing technique when handling the equipment.

High gastric residuals can also be a problem. The definition of a high residual is a return of at least half of the hourly feeding rate. The initial intervention is to hold the feeding for 1 hour and check the residual. This allows time for digestion and for the volume in the stomach to decrease. Repeat this procedure every 1 to 2 hours until the residual volume drops and feedings can be resumed. This reduces the risk for aspiration, abdominal distention, and discomfort.

Fluid and electrolyte imbalance may occur. If this is due to dehydration from inadequate fluid intake, give extra fluid boluses. Electrolytes can also be given through the feeding tube. Hyperglycemia may occur due to increased glucose load (see metabolic complications of parenteral nutrition).

Clogging of Feeding Solution

A clogged feeding tube can delay the administration of nutrients and medications. Crushed tablets may leave a residual that blocks the tube. To prevent clogging, administer liquid medications when available. Flush the tube thoroughly before and after each medication. This will avoid incompatibilities between the medications and feedings and reduce the incidence of clogging. Also flush when turning off feedings for procedures to avoid tube clogging.

Aspiration of Feeding Solution

Aspiration of feeding solution into the lung is a potentially fatal complication. The risk of aspiration can be reduced by maintaining the head of the bed in a 30-degree position and by checking for gastric residuals. Feedings should be discontinued at least 30 minutes before any procedure for which the patient must lay flat. Feeding solutions, particularly gastric feedings, should be colored with food coloring to detect aspiration immediately.

Parenteral Nutrition

There are two types of parenteral nutrition: peripheral and central. Central parenteral nutrition is also called total parenteral nutrition (TPN).

CLINICAL APPLICATION:
Nursing Intervention Guidelines
Reducing the Risk of Aspiration in Enteral Feeding

- Keep the patient's head elevated 30 degrees.
- Stop the feeding 30 minutes before positioning the patient flat for procedures or care.
- Check gastric residuals hourly.

INDICATIONS

Peripheral parenteral nutrition is provided as a supplement for patients whose nutritional and caloric intake is marginal. The accompanying display lists indications for parenteral nutrition. It is recommended that peripheral nutrition be given for no more than 2 weeks. Peripheral nutrition is not recommended for patients with minor injuries who are adequately nourished and expected to resume eating in 5 to 7 days.

When the patient requires long-term nutritional support or has developed protein-calorie malnutrition, TPN is indicated. Parenteral feedings are also indicated for patients with hemodynamic instability because enteral feedings are not recommended when splanchnic blood flow is decreased.

Parenteral nutrition has disadvantages; mainly, it starves the gut and can therefore promote infectious processes. Furthermore, certain necessary nutrients that are normally in an oral diet are missing from TPN, either because they are unstable or poorly soluble in solution. Interestingly, while intravenous nutrition can reduce catabolism, it fails to enhance anabolism significantly in critically ill patients. Patients receiving parenteral nutrition may also experience hunger and food cravings.

SOLUTION

Peripheral Parenteral Nutrition

Peripheral parenteral nutrition provides protein-sparing calories in a solution of dextrose 5% to 10%, amino acids 3.5%, and lipids that are isotonic. In total nutrient admixtures, lipid emulsions are mixed with the amino acid and dextrose solution and administered in a single container through a peripheral vein. The solution is infused over a 24-hour period. The flow rate depends on the calorie needs of the patient. Peripheral nutrition has the potential to reduce infection rates, personnel time, and cost.

CLINICAL APPLICATION:
Assessment Parameters
Indications for Parenteral Nutrition

Malabsorption

Ulcer disease	Protein-losing gastroenteropathy
Chronic diarrhea	
Chronic vomiting	Pancreatitis
Failure to thrive	Diverticulitis
Gastrointestinal obstruction	Alimentary tract fistula
	Alimentary tract anomalies
Granulomatous enterocolitis	Hepatic failure
	Biliary disease
Ulcerative colitis	Short bowel syndrome

Hypermetabolic States

Indolent wounds and decubitus ulcers
Complicated trauma or surgery
Sepsis
Burns

Central Parenteral Nutrition

TPN begins with a solution containing a concentration of 15% to 35% glucose and 3.5% to 5% amino acids. The amount of carbohydrate and protein is determined by the patient's illness and nutritional needs. Special amino acid preparations for renal and hepatic failure are available.

Fat, in the form of lipid emulsions, is included in the nutritional regimen to prevent essential fatty acid deficiency. Fat emulsions also assist in controlling hyperglycemia, because calories obtained from fat do not require the use of insulin for metabolism. These are available in either a 10% solution, which delivers 1.1 kcal/mL or 20% solution, which delivers 2 kcal/mL. A fat emulsion provides up to 40% of the required calories. Lipids are administered through a "Y" connector into the parenteral nutrition line. Because the large fat molecule cannot pass through a filter, the risk of infection is increased. If the serum triglyceride level rises more than 20% above baseline, lipids are usually discontinued until the level returns to normal.

Electrolytes, vitamins, and trace minerals are added daily to the TPN solution. Electrolytes include potassium, sodium, chloride, magnesium, acetate, and phosphorus. Patients who experience unusual electrolyte loss may need additional supplements. A multiple vitamin preparation, including fat-soluble and water-soluble vitamins, is added to the preparation. If vitamin K is necessary to prevent development of prolonged prothrombin time, it can be given in the solution or more commonly, through intravenous or intramuscular injection. The trace elements zinc, copper, chromium, and magnesium are routinely added to solution. Laboratory tests, known as a nutrition or TPN panel, are done on a daily basis to monitor levels. The chemistry and tests for these panels are listed in Table 39–2.

PROCEDURE

The routes for parenteral nutrition are depicted in Figure 39–2. Peripheral parental nutrition requires good venous access, such as the basilic vein. Although peripheral parenteral solutions are isotonic, this vein is too susceptible to irritation and infection for long-term therapy. The use of peripherally inserted central catheter lines increases patient comfort and has improved the ability to provide nutrition through this access.

Parenteral nutrition must be delivered through a central venous catheter when the patient's nutritional requirements are above normal. Because TPN is a high-calorie nitrogen solution, it must be rapidly diluted and dispersed within the blood vessels. The superior vena cava is an excellent site for delivery. Passage of the catheter by way of the subclavian vein is the route of choice, because it allows the patient the greatest freedom of movement without disturbing the site and because the incidence of infection at this level of the body is lower. Jugular veins can be used but are not as comfortable for the patient. Critically ill patients, however, seldom have numerous sites available for intravenous access. The introduction of multiple lumen catheters has greatly facilitated the care of patients who are receiving hyperalimentation therapy. These catheters provide separate infusion channels with exits into different sites in the central vein. Therefore, one channel can be dedicated to exclusive use of TPN, while one or two more remain for the administration of intravenous antibiotics, medications, blood products, and blood sampling.

Parenteral nutrition can be reduced once the patient begins to tolerate enteral feedings. As the enteral feeding rate is increased, parenteral nutrition should be weaned to avoid the complications associated with overfeeding.

COMPLICATIONS

Intravenous feedings can cause mechanical, metabolic, and infectious complications.

Mechanical Complications

Mechanical complications include those associated with central venous catheterization insertion, such as pneumothorax and catheter misdirection. Thrombosis can occur at the tip of the catheter due to the hypertonic solution.

Metabolic Complications

Most metabolic complications result from imprudent formula administration. These can be prevented and corrected by adjustments in the daily formula. Hepatic dysfunction may be seen in patients receiving lipid infusions; this is often related to the amount and flow rate. Respiratory distress can result from overfeeding carbohydrates. To control this problem, the formula can be altered to contain fewer calories from glucose and more calories from fat.

Hyperglycemia, or a blood sugar elevated over 220 mg/dL, can occur if the pancreas does not respond to the increased glucose load. Although it can be caused by either enteral or parenteral feedings, it is more commonly seen in patients receiving parenteral nutrition. Even slightly elevated blood glucose levels can impair the function of lymphocytes, leading to immunosuppression and increased infection risk. Insulin should be administered either through a continuous infusion or subcutaneously to maintain blood glucose levels within normal values.

TABLE 39-2 CLINICAL APPLICATION: Diagnostic Studies
Possible Tests on a Nutritional Panel

Chemistry	Normal Ranges
pH	7.35–7.45
Sodium	135–145 mEq/L
Potassium	3.5–5.3 mEq/L
Chlorides	100–109 mEq/L
Calcium	4.5–5.7 mEq/L
Phosphorus	1.45–2.76 mEq/L
Magnesium	1.4–2.1 mEq/L
Glucose	70–115 mg/dL
BUN	8–22 mg/dL
Creatinine	0.8–1.6 mg/dL
Bicarbonate	22–26 mEq/L
Total protein	5.5–8.0 g/dL

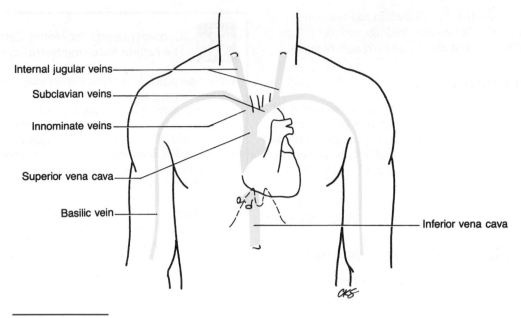

FIGURE 39-2
Venous anatomy for hyperalimentation routes.

Infectious Complications

Both the solution and the indwelling catheter are prime sites for infection. Any break in the system is an entrance for infection.

The solution is an excellent culture medium for many species of bacteria and fungi due to the high glucose content. It should be prepared by a pharmacist under a laminar air-flow hood to to ensure a particle-free environment. The solution bag must be changed every 24 hours. The tubing is changed according to institution policy, generally every 24 to 48 hours.

ASSESSMENT AND MANAGEMENT

Goals of care in nutritional support include the following:

- Provide nutritional support to maintain or improve nitrogen balance.
- Maintain fluid and electrolyte balance.
- Prevent infection and other complications associated with nutritional support.

Meeting these goals involves a multidisciplinary approach that includes the nurse, physician, dietitian, and pharmacist. Regardless of the type of nutritional support, the nurse is responsible for certain interventions. Feeding tube or line site care is of paramount importance to ensure the delivery of nutrients and medications and avoid infection.

Daily Assessments

The nurse evaluates laboratory data, weight, nutritional intake, and changes in patient status daily to determine progress toward goals. The amount of additives needed to maintain the patient's electrolyte balance is based on serial blood tests. Nutritional panel tests should be done on a daily basis to ensure electrolyte balance. When stable, these data can be checked every other day to once a week. Nitrogen balance is monitored by serial blood nitrogen, creatinine, and protein levels.

There is a risk for fluid imbalance, particularly with parenteral nutrition. Intake and output and urine-specific gravity are additional signs to monitor. If the patient is at risk for dehydration, he or she is assessed for excessive thirst, decreased skin turgor, headache, fatigue, nausea, and vomiting. If the patient is at risk for fluid excess, evaluations are made regarding lung congestion, jugular vein distention, and increased central venous pressure or pulmonary artery wedge pressure.

The nurse assesses the patient receiving parenteral therapy for headache, nausea, and lassitude, which are early symptoms that an infusion is too rapid. Edema and excessive weight gain may indicate fluid overload or overfeeding. A rise in temperature, white blood cell count, blood, or urine glucose level may indicate sepsis in a patient who previously tolerated nutritional support. In patients receiving parenteral therapy, these symptoms may indicate catheter sepsis.

The effects, side effects, and interactions of medications are considered in relation to nutrition therapy. This includes interaction with the nutrition solution and for enteral feedings, effects on the gastrointestinal tract.

Asepsis

Asepsis begins with insertion of the catheter under strict sterile technique. The catheter insertion site is a potential portal of entry for organisms. This can be minimized by meticulous catheter care. The risks of infection are reduced when nutrition is provided peripherally as opposed to centrally. Phlebitis is the most frequent complication of peripheral nutrition. If catheter sepsis is suspected, the catheter must be removed and the tip cultured. In addition, when patients who have tolerated enteral feedings complain of gastrointestinal difficulties, it may be an early sign of sepsis.

Dressing Changes

The site is redressed per institution policy, usually every 24 to 72 hours, using either a sterile transparent or gauze dressing. At the time of the dressing change, the site should be examined for signs of leakage, edema, and inflammation. The skin must be cleansed well with an antibacterial solution to remove pathogenic organisms. The presence of a tracheostomy or open and draining wounds near the insertion site requires special precautions to maintain sterility of the site.

Drug Administration Precautions

To maintain sterility of the parenteral nutrition line, do not give intravenous push or piggyback medication in the hyperalimentation solution. Never add steroids, pressor drugs, or antibiotics to the base solution, because they can interact with the fibrin hydrolysate or with one another, forming a precipitate that would not be visible to the naked eye. In addition, if drugs were mixed in the solution, the flow rate might have to be adjusted according to their requirements rather than those of the nutritional hypertonic solution. It is acceptable to add certain medications, such as insulin, to the base solution; however, they cannot be titrated when added to the formula. Instead, select an alternative route for intravenous medication or blood transfusion.

Consistency of Flow

The solution is infused at a constant rate over a 24-hour period to achieve maximum assimilation of the nutrients and to prevent hyperglycemia or hypoglycemia. The aim of treatment is a continuous infusion that meets the caloric requirements of the patient by allowing maximum use of the carbohydrate and protein substrates with minimal renal excretion. Do not increase the flow rate to compensate for interruption or slowing of the infusion, because glycosuria with osmotic diuresis (diuresis from body compartment and cells leading to dehydration) can occur. Never discontinue TPN abruptly. If the solution bag empties and no replacement is available, a solution containing at least 10% dextrose is infused to prevent rebound hypoglycemia.

Volume is given according to established water metabolism levels (2,500 mL/24 h in adults and 100 mL/24 h in infants). If there is renal or cardiac dysfunction, fluid volume must be carefully calculated to prevent cardiopulmonary overload. The patient's signs and symptoms and laboratory test results should be monitored to assess the response to fluid volume.

Family Involvement

Care also includes providing information and emotional support to the patient and family. Examples include explaining the procedure, what to expect, risks, and expected outcomes.

Considerations for Home Care
The Patient Receiving Nutrition Support

- Consider patient's ability to become independent in home care regimen.
- Evaluate support system available in home.
- Identify an in-home caretaker who is willing and able to learn and carry out the home care regimen.
- If the patient does not have a caretaker at home and there are concerns about patient's ability to become independent, reevaluate discharge plan.
- Patient/caregiver learning should include determining procedures and risks, picking up patient and equipment problems early, troubleshooting, and following up with health care provider.
- Refer and communicate with home care services.
- Written instructions are provided for patient.
- If possible, the amount or rate of nutrition support should not be changed on the day of discharge to home.

Exercise

Exercise promotes protein synthesis and preserves joint movement and strength. An exercise program may include range of motion and isotonic exercises, and ambulation.

Clinical Applicability Challenges

Self-Challenge: Critical Thinking

1. *A malnourished, older man with a history of alcoholism, hepatic failure, and diabetes received abdominal injuries in a motor vehicle accident. His injuries were not life threatening. Postoperatively, he is hemodynamically stable, and the physician orders TPN. Explore why TPN may have been ordered, and develop rationale about why this may or may not be appropriate nutrition therapy for this patient.*

Study Questions

1. *One mechanism that explains hyperglycemia during the stress response is*
   a. *increased insulin release from the pancreas.*
   b. *glucagon suppression.*
   c. *increased uptake of glucose in the peripheral tissues.*
   d. *catecholamine release.*

2. *A diagnostic test that reflects low protein mass of internal organs is*
   a. *serum albumin.*
   b. *anthropometric measurements.*
   c. *immunological studies.*
   d. *nitrogen balance.*

3. *A nursing intervention to prevent aspiration of enteral feedings is*
   a. *Trendelenburg position.*
   b. *bolus feedings.*
   c. *gastric residual checks.*
   d. *insertion of large-bore feeding tube.*

4. The most common complication of TPN therapy is
   a. hypomagnesemia.
   b. hypoglycemia.
   c. sepsis.
   d. hypovolemia.

BIBLIOGRAPHY

Anding R: Nutrition support for the critically order patient. Crit Care Nurs Q 19(2):13–22, 1996

ASPEN Board of Directors: Guidelines for the use of parenteral and enteral nutrition in adult and pediatric patients. J Paren Ent Nutr 17(4) Suppl, 1993

DeBiasse MA, Wilmore DW: What is optimal nutritional support? Soc Crit Care Med 2(2):122–130, 1994

Elia M: Changing concepts of nutrient requirements in disease implications for artificial nutrition support. Lancet 345(8960):1279–1284, 1995

Fitzsimmons L, Hadley SA: Nutrition management of the metabolically stressed patient. Crit Care Nurs Q 17(4):79–90, 1995

Gianno S, ST. John RE: Nutritional assessment of the critically ill patient. Crit Care Nurs Clin North AM 5(1):1–15, 1993

Mainous MR, Deitch EA: Nutrition and infection. Surg Clin North Am 74(3):659–876, 1994

Pomposelli JJ, Bistrian BR: Is total parenteral nutrition immunosuppressive? New Horiz 2(2):224–229, 1994

Posa PJ: Nutritional support in the critically ill patient: Bedside strategies for successful patient outcomes. Crit Care Nurs Q 16(4):61–79, 1994

40

Common Gastrointestinal Disorders

OBJECTIVES

Based on the content in this chapter, the reader should be able to:

- Examine the pathophysiological concepts that help define gastrointestinal bleeding and obstruction, hepatitis, cirrhosis, and pancreatitis.
- Compare and contrast the pertinent history, physical examination, and diagnostic study findings for gastrointestinal bleeding and obstruction, hepatitis, cirrhosis, and pancreatitis.
- Discuss six laboratory studies that are useful in diagnosing gastrointestinal bleeding and obstruction, hepatitis, cirrhosis, and pancreatitis.

- Analyze the similarities and differences in caring for patients with gastrointestinal bleeding and obstruction, hepatitis, cirrhosis, and pancreatitis.
- Explore the nursing role in assessing, managing, and evaluating a plan of care for patients with gastrointestinal bleeding and obstruction, hepatitis, cirrhosis, and pancreatitis.

*C*ommon gastrointestinal (GI) disorders affect the esophagus, stomach, intestine, liver, and pancreas. Disorders include acute GI bleeding, intestinal obstruction, hepatitis, cirrhosis of the liver, and acute pancreatitis. The health care goal is to prevent these diseases or, when they do occur, to detect and treat them early in the course of illness. These diseases may worsen, however, and result in complications and critical illness. This chapter focuses on GI disorders that may require critical care.

ACUTE GASTROINTESTINAL BLEEDING

Bleeding in the GI tract is caused primarily by gastric ulcers or gastritis. However, esophageal varices, Mallory-Weiss tears of the gastroesophageal junction, carcinoma of the esophagus or stomach, gastric and duodenal ulcers, ulcerative colitis, polyps, diverticula, hemorrhoids, and hypocoagulable states can erupt in a bleeding episode.

The amount and rapidity of upper GI tract bleeding vary considerably. Gastrointestinal bleeding that is the result of an erosion through an artery is profuse and does not stop with medical management. Bleeding that is caused by gastritis or oozing from granulation tissue at the base of an ulcer is smaller in quantity, transient in nature, and usually responds to medical management. Bleeding that occurs from the lower GI tract is rarely life threatening, usually does not warrant admission to an intensive care unit, or is treated surgically.

Pathophysiological Principles

Peptic ulcer disease is the most common cause of upper GI bleeding. These ulcers are characterized by a break in the mucosa extending through the muscularis mucosae. It is usually surrounded by inflamed cells that, over time, are replaced by granulation and finally scar tissue.

An excess secretion of acid and an inability of the mucosa to secrete mucus for protection are thought to contribute to the development of ulcer disease. Risk factors include family history of ulcer disease and the use of aspirin and nonsteroidal anti-inflammatory drugs. Cigarette smoking is linked with the disease and also impairs healing. The organism *Helicobacter pylori* is implicated in the development of bleeding from peptic ulcers.

Stress ulcers are found in critically ill patients with severe trauma, severe burns, sepsis, or cranial or central nervous system disease and in patients on long-term ventilatory support. Decreased perfusion of the stomach mucosa is probably the main mechanism of ulcer development. This contributes to impaired mucus secretion, low mucosal pH, poor mucosal cell regeneration, and decreased tolerance to acid gastric secretions.

In chronic cirrhosis liver failure, cell death in the liver results in increased portal venous pressure. As a result, collateral channels develop in the submucosa of the esophagus, rectum, and anterior abdominal wall to divert blood

---

⚠ **RED FLAG** **Risk Factors for** Gastrointestinal Bleeding

Upper Gastrointestinal Bleeding
- Esophageal
  Varices
  Inflammation
  Ulcers
  Tumors
  Mallory-Weiss tears
- Gastric
  Ulcers
  Gastritis
  Tumors
  Angiodysplasia
- Small intestine
  Peptic ulcers
  Angiodysplasia
  Crohn's disease
  Meckel's diverticulum

Lower Gastrointestinal Bleeding
- Malignant tumors
- Polyps
- Ulcerative colitis
- Crohn's disease
- Angiodysplasia
- Diverticula
- Hemorrhoids
- Rectal fissures
- Massive upper gastrointestinal hemorrhage

---

from the splanchnic circulation away from the liver. As pressure rises in these veins, they become distended with blood and enlarge. These dilated vessels are called varices and can rupture, resulting in massive GI hemorrhage.

Upper GI hemorrhage results in a sudden loss of blood volume, decreased venous return to the heart, and decreased cardiac output. If the bleeding is significant, it results in decreased tissue perfusion. In response to the decreased cardiac output, the body initiates compensatory mechanisms to attempt to maintain perfusion. These mechanisms account for the major signs and symptoms of acute GI bleeding. If blood volume is not replaced, decreased tissue perfusion results in ischemia. The cells shift to anaerobic metabolism, and lactic acid is formed. Decreased blood flow affects all of the body systems, and without sufficient oxygen supply, they begin to fail.

Assessment

HISTORY AND CLINICAL MANIFESTATIONS

The history includes asking about the signs and symptoms and the presence of precipitating factors, such as stress, infection, dizziness, nausea, vomiting, and generalized discomfort. Ask if the patient has had hematemesis or tarry stools.

The patient may report pain with the GI bleed, and this is thought to arise from gastric acid eating the ulcer crater. Epigastric tenderness is uncommon. The abdomen can be soft or distended. Bowel sounds are most often hyperactive due to the sensitivity of the bowel to blood.

Hematemesis

The patient who is vomiting blood is usually bleeding from a source above the ligament of Treitz (at the duodenojejunal junction). Reverse peristalsis is seldom sufficient to cause hematemesis if the bleeding point is below this area. The vomitus can be bright red or like coffee-grounds in appearance, depending on the amount of gastric contents at the time of the bleed and the length of time the blood has been in contact with gastric secretions. Gastric acid converts bright red hemoglobin to brown hematin, accounting for the coffee-ground appearance of the drainage. Maroon or bright red blood results from profuse bleeding and little contact with gastric juices.

Melena

Tarry stools consistently occur in all people who accumulate 500 mL of blood in their stomachs. A tarry stool may be passed if as little as 60 mL of blood has entered the intestinal tract. Massive hemorrhage from the upper GI tract, along with the increased intestinal motility that occurs, can result in stools containing bright red blood. It takes several days after the bleeding has stopped for melena stools to clear. Gastrointestinal blood loss can also be occult (hidden); it is detected by testing vomitus, nasogastric (NG) drainage, or stool with a chemical reagent called guaiac.

Blood Loss

In the first stage of bleeding—less than 800 mL of blood loss—the person may show signs only of weakness, anxiety, and perspiration. With a significant bleed, the body temperature elevates to 38.4° to 39°C (101°–102°F) in response to the bleeding, and bowel sounds are hyperactive.

If blood loss is moderate to severe (> 800 mL loss), a sympathetic nervous system response causes a release of the catecholamines, epinephrine and norepinephrine. These initially cause an increase in heart rate and peripheral vascular vasoconstriction in an attempt to maintain an adequate blood pressure. With moderate to severe blood loss, signs and symptoms of shock are present.

As the shock syndrome progresses, the release of catecholamines triggers the blood vessels in the skin, lungs, intestines, liver, and kidneys to constrict, thereby increasing the volume of blood flow to the brain and heart. Because of the decreased flow of blood in the skin, the person's skin is cool to the touch. With decreased blood flow to the lungs, hyperventilation occurs to maintain adequate gas exchange.

A change in blood pressure greater than 10 mmHg with a corresponding heart rate increase of 20 beats/min in sitting or standing position indicates blood loss of greater than 1,000 mL. The patient's response to blood loss depends on the amount and rate of blood loss, age, degree of compensation, and rapidity of treatment.

DIAGNOSTIC STUDIES

Common diagnostic findings for the patient with acute GI bleeding are listed in the accompanying display. A hematocrit and hemoglobin are ordered with the complete blood count. It is important to consider that the hematocrit generally does not change substantially during the first few hours after an acute GI bleed because of compensatory mechanisms. Fluids that are administered on admission also can affect the blood count, diluting the hematocrit. The white blood cell count and glucose may be increased, reflecting the body's response to stress. Decreases in potassium and sodium may be found due to the accompanying vomiting.

If the patient has been in shock with decreased blood flow to the liver, metabolic waste products may accumulate in the blood. This, combined with the absorption of decomposed blood from the intestinal tract and a decrease of blood flow through the kidneys, causes an increase in the blood urea level. The blood urea nitrogen (BUN) can be used to follow the course of a GI bleed. A BUN above 40—in the setting of a GI bleed and a normal creatinine level—indicates a major bleed. The BUN will return to normal approximately 12 hours after the bleeding has stopped.

Liver function tests are used to evaluate the patient's hematological integrity. A prolonged prothrombin time can indicate liver disease or concurrent long-term anticoagulant therapy. Respiratory alkalosis is common due to activation of the sympathetic nervous system from the loss of blood. If large amounts of blood are lost, metabolic acidosis occurs as a result of anaerobic metabolism, as described previously. Hypoxemia may also be present because of decreased circulating hemoglobin levels and resultant impairment in oxygen transport to cells.

Endoscopy is the procedure of choice to diagnose the exact site of the bleed, because direct mucosal inspection is

> **CLINICAL APPLICATION:**
> **Assessment Parameters**
> *Diagnostic Findings for Acute Gastrointestinal Bleeding*

Complete blood count
- Decreased hemoglobin
- Decreased hematocrit
- Elevated white blood cell count

Electrolyte panel
- Decreased serum potassium
- Elevated serum sodium
- Elevated serum glucose
- Elevated lactate (severe bleed)

Hematology profile
- Prolonged prothrombin time
- Prolonged partial thromboplastin time

Arterial blood gases
- Respiratory alkalosis
- Hypoxemia

possible with use of a fiberoptic scope. Barium studies also can be done, although they are often not conclusive if there are clots in the stomach or if there is superficial bleeding. Angiography is used if the bleeding source is not accessible by the endoscope.

Management

Caring for the patient with acute GI bleeding is a collaborative endeavor that includes these steps:

- Assess the severity of blood loss.
- Replace a sufficient amount of fluids and blood products to counteract shock.
- Diagnose the cause of bleeding.
- Plan and implement treatment.
- Manage the ongoing plan of care, and monitor progress.

FLUID AND BLOOD PRODUCT RESUSCITATION

The patient with an acute GI bleed requires immediate intravenous access with one or two large-bore intravenous catheters. To prevent progression of hypovolemic shock, fluid is replaced intravenously using solutions such as Ringer's lactate or normal saline. Vital signs are assessed continuously as fluids are replaced. Urinary output is measured hourly. Blood losses of greater than 1,500 mL require blood replacement in addition to fluids. The patient's blood is typed and cross-matched, and packed red blood cells are usually infused to reestablish oxygen-carrying capacity of the blood. Other blood products, such as platelets, clotting factors, and calcium, may also be ordered according to results of laboratory tests and the patient's underlying condition. Calcium replacement may be necessary if large numbers of banked red blood cells are transfused because the preservative (citrate) in the product binds with calcium.

Rarely, vasoactive drugs are used until fluid balance is restored to maintain blood pressure and perfusion to vital body organs. Dopamine, epinephrine, and norepinephrine are drugs that can be ordered to stabilize the patient until definitive treatment can be undertaken.

ENDOSCOPIC THERAPIES

Sclerotherapy is the treatment of choice if the site of the bleed can be found using endoscopy. The bleeding sites are most often sclerosed with a sclerosing agent. These agents traumatize the endothelium, causing necrosis and eventual sclerosis of the bleeding vessel. Thermal methods of endoscopic tamponade include the heater probe, laser photocoagulation, and electrocoagulation. Hemostasis is achieved in 85% of the cases, although it may take four to six sclerosing sessions to obliterate the varices.

In addition, endoscopic variceal ligation may be done. This technique involves the placement of "elastic bands" positioned to strangulate the variceal channel and eliminate

blood flow through the friable vessel. It has been shown to be as effective as sclerotherapy and to improve mortality rates.[1] The placement of a shunt between hepatic vessels (transjugular intrahepatic portosystem stent [TIPS]) to decrease portal pressures may be considered if other methods of managing esophageal varices fail (see complications of cirrhosis).

GASTRIC LAVAGE

Gastric lavage may be ordered during acute bleeding episodes, but it is a controversial treatment modality. Some clinicians believe that lavage disrupts the normal body clotting mechanism over the bleeding site. Other clinicians believe it can help to clear blood from the stomach, assisting diagnosis of the cause of bleeding during endoscopy. If lavage is ordered, 1,000 to 2,000 mL of room temperature sterile normal saline or water is instilled by NG tube. It is then removed by hand with a syringe or placed to intermittent suction until gastric secretions are clear.

Patients with NG tubes and increased intragastric pressures are at risk for aspirating gastric contents. Therefore, they must be monitored closely for gastric distention and positioned with the head elevated to prevent gastric reflux. If this position is contraindicated, place in the right lateral decubitus position that facilitates passage of gastric contents across the pylorus.

ADMINISTRATION OF VASOPRESSIN

If the bleeding from esophageal varices or gastritis cannot be controlled with stomach lavage or sclerotherapy, intravenous vasopressin (Pitressin) may be instituted. This drug lowers portal hypertension and therefore decreases the flow of blood at the site of bleeding. Vasopressin is administered in a dose of 0.2 to 0.4 U/min initially and may be titrated up to 1.0 U/min. Because it is a vasoconstrictor, it is preferable to administer through a central line. Vasopressin must be used with caution because it can cause hypertension and cardiac ischemia. Therefore, patients should have cardiac monitoring during vasopressin therapy to watch for ST segment changes. Nitroglycerin patches or drips may be used to counteract the ischemic changes. However, it is the GI cramping and nausea that most patients notice and that require monitoring for bowel ischemia and perforation.

The drug somatostatin has also been used to decrease portal pressures, although the mechanism by which it achieves this remains unclear. Octreotide, an analogue of somatostatin, has been used and has fewer side effects.

REDUCTION OF GASTRIC ACID

Because gastric acid is extremely irritating to bleeding sites in the upper GI tract, it is necessary to decrease the acidity of the gastric secretions. This is accomplished by the use of the histamine (H_2)-antagonistic drugs. Examples include cimetidine (Tagamet), ranitidine hydrochloride (Zantac), and famotidine (Pepcid). These drugs decrease the production of gastric acid by inhibiting the action of histamine. A single dose decreases acid secretion for up to 5 hours. The intravenous dose of ranitidine is 50 mg diluted in 50 mL D5W every 6 hours. Intravenous cimetidine can be administered in intermittent doses of 300 mg diluted in 50 mL D5W every 6 hours or as a continuous intravenous infusion of 50 mg/h. Best therapeutic results are achieved when a gastric pH of 4 is maintained.

Antacids are also usually ordered. Antacids act as a direct alkaline buffer and are administered to control gastric pH. The nurse is responsible for correctly aspirating gastric contents for pH and monitoring for side effects of therapy. Sucralfate, a basic aluminum salt of sucrose octasulfate, acts locally as a mucosa-protective drug and can be ordered for stress-bleeding prophylaxis.

CORRECTION OF A HYPOCOAGULABLE STATE

It is not unusual to find a patient with severe GI bleeding in a hypocoagulable state that is due to a variety of clotting factor deficiencies. This often happens to patients with liver failure who are unable to manufacture the factors. Other high-risk patients include those who have received prolonged intravenous feedings, have multiple antibiotics, and are subsequently vitamin K deficient. Regardless of the cause, treatment is necessary to correct this situation to try to reduce the amount of bleeding. Vitamin K can be given in the form of phytonadione (AquaMEPHYTON), 10 mg intramuscularly or very slowly intravenously, in an attempt to restore the prothrombin time to normal. If other major factor deficiencies are thought to exist, fresh frozen plasma is ordered to correct the abnormality.

BALLOON TAMPONADE

Esophageal varices should be suspected in the patient who has been addicted to alcohol and who presents with upper GI bleeding. To control the hemorrhage from the varices, if it is not responsive to other therapy, pressure is exerted on the cardia of the stomach and against the bleeding varices by a double-balloon tamponade (the Sengstaken-Blakemore tube; Fig. 40–1).

After the tube is positioned in the stomach, the stomach balloon is inflated with no more than 50 mL of air. The tube is then slowly withdrawn until the gastric balloon fits snugly against the cardia of the stomach. After it is determined by radiograph examination that the gastric balloon is in the right place, at the cardia and not in the esophagus, the gastric balloon can be further inflated—up to the desired amount without surpassing the balloon's capacity. Traction is then placed on the tube where it enters the patient by means of a piece of sponge rubber, as shown in Figure 40-1, or by traction fixed to a head helmet device or foot of bed.

If bleeding continues, the esophageal balloon is inflated to a pressure of 25 to 40 mmHg and maintained at this pres-

CLINICAL APPLICATION: Nursing Intervention Guidelines
The Patient With an Esophagogastric Balloon Tamponade Tube

- Keep the head of the bed elevated to reduce the flow of blood into the portal system and to prevent reflux into the esophagus.
- When a Sengstaken-Blakemore tube is in place, suction saliva frequently from the upper esophagus because the patient is unable to swallow.
  or
- Place a second nasogastric tube above the esophageal ballon to control these secretions and prevent aspiration.
- Suction the esophageal port to control saliva when a Minnesota tube is used.
- Suction the nasopharynx due to increased secretions resulting from irritation by the tube.
- Clean and lubricate the nostrils frequently to prevent tube-caused pressure areas.
- Irrigate the nasogastric port every 2 hours to ensure patency and to keep the stomach empty.
- Teach the patient to avoid coughing or straining, which increases intra-abdominal pressure and predisposes to further bleeding.
- Restrain the arms if necessary of patients who are at risk for pulling the tube. Agitation, confusion, and restlessness are risk factors.

sure for 24 to 48 hours. Although pressure for longer than 24 hours may be needed to control bleeding, it can cause edema, esophagitis, ulcerations, or perforation of the esophagus. After bleeding is controlled, the balloon is maintained and inflated for no longer than 12 to 24 hours to decrease the risk of gastric ischemia and necrosis. Unfortunately, rebleeding often occurs after balloon deflation unless additional therapeutic measures are taken.

With the gastric and esophageal balloons inflated, oral and nasopharyngeal secretions that are normally swallowed and eliminated collect above the esophageal balloon. If these are not removed, the patient may aspirate the secretions into the lungs. Therefore, the Minnesota tamponade tube was developed (see Fig. 40–1). It has a suction port above the esophageal balloon in addition to the usual ports (two balloon, one gastric suction) of the Sengstaken-Blakemore tube. If this tube is not available, an NG tube may be threaded to sit just above the esophageal balloon to collect secretions. See the display of nursing interventions for esophageal tamponade tube.

People with liver damage tolerate the breakdown products of blood in the intestinal tract very poorly. Therefore, blood should *not* remain in the person's stomach, because it will migrate into the intestinal tract. Bacterial action on the blood in the intestinal tract produces ammonia, which is absorbed into the bloodstream. The ability of the liver to convert ammonia to urea is impaired, and ammonia intoxication ensues.

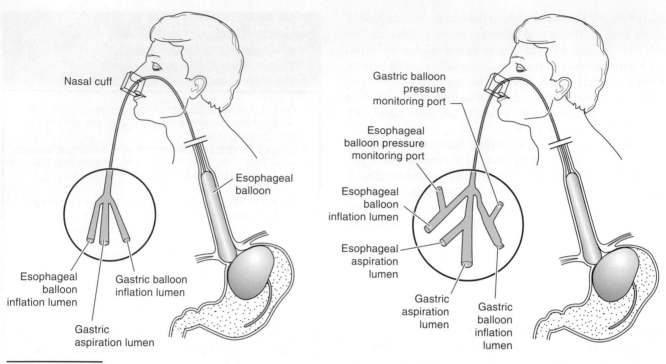

FIGURE 40-1

Comparison of two types of esophageal tamponade tubes. The Sengstaken-Blakemore tube, on the left, is the best known. An additional tube must be placed in the proximal esophagus. The Minnesota esophagogastic tamponade tube, on the right, includes an esophageal aspiration lumen. (From Ignatavicius DD, Workman ML, Mishler MA: Medical Surgical Nursing: A Nursing Process Approach [2nd Ed]. Vol.2. Philadelphia, WB Saunders, 1995)

SURGICAL INTERVENTIONS

Surgery is considered for patients who have massive bleeding that is immediately life threatening and for patients who continue to bleed despite aggressive medical therapies. Surgical therapies for peptic ulcer disease or stress ulcers include gastric resection (antrectomy), gastrectomy, gastroenterostomy, or combined surgeries to restore GI continuity. A vagotomy decreases gastric acid secretion. An antrectomy removes acid-producing cells in the stomach. Billroth I is a procedure that includes a vagotomy and antrectomy with anastomosis of the stomach to the duodenum. A Billroth II involves a vagotomy, a resection of the antrum, and anastomosis of the stomach to the jejunum (Fig. 40–2). A gastric perforation can be surgically treated by simple closure or use of a patch to cover the mucosal hole.

Surgical decompression of portal hypertension can be used in patients with esophageal or gastric varices. In this surgery, called a portal caval shunt, a connection is made between the portal vein and the inferior vena cava that diverts blood flow into the vena cava to decrease pressure.

CLINICAL APPLICATION:
Nursing Intervention Guidelines
Esophageal Tamponade Tube

- Identify and label the tube openings.
- Check each tube opening for patency before insertion.
- Maintain balloon pressure.
- Maintain balloon position.
- Keep scissors readily available at bedside.
- Cut tube immediately to deflate balloon rapidly if gastric balloon ruptures and tube rises into nasopharynx obstructing the airway.
- Cut and remove tube whenever there is a question of respiratory insufficiency or aspiration.

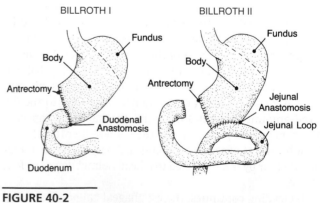

FIGURE 40-2
Billroth I and II procedures.

NURSING INTERVENTIONS

Nursing management of the care plan for patients with GI bleeding includes assessing and monitoring the patient's condition and progress, collaborating with the primary care provider, and carrying out portions of the treatment plan. Nursing is also concerned with the patient's psychosocial response to the illness. These issues need to be incorporated into the plan of care along with physiological issues. Fear and anxiety are responses that often accompany GI bleeding. Patients and families also need information and support during this time. Nurses coordinate plans for the patient's ongoing care.

A patient care study describing Mr. Lane's GI bleeding episode follows. Nursing interventions are presented in the accompanying display.

CLINICAL APPLICATION: Patient Care Study

Mr. Lane is a 45-year-old man admitted from the emergency room to the intensive care unit with an admitting diagnosis of upper GI bleeding. Earlier in the day, he had vomited what he described as a large amount of coffee-ground emesis. He also reported passing one to two maroon-colored stools per rectum. He reported nausea and weakness accompanied by a dull pain in the epigastric region on admission. Mr. Lane reported a history of peptic ulcer disease and has been hospitalized twice in the past 18 months for active GI bleeding. A duodenal ulcer near the pylorus was diagnosed by endoscopy at that time. Both episodes required blood transfusions and were controlled with medical management. Significant risk factors include a family history of peptic ulcer disease, social alcohol use, and a 20-year, one pack per day smoking history.

Admission assessment findings were as follows:

BP lying, 90/60, sitting, 78/50
HR, 120, sinus tachycardia with rare PVCs, no S3, S4
RR, 25/min deep, scattered rhonchi with wheezing anteriorly
Temperature 35.8°C (96.6°F)
Alert; oriented × 3; anxious
Skin: diaphoretic, pale mucous membranes; no edema; peripheral pulses present, equal, thready
GI: abdomen distended with hyperactive bowel sound in all four quadrants; very tender RUQ; liver border WNL

Significant admission laboratory results were as follows:

Hct 25, Hgb 7, WBC 17,000
Coagulation panel and liver function tests, WNL
Na, 145; K, 2; creatinine, 0.8; BUN, 40; glucose, 210
pH, 7.48; PaCO₂, 32; PaO₂, 58; sat, 89%

Three 16-gauge peripheral IVs were inserted, and lactated Ringer's solution was infused at 200 mL/h. A Salem sump nasogastric tube was inserted with an immediate return of 800 mL of coffee-ground, guaiac-positive drainage. Mr. Lane was typed and cross-matched for 8 U of packed red blood cells. Oxygen was delivered at 2 L through a nasal cannula. A 16 Fr indwelling bladder catheter was inserted with an immediate return of 50 mL of dark amber urine. The GI service was consulted for an emergency endoscopy.

INTESTINAL OBSTRUCTION

Intestinal obstruction is the result of a block of the small or large intestine that prohibits normal digestive, absorptive, and elimination processes. The block may be

CLINICAL APPLICATION: Nursing Intervention Guidelines
Potential Complications of Gastrointestinal Bleeding: Hypovolemia

- Monitor for signs and symptoms of shock: vital signs, urinary output, hemodynamic values (PAS, PAD, PAWP, CI, CO, SVR, CVP), oxygen saturation (SaO₂), restlessness, diminished peripheral pulses, cool, pale, or moist skin.
- Monitor fluid status: oral and parenteral intake, urine and gastric drainage.
- Monitor electrolytes, which may be lost with fluids or altered due to fluid shifts.
- Monitor hemoglobin, hematocrit, RBC, PT, PTT, BUN.
- Monitor gastric pH; consult with primary care provider about specific pH range and antacid administration.
- Test gastric drainage or vomitus and stools for occult blood.
- Consult with primary care provider about replacing fluid losses based on findings; administer replacement fluids and blood products as ordered; monitor for adverse reaction to blood products.

paralytic or mechanical. Paralytic obstruction is the result of ineffective intestinal peristalsis, whereas mechanical obstruction results in physical blockage of the intestinal lumen that may be either complete or incomplete. Intestinal obstruction can progress to bowel strangulation, infarction, and perforation and result in potentially life-threatening peritoneal and systemic infection.

Pathophysiological Principles

Obstructions of the small intestine are more common and less problematic than those in the large intestine because the area has fewer sepsis-inducing microorganisms. Obstructions of the small intestine are likely to be caused by abdominal adhesions, whereas obstructions of the large intestine may result from a malignant tumor. Causes of mechanical obstruction are classified according to their organization: *extrinsic* lesions, such as adhesive bands and internal and external hernias; *intrinsic* lesions, such as diverticulitis, carcinoma, and regional enteritis; and closure of the intestinal lumen from such things as gallstones or from intussusception.[2] In some cases, the bowel twists to such an extent that it becomes strangulated, and contents cannot pass. In other cases, the bowel turns in on itself (intussusception), stopping peristalsis and blocking blood flow that leads to ischemia of the affected bowel. If a hernial band or adhesion closes the intestinal lumen at two points, a "closed loop" obstruction is created and often results in severely compromised blood flow to the intestinal wall. Paralytic or adynamic obstructions result from reduced peristalsis anywhere along the GI tract. Adynamic ileus can occur from trauma, handling the bowel during surgery, electrolyte disturbance (hypocalcemia, hypokalemia, and hypomagnesemia), peritonitis, intestinal ischemia, and gram-negative sepsis. Medications that reduce gastric motility (phenothiazines, diphenoxylate [Lomotil], and probanthine) may also contribute to the development of intestinal obstruction. A pathological ileus may develop when the usual mechanisms that slow gastric motility (catecholamines, adrenocorticotropic hormones, inhibitors of smooth muscle) are inappropriately stimulated.

Gas and fluid accumulate above the obstructed segment and result in intestinal distention. Digestive contents join together to form an obstructive mass. Fluid and electrolytes become trapped within the obstructed segment, leak into the peritoneum, and disturb fluid and electrolyte balance. In some cases, the cecum may become so severely distended that it inhibits intramural blood flow and can result in necrosis and gangrene.[3] Obstructions within the small intestine result in the accumulation and absorption of nitrogenous and carbon dioxide gases. Obstructions within the colon result in accumulation of methane and ammonia that are byproducts of bacterial metabolism.[4]

Assessment

HISTORY

The following factors place people at risk for developing intestinal obstruction: recent abdominal surgery or trauma; inflammatory disease, such as diverticulitis, ulcerative co-litis, and Crohn's disease; radiation therapy to the bowel; treatment with vasopressors, benzodiazepines, narcotics, and histamine blockers; stress-induced release of catecholamines; and abdominal discomfort in the patient at risk for Kaposi's sarcoma.

CLINICAL MANIFESTATIONS

The hallmark of intestinal obstruction is abdominal distention. This is most pronounced in colonic obstruction. There is usually little abdominal rigidity. Pain ranges from moderate to severe and often occurs after eating. Temperature does not usually rise above 37.8°C (100°F). A palpable abdominal mass signifies a closed-loop strangulation. Bowel sounds are hypoactive above this type of obstruction and hyperactive, absent, or quiet distal to the obstruction. If rebound tenderness develops, observe for signs and symptoms of shock because perforation is a possibility. Table 40–1 summarizes signs and symptoms of locations and causes of obstructions.

DIAGNOSTIC STUDIES

Laboratory and radiological examinations, along with history and physical findings, aid in diagnosing intestinal obstruction. Hematology, electrolyte, and chemistry panels will reflect the inflammatory, fluid, and electrolyte imbal-

---

TABLE 40-1   CLINICAL APPLICATION: Assessment Parameters
Indications of Intestinal Obstruction

Parameters	Small Intestine Obstruction, Mechanical	Colonic Obstruction, Mechanical	Adynamic Ileus
Pain	Cramping, midabdominal; more severe the higher the obstruction; borborygmi audible during pain episodes Spasmodic; comfortable between episodes Less severe as distention increases *With strangulation,* pain consistent and more localized	Colicky abdominal pain, lower intensity than upper obstructions Stoic patients, older patients may not complain of pain	No colicky pain; discomfort from distention
Vomiting	More profuse the higher the obstruction Usually contains bile and mucus if high in the intestine; more feculent in lower ileal obstruction	Late, if at all Feculent vomitus rare	Frequent, but not profuse Gastric contents and bile, rarely feculent
Obstipation	Unable to pass gas with complete obstruction; may pass stool/gas spontaneously or with enema at onset of obstruction	History of recent changes in bowel habits, failure to pass gas, progressing to constipation	May be complete
Stool	Occasional diarrhea; blood in stool (rare)	Blood in stool (carcinoma, diverticulitis common causes of the obstruction) Ribbon-like stool, diarrhea	
Electrolyte imbalances	Common, less severe in upper bowel; more severe in lower bowel	Rare	

ances common to GI obstruction. Mild leukocytosis is present with simple obstructions, whereas white blood cell elevations from 15,000 to 25,000/µL accompany strangulation. Mesenteric occlusion and perforation will result in white blood cell elevations of 25,000/µL or more.[5] BUN, creatinine, sodium, and osmolality levels reflect the fluid and electrolyte shifts that occur as fluid leaks out of the intestine and electrolytes are either reabsorbed or lost.

Abdominal x-rays are taken with the patient in upright, flat, and side-lying positions. Distended bowel loops will show air and fluid levels to guide in diagnosis. Distention is usually more prominent within the colon for the patients with adynamic ileus, whereas simple obstructions within the small intestine have lower gas levels. Direct visualization (endoscopy, colonoscopy, sigmoidoscopy) and barium studies may confirm the obstruction and aid in determining the type (mechanical, strangulated, paralytic). If colonic obstruction is suspected, a barium enema is used for diagnosis before barium is given by mouth.

Management

When possible, obstructions, especially incomplete obstructions, are treated medically rather than surgically. Oral food and fluid are withheld (ie, nothing by mouth [NPO]), and an NG tube is placed to decompress the stomach or duodenum. Fluid and electrolytes are restored with intravenous lactated Ringer's solution based on central venous pressure readings and electrolyte results. Hyperalimentation may be required.

Patients with paralytic ileus usually do not require surgical intervention. Instead, colonoscopic therapy may be used to decompress the area. Complete obstruction is suspected when the patient fails to pass gas and stool, and gas is not evident in the distal intestine on x-ray.[6] This is accompanied by the risk of a strangulating bowel. Patients with strangulated bowel, early mechanical obstruction, colonic obstruction, and closed-loop obstruction require immediate surgery. Watch all patients with intestinal obstruction closely for signs and symptoms that reflect sepsis, perforation, ischemia, necrosis, or gangrene. Broad spectrum antibiotics are started immediately when strangulation or sepsis is suspected.

Nursing management includes pain and comfort relief measures, monitoring signs and symptoms of obstruction, fluid and electrolyte balance, and detecting complications early.

Complications in Intestinal Obstruction

A strangulated bowel is the major complication of intestinal obstruction. It can lead to ischemia, perforation, sepsis, and multisystem organ dysfunction. Signs and symptoms include changes in hemodynamics, new blood in the stool, increasing abdominal tenderness and pain, changes in x-ray findings, and changes in blood chemistry results.

▬▬ HEPATITIS

Disease processes in the liver can affect the parenchyma, Kupffer's cells, bile ducts, and blood vessels. Severe disease can lead to fulminant liver failure. Causes of liver failure include hepatitis and cirrhotic liver disease. Pathophysiology, assessment, and management of each of these diseases are discussed.

Pathophysiological Principles

Diffuse inflammation of the liver (hepatitis) can be caused by viral infections and by toxic reactions to drugs and chemicals. As inflammation in the liver progresses, the normal pattern of the liver is disturbed. This interrupts the normal blood supply to liver cells, causing necrosis and breakdown of cells. Over time, liver cells that become damaged are removed from the body by the immune system and are replaced with healthy liver cells. Therefore, most patients with hepatitis recover some level of liver function. Causes of hepatic inflammation are listed in the display. Viral in-

---

Selected Causes of Hepatic Inflammation

Infectious Diseases

- Viral hepatitis
- Epstein-Barr
- Cytomegalovirus
- Toxoplasmosis
- Schistosomiasis

Drugs and Toxins

- Alcohol
- Methyldopa
- Methotrexate
- Isoniazid
- Arsenicals
- Oral contraceptives

Inherited or Metabolic Disorders

- Hemochromatosis
- Wilson's disease
- Glycogen storage disease
- Fanconi's syndrome

Other or Unproven Causes

- Sarcoidosis
- Graft-versus-host disease (in bone marrow transplant)
- Chronic inflammatory bowel disease
- Cystic fibrosis
- Jejunoileal bypass
- Diabetes mellitus

fections of the liver parenchyma have been classified according to their specific infecting agent and serology markers. These are hepatitis A, B, C, D, E, and non-A, non-B.

HEPATITIS A

Type A, formerly known as infectious hepatitis, is transmitted by the fecal and oral route. The organism is also food-borne and water-borne; hence, shellfish are also associated with transmission. Type A hepatitis can be epidemic in nature. The clinical course usually runs 1 to 3 months. Recovery is usually complete and does not lead to chronic hepatitis or cirrhosis. In rare instances, type A hepatitis can lead to fulminating liver failure.

HEPATITIS B

Type B hepatitis is spread by contact with blood or blood products. Some of the more common mechanisms of transmission are through the parenteral route, such as through blood transfusions, needlestick injuries in medical personnel, and the use of contaminated needles. However, a significant number of patients contract type B hepatitis through nonparenteral routes. The antigen has been identified in body secretions, such as semen, mucus, and saliva; therefore, sexual exposure to a person with type B hepatitis can result in infection. Maternal perinatal exposure also occurs. It appears that a break in the skin or the mucous membrane is necessary for the transmission to occur.

Chronic active hepatitis is seen in 10% of the patients who have type B hepatitis. They continue to have high levels of surface antigen and can be infective to others. The degree of liver impairment in chronic active hepatitis is variable from mild to serious and can progress to cirrhosis. This type of hepatitis is the leading cause of fulminant liver failure.

NON-A, NON-B HEPATITIS

The transmission and clinical course of non-A, non-B hepatitis are similar to those for type B hepatitis. These patients, however, tend to develop chronic hepatitis with a greater frequency than patients with type B hepatitis. A significant percentage of patients with non-A, non-B hepatitis develop fulminant hepatic failure, but the percentage is less than that of patients with type B hepatitis.

HEPATITIS C

As diagnostic tests have improved, a subset of hepatitis that used to be considered non-A, non-B hepatitis has been identified as hepatitis C. It is a blood-borne virus. More than 90% of the transfusion-related non-A, non-B hepatitis cases have been caused by Hepatitis C.[7] Usually it is transmitted through blood, blood products, shared needles, or transplanted organs from infected donors, although there are indications that it might also be transmitted through perinatal, sexual, household, and occupational exposures.[8] The hepatitis C antibody does not confer immunity, and patients may progress to chronic infection.

DELTA HEPATITIS

Hepatitis D (delta hepatitis) always occurs in the presence of hepatitis B and relies on this virus to spread. Hepatitis D infection may occur as a superinfection in the patient who has chronic hepatitis B, or it may occur along with a hepatitis B infection. It can progress to fulminant hepatitis and chronic disease. It is endemic in the Mediterranean, middle east, and some of South America. In the United States, it occurs primarily among individuals receiving multiple transfusions and those abusing intravenous drugs.

HEPATITIS E

Hepatitis E is transmitted by the oral and fecal route and by contaminated food and water. Hepatitis E has been implicated in epidemics in India, Southeast Asia, Africa, and Mexico and is associated with high fatality rates in pregnant people.

ALCOHOLIC HEPATITIS

Alcohol has a direct toxic effect on the liver that can result in fatty liver disease. The disease may resolve if alcohol intake is stopped, or it can result in severe hepatitis that can eventually lead to hepatic failure and death.

DRUG- AND TOXIN-INDUCED HEPATITIS

This hepatitis results from a toxic reaction to the liver cells caused by a specific drug or toxin or one of its metabolites. The symptoms mimic viral hepatitis clinically and pathologically.

The major drugs involved in toxic reactions include the halogenated anesthetic agents, such as halothane; the antihypertensive medication methyldopa; the antituberculosis medication isoniazid; and the phenytoins, such as Dilantin. Most of these medications cause their toxicity through intermediate metabolites of the drug and rarely by their direct effect on the hepatocytes. There also can be a hypersensitivity reaction to the drug or to one of its metabolites. Acetaminophen and aspirin are other medications that can cause some degree of hepatic toxicity. The acetaminophen toxicity can be overwhelming and fatal because of the toxic effect of its metabolites on the liver cells (see Chapter 52).

Assessment

HEPATITIS A

Early in the course of the disease, there is an incubation period during which the patient is asymptomatic but highly contagious. After symptoms are apparent, the virus can be misdiagnosed because many of the symptoms are similar to those of the flu (see display for symptoms). Some patients seek medical attention because they become jaundiced. Acute symptoms can progress or disappear once jaundice is present. By the time symptoms occur, the virus is no longer shed in the stool, and the patient is generally

Loss of appetite
Nausea and vomiting
Fever
Weakness
Chills
Right upper quadrant pain
Headache
Depression
Irritability
Brown urine
Clay-colored feces

not infectious. Recovery is signaled by liver function tests returning to normal.

Hepatitis A virus (HAV) is diagnosed by the presence of hepatitis A antibodies (anti-HAV) in the blood. These antibodies occur within 2 to 6 weeks and remain in the blood serum indefinitely. These initial antibodies are of the IgM class of immunoglobulins and indicate a current active infection. Later, these are replaced by the IgG class, which indicates immunity to HAV.

HEPATITIS B

Clinical signs and symptoms for hepatitis B virus (HBV) during the acute phase are the same as for HAV, although arthralgia, high fever, and rash are hallmark signs of hepatitis B. There is, however, a greater risk of patients with HBV developing fulminant hepatic failure, which is characterized by sudden degeneration of the liver, loss of all liver functions, and a decrease in liver size.

Three antigens are identified with type B hepatitis: surface antigen, core antigen, and "e" antigen. Hepatitis B surface antigen (HBsAg) is the first to rise in the patient's blood and is usually present at the time the aspartate transaminase (AST) and alanine transaminase (ALT) are rising. As the patient improves, the transaminase levels and the level of HBsAg decrease. Usually as the patient's clinical condition improves, the surface antibody (anti-HBs) rises. Core antigen and core antibody titers are useful in determining a previous infection with type B hepatitis after the surface antigen is negative. "E" antigen (HBeAg) is useful in determining patients who are the most infectious. Patients with "e" antigens usually have very active liver disease that can be either acute or chronic. Those with high antibody to "e" antigen have a tendency to be carriers for a long time.

HEPATITIS C

Fatigue, anorexia, weight loss, and abdominal pain are the more common symptoms of hepatitis C. The presence of hepatitis C virus antibodies and a rise in liver enzymes confirm the diagnosis.

HEPATITIS D

Because this disease coexists with hepatitis B, patients with hepatitis D have symptoms similar to those of acute or chronic hepatitis B but more pronounced. Early in the disease, the hepatitis D antigen (HDVAg) is present in the blood. Later in the disease, antibodies to the hepatitis D virus are present (anti-HDV).

NON-A, NON-B HEPATITIS

Clinical signs and symptoms are similar to those for hepatitis A. There is no specific test for non-A, non-B hepatitis. The diagnosis is made by determining by serological markers that it is not hepatitis A or B, even though the patient has symptoms of acute hepatitis.

ALCOHOLIC HEPATITIS

Assessment parameters for acute, alcoholic, and toxic or drug-induced hepatitis are summarized in Table 40–2. Patients often seek health care because of pain, fever, anorexia, and vomiting. Ecchymosis, fluid retention, jaundice, spider angiomas, and palmar erythema indicate chronic disease. The liver may be swollen and tender or shrunken and difficult to palpate if cirrhosis has developed.

Management

There is no specific treatment for the viral hepatitis infections. Treatment is primarily supportive and includes providing rest and adequate nutrition and preventing further stress on the liver by avoiding hepatotoxic medications and substances. Hospitalization is rarely required. Maintaining adequate nutrition is a priority. A high-carbohydrate diet is recommended to spare protein from being used to meet calorie needs.

Intravenous feedings are needed only if oral intake is limited by nausea and vomiting. Patients with severe fatigue require frequent rest and spacing of activities. If there is severe pruritus from jaundice, a bile salt sequestering agent, cholestyramine, can be used to help alleviate this symptom. Drug- or toxin-induced hepatitis is treated primarily by avoiding the offending agent.

All the hepatitis forms are summarized in Table 40–3. After exposure to HAV, passive immunization can be achieved through the use of immune serum globulin. Most preparations of immune serum globulin contain adequate quantities of anti-HAV. The immune serum globulin may not entirely abort an infection, but it significantly ameliorates the symptoms. It is usually given to intimate contacts of patients with hepatitis A.

Hepatitis B exposure carries a much greater risk to the exposed person. After accidental exposure, such as an inadvertent needlestick, passive immunoprophylaxis can be achieved by using high anti-HBs titer hepatitis B immune globulin. This is a pooled serum containing high titers of the antihepatitis B immune globulin. It is recommended only for postexposure inoculations of high-risk patients.

Fortunately, a vaccine exists for active immunization against hepatitis B (Recombivax-HB, Engerix-B). This vac-

TABLE 40-2 CLINICAL APPLICATION: Assessment Parameters
Acute, Alcoholic, and Toxic or Drug-Induced Hepatitis

Parameter	Acute (Viral)	Alcoholic	Toxic or Drug-Induced
Presenting symptom	Flu-like, fatigue, anorexia, nausea and tiredness; abdominal pain and vomiting	Pain, fever, anorexia, vomiting; fever less than 39.4°C (103°F)	Depends on patient and source hypersensitivity: fever, rash, eosinophilia, 2 wk–2 mo after exposure to agent
Palpation of liver	Smooth, tender, palpable	Enlarged and tender; shrunken if progressed to cirrhosis	
Transaminases, bilirubin	Ten times greater than normal (peak 400–4,000); bilirubin 5–20 mg/dL	Mild increase, AST > ALT; bilirubin 2–10 mg/dL	Slightly elevated to 5,000 IU/L: > 5,000 IU/L, suspect drug injury
Albumin	Normal to low early	Normal to low early, low if late in process (both functional loss and inadequate nutritional intake)	Normal to low early
Prothrombin time	Normal to 1–2 times normal	Prolonged (3–4 times normal)	
Other	Splenomegaly in 20%; leukopenia, lymphopenia and neutropenia Hepatitis A: low-grade fever 38°–39°C (100.4°–102.2°F) Hepatitis B: arthralgia, high fever, urticarial rash Stable hepatitis B with sudden onset of worsening symptoms: suspect hepatitis D superinfection	Splenomegaly in some patients, anemia and leukocytosis, glucose abnormalities If bilirubin and alkaline phosphatase both elevated, consider cholestatic complications found with alcoholic patients May be unresponsive to vitamin K therapy	

TABLE 40-3
Summary of Types of Hepatitis

	Hepatitis A	Hepatitis B	Hepatitis C	Hepatitis D	Hepatitis E	Non-A, Non-B
Incubation	15–45 d	30–180 d	15–160 d	21–90 d	14–60 d	14–180 d
Onset	Acute	Insidious	Insidious	Acute or insidious	Acute	Acute or insidious
Transmission	Fecal/oral Contaminated food, water Rarely blood Rarely sexual	Blood Sexual Perinatal Percutaneous	Blood Maybe sexual	Blood Sexual	Fecal/oral Contaminated food, water	Blood Maybe sexual Maybe perinatal
Severity	Mild	Often severe	Moderate	May be very severe	Virulent, especially in pregnant women	Mild to moderate
Prognosis	Generally good	Worse with age, debility	Moderate	Fair, worse with chronic disease	Good, unless pregnant	Generally good
Diagnosis						
Acute	Anti-HAV IgM	Anti-HBC IGM HB surface Ag	Anti-HCV	HDV Ag	Clinical	Diagnosis of exclusion
Chronic	—	Anti-HBc total HB surface Ag ± HB "e" Ag	Anti-HCV	Anti-HDV	—	—
Prophylaxis (adults)	Immune globulin	Hepatitis B vaccine Immune globulin	?Immune globulin	None available	None available	?Immune globulin
Carrier	No	Yes	?	Yes	No	?

cine, administered prophylactically over a 6-month period, provides active immunization against hepatitis B. It is highly recommended for health care personnel whose risk of infection with hepatitis B is substantial. It is also recommended for people who have had intimate contacts with people already infected with hepatitis B. All nursing personnel who have the potential for needlesticks should be immunized against hepatitis B. Precautions to protect against exposure to blood-borne pathogens must be followed.

CIRRHOSIS OF THE LIVER

Pathophysiological Principles

Cirrhosis of the liver can result from a number of diseases. The most common is alcoholic liver disease. Others include chronic active hepatitis and diseases causing biliary obstruction.

Cirrhosis, which develops over time, can cause severe alterations in the structure and function of liver cells. These changes are characterized by inflammation and liver cell necrosis, which can be focal or diffuse. Fatty deposits within the parenchymal cells may be seen initially. The cause of the fatty changes is unclear, but it may be a response to alterations in enzymatic function responsible for normal fat metabolism. Eventually, all of the liver's metabolic processes are altered.

The enlarged liver cells cause compression of the liver lobule, leading to increased resistance to blood flow. Hypertension in the portal system results. With sufficient back pressure on the portal system, collateral circulation develops and allows blood to flow from the intestines directly to the vena cava. The increased blood flow to the veins leads to esophageal varices, gastric varices, splenomegaly, and hemorrhoidal varices (eg, hemorrhoids). As the disease progresses, portal hypertension also results in cardiac failure.

Necrosis is followed by regeneration of liver tissue but not in a normal fashion. Fibrous tissue is laid down over time, which distorts the normal architecture of the liver lobule. These fibrotic changes are irreversible, resulting in chronic liver dysfunction and eventual liver failure.

Assessment

HISTORY AND PHYSICAL EXAMINATION

The history and physical examination of the patient with cirrhosis will reflect the stage of disease. The liver may be palpable during periods of inflammation but will become nonpalpable in the end stages of liver disease. Early in the disease, there may be bulging flanks and a fluid wave that indicate peritoneal fluid. In later stages, there will be frank ascites. Distended veins may be seen around the umbilicus (caput medusae) due to increased portal pressure. There may be facial and upper chest petechiae, palmar erythema, and gynecomastia in males. Figure 40–3 illustrates clinical effects of cirrhosis.

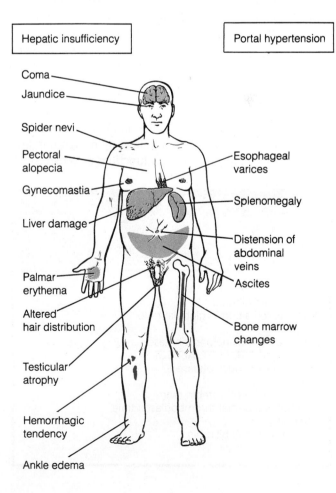

FIGURE 40-3
Clinical effects of cirrhosis of the liver. (Reference: Bullock BL: Pathophysiology: Adaptations and Alterations in Function [4th Ed]. Philadelphia, Lippincott-Raven, 1996)

CLINICAL MANIFESTATIONS

Clinical findings reflect altered liver function. For example, altered carbohydrate metabolism can result in unstable blood sugars. Altered fat metabolism can cause fatigue and decreased activity tolerance. Altered protein metabolism results in a decreased synthesis of albumin. Albumin is necessary for colloid osmotic pressure that holds fluid in the intravascular space. A decrease leads to interstitial tissue edema and decreased plasma volume. Globulin, another protein, is essential for normal blood clotting. This, coupled with a decreased synthesis of many blood clotting factors and decreased metabolism of vitamins and iron, predisposes the patient to hematological complications that range from bruising to hemorrhage. The patient may also develop disseminated intravascular coagulation (see Chapter 48). Portal hypertension and cardiac failure cause signs of jugular vein distention, lung congestion, ascites, and lower extremity edema. Initially, the patient may have hypertension, flushed skin, and bounding pulses. As perfusion to organs falls, hypotension and dysrhythmias are common.

DIAGNOSTIC STUDIES

Loss of the liver's ability to convert ammonia to urea results in impaired ammonia metabolism and elevated ammonia levels. Elevated serum bilirubin reflects the liver's inability to metabolize bile. Generally, jaundice is present with a bilirubin greater than 3 mg/dL. Other indications of liver dysfunction include increased prothrombin and partial thromboplastin time, alkaline phosphatase, 5'-nucleotidase, and hepatocellular enzymes AST (also called SGOT) and ALT (also called SGPT). Diagnostic findings are listed in the display.

Management

Managing the patient with cirrhosis is aimed at preventing further stress on liver function and early recognition and treatment of complications. Liver functions under stress in-

---

CLINICAL APPLICATION:
Assessment Parameters
Diagnostic Findings for Cirrhosis With Impending Liver Failure

Protein
  Decreased albumin
  Decreased albumin globulin ratio
Enzymes
  Increased alkaline phosphatase
  Increased AST/SGOT, ALT/SGPT
  Increased 5'-nucleotidase
Hematology
  Prolonged prothrombin time
  Prolonged partial thromboplastin time
Chemistry
  Increased total bilirubin
  Increased ammonia

CLINICAL APPLICATION:
Nursing Intervention Guidelines
Management Highlights Cirrhosis of the Liver

Rest
Nutrition
Skin integrity
Caution in drug administration
Monitor:
  Fluid intake
  Urinary output
  Electrolyte studies
  Bleeding
  Ascites development
  Neurological changes
Fluid replacement
Bowel cleansing

---

clude nutritional metabolism, clearing drug and metabolic waste products, and formation of clotting factors. Interventions include monitoring nutritional markers and providing nutrition; monitoring fluid balance, urinary output, electrolyte and chemistry studies, drug type, and dose requirements; monitoring bleeding times, platelet function, and hematocrit; and detecting signs of bleeding. Bowel cleansing regimens may be ordered. The early recognition of complications includes detecting signs of impending liver failure: changes in neurological and mental status, increasing ascites, worsening cardiac failure, and hepatorenal syndrome.

The critically ill patient in liver failure is often in some state of unconsciousness with jaundiced skin and sclera. Coagulation times are prolonged, so bleeding is apt to occur from many sources. There is a risk for sores and skin breakdown because of the patient's debilitated state.

Maintaining fluid and electrolyte balance requires ongoing nursing assessment. Imbalance can result from replacement therapy, malnutrition, gastric suction, diuretics, vomiting, diaphoresis, ascites, diarrhea, inadequate fluid intake, and elevated aldosterone levels. The patient may complain of headache, weakness, numbness and tingling of extremities, muscle twitching, thirst, nausea, or muscle cramps and may become confused. Monitor weight and central venous pressure to help determine fluid retention and vascular loading. Monitor for an increase or decrease in urinary output, cardiac dysrhythmias, changes in mental status and level of consciousness, prolonged vomiting or frequent liquid stools, muscle tremors, spasms, edema, or poor skin turgor. See the Collaborative Care Guide regarding cirrhosis of the liver.

Complications in Cirrhosis of the Liver

ASCITES

Impaired handling of salt and water by the kidney and other abnormalities in fluid homeostasis predispose the patient to an accumulation of fluid in the peritoneum (ie, ascites).

COLLABORATIVE CARE GUIDE
for the Patient with Cirrhosis and Impending Liver Failure

OUTCOMES	INTERVENTIONS

Oxygenation/Ventilation

The patient's arterial blood gases will be within normal limits.

The patient has no evidence of pulmonary edema or atelectasis.
Breath sounds are clear bilaterally.

- Monitor pulse oximetry and arterial blood gases, respiratory rate and pattern, and ability to clear secretions.
- Validate significant changes in pulse oximetry with co-oximetry arterial saturation measurement.
- Assist patient to turn, cough, deep breath, and use incentive spirometer q 2 h.
- Provide chest percussion with postural drainage if indicated q 4 h.
- Monitor effect of ascites on respiratory effort and lung compliance.
- Position on side and with head of bed elevated to improve diaphragmatic movement.

Circulation/Perfusion

Patient will achieve or maintain stable blood pressure and oxygen delivery.

Serum lactate will be within normal limits.

Patient will not experience bleeding related to coagulopathies, varices, hepatorenal syndrome.

- Monitor vital signs including cardiac output, systemic vascular resistance, oxygen delivery, and oxygen consumption.
- Monitor lactate q D until it is within normal limits.
- Administer red blood cells, positive inotropic agents, colloid infusion as ordered to increase oxygen delivery.
- Monitor PT, PTT, CBC daily.
- Assess for signs of bleeding (eg, blood in gastric contents, stools or urine); observe for petechiae, bruising.
- Administer blood products as indicated.
- Assist with insertion and manage the esophageal tamponade balloon tube.
- Perform gastric lavage as needed.

Fluids/Electrolytes

Patient is euvolemic.
Patient will not gain weight due to fluid retention.

- Daily weights.
- Monitor intake and output.
- Monitor electrolyte values.
- Measure abdominal girth daily at the same location on the abdomen.
- Monitor signs of volume overload:
    Cardiac gallop
    Pulmonary crackles
    Shortness of breath
    Jugular vein distention
    Peripheral edema
- Administer diuretics as ordered.

Mobility/Safety

Patient is alert and oriented.

Ammonia level is within normal limits.

Patient achieves or maintains ability to conduct ADLs and mobilize self.

No evidence of infection, WBC within normal limits.

- Assess serum ammonia level.
- Administer lactulose as ordered.
- Monitor level of consciousness, orientation, thought processing.
- Assess asterixis.
- Take precautions to prevent falls.
- Consult physical therapist.
- Conduct range of motion and strengthening exercises.
- Monitor SIRS (Systemic Inflammatory Response Syndrome) Criteria: increased WBC, increased temperature, tachypnea, tachycardia.
- Use aseptic technique during procedures and monitor others.

(continued)

COLLABORATIVE CARE GUIDE
for the Patient with Cirrhosis and Impending Liver Failure (Continued)

OUTCOMES	INTERVENTIONS
	• Maintain invasive catheter tube sterility.
	• Change invasive catheters, culture blood, line tips, or fluids, provide site care, etc., according to hospital protocol.
Skin Integrity	
Skin will remain intact.	• Assess skin q 8 h and each time patient is repositioned.
	• Turn q 2 h. Assist or teach patient to shift weight or reposition.
	• Consider pressure relief/reduction mattress.
Nutrition	
Caloric and nutrient intake meet metabolic requirements per calculation (eg, Basal Energy Expenditure).	• Provide nutrition by oral, enteral, or parenteral feeding.
	• Sodium, protein, fat, or fluid restriction may be necessary.
	• Consult dietitian or nutritional support service to evaluate nutritional needs and restrictions.
	• Provide small, frequent feedings.
Evidence of metabolic dysfunction is minimal.	• Monitor albumin, prealbumin, transferon, BUN, cholesterol, triglycerides, bilirubin, aspartate aminotransferase, alanine aminotransferase.
	• Administer cleansing enemas and cathartics if ordered.
Comfort/Pain Control	
Patient will have minimal pain.	• Assess pain and discomfort from ascites, bleeding, pruritis.
Patient will have minimal puritis.	• Administer analgesics cautiously and monitor patient response.
	• Bathe with cool water, blot dry.
	• Lubricate skin.
	• Administer antipruritic medication; apply to skin PRN as ordered.
Psychosocial	
Patient demonstrates decreased anxiety.	• Assess patient's response to illness. Provide time to listen.
	• Assess effect of critical care environment on the patient.
	• Minimize sensory overload.
	• Provide adequate time for uninterrupted sleep.
	• Encourage flexible visiting hours for family.
	• Plan for consistent caregiver.
Teaching/Discharge Planning	
Patient/significant others understand procedures and tests needed for treatment of hepatic dysfunction.	• Prepare patient/significant others for procedures such as paracentesis or laboratory studies.
	• Teach patient and family information regarding sodium, protein, and fluid restrictions. Give written materials.
Patient/significant others are prepared for home care.	• Teach signs and symptoms of progressing hepatic failure (eg, change in mentation, skin coloration, ascites).
	• Teach signs and symptoms of occult bleeding and respiratory infection.
	• Teach home medication regimen.
	• Teach comfort measures.

This complication can be problematic because it can restrict movement of the diaphragm, causing impairment of the patient's breathing pattern. Therefore, monitoring respiratory status is critical. Ascites is managed through bed rest, a low-sodium diet, fluid restriction, and diuretic therapy. Abdominal girth is measured daily, and potential electrolyte imbalance due to diuretic therapy is monitored. Paracentesis is also used to treat ascites; in this procedure, ascitic fluid is withdrawn from the abdomen through a percutaneous needle aspiration. Close monitoring of vital signs is important during this procedure because sudden loss of intravascular pressure and tachycardia can occur.

Peritoneal–venous shunt is a surgical procedure used to relieve ascites that is resistant to other therapies. The Leveen shunt (Fig. 40–4) is inserted by placing the distal end of a tube in the abdominal cavity and tunneling the other end into a central vein (eg, superior vena cava). This allows for ascitic fluid to flow into the central vein. It is not recommended for patients with infected ascites, encephalopathy, or renal failure.

A nonsurgical approach to managing ascites and variceal hemorrhage is the TIPS shunt, illustrated in Figure 40–5. This stent may be used to prevent rebleeding or when other methods of managing esophageal varices fail. Using an angiographic catheter, a guidewire with a dilating balloon is inserted into the internal jugular vein and is advanced through the vena cava into the hepatic vein through the liver parenchyma and into the hepatic vein. A stent is then placed in the liver parenchyma to create a conduit between the hepatic and portal vein that decreases portal pressure (see Fig. 40–5).

HEPATIC ENCEPHALOPATHY

Patients with severe liver disease can progress to hepatic encephalopathy. Clinical manifestations start with cognitive changes, irritability, reversal of day and night schedules,

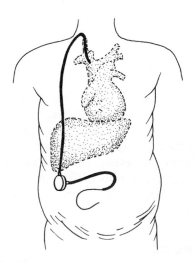

FIGURE 40-4
The Leveen shunt.

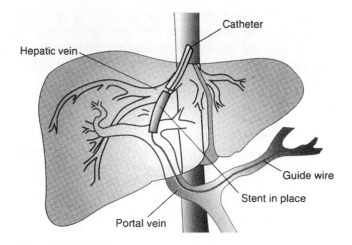

FIGURE 40-5
Transjugular intrahepatic portosystem shunt (TIPS). A stent is inserted through a catheter to the portal vein to divert blood flow and reduce portal hypertension. (Reference: Smeltzer SC, Bare BG: Brunner and Suddarth's Textbook of Medical-Surgical Nursing [8th Ed]. Philadelphia, Lippincott-Raven, 1996)

and somnolence, which can progress to coma. Sometimes patients become very agitated and difficult to manage. Often, they have a characteristic hyperventilation syndrome with a respiratory alkalosis. Asterixis (a flapping tremor, usually of the hands) may occur. To test for this, ask the patient to hold an arm and hand out, with fingers spread, as if stopping traffic and look for involuntary hand "flapping."

The cause of the hepatic encephalopathy and the hyperventilation syndrome is probably related to toxic agents absorbed from the intestinal tract. Elevated serum ammonia and other neurotoxins, such as mercaptens and fatty acids, have been implicated in the development of encephalopathy. *Endogenous* benzodiazepines have also been implicated, and as a result, benzodiazepine inhibitors, such as flumazenil, are used to treat encephalopathy.[9] Unfortunately, bypassing the clearance function of the liver with any kind of stent or shunt may result in decreased clearance and increased accumulation of toxins.

Those with portal systemic shunts can develop hepatic encephalopathy quite rapidly, and they often hemorrhage from esophageal varices or other sites in the GI tract. The hemorrhage produces a significant nitrogenous load to the intestinal tract in the form of blood, from which bacterial deamination produces the ammonia. Normally, this ammonia is detoxified to urea by the liver. If the liver is unable to perform this detoxification or if a good portion of the portal blood is shunted around the liver, the circulating level of ammonia rises. If ammonia and the other toxic agents can be reduced through effective therapy, the encephalopathy gradually clears.

Measures to decrease ammonia production are necessary in the treatment of this disorder. Protein intake is limited to 20 to 40 g/d. Drugs can be administered to reduce bacterial breakdown of protein in the bowel. Lactulose is used to facilitate stools and clearance of nitrogenous products. Neomycin, metronidazole, or oral vancomycin may be given to clear the gut of bacteria, which promotes nitrogenous production. Nursing measures to protect the patient with mental status changes from harm are a priority.

HEPATORENAL SYNDROME

Acute renal failure that occurs with liver failure is called hepatorenal syndrome. The pathophysiology of this disorder is not well understood. Decreased urine output and elevated serum creatinine are clinical signs. The prognosis for the patient is generally poor once renal failure is evident. Management goals include therapies to support liver and kidney functions.

SPONTANEOUS BACTERIAL PERITONITIS

Spontaneous bacterial peritonitis occurs when there is a large accumulation of ascites without an identifiable intra-abdominal source of infection. It may be triggered during endoscopy or when an NG tube, intravenous line, or indwelling bladder catheter are placed.[10] *Escherichia coli*, *Streptococcus*, and *Klebsiella* are the most common causes. When spontaneous peritonitis is suspected, the ascitic fluid is cultured, and the patient is treated with a third-generation cephalosporin until the culture returns. Spontaneous bacterial peritonitis must be differentiated from peritonitis secondary to an abscess or perforation, because the latter needs immediate surgical treatment.

ACUTE PANCREATITIS

Acute pancreatitis has many causes, but gallstone disease and alcohol abuse together account for more than 70% of all cases. Acute pancreatitis usually occurs within a day or two after a large meal or drinking episode. Biliary stones and biliary sludge (cholesterol crystals or calcium bilirubinate granules) are other causes. Many drugs, including diuretics, can precipitate acute pancreatitis either as a result of toxic doses or a drug reaction. High triglyceride levels are another important cause of pancreatitis. Idiopathic pancreatitis is associated with pregnancy, the administration of total parenteral nutrition, or major surgery. Pancreatitis has also occurred following blunt or penetrating abdominal trauma or following endoscopic exploration of the biliary tree. Other possible precipitating factors include infectious processes, such as mumps, *Staphylococcus*, scarlet fever, and viruses. Pancreatitis may occur as an isolated event or repeated attacks. The accompanying display summarizes the major causes of acute pancreatitis.

Pathophysiological Principles

Pancreatic enzymes are normally secreted in an inactive form that prevents autodigestion of the gland. In acute pancreatitis, a chemical inflammatory process begins in and

---

> **RED FLAG** **Major Causes of** Acute Pancreatitis
>
> **Biliary disease**
> Gallstones
> Common bile duct obstruction
> Biliary sludge
> **Alcohol abuse**
> **Drugs**
> Thiazide diuretics
> Furosemide
> Procainamide
> Tetracycline
> Sulfonamides
> **Hypertriglyceridemia**
> **Hypercalcemia**
> **Idiopathic**
> Postoperative
> Ectopic pregnancy
> Ovarian cyst
> Total parenteral nutrition
> **Abdominal trauma**
> **Endoscopic retrograde cholangiopancreatography**
> **Infectious processes**

around the pancreatic gland when these enzymes are prematurely activated. The exact mechanism by which pancreatic enzymes become activated and initiate autodigestion of the gland has been widely studied but remains unknown. As more pancreatic cells are damaged, more digestive enzymes are released. This causes a cycle of increasing pancreatic damage. Trypsinogen, phospholipase A, and elastase are the primary enzymes responsible for the autodigestive process. Pancreatic enzymes, vasoactive substances, and hormones released from the injured pancreas can affect distant organs, such as the lungs, heart, and kidneys.

Acute pancreatitis can be classified by the gradation of lesions found in the pancreas. In the mild form, there are areas of fat necrosis in and around pancreatic cells along with interstitial edema. This can progress to a more severe pancreatitis in which there is extensive fat necrosis in and around the pancreas, pancreatic cellular necrosis, and hemorrhage within the pancreas.

Depending on the degree and extent of pancreatic inflammation, the intensity of the disease ranges from mild to severe. In 85% to 90% of the patients, the disease is self-limiting, and the acute pancreatitis resolves spontaneously within 5 to 7 days. Conversely, severe pancreatitis can affect every organ system in the body. The mortality rate for pancreatitis is 10%; however, this rises to 50% or more when there are complications.[11]

Assessment

The history and physical examination findings in acute pancreatitis can mimic other diseases, such as gastritis, duodenal ulcer, small bowel obstruction, ruptured ectopic pregnancy, sickle cell crisis, and leaking aortic aneurysm. Therefore, laboratory and radiographic studies are particularly important diagnostic tools. Assessment parameters are listed in the display.

HISTORY

Precipitating factors, particularly biliary tract disease and alcohol intake, are explored, and inquiries are made about current medications. A family history includes questions about acute pancreatitis, because in rare cases it is hereditary. Appetite, food intolerance, and character and frequency of bowel movements are included in the history. The patient may report anorexia, weight loss, nausea, vomiting, abdominal distention, and foul smelling, light, frothy, or fatty stools (steatorrhea). Steatorrhea indicates an inability to metabolize fats properly. It is a sign of very poor pancreatic function and advanced chronic disease.

Most patients with acute pancreatitis complain of severe abdominal pain. The pain can be caused by edema and distention of the pancreatic capsule, peritoneal inflammation caused by activated pancreatic enzymes, and obstruction of the biliary system. Location, duration, quality, quantity, and precipitating factors of pain are important. Most often the pain is midepigastric or periumbilical and often radiates to the back. The pain usually begins abruptly, often after a large meal or large intake of alcohol. It may be steady and severe or increase in intensity over several hours. The patient characteristically curls up with both arms over the abdomen in an effort to lessen the pain. Vomiting, caused by irritation of the stomach by the inflamed pancreas, can be persistent and does not relieve the pain. The vomitus consists of gastric and duodenal contents.

Fever is also a common symptom, but it is usually less than 39°C (102.2°F). Persistent fever can indicate complications, such as peritonitis, cholecystitis, or intraabdominal abscess.

PHYSICAL EXAMINATION

Diffuse abdominal tenderness and guarding may be present during abdominal palpation. The upper abdomen may be distended and result in tympany during percussion. The inflammatory process and enzyme activity may reduce intestinal mobility and result in hypoactive or absent bowel sounds. Decreased intestinal mobility may lead to a paralytic ileus.

Patients with more severe pancreatic disease may be slightly jaundiced if pancreatic edema has obstructed the biliary tree. They can also have ascites or palpable abdominal masses. Patients with severe acute hemorrhagic pancreatitis may have signs of dehydration and hypovolemic shock. These signs may worsen when fluid is lost into the bowel lumen due to a paralytic ileus. The presence of a bluish discoloration of the lower abdominal flanks (Grey Turner's sign) or around the umbilical area (Cullen's sign) indicates hemorrhagic pancreatitis and an accumulation of blood in these areas. These signs usually appear 1 to 2 weeks after onset when more of the pancreatic gland has been destroyed. Patients with severe disease may also be confused due to toxicity from the autodigestive processes.

DIAGNOSTIC STUDIES

Serum lipase and amylase are specific test measures for acute pancreatitis because these enzymes are released as the pancreatic cells and ducts are destroyed. However, these values are not always sure indicators of the disease. Serum amylase and lipase levels are usually elevated during the first 24 to 48 hours after the onset of symptoms. In mild pancreatitis, amylase levels can be close to normal. If a few days have elapsed since symptoms began, enzyme values can also be normal even with acute inflammatory processes in the pancreas. In addition, serum amylase can be falsely lowered in patients with elevated serum triglycerides. Because amylase is present in other body tissues, it can be elevated in other diseases. Examples include biliary tract disease, tumors, salivary gland lesions, cerebral trauma, gynecological disorders, and renal failure. Based on these factors, other laboratory studies are needed along with serum amylase to diagnose acute pancreatitis. Elevations of isoenzymes, urinary amylase, and the amylase values of

---

CLINICAL APPLICATION:
Assessment Parameters
Indications of Acute Pancreatitis

History
Alcohol disease
Biliary disease
Nausea and vomiting
Steatorrhea
Urinary discoloration
Hereditary disposition

Clinical Manifestations
Abdominal pain
Abdominal guarding, distention
Paralytic ileus
Fever
Grey Turner's sign
Cullen's sign

Laboratory Findings
Elevated serum and urine amylase
Elevated serum lipase
Elevated WBC count
Hyperglycemia
Elevated bilirubin, AST/SGOT, lactate dehydrogenase (with liver disease)
Elevated alkaline phosphatase (with biliary disease)
Hypertryglyceridemia
Hypocalcemia
Hypoxemia

Diagnostic Studies
Ultrasound
Computed tomography
Magnetic resonance imaging

pleural fluid and paracentesis drainage support the presence of acute pancreatitis.

Other laboratory abnormalities associated with acute pancreatitis include an elevated white blood cell count due to the inflammatory process and an elevated serum glucose due to beta cell damage. Hypokalemia may be present because of vomiting. Hypocalcemia is common with severe disease and usually indicates pancreatic fat necrosis. Elevations in serum bilirubin, AST/SGOT, and prothrombin time are common in the presence of concurrent liver disease. Alkaline phosphatase is elevated with biliary tract disease. Triglycerides can be very high.

Both endocrine and exocrine functions of the pancreas can be impaired and lead to hyperglycemia, hypoglycemia, and nutritional depletion. Arterial blood gas analysis may show hypoxemia and high CO_2 levels, which would indicate respiratory failure.

Ultrasound, computed tomography, and magnetic resonance imaging show the size of the pancreas, the collection of fluid around the pancreas, pancreatic pseudocysts, and abscesses. Intestinal perforation, obstruction of the biliary tree, or masses are also distinguishable. When patients have acute abdominal pain, radiographs of the chest and abdomen are done to rule out intestinal ileus, perforation, pericardial effusion, and pulmonary disease.

Management

No treatment stops the cycle of pancreatic enzyme activation and ensuing inflammation and necrosis. There are efforts, however, to treat the underlying cause of the disease. Priorities for managing acute pancreatitis include the following:

- Replacing fluid and electrolytes to maintain or replenish vascular volume and electrolyte balance
- Resting the pancreas in an effort to prevent the release of pancreatic secretions
- Maintaining the patient's nutritional status
- Controlling pain

Management of the patient with pancreatitis is summarized in the accompanying display.

FLUID AND ELECTROLYTE REPLACEMENT

Fluids

Fluid collects in the retroperitoneal space and peritoneal cavity in all forms of pancreatitis. Initially, most patients have some degree of dehydration. In severe cases, patients may have up to 12 L of fluid sequestration and may be in hypovolemic shock. The goal is to administer enough fluid to obtain a circulating volume sufficient to maintain organ and tissue perfusion and prevent end stage shock. Hypovolemia and shock are major causes of death early in the disease process when aggressive fluid resuscitation fails to reverse the shock process.

Fluid replacement includes colloid and crystalloid solutions, such as Albuminar and lactated Ringer's solution. Pa-

---

CLINICAL APPLICATION:
Nursing Intervention Guidelines
Management Highlights of Acute Pancreatitis

Fluid Replacement
Colloids
Crystalloids
Blood products

Electrolyte Replacement
Calcium
Magnesium
Potassium

Resting the Pancreas
Nasogastric tube to intermittent suction
NPO
Bed rest

Nutritional Support

Pain Management
Nonopiate analgesics
Patient positioning

---

tients with acute hemorrhagic pancreatitis may also need packed red blood cells in addition to fluid therapy to restore volume. Fluid replacement is evaluated by monitoring intake and output and daily weights. Patients with more severe disease may require hemodynamic monitoring. The pulmonary capillary wedge pressure (PCWP) is the most sensitive measure of volume and left ventricular filling pressure. The goal for most patients is to have a PCWP between 6 and 12 mmHg. Central venous pressure readings are also beneficial when patients already have a central venous line in place. The goal is to maintain a central venous pressure between 4 and 6 mmHg.

Patients with severe disease whose hypotension fails to respond to fluid therapy may need medications to support blood pressure. The drug of choice is dopamine, which can be started at a low dose (2–5 µg/kg/min). An advantage of this drug is that at low doses, it maintains renal perfusion while supporting blood pressure.

Urinary output is a sensitive measure of the adequacy of fluid replacement, and it should be maintained at greater then 30 mL/h or 0.6 mL/kg/h. Blood pressure and heart rate are also sensitive measures of volume status. Expected outcomes need to be customized for each patient, but reasonable goals are to maintain mean arterial pressure at greater than 60 mmHg, BP without an orthostatic drop, and heart rate less than 100 beats/min. The presence of warm extremities is one indicator of adequate peripheral circulation.

Electrolytes

Hypocalcemia (< 8 mg/dL) is a common electrolyte imbalance. Patients with severe hypocalcemia should be placed on seizure precautions with respiratory support equipment on hand. The nurse is responsible for monitoring calcium levels, administering replacement solutions, and evaluating the patient's response to any calcium given. Calcium replacements should be infused through a central line, because peripheral infiltration can cause tissue necrosis. The patient also needs to be monitored for calcium toxicity; symptoms include lethargy, nausea, shortening of the Q-T interval, and decreased excitability of nerves and muscles. Hypomagnesemia may also be present, so magnesium may need to be replaced as well. Serum magnesium levels usually need to be corrected before calcium levels can return to normal.

Potassium is another electrolyte that may need to be replaced early in the treatment regimen because it is lost through vomiting and sequestration of potassium-rich pancreatic juices.

Hyperglycemia is surprisingly a less common complication of acute pancreatitis and is related to impaired secretion of insulin by islet cells in the pancreas or release of glucagon by alpha cells. In some cases, hyperglycemia can be associated with dehydration or other electrolyte imbalances. Sliding scale regular insulin may be ordered; it needs to be administered very cautiously, because glucagon levels are only transiently elevated in acute pancreatitis. Successful fluid replacement is marked by return of mental status, urine output, cardiac output, stable hemodynamic values, and a normal serum lactate level.

RESTING THE PANCREAS

In most patients with acute pancreatitis, NG suction is used to decompress the stomach and decrease stimulation of secretin. Secretin, which stimulates production of pancreatic secretions, is released whenever there is acid in the duodenum. Nausea, vomiting, and abdominal pain may also be decreased when an NG tube is placed and connected to suction early in treatment. An NG tube is also necessary in patients with severe gastric distention or a paralytic ileus. Patients should not take anything by mouth until the abdominal pain subsides and serum amylase levels have returned to normal. Starting oral intake sooner can cause the abdominal pain to return and can induce further inflammation of the pancreas by stimulating the autodigestive disease process.

NUTRITION

Total parenteral nutrition is recommended for patients with fulminant pancreatitis who are being kept on prolonged NPO status with NG suction because of paralytic ileus, persistent abdominal pain, or pancreatic complications. Lipids should not be administered, because this can further increase triglyceride levels and exacerbate the inflammatory process. In the patient with mild pancreatitis, oral fluids can usually be restarted within 3 to 7 days with solid food introduced slowly and as tolerated.

Prolonged NPO status is difficult for patients. Frequent mouth care and proper positioning and lubrication of the NG tube are important to maintain skin integrity and maximize patient comfort. Bed rest is prescribed to decrease the patient's basal metabolic rate; this, in turn, decreases the stimulation of pancreatic secretions.

PAIN MANAGEMENT

Pain control is a nursing priority for patients with acute pancreatitis, not only because of the extreme discomfort, but also because pain increases pancreatic enzyme secretion. Pain is related to the degree of pancreatic inflammation, and it can be severe, constant, and last for many days.

Analgesics will be needed to control discomfort. Some analgesics cause spasm of the sphincter of Oddi, which holds the duodenum in place and can thus exacerbate the pain associated with acute pancreatitis. Morphine is one such drug, and therefore non–opiate-containing analgesics, such as levorphanol (Levo-Dromoran) and meperidine (Demerol), have been considered the drugs of choice. Fentanyl citrate (Sublimaze), although an opiate, has also been used successfully to control this type of pain.

Analgesia should be routinely administered at least every 3 to 4 hours to prevent uncontrollable abdominal pain. Use of a pain rating scale is recommended for evaluating the patient's response to medication. An NG tube attached to low intermittent suction can help ease pain considerably. Patient positioning can also relieve some of the discomfort.

PREDICTING PROGNOSIS

After a diagnosis of acute pancreatitis is confirmed, criteria for predicting the prognosis of patients can be reviewed. Ranson's criteria are often used. These criteria have been widely studied, and the number of signs present during the first 48 hours of admission directly relate to the patient's chance of significant morbidity and mortality. These signs are summarized in the display.

In Ranson's research, the mortality rate is 1% for patients with fewer than three signs, 15% for those with three

---

Ranson Severity Criteria of Acute Pancreatitis

Evaluate on Admission or on Diagnosis:

Age > 55 years
Leukocyte count > 16,000/μL
Serum glucose > 200 mg/dL
Serum lactate dehydrogenase > 350 IU/mL
Serum aspartate aminotransferase > 250 IU/dL

During Initial 48 Hours:

Fall in hematocrit > 10%
Blood urea nitrogen level rise > 5 mg/dL
Serum calcium < 8 mg/dL
Base deficit > 4 mEq/L
Estimated fluid sequestration > 6 L
Arterial PaO_2 < 60 mmHg

to four signs, 40% if five to six signs are present, and 100% if seven or more signs are positive. The scale has a 96% accuracy rate and is useful clinically in identifying high-risk patients and those who need early aggressive treatment to prevent complications. The APACHE (Acute Physiology, Age, Chronic Health Evaluation) II score has also been studied and found to be useful in predicting severity. The advantage of these scoring systems is that a patient's risk can be identified within hours of admission. The use of serum markers to prognosticate severity has been tested. The most promising have been quantification of C-reactive protein, leukocyte elastase, and trypsinogen active peptide. False-negative and false-positive responses remain a concern.[11]

Complications in Acute Pancreatitis

Multisystem complications of acute pancreatitis are related to the pancreas' ability to produce many vasoactive substances that affect organs throughout the body. These are listed in the accompanying display.

As pancreatic cells are damaged, more digestive enzymes are released, which in turn cause more pancreatic damage. Local effects of pancreatitis include inflammation of the pancreas, inflammation of the peritoneum around the pancreas, and fluid accumulation in the peritoneal cavity. Hemodynamically significant fluid sequestration is characteristic of the disease in the fulminant form. Another major systemic effect of enzyme release into the circulatory system is peripheral vasodilation, which in turn can cause hypotension and shock.

Major Complications of Acute Pancreatitis

Pulmonary
Atelectasis
Acute respiratory distress syndrome

Cardiovascular
Hypotensive shock
Septic shock
Hemorrhagic shock

Renal
Acute renal failure

Hematological
Disseminated intravascular coagulation

Metabolic
Hypocalcemia
Metabolic acidosis

Gastrointestinal
Pancreatic pseudocyst
Pancreatic abscess
Gastrointestinal bleed

Decreased perfusion to the pancreas itself can result in the release of myocardial depressant factor (MDF). MDF decreases heart contractility and affects cardiac output. Perfusion of all body organs can then become compromised. Early and aggressive fluid resuscitation is thought to prevent the release of MDF. Trypsin activation causes abnormalities in blood coagulation and clot lysis. This promotes the development of disseminated intravascular coagulation with its associated bleeding (see Chapter 48).

The release of other enzymes (eg, phospholipase) is thought to cause the many pulmonary complications associated with acute pancreatitis. These include arterial hypoxemia, atelectasis, pleural effusions, pneumonia, acute respiratory failure, and acute respiratory distress syndrome. Arterial hypoxemia can occur in patients with mild disease without clinical or x-ray findings to support the pulmonary dysfunction. Therefore, arterial blood gases should be drawn every 8 hours for the first few days to detect this complication. Treatment for hypoxemia includes vigorous pulmonary care (eg, deep breathing and coughing) and frequent position changes. Oxygen therapy can also be used to improve overall oxygenation status. Careful fluid administration is also necessary to prevent fluid overload and pulmonary congestion. Patients with acute respiratory compromise may require mechanical ventilatory support.

Acute renal failure is thought to be a consequence of hypovolemia and decreased renal perfusion. Death during the first 2 weeks of acute pancreatitis usually results from pulmonary or renal complications.

Metabolic complications of acute pancreatitis include hypocalcemia and hyperlipidemia, which are thought to be related to areas of fat necrosis around the inflamed pancreas. Hyperglycemia may occur as a result of damage to the cells of the islets of Langerhans; metabolic acidosis can result from hypoperfusion and activation of anaerobic metabolism.

GI complications of acute pancreatitis include pancreatic pseudocyst, pancreatic abscess, and acute GI hemorrhage. Pancreatic pseudocysts occur in up to 20% of all cases of acute pancreatitis and are a part of the necrotizing process. A pseudocyst is a collection of inflammatory debris and pancreatic secretions. The pseudocyst can rupture and hemorrhage or become infected, causing bacterial translocation and sepsis. A pseudocyst should be suspected in any patient who has persistent abdominal pain with nausea and vomiting, a prolonged fever, and elevated serum amylase.

Pancreatic abscess is a walled-off collection of purulent material in or around the pancreas. Signs and symptoms of an abdominal abscess include increased white blood cell count, fever, abdominal pain, and vomiting. Pancreatic infection from an abscess, pseudocyst, or necrotic tissue may be present whenever a patient develops a temperature more than 39°C (102.2°F), tachycardia, leukocytosis > 20,000/mL, or shows other signs of clinical deterioration. Infections usually occur within 8 to 20 hours after onset of pancreatitis and, if untreated, are fatal. Sources of GI hemorrhage include peptic ulcer bleeds, hemorrhagic gastroduodenitis, stress ulcer, and Mallory-Weiss Syndrome.

MANAGEMENT OF SYSTEMIC COMPLICATIONS

In addition to medical interventions to support organ function, peritoneal lavage and surgical therapies have been used in the treatment of acute pancreatitis.

Peritoneal lavage has been used since the 1960s for the treatment of systemic complications. The rationale for this therapy is that it removes the toxic substances released by the damaged pancreas into the peritoneal fluid before systemic effects can be initiated. Lavage may be used if standard therapies have not been effective during the first days of hospitalization.

The procedure for peritoneal lavage involves placement of a peritoneal dialysis catheter. Isotonic solutions with dextrose, heparin, and potassium are added. An antibiotic may also be used in the solution. Two liters of solution are infused over 15 to 20 minutes and then are drained by gravity. This cycle is repeated every 1 to 2 hours for 48 to 72 hours. If peritoneal lavage is effective, the hemodynamic response by the patient is usually immediate.

Respiratory status must be closely monitored during peritoneal lavage, because accumulation of fluid in the peritoneum causes restricted movement of the diaphragm. Hyperglycemia can be another effect of this therapy, because dextrose can be absorbed from the fluid into the bloodstream.

A pancreatic resection for acute necrotizing pancreatitis can be performed to prevent systemic complications of the disease process. In this procedure, dead or infected pancreatic tissue is surgically removed. In some cases, the entire pancreas is removed.

Surgery may also be indicated for pseudocysts; however, it is usually delayed, because some pseudocysts have been known to resolve spontaneously. Surgical treatment of the pseudocyst can be done through internal or external drainage or needle aspiration. Acute surgical intervention may be required if the pseudocyst becomes infected or perforates. Broad-spectrum antibiotics are given to patients suspected of having a pancreatic infection and those who require surgical débridement of necrotic tissue.

Surgery may also be performed if gallstones are thought to be the cause of the acute pancreatitis. A cholecystectomy or endoscopic retrograde cholangiopancreatography and endoscopic sphincterotomy are performed.

See the Collaborative Care Guide concerning the patient with pancreatitis.

CLINICAL APPLICATION: Patient Care Study

Mr. Jackson, a 52-year-old man, was admitted to the emergency room reporting agonizing, knifelike pain in the mid-epigastrium, radiating to his back. His pain began suddenly, about 1 hour after he returned home with his wife from a dinner party. His wife, concerned he was suffering a heart attack, called the ambulance for emergency transport. En route, he became nauseated and vomited several times. This did not relieve the relentless pain.

Admission assessment findings were as follows:

BP 96/40 with 15 mmHg orthostatic drop
Sinus tachycardia (135) with ST segment depression
Temperature, 37.9°C (100.3°F)
RR, 34, diminished breath sound in bases; pulse oximetry, 87%
Alert, oriented to time, place, and person; anxious
Extremities cool, pulses present and equal
Abdomen soft, distended with hypoactive bowel sounds, tender to palpation

Mr. Jackson denied a history of cardiovascular disease, diabetes, or renal disease. He reported a history of cholecystitis with two acute episodes within the last 2 years, which were medically managed. He states he does not smoke and drinks socially.

Intravenous lines were placed and normal saline was infused to maintain MAP greater than 60. A bladder catheter was placed to assist with fluid assessments. Supplemental oxygen was administered to improve oxygenation, and an ABG was drawn. Serum blood counts, chemistries, and cardiac enzymes were also sent to the laboratory. Levorphanol (Levo-Dromoran) was administered for abdominal pain. The nurse helped Mr. Jackson assume a knee-to-chest position, which relieved some of his pain. A chest x-ray and 12-lead ECG were obtained. The patient was scheduled for admission to the intensive care unit.

The initial medical and nursing goals were to assess vital signs and respiratory status. Fluid resuscitation was immediately begun and assessments initiated to monitor hemodynamic status. Serum tests and radiographic studies were done to enable the physician to make a definitive diagnosis. Analgesia was administered, and the patient was positioned to promote optimal comfort.

COLLABORATIVE CARE GUIDE
for the Patient With Pancreatitis

OUTCOMES	INTERVENTIONS
Oxygenation/Ventilation Arterial blood gases are maintained within normal limits.	• Assist patient to turn, deep breathe, cough, and use incentive spirometer q 4 h and PRN. Provide chest physiotherapy. • Assess for hypoventilation, rapid and shallow breathing, and respiratory distress. • Monitor pulse oximetry, end tidal CO_2, and arterial blood gases. • Administer analgesics if splinting is reducing effective ventilation.

(continued)

COLLABORATIVE CARE GUIDE
for the Patient With Pancreatitis (Continued)

OUTCOMES	INTERVENTIONS
The patient's lungs are clear. The patient has no evidence of atelectasis, pneumonia, or adult respiratory distress syndrome.	• Auscultate breath sounds q 2–4 h and PRN. • Suction only when rhonchi are present or secretions are visible in endotracheal tube. • Hyperoxygenate and hyperventilate before and after each suction pass.
Circulation/Perfusion Blood pressure, heart rate, and hemodynamic parameters are within normal limits.	• Monitor vital signs q 1–2 h. • Monitor pulmonary artery pressures and right atrial pressure q 1 h and cardiac output, SVR, and PVR q 6–12 h if pulmonary artery catheter is in place. • Maintain patent IV access. • Administer intravascular volume as indicated by real or relative hypovolemia, and evaluate response.
Serum lactate will be within normal limits.	• Monitor lactate q D until it is within normal limits. • Administer red blood cells, positive inotropic agents, colloid infusion as ordered to increase oxygen delivery.
Patient will not experience bleeding related to acute gastrointestinal hemorrhage, coagulopathies, or disseminated intravascular coagulation (DIC).	• Monitor PT, PTT, CBC daily or PRN. • Assess for signs of bleeding. Observe for Cullen's or Grey Turner's signs. • Administer blood products as indicated.
Fluids/Electrolytes Patient is euvolemic.	• Monitor daily weights. • Monitor intake and output. • Measure abdominal girth q 8 h at the same location on the abdomen. • Monitor electrolytes daily and PRN.
No evidence of electrolyte imbalance or renal dysfunction.	• Assess for signs of lethargy, tremors, tetany, and dysrhythmias. • Replace electrolytes as ordered. • Monitor BUN, creatinine, serum osmolality, and urine electrolytes daily.
Mobility/Safety No evidence of complications related to bedrest and immobility.	• Initiate deep vein thrombosis prophylaxis. • Reposition frequently. • Ambulate to chair when acute phase is past, hemodynamic stability and hemostasis achieved. • Consult physical therapist. • Conduct range of motion and strengthening exercises.
Patient achieves or maintains ability to conduct ADLs and mobilize self. No evidence of infection, WBC within normal limits.	• Monitor SIRS (Systemic Inflammatory Response Syndrome) Criteria: increased WBC count, increased temperature, tachypnea, tachycardia. • Use strict aseptic technique during procedures. • Maintain invasive catheter tube sterility. • Change invasive catheters, culture blood, line tips, or fluids, etc., according to hospital protocol.
Skin Integrity Skin will remain intact.	• Assess skin q 8 h and each time patient is repositioned. • Turn q 2 h. • Consider pressure relief/reduction mattress.
Nutrition Caloric and nutrient intake meet metabolic requirements per calculation (eg, Basal Energy Expenditure).	• Provide parenteral feeding. • Maintain NPO. • Consult dietitian or nutritional support service. • Fat or lipid restriction. • Provide small, frequent feedings.

(continued)

COLLABORATIVE CARE GUIDE
for the Patient With Pancreatitis

OUTCOMES	INTERVENTIONS
Evidence of metabolic dysfunction is minimal.	• Monitor albumin, prealbumin, transferrin, cholesterol, triglycerides, glucose.
Comfort/Pain Control Patient will have minimal pain, < 5 on pain scale.	• Assess pain and discomfort using objective pain scale q 4 h PRN and following administration of pain medication. • Administer analgesics and monitor patient response. • Utilize nonpharmacological pain management techniques, eg, music, distraction, touch, as adjunct to analgesics.
Patient will have minimal nausea.	• Maintain NG tube patency. • Monitor nausea and vomiting. • Administer antiemetic as ordered.
Psychosocial Patient demonstrates decreased anxiety.	• Listen to patient's worries and fears. • Assess patient's response to anxiety. • Support effective coping behaviors. • Teach alternate behaviors for those that are not helpful. • Help patient increase sense of control by providing information and explanation. • Allow choices when possible. • Provide as much predictability in routine as possible.
Teaching/Discharge Planning Patient/significant others understand procedures and tests needed for treatment. Significant others understand the severity of the illness, ask appropriate questions, anticipate potential complications.	• Prepare patient/significant others for procedures such as paracentesis, pulmonary artery catheter insertion, or laboratory studies. • Explain the widespread effects of pancreatitis and the potential for complications such as sepsis or adult respiratory distress syndrome. • Encourage significant others to ask questions related to pathophysiology, monitoring, treatments, etc. • Instruct patient and family in discharge regime that may include wound care, medications, and dietary limitations.

Clinical Applicability Challenges

Self-Challenge: Critical Thinking

1. Develop a teaching plan about the risks of contracting hepatitis. Differentiate the types of hepatitis and methods of transmission related to sexual practices, needle sharing, and blood transfusion.

2. Your patient with cirrhosis and impending liver failure wants to eat the high-protein meal brought in by his family. Compile and organize facts in such a way that he will understand why eating this meal is potentially harmful to him. Then create a response that acknowledges the patient's feelings about not being able to eat this meal.

3. Review the patient care studies for Mr. Lane, who has GI bleeding, and Mr. Jackson, who has acute pancreatitis. Compare and contrast the pathophysiology and management associated with their respective shock states.

Study Questions

1. The most important goal in the initial management of an active upper GI bleed is
   a. preparing the patient for surgery.
   b. administering intravenous vasopressin.
   c. replacing volume losses to stabilize hemodynamics.
   d. administering analgesics to diminish the pain experience.

2. The greatest danger from rupture or sudden deflation of the gastric balloon of the esophogastric tamponade tube is
   a. tearing of the cardiac sphincter.
   b. upward movement of the tube with obstruction of the airway.
   c. excessive pressure on the nares with necrosis.
   d. damage to the esophagus with formation of tracheoesophageal fistula.

3. Strangulated bowel should be treated with
   a. nasogastric suction and pain medication.
   b. endoscopy.
   c. surgical intervention.
   d. enema irrigation.

4. *In a patient with liver failure, which of the following laboratory values is (are) the most specific to hepatocellular damage?*
   a. *Prothrombin time (PT), partial thromboplastin time (PTT)*
   b. *Alkaline phosphatase*
   c. *AST/SGOT, ALT/SGPT*
   d. *Amylase*

5. *When a patient with increasing mentation difficulties is suspected of having hepatic encephalopathy, what laboratory test should be drawn?*
   a. *Amylase*
   b. *PT/PTT*
   c. *Ammonia*
   d. *Hematocrit*

6. *Complications of acute pancreatitis amenable to surgical intervention include*
   a. *abscess.*
   b. *pseudocyst.*
   c. *hemorrhage.*
   d. *All of the above*

7. *The primary goal in the collaborative management of the patient with acute pancreatitis is to*
   a. *conserve nutritional reserves.*
   b. *prevent GI complications.*
   c. *prevent proteolytic enzyme secretions.*
   d. *facilitate diagnostic evaluation.*

REFERENCES

1. Chung R, Jaffe D, Friedman L: Complications of chronic liver disease. Critical Care Clinics 11(2):437, 1995
2. Silen W: Acute intestinal obstruction. Harrison's Principles of Internal Medicine (12th Ed), p 1295. New York, McGraw-Hill, 1991
3. Silen W: Acute intestinal obstruction. Harrison's Principles of Internal Medicine (12th Ed), p 1296. New York, McGraw-Hill, 1991
4. Shelton F: Intestinal obstruction and perforation. Desk Reference for Critical Care Nursing, p 863. Boston, Jones and Bartlett Publishers, 1993
5. Shelton F: Intestinal obstruction and perforation. Desk Reference for Critical Care Nursing, p 864. Boston, Jones and Bartlett Publishers, 1993
6. Silen W: Acute intestinal obstruction. Harrison's Principles of Internal Medicine (12th Ed), p 1297. New York, McGraw-Hill, 1991
7. Tong MJ, El-Farra N, Reikes A, Co RL: Clinical outcomes after transfusion-associated hepatitis C. NEJM 332(22):463, 1995
8. Alter M: Transmission of hepatitis C virus—route, dose and titer. NEJM 330(11):784, 1994
9. Chung R, Jaffe D, Friedman L: Complications of chronic liver disease. Critical Care Clinics 11(2):441, 1995
10. Chung R, Jaffe D, Friedman L: Complications of chronic liver disease. Critical Care Clinics 11(2):447, 1995
11. Forsmark C, Toskes P: Acute pancreatitis: Medical management. Critical Care Clinics 11(2):311–322, 1995

BIBLIOGRAPHY

Angelucci P: TIPS for controlling bleeding . . . transjugular intrahepatic portosystemic shunt. Nursing 25(7):43, 1995
Bouley G, Grinshaw L, Lindewall-Matto D, Kiernan L: Transjugular intrahepatic portosystemic shunt: An alternative. Critical Care Nurse 16(1):23–29, 1996
Huston CJ: Ruptured esophageal varices. AJN 96(4):43, 1996
Levy JF, DeMartinis JE: Trauma-induced severe acute pancreatitis in adults: Conceptual review of pathophysiological events. Gastroenterology Nursing 19(1):18–24, 1996
Rush C: Action STAT! Gastrointestinal bleeding. Nursing 25(8):33, 1995

Endocrine System

41

Anatomy and Physiology of the Endocrine System

OBJECTIVES

Based on the content in this chapter, the reader should be able to:

- Describe the production, action, and regulation of antidiuretic hormone, growth and thyroid hormones, insulin, and glucagon.
- Identify how activated vitamin D, parathyroid hormone, and calcitonin each influence calcium concentrations in the blood.
- Explain how glucocorticoids are secreted.
- Summarize the renin–angiotensin mechanism for regulating mineralocorticoid secretion.
- List the significant effects of glucocorticoid medications.

*C*ommunication between systems in the body is accomplished in three ways. One is the nervous system. The second is the cellular secretion of chemicals in interstitial fluid. Examples include chemicals that trigger a local inflammatory response, such as histamine, complement, and prostaglandins. The third method is the cellular secretion of chemicals that are circulated through the bloodstream. This communication is known more commonly as the *endocrine system*. The secretions of endocrine cells are termed *hormones*.

HYPOTHALAMUS AND PITUITARY

The key to understanding physiology of the hormones of the pituitary gland is in visualizing the anatomy of the gland and its blood supply. The hypothalamus and pituitary together form a unit that controls the state of hydration, the regulation of thirst, the thyroid gland, the adrenal glands and gonads, and growth and metabolism of the organism (Fig. 41–1).

The hypothalamus is a small area at the base of the brain connected to the posterior pituitary gland by a pituitary stalk. This stalk is a direct outgrowth of the neuroectoderm of the base of the brain that drops during development of the gland into the bony sella turcica. This is in direct con-

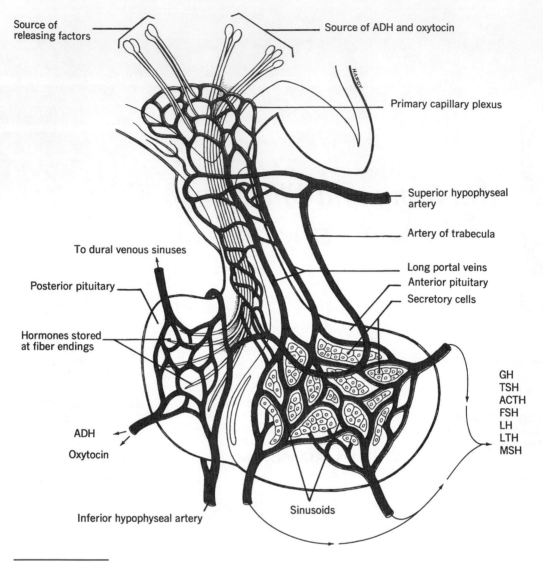

Source of releasing factors

Source of ADH and oxytocin

Primary capillary plexus

Superior hypophyseal artery

Artery of trabecula

To dural venous sinuses

Long portal veins

Anterior pituitary

Posterior pituitary

Secretory cells

Hormones stored at fiber endings

GH
TSH
ACTH
FSH
LH
LTH
MSH

ADH

Oxytocin

Inferior hypophyseal artery

Sinusoids

FIGURE 41-1

Highly diagrammatic and schematic representation of hypophyseal nerve fiber tracts and portal system. Releasing factors produced by cell bodies in hypothalamus trickle down axons to proximal part of stalk, where they enter the primary capillary plexus and are transported via portal vessels to sinusoids in adenohypophysis for control of secretions. ADH and oxytocin, produced by other cell bodies in hypothalamus, trickle down axons for storage in neurohypophysis until needed.

trast to the anterior pituitary gland that rises from the buccal endothelium and develops separately in the same bony structure. Besides being embryogenically separate, their blood supplies differ; this is the other key to the differential regulation of pituitary hormones. The anterior pituitary hormones are controlled by factors that are released from the hypothalamus through a portal venous system that directly links the hypothalamus and the anterior pituitary. This blood may also travel in a retrograde fashion and may be responsible for one level of feedback control of the anterior pituitary and the hypothalamus hormone-releasing factors. The posterior pituitary is a direct neural extension of the hypothalamus, and the controlling factors reside within the neural chiasma of the hypothalamus; they are secreted within those cells into the posterior pituitary gland.

In addition to controlling the pituitary gland through releasing factors, the hypothalamus controls other endocrine roles through releasing factors that control appetite, thirst, emotions, sleep–wake cycles, and cognition.

Posterior Pituitary

The two major hormones of the posterior pituitary gland are the antidiuretic hormone (ADH) and oxytocin (Table 41–1).

ANTIDIURETIC HORMONE

The major action of ADH is to concentrate the urine by permitting only water reabsorption from the hypotonic tubular fluid in the distal nephron. Antidiuretic hormone does

TABLE 41-1
Hormones of the Pituitary Glands and Their Actions

Lobe	Hormone	Action
Posterior	Antidiuretic hormone	Reabsorption of water only
		Maintains body fluid osmolality
		Maintains body fluid volume
	Oxytocin	Stimulates breast milk flow
Anterior	Growth hormone	Growth of bones, muscles, and other organs
	Somatotropin	Increases protein synthesis rate
		Decreases carbohydrate utilization rate
		Increases mobilization and use of fats
	Thyrotropin-stimulating hormone	Increases growth of thyroid gland
		Increases secretion of thyroid hormone
		Controls basic metabolism rate
	Adrenocorticotropic hormone	Increases growth of adrenal cortex
		Increases secretion from adrenal cortex
	Follicle-stimulating hormone	Follicle development
		Estrogen development
	Luteinizing hormone	Secretion of progesterone
		Formation of corpus luteum
		Ovulation
	Prolactin	Secretion of milk
	Melanocyte-stimulating hormone	Pigmentation in skin

not control flow of ions or solutes in this area. The distal convoluted tubule would be impermeable to water without the action of ADH. In the presence of ADH, the tubule and collecting duct are permeable to water, which diffuses from the hypotonic tubular fluid to the hypertonic tissue surrounding the tubules. This concentrates the tubular fluid and ultimately the urine. Antidiuretic hormone binds to specific receptors in the distal renal tubules and acts through binding and activating the induction of adenylate cyclase and the subsequent generation of cyclic adenosine monophosphate (cyclic AMP). This activation of cyclic AMP leads to a cascade of protein kinases to direct the signal from the plasma membrane to the fluid channels.

Metabolic Fate

The half-life of ADH is 18 minutes. It is degraded principally by the liver and kidneys. Metabolic clearance of ADH is augmented from the 10th week of gestation to midterm pregnancy. This phenomenon is the result of an increase in plasma vasopressinase, an enzyme aminopeptidase specific for ADH.

Actions

Antidiuretic hormone acts on the cells of the renal collecting ducts to increase their permeability to water. This results in increased water reabsorption but without electrolyte reabsorption. This reabsorbed water increases the volume and decreases the osmolality of the extracellular fluid (ECF). At the same time, it decreases the volume and increases the concentration of the urine excreted. The term vasopressin originated from the observation that large, su-

praphysiological dosages of ADH act on arteriole smooth muscle to elevate blood pressure. Although this pressor action of ADH does not appear to play a role in the normal homeostasis of blood pressure, it does counteract a fall in blood pressure that results from hemorrhagic or other drastic hypovolemic states.

Regulation

There are three major stimuli for the regulation of ADH secretion. The first is plasma osmolality, which is monitored by osmoreceptors in the anterior hypothalamus. An increase above the normal osmolality of plasma (290 mOsm/kg) results in neural stimuli from these receptors to the ADH-secreting cells, increasing ADH secretion. This increases water retention, thereby diluting the ECF and lowering the plasma osmolality back to normal. Similarly, a fall in plasma osmolality triggers a decrease or cessation in ADH secretion. This allows more water excretion, thereby raising the ECF osmolality. Antidiuretic hormone secretion can be altered by changes in osmolality of less than 1%. This osmoreceptor-mediated reflex arc functions in maintaining osmotic homeostasis of the ECF.

The second stimulus consists of changes in ECF volume. Stretch receptors in the low pressure portion of the cardiovascular system (eg, vena cava, right side of the heart, and pulmonary vessels) monitor blood volume. Stimuli from these receptors are conducted by afferent fibers to the hypothalamus (by way of the brain stem). A decrease in blood volume stimulates ADH secretion. The resultant increase in water retention elevates the blood volume without affecting arterial blood pressure. A rise in blood volume stops ADH secretion. This halts water retention, thereby restoring the normal volume of the ECF compartment. This mechanism alters ADH secretion in response to changes in body position. Movement from the recumbent to the upright position causes a temporary decrease in the stimulation of volume receptors because blood pools in the legs. This results in an increase in ADH secretion. Recumbency increases venous return from the legs. The increased volume triggers a decrease in ADH secretion, thereby increasing the volume of urine excreted.

The third stimulus, changes in arterial blood pressure, also can regulate ADH secretion. The hypothalamus receives information from pressure receptors located in the carotid sinuses and aorta. A fall in arterial pressure increases ADH secretion. The water retention thereby produced increases the plasma volume and pressure. A rise in arterial pressure produces the opposite effect. This mechanism is most important in compensating for large changes in arterial blood pressure (eg, impending or actual shock).

Various other stimuli have been shown to influence ADH secretion. Increased ADH secretion can be prompted by angiotensin II, pain, nausea, hypoglycemia, stress, opiates, nicotine, clofibrate (Atromid-S), chlorpropamide (Diabinese), and barbiturates. Secretion of ADH is inhibited by alcohol and certain opiate antagonists.

OXYTOCIN

Oxytocin is stored as insoluble complexes with specific proteins called neurophysins. These neurohypophysins are specific for the proteins to which they are bound.

Actions and Regulations

This hormone stimulates contraction of the myoepithelial cells that line the milk ducts of the breast. This causes milk to be squeezed into the sinuses, leading to the nipple surface. Oxytocin secretion is triggered by the hypothalamic receipt of afferent impulses from touch receptors around the nipples and also by receipt of afferent optical and aural stimuli. Therefore, suckling by the newborn, manual stimulation of the nipples, or the sight or sound of a crying infant can trigger milk secretion. Oxytocin also causes contraction of the smooth muscles of the uterus. Such con-

tractions play a role in labor and facilitate the transport of sperm from the cervix to the fallopian tubes. During pregnancy, oxytocin secretion is stimulated by cervical dilation and estrogen and inhibited by progesterone and alcohol.

Hypophysiotropic Hormones

Other hypothalamic neurons produce hypophysiotropic hormones that stimulate or inhibit hormonal secretion by the anterior pituitary (adenohypophysis). These hormones are secreted into the capillary plexus near the median eminence that supplies blood to the anterior pituitary. A given hypophysiotropic hormone regulates the secretion of one or two anterior pituitary hormones. Both growth hormone (GH, somatotropin) and prolactin are dually controlled by a stimulatory and an inhibiting hypophysiotropic hormone. Figure 41–2 illustrates the hypophysiotropic regulation of adenohypophyseal secretions.

Such hypothalamic regulation of pituitary functioning can be disrupted by hypothalamic lesions. This can lead to oversecretion or undersecretion of one or more hormones released from the anterior or posterior pituitary. The hypothalamus also receives input from various higher and lower brain centers. These neural connections, together with the influence of the hypothalamus on the pituitary, provide the biological basis for the construction of conceptual models that describe how stress, emotions, environmental stimuli, and perceptions affect endocrine functions.

Anterior Pituitary (Adenohypophysis)

This organ contains five morphologically different types of cells that secrete polypeptide hormones: somatotrophs, which secrete GH (somatotropin); mammotrophs, which secrete prolactin (luteotropic hormone, or LTH); thyrotrophs, which secrete thyroid-stimulating hormone (TSH); corticotrophs, which secrete adrenocorticotropic hormone (ACTH), β-lipotrophin (BLPH), β-endorphin, and melanophore-stimulating hormone (MSH); gonadotrophs, which secrete luteinizing hormone (LH) and follicle-stimulating hormone (FSH).

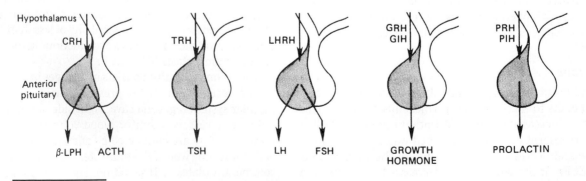

FIGURE 41-2
Effects of hypophysiotropic hormones on the secretion of anterior pituitary hormones.

Each type of cell is separately regulated by hypophys-iotropic hormones (see Fig. 41–2). LTH, LH, and FSH act on cells of the gonads (ovaries and testes) to regulate gamete (sperm and egg) and hormone production. Their function is primarily determined by the timing, relative ratios, and pattern of secretion from the anterior pituitary gland.

The TSH stimulates cells of the thyroid gland to produce and secrete the two thyroid hormones. This and the manner by which these hormones alter TSH output are discussed later in this chapter. The corticotrophs manufacture a long polypeptide chain, of 265 amino acids, called propiomelanocortin (POMC). Before secretion, POMC is separated into shorter fragments. Three of these are readily identified as ACTH, MSH, and BLPH. Part of the BLPH molecule can be further split off to form an endogenous opiate called β-endorphin. Endogenous opiates are further discussed in later chapters.

Melanin is a dark pigment contained in special structures called melanophores within the cells of the skin of lower vertebrates (eg, fish, amphibians, and reptiles). MSH stimulates the dispersion of the melanin granules within these melanophores. This darkens the animal temporarily. Birds and mammals (including humans) have melanin, but it cannot be dispersed and is not contained within melanophores. The normal function of MSH in humans is not known, although there is some evidence that it can cause a darkening of certain areas of skin in humans with Addison's disease. In this condition, excess corticotropin ACTH-releasing hormone stimulates corticotrophs to secrete ACTH. Along with this, the other fragments of POMC, including MSH, are released.

GROWTH HORMONE (SOMATOTROPIN)

The production and secretion of GH occur in the anterior pituitary in response to GH-releasing factor produced in the hypothalamus. Somatotropin release-inhibiting factor inhibits the secretion of GH, resulting in a dual control system for GH secretion.

Metabolic Fate

Growth hormone is degraded primarily in the liver. Other metabolic sites have yet to be uncovered. The half-life of plasma GH is approximately 25 minutes and is primarily controlled in its secretory phase.

Actions

This hormone acts both directly on target cells and indirectly by stimulating the liver and other as yet unidentified tissues to secrete various growth factors termed somatomedins. These growth factors are structurally similar to insulin. Human beings possess two such insulin-like growth factors (IGFs): IGF-I and IGF-II. Direct actions of GH include increasing the breakdown of fats (lipolysis) in adipose cells and releasing the fatty acids produced by lipolysis into the bloodstream (this is termed its ketogenic effect; increasing hepatic glycolysis and thereby increasing plasma glucose levels; increasing the sensitivity of insulin-producing cells to certain stimuli; increasing the cellular uptake of amino acids; and stimulating erythropoiesis.

The various somatomedins exert growth-promoting activity in different types of tissues. Normally, the result of somatomedin-mediated GH activity consists of an increase in the formation of cartilage in the epiphyseal plates, which fosters the growth in length of long bones; an increase in other skeletal growth; and the growth of all other parts of the body (eg, soft tissue and viscera).

All GH actions operate together to produce growth (eg, by cell division) and to provide the materials needed for this growth (ie, amino acids for synthesis of protein cell structure, fatty acids and glucose to provide energy, and erythrocytes to increase the availability of oxygen).

Regulation

Plasma concentrations of GH are controlled by the release of GH-releasing factor and GH release-inhibiting factor from the hypothalamus. Several stimuli influence the secretion of GH. Age is the most important overriding variable, and the actions of many of these other stimuli are influenced by it.

Factors that, at the appropriate age, can stimulate the secretion of GH include hypoglycemia, fasting, exercise, protein meal, glucagon, stress (both physiological and psychological), deeper stages of sleep, and drugs that bind to dopamine receptors. Major stimuli that decrease the output of GH include rapid eye movement sleep (dreaming), elevated plasma levels of glucose or fatty acids, and cortisol. Fluctuations in the levels of GH are dramatic; the average serum level, however, is remarkably similar at all ages. Growth is facilitated by GH, but other factors, such as somatotropins, direct the rate of growth and the organs targeted for growth.

◼ THYROID

This gland is a bilobed, richly vascularized structure. The lobes lie lateral to the trachea just beneath the larynx and are connected by a bridge of thyroid tissue, called the isthmus, that runs across the anterior surface of the trachea. Microscopically, the thyroid is composed primarily of spheroid follicles, each of which stores a colloid material in its center. The follicles produce, store, and secrete the two major hormones: T_3 (triiodothyronine) and T_4 (thyroxine). Table 41–2 summarizes thyroid hormones. If the gland is actively secreting, the follicles are small and contain little colloid. Inactive thyroid tissue contains large follicles, each of which possesses a large quantity of stored colloid. Other cells, the parafollicular cells (C cells), are scattered between the follicles. Parafollicular cells secrete the hormone calcitonin. It and two other hormones directly influence calcium metabolism and are discussed later.

THYROID HORMONES

Manufacture and Secretion

The follicular cells absorb tyrosine (an amino acid) and iodide from the plasma and secrete them into the central colloid portion of the follicle, where they are used in the synthesis of T_3 and T_4. (The subscript refers to the number

TABLE 41-2
Hormones of the Thyroid and Parathyroid Glands and Their Actions

Gland	Hormone	Action
Thyroid gland	Thyroxine (T_4)	Controls basic metabolic rate
	Triiodothyronine (T_3)	Induces growth and development
Parathyroid gland	Parathyroid hormone	Promotes bone resorption
		Increases calcium reabsorption
		Increases calcium blood levels

of iodide molecules that each substance contains.) Two iodide molecules are attached, first one and then the other, to each tyrosine molecule. Two such doubly iodinated tyrosines are combined to form T_4. T_3, which is much more biologically active than T_4 and is the predominant form of thyroid hormone produced, is formed by the combination of a doubly iodinated tyrosine with a singly iodinated one. These hormones are then stored in the colloid until they are needed. When they are to be secreted, the follicle cells transport them from the colloid to the plasma. Because of the role of iodine in the manufacture of thyroid hormones, storage and release of small amounts of radioactive iodine by the thyroid can be used to measure the activity of this gland. Because the thyroid gland is virtually the only tissue of the body that absorbs and stores iodine, larger amounts of radioactive iodine can be used to destroy portions of the thyroid gland as a treatment for hyperthyroidism.

Transport and Metabolic Fate

Less than 1% of the secreted T_3 and T_4 remains free and physiologically active in the plasma. The remainder is bound to plasma proteins. Most is bound to thyroxine-binding globulin, a molecule manufactured by the liver, and the remainder is bound to two types of plasma albumin. Such protein-bound hormone serves as a reservoir to replace free T_3 and T_4 that has been degraded, thereby maintaining stable blood levels of thyroid hormones. The plasma proteins involved in transporting T_3 and T_4 are manufactured in the liver. Consequently, liver damage that decreases the plasma levels of these proteins can produce a condition resembling thyroid hormone excess (ie, hyperthyroidism). Plasma levels of these proteins also can be depressed by glucocorticoids, androgens, and L-asparaginase (an antineoplastic drug). They are elevated during pregnancy, and by estrogens, opiates, clofibrate, and major tranquilizers.

Thyroid hormones are deiodinated and catabolized by the liver, kidneys, and various other tissues. A small amount of degraded hormone is added to the bile secreted by the liver and is excreted in the stool.

An earlier index of thyroid secretion, the protein-bound iodine index, used the protein-bound fraction of secreted thyroid hormones. It measured the iodide contained in the T_3 and T_4 attached to plasma proteins. This index is still used occasionally, although now plasma T_3 and T_4 are measured directly by radioimmunoassay.

Actions

T_3 directly crosses target cell membranes, whereas T_4 is changed into T_3 by target cell membranes before crossing. T_3 binds with receptors on the cell nucleus. Through this interaction with the nucleus, these hormones can alter the cellular synthesis of various enzymes and thereby modify cellular operations. The iodine in these hormones does not seem requisite for their actions because several synthetic non–iodine-containing thyroid hormone analogues exist.

The actions of thyroid hormones are widespread and apparently stem from their stimulation of the basal metabolic rate (BMR) of most tissues (excluding brain, anterior pituitary, spleen, lymph nodes, testes, and lung). The exact manner by which these hormones act on cell metabolism is not clear. T_3, and to a lesser extent, T_4, increase the mitochondrial enzyme systems involved in the oxidation of foodstuffs. The energy released by such oxidation is not efficiently stored in the high-energy bonds of adenosine triphosphate. Much is lost in the form of heat. This increases O_2 consumption of and heat production by these tissues (ie, the BMR). This is termed *calorigenic action*.

Effects secondary to calorigenesis include an increased cellular need for vitamins, increased nitrogen excretion, catabolism of protein and fat stores if the supply of carbohydrates is insufficient, and weight loss. The hepatic conversion of carotene to vitamin A requires thyroid hormone.

T_3 and T_4 have other effects that are independent of their calorigenic ones. The ways in which these effects are produced are even less well understood than calorigenesis. Thyroid hormones are essential for the normal growth and development of many body systems, notably the skeletal and nervous systems. These hormones stimulate the secretion of GH and potentiate its effect on various tissues. The effect of thyroid hormones on the nervous system is best illustrated by the cretinism resulting from congenital thyroid insufficiency. Thyroid hormones are also necessary for normal levels of neuronal functioning. Thyroid insufficiency leads to slowed reflexes, slowed mentation, and decreases in level of consciousness (by way of decreased levels of reticular-reactivating system activity). Hyperthyroidism lowers synaptic thresholds within the central nervous system, causing hyperreflexia and a silky skeletal muscle tremor. Thyroid hormone increases the number of β_1 and β_2 adrenergic receptors in various tissues and the affinity of these receptors for catecholamine. This is why an increased heart rate and sweating often occur in hyperthyroidism. The catabolism of skeletal muscle proteins is increased by thyroid hormones to such a degree that pronounced muscle weakness results from prolonged hyperthyroidism (thyrotoxic myopathy). Thyroid hormones increase the rate of carbohydrate absorption from the small intestine and decrease circulating levels of cholesterol.

Regulation

The secretion of T_3 and T_4 by the thyroid gland is primarily regulated by the secretion of TSH from the anterior pituitary gland. TSH stimulates the manufacture and secretion of T_3 and T_4. A negative-feedback regulatory loop exists whereby increased levels of free (unbound) T_3 and T_4 suppress TSH secretion. Decreased plasma TSH results in decreased thyroid function, which causes a fall in free plasma T_3 and T_4. Low T_3 and T_4 levels stimulate TSH secretion. If a TSH-induced increase in thyroid activity does not raise the plasma levels of free T_3 and T_4, the continued high levels of TSH eventually cause an increase in the size of the thyroid gland (nontoxic goiter). In this case, an enlarged thyroid is not associated with overproduction of hormone.

This feedback loop maintains homeostasis of the daily secretion of TSH and thyroid hormones. In addition to being influenced by circulatory T_3 and T_4 levels, TSH secretion is regulated by a hypothalamic neurosecretory material termed thyrotropin-releasing hormone (TRH). The hypothalamic regulation of TSH and consequently, of thyroid function seems to function in infant thermoregulation. In this process, TRH output is increased in response to cold and decreased in response to heat. The elevated thyroid hormone production presumably increases calorigenesis, which raises the body temperature of the cold infant. Similarly, a heat-provoked decrease in TRH causes a decrease in TSH and thyroid activity. This is thought to decrease calorigenesis, thereby decreasing the temperature of the hot infant. The effect of TRH in thermoregulation of adults is negligible.

Hormonal Influences on Calcium Metabolism

Three hormones exert a major influence on calcium metabolism. Two of these, activated vitamin D, or 1,25-dihydroxycholecalciferol, and parathyroid hormone, elevate plasma calcium levels; one, calcitonin, decreases blood levels of calcium.

1,25-DIHYDROXYCHOLECALCIFEROL

Manufacture

This hormone is produced by the action of the liver and the kidneys on vitamin D. Ultraviolet light changes 7-dehydrocholesterol provitamins in the skin to a group of compounds, collectively called vitamin D. One of these, D_3, can also be obtained from vitamin D–enriched and other foods. The liver converts D_3 to 25-hydroxycholecalciferol, which

is then altered by kidney cells to a more active form, 1,25-dihydroxycholecalciferol.

Transport and Metabolic Fate

Vitamin D is synthesized in the skin, absorbed in the small intestine, and transported into the plasma bound to vitamin D–binding proteins. The metabolism of vitamin D is strictly regulated by phosphate concentration in the kidney and parathyroid hormone. Thus, the effect of a decrease in dietary phosphate or serum phosphate is to increase 1,25-dihydroxycholecalciferol.

Actions

Activated vitamin D acts on intracellular enzymes of intestinal mucosal cells to increase calcium absorption. To a lesser extent, it also increases the active transport of calcium out of osteoblasts into the bloodstream. Both of these actions elevate plasma calcium levels. In vitamin deficiency states, the effect of decreased intestinal absorption outweighs any decrease in the mobilization of calcium from bone to produce an overall hypocalcia and poor mineralization of bone.

Regulation

Plasma calcium and phosphate levels operate in a negative feedback loop to influence the activity of the renal enzyme system, which catalyzes the conversion of metabolically inactive vitamin D to the metabolically active 1,25-dihydroxycholecalciferol. High plasma calcium levels decrease this activation process, whereas low levels increase it. The formation of activated vitamin D is also facilitated by parathyroid hormone and decreased by metabolic acidosis and hypoinsulinemia (diabetes mellitus). The hypocalcemia seen in chronic renal disease results from an activated vitamin D deficiency.

PARATHYROID HORMONE

This hormone is produced by the parathyroid glands. Each lobe of the thyroid gland typically contains two parathyroid glands: one in its superior pole and one in its inferior pole. Individual variation exists with respect to the number and distribution of parathyroid glands. Some people have more or fewer than four. Others have parathyroid tissue in the mediastinum.

Manufacture and Secretion

Parathyroid hormone is a polypeptide produced and secreted by the chief cells of the parathyroid glands. This hormone is stored in secretory granules and released in response to a fall in ionized calcium concentrations. It is cleaved into active form in the kidneys and liver.

Transport and Metabolic Fate

Parathyroid hormone is transported free (unbound) in the plasma, has a half-life of less than 20 minutes, and is metabolically degraded by cells in the liver. A rise in calcium concentration increases parathyroid hormone secretion.

Actions

Parathyroid hormone acts on two target tissues: bone cells and kidney tubules. In bone, it stimulates osteoclast activity and inhibits osteoblast activity. This results in bone reabsorption with consequent mobilization of calcium and phosphate from the bony matrix into the bloodstream. In the kidney, parathyroid hormone increases the reabsorption of calcium by distal tubule cells and decreases the reabsorption of phosphate by proximal tubule cells. The effect of these multiple actions is elevation of plasma calcium levels and lowering of plasma phosphate levels. At the cellular level, parathyroid hormone produces these effects by activating adenylate cyclase after binding to specific membrane receptors, thereby increasing the intracellular levels of cyclic AMP in the target tissues.

Regulation

Plasma calcium levels alter parathyroid hormone secretion by way of a negative-feedback loop. Secretion is inhibited by high plasma calcium levels and stimulated by low blood levels of calcium. The activated vitamin B deficiency-induced hypocalcemia, which occurs in chronic renal failure, typically produces a secondary hyperparathyroidism. Parathyroid gland secretion also is stimulated by hypomagnesemia, adrenergic agonists, and prostaglandins.

CALCITONIN

Manufacture and Secretion

This polypeptide hormone is produced by the parafollicular cells (C cells) of the thyroid gland. It can also be secreted by nonthyroidal tissue (eg, lung, intestine, pituitary, and bladder).

Transport and Metabolic Fate

Calcitonin is transported unbound in the plasma. It has a half-life of 5 minutes and is predominantly metabolized in the kidney.

Actions

Calcitonin lowers plasma calcium and phosphate levels by inhibiting osteoclastic bone reabsorption and increasing urinary phosphate and calcium excretion. Calcitonin levels are elevated during pregnancy and lactation. This suggests that it may help to protect the mother's skeleton from excess calcium loss during these periods of calcium drain.

Regulation

Calcitonin does not function in the normal daily homeostasis of plasma calcium levels. It appears to serve more of an emergency function in that it is secreted only if the plasma calcium level exceeds 9.3 mg/dL. At high blood calcium levels, calcitonin secretion is stimulated by increased levels of plasma calcium. Calcitonin is also released by gastrin, glucagon, and secretion of gastrointestinal hormones.

OTHER HORMONES THAT INFLUENCE CALCIUM METABOLISM

Four hormones bear mention here. T_3 and T_4 are thought by some to produce hypercalcemia, but the mechanism of action is unknown. Estrogens prevent parathyroid hormone from raising plasma calcium by mobilizing calcium from bone. Growth hormone increases urinary calcium excretion while also increasing intestinal calcium absorption. These two effects counterbalance each other, thereby producing no net change in plasma calcium levels. Glucocorticoids tend to lower plasma calcium levels by decreasing intestinal absorption of calcium and increasing renal calcium excretion.

▉ ISLETS OF LANGERHANS

This name refers to the more than 1 million ovoid islands (clusters) of cells that are scattered throughout the pancreas, predominantly in the tail. Because of this distribution of islet cells, acute attacks of pancreatitis, which generally spare the tail, usually spare the islets. Episodes of chronic recurrent pancreatitis, typically involve all of the pancreas. Consequently, these episodes cause islet cell destruction and diabetes mellitus. Each cell cluster is richly supplied with capillaries, into which its hormones are secreted. The islets are composed of four types of cells: alpha cells, which secrete glucagon; beta cells, which secrete insulin; delta cells, which secrete somatostatin; and F cells, which secrete pancreatic polypeptide. Two hormones secreted by the pancreas are summarized in Table 41–3.

INSULIN

Manufacture and Secretion

The precursor of insulin, proinsulin, is manufactured in the granular endoplasmic reticulum. Proinsulin is a necklace of amino acid beads that has one end folded over the other so that it resembles a squashed figure nine. It leaves the reticulum and is stored as secretory granules in another cell structure. Here, two ends of the folded proinsulin neck-

TABLE 41-3 The Pancreas and Its Hormones and Their Actions	
Hormone	**Action**
Insulin	Lowers blood sugar
	Increases carbohydrate utilization
	Decreases gluconeogenesis
Glucagon	Raises blood sugar
	Raises glucogenolysis, gluconeogenesis

lace become attached to one another (by way of disulfide bonds) to form two parallel chains. The two ends are then separated from the center of the necklace. This center chain of amino acids is termed C-peptide. Proinsulin can be found in the plasma as a result of certain islet tumors or overstimulation of the beta cells. C-peptide is secreted into the bloodstream along with insulin. Because there is a 1:1 ratio between C-peptide and insulin, plasma C-peptide levels can be used to measure endogenous insulin secretion or degree of beta cell activity.

Metabolic Fate

Insulin acts only on a few types of tissues. However, the membranes of nearly all types of body cells possess insulin receptors. The possession of insulin receptors by cells on which insulin does not act may be explained by the discovery of the growth factors (IGF-I and IGF-II). The insulin receptors serve as receptors for these growth factors and for insulin.

Binding of insulin to the insulin receptors initiates the physiological action of insulin on the cell. After a molecule of insulin binds to a receptor, the insulin–receptor complex is taken into the cytoplasm of the cell by endocytosis and is destroyed within 14 to 15 hours by lysosomal enzymes. New receptors replace the destroyed ones in the cell membranes. Plasma insulin has a half-life of approximately 5 minutes. About 80% of all circulating insulin is catabolized by liver and kidney cells.

Actions

The mechanism by which insulin exerts its action is unknown. It is known only that insulin does not activate adenylate cyclase. The actions of insulin are summarized in the accompanying display. In addition, insulin facilitates glucose uptake by connective tissue, leukocytes, mammary glands, the lens of the eye, aorta, pituitary, and alpha islet cells. In general, insulin enables glucose to be readily available for aerobic oxidation by the Krebs citric acid cycle in muscle, adipose, and connective tissue cells. Facilitation of the preferential use of glucose as cellular fuel means that the cells do not need to oxidize fatty or amino acids. Instead, these can be conserved. Protein synthesis and fat storage are increased in liver, muscle, and adipose tissue. Breakdown of fats and proteins is decreased. Hepatic gluconeogenesis also is decreased or halted, and glycogen synthesis is increased.

Regulation

Insulin secretion is influenced by a variety of factors as listed in the display. Monosaccharides are the primary regulatory mechanism for insulin secretion. Elevated plasma levels of glucose, fructose, and mannose act in a negative feedback loop to increase the secretion of insulin. Lower levels of these sugars decrease insulin output. Other monosaccharides (eg, galactose, xylose, and arabinose) have no effect on insulin secretion. Glucagon and β-adrenergic-stimulating chemicals increase insulin secretion by stimulating adenylate cyclase, an enzyme that elevates levels of cyclic AMP

Major Actions of Insulin on Fat and Muscle Cells

Muscle Cells	Adipose Cells
Increased glucose entry	Increased glucose entry
Increased K$^+$ uptake	Increased K$^+$ uptake
Increased glycogen synthesis	Increased fatty acid entry and synthesis
Increased amino acid entry	Increased fat deposition
Increased protein synthesis	Increased conversion of glucose to fatty acids
Decreased protein catabolism	Inhibition of lipolysis
Increased ketone entry into cells	

---

within beta cells. Theophylline, which inhibits the degradation of beta cell cyclic AMP, also promotes production. Beta cells are also stimulated to secrete insulin by tolbutamide and other sulfonylurea derivatives; acetylcholine; impulses from vagal nerve branches to the islets; selected amino acids, such as arginine; and beta ketoacids. The mechanisms of action of these stimuli are as yet unclear. Insulin production is inhibited by α-adrenergic-stimulating agents, β-adrenergic blocking agents, diazoxide (Proglycem), thiazide diuretics, phenytoin (Dilantin), alloxan, agents that prevent glucose metabolism (2-deoxyglucose or mannoheptulose), somatostatin, and insulin itself (see the display of factors).

Chronic stimulation of beta cells, such as by a high carbohydrate diet for several weeks, can cause a limited amount of hypertrophy and subsequent increase in the insulin-producing capacity. Overstimulation, however, produces beta cell exhaustion. Stimulation of these exhausted cells produces beta cell death and a depletion in the beta cell reserve. Beta cell activity is also decreased by the administration of exogenous insulin. Such decreased activity enables the cells to rest and results in their being temporarily hyperproductive after the withdrawal of exogenous insulin. The quantity and activity of insulin receptors also can be regulated by various factors. Increased amounts of insulin, obesity, acromegaly, and excess glucocorticoids decrease the receptors' number or activity or both. Exercise and decreased circulating levels of insulin increase the activity of insulin receptors.

GLUCAGON

Secretion

This polypeptide hormone is manufactured and secreted by the alpha islet cells and is stimulated by pure protein meal ingestion that produces an amino acidemia.

Metabolic Fate

The half-life of plasma glucagon is 5 to 10 minutes. The hormone stimulates the synthesis of the gluconeogenic enzyme fructose-1,6-biphosphate. This hormone is degraded mainly by the liver.

Factors Affecting Insulin Secretion

Stimulators	*Inhibitors*
Glucose	Somatostatin
Mannose	2-Deoxyglucose
Amino acids (leucine, arginine, others)	Mannoheptulose
Intestinal hormones (GIP, gastrin, secretin, CCK, glucagon, others?)	α-Adrenergic-stimulating agents (norepinephrine, epinephrine)
β-Keto acids	β-Adrenergic-blocking agents (propranolol)
Acetylcholine	Diazoxide
Glucagon	Thiazide diuretics
Cyclic AMP and various cyclic AMP–generating substances	Phenytoin
β-Adrenergic-stimulating agents	Alloxan
Theophylline	Microtubule inhibitors
Sulfonylureas	Insulin

Actions

The major function of glucagon is to elevate blood sugar levels by influencing enzyme systems within liver, fat, and muscle cells and then to enable this plasma glucose to enter and be used by body cells (eg, muscle) by stimulating the secretion of insulin. By this function, glucagon prevents hypoglycemia between meals, during exercise, during the first few days of fasting, and after a high-protein meal. (Dietary protein stimulates an increase in plasma insulin, which causes a rapid cellular uptake of absorbed dietary carbohydrates.)

To perform this function, glucagon stimulates liver cells to perform glycogenolysis and gluconeogenesis. This increases the glucose concentration within liver cells, and because these cells can dephosphorylate intracellular glucose, this glucose can be released from the liver into the bloodstream. The fatty acids and amino acids needed for gluconeogenesis are supplied by the glucagon-stimulated breakdown of fats in adipose cells and the release of fatty acids into the bloodstream. If the supply of fatty acids is not sufficient, glucagon also stimulates the breakdown of proteins into amino acids in muscle cells and the release of amino acids into the plasma. These fatty acids and amino acids are then taken up by hepatocytes and used as raw materials in gluconeogenesis. Glucagon also elevates plasma ketone levels by increasing hepatic ketone production and promotes the secretion of somatostatin and GH.

Although glucagon opposes the effects of insulin on blood sugar levels, it also stimulates the secretion of insulin. This apparent contradiction is actually a logical second step in the biological function of this hormone. It enables the increased plasma glucose to enter and be used by various tissues. An elevated plasma glucose level stimulates insulin secretion, but this takes a while. The direct action of glucagon on beta cells simply is faster.

At the cellular level, the actions of glucagon on cell enzyme systems are mediated by glucagon-induced elevations in intracellular cyclic AMP. This chemical then acts as a second messenger to alter the enzyme activity of the cell to produce the actions of glucagon. Because of this effect on intracellular cyclic AMP, large amounts of exogenous glucagon increase the inotropic capacity of myocardial tissue. However, lower levels of endogenous glucagon do not seem to have this effect.

Regulation

As is the case with beta cells, alpha cells are stimulated by β-adrenergic agonists, theophylline, elevated plasma levels of dietary amino acids (primarily those used in gluconeogenesis), and vagal (cholinergic) stimulation. Glucagon secretion is also prompted by glucocorticoids (eg, cortisol), CCK, and gastrin. Exercise, physical stress, and infections also increase alpha cell activity. Whereas the effects of exercise on glucagon secretion seem to be mediated by increased β-adrenergic activity, stress and infection probably operate by increasing plasma glucocorticoid levels. Dietary amino acids are believed to enhance glucagon secretion by their effects on CCK or gastrin or both, because intravenous amino acids exert little or no effect on alpha cells.

Elevated plasma glucose operates by a negative-feedback loop to retard or halt the output of glucagon; however, plasma insulin must be present for this mechanism to operate. Like beta cell secretion; alpha cell secretion is inhibited by adrenergic agonists, phenytoin, and somatostatin. Fatty acids and ketone bodies in the plasma can inhibit glucagon secretion, but this inhibition must be weak, because plasma glucagon levels can be quite elevated during diabetic ketoacidosis.

SOMATOSTATIN

Manufacture and Secretion

This tetradecapeptide is produced not only by the delta cells of the pancreas but also by the hypothalamus, where it functions as an inhibitor of anterior pituitary GH secretion;

neurons of the central nervous system, where it probably functions as a synaptic neurotransmitter agent; and delta cells in the gastric mucosa, where it inhibits the secretion of gastrin and other lesser known gastrointestinal hormones. Islet cell somatostatin is secreted into the bloodstream and therefore functions as a hormone.

Metabolic Fate

Little is known of the metabolism of somatostatin because it is so tightly bound with the actions of GH.

Actions

Pancreatic somatostatin inhibits the activity of all other islet cells. The biological significance of this action is not yet known. The only clinical data of relevance concern delta cell tumors. These produce a clinical picture that resembles diabetes mellitus but that is reversible with tumor ablation.

Regulation

The secretion of somatostatin from islet cells is increased by glucose, certain amino acids, and CCK. Factors that inhibit islet somatostatin secretion are unknown.

PANCREATIC POLYPEPTIDE

Not much is known about this islet hormone in humans. Its secretion in humans is enhanced by dietary protein, exercise, acute hypoglycemia, and fasting. Somatostatin and elevated plasma glucose levels decrease the secretion of this polypeptide. No definite actions of this hormone have been established for humans.

ADRENAL GLANDS

An adrenal gland lies at the superior pole of each kidney. Each gland is composed of an inner core, the medulla, surrounded by an outer layer, the cortex. Although they are structurally related, the medulla and cortex are derived from different embryological tissues and function as separate entities. Hormones are summarized in Table 41–4.

Adrenal Medulla

This gland is basically a modified sympathetic ganglion. The axons of preganglionic sympathetic neurons arrive from the thoracic cord by way of splanchnic nerves (see Fig. 31–11 and Table 31–1). They synapse in the adrenal medulla with modified postganglionic cells that have lost their axons and secrete chemicals directly into the bloodstream. Therefore, the adrenal medullas may appropriately be viewed as endocrine extensions of the autonomic nervous system.

Manufacture and Secretion

Four chemicals are produced and secreted by two morphologically different cell types: dopamine, a precursor of norepinephrine; norepinephrine, the typical product of postganglionic sympathetic neurons; epinephrine, a methylated version of norepinephrine; and opioid peptides (enkephalins). The first three chemicals are collectively termed catecholamines. They are stored in granules within the medulla cells. Their secretion is triggered by stimulation of the preganglionic neurons that innervate the medulla. This causes the neurons to release acetylcholine, which in turn prompts the medulla cells to secrete. The specific stimulus for the secretion of opioid peptides has not yet been identified.

Metabolic Fate

The half-life of plasma catecholamines is approximately 2 minutes. These compounds are rapidly degraded by plasma renal and hepatic catechol O-methyltransferase enzymes into vanillylmandelic acid, metanephrine, and normetanephrine, which are excreted in the urine. Only small quantities of nondegraded catecholamines are found in normal urine. The metabolism and fate of the medullary enkephalins are unknown.

Actions

Predictably, the epinephrine and norepinephrine secreted by the adrenal medulla mimic the effects of a mass discharge from sympathetic neurons. Apart from this, however, they produce several metabolic actions. First, they elevate blood sugar levels by activating an enzyme, phosphorylase, that promotes hepatic glycogenolysis. Because liver cells possess the enzyme glucose-6-phosphatase, the glu-

TABLE 41-4
Hormones of the Adrenal Gland and Their Actions

Gland	Hormone	Action
Adrenal gland cortex	Mineralocorticoids	Reabsorption of sodium
		Elimination of potassium
	Glucocorticoids	Responds to stress
		Decreases inflammation
		Alters metabolism of protein and fat
Medulla	Epinephrine	Stimulates sympathetic system
	Norepinephrine	Increases peripheral resistance

cose produced by this glycogen breakdown is able to diffuse out of hepatocytes and into the bloodstream. These hormones also induce muscle cells to participate in elevating blood sugar levels, although this process is less direct. Phosphorylase in muscle cells also is activated by these catecholamines. However, the intracellular glucose thereby produced is unable to exit the muscle cells, because they do not possess glucose-6-phosphatase. Instead, this glucose is catabolized to lactate, which can leave the muscle cells. Lactate then circulates to the liver, where it is converted to glucose that can enter the bloodstream. These hormones can also elevate plasma glucose levels by stimulating the secretion of glucagon and increase the uptake of glucose into body tissues by stimulating the secretion of insulin. Epinephrine and norepinephrine can also produce the opposite effects by stimulating α-adrenergic receptors on islet cells. Because of differential effects of both hormones on α- and β-adrenergic receptors, the result is that epinephrine elevates plasma glucose much more than does norepinephrine.

A second metabolic effect of catecholamines is promotion of lipolysis in adipose tissue. This elevates plasma free fatty acid levels and provides an alternative energy source for many body cells. Circulating catecholamines also increase alertness by stimulating the reticular activating system. Lastly, these hormones produce an increase in the metabolic rate of the body and a cutaneous vasoconstriction, both of which result in an elevation in body temperature. However, the accelerated metabolism requires the presence of the thyroid and adrenal cortex hormones.

The physiological actions of both adrenal medullary dopamine and the enkephalins are unknown. Exogenous dopamine is useful in combating certain shocks because it has a positive inotropic effect on the heart (by way of β-receptors) and produces renal vasodilation and peripheral vasoconstriction. The overall effect of moderate dosages is elevation of systolic blood pressure (without an appreciable increase in diastolic blood pressure) together with retention or restoration of renal output.

Regulation

Stimulation of the adrenal medulla glands is part of a general sympathetic–adrenal medulla (SAM) response to exercise and to perceived threats to biopsychological integrity and survival. (Cannon termed the latter the "fight or flight" response.) Hypoglycemia also stimulates increased adrenal medulla secretion.

The results of the SAM response enable the body to perform vigorous physical exertion optimally. The heart rate and blood pressure are increased (increasing perfusion), and blood flow is shunted away from the skin and gastrointestinal tract to more vital organs for exertion, such as skeletal muscles, brain, and heart. The reticular activating system is stimulated, fostering alertness. Blood glucose and fatty acid levels are raised, thereby increasing the available energy sources for cells. Pupils are dilated, increasing the field of peripheral vision and the amount of light entering the eyes. Sweat glands are stimulated, cooling the body in advance of

and during the time that the body temperature is elevated as the result of the physical exertion. The majority of this SAM response is mediated by sympathetic nerve fibers to various body structures; circulating catecholamines play only a minor role. Furthermore, many tissue responses (eg, those of muscle cells) to such sympathetic demands require the presence of glucocorticoids to enable the tissues to meet the demands of the SAM response, and the SAM response often accompanies the stress-induced secretion of adrenal steroids discovered by Seyle. (This and the endocrine response to physical and psychological stress are discussed in the section on the adrenal cortex.)

The SAM response is initiated by the perception of a stimulus or situation that a person evaluates on the basis of experience and current resources to be a threat to his or her well-being. This response involves the cerebral cortex. Impulses from the cortex travel by way of nerve fibers to the limbic system, where they are involved in generating an emotional response. Additional impulses from the cortex and the limbic system stimulate sympathetic centers in the diencephalon. These centers in turn discharge a specific pattern of impulses down descending fibers to various sympathetic neurons in the cord, bringing about the SAM response.

Adrenal Cortex

This gland is composed of three histologically different layers. Its exterior is covered by a capsule. The outermost layer, the zona glomerulosa, lies just beneath the capsule. It produces and secretes primarily mineralocorticoids, such as aldosterone. The inner two layers, the zona fasciculata and zona reticularis, manufacture and secrete glucocorticoids (cortisol and corticosterone) and adrenal androgens and estrogens. If these inner cortical layers are destroyed, they can be regenerated from zona glomerulosa cells. Because the biosynthetic pathways and metabolic fates for all adrenocortical hormones are interrelated, these are discussed together for all hormones. Actions and regulation are considered separately for mineralocorticoids, glucocorticoids, and sex steroids.

Manufacture and Secretion

Figure 41–3 depicts the metabolic pathways for synthesis of all adrenocortical hormones. Each of these metabolic steps is governed by a specific enzyme. Genetic deficiencies in one or more of these enzymes produce syndromes involving the underproduction or overproduction of various cortical hormones. Drugs that inhibit specific enzymes are used clinically to assess cortical function. One such drug is metyrapone, which inhibits cortisol synthesis.

Metabolic Fate

After secretion, plasma cortisol and to a lesser extent, corticosterone are bound to a plasma globulin called corticosteroid-binding globulin (CBG), or transcortin. Only the unbound hormones are physiologically active. The bound glucocorticoids serve as a hormone reservoir that is used to

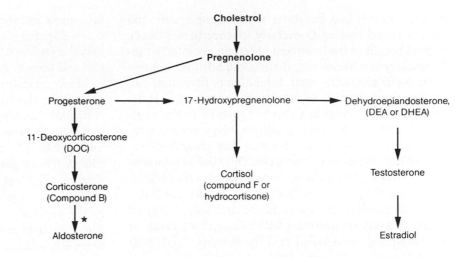

FIGURE 41-3

Biosynthetic pathways for adrenal cortical hormones. Cells in all three layers contain all pathways except that from cortico-sterone to aldosterone: only cells of zona glomerulosa can perform this step (*).

replace degraded unbound hormone. The half-lives of plasma corticosterone and cortisol are roughly 50 and 80 minutes, respectively. CBG is manufactured by liver cells. Therefore, decreased hepatic function (eg, cirrhosis) can lead to subnormal quantities of plasma CBG, resulting in excess quantities of circulating unbound, active glucocorti-coids. Only a small amount of aldosterone is bound to plasma proteins. Its half-life is approximately 20 minutes.

Adrenal steroids are degraded by the liver. Their metabo-lites are converted to a soluble form by the same enzyme system that conjugates bilirubin (ie, the glucuronyltrans-ferase system). The adrenal steroids and bilirubin compete for this system, and an excess of one type of substance can potentially inhibit the degradation of the others. Depressed hepatic function also can retard the degradation of adrenal steroids, thereby producing a clinical picture of hormone excess. The soluble degraded steroid metabolites are ex-creted by the kidneys.

GLUCOCORTICOIDS

Action

The effects of pharmacological dosages of these hor-mones are considered separately from those of normal physiological levels. As the name glucocorticoid suggests, cortisol and corticosterone influence glucose metabolism. They elevate plasma glucose levels by promoting hepatic gluconeogenesis and glycogenolysis. To facilitate gluco-neogenesis, these hormones cause the breakdown of fat and proteins and the release of fatty and amino acids into the bloodstream, which carries them to the liver. Glucocorti-coids enable tissues to respond to glucagon and cate-cholamines; they also prevent rapid fatigue of skeletal mus-cle. The mode by which glucocorticoids produce these effects is not understood, and they go unnoticed in the nor-mal person. One can best appreciate them by observing the result of their absence in adrenalectomized patients and in untreated people who are exposed to perceived threat or stress. These enabling and metabolic effects possibly con-stitute a major portion of the stress resistance provided by the glucocorticoids.

Cortisol and corticosterone also act on the kidneys to permit the excretion of a normal water load in one of three ways: glucocorticoids make distal or collecting tubules more permeable to the reabsorption of water independently of sodium reabsorption; they increase the glomerular fil-tration rate; or they reduce the output of ADH.

The effects of glucocorticoids on plasma components are mixed. They decrease the number of plasma eosinophils and basophils but increase the number of circulating neu-trophils, platelets, and erythrocytes. By suppressing pro-duction and increasing destruction, glucocorticoids de-crease the number of lymphocytes. They also decrease the size of lymph nodes. A major function of lymphocytes is to provide either humoral immunity (with antibodies) or cell-mediated immunity. Stress-induced elevations in glucocor-ticoid secretion and the resulting decrease in lymphocytes may explain the decrease in immunocompetence that often occurs in people who are under psychological or physical stress.

Other effects of physiological levels of glucocorticoids in-clude decreasing olfactory and gustatory sensitivity. People with adrenal insufficiency can detect various chemicals (eg, sugar, salt, urea, and KCl) by either taste or smell with a sensitivity that is 40 to 120 times greater than normal.

In pharmacological dosages, glucocorticoids possess im-munosuppressive anti-inflammatory and antihistaminic ac-tivity. Glucocorticoids suppress the immune system by in-hibiting the production of interleukin-2 by T4 (helper) lymphocytes. Decreases in interleukin-2 reduce the prolif-eration of T8 (suppressor, cytotoxic) T cells and B lympho-cytes. Glucocorticoids act in several ways to suppress the in-flammatory response, including the influx of phagocytes and the activation of complement and kinins. First, they in-hibit the formation of the raw material (arachidonic acid) needed for the manufacture of chemicals that trigger the in-flammatory response (eg, leukotrienes, prostaglandins). Second, they inhibit the release of interleukin-1 from gran-ulocytes. Third, glucocorticoids prevent fibroblasts from acting to wall off an infectious area from the rest of the body. This can be very dangerous to patients with infec-tions, because the inflammatory response destroys invading microorganisms and facilitates the immune system and normal wound healing. Conversely, glucocorticoids can be of great benefit in the treatment of certain noninfective inflammatory conditions (eg, rheumatoid arthritis and systemic lupus erythematosus). Inhibition of fibroblasts can prevent the formation of keloids and postsurgical adhesions. Glucocorticoids can also be beneficial in the treatment of certain allergies (eg, asthma, hives, and minimal change glomerular disease) because they prevent the release of histamines from mast cells. Their use as immunosuppressives enables patients to receive organ transplants. In any case, the potentially deleterious side effects of glucocorticoids usually require that they be used only after other treatments (eg, nonsteroidal anti-inflammatory drugs or antihistamines) have failed or if the benefits clearly outweigh the risks (eg, in renal disease or with organ transplants). In addition to immunosuppression, glucocorticoids trigger the development of all or part of Cushing's syndrome (eg, diabetes, hypertension, protein wasting, and osteoporosis) and inhibit growth in infants and children.

Regulation

Regulation of glucocorticoid secretion is outlined in Figure 41–4. The secretion of glucocorticoids is triggered by the release of corticotropin-releasing factor (CRF), a neurosecretory material released by the hypothalamus. CRF stimulates the cells of the anterior pituitary to secrete ACTH. Without the stimulus of ACTH, the cells of the zona

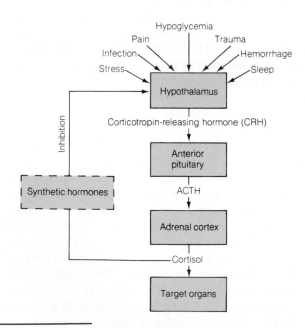

FIGURE 41-4
The hypothalamic–pituitary–adrenal (HPA) feedback system that regulates glucocorticoid (cortisol) levels. Cortisol release is regulated by ACTH. Stress exerts its effects on cortisol release through the HPA system and the corticotropin-releasing factor (CRF), which controls the release of ACTH from the anterior pituitary gland. Increased cortisol levels incite a negative feedback inhibition of ACTH release. Pharmacological doses of synthetic steroids inhibit ACTH release by way of the hypothalamic CRF.

fasciculata and zona reticularis do not secrete glucocorticoids. Elevated plasma glucocorticoid levels function in a negative feedback loop to decrease or halt the secretion of CRF and thereby indirectly ACTH as well.

There is a diurnal rhythm to the secretion of CRF that causes a similar rhythm in the output of ACTH and glucocorticoids. The result is that maximal glucocorticoid secretion occurs between 6:00 and 8:00 AM in people sleeping from midnight to 8:00 AM in a 24-hour day. Tumors that secrete CRF, ACTH, or glucocorticoids do not demonstrate such a rhythm, a fact that is useful in their diagnosis. The biological clock that regulates this and other diurnal, or circadian, rhythms is located in the hypothalamus, just above the area where the optic nerves cross (optic chiasma). Presumably, fibers from this area send impulses to the CRF-secreting area of the hypothalamus to regulate this neurosecretion.

The hypothalamic neurosecretion of CRF is also triggered by neural impulses from higher brain centers (eg, cerebral cortex) in response to psychological stress. This type of stress is defined according to Lazarus' cognitive phenomenological theory as a situation in which demands exceed coping resources. This can occur slowly and deliberately or instantaneously and without the person's being precisely aware that such a phenomenon has occurred. Before the mid-1970s, Selye's proposed general adaptation syndrome was the only existing model for physiological responses to stress. According to this theory, any type of stress, physical or psychological, triggers the release of glucocorticoids by the CRF–ACTH mechanism. Then, in an elegant series of experiments on monkeys that separated psychological from purely physical stressors, Mason and coworkers discovered that glucocorticoids were typically released only in response to psychological stress. These researchers found that physical stressors (eg, cold, and starvation) each induced a different pattern of responses from almost all the endocrine glands. Each type of stressor studied produced a different profile of endocrine responses that continued to change over several days after exposure of the animal to the stress-provoking agent. This work was later confirmed in humans. Thus, the physiological hormone responses to stress can no longer be attributed only to the glucocorticoids. The perception of a potential physical or psychological threat to one's well-being triggers an SAM response. If the demands of this or any other situation are evaluated as exceeding current resources, the CRF–ACTH–glucocorticoid mechanism is activated. The beneficial functions of normal levels of glucocorticoids in enabling tissues to respond to glucagon and catecholamines are more than adequate to meet the needs of the SAM mechanism for a short time. If these needs continue, additional stress-induced glucocorticoid secretion is required. Eventually, if the stress continues unameliorated, exhaustion of the adrenal cortex occurs, glucocorticoid levels drop, tissues are no longer able to meet the demands of the SAM mechanism, muscle fatigue occurs, readily available cell energy sources (eg, plasma glucose and fatty acid) are depleted, and vascular collapse and death result.

MINERALOCORTICOIDS

Actions

Aldosterone and glucocorticoids that have some mineralocorticoid function (eg, 11-Deoxycorticosterone) increase sodium reabsorption by the cells of the collecting ducts and distal tubules of the nephrons. Because of the cation exchange system in the distal tubule cells, such sodium reabsorption can increase potassium secretion and thereby foster potential hypokalemia. The reabsorption of sodium osmotically causes water reabsorption. This expands the volume of ECF. The increase in blood volume causes an elevation in blood pressure. Edema does not usually result, however. Above a certain level of aldosterone-induced sodium reabsorption, the expansion of the ECF compartment can trigger secretion of natriuretic hormone or decreased sodium reabsorption in the proximal tubule. Either of these effects opposes the action of aldosterone and sodium excretion.

Regulation and Secretion

The primary mechanism for this is the renin–angiotensin system. Pituitary ACTH does not stimulate zona glomerulosa cells under normal conditions. Cells of the juxtaglomerular apparatus (JGA) are wedged between the renal afferent arteriole as it enters the glomerulus and the distal tubule as it passes by this area. The JGA contains baroceptor cells that monitor the afferent arteriole blood pressure and other cells that monitor the sodium and chloride concentration in the urine within the distal tubule (the lower the concentration, the slower the formation of filtrate, if all other factors are equal). A fall either in blood pressure or in the concentration of electrolytes stimulates the JGA to secrete the glycoprotein hormone renin. The major classes of stimuli that trigger renin secretion are decreased renal perfusion (eg, cardiac failure, dehydration, and hemorrhage) and low ECF salt concentrations (eg, from excessive use of diuretics).

Renin converts a circulating plasma globulin into angiotensin I. As the blood passes through the lungs (and to a lesser extent in other parts of the circulatory system), angiotensin I is converted to angiotensin II. This physiologically active chemical acts on the zona glomerulosa to promote aldosterone secretion, which leads to retention of salt and water, and vascular smooth muscle, thereby stimulating profound vasoconstriction. The result of both actions of angiotensin II is elevation of systemic blood pressure, which, among other things, improves renal perfusion.

The JGA contains β_2 receptors and can be stimulated by sympathetic fibers. Prostaglandins also stimulate the JGA. All three stimulate the secretion of renin. Therefore, the secretion of renin can be pharmacologically decreased by β_2-blockers (eg, propranolol [Inderal]). Prostaglandin inhibitors (aspirin, nonsteroidal antiinflammatory agents, or indomethacin [Indocin]) can exert a similar action. Captopril (Capoten) prevents the conversion of angiotensin I to angiotensin II. These effects have made captopril and β_2-blockers useful as antihypertensive agents.

Aldosterone secretion is also stimulated by an increase in plasma potassium levels but not by increased sodium levels. The potassium acts by facilitating the conversion of cholesterol to aldosterone in zona glomerulosa cells. Another regulating factor for aldosterone secretion is posture. An upright body position increases aldosterone levels by increasing production and decreasing degradation. How this works is unclear, but because of this, aldosterone levels of bed-ridden patients are slightly subnormal. There also is a poorly understood diurnal rhythm of aldosterone secretion, with highest levels occurring in the early morning hours just prior to the person's awakening. This rhythm is not due to the diurnal CRF–ACTH rhythm because that affects only glucocorticoid secretion.

▋ NATRIURETIC HORMONE

Manufacture and Secretion

Natriuretic hormone is manufactured by cells in the walls of the atria of the heart. For this reason, its other name is atrial natriuretic peptide (ANP). The main stimulus for this secretion is in response to atrial stretch.

Metabolic Fate

The metabolic fate of natriuretic hormones is unknown, but circulating levels of this hormone are elevated in congestive heart failure, cirrhosis, and renal insufficiency and are low in nephrotic syndrome and volume depletion. These results suggest liver and kidney regulation.

Actions

Atrial natriuretic peptide increases renal excretion of salt and water. Some evidence suggests that ANP acts by increasing glomerular filtration. Other evidence indicates that ANP inhibits the membrane active transport mechanism responsible for the reabsorption of sodium by renal tubule cells. Decreased sodium reabsorption decreases the movement of water from the urine in the nephron back into the blood of the peritubular capillaries, thereby increasing the elimination of water and salt from the body. Natriuretic hormone also inhibits the secretion of renin by the juxtaglomerular apparatus of the kidney, thereby lowering plasma angiotensin levels.

Atrial natriuretic peptide also inhibits the membrane active transport mechanism responsible for pumping sodium out of vascular smooth muscle cells. The consequent rise in intracellular sodium inhibits the entry of calcium ions, thereby lowering the intracellular concentration of calcium ions. The decrease in the intracellular free calcium promotes vasodilation and a lowering of the systemic blood pressure.

Regulation

Natriuretic hormone is secreted in response to a rise in ECF volume caused by the ingestion of salt and water. The exact stimulus appears to be a stretch of the muscle fibers in the atrial walls, which results from the increased venous return that is caused by the rise in ECF volume. As the natriuresis causes the ECF volume to fall back to normal, the secretion of natriuretic hormone stops. The capability of ANP to increase the GFR together with its direct effects on the collecting tubules results in a profound natriuresis and diuresis.

Clinical Applicability Challenges

Self-Challenge: Critical Thinking

1. Explore physiological implications when there is faulty regulation of ADH by the posterior pituitary.

2. Compare and contrast the feedback mechanisms that affect the synthesis and production of thyroxine by the thyroid and cortisol by the adrenal cortex.

3. Compare and contrast the mechanisms by which glucagon and insulin regulate the body's glucose level.

Study Questions

1. Side effects of steroid medications include
   1. osteoporosis.
   2. nervousness and insomnia.
   3. peptic ulcer.
   4. hypoglycemia.
      a. 1 and 2
      b. 3 and 4
      c. 1 and 3
      d. 2 and 4

2. At the appropriate age, growth hormone secretion is decreased by
   a. increased plasma glucose levels.
   b. fasting.
   c. exercise.
   d. stress.

3. Blood glucose levels are not affected by
   a. aldosterone.
   b. insulin.
   c. glucagon.
   d. norepinephrine.

BIBLIOGRAPHY

Bullock BL: Pathophysiology, Adaptations and Alterations in Function (4th Ed). Philadelphia, Lippincott-Raven, 1996

Guyton AC: Textbook of Medical Physiology (9th Ed). Philadelphia, WB Saunders, 1996

McCance KL, Huether SE: Pathophysiology. The Biologic Basis for Disease in Adults and Children (2nd Ed). St Louis, Mosby-Year Book, 1994

Porth CM: Pathophysiology: Concepts of Altered Health States (4th Ed). Philadelphia, Lippincott-Raven, 1994

Patient Assessment: Endocrine System

HISTORY

PHYSICAL EXAMINATION

DIAGNOSTIC STUDIES

Laboratory Tests
Total T_4
Free Thyroxine T_4 and Free Thyroxine
Index
Free Triiodothyronine T_3
Thyroid-Stimulating Hormone
(Thyrotropin)

Cortisol (Hydrocortisone)
Cortisol (Dexamethasone)
Suppression
Cortisol Stimulation
Fasting Blood Sugar/Glucose
Insulin
Glucagon
Urine Vanillylmandelic Acid
(Catecholamines)
Urine 17 Ketosteroids and 17
Hydroxycorticosteroids

Urine Specific Gravity
Urine Osmolality
Urine Ketones
Diagnostic Tests
Thyroid Scan and Radioactive Iodine
Uptake Study
Adrenal Scan
Additional Tests

OBJECTIVES

Based on the content in this chapter, the reader should be able to:

- Analyze the relationship between the physiological functions of the endocrine gland and the signs and symptoms that indicate endocrine dysfunction.
- Formulate a plan for collecting history and physical examination data when the patient may have an acute endocrine disorder.
- Differentiate between normal and abnormal findings for specific endocrine disorders.
- Explore laboratory tests used to diagnose acute endocrine disorders.

Endocrine disorders can affect all body systems. Such disorders usually are caused by overproduction or underproduction of hormones.

This chapter gives an overview of the history, physical examination, and diagnostic studies that help diagnose the following specific endocrine disorders: thyroid crisis, myxedema coma, adrenal crisis, syndrome of inappropriate antidiuretic hormone (SIADH), diabetes insipidus (DI), diabetic ketoacidosis (DKA), hyperglycemic hyperosmolar non-ketotic coma (HHNC), and hypoglycemia. It builds on the content presented in Chapter 41, which explored the far-reaching effects of the endocrine system on body functions. This chapter also paves the way for specific applications described in Chapter 43, Common Endocrine Disorders.

HISTORY

When the patient with an acute endocrine disorder arrives in the emergency department in serious condition, the initial history, physical examination, and laboratory tests focus on gathering enough data to begin treatment. After treatment begins, additional history, physical examination, and diagnostic tests will be obtained.

Because endocrine dysfunction is so wide-ranging, the history includes a review of all body systems. The patient's signs and symptoms will depend on the specific gland involved and the degree to which it is underfunctioning or overfunctioning. A history of the presenting signs and symptoms, precipitating events, medical conditions, and current medications provides important clues to diagnosis and direction for additional questions. For example, if the patient has a preexisting endocrine condition, it is important to ask if the patient has been able to take his or her medication. A lapse in taking medication often precipitates an endocrine crisis. Other precipitating factors include illness, infection, trauma, and surgery.

Endocrine disorders characteristically affect the patient's nutrition, hydration, activity level, and mental status. These functions represent multiple body systems, such as the gastrointestinal, renal, cardiovascular, respiratory, and nervous systems. The gastrointestinal system assessment, which begins to give a picture of nutrition, hydration, and gastrointestinal function, includes questions about changes in appetite, fluid intake, weight, bowel function, and the presence of nausea or vomiting. The nurse also asks about problems urinating, and the frequency and amount of urination. Questions about fluid intake and urination may uncover polydipsia and polyuria and potential fluid and electrolyte imbalance.

The nurse asks patients to describe changes in their activity level to ascertain the degree of generalized weakness, fatigue, or tiredness. Adults should discuss work and household activities, and children should be questioned about school and sports or play activities. Changes in sleeping patterns are also important to note. The assessment should also include questions about breathlessness, palpitations, and dizziness, which relate to the cardiovascular and respiratory systems.

The nurse assesses the patient's mental status and level of responsiveness as the interview progresses. Is the patient alert or lethargic? Is the patient oriented? How accurate is his or her recall of recent symptoms? The patient is asked about tremors, heat and cold tolerance, seizures, headaches, numbness, or tingling. Have there been any skin changes, including susceptibility to bruising, purple striae, dry or thick skin, or brittle fingernails and toenails? Has the patient noticed a change in the amount and distribution of body hair? Have there been changes in vision, such as diplopia or blurred vision? Is there a gritty feeling in the eyes?

PHYSICAL EXAMINATION

Thyroid enlargement or nodules can be detected by palpation, and thyroid bruits can be detected by listening over the gland with the bell of the stethoscope. The thyroid gland, however, is the only endocrine gland that can be examined physically. Therefore, the physical examination helps determine the systemic effects of the disease.

If the patient's condition allows, the nurse obtains weight, height, and blood pressure readings while the patient is lying, sitting, and standing. How wide is the pulse pressure? Is there orthostatic hypotension? The nurse takes the patient's temperature and observes and palpates the precordial area to detect heaves and the point of maximal impulse. Heart rate, rhythm, and extra heart sounds are checked. Observation may reveal respiratory effort, pattern, and rate. The nurse listens to the lungs, noting crackles and increased, diminished, or absent breath sounds. Respiratory problems may result from endocrine dysfunction or may precipitate an endocrine crisis.

Observation includes the patient's general appearance, expression, level of consciousness, orientation, appropriateness of responses, mood, posture, and distribution of weight. The patient's speech pattern is noted. Is it slurred, slow, or rapid? The trunk and extremities are examined for skin color, turgor, thickness, hydration, bruises, or other marks or lesions. Is there a saliva pool under the tongue? Are the eyes normal, bulging, or sunken? The thickness of fingernails and toenails and the amount, texture, and condition of the hair are noted. Observation and palpation are used in examining for edema. Deep tendon reflexes, motor tone, and strength are tested.

Findings are integrated by grouping signs and symptoms. Identifying a cluster of symptoms often suggests a particu-

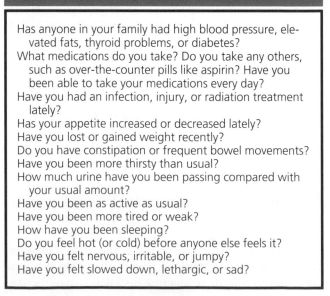

lar endocrine disorder. For example, a patient reports poor appetite, weight loss, nausea, vomiting, diarrhea, thirst, fatigue, and weakness. These symptoms, coupled with the physical findings of irritability, restlessness, lethargy, decreased skin turgor, bronze skin color, tachycardia, and postural hypotension, suggest an adrenal crisis. Another significant cluster of findings includes weight gain, constipation, fatigue, weakness, and lethargy. Additional symptoms of decreased metabolic rate may be evident, such as decreased mentation, low body temperature, bradycardia, and decreased respirations. This cluster strongly suggests a degree of hypothyroidism that can progress to myxedema coma.

A third cluster of symptoms may be signs and symptoms of an increased metabolic rate, including increased appetite, weight loss, thirst, polyuria, extreme weakness and fatigue, and decreased heat tolerance. Physical findings indicate a palpable thyroid, resting tachycardia, hypertension, and a temperature of more than 38°C (100°F). These signs and symptoms suggest impending thyroid storm.

■ DIAGNOSTIC STUDIES

Laboratory Tests

A range of laboratory tests helps diagnose endocrine disorders. The tests that help diagnose acute thyroid and adrenal disorders, SIADH, DI, DKA, HHNC, and hypoglycemia are

described. Table 42–1 summarizes sample tests used in acute endocrine disorders.

TOTAL T_4

Total T_4 measures both the free thyroxine and the portion carried by the thyroid-binding globulin protein. T_4 is increased in hyperthyroidism and decreased in hypothyroidism. Any factor that affects protein binding will affect the results of the total T_4. This includes pregnancy, estrogen or androgen therapy, and taking oral contraceptives, salicylates, or phenytoin. Normal values depend on the laboratory method used. The normal value declines with age and is 16.5 µg/dL in infants. Childhood norms are up to 15 µg/dL. Normal adult values range from 4 to 12 µg/dL and are higher during pregnancy. Older adults have lower values because plasma proteins decrease as people age.

FREE THYROXINE T_4 AND FREE THYROXINE INDEX

Free thyroxine T_4 and free thyroxine index measure the free part of T_4, the part that is not bound to protein. Free T_4 is the metabolically active form of the hormone that can be used by tissues. It makes up a small part of the total thyroxine. The free T_4 test is more useful than the total T_4 in diagnosing hypofunction and hyperfunction of the thyroid gland because it helps diagnose thyroid function when peo-

TABLE 42-1 CLINICAL APPLICATION: Diagnostic Studies
Sampling of Tests Used in Acute Endocrine Disorders

Test	Normal Adult Values	Abnormal Values
Total T_4	4–12 µg/dL	High in hyperthyroidism Low in hypothyroidism
Free thyroxine (FT$_4$)	0.8–2.7 ng/mL	High in hyperthyroidism Low in hypothyroidism
Free thyroxine index (FTI)	4.6–12 ng/mL	High in hyperthyroidism Low in hypothyroidism
Free T_3	260–480 pg/dL	Low in hypothyroidism
Thyroid-stimulating hormone	260–480 pg/dL	High in hypothyroidism (primary) Low in hypofunction of anterior pituitary (secondary hypothyroidism)
Cortisol	8 AM 5–23 µg/dL 4 PM 3–16 µg/dL	High in Cushing's disease (increased ACTH secretion by pituitary) High in stress, trauma, and surgery Low in hyposecretion of ACTH by pituitary and adrenal insufficiency
Cortisol stimulation	Should increase to 18 µg/dL	Low or absent in adrenal insufficiency and hypopituitarism
Urine vanillylmandelic acid (VMA) and catecholamines	VMA up to 2–7 mg/24 h Catecholamines: 270 µg/24 h	High in pheochromocytoma High in hypothyroidism and diabetic acidosis
Urine specific gravity	1.010–1.025 with normal hydration and volume	Low in diabetes insipidus High in diabetes mellitus with dehydration
Urine ketones	Negative	Positive in diabetic ketoacidosis

Sample of Medications That May Interfere With Thyroid Tests

Phenytoin
Propranolol
Corticosteroids
Aspirin
Estrogen
Furosemide
Methadone
Opioids
Lithium
Heparin
Potassium iodide

---

ple have abnormal binding globulin levels. This test can also evaluate thyroid replacement therapy. Radioisotopes can interfere with test results, and heparin can give false high readings. This test can be done by direct assay or by indirect measurement. The direct assay normal value is 0.8 to 2.7 ng/mL, while the free T_4 index is 4.6 to 12 ng/mL.

FREE TRIIODOTHYRONINE T_3

Free triiodothyronine T_3 measures the circulating T_3 that exists in the free state in the blood, unbound to protein. This is one measure to evaluate thyroid function. Decreased values indicate hypothyroidism. Radioisotopes also affect results. Normal adult values are 260 to 480 pg/dL.

THYROID-STIMULATING HORMONE (THYROTROPIN)

This test measures circulating thyroid-stimulating hormone (TSH) from the anterior pituitary. TSH stimulates the release and distribution of the T_3 and T_4 stored in large amounts in the thyroid gland. Measuring TSH helps determine whether the hypothyroidism is due to primary dysfunction of the thyroid gland or secondary to hypofunction of the anterior pituitary gland. High TSH helps diagnose primary hypothyroidism. High doses of corticosteroids and dopamine can suppress TSH. Normal adult values are 260 to 480 pg/dL.

CORTISOL (HYDROCORTISONE)

This test evaluates the ability of the adrenal cortex to produce the glucocorticoid hormone cortisol. Cortisol is elevated in adrenal hyperfunction and decreased in adrenal hypofunction. Adrenal hyperfunction may be caused by an excess secretion of adrenocorticotropic hormone (ACTH) by the pituitary (Cushing's disease), high stress, trauma, and surgery. Adrenal hypofunction may be the result of anterior pituitary hyposecretion, hepatitis, and cirrhosis.

Cortisol secretion is normally higher in the early morning (6:00–8:00 AM) and lower in the evening (4:00–6:00 PM).

This variation is lost in patients with adrenal hyperfunction and in people under stress. Serum samples are drawn between 6:00 and 8:00 AM and 4:00 and 6:00 PM. Normal 8:00 AM values are 5 to 23 µg/dL or 138 to 635 mmol/L and 4:00 PM values are 3 to 16 µg/dL or 83 to 441 mmol/L.

CORTISOL (DEXAMETHASONE) SUPPRESSION

When healthy people receive a low dose of dexamethasone, ACTH production is suppressed. However, people with adrenal hyperfunction and some with endogenous depression continue to produce ACTH and do not have a diurnal variation of cortisol. For this test, dexamethasone is given at bedtime. Blood samples are taken the next day at 8 AM and 4 PM. Medications are discontinued for 24 to 48 hours before this test is started, especially estrogens, phenytoin, and cortisol-related preparations. Radioisotopes should not be given within 1 week of this test.

CORTISOL STIMULATION

This test measures the response of the adrenal glands to an injection of cosyntropin (Cortrosyn, a synthetic ACTH preparation). A fasting 8 AM cortisol level is drawn before cosyntropin is administered, and then blood samples are taken 30 and 60 minutes after it is administered. The adrenal glands normally respond to the cosyntropin by synthesizing and secreting adrenocorticoids. The plasma cortisol level should increase to at least 18 µg/dL. The response to cosyntropin is decreased or absent in adrenal insufficiency and hypopituitarism. Long-term steroid therapy will affect results. This test may be contraindicated in the presence of infections, inflammatory diseases, and cardiac disease.

FASTING BLOOD SUGAR/GLUCOSE

This test provides a foundation for managing diabetes mellitus. Very high blood glucose levels can occur in DKA and HHNC. In addition, elevated glucose levels can occur in Cushing's disease, high stress, pancreatitis, and chronic renal and liver disease. Hypoglycemia can occur in Addison's disease, pancreatic tumors, starvation, and hypopituitary problems. The normal value for adults is 65 to 110 mg/dL. Two-hour postprandial blood glucose testing helps further evaluate carbohydrate metabolism, especially in diabetes mellitus. The normal value is 65 to 139 mg/dL.

INSULIN

This test helps measure abnormal carbohydrate metabolism and diagnose insulinoma, a tumor of the islets of Langerhans. When the glucose tolerance test (GTT) is abnormal, a low insulin level also helps diagnose diabetes mellitus. A fasting blood sample is tested. If the insulin test is done in conjunction with a GTT, blood samples are also drawn at the same time. Oral contraceptives and recent radioisotopes interfere with results. The normal adult value is 6 to 24 µU/mL.

GLUCAGON

This hormone, produced in the alpha cells in the islets of Langerhans, controls the production, storage, and release of glucose. Normally, insulin opposes the action of glucagon. This test measures the production and metabolism of glucagon. A deficiency occurs when pancreatic tissue is lost because of chronic pancreatitis or pancreatic tumors. Increased levels occur in diabetes and acute pancreatitis and when catecholamine secretion is stimulated by such causes as infection, high stress levels, or pheochromocytoma.

Chronic renal failure and cirrhosis of the liver can also raise glucagon levels. Normal fasting values are 50 to 200 pg/mL.

URINE VANILLYLMANDELIC ACID (CATECHOLAMINES)

Urine vanillylmandelic acid (VMA) is a metabolite of catecholamines. It has a high concentration in the urine and is easy to detect. Therefore, this 24-hour urine test is done when a person is suspected of having hypertension due to pheochromocytoma. Catecholamines and VMA levels can be measured. Elevated levels of catecholamines can be found in hypothyroidism, diabetic acidosis, neuroblastomas, and ganglioneuromas. Urine should not be collected when the patient is NPO. Test results are also affected by many drugs and foods, such as tea, coffee, vanilla, and fruit juice. Therefore, some laboratories will restrict certain foods for 2 days before testing and on the day of testing. Drugs may also be discontinued for 4 to 7 days before testing. Normal adult values for VMA are 2 to 7 mg/24 h, and for catecholamines, they are 270 µg/24 h.

URINE 17 KETOSTEROIDS AND 17 HYDROXYCORTICOSTEROIDS

These 24-hour tests reflect adrenal function by measuring the urinary excretion of steroids. They are used infrequently because they have been replaced by serum immunoassays.

URINE SPECIFIC GRAVITY

Specific gravity reflects the kidneys' ability to dilute and concentrate urine. The range depends on hydration, urine volume, and the amount of solids in the urine. It can be measured by using a multiple test dipstick that has a reagent for specific gravity, by a refractometer, or a urinometer. Low specific gravity (1.001–1.010) is seen in DI and is accompanied by a large urine volume. Increased specific gravity (1.025–1.030) is seen in diabetes mellitus with dehydration.

URINE OSMOLALITY

This test is a more exact measure of urine concentration. It is also a more useful test when done in conjunction with serum osmolality. It can be used to diagnose kidney func-

tion, DI, and psychogenic water drinking. It is increased in Addison's disease, SIADH, dehydration, and renal disease. It is decreased in DI and psychogenic water drinking. The normal range is 300 to 900 mOsm/kg/24 h and 50 to 1,200 mOsm/kg in a random sample.

URINE KETONES

Ketones are not normally found in the urine. They are associated with diabetes and other diseases of altered carbohydrate metabolism. Patients with diabetes should test for ketones whenever their urine or blood sugar is high. Because ketones appear in the urine before they can be detected in the blood, this test is often used in the emergency room when screening for acidosis. It is done by dipping a ketone reagent strip in a fresh urine sample.

Diagnostic Tests

THYROID SCAN AND RADIOACTIVE IODINE UPTAKE STUDY

These tests measure the thyroid uptake of radioactive iodine (^{131}I or ^{123}I). After the patient takes the radioactive iodine (by capsule, solution, or intravenous injection), the thyroid is scanned with a gamma camera at specific times during the day. This produces a visual representation of the radioactivity in the thyroid gland, neck, and mediastinum. Scan time is about 20 minutes. Normally the radioactive iodine is evenly distributed in the thyroid gland, and the scan shows a normal size, position, and shape. This test must be done before other radiographic tests using contrast medications (such as gallbladder or intravenous pyelograms).

The thyroid scan may be done in conjunction with a radioactive iodine uptake study. After the patient takes the radioactive iodine, a count is made over the thyroid gland with a scintillation counter at specific times. These tests can indicate areas of increased and decreased function and provide data to diagnose hyperthyroidism, hypothyroidism, nodules, and cancer of the thyroid.

ADRENAL SCAN

This scan is used to identify the site of certain tumors or sites that produce excessive amounts of catecholamines. The radionuclide iobenguane (^{131}I) is injected intravenously, and scans are done on days 2, 3, and 4. Sometimes only 1 day is needed, and other times imaging is needed on days 6 and 7. Normally tumors and sites of hypersecretion are absent.

ADDITIONAL TESTS

Many tests that have been discussed in other chapters must be done to detect the multisystem effects of acute endocrine disorders. Fluid and electrolyte problems accompany many acute endocrine disorders. Therefore, serum sodium, potassium, magnesium, and osmolality are assessed. The blood urea nitrogen and creatinine may also help assess renal involvement (see Chapter 28). Arterial blood gases, bicarbonate levels, and anion gap calculation may be necessary to diagnose acidosis. Electrocardiograms and cardiac monitoring may be needed to diagnose cardiac problems, while a chest x-ray may be necessary to detect pulmonary problems, such as the pleural effusion that can occur in myxedema coma. Computed tomography, magnetic resonance imaging, and ultrasound may be used to localize tumors.

Clinical Applicability Challenges

Self-Challenge: Critical Thinking

1. Compare the history, physical examination, and laboratory findings for adrenal crisis and myxedema coma.

2. Analyze how the history, physical examination, and laboratory data help distinguish the mechanisms that cause decreased consciousness in myxedema coma and DKA.

Study Question

1. In assessing a patient with thyroid storm, indicate the parameter that would be least significant initially.
   a. Temperature
   b. Weight
   c. Apical rate
   d. Blood pressure

BIBLIOGRAPHY

Corbett JV: Diagnostic Procedures with Nursing Diagnosis (4th Ed). Stamford, CT, Appleton and Lange, 1996
Fischbach F: A Manual of Laboratory and Diagnostic Tests (5th Ed). Philadelphia, Lippincott-Raven, 1996
Jacobs DS, Demott WR, Grady HJ, Horvat RT, Huestis DW, Kasten BL: Laboratory Test Handbook (4th Ed). Cleveland, Lexi-Comp Incorporated, 1996
Morton PG: Health Assessment in Nursing (2nd Ed). Philadelphia, FA Davis, 1993
Morton PG, et al: Davis's Clinical Guide to Health Assessment (2nd Ed). Philadelphia, FA Davis, 1995
Reising D: Acute hypoglycemia. Nursing 25(2):33–40, 1995
Reising D: Acute hyperglycemia. Nursing 25(2):41–48, 1995

43

Common Endocrine Disorders

OBJECTIVES

*Based on the content in this chapter, the reader should be
able to:*

- Examine the pathophysiological principles that help explain
  thyroid crises, myxedema coma, adrenal crises, syndrome of
  inappropriate antidiuretic hormone, diabetes insipidus, diabetic ketoacidosis, hyperglycemic hyperosmolar nonketotic
  acidosis, and hypoglycemia.
- Distinguish key precipitating factors, history, and clinical
  manifestations for each disorder.
- Discuss five laboratory studies that are useful in diagnosing
  acute endocrine disorders.

- Analyze the similarities and differences in caring for patients
  with endocrine crises.
- Explore the nursing role in assessing, managing, and evaluating a plan of care for patients with endocrine crises.

*E*ndocrine disorders have multisystem effects. At the
same time, acute illness may lead to hypofunction, and less
commonly, hyperfunction, of the neuroendocrine system.
Patients with acute illness who are at risk for endocrine dys-

function may have a preexisting endocrine disorder. That disorder may be known, but many endocrine dysfunctions are not recognized prior to acute illness. For that reason, endocrine dysfunction should be considered in the assessment and management of *all* critically ill patients.

This chapter presents an overview of pathophysiology, assessment, management, and complications of patients with acute endocrine disorders. These disorders are thyroid dysfunctions, adrenal gland dysfunctions, antidiuretic hormone (ADH) dysfunctions, and diabetic emergencies.

Thyroid Dysfunction

THYROID CRISIS

Thyrotoxic crisis is a severe form of hyperthyroidism often associated with physiological or psychological stress. When the thyroid state worsens critically, it is called thyroid crisis. Rapid deterioration and death can occur if untreated.

The condition may develop spontaneously, but it occurs most frequently in people who have undiagnosed or partially treated severe hyperthyroidism. By definition, hyperthyroidism is a condition in which thyroid hormones' actions result in greater-than-normal responses. Specific diseases that can cause hyperthyroidism include Graves' disease, exogenous hyperthyroidism, thyroiditis, toxic nodular goiter, toxic multinodular goiter, and thyroid cancer. Certain drugs, such as contrast material for radiographic procedures or amiodarone (an antidysrhythmic drug), may precipitate the thyrotoxic state because of their high iodine content.

Pathophysiological Principles

The etiology of thyroid crisis, often referred to as thyroid storm or thyrotoxicosis, is poorly understood. Physiological mechanisms that are thought to induce thyroid crises include the sudden release of large quantities of thyroid hormone, tissue tolerance to T_3 and T_4, adrenergic activity, and excessive lipolysis and fatty acid production. The abrupt release of large quantities of thyroid hormone is thought to produce the hypermetabolic manifestations seen during thyroid crises.

Adrenergic hyperactivity is considered a possible link to thyroid crisis. Although thyroid hormone and catecholamines potentiate each other, catecholamine levels during thyroid crisis are usually within the normal range. It is uncertain whether the effects of hypersecretion of thyroid hormone or increased catecholamine levels cause heightened sensitivity and thyroid overfunction. Thyroid–catecholamine interactions result in an increased rate of chemical reactions, increased nutrient and oxygen consumption, increased heat production, alterations in fluid and electrolyte balance, and a catabolic state.

Another mechanism is excessive lipolysis and fatty acid production. With excessive lipolysis, increased fatty acids will oxidize and produce an overabundance of thermal energy that is difficult to dissipate through vasodilation.

The many different endocrine, reproductive, gastrointestinal, integumentary, and ocular manifestations are caused by increased circulating levels of thyroid hormone and by stimulation of the sympathetic nervous system.

Assessment

Accurate identification of the precipitating factor for thyroid storm allows proper treatment to be initiated. Precipitating factors for people with recognized and unrecognized existing thyroid disease are listed in the accompanying display.

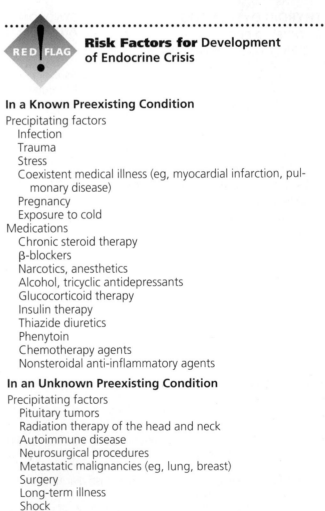

RED FLAG

Risk Factors for Development of Endocrine Crisis

In a Known Preexisting Condition
Precipitating factors
  Infection
  Trauma
  Stress
  Coexistent medical illness (eg, myocardial infarction, pulmonary disease)
  Pregnancy
  Exposure to cold
Medications
  Chronic steroid therapy
  β-blockers
  Narcotics, anesthetics
  Alcohol, tricyclic antidepressants
  Glucocorticoid therapy
  Insulin therapy
  Thiazide diuretics
  Phenytoin
  Chemotherapy agents
  Nonsteroidal anti-inflammatory agents

In an Unknown Preexisting Condition
Precipitating factors
  Pituitary tumors
  Radiation therapy of the head and neck
  Autoimmune disease
  Neurosurgical procedures
  Metastatic malignancies (eg, lung, breast)
  Surgery
  Long-term illness
  Shock
  Postpartum
  Trauma

Data from Halloran T: Nursing responsibilities in endocrine emergencies. Critical Care Nursing Quarterly 13(3):74–81, 1990

Signs and symptoms of hyperthyroidism include sweating, heat intolerance, nervousness, tremors, palpitations, hyperkinesis, and increased bowel sounds. Extremes of these manifestations, specifically a temperature greater than 40°C (104°F) in the absence of an infection, tachycardia, and central nervous system (CNS) dysfunction, indicate thyroid storm. CNS abnormalities include agitation, delirium, seizures, or coma. Signs of thyroid emergencies are listed in Table 43–1.

Older patients may not have the classic signs and symptoms of thyroid crises, so this condition may be overlooked. However, they frequently have suggestive signs and symptoms. In these circumstances, older patients are asked if they have heart disease and what medications they take. This can be important in determining whether there is underlying thyroid disease, because β-blocker medication may mask cardiovascular clues.

DIAGNOSTIC STUDIES

Diagnostic studies may show an elevated total T_4 and free T_3 and T_4. Serum electrolytes, liver function tests, and complete blood counts, although not diagnostic, may help uncover abnormalities that require treatment. They may also help identify the precipitating cause. Electrolyte imbalances due to dehydration, excessive bone resorption, and increased insulin degradation often occur. The serum calcium is often elevated, while potassium and magnesium are decreased, and liver function tests are increased. Diagnostic tests include the radioactive iodine uptake test, which is usually increased. Electrocardiogram (ECG) and cardiac monitoring may show atrial fibrillation, supraventricular

Table 43-1 Indications of Thyroid Emergencies

Thyroid Storm	Myxedema Coma
Tachycardia	Bradycardia
Hyperthermia	Hypothermia
Tachypnea	Hypoventilation
Hypercalcemia	Hyponatremia
Hyperglycemia	Hypoglycemia
Metabolic acidosis	Respiratory and metabolic acidosis
Cardiovascular collapse due to	Cardiovascular collapse due to
Cardiogenic shock	Decreased vascular tone
Hypovolemia	
Cardiac arrhythmias	
Depressed LOC	Depressed LOC
Emotional lability	Seizures, coma
Psychosis	
Tremors, restlessness	Hyporeflexia

LOC, level of consciousness.
Data from Halloran T: Nursing responsibilities in endocrine emergencies. Critical Care Nursing Quarterly 13(3):74–81, 1990

tachycardia, sinus bradycardia, heart block, conduction disturbances, and ventricular dysrhythmias.

Management

Management goals for thyroid crises are fourfold: treating the precipitating factor(s), controlling excessive thyroid hormone release, inhibiting the thyroid hormone biosynthesis, and treating the peripheral effects of thyroid hormone.

Antithyroid drugs are used to control thyroid release or biosynthesis. Propylthiouracil is the preferred agent, although it can be given only orally. Propylthiouracil is preferred because it blocks the conversion of T_4 to T_3 in peripheral tissues and binds iodine to prevent synthesis of the hormone. If the oral route is not possible, methimazole can be given rectally.

Iodine solutions, such as sodium iodide intravenously or oral potassium iodide (SSKI) or Lugol's solution, are given to block the release of thyroid hormone. These agents should not be given until 1 hour after the administration of antithyroid medications. Lithium is the choice for patients who are iodine sensitive. Glucocorticoids may be ordered because they also inhibit thyroid hormone release.

Cardiovascular decompensation, secondary to decreased stroke volume and reduced cardiac output, may be life threatening. β-adrenergic blockers, specifically propranolol, are used to treat the symptoms of the hyperthyroidism rather than the primary thyroid disease. This therapy may be ordered to restore cardiac function by decreasing the catecholamine-mediated symptoms. Carefully monitor the response to β-blockers because intrinsic cardiac disease may worsen as a result of the negative inotropic effects. Digoxin may also be used to treat congestive heart failure or supraventricular tachydysrhythmias. The goal of therapy is to decrease myocardial oxygen consumption, decrease the heart rate (ideally below 100 beats/min), and increase cardiac output.

Management also focuses on monitoring multisystem effects from the hypermetabolism of thyroid crises and the response to treatment. Factors regarding three systems that require close watch are cardiovascular function, fluid and electrolyte balance, and neurological status. Blood pressure, heart rate and rhythm, respiratory rate, and extra heart sounds are assessed every hour. Fluid status and lab-

---

CLINICAL APPLICATION:
Examples of Nursing Diagnoses and Collaborative Problems for the Patient in Thyroid Crisis

Fluid Volume Deficit related to hypermetabolic state
Hyperthermia related to hypermetabolic state
Decreased Cardiac Output related to hypermetabolic state and heart failure
Altered Cerebral Tissue Perfusion related to hypermetabolic state and heart failure

oratory values are evaluated. Body temperature is monitored hourly because the patient is at risk for hyperthermia. Antipyretic agents, particularly acetaminophen, are recommended for fever control. Aspirin is not given because it increases free T_3 and T_4 levels. Tepid baths or a cooling blanket may be needed. Cooling to the point of shivering and piloerection is avoided because this may have a rebound effect of raising body temperature (see "Hypothermia" in Chapter 33). Neurological status is also assessed at least hourly. Seizure precautions and safety measures prevent injury. If the patient's level of consciousness decreases, airway patency and safety issues are assessed. Energy and nutritional needs are heightened because of the hypermetabolism. Interventions include administering glucose-containing solutions and nutritional support.

Complications

Even without preexisting coronary artery disease, untreated thyroid crisis can cause angina pectoris and myocardial infarction, congestive heart failure, cardiovascular collapse, coma, and death.

CLINICAL APPLICATION: Patient Care Study

Mrs. Clark is admitted to the medical ICU with an initial diagnosis of supraventricular tachycardia unresponsive to therapy. Her neurological status is depressed; she is arousable at times but disoriented. She does not recognize her family and cannot remember that she is in the hospital. Mrs. Clark was recently diagnosed with hyperthyroid state due to Graves' disease. She had not been taking her medications. Initial complete blood count and chemistry laboratory values are normal. The physician has ordered an IV of D5/NS to infuse at 100 mL/h. Her initial vital signs are abnormal, temperature of 38.8°C (102°F), heart rate of 165, and a mean arterial blood pressure of 70. The physician orders serum thyroid tests. Propylthiouracil is started as well as acetaminophen for the fever. Cardiac monitoring is also ordered to observe for signs and symptoms of congestive failure.

◼ MYXEDEMA COMA

Myxedema coma is a rare, life-threatening emergency brought on by extreme hypothyroidism. It usually is seen in older patients during winter months.

Pathophysiological Principles

Deficient production of thyroid hormone results in the clinical state termed hypothyroidism. Hypothyroidism, a chronic disease, is 10 times more common in women than in men. It occurs in all age groups but most commonly in those older than 50 years. It is less common than hyperthyroidism.

Hypothyroidism can be primary or secondary. Primary causes include congenital defects, loss of thyroid tissue after treatment for hyperthyroidism, defective hormone synthe-

sis due to an autoimmune process, and antithyroid drug administration or iodine deficiency. Secondary causes include peripheral resistance to thyroid hormone, or infarction, and hypothalamic disorders. Transient hypothyroidism can occur after withdrawal of prolonged T_4 or T_3 treatment.

Hypothyroidism generally affects all body systems. A low basal metabolic rate and decreased energy metabolism and heat production are characteristic. Myxedema results from an alteration in the composition of the dermis and other tissues. The connective fibers are separated by an increased amount of protein and mucopolysaccharides. This binds water, producing nonpitting, boggy edema, especially around the eyes, hands, and feet; it is also responsible for thickening of the tongue and the laryngeal and pharyngeal mucous membranes, resulting in slurred speech and hoarseness.

Assessment

Signs and symptoms of hypothyroidism include fatigue, weakness, decreased bowel sounds, decreased appetite, weight gain, and electrocardiographic changes. Myxedema coma is a rare manifestation of hypothyroidism, characterized by severe depression of the sensorium, hypothermia, hypoventilation hypoxemia, hyponatremia hypoglycemia, hyperreflexia, hypotension, and bradycardia. Myxedema coma patients do not shiver, although temperatures have been reported below 26.6° C (80°F). The diagnosis of myxedema coma depends on recognizing the clinical symptoms and identifying the underlying precipitating factor. The most common precipitating factor is pulmonary infection; others include trauma, stress, infections, drugs (eg, narcotics or barbiturates), surgery, and metabolic disturbances. Symptoms of thyroid emergencies are compared in Table 43–1.

A decrease in T_4 and free T_4 is most common, while sodium is usually decreased and potassium is increased. Arterial blood gases (ABGs) usually show a decreased PaO_2 and increased $PaCO_2$. A chest radiograph will detect pleural effusion. ECG changes include a prolonged PR interval and decreased amplitude of the P wave and QRS complex. Heart block may develop.

Management

The most serious complication of hypothyroidism is a progression to myxedema coma and death, if untreated. A multisystem approach must be used in treating this emergency. Mechanical ventilation is used to control hypoventilation, hypercapnea, and respiratory arrest. Intravenous hypertonic normal saline and glucose will correct the dilutional hyponatremia and hypoglycemia. Fluid administration plus vasopressor therapy may be necessary to correct hypotension.

Pharmacological therapy includes the administration of thyroid hormone and corticosteroids. There are several approaches to this aspect of medical management. Initial drug therapy will include 300 to 500 µg L-thyroxine T_4 intravenously to saturate all protein binding sites and establish a relatively normal T_4 level. Subsequent doses may include 100 µg daily. Intravenous (IV) or oral T_3 is an alternative order. Guidelines to T_3 replacement are 25 µg IV every 8 hours for the first 24 to 48 hours. Oral T_3 doses every 8 hours are also ordered.

Additional interventions include treating abdominal distention and fecal impaction and managing hypothermia by gradual rewarming using blankets and socks. Mechanical devices are not used. The patient is monitored for neurological status and changes in level of consciousness (LOC). Seizure precautions are implemented. When the patient is comatose, care includes preventing complications related to aspiration, immobility, skin breakdown, and infection. Cardiovascular and respiratory function is monitored. Fluid administration must also be monitored because there is a risk for fluid overload. An important aspect of care is to detect early signs of complications. As the patient recovers, interventions focus on patient self-care and education.

Complications

In addition to coma, complications include pericardial and pleural effusions, megacolon with paralytic ileus, and seizures.

Adrenal Gland Dysfunction

▬ ADRENAL CRISIS

Pathophysiological Principles

Adrenal insufficiency is a major life-threatening dysfunction of the adrenal cortex. It also is known as hypoadrenalism or hypocorticism. Adrenal hormone insufficiency can occur with direct involvement of the adrenal gland (primary) or because of lack of stimulation by adrenocorticotropic hormone (ACTH) due to hypothalamic–pituitary disease (secondary).

Primary adrenal insufficiency is termed Addison's disease. The most common cause of primary hypoadrenalism in the industrialized West is autoimmune adrenalitis; the second leading cause is destruction of the gland secondary to *Mycobacterium tuberculosis* infection. Worldwide the latter remains the most common cause of primary adrenal insufficiency. Other causes include bilateral hemorrhage of the glands secondary to bacterial infection with sepsis and shock, metastatic malignancies, and sarcoidosis.

The most common cause of secondary adrenal insufficiency is iatrogenic. Other causes include metastatic carcinomas of the lung or breast, pituitary infarction, surgery or irradiation, and CNS disturbances, such as basilar skull fractures or infections.

Acute adrenal insufficiency or adrenal crisis occurs when there is a change in the chronic condition or massive adrenal hemorrhage. In addition to the chronic disease, an infection, trauma, surgical procedure, or some extra stress occurs, precipitating acute adrenal crisis in the patient.

Assessment

Symptoms of adrenal insufficiency are the same for primary and secondary disease. Weakness, fatigue, anorexia, nausea, vomiting, diarrhea, and abdominal pain may be initial clues to adrenal crisis. These findings are nonspecific until linked with the history of a chronic condition requiring past or present corticosteroid use. Specifically, use of more than 20 mg of hydrocortisone or its equivalent, taken for longer than 7 to 10 days, has the potential for suppressing the hypothalamic–pituitary–adrenal axis. Hyperpigmentation on areas of the elbows, knees, hands, or buccal mucosa is seen in primary adrenal insufficiency. Its presence strengthens the clinical picture of adrenal crisis. The most common physical changes include signs of dehydration, such as weight loss and orthostatic hypotension. Clinical signs and symptoms are listed in the accompanying display.

> ◆ **RED FLAG** **Indications of** Adrenal Crisis
>
> **Aldosterone deficiency**
> - Hyperkalemia
> - Hyponatremia
> - Hypovolemia
> - Elevated BUN
>
> **Cortisol deficiency**
> - Hypoglycemia
> - Decreased gastric motility
> - Decreased vascular tone
> - Hypercalcemia
>
> **Generalized signs and symptoms**
> - Anorexia
> - Nausea and vomiting
> - Abdominal cramping
> - Diarrhea
> - Tachycardia
> - Orthostatic hypotension
> - Headache, lethargy
> - Fatigue, weakness
> - Hyperkalemic ECG changes
> - Hyperpigmentation
>
> *Adapted from Halloran T: Nursing responsibilities in endocrine emergencies. Critical Care Nursing Quarterly 13(3):74–81, 1990*

Laboratory values in acute conditions of glucocorticoid and mineralocorticoid deficiency show hyponatremia, hyperkalemia, decreased serum bicarbonate levels, and elevated blood urea nitrogen (BUN). Metabolic acidosis may occur because of dehydration. Hypoglycemia is generally present. Other abnormal laboratory findings include anemia and lymphocytosis with eosinophilia. Serum cortisol levels and cortisol stimulation (ACTH stimulation) tests are also used to confirm the diagnosis. Cortisol levels are decreased, and the adrenal gland response to the stimulation test is either diminished or absent. A computed tomography scan of the adrenal glands and the head may be done to detect tumors or other pathology of the adrenal and pituitary gland.

Management

The immediate goal of therapy is to administer the needed hormones and restore fluid and electrolyte balance. Hydrocortisone, 100 mg IV, is administered immediately. Fluid resuscitation is also started immediately with normal saline and 5% dextrose solutions. The rate of fluid and electrolyte replacements is dictated by the degree of volume depletion, serum electrolyte levels, and clinical response to therapy. Associated medical or surgical problems may indicate the need for invasive blood pressure and hemodynamic monitoring.

Another management goal is to prevent complications. This includes monitoring signs and symptoms of electrolyte imbalance (hyponatremia and hypercalcemia) and respiratory and cardiovascular function. The nurse looks for changes in blood pressure, heart rate and rhythm, skin color and temperature, capillary refill time, and central venous pressure (CVP). There is a risk for orthostatic hypotension, bradycardia, and dysrhythmias. The nurse also monitors neuromuscular signs, such as weakness, twitching, hyperreflexia, and paresthesia.

Emotional support, a simple explanation, and a quiet environment are effective in assisting the patient emotionally through the physiological crisis. Once the acute crisis is over, patient education is a goal of care. Patient education is necessary because the ultimate prognosis depends on the patient's ability to understand and follow through with self-care. This includes knowing the medication regimen, stress factors and their effect on the disease, and signs of impending crisis; wearing a medical alert tag, bracelet, or carrying a wallet card; and taking medication as prescribed.

Complications

Loss of bilateral adrenal function is fatal if not treated. Death is preceded by dysrhythmia, hypovolemia leading to circulatory collapse, loss of oxygen transport to the tissues, and seizures progressing to coma.

CLINICAL APPLICATION: Patient Care Study

Mr. Cerelo, age 55, was seen in the emergency room with initial symptoms of generalized weakness, fever, orthostatic hypotension, tachycardia, and gastrointestinal complaints. This patient has Addison's disease. A chest radiograph showed multiple infiltrates. Laboratory values indicated decreased serum sodium and increased serum potassium. The initial diagnosis was impending adrenal crisis precipitated by a lung infection.

Fluid resuscitation was started in the emergency room with D5/NS at 200 mL/h. The initial dose of hydrocortisone was also administered. The patient is awake and alert. Initial vital signs are stable; however, the patient remains tachycardic and tachypneic. Chemistry studies will be completed in 2 hours to evaluate any changes in sodium and potassium values. A Foley catheter is inserted to monitor urine output.

Antidiuretic Hormone Dysfunction

Two disorders involve ADH. One is an excess of ADH called syndrome of inappropriate antidiuretic hormone secretion (SIADH). The second is a deficiency of ADH and is called diabetes insipidus (DI). These two disorders are discussed in this section.

SYNDROME OF INAPPROPRIATE ANTIDIURETIC HORMONE SECRETION

Pathophysiological Principles

In SIADH, there may be either increased secretion or increased production of ADH. This increase in ADH occurs even though osmolality is normal. As a result, it causes an increase in total body water. SIADH is considered whenever the patient experiences hypotonic hyponatremia.

The secretion of ADH is considered "inappropriate" in that it continues despite the decreased osmolality of the plasma. Other reasons for the continued secretion of ADH also are lacking. There is no hypokalemia and edema; cardiac, renal, and adrenal function are normal; and there is normal or expanded plasma and extracellular fluid volumes.

Occasionally SIADH is caused by a pituitary tumor, but more commonly it is caused by a bronchogenic (oat cell) or pancreatic carcinoma. These tumors actually secrete ADH but are independent of normal physiological controls (see Chapter 47). Other possible causes of SIADH include head injuries; other endocrine disorders; pulmonary diseases, such as pneumonia, lung abscesses, CNS infections, and tumors; and drugs, such as tricyclics, oral hypoglycemic agents, diuretics, and cytotoxic agents.

Assessment

The symptoms of SIADH are water retention and eventually water intoxication secondary to sustained ADH effect. The hyponatremia in SIADH has two components, an early dilutional component due to increased water and a later, clinically undetectable component, caused by the increased urinary sodium excretion.

Symptoms produced by SIADH are predominantly neurological and gastrointestinal. The most common symptoms are personality changes, headache, decreased mentation, lethargy, nausea, vomiting, diarrhea, anorexia, decreased tendon reflexes, and finally, seizures and coma. Hyponatremia is the clinical focus and probable cause of hospital admission. When the serum sodium falls to less than that of 120 to 125 mEq/L, nausea and vomiting, muscular irritability, and seizures often result. If the condition develops acutely (ie, within 24 hours), a mortality rate of 50% has been reported.[1]

The main laboratory abnormalities in SIADH are a plasma hyponatremia and hypo-osmolality. The urine simultaneously is hyperosmolar and there is a high excretion of urinary sodium. The urine specific gravity is high, usually greater than 1.025. Other laboratory findings include low BUN, creatinine, and uric acid levels; hypocalcemia and hypokalemia; and decreased hemoglobin and hematocrit. The diagnosis can be confirmed by radioimmunoassay of plasma ADH. (See Table 34–3 for a comparison of SIADH and DI.)

Management

There are three categories in the management of SIADH: treatment of the underlying disease, alleviation of excessive water retention, and all the care needed when the patient has a depressed level of consciousness.

The first step in managing SIADH is to restrict fluid intake. In mild cases, fluid restriction is sufficient. A general guideline is that until the serum sodium concentration normalizes and symptoms abate, water intake should not exceed urinary output. In severely symptomatic patients, the administration of 3% hypertonic saline and furosemide is the treatment of choice. Demeclocycline has also been effective because it interferes with the normal ADH effect in kidney tubules.

Fluid and electrolyte balance, especially serum sodium, are monitored. The nurse evaluates intake and output, including hourly urine amounts, and observes for signs of fluid overload. Output should exceed intake.

Neurological status is evaluated. Rapid changes in sodium levels can result in neurological deterioration. When the serum sodium is less than 125 mEq/L, there is significant risk of neurological symptoms, including disorientation and decreasing consciousness. Seizure precautions may be necessary. Complications of SIADH include neurological deterioration leading to seizures, coma, and death.

Patients may find it difficult to limit their fluid intake. Mealtimes may also be difficult because menus will be aimed at meeting nutritional needs without increasing fluid intake. Information, emotional support, and acknowledging the deprivation may help patients through this period.

CLINICAL APPLICATION: Patient Care Study

A 65-year-old woman, Mrs. Perez, was admitted to the ICU with an initial diagnosis of acute mental status changes and severe hyponatremia. Past medical history included recent pneumonia and a history of congestive heart failure related to coronary artery disease. The pneumonia was treated with antibiotics, and Mrs. Perez takes a thiazide diuretic for the congestive heart failure.

Initially, Mrs. Perez's level of consciousness was depressed, and she had decreased deep tendon reflexes. Laboratory tests showed hyponatremia and normal arterial blood gases. Heart and lung sounds were normal, and her extremities were warm, adequately perfused, and without edema. The CT scan did not show any structural defect. Mrs. Perez had a generalized tonic–clonic seizure as she was admitted to the ICU. Laboratory values were as follows:

Na: 115 mEq/L
K: 4.5 mEq/L
Cl: 90 mEq/L
Plasma osmolality: 260 mOsm/kg
Urinary sodium levels were elevated.

■ DIABETES INSIPIDUS

Pathophysiological Principles

In DI, a pathological state, the kidneys excrete great quantities of dilute urine, at times up to 20 L/d. Normally the posterior pituitary releases ADH that acts on the distal renal tubules to promote reabsorption of water. When there is an absence or deficit in ADH, the kidneys lose their ability to reabsorb water and control fluid output (see Chapter 41).

Following surgery, DI may occur in the region of the hypothalamus. It can also occur with head injuries and gunshot wounds that damage the sphenoid bone, maxillofacial injuries, hypothalamic tumors, and nasopharyngeal tumors that invade the base of the skull. DI may also occur because of a primary problem within the hypothalamus or from diseases or drugs that affect the renal collecting tubules. There is also a psychogenic polydipsia, in which excessive water is consumed, resulting in excess output.

Assessment

Polyuria, polydipsia, and dehydration are the hallmarks of DI. When patients are alert, they will experience excessive thirst and excessive urinary output. They will try to increase fluid intake, but this can cause exhaustion and eventually result in dehydration. On the other hand, when people are not alert enough to detect thirst and increase their fluid intake, they can quickly develop hypovolemia because of the fluid loss. If left untreated, this can lead to death.

Recognizing DI may be more difficult when patients are recovering from surgery because the use of steroids and cerebral dehydrating agents used before and during surgery promote diuresis for the first postoperative day or so. If awake, the patient will complain of progressive thirst if DI is present. Urine output will increase and persist despite the amount of fluid intake. Urine specific gravity will fall or remain about 1.001 to 1.005. Plasma osmolality increases, often greater than 300 mOsm/kg. Urine osmolality decreases to 50 to 100 mOsm/kg. The urine sodium will be below normal while the serum sodium will be elevated (see Table 34–3).

Management

The objective of therapy is to prevent dehydration and electrolyte imbalance while treating the underlying cause. Hypotonic IV solutions, such 0.45% sodium chloride, are administered to match the urine output. The volume of replacement fluids will change once ADH therapy has begun. A variety of replacement ADH (vasopressin) therapies are available. Desmopressin acetate (DDAVP) is a synthetic ADH and can be used as an IV or nasal spray therapy. Aqueous vasopressin (Pitressin) may be given as an IV bolus, continuous infusion, or subcutaneously.

Management also focuses on monitoring fluid and electrolyte balance. Fluid excesses or deficits can be detected by evaluating hourly intake and output, serum and urine electrolytes and osmolality results, and urine specific gravity. Changes in blood pressure, pulse, and respirations and the onset of pulmonary crackles, neck vein distention, peripheral edema, and increasing CVP and pulmonary artery wedge pressure are noted. The nurse observes skin turgor and mucous membranes and changes in alertness and cognition. Drowsiness, confusion, and headache may indicate water intoxication. Weight is another indicator of fluid status.

Complications

Major complications are cardiovascular collapse and tissue hypoxia. Seizures and encephalopathy can also result from fluid and electrolyte imbalance.

CLINICAL APPLICATION: Patient Care Study

Mr. Smith is admitted to the intermediate ICU postoperatively after a transsphenoidal pituitary resection. His first postoperative day is uncomplicated. On the second postoperative day, the morning electrolytes show an increased serum sodium, increased serum osmolality, and decreased potassium. The urine output has been 200 mL/h for the past 3 hours. The patient has an increased heart rate.

Diabetic Emergencies

DIABETIC KETOACIDOSIS

Pathophysiological Principles

Diabetic ketoacidosis (DKA) results from severe insulin deficiency that leads to the disordered metabolism of proteins, carbohydrates, and fats. These pathological events lead to hyperglycemia and hyperosmolality, ketoacidosis, and volume depletion. Figure 43–1 outlines these mechanisms and their interrelationships.

HYPERGLYCEMIA AND HYPEROSMOLALITY

The first major consequence of DKA is hyperosmolality due to hyperglycemia (see Fig. 43–1). The central mechanism that protects against hyperosmolality is excretion of glucose by the kidneys.

Glucose is filtered at the kidney glomerulus. With normal circulating blood volume and a normal glucose load, all this glucose is reabsorbed into the bloodstream. However, when the blood sugar exceeds the normal threshold of about 180 mg/dL, glucose begins to escape into the urine because the reabsorption capacity of the tubules is exceeded. As the glucose load to be filtered increases, glucose is lost rapidly in the urine. Eventually, nearly all extra glucose put into the circulation is lost into the urine. The renal

"escape valve" serves as a protective device to prevent extreme accumulation of glucose in blood. Indeed, in people with diabetes whose circulating blood volume is well maintained, it is extremely unusual to find blood sugar levels in excess of 500 mg/dL because of the intense glucose diuresis. Conversely, any patient whose blood sugar is higher than this level has either a severely reduced circulating blood volume, renal damage, or both.

Glycosuria is largely responsible for volume depletion. A vicious cycle occurs in a patient whose diabetes is badly out of control and who cannot take in enough sodium and water to compensate for urinary losses. Hyperglycemia leads to volume depletion, which in turn reduces urinary glucose losses, which again permits the blood sugar to rise even higher.

This hyperosmolality of body fluids probably accounts for the lethargy, stupor, and ultimately the coma that occurs as DKA worsens. Diabetics who have ketoacidosis without hyperosmolality are less likely to have changes in consciousness.

KETOSIS AND ACIDOSIS

The second major consequence of severe insulin deficiency is uncontrolled ketogenesis (see Fig. 43–1). As keto acids enter the extracellular fluid, the hydrogen ion is stripped from the molecule and neutralized by combining with bi-

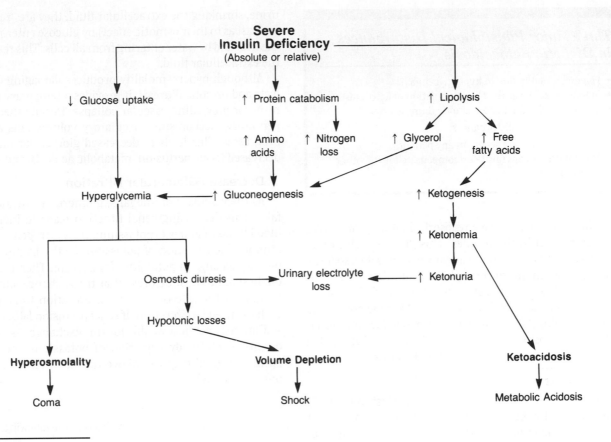

FIGURE 43-1

The pathogenesis of ketoacidosis. The metabolic consequences of severe insulin deficiency and their interrelations leading to diabetic ketoacidosis are depicted. Adapted from Davidson MD: Diabetic ketoacidosis and hyperosmolar nonketotic syndrome. In Diabetes Mellitus: Diagnosis and Treatment, 3rd Ed, pp 175–212. New York, Churchill Livingstone, 1991)

carbonate ion buffer, thus protecting the pH of extracellular fluids and leaving behind keto acid anion residues. The resulting carbonic acid breaks down into water and CO_2 gas, which is exhaled.

As keto acid anions accumulate, they progressively displace bicarbonate from extracellular fluid. The usual laboratory determination of electrolytes does not measure keto acid concentration directly. However, an excess of total measured cations (sodium plus potassium) over total measured anions (chloride plus bicarbonate) provides a clue to the presence of these so-called unmeasured anions. This excess, referred to as the anion gap, can serve as an indirect measure of the quantity of keto acids present (see Chapter 28).

As the keto acids continue to accumulate, the serum bicarbonate falls and the anion gap increases. If this continues, the pH will fall, and the acidosis will become life threatening.

Hyperventilation, a Compensatory Mechanism

Neutrality of body fluids is protected primarily by the bicarbonate buffering system, which determines the pH at all times by the ratio of bicarbonate anion to CO_2 gas in plasma. If bicarbonate anion is lost because of its displacement by keto acid anions, extra CO_2 gas must be driven off at the lung

by hyperventilation in order to keep the ratio at or close to its usual value of 20:1 and to maintain pH close to its physiological value of 7.4. Hyperventilation, which is gradual at first and then rapidly becomes more vigorous and more obvious as arterial pH drops below 7.2, is a characteristic physical finding in DKA. This dramatic increase in ventilation, which occurs more by an increase in the depth than in the frequency of breathing, is known as Kussmaul's respiration. It is associated with the classic "fruity" odor of the breath in DKA. The presence of clear-cut Kussmaul's respiration is a signal that extracellular fluid pH is at or below 7.2, a relatively severe degree of acidosis.

Keto acids are excreted in the urine largely as sodium, potassium, and ammonium salts. This contributes to the third pathophysiological problem of DKA volume depletion.

VOLUME DEPLETION: FLUID AND ELECTROLYTE LOSSES

Osmotic Diuresis

Although loss of glucose through the kidneys helps protect against the ravages of extreme hyperosmolality, the diabetic patient developing ketoacidosis pays a price for this glycosuria. Glucose remaining in the glomerular filtrate

---

Three Major Physiological Disturbances in Diabetic Ketoacidosis

- Hyperosmolality due to hyperglycemia
- Metabolic acidosis due to accumulation of ketoacids
- Volume depletion due to osmotic diuresis

Each of these three disturbances:

- May be more or less severe in any patient
- May interact to aggravate or compensate for the other disturbances

---

after the renal tubules have reabsorbed all they can forces water to remain in the tubules. This glucose-rich filtrate then sweeps out of the body, carrying with it water, sodium, potassium, ammonium, phosphate, and other salts. This rapid urine flow and obligate loss of water and electrolytes is known as an osmotic diuresis. Salts of ketone bodies and the urea resulting from rapid protein breakdown and accelerated gluconeogenesis also contribute to the solute load in the renal tubule, further aggravating the diuresis.

Salt and Water Loss

The average amounts of salts and water lost to the body through osmotic diuresis during the development of DKA have been measured. Overall water loss in a 70-kg adult patient with DKA can be 6 to 7 L, or 15% of total body water.

The fluid lost to the body is slightly hypotonic; it contains a slight excess of water as compared with the volume of salts. This is expected from an osmotic diuresis due to glucose and urea. The fluid losses result from the combination of many different factors, among them the intensity and duration of the hyperglycemia and osmotic diuresis; the amount of water and electrolyte replaced by mouth during this time; the presence of other fluid and electrolyte losses, such as vomiting, diarrhea, or sweating; and the integrity of renal function.

Compensatory Mechanisms

Sodium and water make up the central structure of the extracellular fluid, including the vascular volume. When large quantities of sodium and water are lost in the urine, the body perceives it as a serious threat to the maintenance of the circulation. A variety of compensatory mechanisms are called into play to prevent vascular collapse and shock. For example, an increase in pulse rate usually occurs that helps maintain cardiac output in the face of shrinking intravascular volume.

At least as important, however, is a protective shift in body fluid brought about by the hyperglycemia. Because free glucose is limited almost entirely to the extracellular water, an osmotic pressure gradient is set up across the cell membrane, between the extracellular compartment and the interior of the cells. Therefore, the higher the blood sugar, the more water is drawn out of cells and into the extracellular space. Thus, as sodium and water are lost into the

urine, shrinking the extracellular fluid, they are "replaced" (at least as to their osmotic effect) by glucose entering from the liver and by water entering from all cells. This reexpands the extracellular fluid.

Although hyperosmolality produces damaging CNS effects and osmotic diuresis, it provides a temporary mechanism for preventing vascular collapse. Despite these compensatory mechanisms, circulatory volume falls as DKA progresses. This leads to decreased glomerular filtration, decreased tissue perfusion, metabolic acidosis, and shock.

Decreased Glomerular Filtration

As the vascular volume falls, glomerular filtration also falls. This decreasing renal function leads to increasing blood levels of glucose, potassium, urea nitrogen, and creatinine. The excretion of potassium by the kidney occurs by the exchange of potassium for sodium. Therefore, adequate sodium must be present at the exchange site in the kidney for the rate of potassium excretion to keep pace with the need for excretion. If renal perfusion falls, enough sodium may not be available for this exchange. As a result, despite a total body depletion of potassium, the serum potassium level may rise above normal, even to dangerously high levels.

Decreased glomerular filtration leads to the following:
↑BUN
↑Serum creatinine
↑Blood glucose
↑Serum potassium

Decreased Tissue Perfusion

A second major consequence of diminished vascular volume is generalized decrease in tissue perfusion. Well before the drop in volume has reached the point at which blood pressure actually falls and full-blown shock occurs, blood is shunted away from many tissues, and the perfusion of nearly all tissues suffers. The resulting decrease in oxygen causes those tissues to shift to some degree of anaerobic glucose metabolism. This results in the increased production of lactic acid. The release of lactic acid into the circulation lowers the bicarbonate further, aggravating the already existing metabolic acidosis. Therefore, in patients with DKA, combined lactic acidosis and ketoacidosis is a common finding.

Decreased tissue perfusion leads to the following:
↑Production of lactic acid
↓Bicarbonate
↑Metabolic acidosis

Loss of Phosphate

The loss of phosphate in the urine worsens tissue hypoxia. As body phosphate stores are depleted, circulating plasma phosphate levels fall quite low, depriving the red cells of organic phosphate compounds. Under these circumstances, red cells become depleted of certain key phosphate derivatives, which in turn increases the tightness of oxygen binding to the hemoglobin within these cells. As these cells pass through poorly perfused tissues, less oxygen is given up, and tissue hypoxia worsens.

Shock

Finally, if vascular volume falls low enough, compensation mechanisms fail, blood pressure drops, and true shock supervenes. A rapidly worsening cycle of acidosis, tissue damage, and deepening shock may then occur, leading ultimately to irreversible vascular collapse and death.

The full-blown syndrome of DKA is characterized by major contributions from all three major pathophysiological disruptions, each of which is primarily responsible for one of the major clinical features: coma, shock, and metabolic acidosis (see Fig. 43–1).

Assessment

HISTORY

If ketoacidosis is strongly suspected, an effort is made to establish the diagnosis quickly so that life-preserving therapy can be started. Initial data collection includes an abbreviated history from the family or friends of an unconscious patient, a search for a diabetic identification card, a rapid assessment for clinical clues of volume depletion and Kussmaul's respiration, and blood drawing for initial chemistries. A blood glucose, using a venous sample and glucose meter, and serum ketone measurement at the bedside may confirm the diagnosis. While these preliminary data are collected, an IV line is inserted and volume replacement is started. Then a more considered assessment begins with details of the history and physical examination, a search for precipitating causes, and more complete laboratory tests.

Patients who have completely lost their capacity to secrete insulin can develop DKA without obvious precipitating factors. However, it is very common for stressful events—usually infections but sometimes emotional turmoil—to be precipitating factors. The hormonal responses to stress accelerate catabolic processes and can provide the "last straw" that sets the process in motion. Therefore, look for physiological stressors such as influenza, pneumonia, gastroenteritis, trauma, and myocardial infarction. Interview for emotional stressors as well.

Another precipitating event occurs when diabetics who are completely dependent on insulin stop or skip insulin injections, particularly in the presence of infection or stress. Mismanagement of sick days—improper food intake or insulin administration and failure to report symptoms—is also a precipitating factor. A precipitating cause can be found for most people with DKA.

After asking about the diabetic regimen, medications, and recent changes in health, a systems review is performed. Questions concern appetite, weight change, food and fluid intake, thirst, abdominal bloating and discomfort,

---

Insights Into Clinical Research

Sylvain R, Pokorny ME, English SN, Benson NH, Whitley TW, Ferenczy CJ, Harrison JG: Accuracy of fingerstick glucose values in shock patients. American Journal of Critical Care 4(1):44–48, 1995

Fingerstick blood glucose measurement is used in all health care settings, including emergency rooms and intensive care units. Despite widespread use, there is little research on the clinical situations best suited for this measurement. The purpose of this study was to determine the accuracy of fingerstick blood glucose measurement in patients with poor perfusion.

Inadequate tissue perfusion was defined, and seven signs were identified. The sample included 38 patients who met the study definition of inadequate tissue perfusion and experienced at least three of seven signs. Three glucose measurement techniques were studied: fingerstick blood glucose (drawn from a patient's finger) and analyzed on a glucose meter; venous blood, obtained by venipuncture or from a central catheter and analyzed on a glucose meter; and the remaining venous sample sent to the laboratory for glucose testing. These procedures were defined and standardized for the study. The fingerstick sample was taken within 4 minutes of the venous sample.

Statistical analysis showed that the mean of the laboratory test values was significantly higher than the fingerstick blood glucose results. There was no significant difference between the venous samples tested by the glucose meter or the laboratory. Glucose sliding scale orders were reviewed for each patient. Twelve patients would have received an incorrect insulin dose based on the fingerstick blood glucose results, whereas three would have received an incorrect dose based on venous glucometer results. All patients would have received less insulin based on fingerstick glucose values than if they were based on venous laboratory values. These results suggest that fingerstick blood samples should not be used in patients who have inadequate tissue perfusion.

---

bowel function, and urinary frequency and amount. Cognition and responsiveness can be observed while interviewing.

Possible findings include thirst, frequent urination, poor appetite, nausea and vomiting, abdominal cramps, fatigue, weakness, and drowsiness. The patient may also have symptoms related to urinary tract infection, upper respiratory infection, and chest symptoms because infection is often a precipitating factor.

PHYSICAL EXAMINATION

The physical examination includes blood pressure, heart and respiratory rate, breathing pattern, heart sounds and rhythm, breath sounds, capillary refill, color and warmth of extremities, temperature, signs of hydration (eg, skin turgor, mucous pool under tongue), deep tendon reflexes, LOC, and an abdominal examination. Possible findings include hyperventilation, Kussmaul's respiration and fruity breath, dehydration, abdominal distention, poor perfusion, hypotension, tachycardia, and varying degrees of responsiveness from lethargy to coma.

DIAGNOSTIC TESTS

Diagnostic tests will include blood glucose, chemistries, osmolality, anion gap, pH, ABGs, urine acetone, and glucose. Possible findings include hyperosmolality, increased anion gap (>7 mEq/L), decreased bicarbonate (<10 mEq/L), and decreased pH (7.4). The serum glucose may range from 300 mg/dL to 800 mg/dL or higher. Sodium, potassium, creatinine, and urea nitrogen will all be elevated. Magnesium and phosphate may also be high. Throat, urine, or blood cultures may also be done to determine the presence of infection. Other clues in diagnosis are listed in the accompanying display.

Management

The following are treatment goals for DKA:

- Improve circulatory volume and tissue perfusion
- Correct electrolyte imbalances
- Decrease serum glucose
- Clear the serum and urine of keto acids

SALT AND WATER REPLACEMENT

The immediate threat to life in a critically ill ketoacidotic patient is volume depletion. After establishing an IV line, 0.9% (normal) saline is rapidly infused. The goal is to reverse the worst of the extracellular volume depletion as soon as possible. The first liter may be infused in 1 hour in patients with normal cardiac function. This will replace only one third of the extracellular loss in the average patient.

Fluid replacement continues at roughly 1 L/h until the heart rate, blood pressure, and urine flow indicate that volume is improving. Hypotonic solutions, such as 0.45% normal saline, can be administered at a rate of 150 to 250 mL/h after the intravascular volume has been restored or if the serum sodium level is greater than 155 mg/dL. Other plasma expanders, such as albumin and plasma concentrates, may be necessary if low blood pressure and other clinical signs of vascular collapse do not respond to saline alone.

Rapid infusion of saline in DKA has possible complications. It can dilute plasma proteins and lower the osmotic pressure of the plasma. This allows fluid to leak out of the vascular space through the capillary walls and contributes to the development of pulmonary edema or cerebral edema, particularly in children and older adults. Therefore, observe patients carefully during the first 24 to 36 hours for signs of pulmonary or cerebral edema.

Volume losses will continue throughout the first hours of treatment until the glycosuria and osmotic diuresis are controlled. The next step of fluid replacement can be based on an estimate of the patient's total body fluid loss. About 80% of the fall in blood sugar during treatment of DKA is due to glucose loss into the urine, rather than the result of insulin-induced changes in glucose production and consumption. Therefore, in the earliest phases of treatment, insulin therapy complements fluid and electrolyte replacement.

INSULIN

Insulin is important in treating ketoacidosis for several reasons. It decreases the production of ketones by shutting off the supply of free fatty acids emerging from adipose tissue. It inhibits hepatic gluconeogenesis. This prevents further glucose from being added to the extracellular fluid. Simultaneously, hepatic ketogenesis is further reduced. Insulin also restores cellular protein synthesis. This effect occurs more slowly and permits the restoration of normal potassium, magnesium, and phosphate stores within tissues.

Blood sugar should not fall too fast or too far. Sudden and rapid lowering of the blood sugar with insulin allows water to move very rapidly back into the cells. This can potentially lead to vascular collapse. Instead, early volume replacement should include sodium and water either before or along with insulin therapy.

Low-dose insulin is given by continuous IV infusion rather than by IV bolus or subcutaneous doses. Intramuscular insulin injections are an alternative to IV insulin; however, they should be avoided in hypotensive patients because absorption is unpredictable. Principles for guiding insulin administration are summarized in the display.

POTASSIUM AND PHOSPHATE REPLACEMENT

The initial plasma potassium in patients with DKA can range from very low to very high. Therefore, potassium is not given until the laboratory report is back.

Beginning IV K therapy in the presence of unrecognized hyperkalemia and inadequate renal mechanisms for handling potassium loads can be fatal. Although the ECG can provide clues to the presence of high or low K levels, K therapy should not be based on the ECG alone.

If the initial serum potassium level is low, IV K is generally begun right away. This is particularly important because both insulin and saline drive the K even lower, possi-

---

CLINICAL APPLICATION: Diagnostic Studies
Diabetic Ketoacidosis

- Hyperventilation
- Kussmaul's respiration and "fruity" breath
- Lethargy, stupor, coma
- Hyperglycemia
- Glycosuria
- Volume depletion
- Hyperosmolality
- Increased anion gap (>7 mEq/L)
- Decreased bicarbonate (<10 mEq/L)
- Decreased pH (<7.4)

Principles for Guiding Insulin Administration

- Administer insulin intravenously to the patient with diabetic ketoacidosis to minimize the trauma of repeated injections.
- Use only human regular insulin in intravenous insulin infusions, because it is less antigenic than animal (beef, pork) insulins.
- Administer the insulin infusion through an intravenous infusion pump.
- When the serum glucose level reaches 250 mg/dL, the intravenous fluids should be changed to contain glucose.
- Changes in blood sugar and clinical state should indicate a clear-cut, beneficial response to insulin and fluid replacement. If blood sugar does not drop and blood pressure and urine output do not stabilize, insulin or fluid replacement may not be adequate.

bly to dangerously low levels at which skeletal muscle paralysis and cardiac arrest may occur. If the initial K is normal or high, IV K is generally withheld until the level has begun to drop and urine flow is established. Potassium is usually replaced at concentrations of 20 to 40 mEq/L, depending on the serum potassium level.

Failure of the K to fall can occur for the following reasons:

- Persistent, uncorrected acidosis (which drives K out of cells and into extracellular fluid)
- Hyperosmolality
- Intrinsically impaired renal function
- Insufficient circulating volume

Phosphate levels generally also drop during therapy, aggravating any preexisting tendency of red cells to bind oxygen more tightly. Therefore, many patients receive phosphate in the middle and later phases of therapy. It is usually combined with K replacement in the form of potassium phosphate salts added to the IV infusion. Patients who are receiving IV phosphate therapy should be watched carefully for signs of tetany: tingling around the mouth or in the hands, neuromuscular irritability, carpopedal spasm, or even seizures. Tetany can occur because the phosphate lowers the level of circulating calcium.

BICARBONATE REPLACEMENT

Patients with mild or moderate ketoacidosis who are treated with salt, water, and insulin will eventually excrete and metabolize the ketone bodies remaining in extracellular fluid. As this process continues, more bicarbonate anions are reabsorbed from the renal tubules, and the bicarbonate deficit is slowly repaired. Sometimes the large amounts of chloride administered along with the sodium in IV saline can produce a transient hyperchloremia; this delays the full return of the bicarbonate level to normal for several days.

Bicarbonate is administered to patients with severe acidosis as indicated by an arterial pH of 7.0 or less, whose bicarbonate levels are initially 5 mEq/L or lower. It should also be given when there is cardiac decompensation. The bicarbonate deficit can be calculated and given intravenously over several hours to raise the level at least to the 10 to 12 mEq/L range. Sodium bicarbonate should be administered by slow IV infusion over several hours. It is only administered as a bolus injection in the case of cardiac arrest. Sodium bicarbonate administration can cause a rapid reduction in plasma potassium concentration and sodium overload.

REESTABLISHING GASTROINTESTINAL FUNCTION

Gastric motility is greatly impaired in DKA. Gastric distention with dark, hemipositive fluid (the color of crankcase oil) and vomiting is common. Abdominal pain, tenderness, and a paralytic ileus may also be due to the DKA. The patient may need a nasogastric tube to decompress the stomach. This will increase comfort and decrease the risk of aspiration. Patients should not eat or drink in this phase of illness. Ice chips may decrease thirst. Later, when distention lessens and motility returns, oral intake begins in order to replace the complex nutrition required for recovery.

Metabolic abnormalities should not be corrected too rapidly, especially in patients in whom DKA has been developing for a long time. The key risks during this phase are worsening stupor or coma, hypotension, and hyperkalemia. Osmotic or pH disequilibrium may occur when blood sugar or bicarbonate has been corrected too rapidly. The patient's mental state may worsen even though blood chemistries are improving. Rapid reduction of blood sugar without sufficient sodium and water replacement may be responsible for hypotension. However, sepsis, myocardial infarction, and other causes of shock may also cause hypotension. Hyperkalemia usually results from premature potassium infusion, persistent acidosis, and insufficient volume replacement. However, there may be an early occlusion of the arterial supply to a limb. This can cause large amounts of potassium to leak into the circulation. Therefore, limbs are monitored for asymmetric pallor, coolness, and rubor.

Although patients begin to improve during the initial phase of treatment, recovery usually takes place over 12 days or so. During this time, most metabolic abnormalities are reversed, and body stores of many nutrients (eg, magnesium, protein, phosphate) are replenished. Once recovery is well underway, it is time to think about helping the patient and family understand how to prevent recurrence. See the Collaborative Care Guide.

PATIENT EDUCATION AND SELF-MANAGEMENT

Patients and families who are well informed about diabetes may be more likely to recognize early signs of complications, minimize their development, and seek help if they
(*text continues on page 844*)

COLLABORATIVE CARE GUIDE
for the Patient With Diabetic Ketoacidosis

OUTCOMES	INTERVENTIONS
Oxygenation/Ventilation	
Arterial blood gases are maintained within normal limits.	• Provide chest physiotherapy, turn, deep breath, cough, incentive spirometer q 4 h and PRN.
No evidence of acute respiratory failure.	• Continuously monitor patient's respiratory rate, depth, and pattern. Observe for Kussmaul's respiration, rapid and shallow breathing, and other signs of respiratory distress.
	• Monitor arterial blood gases, pulse oximetry and, if intubated, end tidal CO_2.
	• Provide supplemental oxygen.
	• Prepare for intubation and mechanical ventilation (see Collaborative Care Guide for Patient on Ventilator).
The patient's lungs are clear.	• Auscultate breath sounds q 2 h and PRN.
There is no evidence of atelectasis or pneumonia.	• Take daily chest x-ray.
	• Provide chest physiotherapy q 4 h.
	• Mobilize out of bed as soon as patient is stabilized.
Circulation/Perfusion	
Blood pressure and heart rate are within normal limits. If PA catheter is in place, hemodynamic parameters are within normal limits.	• Monitor vital signs q 1 h and PRN.
	• Assess for dehydration/hypovolemia: tachycardia, decreased CVP and PAWP.
	• Assess for hypervolemia: neck vein distension, pulmonary crackles and edema, increased CVP and PAWP.
	• Administer vasopressor agents if hypotension is related to vasodilation.
Patient is free of dysrhythmias.	• Monitor ECG continuously.
	• Evaluate and treat the cause of dysrhythmias (eg, acidosis, hypoxia, hypokalemia/hyperkalemia).
Fluids/Electrolytes	
Evidence of rehydration without complications:	• Infuse normal saline or lactated Ringer's, then 0.45% normal saline.
—balanced intake and output	
—normal skin turgor	• Monitor serum osmolality, urine output, neurological status, and vital signs closely during rehydration. Observe for complications of DKA (eg, shock, renal failure, decreased LOC and seizures).
—hemodynamic stability	
—intact sensorium	
	• Assess BUN, creatinine, urine for glucose and ketones.
Normal serum electrolytes, mineral levels, and acid–base balance.	• Assess and replace electrolytes, Mg, and PO_4, as indicated.
	• Closely monitor potassium fluctuations as serum glucose is decreased and acidosis reversed.
	• Assess arterial pH and bicarbonate level q 2–4 h during rehydration and insulin administration.
Serum glucose returns to normal range.	• Monitor serum glucose q 30–60 min, then q 1–4 h after level <300 mg/dL.
	• Administer IV insulin bolus then continuous low dose infusion.
	• Infuse D51/2 normal saline or D5W, after glucose is <300 mg/dL.
Mobility/Safety	
The patient will be free of injury related to altered sensorium or seizures.	• Place on seizure and falls precautions.
	• Assess neurological status q 1 h, then q 2–4 h after initial rehydration phase.
Maintain muscle tone and joint range of motion.	• Provide range-of-motion exercises q 4 h.
	• Reposition in bed q 2 h.
	• Mobilize to chair when condition stable.
	• Consult physical therapist.

(continued)

COLLABORATIVE CARE GUIDE
for the Patient With Diabetic Ketoacidosis (Continued)

OUTCOMES	INTERVENTIONS
Skin Integrity	
Skin will remain intact.	• Assess risk for skin breakdown using the Braden Scale. • Initially assess skin and circulation q 1–2 h for 12 h. • If risk for skin breakdown low, assess skin q 8 h and each time patient is repositioned. • Turn q 2 h. • Consider pressure relief/reduction mattress if at risk for skin breakdown.
Nutrition	
Calorie and nutrient intake meet metabolic requirements per calculation (eg, Basal Energy Expenditure).	• Provide parenteral feeding if patient is NPO. • Provide clear, then full liquid diet, and assess patient response. • Progress to diabetic diet. • Consult dietitian or nutritional support service regarding special nutritional needs.
No evidence of metabolic dysfunction.	• Monitor albumin, prealbumin, transferrin, cholesterol, triglycerides, glucose, and protein levels.
Comfort/Pain Control	
Patient will have minimal pain, <5 on pain scale.	• Assess pain and discomfort. If pain present, use objective pain scale q 4 h PRN and following administration of pain medication. • If analgesics are needed, administer cautiously due to risk of respiratory and neurological complications. • Consider nonpharmacological pain management techniques (eg, distraction, touch).
The patient's nausea, vomiting, and abdominal pain or tenderness will resolve.	• Maintain NG tube patency. • Assess bowel sounds q 1–2 h. • Administer antiemetic as ordered. • Provide ice chips and frequent oral hygiene.
Psychosocial	
Patient demonstrates decreased anxiety.	• Provide nonjudgmental atmosphere in which patient can discuss concerns and fears. • Provide patients who are intubated with a method to communicate. • Provide patients with decreased LOC with sensory input. • Provide for adequate rest and sleep.
Teaching/Discharge Planning	
Patient/significant others understand the tests needed for treatment. Significant others understand the severity of the illness, ask appropriate questions, anticipate potential complications.	• Prepare patient/significant others for procedures such as EEG, ECG, and multiple laboratory studies. • Explain the widespread effects of diabetes and the potential for complications of DKA such as seizures, renal failure or vascular collapse. • Encourage significant others to ask questions related to complications, pathophysiology, monitoring, treatments, etc.
Patient/significant others are prepared for home care.	• Teach patient and family information needed to manage diabetes: diabetic diet, skin care, glucose monitoring, insulin administration, signs and symptoms of hypoglycemia and hyperglycemia and appropriate actions. • Discuss sick-day management and factors that can precipitate DKA. • Initiate contacts with diabetic support groups, social services and home health agency.

begin to occur. Although people usually understand the need for insulin injections when they are hungry and eating normally, they may not understand why they need their insulin when they are ill, have no appetite, are not eating, or are vomiting (see accompanying Patient Care Study). The information in the Patient Teaching display along with the sick day plan in the second display will help people with diabetes manage their regimen.

CLINICAL APPLICATION: Patient Care Study

Mr. Oliver, age 31, was admitted to the hospital with the chief complaints of fatigue, cough, nausea, and vomiting for 4 days. He had been diagnosed as having diabetes mellitus 1½ years before admission. Since that time, he had been maintained without incident on 24 U of NPH and 9 U of regular insulin in the morning and 11 U of NPH and 6 U of regular insulin in the evening. Four days before admission, Mr. Oliver began to cough, raising first clear, then brownish, sputum. He soon became fatigued, then experienced some nausea and intermittent vomiting. Two days before admission, he omitted his evening insulin, then took no further insulin the day before and day of admission, "because he was not eating anything." On the day of admission, the patient's wife noted that he had become "less responsive and was breathing fast and deeply" and brought him to the emergency room.

On admission, the patient's rectal temperature was 36.1°C (97°F), pulse was 132, respirations were 28 and deep, and blood pressure was 108/72. He was oriented but lethargic, with coarse rales at both lung bases.

Admission laboratory work revealed a hematocrit of 51.6; white blood cell count of 36,400; and 4+ glucose and ketones on urinalysis. Admission laboratory work included glucose, 910 mg/dL; Na, 128; K, 6.7; Cl, 90; HCO_3, 4; BUN, 43; creatinine, 2.3 mg/dL; serum ketones, 4+ at 1:2 dilution; and trace to 1:32 dilution. Arterial blood pH was 7.06; PaO_2, 112; $PaCO_2$, 13; and HCO_3, 2.5. The admission chest film was negative, but sputum cultured on admission ultimately grew out *Haemophilus influenzae* and *Streptococcus pneumonia*.

Initial therapy consisted of an intravenous infusion of normal saline and 20 U regular insulin by intravenous push, followed by an infusion of insulin at 5 U/h during the first 9 hours. The patient's mental status and sense of well-being improved rapidly. The flow sheet below summarizes the biochemical changes over the first 15 hours.

Mr. Oliver remained afebrile and was treated with antibiotics. By the time of discharge 4 days later, he was eating well, his blood sugars were controlled on his usual doses of NPH insulin, and his cough had improved.

Case Analysis of Clinical Findings

Hyperglycemia and Hyperosmolality. Mr. Oliver presented with the chemical findings of extreme hyperglycemia. As expected in this situation, the BUN and creatinine were elevated, indicating that renal perfusion was reduced, permitting less glucose to escape into the urine and allowing the blood sugar to reach these high levels. The patient's lethargic mental state was the result of the moderately severe hyperosmolality.

Ketosis and Acidosis. For Mr. Oliver, the extremely low initial bicarbonate concentration of 2.5 to 4 signaled the consumption of nearly all the available buffering capacity of plasma, indicating the presence of severe metabolic acidosis. This conclusion was reinforced by the anion gap of $(128 + 7) - (90 + 3) = 42$, about 27 mEq above the usual anion gap upper limit of 15, indicating the presence of 27 mEq of "unmeasured anions." The serum ketones were strongly positive at a dilution of 1:2, confirming the presence of a large quantity of ketone bodies, which could account for most of the unmeasured anions. These findings confirmed the diagnosis of severe DKA.

The patient's deep, rapid breaths represented Kussmaul's respiration, a critically important compensating mechanism that had reduced his arterial CO_2 level ($PaCO_2$) to about one-fourth its usual level and had helped keep his blood pH from falling below its already very low level of 7.06.

Volume Depletion: Fluid and Electrolyte Losses. Mr. Oliver's history of increasing symptoms over at least 4 days suggests that this episode of ketoacidosis had been developing for a substantial period of time, sufficient for osmotic diuresis to produce extensive salt and water losses. Nausea prevented volume replacement by mouth, and vomiting further aggravated the losses. Mr. Oliver failed to realize the need to initiate sick day measures to control his serum glucose level or the need to consult his physician immediately.

The rapid pulse and low blood pressure on admission were further clues to presence of significant hypovolemia. This was confirmed by the elevated BUN and creatinine, reflecting inadequate circulating blood volume to maintain renal perfusion. Finally, the elevated serum potassium ($K^+ = 6.7$ mEq/L, normal = 3.5–4.8 mEq/L) indicated that not enough sodium was being filtered in the kidneys to permit adequate potassium exchange and potassium excretion.

Response to Treatment. Despite severe hyperglycemia, metabolic acidosis, and volume depletion, Mr. Oliver

Biochemical Flow Sheet Indicating Diabetic Ketoacidosis in Mr. Oliver

Time	Sugar	pH	Na	K	Cl	HCO_3	BUN/Creatinine
1:00 PM	710	7.06	128	6.9	90	4	43/2.3
3:00 PM	492		132	6.8	101	6	41/1.7
5:15 PM	375	7.25	137	4.1	106	8	45/1.4
10:00 PM	303		139	4.7	114	15	27/1.2
4:00 AM	304		143	4.3	113	22	22/1.1

PATIENT TEACHING
Self-Management Following Ketoacidosis

- A diabetic person, as any other person, must have insulin, even if no food is being taken in.
- The amount of insulin required when the diabetic person is not eating is about half the total needed when eating.
- The amount of insulin required when a diabetic person is fasting must be spread out as an insulin "trickle" rather than as an insulin "burst."
- Illness generally increases the need for insulin so that even if the diabetic person is not eating, he or she may actually require more than 50% of the usual daily dose.
- There must be enough insulin on hand for daily injections.
- The patient and family members must know how to reach a health care provider for timely phone advice.
- See the Sick Day Plan for Managing Diabetes.

---

responded promptly to volume replacement with saline and low-dose IV insulin. Clinical and chemical signs indicated steady and progressive improvement over the first 15 hours of treatment.

The blood sugar fell from 710 to 304 mg/dL over this time as glucose continued to be lost through the kidneys. The presence of insulin also decreased the hepatic production of glucose. The falling BUN and creatinine indicated that volume replacement had restored renal perfusion. The serum bicarbonate level rose from 4 to 22 mEq/L without the use of IV bicarbonate.

The production of ketones was turned off by insulin; instead, the ketones were metabolized to bicarbonate, which was then reabsorbed by the kidney. Arterial blood pH was restored from its initial very low level of 7.06 to 7.25 as the bicarbonate buffer reappeared in plasma.

Serum potassium fell from 6.9 into the normal range as insulin drove potassium back into cells, pH improved, osmolality returned to normal, and improved renal perfusion permitted exchange of potassium for sodium.

Considerations for Home Care
Sick Day Plan for Managing Diabetes

- Take usual daily dose of insulin or oral hypoglycemic agent.
- Make early call to health care provider to inform him or her of your symptoms and actions.
- Monitor blood glucose every 4 hours or a minimum of four times a day.
- Test urine for ketones every 4 hours if blood glucose is 240 mg/dL or greater.
- Inject small, supplemental doses of short-acting insulin several times daily, if necessary, according to blood glucose test results until glucose levels come under control.
- Drink liberal amounts of fluids, such as water, tea, broth, apple and grape juice, popsicles.
- Eat easily digested carbohydrates, such as custard, pudding, cream soup, saltine crackers, and toast, if unable to eat normal diet.

Finally, the serum chloride rose from the low initial value of 90 mEq/L (normal range, 96–103 mEq/L) to the abnormally high level of 114 mEq/L. The mechanism for this is not entirely understood but is partly due to the IV infusion of large amounts of chloride.

Fortunately, despite Mr. Oliver's severe chemical abnormalities, he was lethargic rather than comatose. This may have been because he was young and otherwise healthy, and the ketoacidosis had developed over a short time. He did not need to be intubated or catheterized, and he tolerated the rapid shifts in volume, pH, and osmolality induced by therapy very well. His rapid response resulted in a brief hospitalization. The slow replenishment of body constituents and readjustment of diabetic regimen—the fourth phase of therapy—could be safely carried out at home with nurse and physician supervision.

Preventing Recurrence. The precipitating causes of the ketoacidosis in Mr. Oliver were classic: the onset of respiratory infection and possibly some initial gastroenteritis and Mr. Oliver's failure to recognize the continuing need for insulin even in the absence of food intake. This episode of ketoacidosis could probably have been prevented if Mr. Oliver had continued to take insulin, perhaps one-half to two-thirds his usual dose, with supplemental short-acting insulin as needed. If the nausea and vomiting had been controlled early, he might also have been able to continue oral fluid and sodium replacement. This situation points out the value of a "diabetes illness plan" and of early contact during an acute illness with a physician or a nurse familiar with diabetes management.

HYPEROSMOLAR HYPERGLYCEMIC NONKETOTIC COMA

Sometimes patients with diabetes develop marked hyperglycemia and hyperosmolality without ketoacidosis. This is the syndrome of hyperosmolar hyperglycemic nonketotic coma (HHNC). Patients are usually middle-aged or older with type II diabetes, sometimes not yet diagnosed. It is not known why some people with diabetes develop this syndrome rather than DKA.

Assessment

The nurse asks the patient about precipitating or associated events. This syndrome can be iatrogenic. It can be induced by some medications, such as glucocorticoids, diazoxide (Proglycem), and diuretics. It can also be caused by hemodialysis against hyperosmolar glucose solutions or by prolonged IV hypertonic glucose infusion, such as those given for total parenteral nutrition.

Often family members will say the patient became a bit drowsy, took in less food and fluid over several days, and slept more until he or she became hard to awaken. They often arrive at the hospital with serious volume depletion and in a stupor or coma. The signs and symptoms are listed in Table 43–2.

Hyperglycemia in HHNC is by definition over 600 mg/dL. In addition to extracellular sodium and water losses, a large additional "free water" deficit exists, probably because the patient did not become thirsty and took in decreasing amounts of fluid. As a result, patients have very high serum levels of sodium and glucose. Glucose can be in excess of 2,000 mg/dL. Serum osmolality is extremely high. Patients may have some degree of ketosis as well. In HHNC, the anion gap attributable to keto acids usually is less than 7 mEq/L.

Management

Therapy for HHNC is directed at controlling hyperglycemia and treating the volume depletion. The volume depletion is usually greater in HHNC than DKA. Patients receive low doses of insulin along with the fluid replacement. Low-dose insulin is given because this population is vulnerable to the sudden loss of circulating blood volume that occurs with higher doses of insulin and a rapid blood sugar reduction.

Older patients who develop HHNC have frequent complications and high mortality rates. They often have difficulty handling the fluid volume shifts that occur during the development and treatment of this syndrome. They are also at risk for intravascular thrombosis and focal seizures that are probably due to the hyperconcentration of the blood and poor circulation.

▬ HYPOGLYCEMIA

Of the two diabetic emergencies, ketoacidosis is far more life threatening than hypoglycemia. The patient, however, usually perceives even mild hypoglycemia as a much greater problem.

TABLE 43-2   CLINICAL APPLICATION: Assessment Parameters
Comparison of Hyperosmolar Hyperglycemic Nonketotic Coma and Diabetic Ketoacidosis

Hyperosmolar Coma	Diabetic Ketoacidosis
• Patient with type II diabetes and may be treated by diet alone, diet and an oral hypoglycemic agent, or diet and insulin therapy	• Patient with type I, insulin-dependent diabetes
• Patient usually more than 40 years of age	• Patient usually less than 40 years of age
• Insidious onset	• Usually rapid onset
• Symptoms include	• Symptoms include
1. Slight drowsiness, insidious stupor, or frequent coma	1. Drowsiness, stupor, coma
2. Polyuria for 2 d to 2 wk before clinical presentation	2. Polyuria for 1–3 d prior to clinical presentation
3. Absence of hyperventilation, no breath odor	3. Hyperventilation with possible Kussmaul's respiration pattern, "fruity" breath odor
4. Extreme volume depletion (dehydration, hypovolemia)	4. Extreme volume depletion (dehydration, hypovolemia)
5. Serum glucose 600 to 2,400 mg/dL	5. Serum glucose 300 to 1,000 mg/dL
6. Occasional gastrointestinal symptoms	6. Abdominal pain, nausea, vomiting, and diarrhea
7. Hypernatremia	7. Mild hyponatremia
8. Failure of thirst mechanism, leading to inadequate water ingestion	8. Polydipsia for 1–3 d
9. High serum osmolality with minimal CNS symptoms (disorientation, focal seizures)	9. High serum osmolality
10. Impaired renal function	10. Impaired renal function
11. HCO_3 level greater than 16 mEq/L	11. HCO_3 level less than 10 mEq/L
12. CO_2 level normal	12. CO_2 level less than 10 mEq/L
13. Anion gap less than 7 mEq/L	13. Anion gap greater than 7 mEq/L
14. Usually normal serum potassium	14. Extreme hypokalemia
15. Ketonemia absent	15. Ketonemia present
16. Lack of acidosis	16. Moderate to severe acidosis
17. High mortality rate	17. High recovery rate

Pathophysiological Principles

Minute-to-minute dependence of the brain on glucose supplied by the circulation results from the inability of the brain to burn long-chain free fatty acids, the lack of glucose stored as glycogen within the adult brain, and the unavailability of ketones. The brain recognizes its energy deficiency when the serum glucose level falls abruptly to about 45 mg/dL. The exact level at which symptoms occur varies widely from person to person, however, and it is not uncommon for levels as low as 30 to 35 mg/dL to occur (eg, during glucose tolerance tests) with no symptoms whatsoever.

Insulin-induced hypoglycemia reactions often occur in the midst of the patient's daily life, which can be at the very least, embarrassing and at worst, dangerous. Even though measurable recovery from hypoglycemia is rapid and complete within minutes after proper treatment, many patients remain emotionally (and possibly physiologically) shaken for hours or even days following insulin reactions. In extreme situations, prolonged or recurrent hypoglycemia, although uncommon, has the potential to cause permanent brain damage and can even be fatal.

Assessment

Occasional reactions happen in even the most stable insulin-dependent diabetic. As long as they are mild, they can usually be tolerated without difficulty and are not cause for alarm or for changes in regimen. Frequently, the precipitating event is clear (eg, a skipped meal or an unusually strenuous bout of exercise).

When hypoglycemic reactions are frequent, recurrent, or severe, it is important to identify the cause and prevent further reactions. Otherwise patients may limit their functional activities and may become unwilling or unable to drive. They may overeat in an effort to prevent reactions. Usually the underlying mechanism can be discovered.

HISTORY

The nurse asks about food intake and exercise because these often contribute to hypoglycemia. Problems with insulin dosage or administration may be noted.

Every detail of insulin therapy should be investigated thoroughly, including insulin purchase, appearance, species, units, and syringes, injection sites, injection technique, and especially any recent change in any part of the regimen. The nurse explores for flaws and inconsistencies in reporting. Prescription errors, mismatched syringe and insulin units, use of new injection sites, and other errors may well emerge.

The administration or withdrawal of other drugs may be the precipitating event for recurrent insulin reactions. For example, salicylates in large doses can reduce blood sugar and, in combination with insulin, can produce hypoglycemia. Also use of glucocorticoid medications should be determined.

Because these medications cause insulin resistance, insulin doses are often raised to meet the increased insulin demand. If the steroids are then tapered without reducing the insulin dose, hypoglycemic reactions can occur. Alcohol often causes hypoglycemia. Not only do patients often eat less when they have a few drinks, but alcohol also shuts off gluconeogenesis by interfering with intermediate biochemical steps within the liver. When combined with injected insulin, this frequently leads to hypoglycemia. Oral hypoglycemia agents can also produce severe and long-lasting hypoglycemia. Patients who experience such episodes tend to be older and undernourished with impaired renal or hepatic function. Nevertheless, any patient on oral agents can become hypoglycemic, especially when potentiated by such agents as salicylates and alcohol.

Another common mechanism that can cause hypoglycemia is an atypical (eg, early or late) response to insulin therapy. Once the response pattern is defined, the insulin regimen can be adjusted, and insulin reactions can be eliminated. Occasionally, when a stable, reaction-free patient begins to experience hypoglycemic episodes, the possibility of insulin sensitivity due to weight loss or the onset of azotemia should be explored.

As blood sugar falls below normal, the CNS responds in two distinct fashions: first, with impairment of higher cerebral functions, and soon thereafter with an "alarm" response in vegetative functions.

Patients most commonly describe the symptoms of mild or early insulin reactions as fuzziness in the head, trouble thinking or concentrating, shakiness, light-headedness, or giddiness. These changes occur when the cerebral cortex is deprived of its main energy supply, usually when the blood glucose has fallen to 50 mg/dL or less or is rapidly declining. This part of the brain is apparently the most sensitive to the loss of glucose.

CLINICAL MANIFESTATIONS

Changes in personality and behavior vary with the person and may not be apparent to them during an insulin reaction. They range from silly, manic, inappropriate behavior to withdrawal, sullenness, or truculence to grumpy, irritable, and suspicious. There may be difficulties in motor function, such as trouble walking and slurred speech, and patients who are well into insulin reactions may closely resemble people who have been drinking alcohol.

Some patients develop aphasia, vertigo, localized weakness, and even focal seizures with their insulin reactions. Such focal changes usually occur when there is prior damage to the specific area of the cortex, such as a head injury or cerebrovascular accident.

Closely following the cortical changes is a series of vegetative neurological responses. The primary response is discharge from the centers that control adrenergic autonomic impulses. This results in the release of norepinephrine throughout the body and epinephrine from the adrenals. Tachycardia, pallor, sweating, and tremor are characteristic signs of hypoglycemia and are important early warning signs for patients who recognize a reaction. Headache can occur, and the stress response can occasionally trigger secondary sequences of symptoms, including angina or pulmonary edema in patients with fragile cardiovascular disease.

As hypoglycemia persists and worsens, consciousness is progressively impaired, leading to stupor, seizure, or coma. This is characteristic of severe hypoglycemia. The vegetative centers controlling fundamental systems, such as respiration and blood pressure, are the most resistant to hypoglycemia and continue to function even when most other cerebral functions are lost.

The more profound the hypoglycemia and the longer it lasts, the greater the chance of transient or even permanent cerebral damage after blood sugar is restored. There does not seem to be a clear duration threshold for such damage, but severe hypoglycemia lasting more than 15 to 30 minutes can result in some symptoms that persist for a time after glucose is given.

Blood sugar measurement, before the administration of glucose if possible, will verify the diagnosis.

Management

Treatment of insulin reactions always is glucose. If the patient can swallow, the glucose is most conveniently given as a glucose- or sucrose-containing drink, because in this form, it probably gets through the stomach and into the absorbing intestine in the fastest possible time. If the patient is too groggy, stuporous, or uncooperative to drink, a bolus of 25 g of 50% dextrose is given intravenously over several minutes. If this route or dosage is unavailable, 1 mg of glucagon given subcutaneously or intramuscularly reverses the symptoms by inducing a rapid breakdown and release of glucose into the bloodstream from hepatic glycogen stores.

The amount of glucose needed to reverse an insulin reaction acutely is not large. The blood sugar can be raised from 20 to 120 mg/dL with less than 15 g (3 tsp) of glucose in an average size adult. Glucose in almost any oral form will serve. Typical treatments for hypoglycemia include 3 glucose tablets, 6 ounces of regular cola, 6 ounces of orange juice, 4 ounces of 2% or skim milk, or 6 to 8 Lifesavers. Starch, as in crackers and cookies, is broken down to free glucose once through the stomach and absorbed so rapidly that blood sugar rises virtually as fast as with free glucose or sucrose.

As an extension of their fears that they might "never wake up" from nocturnal insulin reaction, patients are frequently concerned about what to do if they do not respond to the initial therapy. They must be reassured that if the first bolus of glucose consumed does not seem to work, the sensible thing to do is to take in more. Insulin reactions are always reversible with enough glucose. The response to oral glucose, of course, takes time, perhaps 5 to 15 minutes, whereas the response to IV glucose should occur within 1 or 2 minutes at most.

Failure to respond fully in the appropriate time indicates that not enough glucose has been given, that the diagnosis is incorrect, or that the hypoglycemia has been long and severe enough to produce persistent, although not necessarily permanent, cerebral dysfunction.

Clinical Applicability Challenges

Self-Challenge: Critical Thinking

1. Examine assessment findings for patients with thyroid crisis and myxedema coma. Compare the findings for fluid volume, metabolic state and body temperature, tissue perfusion, and cardiac output. Then construct collaborative interventions for these clinical issues.

2. Compare and contrast fluid volume findings for patients with adrenal crises, SIADH, and DI. Formulate interventions to monitor fluid volume excess or deficit for each. Distinguish differences in interventions for patients with these three endocrine disorders.

3. Analyze the interventions for patients with DKA and HHNC. Distinguish the primary differences.

Study Questions

1. Which of the following pharmacological agents is not recommended for treating thyroid disease?
   a. Aspirin
   b. Propranolol
   c. Glucocorticoids
   d. Propylthiouracil

2. Which of the following symptoms should the nurse recognize as a good indicator of thyroid crisis?
   a. Tachycardia
   b. Neurological dysfunction
   c. Fever
   d. All of the above

3. Myxedema coma is characterized by all but which one of the following symptoms?
   a. Hypotension
   b. Tachycardia
   c. Hypothermia
   d. Hypoventilation

4. DKA is often precipitated by all of the following except
   a. overinsulinization.
   b. stress.
   c. illness.
   d. mismanagement of sick days.

5. Traditional therapy for DKA consists of
   a. fluid replacement with isotonic or hypotonic saline.
   b. a bolus of sodium bicarbonate.
   c. a tracheostomy to assist respirations.
   d. hemodialysis to correct underlying fluid and electrolyte disturbances.

6. During hyperosmolar hyperglycemia nonketotic coma,
   a. the anion gap is usually 8 mEq/L or greater.
   b. ketonemia is present.

c. *serum glucose levels may be 600 to 2,400 mg/dL.*

d. *serum bicarbonate level is less than 10 mEq/L.*

7. *The initial treatment goal of hyperosmolar hyperglycemic nonketotic coma is*

a. *to bring the blood glucose level to a normal range.*

b. *to alleviate ketosis.*

c. *to diurese the patient.*

d. *to rehydrate the patient.*

REFERENCES

1. Isley W: Thyroid disease. In Civetta JM, Taylor RW, Kirby RR (eds): Critical Care, pp 1653–1664 (2nd Ed). Philadelphia, JB Lippincott, 1992

BIBLIOGRAPHY

Anderson S: Seven care types for managing patients with diabetes. AJN 94(9):36–38, 1994

Arbur R: Acute hypoglycemia. Nursing 94 24(1):33, 1994

Bryce J: SIADH. Nursing 94 (4):33, 1994

Davies P: Diabetes insipidus. Nursing 96 26(5):62–63, 1996

Jordon RM: Myxedema coma. Med Clin North Am 79(1):185–194, 1995

Kitabchi A, Wall BM: Diabetic ketoacidosis. Med Clin North Am 79(1):9–37, 1995

Lorber D: Nonketotic hypertonicity in diabetes mellitus. Med Clin North Am 79(1):39–52, 1995

Mc Morrow ME: Emergency! Myxedema coma. AJN 96(10):55, 1996

Reising D. Acute hypoglycemia. Nursing 95 Feb:33–40, 1995

Reising D: Acute hyperglycemia. Nursing 95 Feb:41–48, 1995

Tietgens ST, Leinung MC: Thyroid storm. Med Clin North Am 79(1):169–184, 1995

UNIT VII

Hematological and Immune Systems

44

Anatomy and Physiology of the Hematological and Immune Systems

OBJECTIVES

Based on the content in this chapter, the reader should be able to:

- Describe the blood, its components, and the function of each.
- Delineate the clotting factors and the role each plays in coagulation.
- Describe the anatomy and physiology of the immune system.
- Differentiate between humoral and cell-mediated immunity.

*T*he hematological and immune systems are complex; a change in one system may manifest itself in the other system. Part of the reason for their interrelationship is that both share their origin in bone marrow. The anatomy and physiology of these two systems are discussed separately in this chapter, but the reader should keep in mind their relationship.

Hematological System

Veins, venules, capillaries, arterioles, and arteries constitute an intricate network of conduits for the transportation of blood to and from body tissue. Patency of the conduits and containment of blood within the vasculature depend on the maintenance of the integrity of the transporting conduits.

A delicate balance must be maintained in the vasculature to ensure patency of the vasculature and a liquid state of the blood so that neither thrombosis nor hemorrhage occurs. This delicate balance is provided by the hemostatic and fibrinolytic systems working in concert.

■ BLOOD AND ITS CIRCULATION

Blood is an aqueous solution of colloid and electrolytes that serves as a medium of exchange between body cells and the exterior. Its vital functions are as follows:

- Transport of oxygen and absorbed nutrients to cells
- Transport of carbon dioxide and other waste products to the lungs, kidneys, gastrointestinal system, and skin
- Transport of hormones from endocrine glands to other organs and tissues
- Protection of the body from life-threatening microorganisms
- Regulation of acid–base balance
- Protection from blood loss through hemostasis
- Regulation of body temperature by heat transfer

Blood has distinct characteristics, including variable color (arterial blood is bright red; venous blood is dark red), viscosity (blood is three to four times thicker than water), pH of 7.35 to 7.4, and volume of approximately 70 to 75 mL/kg of body weight (5–6 L). See Chapter 15 for a more detailed discussion of circulation.

■ COMPONENTS OF BLOOD

Plasma

Plasma is the liquid portion of the blood and contains a wide variety of organic and inorganic components (Table 44–1). The concentration of these components is a reflection of diet, metabolic demand, hormones, and vitamins. Plasma is about 90% water and 10% dissolved solutes. The most prevalent substances by weight are the plasma proteins and clotting factors. Serum is plasma that has had clotting proteins removed.

Most plasma proteins, including albumin and fibrinogen, are synthesized by the liver; however, the immunoglobulins are synthesized by B lymphocytes. Albumin is essential for regulation of the colloidal osmotic pressure, which is critical for movement of water and solutes through the microcirculation. It also is a carrier molecule for normal blood components and exogenous agents, such as drugs. Immunoglobulins (antibodies), the products of B lymphocytes, are essential for defense against infectious microorganisms (see section on the immune system later in this chapter for further description).

Lipoproteins, which include the plasma lipids, triglycerides, phospholipids, cholesterol, and fatty acids, are carried through the blood as complexes with the plasma proteins. The electrolytes (sodium, potassium, calcium, magnesium, chloride, bicarbonate, phosphate, and sulfate) maintain the pH and osmolality of the blood. Nutrients, such as glucose, and gases, such as oxygen and carbon dioxide, are circulated to and from the tissues. Waste products are carried to the appropriate organ for excretion.

Cellular Elements

The cellular elements of the blood are the erythrocytes (red blood cells), leukocytes (white blood cells), and platelets. These three elements are summarized in Table 44–2. All the cell types are believed to be derived from a single stem cell, as shown in Figure 44–1. The production of blood cells (hematopoiesis) occurs in the bone marrow. It is a two-stage process that involves mitotic division (proliferation) and maturation (differentiation). Each blood cell type results from pluripotential cells that become committed to a cell line when they receive specific biochemical signals. These signals occur when one or more populations of circulating cells have decreased to a certain level. Mitosis occurs and proliferation continues until the needed number of mature daughter cells has entered the circulation.

ERYTHROCYTES

There are approximately 5 million erythrocytes per cubic millimeter of blood. They are produced in the red bone marrow found in the sternum, ribs, skull, vertebrae, and bones of the hands, feet, and pelvis. Normal cell formation requires such nutrients as iron, vitamin B_{12}, folic acid, and pyridoxine. Reticulocytes are released from the bone marrow and circulate for 1 to 2 days while maturing into adult cells. The average life span of an erythrocyte is 115 to 130 days. Dead red blood cells are eliminated mainly by phagocytosis in the liver and spleen. The erythrocyte is a small disk that has biconcavity and reversible deformability. The flattened, biconcave shape has a surface area to volume ratio that is optimal for the diffusion of gases into and out of the cell. Reversible deformity gives the cell the ability to alter its shape to squeeze through the microcirculation and then return to its normal shape.

Hemoglobin is the iron-containing substance of the erythrocyte. The normal amount of hemoglobin in the body is 12 to 18 g/dL of blood, with a lower level in females and a higher level in males. It is composed of a red compound called heme (which contains iron and porphyrin) and a simple protein called globin. Each red blood cell contains 200 to 300 million molecules of hemoglobin, which combines with oxygen to form oxyhemoglobin. It also combines with carbon dioxide. These characteristics mean that the blood can carry oxygen to the tissues and carbon dioxide to the alveoli of the lungs and from there to the atmosphere. One iron

---

Characteristics of Blood

Color: Arterial blood bright red; venous blood dark red
Viscosity: Three to four times thicker than water
Reaction: pH, 7.35–7.4
Volume: Adults: approximately 70–75 mL/kg of body weight, or 5–6 L

TABLE 44-1
Organic and Inorganic Components of Arterial Plasma

Constituent	Amount/Concentration	Major Functions
Water	93% of plasma weight	Medium for carrying all other constituents
Electrolytes	Total <1% of plasma weight	Maintain water in extracellular compartment; act as buffers; function in membrane ex-citability
Sodium (Na)	142 mEq/L (142 mM)	
Potassium (K)	4 mEq/L (4 mM)	
Calcium (Ca)	5 mEq/L (2.5 mM)	
Magnesium (Mg)	3 mEq/L (1.5 mM)	
Chloride (Cl)	103 mEq/L (103 mM)	
Bicarbonate (HCO_3)	27 mEq/L (27 mM)	
Phosphate (mostly HPO_4^{2-})	2 mEq/L (1 mM)	
Sulfate (SO_4^{2-})	1 mEq/L (0.5 mM)	
Proteins	7.3 g/dL (2.5 mM)	Provide colloid osmotic pressure of plasma; act as buffers; bind other plasma constituents (eg, lipids, hormones, vitamins, metals); clotting factors; enzymes; enzyme precursors; antibodies (immune globulins); hormones
Albumins	4.5 g/dL	
Globulins	2.5 g/dL	
Fibrinogen	0.3 g/dL	
Gases		
Carbon dioxide (CO_2) content	22–20 mmol/L plasma	By-product of oxygenation, most carbon dioxide content from bicarbonate and acts as a buffer
Oxygen (O_2)	PaO_2 80 mmHg or greater (arterial); PvO_2 30–40 mmHg (venous)	Oxygenation
Nitrogen (N_2)	0.9 mL/dL	By-product of protein catabolism
Nutrients		Provide nutrition and substances for tissue repair
Glucose and other carbohydrates	100 mg/dL (5.6 mM)	
Total amino acids	40 mg/dL (2 mM)	
Total lipids	500 mg/dL (7.5 mM)	
Cholesterol	150–250 mg/dL (4–7 mM)	
Individual vitamins	0.0001–2.5 mg/dL	
Individual trace elements	0.001–0.3 mg/dL	
Waste products		
Urea (BUN)	7–18 mg/dL (5.7 mM)	End product of protein catabolism
Creatinine (from creatinine)	1 mg/dL (0.09 mM)	End product from energy metabolism
Uric acid (from nucleic acids)	5 mg/dL (0.3 mM)	End product of protein metabolism
Bilirubin (from heme)	0.2–1.2 mg/dL (0.003–0.018 mM)	End product of red blood cell destruction
Individual hormones	0.000001–0.5 mg/dL	Functions specific to target tissue

From Vander AS, Sherman JH, Luciana DS: Human Physiology: The Mechanisms of Body Function (6th Ed.). New York, McGraw-Hill, 1994

atom is present for each heme molecule. Total body iron ranges from 2 to 6 g. Two thirds of this is in hemoglobin, and the rest is stored in the bone marrow, spleen, and liver. When red blood cells break down, hemoglobin splits into heme and globin factors. The iron is stored by the liver for production of new hemoglobin, and the remainder is converted into bilirubin, which is excreted in feces and urine after conjugation by the liver. This conjugation process is important to the excretion of bilirubin, which causes jaundice when it accumulates in the tissues (see Chapter 40).

LEUKOCYTES

White blood cells (leukocytes), which are transported in the circulation but act primarily in the body tissues, defend the body against microorganisms and remove such debris as dead or injured host cells. There are approximately 5,000 to 10,000 white blood cells per cubic millimeter of blood. The

two major categories of leukocytes are granulocytes and agranulocytes.

Granulocytes comprise about 70% of all white blood cells and include neutrophils, eosinophils, and basophils. They are produced by the bone marrow and function based on the type of enclosed granule. Polymorphonuclear leukocytes (also referred to as PMNs or neutrophils) fight bacterial infections and digest foreign particulate matter or break down products from cells through phagocytosis. PMNs are present during the early acute phase of an inflammatory reaction. After bacterial invasion or tissue injury, they migrate from the capillaries into the inflamed area where they destroy and ingest microorganisms and other debris. They die in 1 or 2 days, releasing digestive enzymes that dissolve cellular debris and prepare the inflamed site for healing.

Eosinophils are particularly important in detoxifying foreign protein. They ingest antigen–antibody complexes, attack parasites, and are elevated during allergic reactions.

TABLE 44-2
Cellular Components of the Blood

Cell	Structural Characteristics	Normal Amounts in Circulating Blood	Function	Life Span
Erythrocyte (red blood cell)	Non-nucleated cytoplasmic disk containing hemoglobin	4.2–6.2 million/mm³	Gas transport to and from tissue cells and lungs	80–120 d
Leukocyte (white blood cell)	Nucleated cell	5,000–10,000/mm³	Bodily defense mechanisms	See below
Lymphocyte	Mononuclear immunocyte	25%–33% of leukocyte count (leukocyte differential)	Humoral and cell-mediated immunity	Days or years, depending on type
Monocyte and macrophage	Large mononuclear phagocyte	3%–7% of leukocyte differential	Phagocytosis; mononuclear phagocyte system	Months or years
Eosinophil	Segmented polymorphonuclear granulocyte	1%–4% of leukocyte differential	Phagocytosis; antibody-mediated defense against parasites, allergic reactions; associated with Hodgkin's disease, recovery phase of infection	Unknown
Neutrophil	Segmented polymorphonuclear granulocyte	57%–67% of leukocyte differential	Phagocytosis, particularly during early phase of inflammation	4 d
Basophil	Segmented polymorphonuclear granulocyte	0–0.75% of leukocyte differential	Unknown, but associated with allergic reactions and mechanical irritation	Unknown
Platelet	Irregularly shaped cytoplasmic fragment (not a cell)	140,000–340,000/mm³	Hemostasis following vascular injury; normal coagulation and clot formation/retraction	8–11 d

From McCance KL, Huether SE: Pathophysiology: The Biologic Basis for Disease in Adults and Children (2nd Ed.). St. Louis, Mosby-Year Book, 1994

Basophils contain cytoplasmic granules with vasoactive amines (histamine, bradykinin, and serotonin), which are thought to play a role in the symptoms of acute systemic allergic reactions. Basophils also contain the anticoagulant heparin.

Agranulocytes (monocytes, macrophages, and lymphocytes) are leukocytes that do not contain lysosomal granules in their cytoplasm. Monocytes (immature macrophages) and macrophages comprise the mononuclear phagocyte system (formerly called the reticuloendothelial system). They are responsible for the phagocytosis of dead leukocytes and erythrocytes in the blood and for the processing of antigenic material. Some of the circulating macrophages migrate out of the blood vessels in response to inflammation or infection, whereas others migrate to fixed sites in lymphoid tissues of the liver, spleen, lymph nodes, peritoneum, or gastrointestinal tract, where they may remain active for months or years.

Lymphocytes are immunocompetent cells that are involved in producing antibodies and maintaining the immune response. The most important classifications are T and B lymphocytes, which are discussed later in the chapter in the section on specific immunity.

PLATELETS

Platelets are disk-shaped cytoplasmic fragments formed from stem cells in the bone marrow, specifically a giant cell called the megakaryocyte. They maintain capillary integrity, accelerate coagulation, and retract clots. There are about 250,000 to 500,000 platelets per cubic millimeter of blood; one third of them reside in a reserve pool in the spleen.

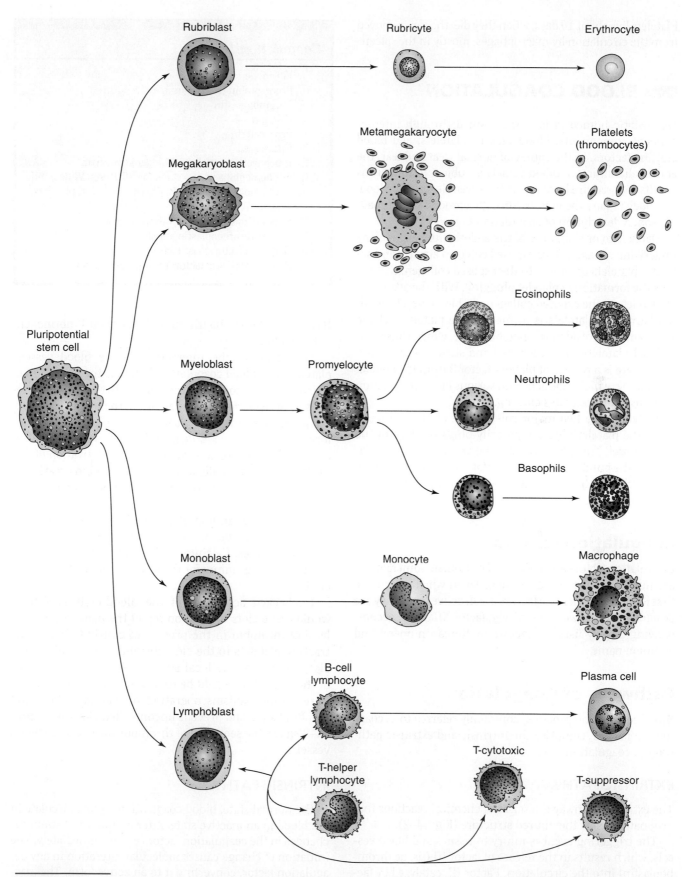

FIGURE 44-1

Components of blood derived from a single stem cell.
(From Belcher AE: Blood Disorders. St. Louis: Mosby-Year Book, 1993.)

Platelets live about 10 days; when they die, they are removed from the circulation by macrophages, mostly in the spleen.

▰ BLOOD COAGULATION

Hemostatic homeostasis is maintained through interdependent components: blood vessels, platelets, and blood clotting factors. In the course of normal wear and tear, the endothelial lining of blood vessels is subject to numerous insults that require local repair to prevent leakage of blood. The body repairs the vessels through a process called coagulation. A description of coagulation follows.

Damage to or sloughing of the endothelium exposes the underlying collagen. This exposed collagen attracts and activates platelets to adhere to the exposed collagen; that begins the formation of platelet plugging. With the attraction of platelets to the exposed collagen of a blood vessel, an initial barrier of platelets is formed. These platelets release small amounts of adenosine diphosphate, which causes additional platelets to be attracted and stick to each other. Then there is a release of platelet factor 3 from the platelet membrane, which interacts with various blood coagulation proteins and accelerates clotting.

Platelets play two major roles in the clotting process. First, the platelet plug temporarily plugs the leak in the blood vessel. This plug provides the architectural foundation for the building of the fibrin clot. The second role is to initiate clotting by way of the intrinsic pathway through the release of platelet factor 3.

Coagulation Factors

Coagulation factors are designated by Roman numerals and are numbered according to the order in which they were first identified. When the factors are in active form, they are designated by a lower case "a" (*eg*, factor XIIa). The accompanying display lists the factors by Roman numeral and common name.

Pathways of Coagulation

Blood coagulation proteins, commonly referred to as coagulation factors, comprise the intrinsic and extrinsic pathways to coagulation.

EXTRINSIC PATHWAY

The extrinsic pathway is a series of chemical reactions that originate outside the injured structure (Fig. 44–2).

The triggering event is injury to tissues and blood vessels, which results in the release of factor III (tissue thromboplastin) into the circulation. Factor III, catalyzed by factor VII (proconvertin), activates factor X (Stuart-Prower). In the presence of calcium ions, factor V (proaccelerin) and platelet factor 3, factor Xa catalyzes the conversion of factor

---

Coagulation Factors
I. Fibrinogen
II. Prothrombin (thrombin in active form–IIa)
III. Thromboplastin
IV. Calcium
V. Proaccelerin
VI. Unassigned
VII. Proconvertin; prothrombinogen; convertin
VIII. Antihemophiliac factor A (factor VIIIR–von Willebrand)
IX. Antihemophiliac factor B; Christmas factor; platelet cofactor II
X. Stuart–Prower factor; prothrombinase
XI. Plasma thromboplastin antecedent
XII. Hageman factor; glass factor
XIII. Fibrin-stabilizing factor; Laki–Lorand factor

II (prothrombin) to IIa (thrombin) and factor I (fibrinogen) to fibrin clot.

The result of the interaction of the blood vessels, platelets, and blood coagulation factors is the formation of factor Xa, which converts prothrombin to thrombin and results in fibrin formation. At factor Xa, the intrinsic and extrinsic pathways merge into a final common pathway to clot formation. Figure 44–2 depicts diagrammatically the sequence of clot formation. Notice that the activation of factor VIII (antihemophilic factor A) by thrombin creates the activation of factor X, resulting in the self-perpetuating effect.

Calcium plays an important role in several steps along the clotting cascade. Many coagulation factors carry two negative charges. Calcium, with its two positive charges, creates a strong affinity for the factors to bind at the site of clotting.

Unchecked activation of the blood-clotting factors would cause clots to form on top of the platelet plug, releasing thrombin in the process of clotting, further attracting platelets to the clot site, and causing additional clots to form at the local site of vessel leak. The result of this activation would be total vessel occlusion if there were no mechanisms operating to maintain the blood in a fluid state and prevent uncontrolled clotting. Figure 44–3 shows the sequence of thrombus formation in blood vessels.

INTRINSIC PATHWAY

In the normal state, blood coagulation factors circulate in the blood in an inactive state. After an initiating stimulus, changes in the coagulation factors occur immediately. The initiation of change causes molecular alteration in any coagulation factor, converting it to an active form. The inactive coagulation factor, known as a proenzyme, is converted to an active state and becomes an active enzyme. The product of this enzymatic reaction activates the next coagula-

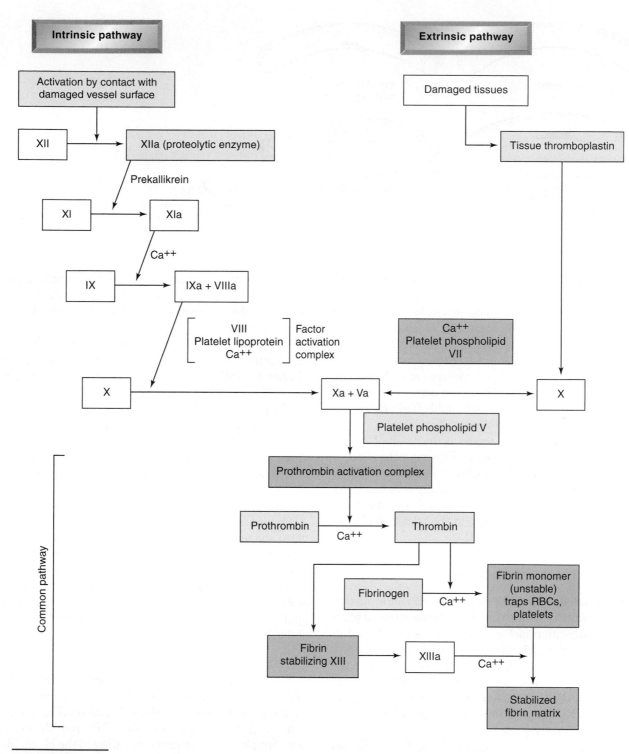

FIGURE 44-2
The coagulation cascade. From McCance KL, SE Huether: Pathophysiology: The Biologic Basis for Disease in Adults and Children (2nd ed.) p. 850. St. Louis, Mosby-Year Book, 1994

tion factor in a chainlike reaction, leading to final clot formation. This chain of chemical reactions is named the intrinsic pathway, which indicates its origin from within the tissue.

When platelet factor 3 is released, it initiates the activation of the intrinsic pathway by activating factor XII (Hage-

man factor); it is also a necessary component for complex reactions at the levels of factors V and VIII. The exposed collagen, phospholipids from injured erythrocytes and granulocytes, antigen–antibody complexes, and endotoxins are thought to be other activators of factor XII. These activators convert inactive factor XII to the active enzymatic form

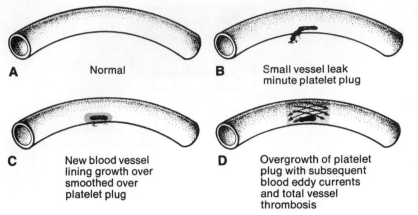

A Normal

B Small vessel leak minute platelet plug

C New blood vessel lining growth over smoothed over platelet plug

D Overgrowth of platelet plug with subsequent blood eddy currents and total vessel thrombosis

FIGURE 44-3
Sequence of thrombus formation in blood vessels.

XIIa, which acts on the next clotting proenzyme, inactive factor XI (antihemophilic factor C), converting it to the active enzyme XIa. Factor XIa is responsible for the activation of factor IX (antihemophilic factor B), which requires calcium ions. The activation of the next factor, factor X, requires factor VII and platelet factor 3. The conversion of factor II to factor IIa (thrombin) requires factor V, platelet factor 3, and calcium ions. Thrombin acts on fibrinogen, converting it to fibrin. This initial soluble fibrin clot is stabilized by factor XIII in the presence of calcium.

A self-perpetuating effect occurs as the result of the ongoing cycle of activation of factor X through the effect of thrombin on factor VIII. Thrombin enhances the activity of factor VIII so that it interacts more rapidly with factor IXa and thus catalyzes the activation of factor X. Thrombin also interacts with platelets, resulting in the release of platelet factor 3, which activates factor XII.

Coagulation Inhibitors

There is a well-controlled balance between clot formation and clot inhibition in humans. Through the action of physiological coagulation factors, the blood is maintained in its fluid state and vessels remain patent. These inhibitors—adequate blood flow, mast cells, antithrombin III, the mononuclear phagocyte system, and the fibrinolytic system—work by limiting reactions that promote clotting and by lysing any clots that do form, thus preventing total occlusion of the vessels.

The maintenance of an adequate blood flow facilitates the quick delivery of dilute activated clotting factors to the liver, where they are cleared from circulation.

Mast cells, which are located in most body tissues, produce heparin, which has a low anticoagulant activity when compared with that of commercially produced heparin.

The liberation of antithrombin III in response to thrombin inactivates the circulating thrombin and neutralizes activated factors XII, XI, and X. This retards the conversion of fibrinogen to fibrin, thus stopping sequential activation of clotting factors.

The mononuclear phagocyte system is composed of tissue macrophages that are located throughout the body. The system inhibits coagulation by clearing activated factors from the blood.

The fibrinolytic system interferes with thrombin at its site of action on fibrinogen. It also involves a chain reaction whereby activation of a series of proenzymes produces lytic enzymes capable of dissolving clots.

The proenzyme plasminogen circulates in the blood. It is believed that the endothelial cells that constitute the endothelial lining of blood vessels release plasminogen activator, converting plasminogen to plasmin. In addition, activated factor XII, thrombin, kallikrein, and substances in the tissues are thought to be involved in the conversion of plasminogen to plasmin.

Plasmin is the dissolving or lytic enzyme that acts to lyse fibrin and attacks factors V, VIII, IX, and fibrinogen. Plasminogen activator levels are found to be transiently elevated in response to exercise, stress, anoxia, and pyrogen.

The lysis of fibrinogen and fibrin results in the liberation of FDPs. These products inhibit platelet aggregation, exhibit an antithrombin effect, and interfere with formation of the fibrin clot.

Fibrinolytic System Inhibitors

Similar to coagulation system inhibitors, there are inhibitors of the fibrinolytic system. These inhibitors prevent inappropriate lysis of needed clot formation. The mononuclear phagocyte system clears the FDPs from the circulation. Antiplasmin, a protein circulating in the blood, binds with plasmin and renders it inactive. The level of circulating antiplasmin far outweighs plasmin concentration, and plasmin is neutralized rapidly.

It is evident that the systems of hemostasis and fibrinolysis in conjunction with their system inhibitors function within a narrow margin to ensure the liquidity of the blood and patency of the vasculature. An upset in these systems may result in clinical evidence of thrombosis, hemorrhage, or the catastrophic event of disseminated intravascular coagulation.

Immune System

The hematological system and the immune system are closely related. In addition to both originating in the bone marrow, blood carries components of the immune system throughout the body. The following are functions of a healthy immune system:

- Protection of the body from destruction by foreign agents and microbial pathogens
- Degradation and removal of damaged and dead cells
- Surveillance and destruction of malignant cells

ORGANS AND CELLS OF THE IMMUNE SYSTEM

The immune system is composed of the following organs and cells: spleen, lymph nodes, thymus, bone marrow, appendix, tonsils and adenoids, B and T lymphocytes, eosinophils, basophils, and phagocytes. The organs of the system are connected with one another and with other bodily organs through a network of lymphatic vessels. Immune cells and foreign particles are conveyed through the vessels in lymph fluid.

IMMUNE RESPONSE

The immune system is responsible for protecting the body or "self" from invasion by "nonself" (also called antigens). Any foreign substance capable of eliciting a specific immune response is referred to as an antigen. Antigens are most often composed of proteins, but polysaccharides, complex lipids, and nucleic acids may sometimes act as antigenic materials; bacteria, viruses, fungi, parasites, and foreign tissue are all antigens. Markers on antigens enable the immune system to identify target cells, against which destructive forces are directed. The intensity of the system's response is affected by the route of invasion, the dosage of the antigen, and its degree of foreignness.

Immunological competence refers to the immune system's capacity to identify and reject foreign materials. The failure of the system to recognize antigens and mobilize effective defenses results in infection or malignancy. Failure to recognize markers of self may result in autoimmune diseases, such as multiple sclerosis, rheumatoid arthritis, or systemic lupus erythematosus. The system's "battle against imaginary enemies," such as pollen or dust, may result in allergies.

Major histocompatibility complex (MHC) is a group of genes contained in a section of chromosome 6 that encode molecules that mark a cell as self. These MHCs vary widely in details of structure from one person to another. Their presence is a factor in transplant rejection, because these markers determine to which antigens one responds and how strongly. They also allow immune cells to recognize and communicate with one another.

The body's protective mechanisms can be divided into two major categories: general immunity and specific immunity.

General Immunity

General immunity is present in all healthy people and forms the first line of defense against illness. A previous exposure to an organism or toxin is not required. These mechanisms do not distinguish among microorganisms of different species and do not alter in intensity on reexposure. General immunities include physical, chemical, and mechanical barriers; biological defenses; phagocytosis; inflammatory processes; and cytokines.

PHYSICAL, CHEMICAL, AND MECHANICAL BARRIERS

Physical barriers prevent harmful organisms and other substances from gaining entrance into the body or body cavities. These barriers include skin, mucous membranes, epiglottis, respiratory tract cilia, and sphincters. Chemical barriers include antibacterial agents, antibodies, and acid solutions that create an environment hostile to many pathogens such as lysozymes in tears, lactic acid in vaginal secretions, and hydrochloric acid in gastric secretions. Mechanical barriers help to rid the body of potentially harmful substances through some action (eg, lacrimation, intestinal peristalsis, urinary flow).

BIOLOGICAL DEFENSES

Under normal conditions, large areas of the human body are colonized with microorganisms. The skin and mucous membranes of the oropharynx, nasopharynx, intestinal tract, and parts of the genital tract each have their own microflora, referred to as normal flora. These microorganisms influence patterns of colonization by competing with more harmful organisms for essential nutrients and by producing substances that inhibit the growth of other microorganisms.

PHAGOCYTES AND PHAGOCYTOSIS

Phagocytosis is a process by which injured cells and foreign invaders are ingested by leukocytes, specifically PMNs (neutrophils) and mononuclear phagocytes (monocytes and macrophages). Both cell types originate from stem cells in the bone marrow and, though structurally different, both approach phagocytosis in a similar manner.

Surface receptors on their cell membranes allow them to attach to foreign substances and then engulf, internalize, and destroy these substances using enzymes present within their cellular interior. Neutrophils provide the "first-wave" cellular attack on invading organisms during the acute inflammatory process. Monocytes spend only a short time in the bloodstream before escaping through the capillary membranes into the tissue. Once in the tissue, they swell to much larger sizes to become macrophages. These macrophages will either attach to certain tissues and destroy bacteria or wander through the tissue phagocytizing foreign matter. These cells are strategically placed throughout the body tissues, where they can exist for months and even years to function as a first line of defense. Macrophages in different tissues differ in appearance because of environmental variations and are known by different names (ie, Kupffer's cells in the liver, alveolar macrophages in the lung, histiocytes in the skin and subcutaneous tissue, and microglia in the brain).

INFLAMMATORY RESPONSES

Inflammation is an acute physiological response of the body to tissue injury caused by such factors as chemicals, heat, trauma, or microbial invasion. It is the primary process through which the body repairs tissue damage and defends itself against infection. There are three stages of the inflammatory response:

- Vascular stage, which is an immediate but short-term vasoconstriction of arterioles and venules and hyperemia and swelling resulting from the secretion of histamine, serotonin, and kinins
- Cellular exudate stage, characterized by neutrophilia, secretion of colony-stimulating factors into the interstitial fluid, and formation of exudate
- Stage of tissue repair and replacement

The most important result of these processes is accumulation of large numbers of PMNs and macrophages at the site of the injury, which inactivate or destroy invaders, remove debris, and begin the initial tissue repair.

CYTOKINES

Cytokines are chemical messengers that enhance cell growth, promote cell activation, direct cellular traffic, stimulate macrophage function, and destroy antigens. They are also called interleukins (IL) because they serve as messengers between leukocytes.

Interleukin-1 (IL-1) augments the synthesis of IL-2, IL-3, IL-4, gamma-interferon, and IL-2 receptors; it can also activate lymphokine-activated killer cells. IL-2 binds to specific receptors on activated T cells and markedly enhances the cytolytic activity of natural killer cells; IL-3 and B-cell differentiation factor provide critical signals for the growth and maturation of antigen-primed B cells. Cytokines can be classified as lymphokines (secreted by lymphocytes) or monokines (secreted by monocytes or macrophages). Interferons (a type of lymphokine) provide some protection to the body against invasion by viruses until more slowly reacting specific immune responses can take over. In addition, interferons appear to be involved in protecting the body against some forms of cancer. These substances have been demonstrated to interfere with cellular division and proliferation of abnormal cells. They also enhance the activity of a specialized group of lymphoid cells called natural killer cells (NKCs). These NKCs act directly, without prior sensitization, to lyse a variety of malignant cells.

Specific Immunity

If a foreign agent persists in spite of general immune responses, activation of specific immune responses occurs. These responses require previous exposure to a foreign agent or organism to be most effective. The cellular components of these types of responses are capable of distinguishing among microorganisms and can alter their intensity and response time significantly on reexposure.

Two types of specific immune response have been identified: humoral immunity and cell-mediated immunity. Most foreign substances stimulate both cellular and humoral immune responses, which results in an overlapping of their reactions and maximum protection against damage from the invading substances.

B AND T LYMPHOCYTES

The B and T lymphocytes originate from stem cells produced in the bone marrow. During fetal development and shortly after birth, primary lymphoid organs are the site where these cells differentiate and mature into the competent cells responsible for humoral and cell-mediated immune responses. For T lymphocytes, this preprocessing occurs in the thymus gland, and for B lymphocytes, it is believed to occur in the bone marrow and possibly the fetal liver. As they develop, both B and T lymphocytes acquire specific receptors for antigens that commit them to a single antigenic specificity for their lifetime. Subsequently, each of these "preprogrammed" T or B lymphocytes (on activation by its specific antigen) is capable of producing tremendous numbers of clones or duplicate lymphocytes. The different types of T cells produced are categorized according to their function, as shown in Table 44–3.

LYMPHOID SYSTEM

After preprocessing in the primary lymphoid organs, B and T lymphocytes migrate to secondary lymphoid tissues where the interaction with antigens and immune responses actually occurs. Secondary lymphatic tissue is located extensively in the lymph nodes. It is also found in special lymphoid tissue, such as that of the spleen, tonsils, adenoids, appendix, bone marrow, and gastrointestinal tract. This lymphoid tissue is placed advantageously through-

TABLE 44-3
Types of T Cells and Their Functions

Cell Type	Function
Cytotoxic T cells (T8)	Direct-attack cells capable of killing many microorganisms; predominant effector cell
	Virus-infected cells, cancer cells, and transplanted cells especially susceptible
Helper-inducer T cells (T4)	Most numerous
	Play pivotal role in overall regulation of immune response
	Often called "master conductor"
	Secrete lymphokines
Suppressor T cells (T8)	Act as negative feedback controllers of T4 cells
	May also limit ability of immune system to attack body tissues
Memory T cells	Sensitized to antigens during specific immune responses
	Remain stored in body
	Capable of initiating far more rapid response by T cells on reexposure to same antigen

out the body to intercept invading organisms or toxins before they can enter the bloodstream and disseminate widely.

CELL-MEDIATED IMMUNE RESPONSE

This type of immunity provides a response to fungi, parasites, and intracellular bacteria. It also plays a major role in rejection or acceptance of certain tissue grafts, the stimulation and regulation of antibody production, and defense against various malignant changes. T lymphocytes contain an antigen receptor that allows for binding of a specific type of antigen. Each of these T cells, on activation by its specific antigen, is capable of producing large numbers of clones. After preprocessing, T cells migrate to lymphoid tissue where they act as effector cells (directly attacking antigens and malignant cells) and regulators of both the humoral and cellular immune response.

The cell-mediated response is initiated by antigenic stimulation of T lymphocytes. This step of the response may be mediated by macrophages that bind to the antigen, facilitating its recognition. The macrophages then produce cytokines, which stimulate T lymphocytes, increase B lymphocyte proliferation, and activate phagocytes.

HUMORAL IMMUNE RESPONSE

This form of immunity is extracellular; that is, it occurs in blood and tissue fluid. It begins in response to most bacteria, bacterial toxins, and the extracellular phase of viral invasion. Humoral immunity involves two types of serum proteins, immunoglobulins (Ig) and complement.

Immunoglobulins are antibody modules made by B lymphocytes that differentiate to plasma cells and memory cells. The plasma cells then secrete antibodies that bind to antigens; the resulting antigen–antibody complexes are ingested by phagocytes. After the complex is eliminated, the

memory cells remain in circulation and in lymphoid tissue to mature into plasma cells when the antigen is encountered again. Immunoglobulins are specific to antigens and are of several types:

- IgA (two types) concentrates in body fluids, such as tears, saliva, and secretions of respiratory and gastrointestinal tracts; it guards entrances to the body.
- IgM tends to remain in the bloodstream where it is effective in killing bacteria.
- IgG (four types) is able to enter tissue spaces and works efficiently to coat microorganisms before phagocytosis occurs.
- IgD is found mostly in the membrane of B cells, where it is believed to regulate the cell's activation.
- IgE is normally present in only trace amounts; it is responsible for symptoms of allergy.

Complement is a nonspecific series of 15 proteins that circulate in inactive form in the bloodstream. These proteins can activate one another in a cascading sequence when the first complement molecule C1 encounters an antigen–antibody complex. The end product of the cascade is a cylinder that lyses the cell membrane, allowing fluids and molecules to flow in and out, which kills the target cell (Fig. 44–4).

Complement also facilitates the interaction of antigens and antibodies and enhances all aspects of the inflammatory process, especially increasing vascular permeability and phagocytosis.

Combined Immune Responses

The specific immune response is complex and involves the interaction of macrophages, complement proteins, and the cellular components of both the cellular and humoral systems (Fig. 44–5). Macrophages initially function to recognize, process, and present the antigen to antigen-specific

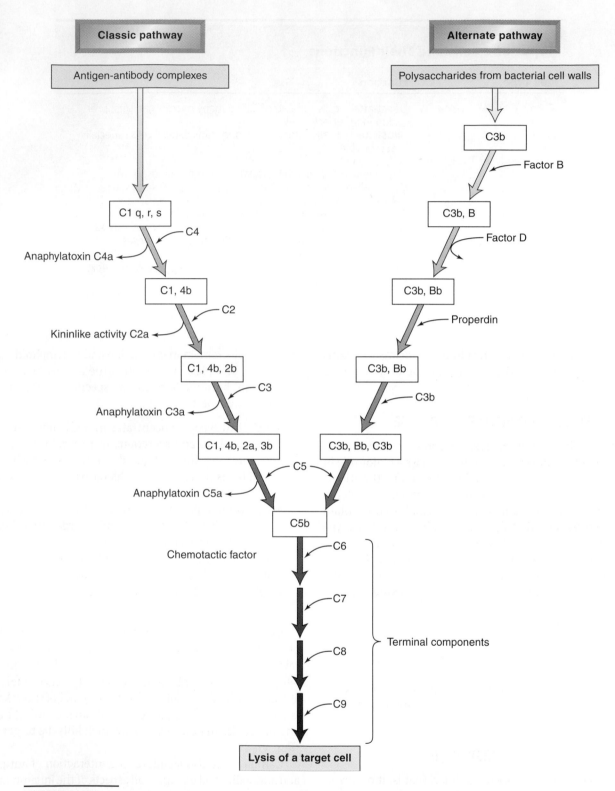

FIGURE 44-4

The complement cascade. The classic pathway is activated by antigen–antibody complexes through component C1. The sequence of action of the initial components is based on their order of discovery (C1, C4, C2, C3, C5, C6, C7, C8, C9); the later acting components are numbered according to their order of reaction. The alternative pathway is activated by numerous agents, such as bacterial polysaccharides. While the complement system is basically a protective mechanism for the body, uncontrolled activation of this system produces inflammation and destruction of body tissues. (Bb is the activated form of factor B.)

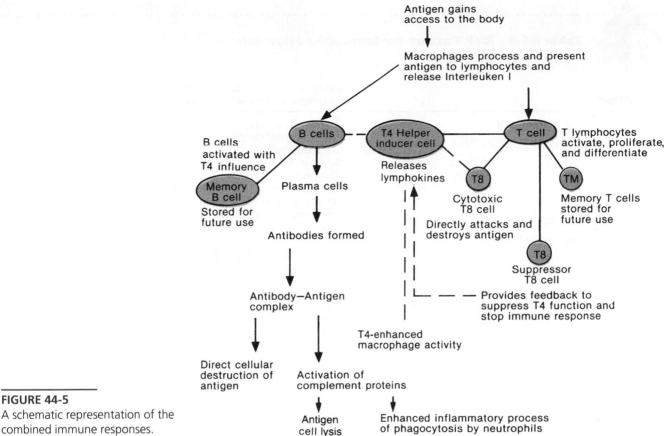

FIGURE 44-5
A schematic representation of the combined immune responses.

T lymphocytes within the lymphoid tissues. Helper-inducer T4 cells subsequently are activated with the help of a chemical factor (IL-1) released by the presenting macrophage. The T4 cells proliferate and produce their own chemical substances, known as lymphokines, which in turn stimulate the activation and proliferation of antibody-producing B lymphocytes, cytotoxic T cells, suppressor T cells, and phagocytic macrophages. The production of antibodies leads to the activation of complement proteins. All of these components work together to destroy the antigen, either through complex processes involving direct attack or through modulation by chemical processes. Suppressor T cells provide feedback to the T4 helper cells to halt these defense reactions when they are no longer needed, and memory cells reactivate them on reexposure to the antigen.

◼ IMPAIRED HOST RESISTANCE

The various components of the immune system provide a complex network of mechanisms that, when intact, function to defend the body against foreign microorganisms and malignant cells. In some situations, however, components of the system can fail, resulting in impaired host resistance. Often the state of immunosuppression is chemically induced by drugs or medications such as corticosteroids and cytotoxic chemotherapeutic agents. People who acquire an

infection because of a deficiency in any of their host defenses are referred to as immunocompromised or immunosuppressed.

The exact effects of and symptoms related to defects in host defense vary according to the part of the immune system affected (Table 44–4). General features associated with compromised host resistance include recurrent infections, infections caused by usually harmless agents (opportunistic organisms), chronic infections, skin rashes, diarrhea, growth impairment, and increased susceptibility to certain cancers.

Clinical Applicability Challenges

Self-Challenge: Critical Thinking

1. *Examine the role of the immune system as it relates to the destruction of hematological components.*

2. *Hypothesize the impact of drugs and diseases on the production and maturation of stem cells in the bone marrow. Determine the implications for patient safety.*

Study Questions

1. *The role of albumin in the blood is to*
   a. *defend against infectious microorganisms.*
   b. *provide colloid osmotic pressure.*
   c. *transport hormones from endocrine glands to other organs.*
   d. *regulate body temperature.*

RED FLAG   **Table 44-4   Risk Factors for Compromised Host Defenses**

Host Defect	Diseases, Therapies, and Other Conditions Associated With Host Defects
Impaired phagocyte functioning	Radiation therapy
	Nutritional deficiencies
	Diabetes mellitus
	Acute leukemias
	Corticosteroids
	Cytotoxic chemotherapeutic drugs
	Aplastic anemia
	Congenital hematological disorders
	Alcoholism
Complement system deficiencies	Liver disease
	Systemic lupus erythematosus
	Sickle cell anemia
	Splenectomy
	Congenital deficiencies
Impaired cell-mediated (T lymphocyte) immune response	Radiation therapy
	Nutritional deficiencies
	Aging
	Thymic aplasia
	AIDS
	Hodgkin's disease/lymphomas
	Corticosteroids
	Antilymphocyte globulin
	Congenital thymic dysfunctions
Impaired humoral (antibody) immunity	Chronic lymphocytic leukemia
	Multiple myeloma
	Congenital hypogammaglobulinemia
	Protein-losing enteropathies (inflammatory bowel disease)
Interruption of physical/mechanical/chemical barriers	Traumatic injury
	Decubitus ulcers/skin defect
	Invasive medical procedures
	Vascular disease
	Skin diseases
	Nutritional impairments
	Burns
	Respiratory intubation
	Mechanical obstruction of body drainage systems, such as lacrimal and urinary systems
	Decreased level of consciousness
Impaired mononuclear phagocyte system	Liver disease
	Splenectomy

2. *Conversion of prothrombin to thrombin occurs prior to*
   a. *injury to tissue and blood vessels.*
   b. *fibrinogen conversion to fibrin clot.*
   c. *tissue thromboplastin's catalyzation by factor VIII.*
   d. *activation of factor X.*

3. *Specific immune responses have all of these characteristics except which of the following?*
   a. *Generally require previous exposure to foreign agent or organism*
   b. *Can alter the intensity and response time on reexposure*
   c. *Use physical, chemical, and mechanical barriers for defense*
   d. *Sometimes responsible for hypersensitivity reactions*

4. *Compromised or impaired host resistance is evidenced by all of the following except*
   a. *autoimmune disorders.*
   b. *recurrent infections.*

   c. *increased susceptibility to certain cancers.*
   d. *opportunistic infections.*

BIBLIOGRAPHY

Baggish J: How Your Immune System Works. Emeryville, CA, Ziff-Davis Press, 1994

Belcher AE: Blood Disorders. St. Louis, Mosby-Year Book, 1993

McCance KL, Huether SE: Pathophysiology: The Biologic Basis for Disease in Adults and Children (2nd Ed). St. Louis, Mosby-Year Book, 1994

Vander AS, Sherman JH, Luciano DS: Human Physiology: The Mechanisms of Body Function (6th Ed). New York, McGraw-Hill, 1994

Workman ML, Ellerhorst-Ryan J, Hargrave-Koertge V: Nursing Care of the Immunocompromised Patient. Philadelphia, WB Saunders, 1993

45

Patient Assessment: Hematological and Immune Systems

OBJECTIVES

Based on the content in this chapter, the reader should be able to:

- Describe physical examination findings pertinent to assessing hematological and immune disorders.
- Differentiate diagnostic tests to assess hematological and immune disorders.
- Use physical examination findings and diagnostic test results to identify hematological and immune disorders.
- Discuss six areas of importance in assessing an immunocompromised patient.

*H*ematological and immune disorders encompass numerous ailments, many of which are life threatening. In general, hematological disorders can be classified as overproduction or underproduction of hematological components or dysfunction of these components. Immune disorders generally are caused by underactivity or overactivity of immune system elements. The hematological and immune systems are closely interrelated; therefore, disorders or dys-

functions of one system will often alter the effectiveness of the other.

HISTORY

Because the physiology of the hematological and immune systems is complex, assessment of the patient with symptoms or a problem related to these systems becomes difficult. In addition, when describing a chief complaint, patients may state symptoms that initially seem unrelated. Assessment of hematological and immune system functions, therefore, involves determining whether deficiencies truly exist in these systems. Following are some questions to guide the history-taking process:

- Has the patient had a history of frequent infections (upper respiratory, lower respiratory, urinary tract, vagina, oral cavity)?
- Has the patient had episodes of bruising or bleeding (epistaxis, bleeding gums, heavy menstruation, unex-

plained bruises, hemoptysis, gastrointestinal disturbances, blood in urine, tarry stools)?
- How does the patient describe his or her energy level and activity tolerance?
- Has the patient experienced frequent headaches, dizziness, visual disturbances, cerebral incidents, or lethargy?
- Has the patient noticed any enlarged lymph nodes or skin eruptions?
- Has the patient experienced fevers, night sweats, or unintentional weight loss?
- Has the patient been exposed to any foreign substances that might cause illness (chemicals, heavy smoke, uncooked foods)?

After obtaining information about the onset and duration of the chief complaint, inquire about the patient's medical history, previous therapies, and family medical history. Table 45–1 summarizes conditions and treatments that may predispose patients to various hematological and immune disorders (see also Chapter 48).

PHYSICAL EXAMINATION

A thorough physical examination is necessary to identify physical signs that may indicate a hematological or immune system disorder. The accompanying display summarizes physical findings that may suggest various disorders of these systems. (Many of these disorders are further described in Chapter 48.) The patient's skin is examined for pallor, jaundice, or facial plethora and for signs of abnormal bleeding. The mucous membranes should also be assessed for abnormal bleeding. The patient's joints should be evaluated for pain, swelling, and limited range of motion, which may suggest hemarthrosis from coagulopathy or sickle cell anemia. Superficial mucocutaneous bleeding and a dependent distribution of petechiae may indicate thrombocytopenia, whereas clusters of palpable, pruritic petechiae may suggest vasculitis. Extensive superficial purpura, deep hematomas, or hemarthroses may indicate a coagulation disorder.[1] Skin rashes, pruritus, and excoriations should also be noted. Extremities should be assessed for areas of redness, tenderness, warmth, or swelling, which may indicate thrombophlebitis. The lips and nail beds should be assessed for cyanosis; digital clubbing may also be present in chronic hypoxemia.

Neurological abnormalities may be present in hematological conditions. Headache and dizziness are symptoms of anemia. These symptoms, along with a sensation of fullness in the head, may indicate polycythemia. Confusion, headache, altered mental status, paresis, aphasia, dysphasia, coma, seizures, paresthesia, and visual problems may be caused by thrombotic thrombocytopenic purpura.[2] An altered level of consciousness, headache, papilledema, vomiting, and bradycardia with widening pulse pressure are signs of increased intracranial pressure, which may be

Table 45-1 Hematological and Immune Disorders to Consider Based on Patient History

Patient History	Potential Disorder
Chronic disease (inflammation, infection)	Anemia
Nutritional deficiencies (iron, folate, B_{12})	Anemia
Endocrine (thyroid, pituitary) dysfunction	Anemia
Hypersplenism	Anemia; thrombocytopenia
Acquired immunodeficiency syndrome	Anemia; neutropenia
Malignancy	Pancytopenia
Chemical exposure	Neutropenia; hemolytic anemia
Prosthetic heart valve or vascular graft	Hemolytic anemia
Collagen vascular disorder	Thrombotic thrombocytopenic purpura (TTP)
Hypersensitivity reaction	TTP
Viral, bacterial, or fungal infection	TTP
Uremia	Coagulopathy
Liver disease	Coagulopathy; thrombosis
Vasculitis	Thrombosis
Tissue necrosis	Thrombosis
Atherosclerosis	Thrombosis
Chronic obstructive pulmonary disease	Polycythemia
Smoking	Polycythemia
Congenital cardiac disease	Polycythemia

Previous Therapies	Potential Disorder
Heparin	Thrombocytopenia
Antibiotics	Agranulocytosis
Alkylating agents	Leukemia; lymphoma; pancytopenia
Blood transfusion	Anemia
Aspirin, nonsteroidal anti-inflammatory agents	Coagulopathy
Irradiation	Pancytopenia
Drugs	Hemolytic anemia (also see Display 48-1)

Family History	Potential Disorder
Sickle cell anemia	Anemia
Thalassemia	Anemia
Congenital hemolytic anemia	Anemia
Polycythemic disorders	Polycythemia vera
Von Willebrand's disease	Bleeding disorder
Hemophilia	Bleeding disorder

caused by intracranial bleeding in a patient with coagulopathy.

Tachycardia and tachypnea may be present in anemia or infection. Dyspnea on exertion and orthostatic changes in blood pressure may be other indications of anemia. Symptoms of intermittent claudication (Chapter 18) and angina pectoris (Chapter 10) indicate problems with oxygen deliv-

RED FLAG

Physical Findings Indicating Possible Hematological or Immune Dysfunction

Pallor
Jaundice
Skin rash, excoriations
Ecchymosis, petechiae, purpura, hematoma
Mucocutaneous bleeding
Thrombophlebitis
Joint pain or swelling
Neurological abnormalities
Fever, night sweats, weight loss
Cyanosis
Digital clubbing
Tachycardia
Tachypnea, dyspnea on exertion
Orthostatic changes in blood pressure
Lymphadenopathy
Splenomegaly
Hepatomegaly
Infection (especially recurrent)

ery in polycythemia. These patients commonly experience hypertension as well.

Lymphadenopathy, splenomegaly, and hepatomegaly are signs of a number of hematological and immune conditions. One should also thoroughly assess for indications of infection, especially in the throat, gingiva, lungs, urinary tract, and perirectal area. Body secretions or fluids (sputum, stool, urine, emesis, or gastric secretions) should be inspected for the presence of blood.

■ DIAGNOSTIC STUDIES

Laboratory tests in hematological and immune disorders determine whether components of these systems are being produced in adequate amounts. Further testing may be required to ascertain if those components are functioning properly. Because patients with severe hematological and immune dysfunctions may be seen in the intensive care unit, tests to differentiate the conditions and their causes are presented here.

Laboratory Tests to Evaluate Anemia

Anemia is a condition in which red blood cell (RBC) mass is decreased. This decrease may be caused by decreased production of RBCs, increased RBC destruction, a combination of these two conditions, or acute blood loss (see Chapter 48). All patients who are being evaluated for anemia should initially have a complete blood count (CBC) with RBC indices, a reticulocyte count, and a peripheral smear analysis. Abnormalities in these tests will indicate subsequent testing required.

COMPLETE BLOOD COUNT

The CBC will give an overall indication of bone marrow production of RBCs, white blood cells (WBCs), and platelets. It also indicates the patient's hemoglobin, hematocrit, RBC indices, and the WBC differential. The anemic patient with low WBCs and platelets has a disorder of blood cell production and requires a bone marrow examination.

RED BLOOD CELL INDICES

The RBC indices indicate characteristics of RBC structure or function.

Mean corpuscular volume is an index indicating the average volume of a single RBC in the blood sample. Anemias are classified as microcytic, normocytic, or macrocytic. Microcytic RBCs indicate a possible iron deficiency anemia, and studies for iron deficiency anemia should be obtained. Macrocytic RBCs require studies of vitamin B_{12} and folate levels (see Chapter 48).

Mean corpuscular hemoglobin (MCH) indicates the average weight of hemoglobin in each RBC. Results are expressed as hypochromic, normochromic, or hyperchromic. An increased MCH (hyperchromic) may indicate macrocytic anemia; a decreased MCH (hypochromic) may indicate iron deficiency anemia.

Mean corpuscular hemoglobin concentration (MCHC) indicates the average hemoglobin concentration in the RBC. A decreased MCHC indicates the RBCs contain less hemoglobin than normal, which may be a result of iron deficiency anemia, macrocytic anemia, or thalassemia. An increased MCHC may indicate hereditary spherocytosis, a condition in which abnormally shaped RBCs are produced.

Red cell distribution width (RDW) is an index that provides a measure of the amount of homogeneity in the RBC width in the blood sample. An elevated RDW may indicate iron, folate, or vitamin B_{12} deficiency or a marked increase in reticulocytes (see below). This is the result of the increased variation in RBC sizes in these conditions. The RDW can also help distinguish thalassemia from iron deficiency anemia. All thalassemia traits result in microcytic RBCs; therefore, the RDW will be normal for these individuals, because the RBCs, although small, are all of similar size.

RETICULOCYTE COUNT

Reticulocytes are immature RBCs that have been recently released from the bone marrow. The reticulocyte count is expressed as a percentage of the RBCs. The bone marrow responds to anemia by increasing RBC production, causing an elevated reticulocyte count. A low reticulocyte count indicates bone marrow underproduction of RBCs.

PERIPHERAL SMEAR

The peripheral smear can indicate disorders of the red cell structure. In Table 45–2, various abnormalities detected by examining the peripheral smear are listed, along with further testing that may be appropriate.

Table 45-2 Peripheral Smear Red Blood Cell (RBC) Abnormalities

Abnormality	Potential Diagnoses	Further Testing
Nucleated RBCs	Acute hemorrhage, hypoxia, megaloblastic anemia	Vitamin B_{12} and folate levels; assess for bleeding; O_2 saturation, ABGs for hypoxia
Spherocytes, elliptocytes	Hemolytic anemia from hereditary spherocytosis, hereditary elliptocytosis	Reticulocyte count, serum bilirubin, serum lactate dehydrogenase, direct Coombs', osmotic fragility
Rouleaux formations	Multiple myeloma	Serum protein electrophoresis, urine for Bence Jones proteins
Target cells, sickle cells, red cell cytoplasmic inclusions	Sickle cell anemia, thalassemia	Hemoglobin studies (hemoglobin electrophoresis, hemoglobin F and A_2)
Schistocytes	Thrombotic thrombocytopenic purpura, mechanical hemolysis	Reticulocyte count, serum lactate dehydrogenase, serum bilirubin, coagulation studies, cardiac auscultation

Nucleated RBCs are not normally present in peripheral blood. They appear in the peripheral smear following profound stimulation, such as acute hemorrhage, hypoxemia, hemolytic anemia, or megaloblastic anemia. If these causes are ruled out, the appearance of nucleated RBCs may be due to infiltrative processes in the bone narrow from malignancy, myelofibrosis, or granuloma. Nucleated RBCs may also be seen in asplenic patients, because the spleen would normally recognize and remove these abnormal cells.[3]

Spherocytes and elliptocytes are abnormally shaped RBCs. They generally appear in patients with a hereditary disorder that causes the RBC membrane defects. These irregular cells are trapped and destroyed in the spleen, causing hemolytic anemia. Testing for red cell osmotic fragility demonstrates that these cells are more likely to lyse than normal RBCs. Serum lactate dehydrogenase and serum bilirubin levels should be ordered if hemolysis is suspected.

The presence of rouleaux formations (the RBCs appear on the peripheral smear as a stack of coins) may indicate multiple myeloma. If clinical findings support this suspicion, serum protein electrophoresis and urine analysis for Bence Jones protein would be the next steps in determining the diagnosis.

The presence of schistocytes in a patient with a prosthetic heart valve may indicate mechanical hemolysis. Schistocytes in a patient with fever, thrombocytopenia, renal dysfunction, and neurological abnormalities require immediate interventions for suspected thrombotic thrombocytopenic purpura (see Chapter 48).

Target cells, sickled cells, and red cell cytoplasmic inclusions on the peripheral smear suggest the need for hemoglobin electrophoresis and hemoglobin F and A_2 levels. The most common anemias diagnosed in this manner are beta-thalassemia and sickle cell anemia.

Laboratory Tests to Evaluate Immune Function

WHITE BLOOD CELLS

The WBC count measures circulating leukocytes. An elevated WBC count usually indicates infection and tends to correlate with the severity of the infection. An elevated WBC should always be assessed in conjunction with the WBC differential and the patient's clinical condition. A low WBC count generally indicates decreased production due to immunosuppressive therapy or a disorder of bone marrow production due to infiltrative processes or bone marrow failure.

The WBC differential describes the ratios of the types of WBCs (neutrophils, eosinophils, basophils, monocytes, and lymphocytes) to the total number of WBCs. See Chapter 44 for a description of the different types of WBCs. There are numerous potential abnormalities in the WBC differential. A *left shift* refers to an increase in the numbers of bands (neutrophil precursors), which generally indicates an infectious process. The presence of blasts (immature granulocytes) in the peripheral blood is always an aberrant finding and suggests the presence of leukemia or a myeloproliferative disorder (see Chapter 48). Table 45–3 summarizes abnormalities of WBC overproduction and potential physiological causes.

Decreases in circulating neutrophils (neutropenia) may be caused by decreased production from bone marrow injury, bone marrow infiltration, nutritional deficiencies, or congenital defects of the stem cells in the bone marrow. Other causes of neutropenia are splenic sequestration and destruction, immune-mediated granulocyte destruction, or overwhelming infection. Lymphocytopenia is most commonly caused by malignancy, followed by collagen vascular disease. Acquired immunodeficiency syndrome (AIDS) and

AIDS-related complex are other notable causes of lymphocytopenia[3] (see Chapter 47).

T AND B CELL COUNTS

As discussed in Chapter 44, lymphocytes are classified as T cells and B cells. T cells are important to the body's ability to distinguish between self and nonself. They comprise 60% to 80% of circulating lymphocytes. B cells comprise 7% to 20% of circulating lymphocytes. Monoclonal antibodies against specific lymphocyte surface proteins are used to identify types of circulating lymphocytes and their subset populations. This can be useful in characterizing hematological malignancies and identifying immunological and autoimmune diseases. A specific example of this is assessing the CD4+ subpopulation of T cells in AIDS patients; a CD4+ count of less than 400 per mm^3 is associated with a poorer prognosis.

When B cells are stimulated by an antigen, they differentiate into plasma cells and produce antibodies. Although plasma cells reside in lymphoid tissue, their antibody production can be evaluated through serum and urine protein electrophoresis. Autoimmune diseases occur when the body produces antibodies directed against its own tissue. These diseases may be organ specific (eg, Graves' disease) or widely disseminated and involve multiple organs (eg, systemic lupus erythematosus). Laboratory testing involves detection of serum antibodies against various tissues. Antinuclear antibody, rheumatoid factor, and erythrocyte sedimentation rate are additional tests used in diagnosing autoimmune disorders.

Laboratory Tests to Evaluate Bleeding and Clotting

Any laboratory testing to evaluate for bleeding and clotting disorders should be guided by the information gathered in the history and physical examination. Family history, underlying clinical conditions, and the duration and type of abnormal bleeding may indicate appropriate testing and diagnostic workup. When evaluating abnormal bleeding, keep in mind that disorders of primary hemostasis occur because of disorders of platelets and small blood vessels, resulting in mucocutaneous bleeding, petechiae, and superficial purpura. Decreased platelets or increased capillary fragility causes the sudden appearance of petechiae, especially in dependent areas, such as the lower extremities. Figure 45–1A overviews the sequence of primary hemostasis. Disorders of secondary hemostasis involve clotting factor deficiencies and are characterized by recurrent oozing of blood and hematoma formation. The onset of these symptoms may be delayed due to the initial plugging of the vessel injury by platelets; however, defective clotting mechanisms fail to provide a stable fibrin clot. Figure 45–1B overviews the sequence of secondary hemostasis.

PLATELET COUNT

The initial test in evaluating primary hemostasis is to obtain a platelet count from the CBC. A platelet count of less than 150,000/mm^3 is abnormal, but bleeding from throm-

RED FLAG

Table 45-3 Potential Causes of Elevated White Blood Cells (WBCs)

Abnormality	Potential Causes
Neutrophilia	Infections, inflammatory disorders, tissue destruction, malignancies, drug induced, hemolysis, diabetic ketoacidosis, myeloproliferative disorders, idiopathic
Eosinophilia	Allergies, hypersensitivity reaction, parasitic infections, immunological disorders, adrenal insufficiency
Basophilia	Myeloproliferative disorders, allergic conditions, myxedema, ulcerative colitis, basophilic leukemia
Monocytosis	Malignancies, infections, recovery from neutropenia, rheumatic disorders, monocytic leukemia, inflammatory bowel disease, cirrhosis, sarcoidosis, drug reactions
Lymphocytosis	Infection (especially viral), pertussis, acute infectious lymphocytosis, immunological disorders, lymphoproliferative disorders

Primary Hemostasis

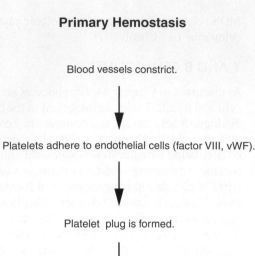

Blood vessels constrict.

↓

Platelets adhere to endothelial cells (factor VIII, vWF).

↓

Platelet plug is formed.

↓

Platelet aggregation initiates coagulation cascade.

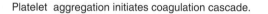

Secondary Hemostasis

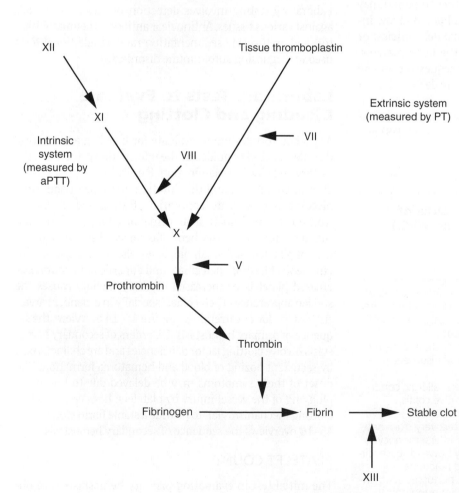

FIGURE 45-1
Mechanisms of primary and secondary hemostasis

Table 45-4 Laboratory Abnormalities in Congenital Bleeding Disorders*

	PT	aPTT	vWF	vWF Antigen	VIII	IX	BT**
von Willebrand's	N	↑	↓	↓	↓	N	↑
Hemophilia A	N	↑	N	N	↓	N	↑
Hemophilia B	N	↑	N	N	N	↓	↑

* Other congenital bleeding abnormalities are rare and not mentioned in this text.
** Bleeding time depends on the severity of the condition; it may be normal in mild cases.
PT, prothrombin time; aPTT, activated partial thromboplastin time; vWF, von Willebrand's factor; VIII, factor VIII; IX, factor IX; BT, bleeding time; N, normal.

bocytopenia alone usually does not happen unless the platelet count falls below 20,000/mm^3. Thrombocytopenia may be caused by decreased bone marrow production, splenic sequestration due to splenomegaly, or peripheral destruction of platelets. Disseminated intravascular coagulation (DIC) and thrombotic thrombocytopenic purpura are serious disorders involving platelet destruction that are discussed in Chapter 48. A peripheral blood smear may reveal megathrombocytes (large platelets), which may be present during premature platelet destruction. A positive platelet antibody screen indicates the presence of immunoglobulin G (IgG) antibodies to platelets. Antiheparin antibody assay (platelet aggregation assay) may be used when evaluating patients with suspected heparin-induced thrombocytopenia.[4] Some patients' platelets will clump when exposed to EDTA (the anticoagulant used in the "purple top" CBC tube). Examination of the peripheral smear will show this clumping, and a repeat CBC in a heparinized "green top" blood collection tube will reveal an accurate platelet count.

An elevated platelet count greater than 400,000/mm^3 indicates increased platelet production or decreased platelet destruction. These platelets may function abnormally, causing aberrant bleeding and clotting tests. Patients with an elevated platelet count may be at increased risk for thrombosis. Primary thrombocytosis is caused by bone marrow disease. Reactive thrombocytosis may be caused by chronic inflammation, infection, malnutrition, acute stress, malignancy, splenectomy, or the postoperative state.

BLEEDING TIME

A bleeding time is done to assess the length of time required for a clot to form at the site of vessel injury. A prolonged bleeding time in a patient with a normal platelet count may indicate a disorder of platelet function that requires further testing. A deficiency in von Willebrand's factor would result in decreased ability of the platelets to adhere to the injured vessel wall. Uremia from renal failure, drugs (especially aspirin), foods, and spices can also cause abnormal platelet function. Platelet aggregation studies are done to detect inherited or acquired disorders in platelet function.

PROTHROMBIN TIME AND ACTIVATED PARTIAL THROMBOPLASTIN TIME

Assessing disorders of secondary hemostasis requires determining whether the disorder is congenital or acquired. A history of excessive or recurrent bleeding in the individual or family members suggests a congenital disorder as the likely cause. The most common congenital bleeding disorders are von Willebrand's disease, hemophilia A, and hemophilia B. Prothrombin time (PT) and activated partial thromboplastin time (aPTT) are ordered for suspected congenital disorders, along with von Willebrand's factor, factor VIII, and factor IX assays. Table 45–4 summarizes the abnormalities that will indicate these congenital disorders.

An acute bleeding problem without a history of chronic bleeding suggests an acquired disorder. Rapid consumption of platelets and coagulation factors occurs in massive trauma, severe bleeding, overwhelming infection, severe liver disease, or DIC.[5] Laboratory testing would vary based on the suspected etiology of the bleeding disorder. In general, testing would include PT, aPTT, thrombin time, bleeding time, liver enzyme and liver function tests, fibrinogen levels, and fibrin degradation products. Table 45–5 summarizes laboratory abnormalities that would indicate some of the acquired coagulation disorders.

A hypercoagulable state causes an increased tendency for thrombosis. Table 45–6 summarizes some of the risk factors for hypercoagulability. Hereditary thrombotic disease is a group of genetic abnormalities causing defects of coagulation, fibrinolysis, or their regulatory systems. Laboratory abnormalities in hereditary hypercoagulability include deficiencies of antithrombin III, protein C, protein S, plasminogen, tissue plasminogen activator, and dysfibrinogen; however, 65% to 70% of the causes remain unknown. Lupus anticoagulant (LA) is an autoimmune disorder in which patients have an elevated aPTT, yet 30% of the patients develop thrombosis. LA is confirmed by the presence of anticardiolipin antibodies, positive platelet neutralization procedure, or positive dilute Russel viper's venom test.[6]

Table 45-5 Laboratory Abnormalities in Acquired Coagulation Disorders

	PT	aPTT	TT	FDP	Plt
Vitamin K deficiency	X	X			
Liver disease:					
Acute hepatitis, early liver disease	X				
Chronic liver disease	X	X	X	X	X
DIC	X	X	X	X	X
Massive transfusion	X	X	X		X

PT, prothrombin time; aPTT, activated partial thromboplastin time; TT, thrombin time; FDP, fibrin degradation products; Plt, platelets; DIC, disseminated intravascular coagulation; X, elevated laboratory result.

Diagnostic Tests to Evaluate Hematological and Immune Disorders

Bone marrow aspiration for biopsy is the most important diagnostic test for determining bone marrow function. It is a means of examining the precursors of the peripheral blood components to determine if hematological abnormalities are due to disorders of blood cell production. Bone marrow examination is useful in detecting infiltrative processes, such as malignancy, that may affect blood cell production. This procedure is also performed to determine response to therapy in patients with hematological malignancies or solid tumor infiltration of the bone marrow.

Tissue biopsy may be performed on skin lesions in which malignancy (eg, cutaneous T cell lymphoma) or an autoimmune process (eg, pemphigus) is suspected. *Lymph node biopsy* is required for lymphadenopathy that does not appear to be caused by an infectious process.

Internal lymph nodes of the chest, abdomen, and pelvis may be evaluated by *computerized tomography (CT) scanning*. A CT scan may be used to determine the presence of masses in suspected malignancy, especially lymphoma. Liver disease, an important factor in coagulopathy, and splenomegaly may also be evaluated through CT scan. *Skeletal survey* (skull, vertebrae, ribs, pelvis, arms, forearms, thighs, and lower legs) is done in suspected multiple myeloma to assess for the typical "punched-out" lytic lesions that occur in that condition.

Intradermal skin testing with various antigens for delayed-type hypersensitivity is used to evaluate cell-mediated immunity. Commonly used antigens include mumps, *Candida*, trichophytin, and tuberculin. Failure to respond to the injected antigens is called *cutaneous anergy* and implies a defect in the patient's cellular immunity. Causes of cutaneous anergy include AIDS; acute leukemia; chronic lymphocytic leukemia; carcinoma; Hodgkin's disease; non-Hodgkin's lymphoma; congenital immune conditions;

Table 45-6 Risk Factors for Hypercoagulability

Physiological	Pathological	Environmental	Iatrogenic
Pregnancy	Malignancy	Smoking	Surgery
Postpartum	Liver disease	Stress	Postsurgical
Venous stasis	Disseminated intravascular	Heat	Oral contraceptives
Age > 40 y	coagulation		Estrogens
Immobilization	Polycythemia		
Varicose veins	Lupus anticoagulant		
Previous venous	Vascular injury		
thromboembolism	Sepsis		
	Heart failure		
	Myocardial infarction		
	Inherited abnormalities		

bacterial, fungal, or viral infections; immunosuppressive medications; cirrhosis; and malnutrition.[7]

ASSESSMENT OF THE IMMUNOCOMPROMISED PATIENT

The ability of the human body to protect itself against disease is described by the term immunocompetence (see Chapter 44). Figure 45–2 illustrates areas to be assessed for immunocompetence. It is essential that immunocompetence be assessed on the critically ill patient at frequent intervals.

Physical and psychological stress from overwhelming illness or trauma in the critically ill patient can depress functioning of the immune system. Invasive procedures, nutritional compromise, and the intensive care environment itself can predispose patients to infections and sepsis. Protective measures, such as handwashing and aseptic technique, are essential to minimize exposure to infectious organisms. The nurse should closely monitor potential sites of infection, changes or fluctuations in body temperature, nutritional status, and laboratory findings for indications of compromised immune function or the onset of infection.

Septic shock is a life-threatening complication that can develop rapidly in immunocompromised patients. Assessment of early septic shock is described in the display (see also Chapter 49).

History

A careful history to identify susceptibility to infection is of major importance in assessing a patient's immunocompetence. The type of infection often provides the first clue as to the nature of the immune defect. For example, patients with defects in humoral immunity may have recurrent or chronic bacterial infections, such as meningitis or bacteremia. Repeated viral or fungal infections may indicate a defect in cell-mediated immunity. (See Chapter 44 for a review of humoral and cell-mediated immunity.)

The patient's chronological age also influences immunocompetence. Immune response may be depressed in the very young owing to the underdevelopment of the thymus gland. In older adults, atrophy of the thymus gland may increase susceptibility to infection.

Nutritional Status

The patient's nutritional status has a major impact on immune function. Inadequate intake of protein and calories can alter immune responses and resistance to infection by decreasing lymphocyte and antibody production and impairing wound healing. A team approach using a nutritionist can assist the nurse in assessing dietary intake and nutritional requirements for the critically ill immunocompromised person.

Chronic Disease

Many chronic diseases are associated with compromised immune functioning. Diabetes, cancer, and aplastic anemia are just a few examples of diseases during the course of which immune deficiencies occur. Because many critically ill patients have underlying chronic disease, the existence of such diseases should be considered contributing factors when the immunocompetence of these patients is assessed.

Immunosuppressed States

Patients with leukemia, lymphoma, multiple myeloma, and other hematological conditions can experience impaired immunity and recurrent infections. Immunodeficiency states can be congenital or acquired. People with congenital immunodeficiencies frequently do not survive childhood. Immunodeficiency syndromes in adults may occur through a spontaneous defect in the immune system or through infection with the human immunodeficiency virus (see Chapter 47).

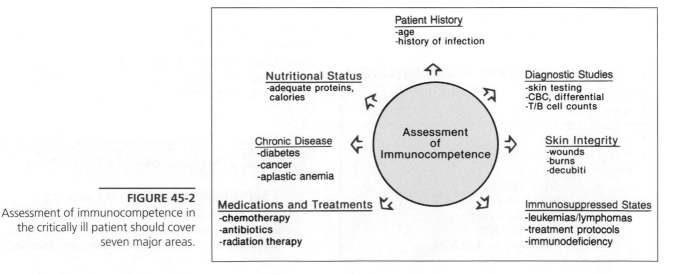

FIGURE 45-2
Assessment of immunocompetence in the critically ill patient should cover seven major areas.

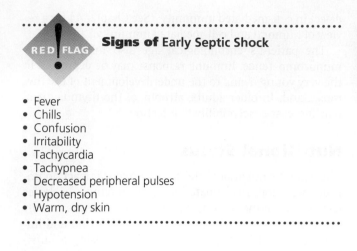

Signs of Early Septic Shock

- Fever
- Chills
- Confusion
- Irritability
- Tachycardia
- Tachypnea
- Decreased peripheral pulses
- Hypotension
- Warm, dry skin

Medications and Treatments

Antibiotics, such as tetracycline and chloramphenicol, impair bone marrow function. Steroids display many immunological effects, including decreased lymphocyte and antibody concentration. Patients placed on treatment regimens with these agents should be monitored for compromise in immune functioning as part of their total response to the therapy.

Treatment protocols for cancer patients can lead to life-threatening complications, such as infection and sepsis. Most chemotherapeutic agents and radiation to the pelvis, spine, ribs, sternum, skull, and metaphyses of the long bones can adversely affect the bone marrow's ability to produce WBCs. The lowest point in WBC levels, or the *nadir*, may not be seen until several days or weeks after the initiation of treatment. The absolute neutrophil count (ANC) is calculated on neutropenic patients to determine the degree of immunosuppression. The method for calculating ANC is given in the display. Usually protective measures, such as those summarized in the accompanying display, are instituted for patients with an ANC of less than 1,000.

Patients who are severely immunosuppressed may not display the typical signs of infection. Fever and redness or pus at sites of infection may be diminished because of the decreased numbers of WBCs required to promote these physical signs.

In addition to chemotherapy and radiation therapy, other cancer treatments also cause immunosuppression. Bone marrow transplantation will cause severe immuno-

---

CLINICAL APPLICATION:
Nursing Intervention Guidelines
Protective Measures for Immunosuppressed Patients*

- Provide a private room or uninfected roommate.
- Use laminar flow or positive pressure room.
- Maintain strict handwashing with antiseptic soap.
- Use no rectal temperatures, enemas, or suppositories.
- Restrict staff and visitors with infections (or require masks).
- Provide patient with mask when he or she goes to other departments or crowded areas.
- Permit cooked foods only.
- Allow no fresh flowers or live plants.
- Avoid sources of stagnant water (vases, water pitchers, humidifiers, denture cups).

* Precautions taken may vary according to institutional policy and the severity of immunosuppression.

---

suppression that can last for weeks or longer (see Chapter 46). Biological therapy with interferon alpha and interleukin 2 can cause leukopenia. Patients who are transfused with RBCs can also demonstrate suppressed immunity.

Skin Integrity

The integumentary system, including skin and mucous membranes, provides a physical barrier to infection. Surgical or traumatic wounds, burn injuries, or pressure sores breach these physical defenses and predispose the critically ill patient to infection. In a critical care setting in which intravenous and intra-arterial catheters, urethral catheters, or endotracheal tubes are used, multiple portals of entry for pathogens can provide simultaneous sites for potential infection. All wounds and portals of entry should be assessed for signs and symptoms of infection.

■ CONCLUSION

Critically ill patients with hematological or immune disorders present challenges for nursing assessment. Consideration of multiple, interacting factors and a thorough evaluation of diagnostic and physical findings are essential when caring for patients with these complex conditions.

Calculating Absolute Neutrophil Count (ANC)

1. Add segs plus bands (from the WBC differential)
2. Multiply the total WBC by the total obtained in #1.
   Example:

   Segs = 42%
   Bands = 10%
   Total WBC = 4,100
   42 + 10 = 52%
   4,100 × .52 = 2,132 ANC

Clinical Applicability Challenges

Self-Challenges: Critical Thinking

1. The nurse assesses all patients for evidence of impaired immune function, especially those with serious illness. Develop an assessment tool that includes the major areas described in this chapter.

2. *A patient with anemia along with other problems has been admitted to your care. List the laboratory tests you would expect to be ordered, giving your rationale and the specific information each test will provide.*

Study Questions

1. *In a patient with a normal platelet count, a prolonged bleeding time could indicate*
   a. *an overproduction of von Willebrand's factor.*
   b. *increased capillary fragility.*
   c. *a disorder of platelet function.*
   d. *defective clotting mechanisms.*

2. *Bone marrow examination is used to*
   a. *determine responses to therapy in hematological malignancy.*
   b. *assess for the presence of antigens in an autoimmune disorder.*
   c. *examine hematopoietic precursor cells.*
   d. *a and c*

3. *Protective measures usually are initiated for patients with an absolute neutrophil count of*
   a. *less than 1,000/μL.*
   b. *less than 2,000/μL.*
   c. *more than 4,000/μL.*
   d. *more than 5,000/μL.*

4. *The ANC usually is calculated to determine the*
   a. *effectiveness of chemotherapy.*
   b. *degree of immunosuppression.*
   c. *bone marrow's ability to produce WBCs.*
   d. *nadir of the WBC count.*

REFERENCES

1. George JN, Kolodziej MA: Excessive bleeding and clotting. In Stein JH (ed): Internal Medicine (4th Ed). St. Louis, Mosby-Year Book, 1994
2. Ellenbberger BJ, Haas L, Cundiff L: Thrombotic thrombocytopenic purpura: Nursing during the acute phase. Dimensions in Critical Care Nursing 12:58–65, 1993
3. Boldt DH: Abnormal nucleated blood cell counts. In Stein JH (ed): Internal Medicine (4th Ed). St. Louis, Mosby-Year Book, 1994
4. Lapka DMV, Wild LD, Barbour LA: Heparin-induced thrombocytopenia and thrombosis: A case study and clinical overview. Oncology Nursing Forum 21:871–876, 1994
5. Hassel KL: Thrombotic thrombocytopenic purpura and hemolytic uremic syndrome. In Wood ME, Bunn PA (eds): Hematology/Oncology Secrets. Philadelphia, Hanley & Belfus, 1994
6. Marlar RA: The hypercoagulable state. In Wood ME, Bunn PA (eds): Hematology/Oncology Secrets. Philadelphia, Hanley & Belfus, 1994
7. Geppert TD, Lipsky PE: Evaluation of cellular immune function. In Stein JH (ed): Internal Medicine (4th Ed). St. Louis, Mosby-Year Book, 1994

BIBLIOGRAPHY

Bush MT, Roy N: Hemophilia emergencies. Journal of Emergency Nursing 21:531–539, 1995

Hull RD, Pineo GF, Raskob GE: Thrombosis and anticoagulation. In Stein JH (ed): Internal Medicine (4th Ed). St. Louis, Mosby-Year Book, 1994

Kajas-Wylie M: Thrombotic thrombocytopenic purpura: Pathophysiology, treatment and related nursing care. Critical Care Nurse 15:44–52, 1995

Payton RG, White PJ: Primary care for women: Assessment of hematologic disorders. Journal of Nurse-Midwifery 40:120–136, 1995

Shelton BK: Disorders of hemostasis in sepsis. Critical Care Nursing Clinics of North America 6:373–387, 1994

White GC: Disorders of blood coagulation. In Stein JH (ed): Internal Medicine (4th Ed). St. Louis, Mosby-Year Book, 1994

Organ and Hemopoietic Stem Cell Transplantation

OBJECTIVES

Based on the content in this chapter, the reader should be able to:

- Analyze the criteria used to evaluate and prepare patients for transplantation.
- Evaluate the principles of organ and hemopoietic stem cell compatibility and immunosuppression.
- Describe the complications related to organ and hemopoietic stem cell transplantation.
- Discuss nursing assessment and management for patients having kidney, liver, heart, pancreas, lung, and hemopoietic stem cell transplants.

Although transplant research began in the early 1900s, it was not until the early 1950s that kidney transplantation became a realistic treatment for chronic renal failure in humans. Heart and liver transplants followed in the 1960s, and since the 1980s have steadily grown as a treatment for end-stage organ failure. Pancreas transplants also began in the mid 1960s and achieved good graft survival rates in the 1980s. The best pancreas transplant survival rate occurs when it is performed simultaneously with a kidney transplant.[1] The number of lung transplants is small primarily

TABLE 46-1
Graft and Patient 1-Year Survival Rates for Organ Transplants Performed in 1993

Organ	Graft Survival	Patient Survival
Kidney		
Cadaveric	83%	94%
Living donor	92%	97%
Heart	82%	82%
Lung	76%	77%
Liver	73%	82%
Pancreas	74%	92%

1995 Annual Report of the U.S. Scientific Registry for Transplant Recipients and the Organ Procurement and Transplant Network—Transplant Data: 1988–1994. UNOS, Richmond, VA and the Division of Transplantation, Bureau of Health Resources Development, Health Resources and Services Administration, U.S. Department of Health and Human Services, Rockville, MD, 1995

due to the lack of medically suitable donors. Survival rates for transplantation are given in Table 46–1.

Hemopoietic stem cell transplantation (HSCT) includes both bone marrow transplants (BMT) and peripheral stem cell transplants (PBCT). Once considered a last resort for treating advanced hematological malignancies, HSCT is now used to treat a broad range of life-threatening hematological, oncological, hereditary, and immunological disorders. Table 46–2 shows disease-free survival at 5 years following HSCT. Advances in histocompatibility matching,

immunosuppression, organ preservation, drugs to combat infections and stimulate hematopoiesis, and surgical techniques have helped increase the success of transplantation.

This chapter includes the major aspects of care for patients having kidney, liver, heart, pancreas, and lung transplants and HSCT. It covers principles that apply to all types of transplantation and discusses content unique to a specific transplant.

■ PATHOPHYSIOLOGICAL PRINCIPLES

Underlying diseases leading to the need for transplantation are covered in respective system-specific units. These units also discuss physiology and pathophysiology of the hemopoietic system and the organ being transplanted and the consequences when they fail to function. The critical care nurse must understand this information and these principles.

■ INDICATIONS FOR TRANSPLANTATION

Many factors influence the indications and patient eligibility for transplantation. Research on patient outcomes, statistics on complications and survival, new developments in techniques, new medications, and the availability of organs and hematopoietic stem cells are some of these factors. Currently, end-stage disease is the primary reason for most

TABLE 46-2
Disease-Free Survival at 5 Years Following Hemopoietic Stem Cell Transplantation

Disease and Stage	Allogeneic (% Survival)	Autologous (% Survival)
Acute myeloid leukemia		
First complete remission	45–65	30–50
Second complete remission	20–45	20–40
Acute lymphoid leukemia		
First complete remission	40–70	30–50
Second complete remission	25–45	15–25
Chronic myelogenous leukemia		
Chronic phase	60–75	0–5
Accelerated phase	30–45	0–5
Blast crisis	10–20	0–5
Hodgkin's and Non-Hodgkin's lymphoma		
First relapse, second remission	40–60	40–60
Advanced disease	10–25	10–25
Breast cancer		
Stage IV	Not done	10–30
Stage II	Not done	70

Data from: Applebaum FR: The use of bone marrow and peripheral stem cell transplantation in the treatment of cancer. CA - A Cancer Journal for Clinicians 46(3):142–164, 1996
Armitage JO: Bone marrow transplantation. N Engl J Med 330(12):827–838, 1994

organ transplants. HSCT is now used when bone marrow is defective or destroyed by a disease process or as a result of treating an underlying disease.

Kidney

Transplantation is indicated for end-stage renal disease (ESRD). Diseases that lead to ESRD include diabetic nephropathy; glomerular disease; acute renal failure; nephrosclerosis; urological diseases, such as chronic infection with nephrolithiasis; systemic disease, such as lupus erythematosus; and hereditary diseases, such as polycystic disease.

Liver

Transplantation is indicated for irreversible liver disease and most liver diseases resulting in end-stage organ failure. Other indications include chronic viral hepatitis, primary sclerosis cholangitis, primary biliary sclerosis, alcoholic cirrhosis, and metabolic disorders, such as α 1-antitrypsin deficiency and Wilson's disease.

Heart

Transplantation is indicated for end-stage heart disease resulting from cardiomyopathy, severe coronary artery disease (CAD), valvular heart disease, congenital heart disease, and myocarditis.

Pancreas

Insulin-dependent diabetes mellitus with end-stage renal disease is the indication for a pancreas transplant either alone or in combination with a kidney transplant.

Lung

Indications include cystic fibrosis, chronic obstructive pulmonary disease, idiopathic pulmonary fibrosis, and emphysema due to antitrypsin deficiency and primary pulmonary hypertension.

Hemopoietic Stem Cell

The indications for BMT and PBCT are malignant disorders, including leukemias, Hodgkin's, and non-Hodgkin's lymphoma; multiple myeloma; and specific solid tumors, such as breast and ovarian cancer and neuroblastoma. Nonmalignant disorders for which BMTs are indicated include hematological disorders, such as aplastic and sickle cell anemias; selected metabolic disorders; and immunodeficiency syndromes.

■ PATIENT EVALUATION AND CONTRAINDICATIONS FOR TRANSPLANTATION

Selecting the ideal candidate for transplantation is an intricate process. For example, in HSCT, care is taken to distinguish patients who can be saved by transplantation from those who may relapse or succumb to the rigors and toxicities of treatment.

A comprehensive multisystem analysis is done to evaluate a patient's suitability for transplantation. This includes both physiological and psychosocial factors that will affect the patient's chance for a successful transplant. During this evaluation phase, newly diagnosed conditions are treated, and plans are made to ensure adequate nutrition, mobility, and muscle strength. The goal is to have the patient in the best possible physical condition for transplantation. When transplants are performed earlier rather than later in the disease process, there are fewer disabilities and a greater chance for survival.

Financial guidance is provided so that patients and families know what their insurance will cover and the nature and amount of their expected out-of-pocket expenses. Costs for transplants range from $39,000 to $250,000.[2-4] Medications after transplant can cost $10,000 a year. Transplant centers may require documentation about the ability to pay prior to accepting a patient for transplantation.

The following general criteria guide the selection for transplantation:

- Age is evaluated individually. Ages may range from newborn (those who may have heart transplantation for hypoplastic left heart syndrome) to 70 years. Those over 55 years may be at increased risk for complications.
- Acute or chronic infection is absent or has been treated. Localized liver infection may be an exception. Inflammatory diseases, such as systemic lupus erythematosus, do not rule out transplantation but should be quiescent at the time of the procedure.
- Severe uncorrectable disease is absent other than in the organ system(s) being transplanted. For the patient with malignancy, HSCT is performed in an attempt to eradicate the underlying malignancy. HSCT is also performed as a marrow *rescue* because of the toxic effects of high-dose chemotherapy and radiation. In nonmalignant diseases, the goal is to replace marrow that is either defective or has failed. Organ-specific criteria for transplantation are listed in Table 46–3.

In general, evaluation common to all transplants includes the following:

- ABO typing
- Tissue typing, human leukocyte antigen (HLA) matching, mixed lymphocyte culture (MLC) matching
- Transfusion history
- Infectious disease screening (tuberculin skin test, human immunodeficiency virus [HIV], hepatitis B surface antigen, hepatitis C virus, Epstein-Barr virus, cytomegalovirus [CMV], toxoplasmosis titers, herpes simplex, varicella virus, venereal disease)
- Liver function studies
- Renal function studies
- Complete blood count
- Coagulation studies
- Gastrointestinal evaluation (depending on age and history)

TABLE 46-3

Criteria, Contraindications, and Evaluations in Transplantation

Organ	Specific Criteria	Contraindications	Specific Evaluation
Kidney	• End-stage or near end-stage renal failure Defined as a glomerular filtration rate of <10 mL/min Pre–end stage preferable for some patients (ie, children, patients with diabetes mellitus, and those for whom there is a living donor)	• Severe or uncorrectable coronary artery disease, peripheral vascular disease, or pulmonary disease • Severe cardiomyopathy	• Voiding cystourethrogram to evaluate for obstruction or reflux (medical history dependent) • Cardiac evaluation (age and medical history dependent)
Liver	• Malnutrition • Severe blood clotting abnormalities • Variceal bleeding • Hepatic encephalopathy • Severe, intractable ascites • Severe, intractable pruritus	• Multiple uncorrected congenital anomalies • Advanced cardiopulmonary disease • Severe pulmonary hypertension	• Abdominal CT scan (to detect hepatoma) • Doppler ultrasound (to identify patency of portal vein) • Liver disease studies and autoimmune markers, such as ceruloplasmin, CEA, AFP, antimitochondrial and antinuclear antibody • ERCP/Cholangiogram (if indicated, usually for patients with cholestasis) • Liver biopsy (if indicated) • Upper and lower endoscopy (if indicated)
Pancreas	• End-stage renal failure (combine kidney and pancreas transplant) • Absence of (or corrected) coronary artery disease	• Uncorrectable coronary artery disease • Previous major amputation • Blindness (not absolute contraindication) • Same as kidney	• Thallium Stress Test or Coronary Angiogram • Cardiology consult • Gastric emptying study • Ophthalmology evaluation • Endocrine studies: glycosylated hemoglobin, serum amylase and lipase, islet cell antibody, urine and serum peptide measurements
Heart	• Cardiac disease, New York Heart Association Class IV (or advanced III) • Condition not amenable to other forms of medical or surgical therapy • End-stage cardiac disease with less than a 25% likelihood of survival at 1 year without a transplant • Patients with potentially fatal arrhythmia not amenable to other therapies	• Fixed pulmonary hypertension with pulmonary vascular resistance: > 6–8 wood units (> 480–640 dyns/sec/cm^{-5} or pulmonary arteriolar gradient >15 mm) • Recent unresolved pulmonary infarct (increased post-transplant risk of pulmonary infection) • Advanced or poorly controlled diabetes mellitus	• Right heart catheterization; full cardiac catheterization if indicated • Cardiopulmonary exercise testing (MVO$_2$) • Pulmonary function tests, including diffusion capacity (DL$_{CO}$) • Cardiac rehabilitation consultation • MUGA or echocardiogram
Lung	• Untreatable end-stage pulmonary disease (parenchymal or vascular) • Medical therapy ineffective • Estimated survival (without lung transplant) less than probability of survival with lung transplant	• Significant coronary artery disease • Poor nutritional status (ie, <10–15% of ideal body weight) • Previous cardiothoracic surgery • Corticosteroid use >15 mg/d • Ventilation dependency	• Quantitative ventilation/perfusion (V/Q) scan • Cardiac evaluation • Full pulmonary function testing, including DL$_{CO}$, arterial blood gases, lung volume • 6-min walk test (rehabilitation assessment) • Nutritional assessment

(continued)

TABLE 46-3
Criteria, Contraindications, and Evaluations in Transplantation (Continued)

Organ	Specific Criteria	Contraindications	Specific Evaluation

BMT/PBCT	• Malignant disorders: "rescue" to compensate for the marrow toxic effects of high-dose chemotherapy with or without radiation
	• Nonmalignant diseases: replacement of marrow that is either defective or that has failed
		• Poor or no response to conventional-dose therapy for malignant disorders
		• Poor performance status (using the Karnofsky Performance scales to assess physical functioning)
		• Advanced cardiopulmonary disease (LVEF <50%, DL$_{CO}$ <50%)
		• Renal impairment (creatinine clearance < 60 mL/min
		• Brain metastasis
		• Age >70 years
		• Absence of available support systems post-transplantation
			• Evaluation of underlying disease:
			  • Bone marrow aspirate and biopsy/flow cytometry/cytogenetics
			  • Diagnosis specific CT/bone scans/lumbar puncture
			  • Immunoglobulins for specific diagnoses
			• Pulmonary function tests including DL$_{CO}$
			• MUGA scan

CEA, carcinoembryonic antigen; AFP, alpha-fetoprotein; ERCP, endoscopic retrograde cholangiopancreatography; DL$_{CO}$, diffusion capacity of lungs, with carbon monoxide; MUGA, Multigaited Acquisition scan) (evaluates cardiac wall motion and ventricular ejection fractions); LVEF, left ventricular ejection fraction

• Gynecological examination
• Electrocardiogram
• Chest x-ray
• Dental examination to rule out infection
• Social history, review of patient motivation, and ability to follow postoperative regimen; possible psychological evaluation

See the summary of organ-specific evaluation listed in Table 46–3.

Contraindications are based on conditions and behaviors that decrease the chance of survival. For organ transplantation, these include serious active infection or sepsis, recent cancer (unless that is the reason for transplant), current substance abuse, HIV infection, severe cachexia, active peptic ulcer disease, psychiatric disorders that impair the ability to give informed consent or adhere to the treatment regimen, and repeated noncompliance. Table 46–3 lists these contraindications.

DONOR SELECTION

After a person is selected as a recipient for transplantation, a donor source must be selected. If a living donor is selected, the donor transplant is scheduled. When a cadaveric donor is needed, the recipient is placed on the national waiting list.

Determining Compatibility

Histocompatibility testing (ie, tissue typing) is performed for both organ transplants and BMT to determine the compatibility between donor and recipient. Compatibility improves the chances of graft acceptance.

Antigens that comprise a person's tissue type are coded by the major histocompatibility complex genes. These genes contain genetic information for cell surface antigens that differentiate self from nonself. These antigens (referred to as HLAs) are found on the surface of lymphocytes. Lymphocytes isolated from peripheral blood, lymph nodes, or the spleen may be used to identify these antigens.

The major histocompatibility complex that is important in transplantation includes A, B, and DR (D-related) antigens. Each person has two A, B, and DR locus antigens that are inherited as a haplotype (ie, a single unit) from each parent. Many possible antigens may occur at each locus, resulting in a large number of HLA combinations. Therefore, it is rare for people who are unrelated to have identical antigens.

The greatest potential for a successful transplant exists when the donor and recipient have inherited identical antigens from their parents. Other possible matches include a one-haplotype match, in which half of the antigens in the donor and recipient are identical; a no-antigen match, in which there are no shared haplotypes or antigens; or a range of matches between one and six.

ORGAN TRANSPLANT COMPATIBILITY

There are several requirements for selecting donor–recipient pairs. The first requirement is red blood cell compatibility (ABO type). This is essential in avoiding reactions that could cause organ loss. An exception is liver transplantation in which compatibility is preferred but not essential. Once ABO compatibility is determined, the next step is tissue testing, followed by cross-matching blood for antibodies.

In renal transplantation, because of the number of possible antigen combinations, most centers try to match at the B and DR locus. The Organ Procurement and Transplantation Network allocates kidneys and pancreata based on the degree of HLA matching. HLA matching has less priority in other organ transplants primarily because of time constraints.

In addition to determining ABO and HLA compatibility, the donor's and recipient's blood are cross-matched. This test screens the recipient's serum for preformed antibodies to donor antigens that are present on donor lymphocytes. The recipient may have produced antibodies as a result of prior exposure to antigens because of pregnancy, transfusion, or previous transplantation. A positive cross-match is a contraindication to renal, heart, and lung transplantation because the potential recipient has an antibody that will attack the donor graft and cause hyperacute rejection. Because hyperacute rejection is rare in liver transplantation, a negative cross-match is not mandatory, and many centers do not require cross-matching before liver transplant.

Blood transfusions are avoided in patients waiting for organ transplantation because of the risk of sensitization and a resulting positive cross-match between donor and recipient. If transfusions are necessary, leukocyte-filtered blood should be given.

HEMOPOIETIC STEM CELL TRANSPLANT COMPATIBILITY

Donor selection is based on the type and stage of disease, the condition of the patient's bone marrow, the patient's age and ability to perform activities of daily living, and the availability of an appropriate donor who is HLA and MLC matched.

For patients who receive another person's bone marrow (ie, an allogeneic transplant), donor selection is based on the availability of a donor who is HLA and MLC matched. The best donor choice is a syngeneic donor. This is an HLA-identical twin of the patient. The next best choice is an HLA-matched sibling donor. Patients who lack a matched sibling donor may use a less-than-perfect mismatched related donor. Another option is to use a matched unrelated donor. Unrelated donors may be identified through the National Marrow Donor Program or the American Bone Marrow Registry (see display). Once potential HLA-matched donors are identified, an MLC is done to observe for interaction between the potential donor cells and recipient cells. Low reactivity indicates greater compatibility.

Living Donors

A living donor is used exclusively in BMT. Living donors are increasingly being used for kidney, liver, pancreas, and lung transplants. Although there is an increase in the use of living organ donors, there is a dire shortage of organs for transplantation. This is due to a growing number of transplant candidates and a relatively constant number of cadaveric organ donors.

> ### *Bone Marrow Registries*
>
> The National Marrow Donor Program (NMDP) is a federally funded registry established in 1986 to coordinate the donor search and matching process. The program was initially formed by bone marrow transplant family members. There are more than 2 million donors at 102 centers in the United States, and NMDP works with the American Red Cross and international organizations. The office of patient advocacy is reached at 1-800-MARROW-2.
>
> The American Bone Marrow Donor Registry is a private registry with more than ½ million donors. It also coordinates international searches.
>
> *Data from Stancek D, Bartsch G, Perkins HA,* et al: *The national marrow donor program. Transfusion 33:567–577, 1993*
>
> *Bone Marrow Transplantation and Peripheral Stem Cell Transplantation. Office of Cancer Communications, National Cancer Institute. NIH Publication Number 95-1178, 1994*

Once identified, a potential donor has a thorough medical evaluation to determine that the organ functions normally, there is no underlying disease, and donation would not in any obvious way jeopardize the donor's well-being. Once this evaluation is completed successfully, a living donor transplant may be performed.

KIDNEY DONOR

Living donors historically have been blood relatives because tissue matching was considered more likely. More recently, however, living kidney donors have been spouses and friends, and the results have been comparable to living blood-related donors.[5] Although either kidney may be used for transplant, the left is preferred because the left renal vein is longer than the right.

LIVER DONOR

Currently, a lobe of the liver from a parent can be transplanted in children. This technique and another in which an adult cadaveric liver is divided for transplant into two recipients, were developed because a high number of children were dying before a cadaveric donor with a liver of the correct size became available. Graft and patient survival in one series of living donor recipients is 94% at 1 year.[4,6,7]

PANCREAS DONOR

Transplanting part of the pancreas from a living person is controversial. The donor must not be at risk for diabetes.

LUNG DONOR

Recently, the use of living related donors in lung transplantation has been successful.[8] Either the lobe of one lung from one parent is transplanted into the child or one lobe from each parent is used for a bilateral lobar transplant. The major advantage of lung lobe transplantation is that it enables children to have the transplant either when they are in the best condition, or if they become critically ill and a cadaveric donor is unavailable.

Ethical questions continue to be raised about the use of living donors. Long-term studies of living donors have shown that the risks and adverse effects of donation are rare, and, in fact, some donors report beneficial psychological effects from donating. However, some question the risk of coercion in living donors, especially when the donor is the parent of a child who will die without a transplant. To ensure freely given and informed consent, there may be an assessment by a psychiatrist, involvement of a non–transplant-related physician, and education of the donor.

Cadaveric Donors

In addition to the exclusive use in heart transplants, cadaveric donors continue to be the most frequent donor source for organ transplants. See the display about the United Network for organ sharing.

Despite the increasing frequency of living donor transplants, the supply of organs does not meet the demand. In 1996, the national waiting list for organ transplants reached 49,000. In the previous year, there were 5,104 cadaveric organ donors in the United States.[8] Estimates based on age, cause of death, and other criteria indicate that 14,000 of the 2.2 million Americans who die each year could be organ donors.[9] Clearly, there is a large discrepancy between the number of potential versus actual organ donors. The reasons for this discrepancy are varied and include lack of information on the part of the public. Polls, however, show that 84% of those surveyed approve of organ donation; almost 75% would want their own organs donated after death.[10]

Another reason for the lack of donors is that health care professionals often do not inform families of potential donors about the option of donation. Lack of knowledge about donation and how to discuss donation with the family often are cited as reasons for not addressing this matter with families. As a result, routine inquiry (or required request) legislation has been implemented. This legislation requires that families of appropriate potential organ donors

be given the opportunity to donate organs. In an effort to decrease the reluctance to discuss donation with families, some laws also require training for those who are in the position to speak with families about the option of donation.

Identification of Potential Cadaveric Organ Donors

Any health care professional can identify a patient as a potential cadaveric organ donor. Potential donors often are victims of trauma or cerebral aneurysm or a variety of other circumstances. Criteria for organ donation vary widely. Therefore, it is recommended that any patient for whom the possibility of donation is considered be referred to the local Organ Procurement Organization.

Insights Into Clinical Research

van Pohle WR: Obtaining organ donation: Who should ask? Heart Lung 25(4):305–308, 1996

The purpose of this study was to find out the rate of organ donation when a decoupling process was used to present the option of donation. A decoupling presentation means that there is a 1- to 2-hour delay between notifying the patient's significant other of the patient's death and presenting the option of organ donation.

Data was gathered by a retrospective record review of 96 patients who were declared dead by neurological criteria in 1992 and 1993. Eighty-one patients were suitable for organ donation. There were 10 patients whose records did not indicate why their significant others were not presented the option of donation. The significant others of 71 patients were presented the option of donation. Of these, 44 were presented using the decoupling process, 24 were not, and three presentations were unknown. For the 44 for whom the decoupling process was used, 38 agreed to donation; for the 24 for whom the process was not used, 6 agreed to donation.

There was a greater number of organ donations when the decoupling process was used to inform the significant other of death.

Personnel presenting the option of donation were an RN representative from an organ procurement organization, physicians, RNs, and social workers. In this study, the organ procurement organization representative also spends whatever time is needed to explain the process, the need for donation, and the outcomes and to ensure that there is no cost for the process and that it does not delay funeral arrangements.

The RN representative made 36 presentations to significant others using the decoupling process, which resulted in 32 donations. Physicians made 29 presentations. They used the decoupling process in three presentations and yielded one donation. Nurses and social workers made the remaining small number of presentations. In this study, a greater number of organ donations occurred when the presentation was carried out by an organ procurement organization RN representative who used a decoupling process.

United Network for Organ Sharing

Federal legislation in 1984 mandated the formation of the Organ Procurement and Transplantation Network. The United Network for Organ Sharing (UNOS) is the federally funded organization that coordinates organ sharing among organ procurement organizations. UNOS maintains a computer network for matching donors and recipients and has organ allocation policies based on the ethical principles of justice and equity.

Determination of Death

With current technology, death can be determined in two ways. The absence of cardiopulmonary function is the better-known method; however, the absence of brain function (brain death) also is a common method of determining death (see Chapter 32 for neurological criteria for determining death). Most patients who are organ donors are pronounced dead based on the absence of brain function. The critical care nurse should be familiar with the laws in his or her state related to "brain death" and with the institutional policies for the determination of death.

The Nurse's Role

Critical care nurses are an integral part of the organ donation team. Almost all organ donors die in critical care units; thus, the critical care nurse is a key person in identifying potential donors. Moreover, the nurse plays an important role as advocate by making certain that all efforts are made to determine and act on the patient's wishes regarding donation. Nurses also play a vital role in supporting the family psychologically, particularly when they are trying to accept the donor's death. When a decision is made for organ donation, the nurse also plays an important role in supporting the donor psychologically.

When caring for a potential donor, it is essential to maintain hemodynamic stability so that vital organs are perfused adequately. To do this, hypotension is first treated by administering fluids and plasma volume expanders. Next, if vasopressors are necessary, dopamine is administered in doses less than 10 μg/kg to maintain systolic blood pressure above 100 mmHg. If dopamine is not maintaining blood pressure, other vasopressors can be used. However, as more vasopressors are added, the possibility for multiorgan recovery decreases.

It is also essential to assess urine output hourly to detect diabetes insipidus. This is common in organ donors and is due to failure of the posterior pituitary to produce or release antidiuretic hormones. Aqueous vasopressin or desmopressin acetate may be ordered to reduce urine output and help maintain fluid balance.

Laboratory results, such as electrolytes, complete blood count (CBC), liver and renal function tests, and arterial blood gases (ABGs), are necessary to assess organ function and determine appropriate intervention. An electrocardiogram (ECG) and echocardiogram are required for heart donation, whereas serial chest x-rays, sputum for Gram stain, bronchoscopy, and visual inspection at the time of organ procurement are required for lung donation.

Preservation Time

There is a broad range of acceptable preservation times for organs. The goal, however, is to transplant organs as soon as possible. Kidneys can be stored for up to 48 hours using pulsatile perfusion preservation and for 24 to 36 hours using cold storage. Livers can be stored for up to 20 hours, pancreata up to 12 hours, and hearts and lungs for 4 to 6 hours. Organs are stored in cold solution specifically designed to decrease cellular injury. Solutions are different for each organ and are based on the metabolic needs of the organ. The focus of preservation is to protect the organ from ischemic injury.

The Transplant Coordinator's Role

The role of the transplant or donation coordinator has evolved as a result of the need to make organs available for transplantation. Although kidneys are the most commonly transplanted organs, the coordinator is involved in the coordination and procurement of all transplantable organs. A person may donate kidneys, heart, lungs, liver, pancreas, corneas, skin, bone, and perhaps other organs or tissue. The role of the transplant coordinator usually includes ensuring that the family has the information necessary to give informed consent and providing them with access to bereavement support. They also serve as a resource for the health care team and as a liaison between the transplant program and the critical care area. Cooperation between the critical care staff and the transplant program will help ensure that the option of donation is offered to families of all potential donors.

ASSESSMENT AND MANAGEMENT IN ORGAN TRANSPLANTATION

Preoperative Phase

The immediate preoperative phase, which is usually only a matter of hours, includes comprehensive laboratory studies, chest x-ray, electrocardiogram, and for kidney transplant recipients, dialysis within 24 hours of transplantation. Laboratory studies usually include CBC, prothrombin time (PT), partial thromboplastin time (PTT), electrolytes, blood sugar, blood urea nitrogen (BUN), creatinine, liver function tests, type and cross-match, and urinalysis.

The Surgical Procedure

KIDNEY

Typically, the kidney is placed retroperitoneal in the iliac fossa. The hypogastric or internal artery and the external iliac vein are usually used for anastamosis. When it is mechanically difficult to access these vessels, as with children, it may be necessary to anastomose the renal vessels to the inferior vena cava and aorta.

Two common types of ureteral anastomoses can be performed. In the first, the donor ureter is implanted into the recipient's bladder by a vertical cystotomy and a submucosal antireflux tunnel, because the ureter will lack enervation and normal peristalsis. In the second type, used less frequently, the donor kidney is anastomosed at the ureteropelvic junction to the recipient ureter. An indwelling catheter is used for both types of anastomoses, and occasionally a ureteral stent may be used. In either case, hema-

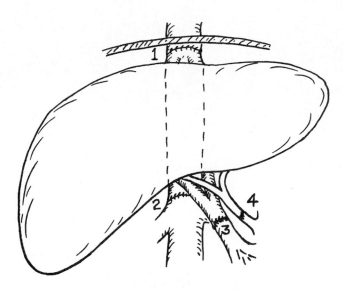

FIGURE 46-1

Diagram representing vascular anastomoses in liver transplantation. 1, suprahepatic vena cava; 2, infrahepatic vena cava; 3, portal vein; 4, hepatic artery.

turia will be present for several days. In the more common procedure, clots may be seen in the urine, because of the vascular nature of the bladder. In the latter procedure, the urine will change to pink within the first postoperative day because there are no sutures in the bladder.

LIVER

The liver is transplanted orthotopically, that is, in its normal position after the native liver is removed. Four vascular anastomoses must be done: the suprahepatic vena cava, the infrahepatic vena cava, the portal vein, and the hepatic artery (Fig. 46–1). Then the liver is reperfused, and the bile duct is anastomosed, usually to the recipient bile duct. A T tube is usually inserted. During liver transplantation, a rapid infusion system is used for administering blood and blood products, a cell saver is often used to limit the amount of banked blood required, and a pump for veno-venous bypass is often used in adults to return blood to the heart. This is done by inserting a catheter into the saphenous or femoral vein and another into the axillary vein (usually on the left side), which allows blood to circulate from the lower extremities back to the heart. Surgery usually takes between 8 and 16 hours.

HEART

Orthotopic Transplantation

Orthotopic transplantation is performed most commonly. The recipient's heart is excised, and the donor heart is implanted in its place. A median sternotomy incision is made, cardiopulmonary bypass is initiated, and the recipient's heart is removed by incising the left and right atria, pulmonary artery, and aorta. The atrial septum and posterior and lateral walls of the recipient's atria are left intact,

including the areas of the sinoatrial (SA) node, inferior and superior venae cavae to the right atrium, and pulmonary veins to the left atrium. The remnant atria serve as anchors for the donor heart.

The donor atria are trimmed to preserve the anterior arterial walls, SA node, and internodal conduction pathways. Then anastomoses are made between the recipient and donor left and right atria, the pulmonary arteries, and the aortas. Atrial and ventricular pacing wires are placed at the time of surgery so that temporary pacing can easily be initiated. Cardiopulmonary bypass is weaned off, and the donor heart assumes the role of providing the cardiac output (Fig. 46–2).

Heterotopic Transplantation

An infrequently used technique is heterotopic transplantation, or piggyback procedure, in which the recipient's heart is left in place, and the donor heart is placed next to it in the right chest. The two hearts are connected in parallel by anastomoses made between the donor and recipient left and right atria, aortas, and pulmonary arteries using a synthetic tube graft. By allowing blood to flow through either or both hearts, two functional hearts work together to provide the cardiac output (Fig. 46–3).

Heterotopic transplantation can be used in patients with pulmonary hypertension in whom the donor heart alone would not have a strong enough right ventricle to pump against the increased pulmonary vascular resistance. It can also be used as a life-saving procedure in urgent cases if the only available donor heart is too small for the size of the recipient. Limitations of heterotopic transplantation include thromboembolism from the native heart with need for anticoagulation, limited space in the chest cavity, and, in ischemic heart disease, ongoing angina and the possibility of ischemia-induced dysrhythmias in the native heart. The survival rates are less favorable for heterotopic transplantation than for orthotopic transplantation.

PANCREAS

The most frequent surgical technique is to transplant the entire pancreas. This is often done in combination with a kidney transplant because recipients have ESRD secondary to diabetes mellitus. The organs may be transplanted at the same time or months apart. Segmental pancreas and islet cell transplantations are done less often.

The pancreas is placed into a heterotopic position, usually the right iliac area. Techniques vary for vascular and exocrine anastomoses. The most controversial aspect of the surgical technique is the approach for draining exocrine secretions. The exocrine duct may be occluded, or exocrine secretions may drain either into the small bowel or bladder. There is no consensus about the best approach, and all have advantages and disadvantages.[11,12]

LUNG

Both single and double lung transplants are done. In single lung transplants, the left lung is preferred because the main

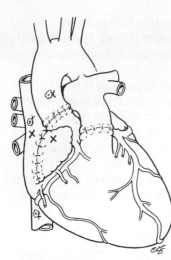

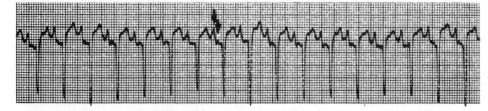

FIGURE 46-2
Orthotopic method of transplantation. Both the donor and the recipient SA nodes are intact (**X**). This results in an ECG tracing as shown. Note the double P wave at independent rates.

stem bronchus is longer, which makes the procedure easier technically. Anastomoses are made at the main stem bronchus, pulmonary artery, and at the cuff of atrium containing pulmonary veins. Cardiopulmonary bypass is not always necessary and depends on the patient's pulmonary artery pressure, blood pressure, and gas exchange. The single lung transplant incision is made at the fifth intracostal space using a posterior lateral thoracotomy, whereas a me-

dian sternotomy incision is made for the double lung procedure. Surgeons telescope the recipient's bronchus into the donor or vice versa, or perform an end-to-end anastomosis with omentopexy in which an omental flap is wrapped around the tracheal anastomosis to increase blood supply to the area.[13,14]

Postoperative Phase

Immediately after surgery, the transplant recipient is cared for in a closely monitored area until stable. Kidney transplant patients often go to a postanesthesia care unit and then directly to a transplant unit. Other organ recipients go to an intensive care unit (ICU) from the operating room. As the patient arrives in the postanesthesia or intensive care area, the following assessments are made:

- Blood pressure, heart rate, respirations, oxygenation and ventilator settings, temperature, central venous pressure, and cardiopulmonary hemodynamics. In renal transplant patients, blood pressure should be taken on an extremity that does not have a functioning vascular access site, because even momentary interference with arterial blood flow may lead to access malfunction.
- Patient's level of consciousness and degree of pain
- Number of intravenous and arterial lines, noting the site, type of solution, and flow rate
- Abdominal or chest dressing for drainage, noting the presence of drains and amount and type of drainage
- Presence of bladder and possible ureteral catheters and patency and urinary drainage

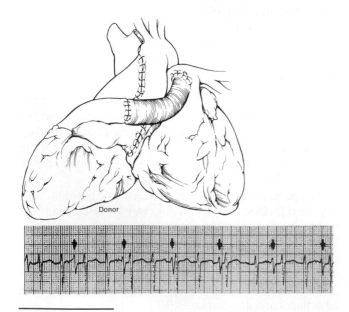

FIGURE 46-3
Heterotopic method of transplantation. The donor heart is anastomosed with a Dacron graft to the recipient's heart. This results in an ECG tracing as shown. Note the "extra" QRS at an independent rate.

- Attachment of nasogastric tube to appropriate drainage system and amount and character of drainage
- Most recent hemodynamic and intraoperative laboratory results

KIDNEY

Care of the kidney transplant recipient is centered around assessing renal function and administering immunosuppressive therapy. Therefore, answers to the following questions will help guide care:

- Are the patient's own kidneys present in addition to the graft, and if so, how much urine do they produce daily? This information will help determine how much urine is from the transplanted kidney.
- What are the preoperative results of laboratory tests (urea nitrogen, creatinine, hematocrit)?
- How much and what kind of intravenous fluid has the patient received?
- What immunosuppressive drugs were given preoperatively or intraoperatively? What immunosuppressive therapy should be given postoperatively?

In addition, the vascular access is located and its patency determined by placing either fingers or a stethoscope directly over the access site and feeling or listening for a characteristically loud, pulsating noise called a *bruit*. If the patient has been maintained on peritoneal dialysis and the catheter is in place, the catheter system must be sterile and capped.

Nursing responsibilities revolve around the following:

- Observing the function of the transplanted kidney
- Monitoring fluid and electrolyte balance
- Helping the patient avoid sources of infection
- Detecting early signs of complications
- Supporting the patient and family through the recovery phase

Renal Graft Function

The amount of urine produced by the transplanted kidney varies from a large amount (200–1,000 mL/h) to small amounts (<20 mL/h). The degree of renal function is related to ischemic injury in the donor kidney, usually from either hypotensive periods in a cadaveric donor or from the time the kidney is stored outside the body (preservation time). Renal function is better when kidney preservation time is kept under 24 hours. Most posttransplant dysfunction is reversible but may take up to 4 weeks to return to normal.

Renal function is assessed by periodic serum urea nitrogen and creatinine levels and in some centers by a β-microglobulin test. This low-molecular-weight globulin is filtered readily by the glomerular basement membrane and is reabsorbed and metabolized almost completely by the proximal renal tubules.

A renal scan is a radionuclitide test used to determine renal perfusion, filtration, and excretion. It is usually done in the first 24 hours for baseline data and periodically thereafter when laboratory values or clinical changes suggest an alteration in renal function.

Urinary Drainage Problems

When a change in urinary output occurs, such as a large volume one hour and a diminished amount the next, mechanical factors that interfere with urinary drainage should be suspected. Clotted, kinked, or compressed tubing in the urinary drainage system may be the cause of the decreased output. When the catheter is occluded by a clot, the patient may complain of pain, feel an urgency to void, or have bloody leakage around the catheter. Milking is the preferred way to dislodge clots because irrigation, even under aseptic conditions, increases the risk of infection. Gentle irrigation with strict aseptic technique may be necessary, however. Small amounts of irrigant (no more than 30 mL) are recommended because recipients commonly have small bladders. Vigorous irrigation also could cause extravasation at the ureteral anastomosis site.

Urinary Leakage

Urinary leakage on the abdominal dressing and severe abdominal discomfort or distention may indicate retroperitoneal leakage from the ureteral anastomosis site.

Decreased urinary output or severe abdominal pain in the presence of good renal function and adequate pain medication should be reported because technical and surgical complications can result in loss of graft function.

Hyperkalemia

The most frequent electrolyte disturbance in the acute postoperative phase is hyperkalemia. If the graft functions and excretes a high volume of urine, it generally also is able to excrete the excessive serum potassium created by surgical tissue damage. If the patient is oliguric or anuric after surgery, the serum potassium may increase to unacceptable levels. Interventions include administration of glucose and insulin to transport potassium into the cell and administration of oral polystyrene sulfonate.

LIVER

Immediate postoperative care is focused on hemodynamic stability, adequate oxygenation, fluid and electrolyte balance, adequate hemostasis, and graft function. An arterial line and pulmonary artery catheter are in place. The pulmonary artery catheter readings help monitor cardiac function and fluid status because high cardiac output and low systemic vascular resistance related to the effects of end-stage liver disease continue immediately postoperatively.

Vasopressors and additional fluid boluses may be required in the first 24 to 36 hours. Central venous pressure should be maintained at greater than 10 cm H_2O to balance the importance of good cardiac function against the risk of passive congestion of the liver.

Oxygenation

Adequate ventilation is crucial for graft perfusion and helps reduce the risk of pulmonary complications. Ventilator settings are determined by the critical care team, and SaO_2 and SvO_2 are monitored. Pulse oximetry may be used, but severe jaundice may interfere with saturation measurements. Pleural effusion is common postoperatively due to the presence of ascites and risk of injury to the diaphragm during surgery. A chest tube may be required for drainage.

Ventilator support is usually withdrawn when the patient is fully awake. However, if the patient is going to receive a monoclonal antibody, such as muromonab-CD3, the first dose should be given before extubation because there is a risk of pulmonary edema as a reaction to the medication.

Coagulation

Abnormal clotting factors, anastomosis site bleeding, and decreased graft function can all contribute to problems with hemostasis. Therefore, PT, PTT, fibrinogen, and factor V level are monitored along with the amount, color, and consistency of bleeding from the incision and drainage tubes.

The patient may need infusions of platelets, red blood cells, or cryoprecipitate. Blood products should be filtered to avoid introduction of CMV, especially if the patient is CMV negative. Care is taken to avoid overcorrecting coagulation deficiencies, which could lead to vascular thrombosis of the extremities or the graft. As a result of the veno-venous bypass system, there is also a risk of phlebitis or thrombosis in the femoral and axillary access site. This may be indicated by ipsilateral swelling in these extremities. Anticoagulation or an inferior vena cava filter may be necessary if deep vein thrombosis develops.

Electrolyte Balance

Hyperglycemia, hyperkalemia, metabolic alkalosis, and calcium, phosphorus, and magnesium disorders may occur. Hyperglycemia is an indication that the liver is able to store glycogen and convert it to glucose. Hyperkalemia can indicate nonfunctional hepatocytes and in turn, a nonfunc-

tional graft. Metabolic alkalosis is related to the citrate in stored blood (metabolized to bicarbonate), hypokalemia, diuretic therapy, and the administration of large volumes of fresh, frozen plasma. This usually resolves spontaneously, but the hypoventilation in response to the alkalosis may slow weaning from mechanical ventilation. Calcium, phosphorus, and magnesium disturbances are primarily due to the administration of fluid and blood products.

Some degree of renal dysfunction is also common postoperatively due either to hepato-renal syndrome or hypotension during surgery. In addition, some immunosuppressive medications are nephrotic. This can affect fluid and electrolyte balance. On occasion, when dialysis is needed, continuous arteriovenous or veno-venous hemofiltration are used because they interfere the least with hemodynamic stability.

Liver Function

Function of the transplanted liver can range from excellent to primary nonfunction. Although the cause of primary nonfunction is not known, it is believed to be related to preservation injury, and it requires retransplantation. Liver function is assessed by bile production, coagulation factors, and later by liver function tests. Measuring bile production from the biliary drainage tube helps assess the excretory function of the liver and is a good early indicator of graft function. Transaminases (alanine aminotransferase and aspartate aminotransferase) provide a measure of the synthetic function of the liver and information about the degree of hepatic injury related to preservation. Liver function is also assessed by improvement in the clearance of lactate, encephalopathy, and glucose metabolism. All liver function tests will be elevated initially and gradually will decrease.

HEART

Postoperative care of the heart transplant patient is similar to that for any person undergoing cardiac surgery; however, there are several major differences, including changes in cardiac rhythm and function caused by denervation of the donor heart and the potential for right ventricular failure. Only the more common orthotopic transplant is discussed here.

Remnant P Waves

Because the recipient SA node and portions of the recipient atria are left intact at the time of surgery, two P waves are usually seen on the ECG. The recipient SA node initiates an impulse that depolarizes the remnant recipient atria; however, this depolarization wave usually does not cross the atrial suture line. The donor SA node initiates the impulse that causes depolarization of the entire donor heart and elicits the QRS complex. Because the two sets of atria beat independently of each other, two different P waves appear on the ECG. Remnant P waves can be identified by their dissociation or lack of relationship to the QRS complexes. They usually occur at a slower rate than the donor P waves, and their rate can speed up or slow down because the remnant P waves are still under autonomic nervous system influence, whereas the donor P waves are denervated. The two sets of atria can also be in different rhythms. For example, the recipient atrial remnants can be in atrial fibrillation, while the donor heart is in normal sinus rhythm.

Effects of Denervation

During donor heart removal, the nerve supply is severed, resulting in no autonomic nervous system innervation of the transplanted heart. Because of the loss of vagal influence, the resting sinus rate is higher than normal—usually between 90 and 110 beats/min—and heart rate variations due to respiration do not occur.

Decreased donor SA node automaticity can also occur after transplant as a result of injury to the node during procurement, transport, surgical procedure, or postoperative edema of the atrial suture line. Generally, these problems resolve within 1 to 2 weeks posttransplant, but isoproterenol (Isuprel) or temporary pacing may be needed to maintain an adequate heart rate. Atropine, which blocks vagal stimulation, is ineffective in treating bradyarrhythmias in the transplanted heart because there is no parasympathetic innervation. If the sinus rate is reduced, junctional rhythms can occur earlier than normal because of the loss of vagal tone.

Normal cardiovascular reflexes are also removed by denervation. In the normal heart, increased body metabolic demands cause direct compensatory stimulation of the heart by the sympathetic nervous system, which immediately increases heart rate, contractility, and cardiac output. Because direct sympathetic nervous system stimulation of the transplanted heart is absent, this response is mediated through release of circulating catecholamines from the adrenal medulla. Therefore, increases in heart rate, contractility, and cardiac output occur much more slowly than normal. With exercise, heart rate and cardiac output increase gradually over 3 to 5 minutes and remain elevated longer after exercise. Prolonged warm-up before and cool down after exercise help compensate for these changes.

Orthostatic hypotension can occur because the normal, immediate reflex tachycardia, which compensates for venous pooling with position change, does not occur. When patients begin ambulating, they should be cautioned to change position gradually to prevent orthostatic hypotension.

Because of denervation, the cardiac effects of medications normally mediated by the autonomic nervous system are abnormal. Atropine, which increases heart rate by blocking parasympathetic influence, is ineffective. Instead, pharmacological management of symptomatic bradyarrhythmias is achieved with isoproterenol, because it stimulates myocardial β-receptors directly.

Digitalis preparations are ineffective in decreasing the heart rate or increasing the atrioventricular nodal refractory period, because these effects are mediated primarily by the parasympathetic nervous system. Digitalis does increase myocardial contractility by its direct action on myocardial cells. β-blocking drugs or calcium channel blockers (eg, verapamil) can be used to control supraventricular tachy-arrhythmias in the transplanted heart; carotid sinus pressure, the Valsalva maneuver, and digitalis are ineffective.

Finally, denervation prevents transmission of pain impulses from ischemic myocardium to the brain, so the patient does not experience angina. Severe myocardial ischemia or infarction can go unnoticed. For this reason, ECG stress testing and annual coronary angiography or coronary vascular ultrasound are usually performed.

Potential for Ventricular Failure

Posttransplant ventricular failure, causing decreased cardiac output, occurs for the same reasons as in other cardiac surgical procedures. In addition, a prolonged ischemia time, inotropic support of the donor, or rejection can cause myocardial depression in a transplant recipient.

Right ventricular failure is more common after transplant. Often, there is some degree of pulmonary hypertension because of chronic left ventricular failure. Postoperative changes in pH or ABGs can cause pulmonary vascular spasm, compounding the problem. Both pulmonary hypertension and spasm increase the pulmonary vascular resistance or resistance to ejection of blood by the right ventricle. The normal right ventricle of the donor heart may be unable to increase its output acutely to overcome a high preexisting pulmonary vascular resistance. Signs of acute right ventricular failure include elevated central venous pressure and jugular venous distention. Left ventricular cardiac output decreases as the right ventricle is unable to pump enough blood through the lungs.

A good drug for treating ventricular failure in the transplanted heart is isoproterenol. It directly stimulates β_1-receptors of the denervated heart, increasing contractility. It also stimulates β_2-receptors in the lungs, decreasing pulmonary vascular resistance; nitroglycerin, nitroprusside, prostacycline, or amrinone may be successful. Other drugs that can increase contractility of the denervated heart are epinephrine, dobutamine, and amrinone.

PANCREAS

Pancreas transplant recipients may been cared for briefly in the critical care setting. Their care is somewhat similar to patients having had abdominal surgery. The differences relate to pancreatic function, the type of surgical procedure, and secondary effects of diabetes mellitus.

Blood glucose response usually returns within the first few postoperative hours; however, an insulin drip may be required until it is normal. Pancreatic function is monitored by glucose levels before and after meals and by the results of glycosylated hemoglobin and sometimes glucose tolerance testing. Even minor abnormalities can indicate rejection or vascular thrombosis of the graft.

Preventing infection is particularly challenging when a section of duodenum is used for exocrine drainage. As a result, antibiotics are usually administered until the intraoperative culture of the duodenum is reported.

When the bladder is used for exocrine drainage, bicarbonate wasting in the urine may occur. Therefore, intravenous and oral sodium bicarbonate are given to help maintain normal bicarbonate levels.[15] With this surgical approach, an indwelling catheter is placed to prevent bladder distention, which can result in stress on suture lines and pancreatitis. Depending on the patient's ability to void, the catheter may be needed for several days or possibly weeks if there is long-standing neurogenic bladder dysfunction secondary to diabetes mellitus.

A nasogastric tube is kept in place until bowel activity returns. If diabetic gastroparesis is present, this may take 3 to 5 days.[16] If it continues, enteral or parenteral feedings may be needed until bowel activity returns.

LUNG

The lung transplant patient will be anesthetized, intubated, and mechanically ventilated on arrival to the ICU. Generally, extubation occurs 24 to 36 hours postoperatively. Patients with emphysema and a single lung transplant are generally extubated more quickly than patients with pulmonary hypertension who may need a longer intubation period.

The post–lung transplant patient will not have a cough reflex because of denervation. Therefore, when suctioning, avoid inserting the catheter where it can cause damage. A common problem in the immediate posttransplant period is pulmonary edema due to a phenomenon known as "pulmonary reimplantation" injury. As a result, the patient is maintained in a relatively hypovolemic state for the first few days. Diuresis is started when the patient is hemodynamically stable. The goal is to obtain the patient's pretransplant weight.

Because the lungs are constantly exposed to the outside world, preventing infection is especially important after lung transplant. Antibiotics are given prophylactically and are determined by donor cultures, preoperative serology results, and sputum samples. Patient care measures to prevent infection include giving oral care, encouraging physical activity early in the postoperative course, and performing daily respiratory and chest physiotherapy. Continuous pulse oximetry is used to monitor oxygen saturation, and daily chest x-rays help monitor progress. Infection control measures by staff include washing hands, wearing masks, and using aseptic suctioning technique.

marrow or peripheral blood) may be taken from another person (allogeneic) or from the recipient (autologous). Stem cells from an identical twin are syngeneic.

Peripheral stem cell transplantation is an important advance in restoring bone marrow that has been destroyed by high-dose chemotherapy and radiotherapy. Because stem cells are not abundant in the peripheral blood circulation, most centers give high-dose chemotherapy in conjunction with a bone marrow stimulant, such as granulocyte colony-stimulating factor to induce the progenitor cells into the peripheral circulation. This rapid movement of progenitor cells into the bloodstream results in a larger volume of stem cells available for collection. Peripheral blood stem cells may serve as an alternative or a supplement to BMT. Although PBCTs may be allogeneic, syngeneic, or autologous, currently most are autologous.

Peripheral blood stem cells are increasingly used instead of bone marrow because recovery often is faster and with fewer complications. Umbilical cord blood has also been investigated as a source of progenitor stem cells. The major limitation in using cord blood is collecting a volume of cells large enough to replace the recipient's marrow.

Procuring Progenitor Cells From Bone Marrow

After the patient's underlying disease has been reduced or eradicated and the source of progenitor cells has been determined, the progenitor cells are collected. Bone marrow progenitor cells are harvested from the patient or donor in the operating room under general or spinal anesthesia. The marrow is collected from the posterior iliac crest and sometimes from the anterior iliac crest or sternum. Large-bore needles are used to collect a series of 1- to 5-mL aspirations until a total of 2 to 3×10^8 nucleated cells per kilogram of body weight are harvested. The total volume collected ranges from 1 to 2 L. The marrow is mixed with tissue culture medium and heparin and then filtered through mesh screens to remove bone spicules, fat, and clots. In allogeneic and syngeneic transplants, the cells are taken directly to the recipient's room for infusion.

Pressure dressings are applied to the aspirate sites, and the donor is usually admitted for overnight observation and

---

ASSESSMENT AND MANAGEMENT IN HEMOPOIETIC STEM CELL TRANSPLANTATION

An HSCT involves replacing diseased or nonfunctioning bone marrow with healthy *progenitor* cells, also called *stem* cells, which are primitive cells capable of self-renewal and maturation. Stem cells can be obtained from the bone marrow or from the peripheral blood. Stem cells (from bone

---

Considerations for the Pediatric Patient
Organ and Hemopoietic Stem Cell Transplant

- Growth and development
- Education, play, and socialization
- Response to illness, hospitalization, treatment, and sequelae
- Body image and self-esteem
- Family role and relationships
- Effect of child's illness on parents (ie, fear of child's death, separation, sick role issues, financial concerns)

replacement of fluid and blood products. The harvest sites may be mildly uncomfortable.

Procuring Progenitor Cells From Peripheral Blood

Leukapheresis is a method of selecting progenitor stem cells from the peripheral blood. A commercial cell separator machine collects the progenitor stem cells and returns the plasma and erythrocytes to the donor. This is done through a wide-bore double lumen central or femoral catheter over 3 to 4 hours. The number of leukapheresis procedures required is determined by the number of stem cells harvested at each session. The goal is to collect 5 million CD 34+ cells per kilogram of body weight. CD34+ cells are cell surface markers that identify progenitor cells. With autologous PBCTs, the cells are immediately cryopreserved and stored in liquid nitrogen until the recipient is prepared for reinfusion. The donor may have a transient hypocalcemia reaction with chills, fatigue, tingling in the extremities, and vertigo resulting from the citrate infusion, which is used to prevent clotting of the blood during the procedure. The symptoms usually resolve by taking a calcium supplement, such as Tums.

Preconditioning Regimen

After the progenitor cells have been obtained, the patient begins the preconditioning regimen. This procedure destroys any residual tumor cells and, in allogeneic transplants, provides enough immunosuppression to permit donor cells to be accepted so that engraftment can occur. Alkylating agents (cyclophosphamide, carboplatin, busulfan, thiotepa, cisplatin, melphalan, carmustine), etoposide, cytarabine, and sometimes total body irradiation are used to destroy the bone marrow function. This is also called ablative therapy. The regimen is administered over 4 to 8 days. The patient is then allowed one to two rest days to clear the chemotherapy from the system prior to the infusion of stem cells. Bone marrow aplasia occurs within days after the regimen is completed, while the acute toxicity from the regimen lasts for weeks until engraftment occurs.

Infusion

In allogeneic or syngeneic transplant, the stem cells are infused immediately after they are collected. Autologous stem cells that were previously collected and cryopreserved must be thawed in a warm normal saline bath before reinfusion. The bone marrow or peripheral blood stem cell product is administered over 2 to 3 hours in a manner similar to a blood transfusion. The volume of a peripheral blood stem cell infusion is generally less than a bone marrow infusion. Patients are usually premedicated with acetaminophen, hydrocortisone, and diphenhydramine and prehydrated to maintain renal perfusion. Antihypertensives, diuretics, and mannitol

may be required to prevent fluid overload and manage hemodynamic changes during infusion. Vital signs are monitored, and oxygen and cardiac monitoring are readily available. Except for renal toxicity, which results from red blood cell contamination, complications are rare but may include fluid overload, pulmonary insufficiency caused by microemboli, sepsis caused by contamination of the marrow, and hypersensitivity reactions exhibited by fever and urticaria. Common reactions may include hemoglobinuria, hematuria, dysrhythmias, tachycardia, and elevated serum bilirubin and creatinine levels. The patient may experience fever, chills, or nausea from the cryoprotectant, dimethylsulfoxide. Nursing considerations include evaluating fluid balance, renal function, reactions to the reinfusion, and potential toxicity.

Recovery (Engraftment)

Engraftment occurs when the transplanted progenitor cells begin to grow and manufacture new hemopoietic cells in the recipient's bone marrow. The rate of engraftment depends on the source of the progenitor cells, the use of colony-stimulating factors, and the choice of prophylaxis against graft-versus-host disease (GVHD) in allogeneic transplants. In BMT, the recovery usually occurs within 3 weeks after infusion. The recovery is more rapid with PBCTs and usually occurs by day 12. However, the use of methotrexate for GVHD prophylaxis delays recovery. Exogenous recombinant cytokines and growth factors may be used to stimulate engraftment.

The stage of hemopoietic and immune system recovery serves as a basis for nursing and medical management. In the pre–engraftment period, the patient is neutropenic. During the early engraftment stage, cell production begins, and in the late recovery phase, engraftment is well underway. Complete recovery of the immune system can take 6 to 24 months (see the Collaborative Care Guide).

▆▆▆ IMMUNOSUPPRESSIVE THERAPY

The transplanted organ or allogeneic stem cells are foreign antigens, and eventually, the recipient's body will recognize it and mobilize its defense system to try to get rid of it. Therefore, immunosuppressive therapy is necessary to suppress the immune response so the transplanted organ or stem cells will be accepted. In allogeneic HSCT, because the immune system is generated from donor cells, immunosuppressive therapy is also used to prevent GVHD in which donor T lymphocytes attack the recipient's cells. See GVHD under the section "Complications."

The challenge of immunosuppressive therapy is to provide the recipient with adequate suppression without undue toxicity, unfavorable reactions, and gross susceptibility to opportunistic infections.

(text continues on page 896)

COLLABORATIVE CARE GUIDE
Allogeneic Bone Marrow Transplant Care Path: In-Patient Admission

Diagnosis:
BMT Contact:
Phone:
Date:

Patient:
Case Number:

Hospital Day	1	2–9	10	11–17	18–24	25–40	Discharge Planning
Transplant Day	Admission	−8 – −1	0	+1–+7	+8–+14	+15–+30	
Treatment plan	Preparation for high-dose chemotherapy (+/−radiation per protocol) Routine consults; dietary, social work, etc. Continue patient/family teaching Discharge planning	High dose chemotherapy (+/−radiation) per protocol Dietary assessment and management	Reinfusion of bone marrow Nutritional support –oral supplements –TPN	Patient neutropenic (ANC <500 cells/µL) Neutropenic precautions, –Low bacterial diet –Isolation routines Fever management; evaluation of cultures	Evidence of engraftment: WBC, ANC increasing. Pt. neutropenic until ANC >500/µL 48° Dietary assessment; calorie count. Treating mucositis Assess for GVHD Continue neutropenic precautions Continue fever management	Continued engraftment Increase oral calories, decrease TPN Possible bx, r/o GVHD	Criteria for discharge; ANC >500 cells/µL for 48° Afebrile off antibiotics for 48° Adequate caloric intake Transfusion needs manageable as outpatient GVHD and medication prophylaxis stabilized Determine frequency of BMT center visits and need for home-care referral
Medications	1. Prophylactic antibiotics, antivirals, antifungals 2. Hydration	1 & 2 continue 3. Antiemetics/antianxiety agents prn 4. Possible parenteral nutrition (TPN) 5. GVHD prophylaxis 6. Ulcer prophylaxis	1,2,3,4,5,6 continue 7. Prophylaxis for potential allergic reaction (eg, antihistamine and anti-inflammatory medications) 8. Begin CSF per protocol	1,2,3,4,5,6,8 continue 9. Broad-spectrum antibiotics with first fever >100.5°F (or neutropenia) 10. Pain meds for mucositis 11. Antihistamine and/or anti-inflammatory medications prn for blood product reactions 12. K+ and Mg+ IV supplements common prn	1. Continue (antiviral drugs may be stopped during engraftment) 2,3,4,5,6,8,10,11,12 continue 9. Continue with changes as indicated	1,2,3,4,5,6,8,11,12 continue 8. DCd per protocol 9. DCd as ANC increases or therapy completed 10. DC when mucositis resolves	1. Some prophylactic antimicrobials may be continued at home 5. Begin tapering schedule if GVHD stable 6,11 continue prn 12. K+, Mg+ supplements may be indicated either oral or IV
Daily schedule/other	1. Daily/bid weight 2. I&O q shift 3. Central line care 4. Oral and skin care routines 5. Incentive spirometer 6. Hematest all specimens 7. Chest x-ray q week and prn	1–7 continue 8. Cardiac monitor or EKG with some chemo drugs	1–7 continue 8. Possible EKG after reinfusion if clinically indicated	1–7 continue 9. Consult GI service, infectious disease, pulmonary as needed	1–7,9 continue Other diagnostic tests as indicated	Continue weekly chest x-rays Increase activity/self care Other diagnostic tests as indicated	Continued patient teaching re: outpatient guidelines; CSFs, GVHD, medication compliance, central line care, medications, and homecare needs as appropriate

(continued)

COLLABORATIVE CARE GUIDE
Allogeneic Bone Marrow Transplant Care Path: In-Patient Admission (Continued)

Diagnosis:
BMT Contact:
Phone:
Date:

Patient:
Case Number:

Hospital Day	1	2–9	10	11–17	18–24	25–40	Discharge Planning
Transplant Day	Admission	–8 – –1	0	+1 – +7	+8 – +14	+15 – +30	
Labs	1. CBC, diff, plt qd 2. Electrolytes qd 3. SMA-20 twice weekly 4. Baseline ABG's 5. PT/PTT q week 6. Type and cross-match	1,2,3 continue	1,2,3,5 continue	1,2,3,5 continue 6. 2x week 7. Monitor antibiotic drug levels 8. Monitor CSA levels	1,2,3,5 continue 7. Continue until antibiotics DCd 8. Continue as ordered	1,5,6,7,8 continue 2. Continue biweekly 3. Continue weekly	Frequency of lab draws based on stability of blood counts and need for transfusions CSA levels per protocol
Cultures	Baseline surveillance cultures; blood, nose, throat, urine CMV surveillance		Baseline culture on bone marrow product	Blood cultures with fever spike once q24h Culture urine, stool, and new skin/oral lesions	Cultures with new fever spike	Continue cultures as needed and indicated	Surveillance CMV culture Other cultures decrease unless S/S of infection develop
Blood products	Ø	Ø	Ø	Irradiated CMV screened if patient seronegative Leukocyte poor filter may be used Transfuse RBC for Hg <9.0 Transfuse platelets if <20K	RBC, platelets	Possible RBC, platelet	Continue RBC and platelet transfusions
Possible Complications	Unexpected fever related to possible infection Abnormal (unexpected) lab results Problems need to be resolved/explained before proceeding with high-dose therapy	Fluid overload Electrolyte imbalance Nausea/vomiting Anorexia Diarrhea Cardiac toxicity from some chemotherapeutic drugs Hemorrhagic cystitis from some chemotherapy Tumor lysis syndrome	Fluid overload Transfusion reaction to donor marrow: SOB; flushing; chest tightness, Renal failure Nausea/vomiting	Mucositis Nausea/Vomiting Fatigue Diarrhea–r/o infection Neutropenic sepsis Hemorrhage Hemorrhagic cystitis Veno-occlusive disease Acute GVHD Renal failure Electrolyte imbalance	Fungal infection Interstitial pneumonia Veno-occlusive disease Alopecia Prolonged N/V Acute GVHD Renal Failure Electrolyte imbalance	Mucositis resolving Neutropenia resolving Fungal infection Interstitial pneumonia Veno-occlusive disease resolving Alopecia N/V resolving Acute GVHD Graft Failure Electrolyte imbalance Renal Failure	New fever may delay discharge pending evaluation and diagnosis Unresolved complications New or increase in symptoms of GVHD will delay discharge Evidence of graft failure (pt. remains neutropenic/thrombocytopenic) Inadequate nutrition may require home TPN Renal Failure Electrolyte imbalance

Key: GVHD, Graft-versus-host disease; CSA, cyclosporine; CSF, colony-stimulating factor; ANC, absolute neutrophil count; °, hour; TPN, total parenteral nutrition; WBC, white blood cells; IV, intravenous; CSF, cerebrospinal fluid; CMV, cytomegalovirus; SMA, sequential multiple analysis; ABG, arterial blood gases; DC, discontinue; s/s, signs and symptoms; SOB, shortness of breath; r/o, rule out. © Copyright Coram Healthcare 1995

Medications

The medications given to control the immune response are methylprednisolone (Solu-Medrol), prednisone, azathioprine (Imuran), cyclosporine (Sandimmune), tacrolimus (Prograf, FK506), muromonab-CD3 (Orthoclone OKT3), antilymphocyte globulin (ALG) or antithymocyte globulin (ATG), cyclophosphamide (Cytoxan), mycophenolate mofetil (Cellcept), and methotrexate. Major points about these drugs are summarized in Table 46–4.

Steroids

Steroids are used both to prevent and reverse rejection. These anti-inflammatory agents also decrease the production of activated T-helper cells and cytotoxic cells, which help decrease the antigenic activity of the graft. Schedules and doses vary among centers. The disadvantage of steroids is the numerous side effects. Some centers avoid steroids for 2 weeks after lung transplant to help promote bronchial healing. Induction therapy in the form of ATG or muromonab-CD3 is used instead. Some centers withdraw all steroids after a defined amount of time.

Azathioprine

Azathioprine, one of the first drugs developed for immunosuppression, is an antimetabolite. It interrupts DNA synthesis and inhibits cellular division of immunocompetent cells. In doing so, the growth of activated B lymphocytes and cytotoxic T cells is inhibited. Azathioprine may be added to an immunosuppressive regimen during or after periods of rejection. The dose, however, is not increased to treat rejection because it suppresses bone marrow and can cause leukopenia and neutropenia.

Cyclosporine

Cyclosporine, a fungal metabolite is used to prevent rejection rather than to reverse acute rejection. It is much more specific than steroids and azathioprine. It acts on T-helper cells, preventing them from secreting interleukin-2 (IL-2) and IL-1 from macrophages. This prevents maturation of helper and cytotoxic T cells. Cyclosporine also suppresses humoral immunity to the extent it is dependent on T-helper cells.

Because cyclosporine selectively inhibits T cells, T cell–independent humoral immunity remains intact, the bone marrow is not suppressed, and neutrophils remain viable. This selective immunosuppression reduces the risk of infection compared with the broad suppression of other medications.

The usefulness of cyclosporine in transplantation is limited by its adverse effects. Nephrotoxicity is a common side effect, and patients with impaired renal function before transplant are at increased risk for posttransplant cyclosporine-induced renal failure. BUN and creatinine levels are monitored daily in the immediate posttransplant period, and if nephrotoxicity is developing, the dose of cyclosporine can be reduced. Doses are determined by daily trough blood levels to find the therapeutic "window" between organ rejection and cyclosporine toxicity.

> Many drugs interact with cyclosporine and tacrolimus, including several antibiotics, antifungals, calcium-channel blockers, anticonvulsants, and antituberculosis drugs. In addition, antacids should be avoided because they alter the bioavailability of the medication.

Tacrolimus

Tacrolimus (Prograf, FK506) decreases the production of IL-2 and other lymphokines that help T cells proliferate. Although the best method of using tacrolimus has yet to be determined, it is usually used in combination with at least one other immunosuppressant, often steroids. The method of action is similar to cyclosporine's so the two are not usually given together. The dose is determined by trough levels. Tacrolimus has been an effective immunosuppressive agent both as primary immunosuppression and for "rescue therapy."

Muromonab-CD3

Muromonab-CD3, or OKT3, is a monoclonal antibody specifically directed against the T lymphocyte. As a monoclonal antibody, it has a number of advantages: homogenicity, specificity, consistent potency, and predictable adverse reactions and efficacy. Muromonab-CD3 is administered as an intravenous bolus drug as a prophylaxis for rejection. It is also used in the treatment of acute rejection episodes as rescue therapy when rejection has failed to respond to other efforts.

Muromonab-CD3 removes most T lymphocytes from circulation. Those remaining are rendered unresponsive to the antigenic stimulation of the graft. A reaction to the first dose may be severe, including anaphylactic shock, pulmonary edema, high fever, chills, and aseptic meningitis. Antibodies may also develop after receiving the drug, so there is a risk of serious reaction with an additional course of treatment.

Antilymphocyte and Antithymocyte

Antilymphocyte globulin (ALG), antithymocyte globulin (ATG), antilymphocyte serum (ALS), and antithymocyte serum (ATS) are used in a number of centers in an effort to prevent rejection by providing the patient with antibodies against lymphocytes or thymocytes, which are the cells responsible for rejection. These polyclonal antibodies are produced by injection of human lymph or thymus cells into an animal (horse, rabbit, or goat), which then produces antibodies against these cells. These antibodies against human T cells are administered for 14 to 21 days, either intravenously or intramuscularly. Sensitivity against the agent usually develops after one course, and the drug cannot be reintroduced unless the animal source used to produce the drug is different.

(text continues on page 900)

TABLE 46-4   CLINICAL APPLICATION: Drug Therapy
Immunosuppressive Drugs Used in Transplantation

Drug	Adverse Reactions	Dosage	Comments
Methylprednisolone (Solu-Medrol) (IV) Prednisone (PO)	Increased susceptibility to infection Masks symptoms of infection Peptic ulcer, GI bleeding Increased appetite, weight gain Increased sodium and water retention, which exaggerate hypertension Delayed healing Negative nitrogen balance Adrenal gland suppression Behavior and personality changes Diabetogenic effect Muscle weakness Osteoporosis with long-term therapy Skin atrophy, striae Easy bruising Glaucoma, cataracts Hirsutism Acne Avascular/aseptic necrosis	Initial: 0.5–3 mg/kg of body weight, tapered to an adequate oral maintenance dose During rejection: methylprednisolone may be given in IV boluses up to 1 g/dose	An antacid and H_2 blockers are given while patient is on steroids to reduce the risk of gastric irritation and ulceration; cimetidine may also be used to decrease ulcerogenic tendencies. Cardiac arrest can occur if IV bolus of 1 g is given rapidly. Sodium restriction may be necessary when steroid dosage is high or when fluid retention increases.
Azathioprine (Imuran) (IV or PO)	Bone marrow suppression: leukopenia, thrombocytopenia, anemia, pancytopenia Rash Alopecia Liver damage, jaundice Increased susceptibility to infection	Regulated to keep WBC 5,000–10,000; drug usually stopped when WBC 3,000 or less Initial 2–5 mg/kg of body weight Maintenance: 2–3 mg/kg of body weight During rejection: maximum of 3 mg/kg of body weight, dose not usually increased with rejection	The dose is lowered when allopurinol is added to medication regimen because allopurinol delays metabolism of azathioprine (allopurinol and azathioprine are synergistic).
Cyclosporine (Sandimmune) (IV or PO) Neoral (PO, microemulsion)	Nephrotoxicity Hepatotoxicity	Initial: 4 mg/kg/d (IV) Maintenance: 5–15 mg/kg/d PO may be used as part of triple-therapy regimen (prednisone, azathioprine, cyclosporine), or quadruple-therapy regimen (same as triple therapy plus ALG or OKT3)	Initially, nephrotoxicity and hepatotoxicity seem to be dose related and respond to dose reduction.

(continued)

TABLE 46-4   CLINICAL APPLICATION: Drug Therapy (Continued)
Immunosuppressive Drugs Used in Transplantation

Drug	Adverse Reactions	Dosage	Comments
Cyclosporine (Sandimmune) **(continued)** (IV or PO) Neoral (PO, microemulsion)		The dose for Sandimmune® and Neoral® are not interchangeable due to differences in bioavailability. When preparations are changed, dose adjustments are based on blood levels. Dosage altered by monitoring drug levels at least during initial period	Long-term nephrotoxicity is a major concern. Nephrotoxicity is sometimes difficult to differentiate from rejection or ATN in renal patients. Metabolized by cytochrome P-450 enzymes. Drugs that are inducers or inhibitors for P-450 enzymes may increase or decrease cyclosporine concentrations. Trough levels done to monitor and titrate dosage. Drug interactions can raise or lower blood levels.
	Hypertension Hirsutism Gum hyperplasia Malignancy Nausea, vomiting, diarrhea Tremors/seizures Diabetogenic effects Anaphylactic reactions have been seen with IV administration		Risk of anaphylaxis is reduced if slow continuous infusion is given.
Tacrolimus (Prograf, 7K506)	Infection Nephrotoxicity Neurotoxicity Hypertension Diabetogenesis Tremors	Dosage varies 0.10 mg/kg/d IV 0.05–0.2 mg/kg/d PO (given in divided doses)	Dose based on trough levels. May be able to discontinue steroids. Monitor renal and liver function. Drug interactions and liver function can affect blood levels. P-450 enzyme system is affected.
Muromonab-CD3 (Orthoclone OKT3)	Febrile reactions; fever, chills, tremor Respiratory: dyspnea, chest pain, wheezing, pulmonary edema GI: nausea, vomiting, diarrhea Anemia, thrombocytopenia	2.5–5 mg/d IV bolus over 30–60 s, for 10–14 d	Reactions are greatest with first dose and occur within 30–60 min. To minimize first dose reaction, pretreat with methylprednisolone, acetaminophen, and diphenhydramine hydrochloride. Monitor vital signs q15min for 2h, then q30min first two doses. Have emergency equipment and cooling blanket available. Repeat administrations may cause serious reactions if antibodies develop.

(continued)

TABLE 46-4 CLINICAL APPLICATION: Drug Therapy (Continued)
Immunosuppressive Drugs Used in Transplantation

Drug	Adverse Reactions	Dosage	Comments
Antilymphocyte globulin (ALG) Antithymocyte globulin (ATG) Antilymphocyte serum (ALS)	Anaphylactic shock due to hypersensitivity to animal serum Fever (up to 105°F or 40.6°C) and chills Increased susceptibility to infections due to decreased lymphocytes	Skin test for hypersensitivity to animal serum performed before initial dose Dosage may vary	Lymphocytes or platelets decrease sharply with drug administration; therefore, blood work for lymphocyte and platelet counts should be drawn before infusion is started.
Antithymocyte serum (ATS) (usually IV, IM, or deep SC)	IM or deep SC injection site swollen, red, and painful, with abscess formation Difficulty walking if IM or SC injection given in thigh		Usually given only for short period of time either to prevent or treat rejection; not a long-term immunosuppressant.
Cyclophosphamide (Cytoxan)	Leukopenia, thrombocytopenia Increased susceptibility to infections Metabolites direct irritants to bladder mucosa and may cause hemorrhagic cystitis	1–2 mg/kg (or ½ to ⅔ of azathioprine dosage)	Given in place of azathioprine when it causes hepatotoxicity. Administer on awakening to avoid accumulation of metabolites in bladder while sleeping. Observe for hematuria. Fluid intake should be encouraged to dilute metabolites.
Mycophenolate mofetil (Cellcept)	Alopecia Nausea Vomiting Diarrhea Dyspepsia	Usual dosage 1 g bid (250-mg capsules)	GI symptoms may be dose related and may improve with decrease. Preferable to take on an empty stomach unless GI symptoms are intolerable.
Methotrexate	Myelosuppression Mucositis Hepatotoxicity	15 mg/m² day 1, then 10 mg/m² day 3, 6, 11	No other regimen has proven superior to a methotrexate/cyclosporine combination for prevention of GVHD in allogeneic BMT patients. The consequences of MTX exposure can be reversed by leukovorin if it is administered before irreversible changes lead to cell death (usually when plasma levels are greater than 4×10^{-8}) Most of the drug is excreted through the kidney, with a small fraction excreted through the bile. Standard doses in patients with good renal function, bili less than 10 and without effusions or ascites are not likely to produce serious toxicity

The incidence of CMV infection is increased with the use of ATG as well as muromonab-CD3; therefore, prophylaxis for CMV is indicated when these medications are given.

Cyclophosphamide

Cyclophosphamide decreases serum immunoglobulins and destroys proliferative lymphoid cells. Rarely used since the addition of cyclosporine to immunosuppressive regimens, clyclophosphamide may replace azathioprine when hepatotoxicity develops. Cyclophosphamide is inferior to azathioprine in prolonging graft survival and can cause such serious side effects as hemorrhagic cystitis and bladder fibrosis.

Myclophenolate Mofetil

Mycophenolate mofetil (Cellcept), formerly known as RS-61443, predominantly acts on lymphocytes. It inhibits purine synthesis, T and B cell proliferation, and the activation of leukocytes to inflammatory sites. Two major disadvantages of this medication are its cost and the number of pills per day a patient has to take because it is only available in 250-mg capsules, and the daily dose for adults is 1 to 2.5 g.

Methotrexate

Methotrexate is commonly used in allogeneic HSCT and occasionally in heart transplantation. It is an antimetabolite that inhibits synthesis of thymidine and purine, which are essential for DNA synthesis. Patients must have good renal function because methotrexate is excreted in the urine.

Regimens

A single medication usually cannot suppress all of the necessary immune responses. Therefore, immunosuppressive regimens include medications that complement each other and increase the effectiveness of the immunosuppression. The foundation of most immunosuppressant regimens is triple-drug therapy, although the combination of drugs used for organ transplant and HSCT may differ.

Triple therapy is a combination of low-dose prednisone, azathioprine, and cyclosporine or tacrolimus. These drugs are used in lower dosage so patients experience fewer side effects than they would from any one agent. For example, the risk of aseptic necrosis, diabetes mellitus, cataracts, and gastrointestinal complications attributed to chronic steroid therapy is greatly reduced. Because the dosage of azathioprine is low, the potential for hepatotoxicity and leukopenia is less. Problems associated with higher doses of cyclosporine, including lymphoma, hirsutism, hepatotoxicity, gingival hyperplasia, seizures, or gastrointestinal disturbances, rarely are seen.

In allogeneic HSCT, patients receive prophylaxis treatment for GVHD consisting of methotrexate, cyclosporine, and methylprednisolone. Another advantage includes greater flexibility in altering dosage if problems occur with any one medication. For example, the specific drug causing a problem can be reduced in dosage and the others slightly increased to maintain optimal immunosuppression. A final advantage is that cyclosporine, which is very costly, is used with two other agents, allowing it to be given in smaller, less expensive doses.

Quadruple or sequential therapy uses the same three agents as in triple therapy, plus antithymocyte antibody preparations or monoclonal antibody, monomurab-CD3. Cyclosporine may not be added to the regimen until renal function is present. All four drugs are given for several days, after which the polyclonal or monoclonal antibody preparation is discontinued. A triple-drug regimen is used for maintenance therapy. The primary advantage of quadruple therapy is that cyclosporine can be withheld in the absence of renal function. Because of cyclosporine's nephrotoxicity and its cumulative effect in the absence of renal function, both broad and specific immunosuppression can be accomplished without it. The disadvantage of quadruple therapy is the potential inability to use the polyclonal or monoclonal antibody preparation for treatment of rejection or rescue therapy. These regimens demonstrate the increasing options available to individualize immunosuppression based on each patient's needs.

▰▰ COMPLICATIONS OF TRANSPLANTATION

Complications after organ and bone marrow transplantation are usually due to graft function and problems with immunosuppression or the transplant preconditioning regimen. Organ rejection, failure of the stem cells to engraft, and infection are common complications.

Organ Rejection

Because the transplanted organ is not immunologically identical to the recipient, it acts as an antigen or foreign substance and triggers the immune system to reject it. Rejection can vary in degree from mild to severe and may be irreversible. Rejection can occur at any time, but the risk is highest in the first 3 months after organ transplant. The earlier and more severe the rejection episode, the worse the

RED FLAG

Complications of Organ Transplantation

- Rejection
- Infection
- Bleeding
- Cardiovascular disease
- Gastrointestinal problems
- Malignancy

prognosis for graft survival. Biopsy of the transplanted organ is usually needed to diagnose rejection definitively.

Four types of rejection are defined: hyperacute, accelerated, acute, and chronic, although all types do not occur in all transplanted organs. Acute and chronic are the most common types of rejection.

HYPERACUTE REJECTION

This occurs in the operating room immediately after the transplant. It is a humoral immune response in which the recipient has preformed antibodies that immediately react against antigens of the donor organ. Vascular damage occurs, resulting in severe thrombosis and graft necrosis. In kidney and heart transplantation, hyperacute rejection always results in graft failure and removal of the organ. Fortunately, hyperacute rejection is uncommon and can usually be prevented by pretransplant cross-matching.

ACCELERATED REJECTION

This type of rejection is only defined in kidney transplantation, and it occurs within 1 week after transplant. It is due to either preformed antibodies against the donor antigens in the recipient's blood or to lymphocytes in the recipient that are already sensitized to some of the donor antigens. Accelerated rejection, like hyperacute rejection, is seen infrequently because of improved tissue typing and cross-matching. It is treated aggressively with immunosuppressants and usually results in loss of the transplanted kidney.

ACUTE REJECTION

Acute rejection occurs within the first 3 months after transplant. This is the most common type of rejection, and most patients experience at least one episode. It also is the type that responds best to immunosuppressive therapy. Acute rejection occurs when antigens on the donor organ trigger lymphocytes to mature into helper T cells. The helper T cells increase the production of cytotoxic killer T cells, which bind to the transplanted organ and damage it by secreting lysosomal enzymes and lymphokines.

CHRONIC REJECTION

Chronic rejection is not fully understood, but most likely it is a combination of a cell-mediated response and a response to circulating antibodies. It usually occurs from 3 months to years after transplant and is accompanied by deteriorating organ function.

Kidney

Acute rejection occurs after the first postoperative week. It is the most frequently seen form of rejection and the type that responds best to therapy. Changes in laboratory values are the earliest and most reliable indicators that graft function is deteriorating. Clinical manifestations of rejection are more subtle and may not be seen. The patient may experi-

---

> ### *Kidney Rejection*
>
> Changes in laboratory values and tests are the best indicators of rejection.
> ↑ Serum creatinine
> ↑ β_2 microglobulin
> ↑ Blood urea nitrogen
> ↓ Creatinine clearance
> ↓ Urine creatinine and possibly urine sodium
> ↓ Blood flow on renal scan

ence any, all, or none of the following during an acute rejection episode.

Laboratory Findings

- Increased serum creatinine, BUN, serum β_2 microglobulin
- Decreased creatinine clearance
- Decreased urine creatinine
- Possibly decreased urine sodium
- Decreased blood flow on renal scan

Clinical Manifestations

- Decreased urine output
- Weight gain
- Edema
- A temperature of 37.8°C (100°F) or greater
- Tenderness over the graft site with possible swelling of the kidney
- General malaise
- Increased blood pressure

Chronic rejection is the result of repeated episodes of acute rejection in which the vessels become infarcted due to the vasculitis, and the renal tissue becomes scarred. This gradually leads to deteriorating kidney function. The symptoms are similar to acute rejection except for fever and graft enlargement. Laboratory findings are similar to those of acute rejection but also include signs of chronic renal failure, such as a declining hematocrit and calcium–phosphorus imbalance. The rate of deterioration can vary from months to years. A transplant nephrectomy is not usually required unless the kidney becomes necrotic and life threatening.

Liver

Acute rejection in liver transplantation is suspected when liver function tests, specifically transaminases, alkaline phosphatase, and total bilirubin, are increased. Clinical signs, such as decreased bile production and perigraft tenderness, are absent or nondistinct. Chronic rejection is not completely understood and believed to be due to multiple acute rejection episodes or a positive cross-match. A definitive diagnosis is made when a biopsy shows portal and bile duct inflammation and the presence of inflammatory cells, such as T lymphocytes.[17]

Heart

Although acute rejection is often asymptomatic, subtle signs and symptoms may include decreased cardiac output, atrial flutter or fibrillation, elevated white blood cell (WBC) count, and low-grade fever. Endomyocardial biopsy is performed weekly for the first month and then less frequently to diagnose rejection. Acute rejection is a major cause of death within the first year after transplantation.

CLINICAL APPLICATION: Patient Care Study

Mrs. Franklin is a 37-year-old woman who had a heart transplant 4 months ago. This was necessary because of idiopathic cardiomyopathy. She also developed intractable ventricular dysrhythmias for which she had an automatic implantable cardioverter defibrillator (AICD).

Her pretransplant serology showed the following:

Negative: Hepatitis B surface antigen, CMV antibody, toxoplasmosis, HIV

Positive: Epstein-Barr virus

Normal: Renal and liver function tests

Minor: Anemia (hematocrit = 35.2)

Mrs. Franklin waited 5 months for her heart transplant. During that time, her AICD discharged five times, and she was hospitalized twice for congestive heart failure, pulmonary edema, and ventricular tachycardia. At the time of her transplant surgery, she was taking amiodarone, quinidine, furosemide, digoxin (Lanoxin), and potassium supplements. Her transplant surgery lasted approximately 4 hours, and she was in the cardiothoracic ICU for 4 days. Immunosuppression therapy included methylprednisone, azathioprine, and cyclosporine. She recovered without complications, and the first endomyocardial biopsy showed ischemic changes but no evidence of rejection.

On the 14th postoperative day, she experienced fatigue, and her liver function tests and WBC were elevated. An echocardiogram showed a dilated right ventricle with poor contractility and a hypokinetic left ventricle. She was transferred to the ICU where isoproterenol (Isuprel) was started and a Swan-Ganz catheter was inserted. An endomyocardial biopsy on the following day showed moderate acute rejection. She was started on muromonab-CD3 (OKT3) after a chest x-ray showed that her lungs were clear. After a severe reaction consisting of flulike symptoms, fever, and muscle aches, she tolerated 14 days of treatment with OKT3. Future biopsies showed resolving rejection; however, she continued to need isoproterenol. A pacemaker was inserted. She improved and was transferred out of the ICU. She had two more episodes of rejection, which were treated with intravenous methylprednisolone. She was also switched from azathioprine to mycophenolate mofetil.

Fifty days after surgery, her fever returned, and her liver function tests increased. The fever was believed to be due to CMV infection because she was CMV negative pretransplant and had received immunosuppressive treatment for several rejection episodes. A CMV early antigen test and her endomyocardial biopsy showed CMV myocarditis. It was treated with intravenous ganciclovir. Her condition improved over the next 2 weeks, and she was discharged. She continued to take prednisone, cyclosporine, mycophenolate mofetil, trimethoprim, sulfamethoxazole, acyclovir, furosemide, and vitamins.

She felt well for 2 months, although she had one rejection episode. Then she was admitted to the hospital with fever and malaise, along with elevated liver function tests and a positive early CMV antigen test. Intravenous treatment with ganciclovir was started, and plans were made with a home care agency to continue treatment at home.

Chronic rejection may occur from 3 months to years after transplant. It is characterized by diffuse, rapidly progressing CAD that causes ischemic myocardial damage and progressive loss of heart function. Chronic rejection is a major factor limiting long-term survival, because 5 years after transplant, the incidence of CAD is 40% to 50%.[18] Because the heart is denervated, angina cannot be used as a warning sign for CAD. Instead, decreased exercise tolerance during stress testing and annual coronary angiography or intravascular ultrasound are used for diagnosis.

Pancreas

Rejection is a major cause of graft loss in pancreas transplantation. This may be attributed to the difficulty in diagnosing rejection. Elevated blood glucose is a late sign of rejection and may occur too late to initiate successful treatment. When the bladder is used for exocrine drainage, urinary amylase levels will reflect rejection earlier than hyperglycemia becomes obvious. In combined kidney–pancreas transplantation, an elevated serum creatinine may indicate rejection, although rejection can occur in one organ and not the other. Less is known about chronic pancreas rejection, and some say that it may not occur in kidney and pancreas transplants. A needle biopsy during cystoscopy is used for definitive diagnosis.

Lung

The signs and symptoms of lung transplant rejection are difficult to distinguish from pulmonary infection. For example, decreased lung function (ie, forced expiratory volume), dyspnea, cough, decreased breath sounds, fever, and tachypnea may occur in both rejection and infection. Immediately postoperatively, rejection may also be confused with volume overload, reperfusion injury, or ischemic injury secondary to preservation. Chest x-rays showing interstitial and perihilar edema can be signs of rejection and signal the need for biopsy. Even so, biopsies must be carefully interpreted to rule out infectious complications, such as CMV or *Pneumocystis carinii*, which can have histology findings similar to acute rejection.[19]

Chronic rejection is known as obliterative bronchiolitis (OB) and occurs in approximately 15% to 25% of lung transplant recipients. Acute rejection and infection are believed to play a role in OB.[20]

Hemopoietic Stem Cell Graft Failure and Rejection

To survive after ablative therapy, the patient must be given a new hemopoietic system, and it must engraft. Grafting is considered a failure when bone marrow function does not return or when it is lost after a period of recovery.

RED FLAG

Long-Term Complications of Hemopoietic Stem Cell Transplant

- Chronic graft-versus-host disease
- Infection
- Cataracts
- Gonad dysfunction
- Growth failure
- Hypothyroidism
- Secondary or recurrent malignancy
- Psychosocial issues related to long-term illness

The overall incidence of failure is less than 5% and occurs most often in patients with aplastic anemia or those receiving unrelated donor transplants.[21] Failure to engraft is rare in allogeneic transplants and almost never occurs in PBCT. Long-term complications of HSCT are listed in the display.

Rejection is one cause of graft failure. It can occur when the preconditioning regimen did not eliminate all of the recipient's immune cells; when there is a disparity in HLA matching, including mismatched HLA-D antigens; and when patients who received a high number of pretransplant blood transfusions produce antibodies. HSCT failure may also result from the following situations:

- The cells were damaged by treatment or preparation for transplant before the autologous stem cells were collected.
- Autologous stem cells have been damaged after collection either during the cleansing (ie, purging of cancer cells) or the cryopreservation process.
- The allogeneic donor's stem cells were damaged after collection and before infusion during the T cell depletion process. Donor T cells are destroyed or removed to prevent GVHD.
- The recipient's cells are damaged after transplant due to viral infection or marrow-toxic drugs, such as ganciclovir and sulfamethoxazole (Bactrim).

Failure to engraft is reflected by a hypocellular marrow, which results in hemorrhage, anemia, and life-threatening infection. If the bone marrow does not engraft, the patient will die. Persistent graft failure may be treated with a second transplant usually without the preparatory ablative regimen if a stem cell product is available.

Infection

Infection is a major cause of morbidity and mortality after organ and stem cell transplantation. Prevention, detection, and early treatment are primary nursing care goals.

The pathogens include bacterial, fungal, viral, and even protozoan organisms. The last three groups of organisms are referred to as *opportunistic* pathogens. Normally harmless and found in humans and in the environment, they pose serious threats to patients with compromised immune sys-

tems. They take advantage of the decreased host defenses—thus, the term "opportunistic." Some examples of opportunistic infections include herpes simplex and herpes zoster viruses, CMV, *Candida albicans, Pneumocystis carinii, Aspergillus fumigatus,* and *Cryptococcus neoformans.*

Organ transplant recipients are at high risk for infection during the first 3 months posttransplant because they have received high dosages of immunosuppressants. Infections in the post–stem cell transplant period generally follow a predictable pattern based on the recovery of the immune system. Therefore, HSCT recipients are at high risk for infection during the first month, which is the pre–engraftment phase, because of neutropenia. They are also at risk 30 to 60 days after transplant, in the early engraftment phase, if they have received immunosuppressive medications to prevent or treat GVHD. Figure 46–4 illustrates the sequence of complications following HSCT.

All transplant recipients are at risk for bacterial infections due to intravascular lines and urinary drainage catheters, but organ transplant patients can also develop postoperative wound and lung infections. Usually broad-spectrum antibiotics are given prophylactically for 48 hours after organ transplant or until invasive lines and drains are removed. HSCT patients receive antibiotics prophylactically for months posttransplant.

During the first month, the predominant fungal infection for HSCT patients is *Candida albicans*, for which amphotericin B and fluconazole are used prophylactically. The most frequent viral infection is the herpes simplex virus, and 80% of the patients who were seropositive before transplant will experience a reactivation of the virus unless they receive acyclovir prophylactically.[22]

After the first month, CMV is the most common infection for all transplant patients.[22] To prevent CMV, patients who are CMV seronegative should receive only CMV-negative blood products. Many centers require that all blood transfusions be filtered. Patients who are CMV seropositive and symptomatic and those receiving increased immunosuppression for an episode of acute organ rejection can be treated with ganciclovir. Prevention is important for heart transplant patients because there is a connection between CMV and CAD.[23] CMV can affect many organ systems, so there may be signs and symptoms of hepatitis, retinitis, enteritis, pneumonitis, fever, chills, and malaise.

A small number of HSCT patients develop severe and potentially fatal infections 3 months or more posttransplantation during the late recovery phase due to cellular immune deficiencies. These infections are caused most frequently by pyrogenic *Pneumococcus, Staphylococcus aureus, Candida*, and varicella zoster virus.

Six months following HSCT, *Pneumocystic carinii* pneumonia may occur and is associated with an 89% mortality rate. When it occurs more than 6 months after HSCT, mortality drops to 40%.[24]

If infection develops in the immunosuppressed patient, the usual signs and symptoms may be absent. For these patients, even a small rise in temperature, such as 37.2°C (99°F), can be significant. The WBC count is monitored

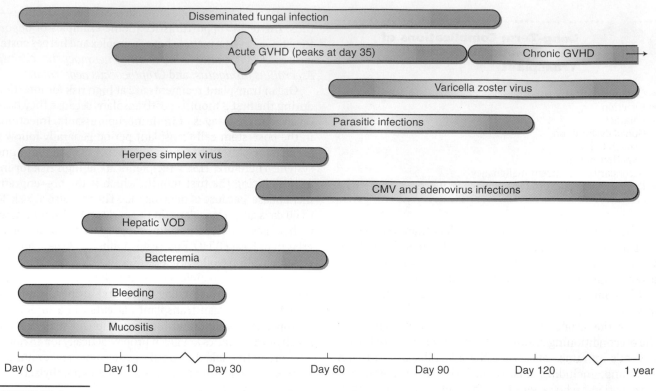

FIGURE 46-4
Sequence of complications following hematopoietic stem cell transplantation.

daily. After organ transplant, the leukocyte count is usually slightly elevated due to surgery and steroid treatment. However, infection may be present if the elevation persists, a rapid elevation occurs after a decline, or there is an increase in immature WBCs (bands).

In kidney and pancreas transplantation, immunosuppressive drugs may be discontinued in the presence of a severe infection so the patient's immune system can be mobilized. Consequently, the graft may be lost to save the patient. In heart, lung, and liver transplantations, immunosuppression is decreased but must be continued.

Additional preventive measures for HSCT patients include protective isolation precautions, air filtration systems, gut and skin decontamination, a low microbial diet, and the use of colony-stimulating factors.

Bleeding

Bleeding, oozing from the surface of the transplanted organ, and development of a hematoma or lymphocele may occur postsurgery. The heart transplant patient is at risk of bleeding because the pericardial sac has stretched to accommodate an enlarged heart. When a smaller, healthy heart is implanted, the larger pericardial sac becomes a reservoir that can conceal postoperative bleeding. This may result in cardiac tamponade. Long-term coagulation therapy and liver congestion from pretransplant heart failure also increase the risk for bleeding.

After liver transplantation, bleeding may occur as a result of coagulopathy due to liver dysfunction or from small vessels that continue to bleed postoperatively. Pancreas

transplant recipients who have had the bladder drainage technique for exocrine drainage may develop postoperative hematuria when the transplanted duodenal segment becomes ulcerated or if cystitis develops. Electrocautery using cystoscopy may be required for severe bleeding.

Recipients of HSCT are at high risk for bleeding and severe anemias. Because of the preparative regimen, which causes pancytopenia, HSCT patients require both platelet and red blood cell infusions until the cells engraft and the blood counts improve.

Gastrointestinal Complications Related to Steroid Therapy

Chronic steroid therapy increases the risk of peptic ulceration and erosive gastritis because it increases the secretion of hydrochloric acid and pepsinogen. Massive gastrointestinal bleeding may occur not only from steroid therapy, but also from stress and decreased tissue viability caused by long-term protein restriction.

For these reasons, patients usually are given antiacids (H_2 antagonists). The degree of renal function dictates which antacid is selected. Liquid preparations are considered more effective. Histamine antagonists, such as cimetidine or ranitidine, may also be prescribed to prevent ulceration.

Other serious gastrointestinal complications include acute pancreatitis, diverticulitis, *Candida*, esophagitis, obstruction from bowel adhesions, and ulcerative colitis. Infection becomes an added risk if the patient has an intestinal perforation. Ischemic bowel disease has been observed in the early posttransplantation period as a result of dehydration or ischemia due to low cardiac output.

More than one complication may occur simultaneously. In addition, signs and symptoms of gastrointestinal bleeding or perforation may be obscured by the antiinflammatory effects of steroids. Therefore, complaints and changes in the patient's progress require thorough and prompt assessment.

The gastrointestinal tract of the HSCT patient may also be affected by the total body irradiation and chemotherapy used in the preparatory regimen. Symptoms may include mucositis, nausea, vomiting, diarrhea, cramping, dyspepsia, anorexia, taste changes, and xerostoma.

Other Hemopoietic Stem Cell Transplant Complications

GRAFT-VERSUS-HOST DISEASE

When the donor's T lymphocytes recognize the recipient's cells as foreign and attack them, producing inflammatory and fibrotic changes in specific tissues, GVHD occurs. GVHD primarily affects the skin, gastrointestinal system, and liver.

Graft-versus-host disease occurs primarily in allogeneic transplants. In fact, the incidence ranges between 40% to 50% in allogeneic transplants. The greatest risk factor is histoincompatibility. Other risk factors include opposite sex donor and recipient (especially female donor to male recipient) and recipients who are over age 30, have had high numbers of blood transfusions, have infection, have a diagnosis of chronic myelogenous leukemia or acute lymphocytic leukemia, and receive donor T-cell infusions posttransplant.

Therapy

One of the primary tasks in allogeneic transplantation is to prevent acute GVHD. Immunosuppresive therapy is aimed at inactivating T lymphocytes that attack the target systems. Patients undergoing allogeneic BMT typically receive triple immunosuppressive treatment with cyclosporine, methotrexate, and methylprednisolone prophylactically. T-cell depletion appears to decrease the frequency of acute GVHD but may also result in failure to engraft, disease relapse, and secondary malignancies. Psoralen with ultraviolet irradiation is used to inactivate T lymphocytes in hopes of preventing both GVHD and graft rejection. In some studies, intravenous immune globulin has decreased the incidence of GVHD.[25] Once acute GVHD develops, it can be treated with steroids, ATG, and monoclonal antibodies.

Chronic and Acute Graft-Versus-Host Disease

Chronic GVHD usually occurs in patients who have had acute GVHD, although it can occur without an episode of acute GVHD. A combination of cyclosporine and methotrexate may decrease the development of chronic GVHD. Once developed, chronic GVHD is usually treated with steroids, cyclosporine, azathioprine, and other immunomodulary agents like thalidomide.

Acute GVHD can occur as early as 7 to 21 days posttransplant but peaks at 30 to 40 days. It targets the skin, liver, and gastrointestinal system. Skin reactions often occur first and include an itchy maculopapular erythematous rash on the palms, soles, ears, and trunk. It may resolve at this point or progress to generalized erythroderma and desquamation. An enlarged liver, right upper quadrant pain, jaundice, and elevated bilirubin and alkaline phosphatase may occur. Gastrointestinal symptoms include nausea, vomiting, anorexia, abdominal cramping, and diarrhea. The diarrhea is characteristically green and watery and in large amounts, and there may be guaiac-positive stool as a result of intestinal mucosa sloughing. Clinical stages of acute GVHD are summarized in Table 46–5.

Chronic GVHD typically occurs 100 to 400 days after transplant, and clinical manifestations may be limited or extensive. In addition to the clinical manifestations mentioned in acute GVDH, chronic GVHD includes scleroderma-like features, such as dermal thickening, fibrosis, dyspigmentation, and dryness. The patient may develop contractures and loss of function. Esophageal involvement can result in difficult and painful swallowing and retrosternal pain from acid reflux. These can result in poor nutrition and weight loss.

PATIENT AND FAMILY TEACHING

Symptoms Hemopoietic Stem Cell Transplant Patients Should Report Following Hospital Discharge

- Temperature above guideline
- Chills, shortness of breath, cough, congestion
- Change in central line site appearance
- Skin rash, "cold sores," mouth sores
- Decreased appetite, trouble swallowing, nausea, vomiting, diarrhea
- Change in color of urine
- Fatigue, pain, bleeding
- Change in level of consciousness
- Inability to take prescribed medications

TABLE 46-5
Clinical Stages of Acute Graft-Versus-Host Disease

Stage	Skin	Liver	Gut
+ (mild)	Maculopapular rash <25% body surface	Bilirubin 2–3 mg/dL	Diarrhea 500–1,000 mL/d
++ (moderate)	Maculopapular rash 25%–50% body surface	Bilirubin 3–6 mg/dL	Diarrhea 1,000–1,500 mL/d
+++ (severe)	Generalized erythroderma	Bilirubin 6–15 mg/dL	Diarrhea >1,500 mL/d
++++ (life threatening)	Desquamation and bullae	Bilirubin >15 mg/dL	Pain or ileus

Data from Armitage JO: Bone marrow transplantation. N Engl J Med 330(12):830, 1994
Buchsel PC: Bone marrow transplantation. In Groenwald SL, Frogge MH, Goodman M, Yarbro CH (eds): Cancer Nursing: Principles and Practice (3rd Ed). Jones and Bartlett, Boston, 1993
Moore JG, Szekley S: Marrow transplantation. In Otto S (ed): Oncology Nursing (2nd Ed). p 576, 1994

HEPATIC VENO-OCCLUSIVE DISEASE

Veno-occlusive disease (VOD) of the liver is a common and often fatal complication of high-dose chemotherapy or radiotherapy that may develop in the first 2 weeks following HSCT. Hepatic VOD is a fibrous obliteration of hepatic venules that leads to portal hypertension, liver congestion, and destruction of liver cells. It may range from mild disease to severe liver failure. Mild VOD persists until hepatic tissue heals and resumes normal function, usually 10 to 14 days after onset, while severe disease can result in multisystem failure. Some studies report an incidence of 25% and a mortality rate close to 50%.[26]

Clinical manifestations include a progressive weight gain, a rise in bilirubin, an elevated alanine aminotransferase, abdominal pain, ascites, hepatomegaly (usually painful), and eventually hepatic encephalopathy. Treatment is supportive and focuses on maintaining intravascular volume and renal perfusion while minimizing fluid accumulation. Sodium is restricted, and spironolactone is given to decrease extravascular accumulation. Mechanical ventilation and pulmonary artery monitoring may be required if excess fluids accumulate in the lungs. There have been attempts to hypertransfuse the patient with packed red blood to increase the intravascular volume and maintain a high osmotic pressure within the vascular space.

■ LONG-TERM CONSIDERATIONS

Organ transplantation can lead to long-term survival. Increasing numbers of recipients lead healthier and longer lives. Complications, however, can occur long after transplantation.

Long-term care focuses on monitoring the patient's progress and adhering to the health care regimen. A major cause of graft loss in the long term occurs because patients do not adhere to the medication regimen. Patients must also be monitored for the development of late complications, including hypertension and cardiovascular disease, chronic rejection, and recurrence of the original disease, such as hepatitis in liver transplantation and recurrent glomerulonephritis in kidney transplantation. There is also increased incidence of malignancy in patients who are immunosuppressed.

Weight gain can be a significant complication posttransplantation as a result of corticosteroid use or because of general improved well-being related to the organ transplantation. Osteoporosis is also a long-term issue for organ transplant recipients, more often for heart and liver than kidney transplant recipients.

The refinement and success of HSCT has resulted in a large population of patients who have achieved a long-term remission of their underlying disease. They must often deal, however, with long-term sequelae and late effects of the HSCT process. In addition to chronic GVHD and infectious processes, this can include cataract formation, thyroid and

---

❀ **Considerations for Home Care Following Hemopoietic Stem Cell Transplant**

- Medication regimen: actions, schedule, and side affects
- Central venous catheter care
- Neutropenic precautions
- Signs and symptoms of infection
- Signs and symptoms of graft-versus-host disease
- Signs and symptoms of other complications
- Daily living activities
- Ongoing health care follow-up
- Surveillance cultures, blood and urine tests
- Access to health care provider to report changes in condition
- Referral to home health care for ongoing education, assessment, and intervention

gonadal dysfunction, growth failure, and secondary malignancies. Total body irradiation may also result in endocrine dysfunction, cataracts, cognitive changes, and secondary malignancies.

Clinical Applicability Challenges

Self-Challenge: Critical Thinking

1. *Analyze the similarities and differences in the care of transplant recipients with other postoperative patients.*

2. *Based on the Patient Care Study in this chapter, determine Mrs. Franklin's strengths and risks during her preoperative and postoperative course. Develop a care plan for her based on your analysis.*

Study Questions

1. *Which of the following factors do not affect the decision about a patient's physical readiness for transplantation?*
   a. Degree of organ failure
   b. Past medical history
   c. Ability to pay
   d. Current infection

2. *In which two types of transplants is HLA matching the most important?*
   a. Heart and lung
   b. Liver and kidney
   c. Kidney and bone marrow
   d. Bone marrow and liver

3. *HSCT differs from organ transplantation in which of the following ways?*
   a. Survival is better with HSCT than organ transplantation.
   b. The goal of immunosuppression in organ transplantation is to prevent rejection of the organ, while the goal in HSCT is to prevent rejection of the host by the donor cells.
   c. Matching donors with recipients is not important.
   d. HSCT has fewer complications.

4. *Which of the following medications are monitored by following drug levels?*
   a. Prednisone and azathioprine
   b. Tacrolimus and prednisone
   c. Cyclosporine and prednisone
   d. Cyclosporine and tacrolimus

REFERENCES

1. 1995 Annual Report of the U.S. Scientific Registry for transplant recipients and the organ procurement and transplant network—Transplant Data: 1988–1994. UNOS, Richmond, VA, and the Division of Transplantation, Bureau of Health Resources Development, Health Resources and Services Administration, U.S. Department of Health and Human Services, Rockville, MD, 1995
2. Evans RW, Manninen DL, Dong FB: An economic analysis of heart-lung transplantation. Costs, insurance coverage, and reimbursement. J Thorac Cardiovasc Surg 105(6):972–978, 1993
3. Evans RW, Manninen DL, Dong FB: An economic analysis of liver transplantation. Costs, insurance coverage, and reimbursement. Gastroenterol Clin North Am 22(2):451–473, 1993
4. Eggers PW, Kucken LE: Cost issues in transplantation. In Kahan BD (ed): The Surgical Clinics of North America: Horizons in Organ Transplantation 74(3):1259–1267, 1994
5. Terasaki PI, Cecka JK, Gjertson DW, Takemoto S: High survival rates of kidney transplants from spousal and living unrelated donors. N Engl J Med 333(6):333–336, 1995
6. Shaffer S, Wilson JN: Bone marrow transplantation: Critical care implications. Critical Care Nursing Clinics of North America 5(3): 531–550, 1993
7. Heffron TG, Emond JC: Living related liver transplantation. In Busuttil RW, Klintmalm GB (eds): Transplantation of the Liver, pp 518–528. Philadelphia, WB Saunders, 1996
8. Starnes VA: Lobar transplantation: Indications and outcome. Journal of Heart and Lung Transplant 12(suppl):594 (abstract), 1993
9. United States Department of Health and Human Services: The Surgeon General's Workshop on Increasing Organ Donation, p 233. Rockville, MD, United States Department of Human Services, 1991
10. Kleiger J, Nelson K, Davis R, et al: Analysis of factors influencing organ donation consent rates. Journal of Transplant Coordination 4(3): 132–134, 1994
11. Sollinger HW, Geffner SR: Pancreas transplantation. In Kahan BD (ed): The Surgical Clinics of North America: Horizons in Organ Transplantation, 74(5):1183–1195, 1994
12. McCullough CS: Pancreas transplantation. In Flye MW (ed): Atlas of Organ Transplantation, pp 197–206. Philadelphia, WB Saunders, 1995
13. Egan TM, Cooper JD: Surgical aspects of single lung transplantation. Clinical Chest Medicine 11:195–205, 1990
14. Calhoun JH, Grover FL, Gibbons WJ, et al: Single lung transplantation: Alternative indications and techniques. J Thorac Cardiovasc Surg 101: 816–825, 1991
15. Bartucci MR: Combined kidney and pancreas transplantation. AACN Clinical Issues 6(1):143–152, 1995
16. Villagomez E: Pancreas transplantation. Critical Care Nursing Quarterly 17(4):15–26, 1995
17. McVicar JP, Kowdley KV, Bacchi CE: The natural history of untreated focal allograft rejection in liver transplant recipients. Liver Transplantation and Surgery 2(2):154–160, 1996
18. Kapoor AS: Complications after heart and lung transplantation. In Kapoor AS, Laks H (eds): Atlas of Heart-Lung Transplantation. McGraw Hill, 1994
19. Starnes VA, Lewiston N, Theodore J, et al : Cystic Fibrosis target population for lung transplantation in North America in the 1990s. J Thoracic Cardiovascular Surg 103:1008–1014, 1992
20. Sharples LS, Tamm M, McNeil K, et al: Development of bronchiolitis obliterans syndrome in recipients of heart-lung transplantation—early risk factors. Transplantation 61(4):560–566, 1996
21. Crouch MA, Ross JA: Current concepts in autologous bone marrow transplantation. Seminars in Oncology Nursing 10(1):28–41, 1994
22. Wujcik D, Ballard B, Camo-Sorrell D: Selected complications of allogeneic bone marrow transplantation. Seminars in Oncology Nursing 10(1):28–41, 1994
23. Grattan MT, Moreau-Cabral EC, Starnes VA, et al: CMV infection is associated with cardiac allograft rejection and atherosclerosis. JAMA 261:3561, 1989
24. Hoyle C, Goldman JM: Life-threatening infections occurring more than three months after BMT. Bone Marrow Transplantation 14: 247–252, 1994
25. Hudson JG, Lawlor M, Pamphilon DH: Ultraviolet irradiation for the prevention of GVHD and graft rejection in bone marrow transplantation. Bone Marrow Transplantation 14:511–516, 1994
26. Baglin TP: Veno-occlusive disease of the liver complicating bone marrow transplantation. Bone Marrow Transplantation 13:1–4, 1994

BIBLIOGRAPHY

Martin SA: Assessing and caring for the infant liver transplant recipient. Critical Care Nurse 16(3):74–88, 1996

47

Common Immunological Disorders

OBJECTIVES

Based on the content in this chapter, the reader should be able to:

- Describe the etiology and immunopathology associated with human immunodeficiency virus (HIV) infection and acquired immunodeficiency syndrome (AIDS).
- Discuss the use of nucleoside reverse transcriptase inhibitors and protease inhibitors in the treatment of HIV infections and AIDS.

- Explain standard precautions and transmission-based precautions and their implementation in the intensive care unit.
- Describe the pathophysiological processes of eight oncological emergencies.
- Identify appropriate assessment data for each oncological emergency derived from patient history and physical examination, clinical manifestations, and diagnostic studies.
- Explain the anticipated medical management and rationale for the treatment of selected oncological emergencies.
- Describe relevant aspects of nursing management for each of the oncological emergencies.

*N*ormally an intact immune system provides protection from disease. When one or more components of this system is weakened or adversely altered, the individual becomes susceptible to disease.

An immunodeficiency that is congenital or inherited is classified as primary. If acquired later in life, the immunodeficiency is referred to as secondary. Examples of secondary immunodeficiency are human immunodeficiency virus (HIV) infection, acquired immunodeficiency syndrome (AIDS), any form of neoplastic disease, or immunosuppression as a result of drug therapy, such as cortisone or cyclophosphamide.

This chapter deals with two areas of secondary immunodeficiency: HIV infections and AIDS and emergent situations precipitated by commonly occurring neoplastic disorders. The reader is encouraged to review Chapter 44, Anatomy and Physiology of the Hematological and Immune Systems. Especially important is the material relating to the immune mechanisms (humoral and cell-mediated immunity, the complement system, and phagocytosis). This review will help the reader appreciate the pathophysiological changes occurring in the conditions discussed in this chapter.

Human Immunodeficiency Virus (HIV) Infection

AIDS was first recognized in 1981. In 1982 AIDS was defined by the Centers for Disease Control and Prevention (CDC), and in 1993 the case definition for AIDS was expanded and updated to include the latest research. An as-yet incurable disease caused by HIV, its hallmark is impaired cellular immunity. The display details the AIDS indicator conditions for surveillance purposes.

Currently, HIV infection appears to be a uniformly fatal disease. It is considered a chronic illness because of the length of time people are living with the infection. Length of survival has improved because of advances in the area of antiretroviral therapy and in the treatment of opportunistic infections that plague this population.

Most patients require sophisticated medical and nursing care during the course of the illness. The person with HIV infection may be admitted to the intensive care unit (ICU)

for the HIV infection itself; for a completely unrelated problem, such as trauma; or for a surgical procedure. It is imperative that critical care nurses understand the disease process and the multisystem complications that may occur.

Epidemiology

It is estimated that 11 to 13 million people worldwide are HIV positive. Of these individuals, 1½ to 2 million are in the United States and Western Europe, about 8 million are in sub-Saharan Africa, and about 2 million are in Latin America. Within the United States, most cases of HIV disease are reported in urban areas. The five metropolitan areas with the highest cumulative totals of reported AIDS cases, in descending order, are New York City, Los Angeles, San Francisco, Miami, and Washington, DC.[1]

RED FLAG **AIDS Indicator Conditions**

Case Definition for Surveillance Purposes

- Candidiasis of bronchi, trachea, or lungs
- Candidiasis, esophageal
- Cervical cancer, invasive*
- Coccidioidomycosis, disseminated or extrapulmonary
- Cryptococcosis, extrapulmonary
- Cryptosporidiosis, chronic intestinal (>1 month's duration)
- Cytomegalovirus disease (other than liver, spleen, or nodes)
- Cytomegalovirus retinitis (with loss of vision)
- Encephalopathy, HIV-related
- Herpes simplex: chronic ulcer(s) (>1 month's duration); or bronchitis, pneumonitis, or esophagitis
- Histoplasmosis, disseminated or extrapulmonary
- Isosporiasis, chronic intestinal (>1 month's duration)
- Kaposi's sarcoma

- Lymphoma, Burkitt's (or equivalent term)
- Lymphoma, immunoblastic (or equivalent term)
- Lymphoma, primary, of brain
- *Mycobacterium avium* complex or *Mycobacterium kansasii,* disseminated or extrapulmonary
- *Mycobacterium tuberculosis,* any site (pulmonary* or extrapulmonary)
- *Mycobacterium,* other species or unidentified species, disseminated or extrapulmonary
- *Pneumocystis carinii* pneumonia
- Pneumonia, recurrent bacterial*
- Progressive multifocal leukoencephalopathy
- *Salmonella* septicemia, recurrent
- Toxoplasmosis of brain
- Wasting syndrome due to HIV
- CD4 count of 200 or less cells/μL.*

---

* Added in the 1993 expansion of the AIDS surveillance case definition.

From Centers for Disease Control: 1993 Revised Classification System for HIV Infection and Expanded Surveillance Case Definition for AIDS Among Adolescents and Adults. MMWR 41, No. RR-17, December 18, 1992

About 51% of the total number of reported AIDS cases in the United States and Western Europe occur among gay and bisexual men. The rate of new HIV infection in this population, however, has dropped to about 1%. The drop is due mostly to the changes in sexual practice within the gay and bisexual community. Women represent about 14% of the total number of AIDS cases, with the majority being caused by intravenous (IV) drug use, while children under 13 years of age account for 1.3% of the total number of reported AIDS cases.[1] Women and IV drug users are the two groups showing the fastest increase in the incidence of HIV infection.

Pathophysiological Principles

Immune defects seen in HIV infection are caused by a viral agent (HIV) from the group of viruses known as retroviruses. Retroviruses are transmitted by blood and intimate contact (sexual) and have a strong affinity for T lymphocytes.

VIRAL REPLICATION

A retrovirus is composed of a small outer envelope, an inner core of genetic material (RNA), and three enzymes necessary for reproduction: reverse transcriptase, integrase, and protease. Like all retroviruses, HIV cannot reproduce on its own. It must invade other cells, in this case the T4 lymphocytes, to reproduce. The process of viral replication is illustrated in Figure 47–1.

HIV enters the recipient's bloodstream, attaches to a T lymphocyte, and then sheds its outer envelope. Viral RNA is then translated into DNA by way of the enzyme, reverse transcriptase. The viral DNA is then incorporated into the T lymphocyte's DNA, in essence tricking the T lymphocyte into making components for more virus. At this point, the cell can remain dormant for an extended time, or it can begin to reproduce. It is unclear why some cells remain dormant and others reproduce virions (structurally intact and infectious virus particles) at a rapid pace. The new virions undergo a process of coating and are then expelled from the host cell by way of budding, a process whereby rather than dividing, the parent cell releases a daughter cell with its share of cytoplasmic material, which begins existence as a separate cell. These daughter cells disseminate through the bloodstream and infect other cells. At some point, the T lymphocyte becomes so engorged that it ruptures, destroying itself and releasing many virions into the system. Figure 47–2 schematically depicts consequences of viral infection.

IMMUNE DEFECTS

Patients with HIV infection exhibit impaired activation of both cellular and humoral immunity. HIV infects the T4 helper cell of the immune system primarily. As discussed in Chapter 44, the T4 helper cell plays a major role in the overall immune response. Infection of the T4 helper cell with HIV

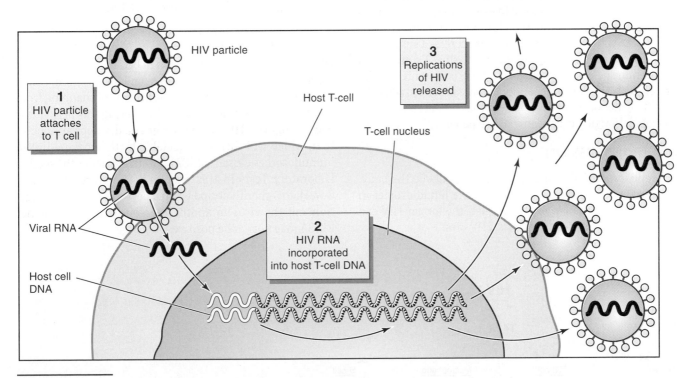

FIGURE 47-1

Process of viral replication. *1,* Human immunodeficiency virus (HIV) attaching itself to a host cell, most often a T cell, and injecting its genetic material (RNA). *2,* The genetic material for HIV becomes part of the cell's genetic material. This changes the host cell into an HIV-producing machine. *3,* Many new copies of HIV are produced from the host T cell. These new copies infect even more T cells. This is replication. (Redrawn from GlaxoWellcome: HIV: Understanding the disease. Research Triangle Park, NC, 1995, with permission.)

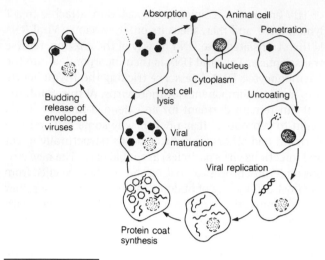

FIGURE 47-2
Schematic representation of the many possible consequences of viral infection of host cells, including cell lysis and continuous release of byudding viral particles.

results in profound lymphopenia with decreased functional abilities, including decreased response to antigens and loss of stimulus for T and B cell activation. In addition, the cytotoxic activity of the T8 killer cell is impaired. Functional abilities of macrophages also are affected, with decreased phagocytosis and diminished chemotaxis. In humoral immunity, there is diminished antibody response to antigens, along with deregulation of antibody production. In essence, serum antibodies are increased, but their functional abilities are decreased. The total effect of these immune defects is increased susceptibility to opportunistic infections and neoplasms. A summary of the immune defects associated with AIDS is presented in Figure 47–3. In HIV infection, antibodies are produced against a specific lymphocyte surface protein that produces the CD4+ subpopulation of T cells seen in these patients.

HIV TRANSMISSION

A fragile virus, HIV cannot survive long outside the body. Survival time depends on the size of the liquid droplet in which it exists; the larger the droplet, the longer HIV can remain alive. As the droplet dries, HIV dies.

HIV has been isolated from all types of body fluids and tissues as listed in the accompanying display. Not all body fluids, however, have been implicated in the transmission of HIV. The four fluids from which large amounts of virus have been isolated and which have been implicated in transmission include blood, semen, vaginal fluid, and breast milk.

The infectiousness of a fluid depends on the amount of virus present in the fluid and the ability of that fluid to reach the target cell, in this case the T lymphocyte. Even though HIV has been isolated in all the fluids listed in the display, the amount of virus present is very low (except in the four fluids associated with HIV transmission). Also, for HIV to cause infection, it must leave the infected individual's body, travel to another person's body, penetrate the skin barrier, enter the bloodstream, and attach itself to a T lymphocyte. The likelihood of all this occurring is low, especially because a certain amount of virus is required to cause an infection. Small tears in the anus or vagina provide a portal of entry for virus present in blood, semen, and vaginal fluid. The virus in breast milk can enter through cuts or irritation in the gastrointestinal tract of the infant.

There are three known modes of transmission of HIV:

- Unprotected vaginal or anal sexual contact with an infected person
- Inoculation with infected blood or blood products
- Pregnancy, delivery, or breastfeeding

One does not become HIV positive immediately after HIV enters the body. In fact, it can take 6 weeks to 3 months after exposure for seroconversion to begin. (Seroconversion is the development of antibodies from HIV infection, which can be detected in the blood—the process of changing from a negative to a positive test result.) During this period, the body recognizes HIV as an invader and develops antibodies to it, which will then be detectable by the enzyme-linked immunosorbent assay (ELISA) (discussed under the section Laboratory Tests in this chapter). Therefore, there is a 6-week to 3-month period when a person can unknowingly transmit the virus to another person because his or her ELISA may not yet be positive.

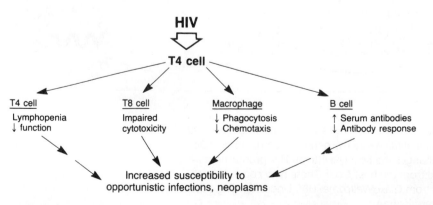

FIGURE 47-3
Summary of immune defects in AIDS.

Potentially Infected Body Fluids

RED FLAG

Blood*   Pleural fluid
Semen*   Nasal secretions
Vaginal fluid*   Pericardial fluid
Breast milk*   Peritoneal fluid
Saliva   Cerebrospinal fluid
Tears   Synovial fluid
Sweat   Amniotic fluid
Bronchial secretions   Soft-tissue fluid

_____

* These fluids have been associated with transmission of HIV.

The risk of transmission to health care workers is low if the Standard Precautions (see display) and Transmission-Based Precautions (see display) are followed. (These guidelines replace the well-known Universal Precautions and Body Substance Isolation procedure previously issued by the CDC.)

Since 1978, 51 health care workers have acquired HIV infection through occupational exposure, and 108 health care workers have acquired HIV through a *possible* occupational exposure. All seroconversions in health care workers have been the result of exposure to blood or bloody fluids or in laboratory personnel working with high concentrations of HIV.[1] The seroconversion rate with percutaneous exposure (needlestick) is reported to be 0.25% to 0.3%.[2]

Summary of Recommended Practices for Standard and Transmission-Based Precautions

RED FLAG

Standard Precautions

- Wash hands after touching blood, body fluids, secretions, excretions, and contaminated items, regardless of whether gloves are worn. Wash hands immediately after gloves are removed, between patient contacts, and whenever indicated to prevent transfer of microorganisms to other patients or environments. Use plain soap for routine handwashing and an antimicrobial or waterless antiseptic agent for specific circumstances.
- Wear clean nonsterile gloves when touching blood, body fluids, excretions or secretions, contaminated items, mucous membranes, and nonintact skin. Change gloves between tasks on the same patient as necessary, and remove gloves promptly after use.
- Wear mask, eye protection, or face shield during procedures and care activities that are likely to generate splashes or sprays of blood or body fluids. Use gown to protect skin and prevent soiling of clothing.
- Ensure that used patient-care equipment that is soiled with blood or identified body fluids, secretions, and excretions is handled carefully to prevent transfer of microorganisms, or cleaned and appropriately reprocessed if used for another patient.
- Use adequate environmental controls to ensure that routine care, cleaning, and disinfection procedures are followed.
- Handle, transport, and process linen soiled with blood and body fluids, excretions, and secretions in a manner that prevents skin and mucous membrane exposures, contamination of clothing, and transfer of microorganisms.
- Use previously identified techniques and equipment to prevent injuries when using needles, sharps, and scalpels, and place these items in appropriate puncture-resistant containers after use.

Transmission-Based Precautions

The following precautions are recommended in addition to Standard Precautions:

Airborne Precautions

- Place patient in private room that has monitored negative air pressure in relation to surrounding areas, 6 to 12 air changes per hour, and appropriate discharge of air outside or monitored filtration if air is recirculated. Keep door closed and patient in room.
- Use respiratory protection when entering room of patient with known or suspected tuberculosis. If patient has known or suspected rubeola (measles) or varicella (chickenpox), respiratory protection should be worn unless person entering room is immune to these diseases.
- Transport patient out of room only when necessary, and place a surgical mask on the patient if possible.
- Consult Centers for Disease Control and Prevention Guidelines for additional prevention strategies for tuberculosis.

Droplet Precautions

- Use a private room, if available. Door may remain open.
- Wear a mask when working within 3 ft of patient.
- Transport patient out of room only when necessary, and place a surgical mask on the patient if possible.

Contact Precautions

- Place the patient in a private room if available.
- Change gloves after having contact with infective material. Remove gloves before leaving the patient environment, and wash hands with an antimicrobial or waterless antiseptic agent.
- Wear a gown if contact with infectious agent is likely or patient has diarrhea, an ileostomy, colostomy, or wound drainage not contained by a dressing.
- Limit movement of the patient out of the room.
- When possible, dedicate the use of noncritical patient-care equipment to a single patient to avoid sharing equipment.

_____

Centers for Disease Control and Prevention: Guideline for isolation precautions in hospitals. Part II: Recommendations for isolation precautions in hospitals. Am J Infect Control 24(1):32–52, 1996

Zidovudine (ZDV, formerly AZT) has been shown to reduce seroconversion fivefold in health care workers exposed on the job. ZDV should be started within 72 hours of exposure or earlier if possible (preferably within 1 to 2 hours postexposure). The decision for initiating postexposure prophylaxis (PEP) should be based on the type of exposure, risk assessment of the incident, and the risk assessment for HIV. The recommended dose of ZDV is 200 mg PO three times a day. Additional drugs may be started, such as lamivudine (3TC), ritonavir, or indinavir, depending on results of the risk assessment.[2] The optimal duration of PEP is unknown, but 4 weeks of ZDV appeared protective in one study and should probably be continued for this period if tolerated.[3]

Assessment

HISTORY AND PHYSICAL EXAMINATION

The patient with AIDS typically gives a history that includes weight loss, fever, night sweats, lymphadenopathy, diarrhea, and a persistent nonproductive cough.

The spectrum of clinical findings ranges from asymptomatic infection with HIV, to a variety of infections and symptoms of decreasing immunocompetence, to unquestionable AIDS. Patients with HIV disease can become seriously ill, thus requiring frequent hospitalizations and care in the ICU. The critical care nurse more often encounters patients with AIDS when they have life-threatening opportunistic infections. It is not uncommon for patients to be admitted to the ICU for an opportunistic illness and be diagnosed as HIV positive at the same time. The most common opportunistic infection requiring admission to the ICU is *Pneumocystis carinii* pneumonia (PCP), an interstitial pneumonia caused by a protozoan. (Recent reports that PCP may be caused by a fungus or algae have not been confirmed scientifically.) PCP is the most common AIDS-defining condition. This pneumonia is accompanied by dyspnea, tachypnea, cyanosis, a nonproductive cough, and initial respiratory alkalosis.

The major indication for critical care of AIDS patients is impending or actual respiratory failure due to PCP. Symptoms of respiratory compromise often are more severe than diagnostic studies such as chest x-rays and blood gas values indicate. Therefore, early aggressive therapy with IV trimethoprim, sulfamethoxazole (Bactrim, Septra), and corticosteroids is the treatment of choice for the person with diagnosed or suspected PCP. Corticosteroids are given to reduce the inflammation caused from the death of PCP in the lungs. Even with urgent, aggressive treatment, many patients require mechanical ventilation for progressive alveolar hypoventilation.

Although single infections may develop in critically ill patients with AIDS, patients often have multiple infections occurring simultaneously and requiring a variety of treatment strategies.

CLINICAL MANIFESTATIONS

No organ system escapes involvement of the HIV infection. The multisystem manifestations that develop are due to the decrease in immune system functioning and an increase in opportunistic infections. These clinical manifestations are detailed in Table 47–1.

TABLE 47-1 CLINICAL APPLICATION: Assessment Parameters
Clinical Manifestations of AIDS

Possible Causes	Possible Effects
Oral Manifestations	
Lesions due to *Candida,* herpes simplex, Kaposi's sarcoma; papillomavirus oral warts; HIV gingivitis or periodontitis; oral leukoplakia	Oral pain leading to difficulty in chewing and swallowing, decreased fluid and nutritional intake, dehydration, weight loss and fatigue, disfigurement
Neurological Manifestations	
AIDS dementia complex due to direct attack of HIV in nerve cells	Personality changes; impaired cognition, concentration, and judgment; impaired motor ability; weakness; assistance needed with ADL or unable to perform ADL; unable to talk or comprehend; paresis and/or plegia; incontinence; caregiver burden; inability to comply with medical regimen; inability to work; social isolation
Acute encephalopathy due to therapeutic drug reactions; drug overdose; hypoxia; hypoglycemia from drug-induced pancreatitis; electrolyte imbalance; meningitis or encephalitis resulting from *Cryptococcus,* herpes simplex virus, cytomegalovirus, *Mycobacterium tuberculosis,* syphilis, *Candida, Taxoplasma gondii*; lymphoma	Headache, malaise, fever; full or partial paralysis; loss of cognitive ability, memory, judgment, orientation or appropriate affect; sensory distortion; seizures, coma, death

(continued)

TABLE 47-1   CLINICAL APPLICATION: Assessment Parameters
Clinical Manifestations of AIDS (Continued)

Possible Causes	Possible Effects
Cerebral infarction resulting from vasculitis, meningovascular syphilis, systemic hypotension, and marantic endocarditis	
Neuropathy due to inflammatory demyelination resulting from direct HIV attack; drug reactions; Kaposi's sarcoma lesions	Loss of motor control; ataxia; peripheral numbness, tingling, burning sensation; depressed reflexes; inability to work; caregiver burden; social isolation
Gastrointestinal Manifestations	
Diarrhea due to *Cryptosporidum, Isopora belli, Microsporidium, Strongyloides stercoides,* cytomegalovirus, herpes simplex, enterovirusus, adenovirus, *Mycobacterium avium intracellulare, Salmonella, Shigella, Campylobacter, Vibrio parahaemolyticus, Candida, Histoplasma capsulatum, Giardia, Entamoeba histolytica,* normal flora overgrowth, lymphoma, and Kaposi's sarcoma	Weight loss, anorexia, fever; dehydration, malabsorption; malaise, weakness and fatigue; loss of ability to perform social functions due to inability to leave house; incontinence and caregiver burden
Hepatitis due to *M. avium intracellulare; Cryptococcus;* cytomegalovirus; *Histoplasma; Coccidiomycosis; Microsporidium;* Epstein-Barr virus; hepatitis A, B, C, D (delta agent), and E viruses; lymphoma; Kaposi's sarcoma; illegal drug use; alcohol abuse; and prescribed drug use (particularly sulfa drugs)	Anorexia, nausea, vomiting, abdominal pain, jaundice; fever, malaise, rash, joint pain, fatigue; hepatomegaly, hepatic failure, death
Biliary dysfunction due to cholangitis from cytomegalovirus and *Cryptosporidum;* lymphoma and Kaposi's sarcoma	Abdominal pain, anorexia, nausea, vomiting, and jaundice
Anorectal disease due to perirectal abscesses and fistulas, perianal ulcers and inflammation resulting from infections with *Chlamydia, Lymphogranulum venereum,* gonorrhea, syphilis, *Shigella, Campylobacter, M. tuberculosis,* herpes simplex, cytomegalovirus, *Candida albicans* obstruction from lymphoma; Kaposi's sarcoma and papillomovirus warts	Difficult and painful elimination; rectal pain, itching, diarrhea
Respiratory Manifestations	
Infection due to *Pneumocystis carinii, M. avium intracellulare, M. tuberculosis, Candida, Chlamydia, Histoplasma capsulatum, T. gondii, Coccidioides immitis, Cryptococcus neoforms,* cytomegalovirus, influenza viruses, *Pneumococcus, Strongyloides*	Shortness of breath, cough, pain; hypoxia, activity intolerance, fatigue; respiratory failure and death
Lymphoma and Kaposi's Sarcoma	Same as above
Dermatologic Manifestations	
Staphylococcal skin lesions (bullous impetigo, ecthyma, folliculitis); herpes simplex virus lesions (oral, facial, anal; vulvovaginal); herpes zoster; chronic mycobacterial lesions appearing over lymph nodes or as ulcerations or hemorrhagic macules; other lesions related to infection with *Pseudomonas aeruginosa, Molluscum contagiosum, C. albicans,* ringworm, *Cryptococcus, Sporotrichosis;* xerosis-induced dermatitis, seborrheic dermatitis; drug reactions (particularly from sulfa-based drugs); lesions from parasites such as scabies or lice; Kaposi's sarcoma; decubiti and impairment in the integrity of the skin resulting from prolonged pressure and incontinence	Pain, itching, burning, secondary infection and sepsis; disfigurement and altered self-image
Sensory System	
Vision: Kaposi's sarcoma on conjunctiva or eyelid; cytomegalovirus retinitis	Blindness
Hearing: Acute external otitis and otitis media; hearing loss related to myelopathy, meningitis, cytomegalovirus, and drug reactions	Pain and hearing loss

Reproduced by permission from Grimes DE: Infectious Diseases. St. Louis, Mosby-Year Book, 1991

CLASSIFICATION OF HIV DISEASE

Initially it was believed that individuals were exposed to HIV, became HIV positive, developed AIDS, and died within a very short period of time. Now we know that individuals who are HIV positive can survive for 10 to 15 years or longer after being infected with the virus.

In 1992, the CDC developed a classification system for identifying in which clinical category a particular individual fits while progressing along the disease continuum from HIV positive to AIDS. The classification system, shown in Table 47–2, is divided into three clinical categories and three CD4 cell categories. When an individual develops one of the clinical conditions in category C or develops a CD4 lymphocyte count less than 200 cells/mm³, then the diagnosis of AIDS is made. If, however, the individual falls within category A1, A2, B1, or B2, then he or she is considered HIV positive.

The AIDS indicator conditions in category C are divided into viruses, fungi, parasites, bacteria, and cancers. The Red Flag display at the beginning of the chapter gives a detailed list of these conditions. All of these agents are always present in the environment. In the immunocompetent person, the immune system keeps these opportunists under control, but in the immunosuppressed individual, such as one who is HIV positive, the immune system loses this ability. Depletion of T4 cells and the resultant increase in opportunistic infections lead to overwhelming problems and ultimately death in this patient population. Table 47–3 illustrates the correlation between CD4 cell counts and various infections and noninfectious complications seen in HIV infection.

DIAGNOSTIC STUDIES

Laboratory Tests to Detect HIV

Several serological tests are used to determine if a person has been exposed to HIV. The most widely used test is the ELISA, which determines the presence of antibodies for HIV. This is a rapid and inexpensive test, with results being available in a few hours. The ELISA has a sensitivity index of 99% and a specificity index of 99%.[4] Unfortunately, the presence of other antibodies can lead to a false-positive result. For this reason, anytime an ELISA is determined to be positive, it is always repeated. If the second ELISA is also positive, a more confirmatory test is performed. The frequency of false-negative results is low, with reports ranging from 1:40,000 to 1:150,000.[5]

The Western blot analysis is the most widely used confirmatory test and is more specific than the ELISA in that it identifies the presence of antibodies to individual viral components. A false-positive Western blot test is possible, but it occurs less frequently than a false-positive ELISA. The Western blot is more expensive and requires more skill in interpretation than the ELISA.

There are several other tests for determining the presence of HIV, but usually they are not used as screening tests for adults. These include the p24 antigen, polymerase chain reaction (PCR), and viral culture. The core protein of HIV is *p24*. Initially, it can be detected in the blood; however, p24

TABLE 47-2   CLINICAL APPLICATION: Assessment Parameters
Classification of HIV Disease

	Clinical Categories		
CD4 Cell Categories	*A* *Asymptomatic,* *or PGL[†] or Acute* *HIV Infection*	*B* *Symptomatic*** *(not A or C)*	*C** *AIDS Indicator* *Condition (1987)*
1) >500/mm³ (≥29%)	A1	B1	C1
2) 200–499/mm³ (14%–28%)	A2	B2	C2
3) <200/mm³ (<14%)	A3	B3	C3

  * All patients in categories A3, B3 and C1–3 (shown in grey) are reported as AIDS, based on the AIDS-
    indicator conditions and/or a CD4 cell count <200/mm³.
  † PGL, persistent generalized lymphadenopathy
** Symptomatic conditions not included in Category C that are 1) attributed to HIV infection or indicative of
    a defect in cell-mediated immunity, or 2) considered to have a clinical course or management that is com-
    plicated by HIV infection. Examples of B conditions include but are not limited to bacillary angiomatosis;
    thrush; vulvovaginal candidiasis that is persistent, frequent, or poorly responsive to therapy; cervical dys-
    plasia (moderate or severe); cervical carcinoma in situ; constitutional symptoms such as fever (38.5°C) or
    diarrhea >1 mo; oral hairy leukoplakia; herpes zoster involving two episodes or >1 dermatome; ITP;
    listeriosis; PID (especially if complicated by a tubo-ovarian abscess); and peripheral neuropathy.

From Centers for Disease Control and Prevention: 1993 Revised Classification System for HIV Infection and Expanded Surveillance Case Definition for AIDS Among Adolescents and Adults. MMWR 41 (RR-17), 1992

TABLE 47-3   CLINICAL APPLICATION: Diagnostic Studies
Correlation of Complications With CD4 Cell Counts

CD4 Cell Count*	Infections	Noninfectious Complications†
>500/mm³	Acute retroviral syndrome Candidal vaginitis	Persistent generalized lymphadenopathy (PGL) Guillain-Barré syndrome Myopathy Aseptic meningitis
200–500/mm³	Pneumococcal and other bacterial pneumonia Pulmonary tuberculosis (TB) Herpes zoster Thrush Candidal esophagitis Cryptosporidiosis, self-limited Kaposi's sarcoma Oral hairy leukoplakia	Cervical intraepithelial neoplasia (CIN) Cervical cancer B-cell lymphoma Anemia Mononeuritis multiplex Idiopathic thrombocytopenic purpura Hodgkin's lymphoma Lymphocytic interstitial pneumonitis
<200/mm³	*Pneumocystis carinii* pneumonia Disseminated/chronic herpes simplex Toxoplasmosis Cryptococcosis Disseminated histoplasmosis and coccidioidomycosis Cryptosporidiosis, chronic Microsporidiosis Miliary/extrapulmonary TB Progressive multifocal leukoencephalopathy (PML) Candidal esophagitis	Wasting Peripheral neuropathy HIV-associated dementia Central nervous system lymphoma Cardiomyopathy Vacuolar myelopathy Progressive polyradiculopathy Immunoblastic lymphoma
<50/mm³	Disseminated cytomegalovirus Disseminated *Mycobacterium avium* complex	

* *Most complications occur with increased frequency at lower CD4 counts; lymphomas may occur at any CD4 cell count but are most frequent with counts <200/mm³.*
† *Some conditions listed as "noninfectious" are probably associated with transmissible microbes: lymphomas, cervical cancer, and CIN.*
From Bartlett JG: Medical Management of HIV Infection, p 14. Glenview, IL, Physicians & Scientists, 1996

drops to very low levels during the latent phase of the disease. As the virus becomes more active, p24 again becomes detectable in the blood. Some clinicians monitor p24 antigen to determine how rapidly the virus is multiplying. *PCR* is expensive and actually looks inside the DNA strain to determine if HIV has been incorporated into the genetic makeup. This test's greatest clinical use is in neonates born to HIV-positive women. About 50% of infected neonates can be identified after birth by PCR. It is an important test to perform because maternal antibodies can be present in the neonate for up to 18 months. *Viral culture* is used to grow HIV. It is expensive and used mainly in research.

Tests to Evaluate Progression of HIV Infection

Several tests used to evaluate the progression of HIV infection include CD4 cell count and percentage (most widely used), beta-2 microglobulin, neopterin, and p24 antigen (Table 47–4). The CD4 count and percentage is an important evaluation tool used to stage the disease and to make decisions concerning the initiation of antiviral therapy and prophylactic treatment for opportunistic organisms. The normal CD4 count is about 1,000 cells/mm³ and declines over time in the person with AIDS (Fig. 47–4).

Other tests used to evaluate HIV infection include the complete blood count, rapid plasma reagin, chest x-ray, serum chemistries, Pap smears in women, purified protein derivative skin test, hepatitis serology, toxoplasmosis serology, and cytomegalovirus antibody serology.

Management

Management of the patient with HIV infection involves a complex, multisystem disease process, multiple hospitalizations, and invasive diagnostic testing. The prognosis is related to the nature of the secondary disease that develops and the degree of immunocompromise. Patients with multiple opportunistic infections tend to be more seriously immunosuppressed and have a poorer prognosis.

CONTROL OF OPPORTUNISTIC INFECTION

The primary goal of management for the critically ill patient with HIV infection is the prevention or resolution of opportunistic infections and nosocomial infections. Management of opportunistic infection(s) is aimed at support of the involved system(s). Because opportunistic infections are the leading cause of death in the patient with HIV infection,

TABLE 47-4 CLINICAL APPLICATION: Diagnostic Studies
Laboratory Markers of Human Immunodeficiency Virus Disease Progression

Test	Description
CD4 cell count	Most widely used test for recognizing HIV disease progression and is recognized as the "gold standard"
	Pivotal for staging and making decisions regarding prophylaxis for opportunistic illnesses and treatment with antiviral agents
	Decreases as disease stage progresses
	Normal, 800–1,050 cells/mm³
CD4 percent	Identifies the percentage of lymphocytes that have the CD4 antigen on its surface
	Less variability than absolute CD4 cell count
P24 antigen	Measures the amount of free viral core antigen
	Not routinely used in practice because of highly variable levels and inconsistence in correlating with disease progression
	Qualitative PCR and bDNA replaced p24 for therapeutic monitoring
B₂-microglobulin	Indicator of cellular stimulation
	Increased levels—cell destruction and generalized immune system activation
	Nonspecific marker of immune system stimulation
Neopterin	Produced by macrophages following activation of immune system
	Nonspecific marker of immune system stimulation
Quantitative RNA PCR	Not approved by FDA
	Assesses viral load
	Good reproducibility
	Detects cell-free or cell-associated viral RNA
	Does not indicate if RNA is from actively reproducing virus or from replication defective virus
Quantitative bDNA	Not approved by FDA
	Used for therapeutic monitoring and staging

prevention is the cornerstone of treatment. Standards of care have been developed for prophylaxis against several organisms associated with opportunistic infections. The current organisms for which prophylaxis is strongly recommended include *P. carinii, Mycobacterium tuberculosis*, and *Toxoplasmosis gondii*. Organisms that should be considered for prophylaxis include *Streptococcus pneumoniae*, *Mycobacterium avium* complex, hepatitis B, and influenza. Organisms and the preferred choice for prophylaxis are listed in Table 47–5. Safe infection control measures to prevent bacterial contamination and complications must be maintained for the patient with AIDS in the ICU.

ANTIRETROVIRAL THERAPY

Two classifications of drugs are used to manage the patient with HIV disease. These include the nucleoside reverse transcriptase inhibitors and the protease inhibitors.

The *nucleoside reverse transcriptase inhibitors* include ZDV, didanosine (ddI), zalcitabine (ddC), stavudine (d4T), and 3TC and remain the mainstay of treatment for HIV infection[6] (Table 47–6). Nucleoside analogs block the conversion of viral RNA to viral DNA through inhibition of the enzyme reverse transcriptase. Initially, drugs were used individually to slow down the progression of the virus; however, monotherapy is now outdated, and combination therapy has gained favor. The advantage of combination therapy

is that the virus can be attacked at different stages in its life cycle, potentially eliminating it from the body. Compared with monotherapy, combination therapy has been shown to delay the progression to AIDS and death.[2]

AZT (now known as ZDV) was the first drug approved to treat HIV infection by the Food and Drug Administration (FDA) in 1987, and it remains the first drug of choice among the antiretroviral drugs. Frequently experienced side effects of ZDV include headache, nausea, vomiting, malaise, myalgia, myopathy, and insomnia. However, with continued use of the drug or a decrease in dosage, most side effects are reduced or resolve. The most serious side effect of ZDV is bone marrow suppression with anemia and neutropenia. When these occur, the dose is reduced or discontinued, and a different nucleoside analog is initiated.

ddI was approved by the FDA in 1991 for patients with advanced HIV disease who were progressing along the continuum despite ZDV therapy or for individuals who were intolerant of ZDV. The most serious side effects of ddI are pancreatitis and peripheral neuropathy, which usually resolve when the drug is discontinued.

ddC was approved in 1992 to be used only in combination with ZDV in patients with advanced disease (CD4+ cell counts <300).[7] The most common side effect is peripheral neuropathy, which occurs in about 17% to 31% of patients. This will usually resolve when the drug is discontinued. The

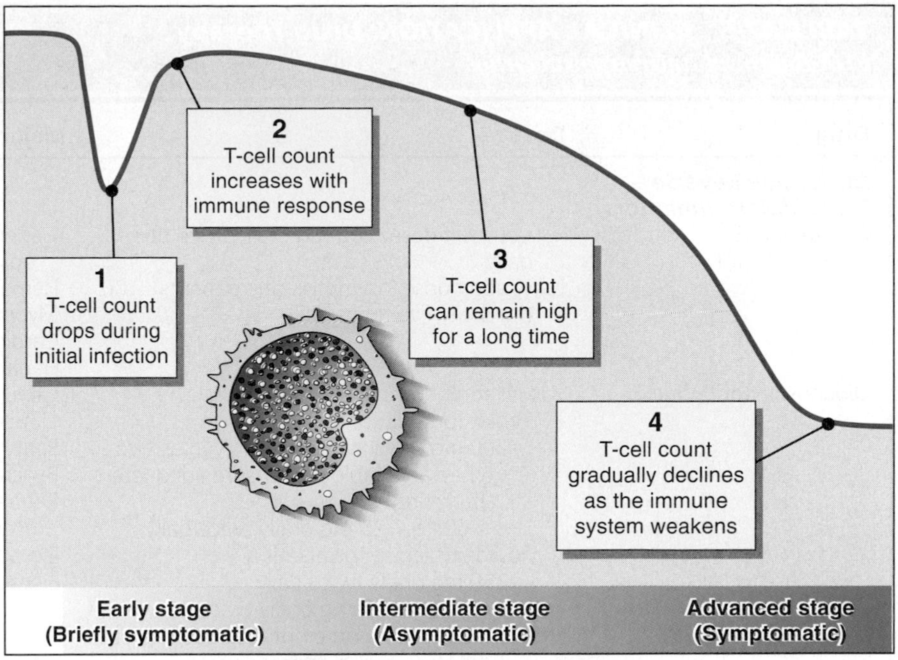

FIGURE 47-4
Use of T-cell count (CD4) to stage HIV infection. *1,* The T-cell count drops during initial infection because the virus is destroying the T cells. *2,* Once the immune system starts to fight back, the T-cell count increases. T-cell counts can go up and down at different times during HIV disease, but they do not return to where they were before infection. *3,* T-cell counts can remain fairly high for a long time—sometimes for years—but steadily lose ground. (Redrawn from Glaxo/Wellcome. HIV: Understanding the disease. Research Triangle Park, NC, 1995, with permission.)

drug is then restarted at half the original dose. Other side effects of ddC include stomatitis, esophageal ulcers, pancreatitis, and hepatitis.

d4T was approved in 1994. Its primary side effects are peripheral neuropathy and elevations in hepatic transaminases. Other side effects are similar to those of ZDV; however, it does not result in the bone marrow suppression associated with ZDV.[8]

3TC was approved in 1995 and has side effects of headaches, nausea, diarrhea, abdominal pain, and insom-

nia, which are all infrequent. It was approved to be used in combination with AZT and not as a monotherapy agent. The most common side effects when given a combination with AZT include headache (35%), nausea (18%), peripheral neuropathy (12%), neutropenia (7%), and anemia (3%).[2]

Nevirapine, which was approved by the FDA in 1996, is the only *non-nucleoside reverse transcriptase inhibitor* available. The primary side effect of nevirapine is rash. With a lower initial dose and continued therapy, however, the rash typically resolves. Other side effects include headache,

---

TABLE 47-5 CLINICAL APPLICATION: Drug Therapy
Organisms Strongly Recommended for Prophylaxis and Preferred Pharmacological Agents

Organism	Patients at Risk	Preferred Agent
Pneumocystis carinii	CD4 count <200 mm³, prior PCP, or HIV-associated thrush, or FUO for 2 wk	Trimethoprin-sulfamethoxazole 1 DS/d
Mycobacterium tuberculosis	Positive PPD (>5 mm induration) or prior positive PPD without treatment or contact with active case	INH 300 mg PO qd plus pyridoxine 50 mg po qd for 12 mo
Toxoplasma gondii	CD4 count <100/mm³ plus positive serology for *T. gondii*	Trimethoprin-sulfamethoxazole 1 DS/d
Streptococcus pneumoniae	All patients	Pneumovax 0.5 mL IM once
Mycobacterium avium complex	CD4 count <75 mm³ or <50 mm³	Rifabutin 300 mg po qd
Hepatitis B	Negative anti-HBc screening test plus high-risk category	Recombivax HB 10 mg IM × 3 or Energix-B 20 mg IM × 3
Influenza	All patients annually	Influenza vaccine 0.5 mL IM each year between October and November

PCP, Pneumocystis carinii pneumonia; FUO, fever of unknown origin; DS, double strength; PPD, purified protein derivative
Adapted from Bartlett JG: Medical Management of HIV Infection, pp 41–42. Glenview, IL, Physicians & Scientists, 1996

TABLE 47-6 CLINICAL APPLICATION: Drug Therapy
FDA-Approved Antiretroviral Drugs

Drug	Dosage	Major Toxicities
Nucleoside Reverse Transcriptase Inhibitors		
Zidovudine (ZDV, Retrovir; formerly AZT)	Usual adult dose: 200 mg orally three times daily Low adult dose (asymptomatic patients): 100 mg orally five times daily	General: transient headache, gastrointestinal upset, fatigue, nail pigmentation Hematological: anemia common, neutropenia Myopathy (prolonged use) Cardiomyopathy (prolonged use; rare) Hepatic dysfunction (can be fatal; rare)

Didanosine (ddI, Videx)	Usual adult dose:
	Tablet formulation:
	  200 mg orally twice daily (given as two chewable tablets to ensure adequate buffering)
	  If <60 kg: 125 mg orally twice daily
	Powder (sachet) formulation
	  250 mg orally twice daily
	  If <60 kg: 167 mg orally twice daily
	Note: administer on empty stomach at least 1 h before or 2 h after meals.
		General: gastrointestinal upset, diarrhea, headaches
		Peripheral neuropathy
		Pancreatitis (can be fatal)
		Retinal depigmentation (only reported in children; rare)
		Elevated transaminases (hepatic failure, rare)
		Elevated uric acid, triglycerides

Zalcitabine (ddC, Hivid)	Usual adult dose: 0.75 mg orally three times daily Approved for use in combination with ZDV	General: rash, stomatitis (includes esophageal ulcer, rare) Peripheral neuropathy Hematological (anemia, leukopenia; uncommon) Pancreatitis (rare) Cardiomyopathy (rare)

Stavudine (d4T, Zerit)	Usual adult dose:
	  40 mg orally twice daily
	  If <60 kg: 30 mg orally twice daily
		Peripheral neuropathy
		Hepatic toxicity
		Pancreatitis (rare)
		Hematological (anemia, leukopenia; rare)

Lamivudine (3TC, Epivir)	Usual adult dose: 150 mg orally twice daily Approved for use in combination with ZDV	General: mild and transient headache, diarrhea, nausea, fatigue Pancreatitis (rare, reported in children with advanced disease) Hematological (leukopenia; uncommon, primarily with high doses)
Non-Nucleoside Reverse Transcriptase Inhibitors		
Nevirapine (NVP, Viramune)	Usual adult dose: 200 mg qd for 2 wk, then 400 mg qd	General: rash (common, can be severe), headache, diarrhea, fatigue, fever, chills, vomiting, nausea, joint/muscle ache, insomnia Hematological: leukopenia Hepatitis

Adapted from Moffenson LM: The role of antiretroviral therapy in the management of HIV infection in women.
Clin Obstet Gynecol 39(2):364, 1996

diarrhea, fatigue, fever, nausea, vomiting, chills, joint/muscle ache, insomnia, leukopenia, and hepatitis.

Another group of drugs proving to be of great benefit in the treatment of HIV infection are the *protease inhibitors*. These drugs provide an even greater increase in antiretroviral activity. Protease is an enzyme necessary for breaking down large polyproteins into smaller viral proteins that are necessary for viral assembly, maturation, and budding. Protease inhibitors bind with protease and block this process, resulting in viral particles that are immature and noninfec-

tious. Currently, three protease inhibitors have been approved by the FDA: saquinavir, indinavir (IDV), and ritonavir. IDV is more potent than saquinavir and seems to have fewer short-term side effects and fewer drug interactions than ritonavir.[9]

VACCINES AND IMMUNE RECONSTRUCTION

Since the causative agent in HIV infection and AIDS was isolated, vaccine development has been actively researched. Attempts at immune reconstruction also are being studied with such agents as interferon. Future research no doubt will develop additional drugs and protocols for the treatment of this disease.

CLINICAL APPLICATION: Patient Care Study

Arthur Jacobs is a 33-year-old man with human immunodeficiency virus (HIV) disease. His social history involves homosexuality and intravenous drug use (IVDU) risk behaviors. He converted to HIV positive in 1989 and was diagnosed with acquired immunodeficiency syndrome (AIDS) in 1990. He has a steady partner and denies IVDU since 1991. He has been involved in various HIV treatment protocols with both ZDV and ddI. Currently he is on ZDV.

Mr. Jacobs presented to the emergency department with complaints of increasing shortness of breath, fever, and pain. He was emaciated (50 kg) and had Kaposi's sarcoma on his face, arms, and trunk. Chest radiography revealed dense infiltrates in all lobes. Arterial blood gases (ABGs) were pH, 7.27; PO_2, 45 mmHg; PCO_2, 50 mmHg; HCO_3, 25 mEq; and SaO_2, 85%. He was placed on humidified oxygen through nonrebreather mask and admitted to the medical intensive care unit (ICU) with diagnosis of R/O *Pneumocystis carinii* pneumonia. He was started on pentamidine, 200 mg daily (due to a Bactrim/sulfa allergy) and was closely monitored and treated with aggressive respiratory therapy.

After 12 hours in the ICU, Mr. Jacob's condition deteriorated. His ABGs revealed worsening gas exchange with a pH of 7.22; PO_2, 40 mmHg; PCO_2, 60 mmHg; and HCO_3, 23 mEq. Mr. Jacobs had decided previously on no cardiopulmonary resuscitation in the event of a cardiac arrest but had stated that he would like to have his pulmonary status aggressively managed until it seemed evident that this episode would not resolve. He did not want to be "lingering on a respirator." The medical team intubated Mr. Jacobs, and he was placed on a ventilator. His postintubation ABGs showed pH, 7.33; PO_2, 60 mmHg; PCO_2, 36 mmHg; and HCO_3, 18. Chest radiography showed the endotracheal tube in good position.

Mr. Jacobs required suctioning every 1 to 2 hours, frequent positioning for postural drainage, and aggressive respiratory therapy. He was receiving 200 mg intravenous pentamidine every day. During his pentamidine therapy, his blood pressure remained stable; however, his blood sugar frequently fell and usually was treated with 50% dextrose when symptomatic. The nurses placed Mr. Jacobs on a specialty bed to provide continuous lateral rotation and to maintain his skin integrity. He was medicated with morphine sulfate for pain (secondary to his Kaposi's sarcoma). His family and significant other (SO) visited often and were appropriately concerned yet remained optimistic. Mr. Jacobs was able to communicate by writing, but as he became weaker, this became more difficult.

On hospital day 6, Mr. Jacobs was showing no improvement. His respiratory status was unchanged, and his white blood cell count dropped to 700 (secondary to the pentamidine/ZDV therapy). Mr. Jacobs' electrolytes were abnormal, and he required frequent potassium boluses to maintain a therapeutic potassium level. Mr. Jacobs' mental status fluctuated between obtunded and confused, and he was no longer able to communicate coherently with his family and SO.

His clinical picture deteriorated further on hospital day 7 when he began showing signs of sepsis and septic shock. His resuscitation status was readdressed with his family and SO. They and the health care team agreed that in light of this clinical development (septic shock), it would be unlikely that Mr. Jacobs would survive this hospitalization. The decision was made to limit his care to supportive and comfort measures. He remained ventilated and received morphine, and within 6 hours, he suffered a cardiac arrest and died without medical resuscitation efforts.

CONCLUSION

As progress toward a cure for AIDS continues, critical care nurses are challenged to use their expertise in assessment, nursing diagnosis, and research to contribute to the understanding and success of future therapies and management strategies to combat AIDS.

CLINICAL APPLICATION:
Examples of Nursing Diagnoses for the Patient With HIV Infection

Risk for Infection related to HIV immunodeficiency and malnutrition

Risk for Impaired Gas Exchange related to alveolar–capillary membrane changes with *Pneumocystis carinii* pneumonia infection

Risk for Fluid Volume Deficit related to diarrhea, dysphagia

Risk for Infection Transmission related to AIDS

Anxiety related to critical illness, fear of death

Knowledge Deficit related to illness and impact on patient's future

Risk for Altered Thought Processes related to HIV or opportunistic infection of central nervous system

Oncological Emergencies

As many as 20% of people diagnosed with cancer develop at least one oncological emergency during the course of their disease. The incidence of these emergencies increases as more patients survive longer. The most commonly occurring oncological emergencies are cardiac tamponade, carotid rupture, hypercalcemia, obstruction of the superior vena cava, sepsis, spinal cord compression, syndrome of inappropriate antidiuretic hormone (SIADH), and tumor lysis syndrome.

Before treatment is initiated, several factors must be considered by the clinician, including existing signs and symptoms, the natural history of the primary tumor, efficacy of available treatment, and treatment goals. Management factors in evaluation and treatment of an oncological

Symptoms and Signs

1. Are the symptoms and signs due to the tumor or to complications of treatment?
2. How quickly are the symptoms of the oncological emergency progressing?

Natural History of the Primary Tumor

1. Is there a previous diagnosis of malignancy?
2. What is the disease-free interval between the diagnosis of the primary tumor and onset of the emergency?
3. Has the emergency developed in the setting of terminal disease?

Efficacy of Available Treatment

1. Has there been no prior therapy or extensive pretreatment?
2. Should treatment be directed at the underlying malignancy or the urgent complications?
3. Will the patient's general medical condition influence the ability to administer effective treatment?

Treatment and Goals

1. What is the potential for cure?
2. Is prompt palliation required to prevent further debilitation?
3. What is the risk versus benefit ratio of treatment?
4. Should treatment be withheld if there is a minimal chance of response to available antitumor therapies?

Used with permission from Murphy GP, Lawrence W, Lenhard RE: Clinical Oncology, p 597. Atlanta, GA, American Cancer Society, 1995

emergency are summarized in the display. Aggressive management of most oncological emergencies is indicated if a histological diagnosis of cancer has not been established; if the patient has a good prognosis with treatment or the possibility of cure or prolonged palliation; or if there is the possibility of restoring functional status. The generally accepted approach to the management of oncological emergencies is to treat the underlying disease with the goal of preventing complications or permanent disability. For terminally ill patients, treatment may be withheld and intervention focused on symptom management.

CARDIAC TAMPONADE

Cardiac tamponade is the result of the formation of pericardial fluid or the presence of a tumor that compresses the heart and causes life-threatening changes in cardiac function. The consequence of the compression is limited filling of the heart with blood in diastole, resulting in lowered cardiac output. At autopsy, as many as 20% of individuals with cancer are found to have cardiac or pericardial metastases. Cancers of the esophagus or lung grow by direct extension into the pericardium, whereas distant primary cancers metastasize to the pericardium through the bloodstream. The most common primary tumors associated with pericardial effusion are outlined in the accompanying display. Radiation pericarditis may be a causative factor, especially if the patient's heart was in the treatment field and if the total dose of radiation therapy (RT) to this field exceeded 4,000 rad (40 Gy).

Pathophysiological Principles

The pericardium is a double-walled sac that surrounds the heart and great vessels. A visceral layer lines the surface of the heart and the parietal layer (or outer layer) moves freely (Fig. 47–5). The pericardial cavity lies between the two layers. It contains approximately 10 to 50 mL of serous fluid. The function of the pericardium is to support the heart in a stable position and to provide a frictionless sac for cardiac contractions.

Neoplastic cardiac tamponade results from the formation and accumulation of excessive amounts of fluid in the pericardial sac. Encasement of the heart by tumor or postirradiation pericarditis can mimic this emergency condition. The severity of the tamponade is in direct proportion to the rate of fluid formation and the volume of fluid accumulated. Slow accumulation may stretch the pericardium so that cardiac contractility is not adversely affected. Normal diastolic filling is impaired by elevated pericardial pressures, and stroke volume is reduced. As stroke volume continues to fall, hypotension, compensatory tachycardia, and equalization and elevation of the mean left atrial, pulmonary arterial and venous, right atrial, and vena caval pressures occur. In an attempt to maintain arterial pressure, increase blood volume, and improve venous return, tachycardia and peripheral vasoconstriction develop. If the tamponade goes undiagnosed or untreated, circulatory collapse ensues.

Assessment

CLINICAL MANIFESTATIONS

Signs and symptoms presented by the patient reflect the rapidity with which the fluid accumulates in the pericardial sac and are mainly those of right-sided heart failure. Signs of

RED FLAG — **Risk Conditions for** Cardiac Tamponade

- Esophageal or pulmonary carcinoma
- Breast carcinoma
- Leukemia
- Lymphoma
- Melanoma
- Gastrointestinal carcinomas
- Sarcomas
- Radiation therapy exceeding 4,000 rads (40 Gy) in vicinity of the heart (radiation pericarditis)

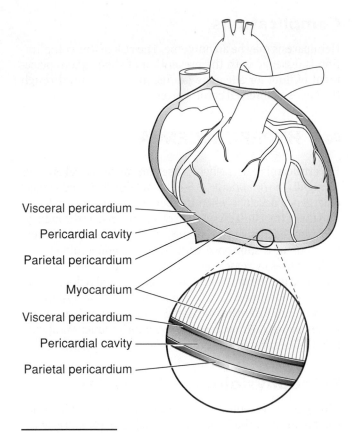

Visceral pericardium

Pericardial cavity

Parietal pericardium

Myocardium

Visceral pericardium

Pericardial cavity

Parietal pericardium

FIGURE 47-5
The pericardium is a double-walled sac that surrounds the heart. The pericardial cavity lies between two layers: visceral layer, which lines the surface, and parietal layer, which is the outer layer.

tamponade include rapid, weak pulse; distant heart sounds; distended neck veins during inspiration (Kussmaul's sign); pulsus paradoxus (inspiratory decrease in arterial blood pressure of more than 10 mmHg from baseline); ankle or sacral edema; pleural effusion; edema; ascites; hepatosplenomegaly; hepatojugular reflex; lethargy; and altered level of consciousness. The patient may complain of dyspnea, cough, and retrosternal pain that is relieved by leaning forward. On occasion, a patient with a large effusion develops epigastric pain, hiccups, hoarseness, nausea, and vomiting.

DIAGNOSTIC STUDIES

A variety of studies are used to determine the presence and severity of cardiac tamponade. A chest film is used to determine the presence of cardiac enlargement, mediastinal widening, or hilar adenopathy. Electrocardiogram may show nonspecific abnormalities, including low QRS voltage in limb leads, sinus tachycardia, ST elevations, and T-wave changes. Echocardiogram is the most sensitive and most specific noninvasive test for the presence of tamponade and is used routinely in most settings. Two distinct echoes may be identified: one from effusion and the other from the posterior heart border. Spaces between these echoes indicate the size of the effusion or thickness of the pericardium.

Right heart catheterization will reveal pericardial tamponade or constriction but is performed infrequently because echocardiograms are routinely available. Pericardiocentesis provides a positive cytological test result in the patient with metastatic cancer. Pericardial biopsy reveals malignant cells.

Management

Emergency *pericardiocentesis* is the intervention of choice if the patient develops any of the following:

- Cyanosis, dyspnea, impaired consciousness, or shock
- A pulsus paradoxus greater than 50% of the pulse pressure
- A decrease of more than 20 mmHg in pulse pressure
- Peripheral venous pressure above 13 mmHg

Oxygen should be administered. Although they are not curative interventions, isoproterenol and volume expansion may be prescribed for administration prior to the procedure to improve cardiac contractility and filling.

Sclerosis can be used to control tamponade. The procedure involves the insertion and maintenance of an indwelling pericardial catheter until drainage stops. Tetracycline (500–1,000 mg) is then instilled through the cannula, after which the line is flushed with normal saline. This protocol is repeated every 2 to 3 days until there is a 24-hour period without fluid drainage. The intrapericardial tetracycline causes an inflammatory response and fibrosis, which obliterate the space between the visceral and parietal pericardia, thus preventing the formation of fluid. Another effective sclerosing agent is bleomycin. A single dose (30 or 60 mg) is instilled after a 24-hour period without fluid drainage. The catheter is then clamped for 10 minutes, after which it is withdrawn. Bleomycin may cause fewer side effects for the patient than does tetracycline, especially less pain.

Inferior pericardiotomy may be performed under local anesthesia. In this procedure a pleural–pericardial window is created, which provides immediate relief of cardiac compression and tissue specimens for histological diagnosis. Less than 5% of patients have recurrence of symptoms.

If the tumor is sensitive to its effects, *RT* may be used. RT has been reported to control more than 50% of malignant pericardial effusions.[10]

Pericardiectomy is used if radiation-induced pericardial disease is not responsive to conservative medical management. This procedure should not be performed if an extensive pericardial tumor is present, because surgical morbidity and mortality rates are high.

Tamponade is likely to recur in 24 to 48 hours if treatment to prevent pericardial fluid reaccumulation is not initiated quickly. Factors to be considered when selecting a therapeutic option include the sensitivity of the primary tumor to specific treatment modalities, previous treatment, and the patient's life expectancy. If effective drugs are available (eg, as in lymphoma and small cell lung cancer), then *systemic chemotherapy* may be initiated after the patient is clinically stable. This treatment may also be effective in patients with leukemia, lymphoma, and breast cancer who develop pericardial effusion.

CAROTID RUPTURE

Carotid artery rupture (or blowout) results in the loss of large amounts of blood, which proceeds, without rapid intervention, to life-threatening bleeding. Patients at risk for this oncological emergency are listed in the accompanying display.

Pathophysiological Principles

Rupture of a carotid artery is likely to occur when that vessel is weakened by invasion of tumor or by surgical manipulation. Other causes of vessel weakness include simultaneous infection or skin flap necrosis.

Assessment

CLINICAL MANIFESTATIONS

The rupture of the artery may occur suddenly with forceful expulsion of large volumes of blood from the damaged vessel; however, the usual first sign of blowout is a small trickle of blood from the neck area. If the skin over the artery is intact, the patient may evidence change in color of the tissue, that is, darkened or eccyhmotic; swelling; and difficulty swallowing or breathing or both.

Management

Digital pressure is the initial intervention in the presence of carotid blowout. A saline-soaked cotton dressing is wrapped around the two middle fingers and constant digital pressure is applied directly to the area over the artery. The nurse must not lessen pressure to see whether the bleeding has stopped nor attempt to apply a hemostat. Either of these steps increases the likelihood of further blood loss. Maintenance of the patient's airway is essential. When help arrives, blood is drawn and sent to the blood bank for typing and cross-matching. An IV infusion line is initiated. Only after the patient is in the operative suite and the operative area has been prepared can the pressure be released. The surgical treatment of choice is ligation of the damaged artery. Chapter 21 contains a detailed discussion of carotid artery surgery with assessment and nursing care.

Risk Conditions for Carotid Artery Rupture

- Invasive tumor of head or neck
- Previous head or neck surgery for carcinoma

Complications

Hemiparesis may be an outcome. The risk of this complication is lessened with the prevention of shock and replacement of fluid for adequate perfusion of the brain through the opposite internal carotid artery.

HYPERCALCEMIA

Hypercalcemia exists when the serum calcium level is above 11 mg/dL (normal range, 8.5–10.5 mg/dL). This oncological emergency develops when the bones release more calcium into the extracellular fluid than can be filtered by the kidneys and excreted in the urine. Some tumors produce parathyroid hormone or a substance with the same endocrine effects, which causes increased resorption of calcium from the bone, increased intestinal absorption of calcium, and reduced renal excretion. However, destruction of the bone by metastatic invasion is believed to be the most common cause of malignant hypercalcemia. Other causes are tumor production of vitamin D–like substances and osteoclast-activating factors.

Pathophysiological Principles

Ninety-nine percent of the calcium in the body is in an insoluble form in the bones. The remaining 1% is freely exchangeable calcium. The calcium of importance is the ionized calcium, which must be maintained within a precise range. Serum calcium levels are regulated by parathyroid hormone and calcitonin. The release of parathyroid hormone from the parathyroid glands stimulates an increase in serum calcium levels, whereas the release of calcitonin produces a decrease in serum calcium levels. See Chapter 41 for a more detailed discussion of the hormonal balance of calcium.

Twenty percent of patients with solid tumors usually associated with hypercalcemia do not show evidence of bony involvement. Certain humoral substances, such as parathyroid hormone–like substances or osteolytic prostaglandins, are secreted by tumor cells. Patients with multiple myeloma have osteoclast activating factor (OAF) produced by the abnormal plasma cells; however, these patients do not develop hypercalcemia unless they have inadequate renal function. Patients with adult T-cell lymphoma have severe hypercalcemia related to the ectopic production of OAF, colony-stimulating factor, interferon gamma, and an active vitamin D metabolite.

As many as 40% to 50% of women with metastatic breast cancer develop hypercalcemia. Estrogen and antiestrogens stimulate breast cancer cells to produce osteolytic prostaglandins and to increase bone resorption. Hypercalcemia resulting from hormonal therapy must be treated before the medication can again be prescribed.

Assessment

CLINICAL MANIFESTATIONS

The severity of signs and symptoms of hypercalcemia often correlates with the serum calcium level. Risk conditions for hypercalcemia are given in the accompanying display.

Risk Conditions for
Hypercalcemia

- Multiple myeloma
- Carcinomas of
  Breast
  Lung
  Kidney
  Head and neck
  Esophagus
  Thyroid
- Lymphomas
- Immobilization
- Dehydration

DIAGNOSTIC STUDIES

The following laboratory study results are elevated: ionized serum calcium, alkaline phosphatase, and immunoreactive parathyroid hormone. Serum phosphate and serum potassium are decreased in the patient with hypercalcemia.

Management

Medical management involves the use of IV fluids and drug therapy to enhance renal excretion of calcium and to decrease bone resorption. Acute hypercalcemia is initially treated with IV normal saline to increase urinary calcium excretion. When hypercalcemia is life threatening, aggressive hydration (250–300 mL/h) and IV furosemide (Lasix) are prescribed.

Most patients are effectively treated with hydration, mobilization, appropriate antitumor therapy, and slowly tapered doses of plicamycin, calcitonin, or corticosteroids. Patients who are not responsive to or do not have the option of chemotherapy must be maintained on hypocalcemic therapy indefinitely, with the serum calcium level monitored at least twice a week. The drugs used most frequently for treating hypercalcemia are detailed in Table 47–7.

IV phosphate, which is effective in rapidly decreasing the serum calcium level, is rarely used because of the incidence of severe complications, such as hypocalcemia, hypotension, and renal failure. Oral phosphates (1–3 g of sodium acid phosphate daily) are safe and effective in controlling mild hypercalcemia.

TABLE 47-7   CLINICAL APPLICATION: Drug Therapy
Most Common Drug Therapy for Hypercalcemia

Drug	Action	Dose	Comment
Plicamycin (Mithracin) (chemotherapeutic antibiotic)	• Reduces number and activity of osteoclasts • Most effective in patients with bone metastasis or bone resorption from ectopic humoral substances • Response within 6–48 h of initial dose; if no response within 48 h, second dose given	Given as bolus through fresh IV line; 15–25 µg/kg/d over 4–6 h for 3–4 d	• Patients rarely develop side effects because low doses are used but the potential exists for serious toxicity. • With chronic use, injections can be given less frequently.
Corticosteroids	• Block bone resorption caused by osteoclast activating factor • May ↑ urinary Ca excretion, inhibit vitamin D metabolism, ↓ intestinal absorption of Ca.	40–100 mg prednisone qd for several days and then taper to lowest effective dose	• Negative Ca balance can be produced in bones after long-term use.
Calcitonin	• Inhibits bone resorption • Causes ↓ Ca level within hours	4–8 units/Kg IV qd or IM or SQ BID. Injection interval can be slowly increased from 12–24 h	• Glucocorticoid is given in conjunction to avoid tachyphylaxis.
Gallium nitrate (Ganite)	• Inhibits Ca⁺ resorption from bone	200 mg qd as continuous 24-h infusion for 5 consecutive days or until Ca level returns to normal	• Adequate hydration is necessary before initiating therapy.
Pamidronate	• Inhibits bone resorption	60–90 mg over 2–4 h or as 24-h infusion	• Response occurs within 24–48 h • Most patients are treated with these diphosphonates.
Etridronate (Didronel)	• Inhibits bone resorption	7.5 mg/Kg body weight in 300 mL saline over 3 h	• Same as pamidronate

Patients should ambulate if possible to prevent osteolysis. Constipation, usually caused by an increased level of calcium in the blood, should be eliminated. Reduced oral intake of calcium may be of some help. Medications such as thiazide diuretics and vitamins A and D should not be prescribed, as these elevate the calcium level.

The patient and family should be taught the signs and symptoms of hypercalcemia so that it can be detected early and treatment initiated before serious problems develop.

Fluid status must be closely monitored because patients may receive up to 10 L of IV fluids daily. Intake and output should be carefully measured. The patient should be carefully observed for signs of overhydration. Potassium supplements may be prescribed.

Complications

Patients with prolonged hypercalcemia may develop permanent renal tubular abnormalities. Sudden death from cardiac dysrhythmias may result from an acute rise in the serum calcium level.

CLINICAL APPLICATION: Patient Care Study

Joe Bell is a 60-year-old man with a history of squamous cell cancer of the lung being treated with radiation. He was brought to the emergency department by his family because of his increasing lethargy. Over the past 10 days, he had lost his appetite, and 2 days ago became drowsy and difficult to arouse and was vomiting after consuming food or fluids. When examined by the nurse, he appeared to be cachectic and chronically ill. His blood pressure was 130/90 mmHg, and his pulse was 90 beats/min. His mucous membranes were dry. Bronchial breath sounds and dullness were noted in the left lung base. He fell asleep several times during the examination.

His laboratory values were as follows:

Serum calcium, 14.4 mg/dL
Serum phosphorus, 3.5 mg/dL
Potassium, 3.6 mEq/L
Urea nitrogen, 45.0 mg/dL
Creatinine, 2.2 mg/dL

Treatment included intravenous fluids, 0.9% sodium chloride 100 to 250 mL/h to correct volume depletion, followed by continued administration at a slower rate as needed to promote renal calcium excretion and hydration. Pamidronate disodium 60 mg IV over 24 hours was ordered. A Foley catheter was inserted, and an accurate intake and output record was maintained. Safety precautions included side rails up at all times and frequent assessment of Mr. Bell's level of consciousness.

Mr. Bell's serum calcium level was 10.5 mg/dL within 24 hours. He was eating well, drinking adequate amounts of fluid, and had no further vomiting. He was alert, oriented, had sufficient urinary output and clear breath sounds, and had begun to ambulate. Plans were made for resumption of radiation therapy treatments. Mr. Bell was encouraged to maintain a program of moderate exercise, avoid bed rest, and eat a diet adequate in sodium. Family members were taught early signs and symptoms to report to Mr. Bell's physician.

◼ OBSTRUCTION OF THE SUPERIOR VENA CAVA

Obstruction of the superior vena cava (superior vena cava syndrome, SVCS) by an adjacent, expanding mass results in venous blockage that produces pleural effusion and facial, arm, and tracheal edema. Severe obstruction may result in impaired cardiac filling and brain edema.

Pathophysiological Principles

The superior vena cava is a thin-walled, low-pressure blood vessel within the mediastinal cavity. It collects blood from the venous vessels that drain the head and neck and the upper thoracic cavity. The mediastinum is a rigid anatomical structure that contains the trachea, the vertebral column, the sternum and ribs, and the lymph nodes.

Most cases of SVCS are caused by mediastinal tumors, which may be an extrinsic mass or invasive tumor. More than 75% are secondary to small cell or squamous cell lung cancers; 10% to 15% are secondary to mediastinal lymphomas. Breast cancer and gastrointestinal tract metastases may also cause SVCS. Obstruction of the vessel lumen by a neoplastic thrombus may occur. The most common nonmalignant cause of SVCS is thrombus in a central venous catheter. Other causes of SVCS are listed in the accompanying display.

Assessment

CLINICAL MANIFESTATIONS

Signs and symptoms of SVCS depend on the rapidity of compression of the superior vena cava. If it is compressed gradually and collateral circulation develops, indications of the syndrome may be more subtle. Initial symptoms occur in the early morning; they include periorbital and conjunctival edema, facial swelling, and Stokes' sign (tightness of the shirt collar). These signs disappear after the patient has been upright for a few hours.

The patient may also complain of visual disturbances and headache. Altered consciousness and focal neurological signs may result from brain edema and impaired cardiac filling. Late signs and symptoms include distention of the veins of the thorax and upper extremities, dysphagia, dyspnea, cough, hoarseness, and tachypnea.

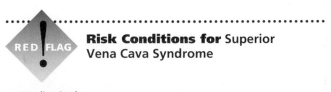

RED FLAG   **Risk Conditions for** Superior Vena Cava Syndrome

- Mediastinal tumors
- Small-cell and squamous-cell lung carcinomas
- Breast cancer metastases
- Gastrointestinal cancer metastases
- Neoplastic thromboses
- Central venous catheter thromboses

DIAGNOSTIC STUDIES

Venography and radionuclide scans will demonstrate compression of the superior vena cava. Chest computed tomography (CT) with IV contrast or magnetic resonance imaging (MRI) will provide anatomical detail and definition of radiation portals. Radionuclide vena cavagrams or angiography will reveal complete obstruction of the superior or inferior vena cava.

Biopsy or cytological tests may be ordered to establish a diagnosis, because many patients with SVCS do not present with a histological diagnosis of cancer. These may include sputum cytology, bronchoscopy with brushings and washings, and node biopsy.

Management

The primary treatment of choice for SVCS caused by a tumor is RT. Dosage depends on the size of the tumor and its radiosensitivity. RT is initially given in high daily fractions (total dose of 30–50 rads) with symptom relief in 7 to 14 days.

Patients with locally advanced non–small-cell lung cancer will have irradiation of the mediastinal, hilar, and supraclavicular lymph nodes and any adjacent parenchymal lesions. RT is palliative for SVCS in 70% of patients with lung cancer and for more than 95% of patients with lymphoma.

Corticosteroids are administered for 3 to 7 days to decrease the edema associated with radiation-induced tumor necrosis.

When SVCS is caused by a thrombus around a central venous catheter, treatment may include antifibrinolytics or anticoagulants and possibly surgical removal of the catheter.

If signs and symptoms continue to be present after RT, there may be tumor outside the treatment portals; if this is the case, invasive diagnostic procedures, such as contrast venography, may be needed.

Chemotherapy may be the treatment of choice in patients with disseminated disease, such as small cell anaplastic carcinoma or lymphoma. The agents used most often are cyclophosphamide (Cytoxan), methotrexate, and nitrogen mustard.

Supportive care of the patient is essential. Maintenance of a patent airway is of the highest priority. Oxygen therapy, diuretics, steroids, and heparin may be prescribed and must be administered with careful observation of patient response. The patient should be taught not to bend over and to avoid Valsalva maneuvers. When the patient is in bed, the head should be at least in a semi-Fowler's position. Elevation of the patient's arms on pillows will help to alleviate swelling; however, the legs should not be elevated because this increases fluid volume in the torso.

▉ SEPSIS AND SEPTIC SHOCK

Bacterial invasion of the circulatory system results in inadequate tissue perfusion. Normal cellular metabolic processes are disrupted with adverse consequences in every major organ system. Sepsis is the most common cause of death in immunocompromised patients.

Pathophysiological Principles

This oncological emergency is seen most often in the neutropenic patient whose immune response is weakened by a decreased number of functional neutrophils. The most common causative agent is gram-negative bacteria. Sepsis results from the release of an endotoxin from dead bacteria. This endotoxin causes secretion of various vasoactive substances, which produce dilation of arterial and venous systems. If the disease is not treated, more endotoxin is released, which stimulates the release of bradykinin and histamine. These substances produce increased capillary permeability and leakage, which in turn causes stagnation of the blood, lactic acidosis, decreased circulating blood volume, and decreased cardiac output. (See Chapter 49 for a detailed discussion of septic shock.)

Assessment

CLINICAL MANIFESTATIONS

Signs and symptoms of sepsis include those of warm shock: chills, fever, restlessness, confusion, flushed and warm skin, tachycardia, tachypnea, and decreased PO_2. If the patient is not treated, progression into cold shock will occur: cool and clammy skin, tachycardia, hypotension, tachypnea, pulmonary congestion, hypoxemia, decreased pulses, decreased urinary output, and bleeding from one or more sites (may be secondary to disseminated intravascular coagulation).

DIAGNOSTIC STUDIES

Blood cultures are positive for gram-negative bacteria. Chest film may reveal infiltrates. The white blood cell count may be either high or low. An arterial blood gas analysis indicates metabolic acidosis. Prothrombin time and partial thromboplastin times are prolonged.

Management

The acronym VIP is used to describe the treatment of septic shock:

- V—Ventilate using oxygen and mechanical ventilation as required.
- I—Infuse with crystalloid and colloid solutions to maintain an adequate blood pressure.
- P—Perfuse with dopamine, which is the most commonly used vasopressor because it improves cardiac output and maintains renal perfusion.

Antibiotics are prescribed empirically and usually include a penicillin, an aminoglycoside, and a cephalosporin.

Supportive care includes monitoring the patient's temperature and reducing fever with antipyretics, ice packs, a hypothermia blanket, and other appropriate techniques; administering fluid volume replacement; monitoring vital signs, urinary output, arterial blood gas values, and hemodynamic stability; and performing blood cultures as needed.

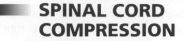

SPINAL CORD COMPRESSION

Spinal cord compression, a grave oncological emergency, results when a tumor in the epidural space exerts pressure on the cord, which may result in permanent dysfunction (including paralysis) if not diagnosed and treated promptly. Tumors most likely to cause cord compression are noted in the display. At autopsy, more than 5% of patients with metastatic disease have been found to have epidural tumors.

Pathophysiological Principles

Epidural tumors usually arise within the vertebral body and grow along the epidural space anterior to the spinal cord. Patients with paraspinal tumors may develop epidural metastases when the tumor grows through the intervertebral foramina from adjacent lymph nodes.

In addition to cord compression caused by metastatic cancer, vertebral collapse from destructive bony metastases can cause both spinal cord and nerve root compression. Permanent neurological damage can also occur if vascular compromise results in prolonged ischemia or hemorrhage. Other disorders producing signs and symptoms of cord compression are paraneoplastic syndromes, radiation myelopathy, herpes zoster, pain from a pelvic or long bone metastasis, or cytotoxic drug effects.

Assessment

CLINICAL MANIFESTATIONS

When a primary tumor presses on the spinal cord, signs and symptoms generally develop slowly. Problems develop more rapidly with metastatic disease. The majority of patients with spinal cord compression complain of progressive central or radicular back pain that often is aggravated by weight bearing, lying down, coughing, sneezing, or performing the Valsalva maneuver and is relieved by sitting.

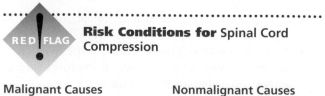

Risk Conditions for Spinal Cord Compression

Malignant Causes	Nonmalignant Causes
• Breast cancer	• Radiation myelopathy
• Lung cancer	• Herpes zoster
• Prostate cancer	• Cytotoxic drug effects
• Multiple myeloma	
• Lymphoma	

The earliest neurological symptoms are sensory changes, such as numbness, paresthesia, and coldness. Compression occurs most often in the thoracic section of the spinal cord, causing neurogenic bladder with urinary retention and incontinence. The patient may also lose the urge to defecate and be unable to bear down. Men on occasion lose the ability to have or maintain an erection. Metastases to the cauda equina frequently produce impaired urethral, vaginal, and rectal sensations; bladder dysfunction; decreased sensation in the lumbosacral dermatomes; and saddle anesthesia. (See Figure 31–10 to review autonomic nervous system innervation.)

The level of cord compression can be determined by the patient's report of pain during straight leg raising, neck flexion, or vertebral percussion. The upper limit of the sensory level is usually one or two vertebral bodies below the site of compression. Lessened rectal tone and perineal sensation are observed with autonomic dysfunction. Deep tendon reflexes can be brisk with cord compression and diminished with nerve root compression.

Once the patient experiences pain, motor weakness and ataxia often follow. The patient may complain that the arms or legs feel heavy. Some patients lose the ability to sense light touch, pain, and temperature. Over time, weakness may progress to spasm, paralysis, and muscle atrophy; the sensations of deep pressure and position may disappear.

DIAGNOSTIC STUDIES

Myelogram or CT scan often reveals a spinal tumor. MRI, which is the procedure of choice, demonstrates complete or partial block of the spinal cord with epidural deposits at other levels. Malignant cells are seen in cerebrospinal fluid obtained by lumbar puncture.

Management

Factors considered in the selection of the best therapeutic option are the level of cord compression, the rate of neurological deterioration, and the patient's previous treatment with radiotherapy. Radiation therapy is used when the tumor is determined to be radiosensitive and should be initiated as soon as the diagnosis of cord compression has been confirmed. Radiation portals include the entire area of blockage and two vertebral bodies above and below this area. More than 50% of patients with rapid neurological deterioration improve with RT. However, patients with autonomic dysfunction or paraplegia have a poor prognosis with either RT or surgery.

Immediate decompression of the spinal cord and nerve roots can be achieved with posterior laminectomy. It is difficult, however, to remove the tumor because most metastases arise in the vertebral bodies anterior to the spinal cord; therefore, postoperative RT is used to shrink residual tumor, relieve pain, and improve the patient's functional status. Surgery is contraindicated if there is a collapsed vertebral body or if there are several areas of cord compression. If there is no previous histological diagnosis of cancer or if infection or epidural hematoma must be ruled out, then laminectomy can be used for both diagnosis and treatment.

If high cervical cord compression precludes surgery, the patient's neck should be stabilized in halo traction to prevent respiratory paralysis. If, despite high doses of steroids and RT, the patient continues to deteriorate neurologically, then emergency decompression should be attempted.

Peritumoral edema and neurological dysfunction can be lessened with corticosteroids. Dexamethasone 10 mg is administered to patients with neurological symptoms before emergency diagnostic procedures are performed and is continued during RT (4–20 mg every 6 hours) and then tapered. It is not clear whether such steroid therapy affects the final patient outcome.

If the tumor is sensitive to it, chemotherapy may be administered concurrently with or soon after completion of RT or surgery. It may also be effective in patients with multiple myeloma who have had previous RT. Systemic chemotherapy or hormonal therapy may be used with certain types of tumors, for example, lymphoma or prostatic cancer.

Pain management should include administration of appropriate analgesics, bed rest, and patient support during position changes and transfer. Range-of-motion exercises are of value to those patients with motor and sensory deficits. Bowel retraining and intermittent urinary catheterization may be needed by the patient. Frequent skin care is essential.

SYNDROME OF INAPPROPRIATE ANTIDIURETIC HORMONE

When thoracic or mediastinal tumors press on major cardiac vessels, the obstruction may impede cardiac output. The posterior pituitary gland perceives this to be a fall in circulatory volume and compensates by inappropriately secreting ADH, which in turn suppresses urinary output. The resulting volume expansion does improve cardiac output but leaves the patient with a relative sodium deficit (dilutional hyponatremia).

The posterior pituitary gland releases ADH in response to changes in plasma osmolality (concentration of solutes) and circulating blood volume. Under normal circumstances, when there is hypotonic plasma or increased blood volume, ADH release is decreased. When there is hypertonic plasma or decreased blood volume, ADH release is increased. Normally ADH release is stimulated by the presence of pain, stress, traumatic hemorrhage, and certain drugs. ADH has its major effects in the collecting duct and distal tubule of the nephron. ADH release causes decreased urine production and volume and increased water resorption.

Pathophysiological Principles

In addition to the pressure of thoracic or mediastinal tumors on cardiac vessels, SIADH can also be precipitated by the cancers and nonmalignant factors detailed in the ac-

---

RED FLAG   **Risk Conditions for** SIADH

Malignant Causes
- Hodgkin's and non-Hodgkin's lymphoma
- Thymoma
- Carcinomas of
    Prostate
    Esophagus
    Head and neck
    Colon
    Pancreas
    Lung (small cell)

Nonmalignant Causes
- Chemotherapy agents:
    Cyclophosphamide
    Vincristine
- Morphine
- Viral or bacterial pneumonia
- Neurological trauma
- Hypotension
- Dehydration

---

companying display. Small-cell lung cancers release an ADH-like substance. Certain chemotherapeutic agents, such as cyclophosphamide (Cytoxan) and vincristine (Oncovin), as well as morphine, may stimulate ADH release or potentiate its effects on the kidneys.

Assessment

CLINICAL MANIFESTATIONS

Signs and symptoms of SIADH are the same as those of water intoxication. When the serum sodium level drops to 120 to 130 mEq/L, the patient usually complains of anorexia, nausea and vomiting, diarrhea, weakness, lethargy, headaches, and irritability. When the sodium level falls below 120 mEq/L, confusion and psychotic behavior may become evident. There is also loss of reflexes and positive Babinski's sign. Other manifestations may include anasarca (total body edema), weight gain, dyspnea, and rales. Further decreases in the serum sodium level result in the patient's loss of deep tendon reflexes, convulsions, and coma. If not treated, the patient usually dies.

DIAGNOSTIC STUDIES

Normal plasma osmolality is 280 to 295 mOsm/kg of water; in SIADH, it is less than 280 mOsm/kg. Normal serum sodium is approximately 140 mEq/L; in SIADH, it is less than 125 mEq/L. Normal urine sodium is 10 to 20 mOsm/kg; in SIADH, it is greater than 20 mOsm/kg. Other abnormalities include decreased blood urea nitrogen and creatinine and increased urine osmolality, hypokalemia, and hypocalcemia.

Management

Treatment of the underlying condition is of primary importance, for example, combination chemotherapy for small-cell lung cancer. Fluid intake is limited to 500 to 1,000 mL/d, which should result in a corrected fluid balance in 7 to 10 days. Demeclocycline (Declomycin), an antibiotic that inhibits ADH secretion, may be prescribed. Adverse effects include diarrhea, nausea, dysphagia, and photosensitivity.

Steroids and RT may be ordered if the SIADH is linked to brain metastases. Diuretics are not ordered except in severe circumstances, because they may produce additional electrolyte imbalances. However, the patient who is comatose or convulsing is given 3% IV hypertonic saline and a diuretic, such as furosemide or ethacrynic acid (Edecrin). In patients with chronic SIADH, demeclocycline 900 to 1,200 mg/d may be prescribed.

The nurse should maintain an accurate record of intake and output, check urine-specific gravity at least every 8 hours, obtain daily weight, restrict fluids as prescribed, monitor laboratory reports of fluid and electrolyte balance, and protect weak and confused patients from injury. Skin and mucous membranes should be assessed for turgor and moistness. (See Chapter 43 for further discussion of SIADH.)

TUMOR LYSIS SYNDROME

Tumor lysis syndrome (uric acid nephropathy) is a metabolic imbalance caused by rapid cancer cell death, which results in uric acid nephropathy.

Insights Into Clinical Research

Silliman CC, Haase GM, et al: Indications for surgical intervention for gastrointestinal emergencies in children receiving chemotherapy. Cancer 74(1):203–216, 1994

Clinical decision making about if and when surgical intervention is required in children with abdominal pain is compounded when the child is receiving chemotherapy for cancer and has an altered immunity. This retrospective study looked at the clinical, laboratory, and radiographic data of 68 out of 1,090 children who developed abdominal complaints that required hospitalization while undergoing treatment for cancer.

Nineteen patients had exploratory laparotomy, and the other 49 were just observed. Between the operative and the nonoperative group, no significant differences were noted in hematological parameters, treatment with corticosteroids or vincristine, or the phase of chemotherapy. Seventeen (89%) of the laparotomies were positive based on the operative report and the surgical pathology. There was a significant correlation between peritoneal signs on physical examination or intestinal air on abdominal x-rays with positive surgical findings. The authors concluded that in the immunocompromised pediatric oncology patient, peritoneal signs and intestinal air on abdominal films were specific for the presence of acute surgical disease of the abdomen.

This information will be useful in the assessment and management of a child receiving chemotherapy who presents with a complaint of abdominal pain.

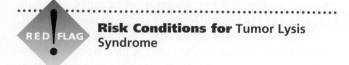

Risk Conditions for Tumor Lysis Syndrome

- Chemotherapy*
- Radiation therapy*
- Hodgkin's lymphoma
- Leukemia
- Chronic myeloproliferative syndrome
- Multiple myeloma
- Squamous-cell carcinoma of head and neck

---

* Precipitate most episodes of tumor lysis syndrome

Pathophysiological Principles

The presence of bulky tumors that have a high growth fraction increases a patient's risk of developing this syndrome, which usually begins 1 to 5 days after initiation of chemotherapy. Patients with conditions listed in the accompanying display have been reported as experiencing this syndrome.

Rapid malignant cell death, with the release of intracellular contents, increases the amount of uric acid in the blood. The increased uric acid results in hyperuricemia and deposition of uric acid crystals throughout the urinary tract, because the kidneys cannot excrete the intracellular metabolites quickly enough. Most episodes are associated with chemotherapy or RT, but spontaneous nephropathy has been noted. The incidence and severity of tumor lysis syndrome have been reduced by the use of allopurinol, aggressive hydration, and urine alkalinization.

Assessment

CLINICAL MANIFESTATIONS

Signs and symptoms of tumor lysis syndrome include oliguria, anuria, urine crystals, flank pain, hematuria, nausea and vomiting, cardiac dysrhythmia, muscular cramps, tetany, lethargy, and confusion.

DIAGNOSTIC STUDIES

Elevated serum uric acid, blood urea nitrogen, creatinine, and serum phosphate are reported. Serum calcium is decreased; urinary uric acid-to-creatinine ratio is greater than one. Renal ultrasound is used to exclude ureteral obstruction.

Management

The goal of cancer treatment is to prevent tumor lysis syndrome. Patients at risk should receive allopurinol, aggressive hydration and urinary alkalinization for at least 48 hours before receiving chemotherapy. Drugs that block tubular reabsorption of uric acid should be avoided, that is, aspirin, radiographic contrast, probenecid, and thiazide diuretics. The goal is to keep the serum uric acid level within normal limits and the urine pH above 7.

Serum potassium and magnesium levels should be monitored closely and allopurinol administered in doses ranging from 300 to 800 mg/d. IV fluids are given to ensure a urine volume of more than 3 L/d. IV sodium bicarbonate (4 g initially, then 1–2g q4h) is administered to alkalinize the urine. If oliguria or anuria develops, ureteral obstruction must be excluded. Once this is done, mannitol or high-dose furosemide should be given in an effort to restore urine flow. Usually a Foley catheter is inserted into the bladder to measure urine output more accurately.

If diuresis does not occur within a few hours after the initiation of treatment, hemodialysis is needed. Within 6 hours of beginning this therapy,, the patient's uric acid levels usually fall by 50% Most patients require 6 days of dialysis before the hyperuricemia resolves and renal function returns to normal. A low-calcium dialysate is used to prevent calcium phosphate precipitation. Aluminum hydroxide antacids may be useful in reducing gastrointestinal phosphate absorption. If peritoneal dialysis is used, albumin is added to the dialysate to increase uric acid protein binding and removal.

The focus of nursing care is on careful monitoring of fluid therapy, intake and output, and electrolyte balance. Allopurinol should be administered as prescribed and the patient's urine tested at frequent intervals for specific gravity and hematuria.

■■■ CONCLUSION

With earlier diagnosis and increased survival time of patients with cancer, emergent oncological problems may be seen with more frequency in the intensive care setting. Understanding the indications for aggressive management and recognition of those patients most at risk for a particular oncological complication will enable the nurse to provide knowledge-based quality care.

Clinical Applicability Challenges

Self-Challenge: Critical Thinking

1. Describe how P. carinii pneumonia results in the arterial blood gas alterations experienced by Mr. Jacobs in the patient care study.

2. Patients and families often are surprised by an oncological emergency. Develop teaching plans that emphasize early signs and symptoms of each emergency using a format that is both informative and easy to display.

3. Explore the ethical dimensions of treating patients with advanced cancer who present to the emergency department with an oncological emergency.

Study Questions

1. The test most widely used to evaluate HIV disease progression is
   a. beta-1 microglobulin.
   b. CD4 count and percentage.
   c. P24 antigen.
   d. neopterin.

2. The average time from exposure to HIV and conversion to seropositivity is
   a. 2 to 6 weeks.
   b. 6 weeks to 3 months.
   c. 6 months to 12 months.
   d. 8 months to 18 months.

3. The four body fluids that have been implicated in the transmission of HIV are
   a. tears, saliva, urine, sweat.
   b. blood, saliva, semen, vaginal fluid.
   c. blood, semen, vaginal fluid, breast milk.
   d. urine, semen, vaginal fluid, breast milk.

4. The patient with the greatest risk of developing hypercalcemia is the one with a diagnosis of
   a. leukemia.
   b. skin cancer.
   c. brain tumor.
   d. multiple myeloma.

5. Which position is safest for the patient with SVCS?
   a. Sims'
   b. Prone
   c. High Fowler's
   d. Supine

REFERENCES

1. Centers for Disease Control and Prevention: HIV/AIDS Surveillance Report 8(1), 1996
2. Bartle JG: Medical Management of HIV Infection, 1996 edition. Glenview, IL, Physicians Scientists Publishing, 1996
3. Centers for Disease Control and Prevention: Case-control study of HIV seroconversion in health-care workers after percutaneous exposure to HIV-infected blood—France, United Kingdom, and United States. January 1988–August 1994. MMWR 44:929–933, 1995
4. Grady C: Laboratory method for diagnosing and monitoring HIV infection. Journal of the Association of Nurses in AIDS Care 4(2):11–23, 1993
5. Barrick B, Vogel S: Application of laboratory diagnostics in HIV nursing. Nurs Clin North Am 31(1):41–56, 1996
6. Moffenson LM: The role of antiretroviral therapy in the management of HIV infection in women. Clin Obstet Gynecol 39(2):361–385, 1996
7. Ungvarski P: Treatment review: Zalcitabine. Journal of the Association of Nurses in AIDS Care 4(3):53–55, 1993
8. Porche DJ: Treatment review: Zerit. Journal of the Association of Nurses in AIDS Care 6(5):50–52, 1995
9. Anonymous: New drugs for HIV infection. The Medical Letter on Drugs and Therapeutics 38:35–37, 1996
10. Personal communication with staff of University of Maryland Cancer Center, 1996

BIBLIOGRAPHY

Bach F: Metastatic spinal cord compression. Topics on Supportive Care in Cancer 3:4–5, 1993
Bechtel-Boenning C: State of the Art Antiviral treatment of HIV infection. Nurs Clin North Am 31(1):1–13, 1996
Casey KM, Cohen F, Huges A: ANAC's Core Curriculum for HIV/AIDS Nursing. Philadelphia, Nursecom, 1996

Centers for Disease Control and Prevention: Guideline for isolation precautions in hospitals. Am J Infect Control 24:24–52, 1996

Centers for Disease Control and Prevention: Update: Provisional public health service recommendations for chemoprophylaxis after occupational exposure to HIV. MMWR 15(22):468–472, 1996

Flaskerud J, Ungvarski P: HIV/AIDS: A Guide to Nursing Care (3rd Ed). Philadelphia, WB Saunders, 1995

Gucalp R, Thevault R, Gill I, Madajewicz S, Chapman R, Navari R, Ahmann F, Zelenakas K, Heffernan M, Knight RD: Treatment of cancer-associated hypercalcemia: Double-blind comparison of rapid and slow intravenous infusion regimens of pamidronate disodium and saline alone. Arch Intern Med 154:1935–1944, 1994

Kattan J, Culine S, Tavakoli-Razavi T, Kramar A, Droz J-P: Acute tumor lysis syndrome in poor-risk germ cell tumors: Does it exist? Support Care Cancer 2:128–131, 1994

Larson E: APIC guidelines for handwashing and hand antisepsis in health care settings. Am J Infect Control 23(4):251–269, 1995

McCorkle R, Grant M, Frank-Stromborg M, Baird S: Cancer Nursing. Acomprehensive Textbook. Philadelphia, WB Saunders, 1996

Murphy GP, Lawrence W, Lenhard RE: American Cancer Society Textbook of clinical oncology. Atlanta, The American Cancer Society, 1995

Rossoff L, Borenstein M, Isenberg H: Is hand washing really needed in an intenve care unit? Crit Care Med 23(7):1211–1216, 1995

Tattersall MHN: Hypercalcaemia: Historical perspectives and present management. Support Care Cancer 1:19–25, 1993

Zeller JM, McCain NL, Swanson B: Immunological and virological markers of HIV disease progression. Journal of the Association of Nurses in AIDS Care 7(1):15–27, 1996

48

Common Hematological Disorders

OBJECTIVES

Based on the content in this chapter, the reader should be able to:

- Describe basic management principles for hematological disorders.
- Discuss two methods of therapeutic manipulation of the immune system in the treatment of hematological disorders.
- Describe the pathophysiological process of disseminated intravascular coagulation (DIC).
- List the abnormal laboratory findings associated with DIC.
- Explain the anticipated medical management and rationale for the treatment of DIC.
- Describe four nursing diagnoses and interventions for DIC.

*A*lthough categorizing either the hematological or immune system alone is somewhat artificial, for purposes of organization and general orientation, discussion of the two systems has been separated in this unit. Full recognition of the reciprocal role of each system must be given in conditions of the other system. Disorders of the immune system are discussed in Chapter 47; disorders of the hematological system are discussed in this chapter.

Topics in this chapter are divided into disorders of red blood cells (RBCs), white blood cells, bone marrow failure, and hemostasis. Considerable discussion is given to disseminated intravascular coagulation (DIC), a major hematological and life-threatening problem.

Disorders of Red Blood Cells

This discussion of RBCs includes summaries of hemolytic, iron deficiency, and megaloblastic anemias; anemia resulting from chronic disease; and polycythemia.

■ HEMOLYTIC ANEMIAS

Hemolytic anemias are those resulting from destruction of RBCs. They may be congenital or acquired and can vary greatly in the degree to which the anemia is experienced.

Congenital Hemolytic Anemia

The most common types of congenital hemolytic anemias are caused by enzyme defects or red cell membrane defects. Table 48–1 lists these congenital hemolytic anemias and their primary interventions. RBCs with a membrane enzyme defect will lyse when exposed to certain stressful conditions, such as drugs, chemicals, infections, surgery, or pregnancy. Substances to which individuals may be susceptible are listed in the display. Hydration and avoiding causative agents is standard treatment for hemolytic anemia from glucose-6-phosphate dehydrogenase enzyme defect. Transfusion and splenectomy may be required in pyruvate kinase deficiency.

Hemolytic anemia from hereditary spherocytosis or elliptocytosis is caused by an RBC membrane defect that gives the RBC an abnormal shape. These RBCs are sequestered in the spleen and destroyed. Splenectomy and folic acid supplements are usually required in hereditary spherocytosis. Most anemias from hereditary elliptocytosis are not as severe; usually no treatment is required other than folic acid supplements.

Acquired Hemolytic Anemia

Acquired hemolytic anemias can be caused by several different factors, as listed in Table 48–2. In microangiopathic hemolytic anemia, RBCs are fragmented by abnormal microvasculature, abnormal cardiac valves, arteriovenous malformations, or DIC. These RBC fragments are called schistocytes and are seen on the peripheral smear. Treatment focuses on removing the causative factor, such as replacing the abnormal heart valve or repairing the arteriovenous shunt. If this is not possible, the patient may be maintained on iron and folate supplements and periodic transfusions of RBCs.

Infectious agents may cause hemolytic anemia indirectly by causing splenomegaly or directly by invading the RBC and destroying its membrane. Malaria is an example of the latter. These patients are treated with transfusion support and anti-infective agents to address the underlying cause.

Abnormally shaped RBCs are frequently noticed in patients with liver disease. These patients may also have congestive splenomegaly, which causes sequestration and destruction of RBCs. In severe hemolysis, splenectomy and supportive RBC transfusions may be required.

Numerous drugs, chemicals, and toxins can induce a hemolytic reaction. These substances are listed in the previous display. Some of these reactions can be severe, necessitating RBC transfusions. Treatment of the underlying cause will vary according to the type of agent that has caused the reaction.

TABLE 48-1 CLINICAL APPLICATION:
Nursing Intervention Guidelines
Management Highlights: Congenital Hemolytic Anemias and Primary Interventions

Type of Defect	Primary Interventions
Enzyme defects	
Glucose-6-phosphate dehydrogenase	Avoidance of agents that trigger hemolysis; hydration
Pyruvate kinase deficiency	Transfusion; splenectomy
Red-cell membrane defects	
Hereditary spherocytosis	Splenectomy; folic acid supplements
Hereditary elliptocytosis	Usually no treatment required; folic acid supplements

---

RED FLAG **Substances That May Cause**
Hemolytic Anemia in Susceptible Individuals

Congenital Hemolytic Anemia	Acquired Hemolytic Anemia
Acetanilid	Chloramines
Nalidixic acid	Nitrobenzenes
Nitrofurantoin	Isobutyl nitrates
Phenylhydrazine	Aniline dyes
Sulfanilamide	Arsine gas
Toluidine blue	Sodium chlorate
Methylene blue	Potassium chlorate
Naphthalene	Wasp and bee stings
Pamaquine	Spider bites
Sulfacetamide	Snake bites
Sulfapyridine	Copper
Trinitrotoluene	Lead
Primaquine	Paraquat
Niridazole	
Pentaquine	
Sulfamethoxazole	
Thiazolesulfone	

TABLE 48-2 CLINICAL APPLICATION:
Nursing Intervention Guidelines
Management Highlights: Acquired Hemolytic
Anemias and Potential Interventions

Acquired Hemolytic Anemia	Interventions
Microangiopathic	Removal of causative factor; iron and folate supplements; transfusion
Infectious agents	Treatment of underlying infection; transfusion
Liver disease	Splenectomy; transfusion
Autoimmune	
Warm antibody	Glucocorticoids; splenectomy; immunosuppressive agents; transfusion
Cold-reactive	Avoidance of exposure to cold; transfusion; plasma exchange
Drug-induced	Discontinuation of drug; transfusion

Some patients can experience autoimmune hemolytic anemias. Warm autoimmune hemolytic anemia is the most common of these types. Immunoglobulin G (IgG) is the autoantibody that attaches to the RBC membrane, resulting in its destruction by macrophages in the peripheral circulation and the spleen. The peripheral smear will reveal microschistocytes due to incomplete RBC destruction. The Coombs' test will be positive for autoantibody on the RBC surface. The reticulocyte count and the indirect bilirubin level will be elevated. Primary therapy is oral glucocorticoids to suppress the immune system. Patients who do not respond to glucocorticoids or require high doses are candidates for splenectomy. Patients who undergo splenectomy will generally still require low maintenance doses of glucocorticoids. If no response is noted following these interventions, immunosuppressive agents, such as azathioprine, cyclophosphamide, or vinca alkaloids, may be used.[1]

Cold-reactive autoimmune hemolytic anemia is a disorder in which exposure to cold triggers complement-fixing IgM antibodies to attach to RBCs in susceptible individuals, causing agglutination and hemolysis. Agglutination in the blood vessels is thought to produce the characteristic acrocyanosis of fingers, toes, ear lobes, and nose. Often these patients have an underlying lymphoproliferative disorder; others may have *Mycoplasma pneumoniae* infection, infectious mononucleosis, or hepatitis. The peripheral smear shows spherocytes, and the reticulocyte count, serum lactate dehydrogenase, and indirect bilirubin are elevated. Susceptibility to cold varies among individuals and correlates with the severity of hemolysis. If these patients require transfusion, a blood warmer and measures to keep the patient warm are recommended. Steroids and splenectomy are ineffective in this disorder; intervention focuses on avoiding exposure to cold. Because IgM is entirely in the intravascular space, plasma exchange may be beneficial.[2]

Hemolytic anemia can be induced by exposure to various drugs. Some drugs, such as penicillin, bind to the RBC membrane and cause antibodies to react against the drug itself. The RBC is incidentally destroyed during this reaction. Other drugs (sulfonamides, phenothiazines, quinine) may bind to antibodies in the patient's plasma, then attach to the RBC, causing its complement-mediated destruction. Finally, a drug, such as methyldopa, may induce the formation of autoantibodies against the RBCs. All of these mechanisms cause a positive direct Coombs' test. Treatment is discontinuation of the suspected drug and RBC transfusions, if required.

OTHER ANEMIAS

Table 48–3 lists common anemias other than hemolytic anemias.

Iron Deficiency Anemia

Iron deficiency is the most common cause of anemia. It occurs when there is excessive loss of iron through chronic bleeding or by inadequate iron intake or absorption. Treatment is to correct the underlying bleeding, if possible, and replace iron using oral supplements. An increase in the patient's hemoglobin will be noticed over a period of weeks. If an increase does not occur, the patient may be noncompliant with therapy or have malabsorption of iron from the gastrointestinal system. Parenteral iron may be given to patients with malabsorption or poor tolerance for oral iron. Severe anaphylactic reactions may occur with this treatment. Intramuscular iron injection may be painful and stain the patient's skin. Instead, intravenous injection with close patient observation is recommended.

Megaloblastic Anemia

Megaloblastic anemias are a group of anemias, most of which are caused by a deficiency of vitamin B_{11} (cobalamin), folate, or both. Once the particular vitamin deficiency is as-

TABLE 48-3 CLINICAL APPLICATION:
Nursing Intervention Guidelines
Management Highlights: Common Anemias and
Primary Interventions

Type of Anemia	Primary Interventions
Iron deficiency	Iron supplements; correction of underlying stressor
Megaloblastic	Vitamin B_{12} replacement; folic acid supplement
Anemia of chronic disease	Transfusion; recombinant erythropoietin; correction of underlying disorder

Insights Into Clinical Research

Crosby L, VA Palarski, et al: Iron supplementation for acute blood loss anemia after coronary artery bypass surgery: A randomized, placebo-controlled study. Heart Lung 23(6):493–499, 1994

In a controlled, double-blind, randomized clinical trial, 121 postoperative coronary artery bypass patients were studied to determine if oral iron supplements were effective in treating postoperative blood loss anemia. Patients were randomly assigned to a control, low-dose, usual-dose, and placebo group. The usual-dose group took 200 mg elemental iron (Feosol) and the low-dose group took 50 mg elemental iron and 60 mg ascorbic acid in a multivitamin daily for 8 weeks postoperatively. Preoperative hemoglobin and hematocrit levels were within normal limits, as were preoperative iron stores.

At 6 days postoperative, all patients showed a decrease in hemoglobin to a mean of 9.5 g/dL and a hematocrit of 28%. At 8 weeks postoperative, hematocrit and hemoglobin had returned to normal in all patients. No significant differences were found among the four groups in hematocrit and hemoglobin levels. Significantly more patients in the usual-dose group reported gastrointestinal side effects.

It appears that if patients have normal iron stores, very little supplemental iron is absorbed, and iron supplementation does not restore hemoglobin levels in acute blood loss anemia following surgery.

certained, the treatment is to correct the deficiency. Cobalamin is poorly absorbed from the gut, and intramuscular or subcutaneous injection is required. The majority of patients will require maintenance injections monthly for the remainder of their lives. Body stores of folate can be restored with oral folate supplement given daily for approximately 4 weeks. Once the deficiency is corrected, maintenance therapy is rarely necessary. An increase in the hematocrit should be noticed by the second week, with a normal hematocrit being achieved by 8 weeks. A suboptimal response may be related to iron deficiency, renal disease, infection, inflammation, thyroid disorders, excessive oxygen administration, or trimethoprim-sulfamethoxazole.[3]

Anemia of Chronic Disease

Finally, anemia is seen with a number of chronic disorders, including renal failure, infections, malignancies, and connective tissue diseases, such as rheumatoid arthritis. Several mechanisms cause anemia of chronic disease. One defect is the apparent inability of the mononuclear phagocyte system to recirculate iron from phagocytosed, senescent RBCs. This causes a decrease in the iron stores available for erythropoiesis. A significant increase in macrophage production also occurs. These cells release cytokines (interleukin-1 alpha, tumor necrosis factor, and interferon) that directly suppress RBC production. Other factors are a decreased RBC survival time and low serum erythropoietin

levels.[4] Treatment involves correcting the underlying cause, if possible. Transfusion may be of temporary benefit, although the survival of the transfused RBCs will be reduced. Recombinant erythropoietin (rEPO) may be the treatment of choice for many individuals. Cost of rEPO and adequate iron stores are important considerations prior to beginning therapy. Potential complications are seen mostly in renal dialysis patients and include hypertension, seizures, arteriovenous shunt thromboses, and increased blood viscosity.

■ POLYCYTHEMIA

Polycythemia is a disorder of increased RBC production indicated by a high hematocrit and an increased RBC mass. This results in increased blood viscosity, vascular insufficiency, decreased tissue oxygenation, and risk of thrombosis. Polycythemia vera is a myeloproliferative disorder of uncontrolled RBC production that is independent of erythropoietin. These patients may also have leukocytosis, thrombocytosis, splenomegaly, and hypercellular bone marrow. Table 48–4 lists additional clinical findings in polycythemia vera.

Patients 40 years old or younger who do not have vascular disease may be maintained by phlebotomy alone. The disadvantage of phlebotomy is that it stimulates bone marrow production, which leads to increased numbers of defective, sticky platelets. Antiplatelet aggregating agents, such as aspirin or dipyridamole, do not reduce thrombotic events and may increase the risk of bleeding.[5] Older patients

**TABLE 48-4   CLINICAL APPLICATION:
Assessment Parameters**
*Clinical Findings and Related Causes in
Polycythemia Vera*

Clinical Finding	Cause
Dizziness, headache	Increased blood viscosity
Thrombosis	Increased blood viscosity, thrombocytosis, platelet defects
Pruritus	Elevated blood levels of histamine and/or increased skin mast cells
Bleeding tendency	Increased RBC-to-fibrin ratio; engorged capillaries and venules due to increased blood volume
Epigastric distress	Engorgement of gastric mucosa; increased blood histamine levels
Numbness and burning of toes	Peripheral vascular insufficiency
Cardiovascular insufficiency	Impaired tissue oxygenation due to increased blood viscosity

with vascular disease are at high risk for thrombosis and require bone marrow suppression with alkylating agents (chemotherapy) in addition to phlebotomy. Hydroxyurea is the agent of choice, because it has not been shown to increase the incidence of acute leukemia, as has been the case with some other alkylating agents.

Secondary polycythemia is caused by elevated levels of serum erythropoietin. This may be a result of chronic hypoxia or autonomous erythropoietin production. Causes for autonomous erythropoietin production include renal lesions, such as renal cysts, renal artery stenosis, or hydronephrosis, and exogenous production by malignant or benign tumors. Treatment is to correct the underlying cause with long-term oxygen therapy, smoking cessation, or surgical intervention as indicated. If this is ineffective, repeated phlebotomy to maintain a hematocrit of 45% or less is required.

NURSING INTERVENTIONS

Anemias in the ICU are most commonly seen in the patient admitted to the unit for other acute illnesses. Nursing interventions primarily are supportive of treatment protocols and of measures to identify the underlying cause. Other important actions include assessing for adverse effects of replacement therapy and for signs and symptoms indicative of decreased perfusion secondary to anemia, such as tachycardia, chest pain, dyspnea, and dizziness.

The patient with p. Vera is at increased risk for thromboembolic events due to the hyperviscosity, especially myocardial and cerebral infarction, deep vein thrombosis, and pulmonary embolism. Measures to prevent thromboembolic complications, such as lower extremity compression devices or facilitating ambulation if the patient's condition permits, should be instituted.

Disorders of White Blood Cells

The following discussion of white blood cells includes neutropenia and lymphoproliferative and myeloproliferative disorders.

NEUTROPENIA

Neutropenia refers to an abnormally small number of neutrophil cells in the blood. Neutropenia can be caused by infection, autoimmune disorders, splenomegaly, or bone marrow suppression. These patients are susceptible to overwhelming infection and sepsis. Treatment involves managing the underlying cause, and the use of anti-infectives and recombinant granulocyte colony-stimulating factor (rG-CSF). rG-CSF stimulates bone marrow production of neutrophils and enhances the activity of circulating neutrophils. Intravenous immunoglobulin and steroids may be used to treat immune-related neutropenia.

LYMPHOPROLIFERATIVE DISORDERS

Lymphoproliferative disorders (disorders in which lymphoid tissue increases by reproducing itself) may originate in the bone marrow or the lymph nodes and thymus. The latter are lymphomas and will not be discussed in this section. Lymphoproliferative disorders of the bone marrow are leukemias.

Chronic Lymphocytic Leukemia

Chronic lymphocytic leukemia (CLL) is a disorder in which there is an increase in the well-differentiated lymphocytes in the bone marrow and peripheral blood. In the majority of cases, the lymphocytes will be B cells derived from a single clone. These B cells function poorly, resulting in progressive humoral immunodeficiency. The T-cell pool in the peripheral blood expands, but most of these cells are helper/suppressor T cells, causing further immunosuppression. Other clinical findings include bulky lymphadenopathy, anemia, thrombocytopenia, and hepatosplenomegaly.

Chronic lymphocytic leukemia is incurable, so therapy focuses on controlling the disease and managing recurrent infections. Early-stage CLL does not require treatment; progressive disease requires treatment with an alkylating agent, such as chlorambucil or fludarabine. Patients experiencing recurrent bacterial infections may respond to treatment with intravenous immunoglobulin. Death most commonly occurs from infectious complications caused by the disease itself or immunosuppressive therapy. CLL can transform into acute leukemia or immunoblastic sarcoma.

Acute Lymphoblastic Leukemia

When a lymphoid cell transforms into a leukemic cell, the result is adult acute lymphoblastic leukemia (ALL). The leukemic clones proliferate and infiltrate normal tissues, especially the bone marrow. A diagnosis of ALL depends on the presence of 30% or more lymphoblasts in the patient's bone marrow. Anemia, thrombocytopenia, and granulocytopenia are common. Patients experience weakness, fatigue, easy bruising, weight loss, and frequent infections. The spleen, liver, thymus, and lymph nodes are usually enlarged. Five to ten percent of patients experience meningeal involvement with cranial dysfunction.[5]

Treatment involves induction chemotherapy for weeks to months to eradicate the leukemic cells and achieve remission. If this is successful, the next step is to prolong the remission through cyclic administration of chemotherapy in the consolidation phase. Lower doses of drugs may be given over months or years in the maintenance phase. The central nervous system is prophylactically treated following remission with cranial irradiation and intrathecal methotrexate. Approximately 90% of adults who undergo intensive therapy achieve complete remission, and 40% are disease-free at 5 years.[5] Relapsed ALL has a poor response to secondary chemotherapy and requires bone marrow transplantation (BMT). BMT may be indicated for high-risk patients in first remission. Other practitioners consider all patients high risk for relapse and recommend BMT to patients in first remission.

■ MYELOPROLIFERATIVE DISORDERS

Myeloproliferative disorders encompass numerous defects in bone marrow production, as listed in the accompanying display. Some of these disorders are discussed in other sections of this chapter. Chronic and acute myelogenous leukemias are discussed here.

Chronic Myelogenous Leukemia

Chronic myelogenous leukemia (CML) is caused by a chromosomal abnormality that results in the proliferation of mature and immature granulocytes, along with splenomegaly. The chronic phase of CML lasts for several years. In addition to leukocytosis and splenomegaly, many patients experience fatigue and weakness. Less common symptoms are bleeding, bone and joint pain, fevers, sweating, and weight loss. The acute phase of CML is called a blast crisis, and in most instances is similar to acute myelogenous leukemia (AML). Twenty percent of the cases, however, may resemble ALL.

Types of Myeloproliferative Disorders

Chronic myeloproliferative disorders
- Chronic myelogenous leukemia
- Idiopathic myelofibrosis
- Essential thrombocytosis
- Polycythemia vera

Acute myeloproliferative disorders
- Acute myelogenous leukemia

Myelodysplastic syndromes
- Refractory anemia
- Refractory sideroblastic anemia
- Chronic myelomonocytic leukemia
- Refractory anemia with excess blasts
- Refractory anemia with excess blasts in transformation

The transformation may be gradual or abrupt. It is characterized by worsening of the above symptoms, as well as increasing numbers of blasts in peripheral blood and bone marrow, and increasing myelofibrosis.

The chronic phase of CML is often well controlled with oral chemotherapy, such as hydroxyurea or busulfan. More aggressive chemotherapy in this phase has not produced satisfactory results. Recombinant alpha interferon can produce remissions in the chronic phase and has shown improved survival rates, especially for patients ineligible for BMT or in later phases of CML. BMT may be performed on good-risk patients in the chronic or accelerated phase with 60% and 40% 5-year survival rates, respectively. Patients with a myeloid transformation who do not receive BMT have a poor prognosis. The blast crisis is less responsive to chemotherapy than AML, and median survival is approximately 18 weeks. A lymphoid transformation is treated with the same agents one would use for ALL. Approximately 60% will achieve a second chronic phase that may be sustained for months to years.[6]

Acute Myelogenous Leukemia

A malignant disorder of hematopoietic stem cells, AML causes abnormal production of the myeloid cell lines (erythrocyte, neutrophil, megakaryocyte, macrophage). The malignant clones proliferate but do not differentiate into mature, functional cells. These cells, which are primarily blasts, circulate in peripheral blood and infiltrate the bone marrow and other body tissues. The proliferation of immature cells and bone marrow infiltration results in anemia, neutropenia, and thrombocytopenia; patient symptomatology is related to these conditions. Splenomegaly is present in approximately one third of patients. Approximately 25% of patients with AML will have a history of myelodysplasia. Nucleated RBCs are often present in the peripheral smear, which is usually due to the presence of blasts. The bone marrow is hypercellular with predominantly blasts present. Patients may require immediate interventions at the time of diagnosis for infections, for anemia, or to achieve hemostasis.

The goal of treatment is to eradicate the leukemic clone and restore normal bone marrow function. Induction therapy with one to two cycles of chemotherapy results in a complete remission rate of 60% to 80%. Intensification, consolidation, and maintenance therapies are given to prolong the remission. Intensification therapy consists of chemotherapy given in higher doses than used for induction, possibly followed by BMT. This has resulted in long-term disease-free survival rates of 40% to 60%.[7] Up to 50% of patients who relapse following first remission may achieve a second remission. Results will depend on the intensity of treatment given for the initial remission, length of time to relapse, and whether BMT was done in first remission.

NURSING INTERVENTIONS

The major goals of nursing care for the patient with leukemia include preventing infection and preventing and managing bleeding related to associated disorders of disseminated intravascular coagulation (DIC), thrombocytopenia, or leukostasis. Nursing interventions are guided by the treatment modality (eg, chemotherapy, radiation, bone marrow transplantation; see Chapter 46). Meticulous attention to infection control procedures and vigilant surveillance of invasive lines and equipment are mainstays of care. Assessment for early indications of infection (fever, chills, tachycardia, tachypnea, etc.) may allow for prompt and aggressive initiation of pharmacological therapies to reduce morbidity and mortality associated with infection in patients with white blood cell disorders.

Disorders of Bone Marrow Failure

Bone marrow failure describes numerous conditions in which the marrow fails to produce precursor cells for the peripheral components, resulting in cytopenias. This section discusses aplastic anemia, myelodysplastic syndrome (MDS), and myelofibrosis.

APLASTIC ANEMIA

Aplastic anemia is a condition of pancytopenia of the peripheral blood and bone marrow. Bone marrow is hypocellular and mostly replaced by fat. In many cases, the cause of aplastic anemia is unknown. Possible factors include drugs, chemicals, viruses, and immunological and congenital disorders. A list of factors is given in the accompanying display. An immunological mechanism appears to be responsible in about 50% of cases. In some patients, aplastic anemia is thought to result from replacement of normal cells by clones of cells that are incapable of normal hematopoiesis. Aplastic anemia causes anemia, neutropenia, and thrombocytopenia; clinical features are related to these conditions.

Mild aplastic anemia is treated by removing any known causative agents and administering supportive care (ie, transfusions) as indicated. Oral androgens and glucocorticoids may be of some benefit. Hematopoietic growth factors may be of temporary benefit in patients who still have some residual bone marrow function. Most patients with mild aplastic anemia will spontaneously recover; however, others may experience mild aplasia for years, which may progress to severe aplastic anemia in some cases.

Severe aplastic anemia is treated with transfusion support, immunosuppressive agents, and BMT. Drugs to stimulate marrow function are of no benefit in this condition. BMT can produce disease-free survival in 70% to 80% of patients 50 years old or younger with histocompatible donors.[8] These patients should be considered for immediate transplantation and should not receive any transfusions or drug therapy prior to transplant, if possible. Immunosuppressive therapy should be used for patients who are not candidates for BMT. Immunosuppressive therapy with antithymocyte globulin or cyclosporine may benefit 50% of patients. Combined therapy with these two agents produces a 60% to 80% 3-year survival rate.[8] BMT may be used for patients who fail immunosuppressive therapy, although the results are not as successful.

MYELODYSPLASTIC SYNDROME

In a group of clonal hematopoietic diseases called MDS (see display in the earlier section on Myeloproliferative Disorders), the precursor cells do not mature, resulting in peripheral cytopenias. Unlike acute leukemia, the abnormal clone expands slowly and retains the ability to differentiate.

> **RED FLAG** **Risk Factors for** Aplastic Anemia
>
> Idiopathic
> Irradiation
> Drugs:
> - Chloramphenicol
> - Phenylbutazone
> - Quinine derivatives
> - Sulfonamides
> - Cimetidine
> - Gold salts
> - Hydantoins
> Chemicals:
> - Benzene and benzene derivatives
> - Insecticides
> - Cleaning solvents
> Viral
> - Non-A, non-B hepatitis
> - Epstein-Barr virus
> - Human immunodeficiency virus
> Immunological
> - Graft-versus-host disease
> - Systemic lupus erythematosus
> - Thymoma
> Pregnancy
> Congenital
> - Fanconi's anemia
> - Schwakman-Diamond syndrome

Over time, however, the abnormal clone suppresses normal bone marrow function, causing severe and fatal pancytopenia or an acute leukemia–like condition. In most cases, the cause of MDS is unknown. Known causative agents include alkylating agents, irradiation, and benzene. Symptoms are related to bone marrow failure and include pallor, fatigue, infection, bruising, and bleeding. The peripheral blood shows pancytopenia, often with monocytosis and abnormal cells from all three cell lines.

The only curative treatment for MDS is BMT, which has a long-term disease-free survival of 40% to 50%. Glucocorticoids and androgens are of very little benefit. Intensive chemotherapy, similar to therapy in AML, produces a 30% to 60% complete response, but the duration of the response in most patients in less than 12 months.[8] Patients will require transfusion support and treatment of infectious complications. Hematopoietic growth factors have improved neutrophil and RBC counts in some patients. Survival for MDS ranges from 1 to 10 years; patients eventually die from progressive pancytopenia or develop acute leukemia.

MYELOFIBROSIS

Myelofibrosis is fibrosis of the bone marrow that occurs as a result of hematological disease or as a response to other disorders, such as malignant infiltration of bone marrow, infectious agents, or granulomatous disorders. Primary myelofibrosis, also known as idiopathic myelofibrosis (IMF) is caused by clonal proliferation of an abnormal hematopoietic progenitor and is considered a myeloproliferative disorder (see previous display under Myeloproliferative Disorders). The abnormal hematopoietic clone may produce a substance that results in the proliferation of fibroblasts in the bone marrow.[8] Patients experience a slowly progressive anemia due to ineffective RBC production and low-grade hemolysis. Thrombocytopenia occurs as IMF worsens, and immature myeloid precursors are noted in the peripheral blood smear. Other clinical findings are pallor, fever, night sweats, anorexia, fatigue, and hepatosplenomegaly. No aspirate is usually obtained from the bone marrow, and biopsy shows fibrosis and osteosclerosis.

Asymptomatic IMF requires no treatment. Symptomatic anemia is treated with transfusion; some patients also respond to androgens. Corticosteroids are used if hemolysis is present. Thrombocytopenia is treated with platelet transfusions, but long-term management is difficult because of hypersplenism and alloimmunization. Hypersplenism may be treated with irradiation, splenectomy, busulfan, or alpha-interferon. Few patients have received BMT. Survival averages approximately 5 years. Most patients with IMF develop refractory thrombocytopenia and neutropenia, and death results from bleeding or infection.

NURSING INTERVENTIONS

Nursing interventions for the patient with a disorder of the bone marrow is dependent on choice of treatment and seriousness of the illness. Prevention of infection, assessment for signs and symptoms of bleeding, and institution of bleeding precautions are paramount. Most patients in the ICU setting are seen as a result of bone marrow transplantation, which is the curative treatment for a majority of these disorders. Nursing care of these patients is discussed in detail in Chapter 46.

Disorders of Hemostasis

Disorders of hemostasis include bleeding disorders, immune thrombocytopenic purpura (ITP), and thrombotic thrombocytopenic purpura (TTP).

BLEEDING DISORDERS

Management of bleeding disorders involves correcting the coagulation factor deficiency and treating sequelae that occur as a result of abnormal bleeding. Bleeding disorders vary greatly in their severity; not all patients with a bleeding disorder will require intervention. Treatment of most bleeding disorders is administered by the patient at home at the start of the bleeding episode. However, more recent evidence suggests that complications in hemophilia, such as hemarthroses, may be minimized with regular, prophylactic administration of factor. Patients with mild hemo-philia A and mild von Willebrand's factor deficiency may respond to intravenous or nasal spray administration of desmopressin acetate, a hormone that temporarily stimulates the release of factor VIII to control bleeding.[9]

More severe cases of hemophilia A or active bleeding require intravenous infusion of factor VIII concentrate. Bleeding in hemophilia B is controlled with intravenous infusions of factor IX concentrate. Patients with more severe presentations of von Willebrand's disease will require factor VIII concentrate that contains von Willebrand factor. Von Willebrand's factor is also found in cryoprecipitate, and factors VIII and IX are in fresh frozen plasma. Epsilon-aminocaproic acid is an antifibrinolytic agent used in bleeding disorders to control mucous membrane bleeding in the mouth and nose.

Numerous complications can occur as a result of bleeding disorders. These are listed in Table 48–5. Additional problems experienced by patients with bleeding disorders

Table 48-5 Complications in Bleeding Disorders

Bleeding Site	Complication
Abdomen	Hypotension, hypovolemic shock
Muscle	Compartment syndrome
Joint	Hemarthrosis with destruction of bone and cartilage in joint capsule
Intracranial	Increased intracranial pressure
Retropharyngeal	Airway obstruction
Urinary tract	Clots in ureters (especially after factor administration)

include the high cost of factor replacement therapy, intravenous access, transfusion-associated hepatitis, and chronic pain from joint destruction.

IMMUNE THROMBOCYTOPENIC PURPURA

There are two distinct forms of ITP. The acute form typically occurs in childhood and may resolve spontaneously in several weeks. Autoimmune platelet destruction appears to be stimulated following a viral illness. Chronic ITP generally occurs in adults. The platelet membrane is coated with an autoantibody (usually IgG), and the sensitized platelets are destroyed in the reticuloendothelial system of the spleen and liver. At least half the cases of ITP have no known causative agent; other patients may have underlying autoimmune, rheumatic, or lymphoproliferative diseases or human immunodeficiency virus infection. The main clinical feature of patients with ITP is bleeding that may have a gradual or abrupt onset. Bone marrow examination shows increased megakaryocytes, but this is typical for other thrombocytopenic disorders as well. The sensitivity of antiplatelet antibody tests is highly variable. ITP is diagnosed by ruling out other disorders of platelet destruction, including DIC, TTP, and drug-induced thrombocytopenia.

Patients with mild to moderate thrombocytopenia without bleeding require no treatment. The severity of thrombocytopenia in these patients can be exacerbated, however, by even mild viral infections. Initial therapy for ITP may be immunosuppression with corticosteroids. A short course of prednisone may be sufficient to induce a remission, but only 10% to 30% obtain long-term remission with steroids alone. Patients refractory to steroids or unable to tolerate steroid tapering may require splenectomy, which has a sustained remission rate of approximately 60%.[10] Intravenous immunoglobulin (IV IgG) is a highly successful treatment in patients at high risk for bleeding who require intervention. IV IgG is also used in thrombocytopenic patients who have undergone splenectomy.

Patients refractory to the previous interventions may receive treatment with drugs such as azathioprine, vincristine, cyclophosphamide, colchicine, and danazole. Plasmapheresis may be used to remove alloantibodies and prolong the survival of transfused platelets.

THROMBOTIC THROMBOCYTOPENIC PURPURA

In TTP, a rare, acute, often fatal disorder, platelets become sensitized and clump in blood vessels, causing occlusion. This process causes the following:

- Thrombocytopenia due to increased consumption of platelets
- Microangiopathic hemolytic anemia due to rupture of RBCs as they try to pass through partially occluded blood vessels
- Fluctuating and often bizarre neurological abnormalities due to interrupted blood flow to the brain
- Renal dysfunction due to obstruction of intraglomerular capillaries and infarction of the renal cortex
- Fever, which is possibly due to hemolysis or vascular infarction of the hypothalamus[11]

Not all five characteristics must necessarily be present. Clinical features are described further in Table 48–6. Initiation of the disease process may be related to immune-

TABLE 48-6   CLINICAL APPLICATION: Assessment Parameters
Clinical Manifestations of Thrombotic Thrombocytopenic Purpura

Abnormality	Findings
Thrombocytopenia	Bleeding, ecchymosis, purpura at various sites
Hemolytic anemia	Schistocytes, reticulocytosis, elevated serum lactate dehydrogenase and bilirubin, jaundice, pallor, weakness
Neurological abnormalities	Headache, mental changes, confusion, visual problems, seizures, coma, aphasia, dysphasia, paresthesias
Renal dysfunction	Proteinuria, microscopic hematuria, elevated blood urea nitrogen and creatinine, renal failure
Fever	Persistent elevation of temperature during acute phase
Other	Abdominal pain, malaise, nausea, vomiting, weakness, ECG changes

mediated endothelial damage, causing platelet aggregation. Autoimmune disorders, viral and bacterial infections, toxic agents, and genetic predisposition may also be involved in the development of TTP.

Primary treatment of TTP is based on the knowledge that patients with TTP have absent or decreased levels of platelet-aggregating factor inhibitor, which is normally present in plasma.[12] Plasma exchange, in which plasmapheresis is used to remove 2 to 3 L of the patient's plasma and an equal amount of fresh plasma is given as replacement, is initiated as quickly as possible and repeated daily for 5 to 10 days. Administration of fresh frozen plasma or cryosupernatant plasma alone has also improved patient conditions, possibly because the patient's own plasma may be missing a necessary regulatory factor. To protect the endothelium from further damage, prednisone is also initiated immediately. Antiplatelet agents, such as aspirin and dipyridamole, may be used to inhibit platelet aggregation. Intravenous immunoglobulin and splenectomy may be used if TTP relapses after the initial response; vincristine may also be given as an immunosuppressive agent. Platelet transfusion is contraindicated even in severe thrombocytopenia, because it may exacerbate the thrombotic process. Despite the previous interventions, acute, severe TTP has a mortality rate of 30% to 40%. Early recognition and prompt initiation of treatment may improve patient survival. Long-term follow-up of patients with TTP is required; 20% to 40% relapse following the initial remission.[13]

■ NURSING INTERVENTIONS

As illustrated in the following Patient Care Study, patients with bleeding disorders may be critically ill. Assessment of the extent of bleeding or the risk for bleeding is a primary nursing intervention. The risk of bleeding increases exponentially when the platelet count drops below 20,000/mm³. Platelet counts below 5,000/mm³ are associated with GI bleeding and the possibility of spontaneous intracranial hemorrhage. Avoidance of trauma is essential and may even preclude the placement of central venous catheters in some situations.

If platelet transfusions are indicated, the patient must be monitored for allergic reactions, anaphylaxis, and volume overload. Evaluation of continued blood loss and assessment of laboratory data for adequacy of the platelet count are important measures. Further nursing interventions are dictated by other treatment protocols such as the use of immunosuppressive drugs and plasmapheresis.

CLINICAL APPLICATION: Patient Care Study

M.C. is a 37-year-old African American woman with a history of systemic lupus erythematosus. She presented to the emergency department complaining of worsening fatigue, bruising, and persistent vaginal bleeding. Her responses during the history and physical examination were vague and disorganized, and she complained of blurred vision and a persistent headache.

Lab Results

Hgb, 6.2 g/dL
Hct, 18.1%

platelets, 8,000/mm³
reticulocytes, 5.9% peripheral blood smear; schistocytes
serum LDH, 997 U/L
serum bilirubin, 4.3 mg/dL
BUN, 32 mg/dL
serum creatinine, 1.4 mg/dL
urine RBCs: many; urine WBCs: few; urine protein: 1+

Physical Findings

Vital signs: pulse, 112; respirations, 26; blood pressure, 100/64 mmHg; temperature, 37.1°C (98.8°F)
Skin/mucous membranes: multiple ecchymoses, gingival oozing, bright red vaginal bleeding, jaundiced sclera
Neurological: cranial nerves intact, pupils equal and reactive to light; blurred vision, alert, altered mental processes
Lungs: clear to auscultation
Heart: tachycardia, regular rhythm, no S_3 or S_4
Abdomen: soft, slight epigastric discomfort, active bowel sounds, Hemoccult-positive stool on digital rectal examination

Based on the evidence of thrombocytopenia, microangiopathic hemolytic anemia, neurological changes, and renal dysfunction, a diagnosis of thrombotic thrombocytopenic purpura (TTP) was made, and the patient was admitted to the intensive care unit (ICU).

The patient's mental status quickly deteriorated in the ICU; she became agitated and confused and required restraints to prevent injury to herself. A computed tomography of the brain was normal; the mental status changes were thought to be due to transient ischemia from microvascular thrombi in the intracranial arterioles. Oxygen therapy was begun at 5 L/min and titrated according to oxygen saturation levels. Prednisone 2 mg/kg daily was initiated, along with ranitidine to prevent gastrointestinal bleeding. Two units of packed red blood cells were transfused. Repeat transfusions of packed red cells were required on days 2, 4, 6, and 10. Arrangements were made for plasmapheresis and plasma exchange. Because this treatment was not immediately available at the hospital, cryosupernatant plasma was administered. Several hours later, the necessary equipment and personnel had arrived, and plasmapheresis and exchange of 2 L of plasma daily was begun and ordered to continue for the next 10 days.

M.C. continued to demonstrate a mild proteinuria over the next 10 days, but her BUN and creatinine remained stable during this time. The patient's blood sugar ranged between 280 and 320. This was thought to be due in part to the prednisone, but thrombotic lesions of the pancreatic islet cells could not be ruled out. The hyperglycemia was covered with sliding scale insulin and returned to normal as the steroids were tapered. M.C.'s platelet count initially rose to 32,000/mm³. Vincristine was administered for further immune suppression, and aspirin and dipyridamole were added to decrease platelet aggregation. This resulted in a platelet count of 62,000/mm³ by day 12. Plasmapheresis and exchange were extended through day 14, then decreased to every other day for the next week, then twice weekly for a month.

M.C. experienced noticeable improvement in her neurological status by day 7. Her serum LDH and bilirubin had returned to near normal by day 14, although schistocytes remained on her peripheral blood smear for a month. This was thought to be due to ineffective clearing of the ruptured RBCs by the reticuloendothelial system, because her hematocrit remained stable. Two months after her discharge, M.C. returned to the hospital with relapsed TTP following a viral illness that was detected on routine complete blood count. This was treated promptly with prednisone, plasmapheresis and exchange, and antiplatelet agents and was resolved without incident by day 11.

Disseminated Intravascular Coagulation

States of physiological disequilibrium that increase permeability or weakening of the vessel walls may lead to leaking of blood outside the vasculature. Hemorrhage is the result. If the response of the hemostatic system to this threat is too great, thrombus formation that occludes the vasculature may result. Thus, transportation of blood is inhibited. (Refer to Chapter 44 for a review of the anatomy and physiology of the hematological system.)

Pathophysiological Principles

Disseminated intravascular coagulation syndrome has the distinction of being the oldest universally accepted hypercoagulable clinical state known. As a syndrome of transient coagulation, DIC causes transformation of fibrinogen to fibrin clot and is associated with acute hemorrhage. Microvascular thrombosis, hyperfibrinolysis, hemorrhage, and biochemical evidence of end-organ dysfunction are characteristic hallmarks of this catastrophic coagulopathy.

The syndrome is triggered by a host of diverse states of physiological disequilibrium, resulting in systemic activation of coagulation and fibrinolysis. Usually DIC is associated with clearly defined pathological conditions. The accompanying display outlines malignant and nonmalignant states of physiological disequilibrium that are precipitating factors in DIC.

RED FLAG

Disease States Associated With Disseminated Intravascular Coagulation

Nonmalignant
Bacterial infections
   Gram-negative
   Gram-positive
Viremias
   HIV
   Cytomegalovirus
   Hepatitis
Burns
Crush injuries and necrotic
   tissue
Obstetrical complications
   Amniotic fluid embolism
   Missed abortion
   Eclampsia
   Placental abruption
Intravascular hemolysis
   Hemolytic transfusion reactions
   Massive blood replacement
   therapy
Acute liver disease
Intravascular prosthetic
   devices

Malignant
Leukemia
   Acute promyelocytic
   Acute myelomonocytic
   Others
Metastatic diseases
   Lung cancer
   Breast cancer
   Hepatic cancer
   Colon cancer
   Prostate cancer
Chemo-radiation therapy

Further descriptions of DIC are fulminant (acute) and low grade (compensated or chronic). The fulminant state typifies the clinical picture often associated with this disorder: acute hemorrhage leading to hypovolemia, abnormal coagulation studies, perfusion deficits related to the obstructive nature of the thrombotic process, and multiple organ dysfunction. Patients with low-grade DIC present with subacute bleeding, diffuse thromboses, and normal coagulation studies.

In all of these states, the presence of injured or lysed cells causes the release of tissue phospholipid into the bloodstream, which can then trigger activity of the intrinsic pathway. Prolonged low cardiac output states, such as seen with prolonged cardiopulmonary bypass or hemorrhagic shock, result in injury to the vascular endothelial lining. This also can trigger intrinsic pathway activity. Abnormalities of vascular endothelium secondary to such conditions as burns, vasculitis, sepsis, and major surgical interventions also can trigger DIC.

Regardless of the precipitating event in DIC, the triggering stimulus initiates systemic coagulation activity, resulting in diffuse intravascular fibrin formation and deposition of fibrin in the microcirculation. The result is the accumulation of clot in the body's capillaries, the total length of which exceeds 100,000 miles in the average adult. The amount of blood clot sequestration in the capillaries due to DIC is enormous. Because of the rapidity of intravascular thrombin formation, clotting factors are used up in the capillary clotting process at a rate exceeding factor replenishment. Circulating thrombin persists in the extravascular space waiting for its substrate, fibrinogen, to arrive. The availability of the inhibitor, antithrombin III, is greatly reduced by the excessive thrombin formation.

Activation of coagulation mechanisms also activates the fibrinolytic system. (Activated factor XII, thrombin, endothelial cells, and tissue substances stimulate the release of plasminogen activators.) The breakdown of fibrin and fibrinogen results in fibrin degradation products (FDPs) that interfere with platelet function and the formation of the fibrin clot. Thus, the patient has a simultaneous, self-perpetuating combination of thrombotic and bleeding activity occurring in response to the precipitating event.

Almost uniformly, there is arterial hypotension, often associated with activation of the kallikrein and complement systems. Kallikrein perpetuates the activation of factor XII to XIIa, further enhancing clotting activity. In addition, kallikrein releases kinins that increase vascular permeability and vasodilation, increasing hypotension. The activation of the complement system results in an increased vascular permeability and lysis of erythrocytes, granulocytes, and platelets. This activity produces phospholipids, which provide fuel for accelerating clotting activity by activating factor XII.

Arteriole vasoconstriction and capillary dilation ensue as the result of activation of the kallikrein and complement systems. Blood is then shunted to the venous side, bypassing dilated capillaries owing to the opening of arteriovenous (AV) shunts. The dilated capillaries now contain stagnant blood, in which metabolic by-products accumulate that render the blood acidotic. Three concomitant procoagulating conditions are now present in the capillary blood: acidosis, blood stagnation, and the presence of coagulation-promoting substances. Figure 48–1 depicts the effect of AV shunting.

The DIC patient bleeds not only because of increased clotting, which results in consumption of clotting factors, but also because of increased fibrinolysis and diminished antithrombin III. As mentioned, the thrombin concentration is regulated by antithrombin III, and in DIC, antithrombin III cannot keep up with the excessive generation of thrombin. This circulating thrombin continues to activate the conversion of plasminogen to plasmin, which compounds the bleeding diathesis. Figure 48–2 depicts the self-perpetuating cycle of thrombosis and bleeding in DIC.

Assessment

All critically ill patients are at risk for development of DIC because many are in the state of physiological disequilibrium characterized by hypovolemia, hypotension, hypoxia, and acidosis, all of which have procoagulant effects. Increased awareness of DIC as a potentially catastrophic complication in the critically ill patient has resulted in earlier recognition and intervention. The critical care nurse who is armed with a knowledge of physiological norms and who uses a systemic approach

NORMAL

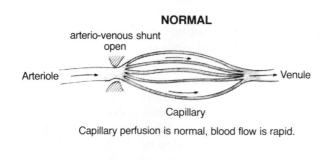

Capillary perfusion is normal, blood flow is rapid.

DIC

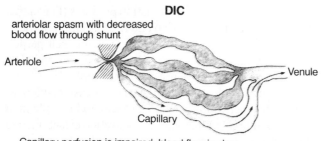

Capillary perfusion is impaired, blood flow is slow, intracapillary thrombosis occurs with blood stagnation and acidosis. Cells nourished by capillaries die of ischemia due to blood clotting.

FIGURE 48-1

Arteriole–capillary–venule relationship in normal circulation as opposed to the disseminated intravascular coagulation (DIC) patient. The diagram shows the effect of arteriovenous shunting in DIC.

to assessment may be the first person to identify the early signs of coagulation dysfunction and its probable trigger.

CLINICAL MANIFESTATIONS

Patients with DIC exhibit a varied constellation of problems and have the potential for development of more. The critical care nurse will be confronted with a patient bleeding from the nose, gums, gastrointestinal tract, surgical sites, injection sites, and intravascular access sites. The patient will present with hematuria, acral cyanosis, petechial rashes, and purpura fulminans.

Assessment of the patient with possible DIC centers around several priorities. First, the patient will have a history of a possible triggering event, such as a crush injury, coupled with bleeding. Bleeding often is observed as oozing from venipuncture sites. Petechiae development, bleeding from mucous membranes, or occult blood present in gastric contents or stool are observed.

Hypovolemic shock may develop in patients who are bleeding; therefore, DIC patients must be monitored closely for signs and symptoms of onset of shock. (Refer to Chapter 49 for a discussion of hypovolemic shock.) Nurses also should be vigilant in preventing severe anemia. All organs can become dysfunctional because of bleeding into tissue spaces or because of ischemia caused by thrombosis. Ongoing assessment of cerebral, pulmonary, renal, and hepatic function is vitally important.

DIAGNOSTIC STUDIES

Table 48–7 outlines studies that are commonly used to assess DIC. Prothrombin time (PT) and partial thromboplastin time (PTT) are generally unreliable and are of minimal usefulness in evaluating DIC. PT and PTTs are within normal limits in about 50% of patients with DIC.

Management

ELIMINATION OF CAUSE

The backbone of therapy for DIC is elimination of the cause. The factor that activates the clotting factors must be "turned off." If the initiating state of physiological disequilibrium is septic shock, volume must be restored and antibiotic therapy initiated to eliminate the precipitating event.

MINIMIZATION OF FURTHER BLEEDING

A second management priority is to minimize the risk of further bleeding by protecting the patient from trauma or traumatic procedures, if possible. The third management priority will be to correct the clotting deficiencies by administering component therapy.

Attention also should be directed to correction of hypovolemia, hypotension, hypoxia, and acidosis, all of which have procoagulant effects. Correction of these imbalances must be the focus of the treatment of bleeding patients with DIC. Additionally, correction of hemostatic deficiencies that compromise the clotting mechanisms is necessary.

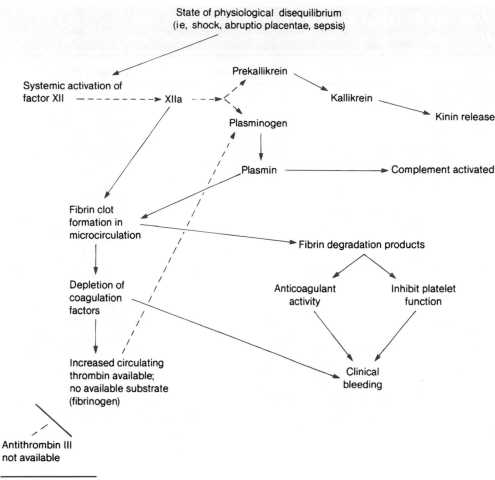

State of physiological disequilibrium
(ie, shock, abruptio placentae, sepsis)

Prekallikrein

Systemic activation of
factor XII ------→ XIIa --→

Kallikrein

Kinin release

Plasminogen

Plasmin ————→ Complement activated

Fibrin clot
formation in
microcirculation

Fibrin degradation products

Depletion of
coagulation
factors

Anticoagulant
activity

Inhibit platelet
function

Increased circulating
thrombin available;
no available substrate
(fibrinogen)

Clinical
bleeding

Antithrombin III
not available

FIGURE 48-2
Self-perpetuating cycle of thrombosis and bleeding in disseminated intravascular coagulation.

REPLACEMENT OF DEPLETED FACTORS

Continued bleeding despite treatment of the underlying cause may indicate depletion of the coagulation factors. Some authorities advocate administration of depleted factors only *after* heparin therapy is initiated so that the infused fibrinogen present in whole blood or fresh frozen plasma does not add "fuel to the fire" of circulating thrombin waiting for its substrate. Others do not support this rationale, but advocate the administration of depleted factors as the patient's condition dictates.

HEPARIN THERAPY

If the underlying cause of DIC cannot be eliminated, it can be controlled by stopping the cycle of thrombosis–hemorrhage with heparin administration. Heparin helps prevent further thrombus formation, but it does not alter clots that already have formed. Heparin also slows coagulation and permits restoration of coagulation proteins. It does this by combining with antithrombin III and, in the presence of thrombin, forming a reversible combination in which thrombin is inactivated. In addition, this combination of heparin and antithrombin III neutralizes activated factors XII, XI, IX, and X, thus blocking the progression of the sequential activation of coagulation factors. Furthermore, heparin inhibits thrombin-mediated platelet aggregation by neutralizing the effects of thrombin. The administration of heparin, therefore, inhibits thrombin generation, thrombin–fibrinogen interactions, and platelet aggregation.

The dose of heparin required to treat DIC must agree with the clinical status and individual needs of the patient. There are advocates for both the subcutaneous and the intravenous routes of administration. Those who advocate intravenous administration favor continuous infusion of doses ranging up to 20,000 to 30,000 U/24 hours. Proponents of subcutaneous heparin favor low doses that range from 2,500 to 5,000 U every 4 to 8 hours. Sequential coagulation studies must be conducted to regulate the heparin dose and to determine the patient response to the heparin. Heparin should be continued until the primary precipitating cause has been removed and the clinical and laboratory data suggest that the patient is on the way to recovery.

MEDIATOR MODULATION

Chemical mediators are released by a variety of mechanisms ranging from trauma to decreased perfusion states. These mediators are involved in impairing microcirculation by in-

---

TABLE 48-7 CLINICAL APPLICATION: Diagnostic Studies
Laboratory Findings in Acute Disseminated Intravascular Coagulation (DIC)

Test	Normal Value	Value in DIC
Prothrombin time	11–15 sec	Prolonged
Partial thromboplastin time	39–48 sec	Prolonged
Thrombin time	10–13 sec	Usually prolonged
Fibrinogen level	200–400 mg/100 mL	Decreased
Antithrombin III levels	89%–120%	Decreased
Platelet count	150,000–400,000/mm³	Decreased
Fibrin degradation products	<10 µg/mL	Increased
Plasminogen levels		Decreased
D-dimer assay		Increased (most specific)
Plasmin-alpha2-plasmin inhibitor complex assay		Increased
Platelet factor 4		Increased
Beta-thromboglobulin		Increased

---

ducing coagulopathy, leading to DIC, and stimulating the inflammatory immune response (IIR). It is generally accepted that mediators, such as tumor necrosis factor, platelet aggregating factor (PAF), cytokines, oxygen free radicals, and arachidonic acid metabolites, can activate the intrinsic and extrinsic pathways. Clinicians are awaiting the results of the use of investigational monoclonal antibodies, PAF inhibitors, oxygen free radical scavengers, and IIR modulators. Thus far, the studies have been favorable. Perhaps in the future, there will be a wide variety of pharmacological agents available to treat DIC.

Complications

A patient with DIC is vulnerable to a wide variety of complications, all of which are related to bleeding or thrombosis.

RELATED TO BLEEDING

A serious bleeding-related complication is intracranial hemorrhage, which may manifest as headache, loss of motor or sensory function, altered level of consciousness, and changes in pupil reactions. Gastrointestinal hemorrhage may become evident in the patient who complains of abdominal pain and has distention, vomiting, signs of hypovolemia, and the presence of occult or frank blood in stool or emesis. Bleeding into the skin will manifest as petechiae and ecchymoses.

RELATED TO THROMBOSIS

Thrombus formation in the microcirculation can cause problems related to ischemia. Cerebrovascular ischemia most likely will be manifested by changes in the level of consciousness, sensory abnormalities, visual disturbances, or motor weakness. Ischemia in the gastrointestinal tract can cause necrosis, resulting in severe abdominal pain, absent bowel sounds, and vomiting. Microthrombus in the renal vascular bed impairs normal renal function and could result in renal failure when prolonged hypotension or shock is present. Another danger is the formation of deep venous thromboses, which could embolize to the lungs. Pulmonary embolus is a catastrophic event that presents with hyperventilation, hemoptysis, chest pain, hypoxia, cyanosis, hypotension, and extreme apprehension in the patient.

CLINICAL APPLICATION: Patient Care Study

R.P. is a 62-year-old man receiving care in the intensive care unit after an abdominal aortic aneurysm repair. His aneurysm was located above the superceliac artery, and aortic cross-clamp was required for 62 minutes. He is 1 day postoperative. He is being mechanically ventilated. His abdomen is distended, tender to touch, and he has no bowel sounds. His temperature is 40°C (104°F). Dopamine hydrochloride, 10 µg/kg/min, is being used to support his blood pressure. He has had several hypotensive episodes that have responded to fluid boluses with normal saline. The nurse caring for R.P. notices that slow but constant bleeding has developed from his abdominal wound and from his central venous line insertion site. His blood is cultured for possible pathogens and screening for suspected disseminated intravascular coagulation (DIC) is obtained. His laboratory values are as follows:

Packed cell volume, 36%
Platelet count, 95,000/mm³
Prothrombin time, 36 seconds
Partial thromboplastin time, 57 seconds
Fibrinogen level, 100 mg/dL

His hemodynamic status continues to deteriorate, and his abdomen continues to enlarge and is increasingly tender. Peripheral perfusion is poor, and petechiae are starting to develop. A repeat platelet count shows platelets to be decreased to 80,000/mm³. A repeat fibrinogen gives a value of 78 g/dL. His oxygenation has deteriorated, probably related to microthrombus in the pulmonary vascular bed. Currently, his PaO_2 has fallen to 70 mmHg on 80% oxygen.

Studies indicate consumption of coagulation factors, fibrinogen, and platelets. The trigger for this process seems to be a portion of the bowel that became ischemic after a prolonged aortic cross-clamp during resection of his aneurysm.

The patient is treated with antibiotics because the possibility of a bowel perforation is not totally ruled out. He also is given platelets, cryoprecipitate, and fresh frozen plasma. After administration of these blood components, his laboratory studies improve as follows:

Platelet count, 110,000/mm³
Prothrombin time, 25 seconds
Partial thromboplastin time, 54 seconds
Fibrinogen level, 170 mg/dL

A decision is made to proceed with an emergency exploratory laparotomy. The patient is discovered to have a 4- to 5-in segment of colon that is necrotic, with evidence of a small perforation. This segment is removed along with adjoining ischemic tissue. The remainder of the bowel appears to be healthy.

R.P. required treatment with antibiotics for 6 days and coagulation factor replacement for 2 days after the bowel

resection. After removal of the trigger for the DIC, his coagulation status gradually normalized. His pulmonary function also improved, and he was extubated on the fifth postoperative day. Although his ischemic bowel and subsequent DIC were life threatening, he made a gradual, successful recovery.

The patient with DIC presents the ultimate challenge to the critical care nurse—the use of the intellect for assessment and the integration of psychomotor skills for interventions, blended with compassion. A Collaborative Care Guide for the patient with DIC follows.

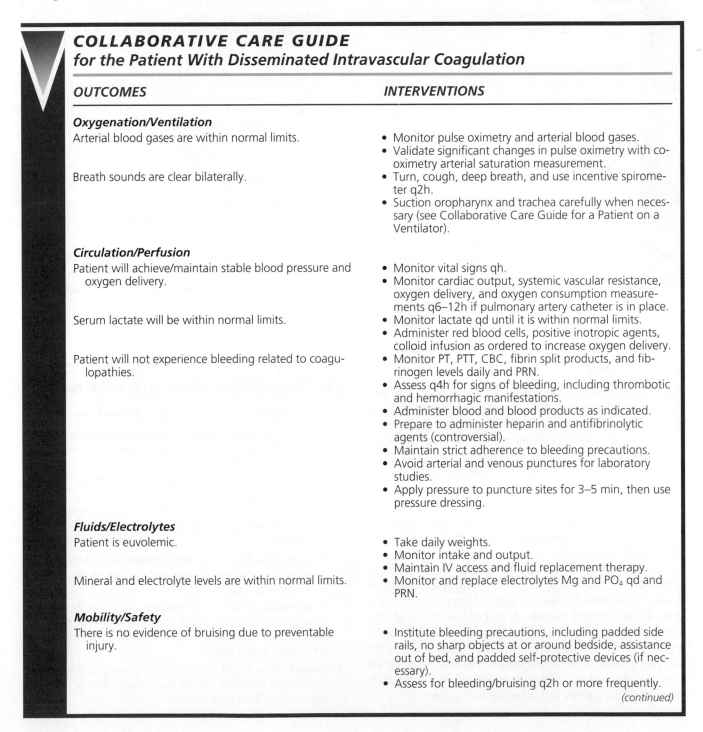

COLLABORATIVE CARE GUIDE
for the Patient With Disseminated Intravascular Coagulation

OUTCOMES	INTERVENTIONS
Oxygenation/Ventilation	
Arterial blood gases are within normal limits.	• Monitor pulse oximetry and arterial blood gases. • Validate significant changes in pulse oximetry with co-oximetry arterial saturation measurement.
Breath sounds are clear bilaterally.	• Turn, cough, deep breath, and use incentive spirometer q2h. • Suction oropharynx and trachea carefully when necessary (see Collaborative Care Guide for a Patient on a Ventilator).
Circulation/Perfusion	
Patient will achieve/maintain stable blood pressure and oxygen delivery.	• Monitor vital signs qh. • Monitor cardiac output, systemic vascular resistance, oxygen delivery, and oxygen consumption measurements q6–12h if pulmonary artery catheter is in place.
Serum lactate will be within normal limits.	• Monitor lactate qd until it is within normal limits. • Administer red blood cells, positive inotropic agents, colloid infusion as ordered to increase oxygen delivery.
Patient will not experience bleeding related to coagulopathies.	• Monitor PT, PTT, CBC, fibrin split products, and fibrinogen levels daily and PRN. • Assess q4h for signs of bleeding, including thrombotic and hemorrhagic manifestations. • Administer blood and blood products as indicated. • Prepare to administer heparin and antifibrinolytic agents (controversial). • Maintain strict adherence to bleeding precautions. • Avoid arterial and venous punctures for laboratory studies. • Apply pressure to puncture sites for 3–5 min, then use pressure dressing.
Fluids/Electrolytes	
Patient is euvolemic.	• Take daily weights. • Monitor intake and output. • Maintain IV access and fluid replacement therapy.
Mineral and electrolyte levels are within normal limits.	• Monitor and replace electrolytes Mg and PO_4 qd and PRN.
Mobility/Safety	
There is no evidence of bruising due to preventable injury.	• Institute bleeding precautions, including padded side rails, no sharp objects at or around bedside, assistance out of bed, and padded self-protective devices (if necessary). • Assess for bleeding/bruising q2h or more frequently.

(continued)

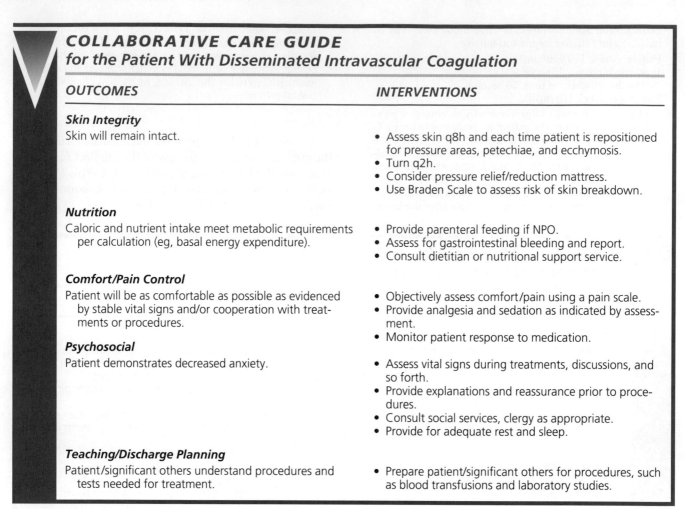

COLLABORATIVE CARE GUIDE
for the Patient With Disseminated Intravascular Coagulation

OUTCOMES	INTERVENTIONS
Skin Integrity Skin will remain intact.	• Assess skin q8h and each time patient is repositioned for pressure areas, petechiae, and ecchymosis. • Turn q2h. • Consider pressure relief/reduction mattress. • Use Braden Scale to assess risk of skin breakdown.
Nutrition Caloric and nutrient intake meet metabolic requirements per calculation (eg, basal energy expenditure).	• Provide parenteral feeding if NPO. • Assess for gastrointestinal bleeding and report. • Consult dietitian or nutritional support service.
Comfort/Pain Control Patient will be as comfortable as possible as evidenced by stable vital signs and/or cooperation with treatments or procedures.	• Objectively assess comfort/pain using a pain scale. • Provide analgesia and sedation as indicated by assessment. • Monitor patient response to medication.
Psychosocial Patient demonstrates decreased anxiety.	• Assess vital signs during treatments, discussions, and so forth. • Provide explanations and reassurance prior to procedures. • Consult social services, clergy as appropriate. • Provide for adequate rest and sleep.
Teaching/Discharge Planning Patient/significant others understand procedures and tests needed for treatment.	• Prepare patient/significant others for procedures, such as blood transfusions and laboratory studies.

Conclusion

In DIC, localization of clotting and clot lysis has failed. Successful management of DIC requires that the inciting cause be recognized and treated. Treatment of the cause is the mainstay of therapy. Once this is accomplished, the whole bleeding process will begin to correct. If the precipitating factor cannot be corrected, patient survival is unlikely. Until total correction is achieved, a second major focus of management will be protection of the patient from further bleeding and the replacement of consumed clotting factors so that fibrin can be produced and clotting returned to a more physiological state.

Hematological disorders continue to present challenges in assessment and management. Ongoing research is continuing to expand knowledge and interventions in these areas. Careful patient assessment and interpretation of diagnostic tests are essential to improved patient outcomes. Potentially fatal complications can result from required interventions for these disorders or from the disease process itself. Intensive observation and follow-up are essential in the management of the patient with a hematological disorder.

Clinical Applicability Challenges

Self-Challenge: Critical Thinking

1. An option for treating some hematological disorders is BMT. Evaluate the factors that need to be considered when determining if this is an appropriate intervention for leukemias, aplastic anemia, and myelodysplastic syndromes.

2. Some disorders of the hematological and immune systems are treated by immunosuppression. Compare and contrast potential benefits with possible long-term risks of immunosuppressive therapy.

3. A variety of malignant factors can cause DIC. Distinguish between factors that initiate the intrinsic versus the extrinsic pathways of coagulation.

4. Biochemical mediators are implicated in the activation and acceleration of the IIR, which can precipitate DIC. Develop a plan of care directed to reducing the inflammatory response in a multiple trauma patient.

5. Today's rising health care costs place many constraints on health care providers. Assess the impact patients with DIC have on health care institutions.

Study Questions

1. Anemia of chronic disease is best managed by
   a. cobalamin and folate.
   b. transfusion and rEPO.
   c. iron supplements.
   d. hydroxyurea.

2. Severe aplastic anemia is managed by all of the following except
   a. immunosuppressive drugs.
   b. BMT.
   c. drugs that stimulate bone marrow function.
   d. transfusion.

3. A 29-year-old man with hemophilia B notices a "bubbling" sensation in his knee, followed by progressive pain and decreasing range of motion. He should
   a. report immediately to the nearest emergency department.
   b. schedule an appointment with a hematologist.
   c. elevate his knee and apply ice for 24 hours.
   d. self-administer factor IX at home.

4. Normal inhibitors of coagulation include all but the following:
   a. Adequate cardiac output, which dilutes activated factors
   b. Antithrombin III, which inactivates thrombin
   c. Tissue thromboplastin, which interferes with fibrin formation
   d. Plasminogen converting to plasmin

5. An early indication of a DIC process is bleeding associated with
   a. a decreased platelet count.
   b. a decreased prothrombin time.
   c. decreased levels of FDPs.
   d. increased fibrinogen.

6. Patients with DIC, a hypercoagulable syndrome, bleed because of all of the following except
   a. depleted clotting factors.
   b. increased levels of fibrin degradation products.
   c. diffuse microthrombosis.
   d. decreased plasminogen levels.

REFERENCES

1. Roodman GD: Hemolytic anemia. In Stein JH (ed): Internal Medicine (4th Ed). St. Louis, Mosby-Year Book, 1994
2. Kelton JG, Crowther MA: Autoimmune hemolytic anemia. In Brain MC, Carbone PP (eds): Current Therapy in Hematology/Oncology (5th Ed). St. Louis, Mosby-Year, 1995
3. Solanki DL: Megaloblastic anemia. In Brain MC, Carbone PP (eds): Current Therapy in Hematology/Oncology (5th Ed). St. Louis, CV Mosby, 1995
4. Lipschitz DA: Iron deficiency anemia, the anemia of chronic disease, sideroblastic anemia, and iron overload. In Stein JE (ed): Internal Medicine (4th Ed). St. Louis, Mosby-Year, 1994
5. Hutton JJ: The leukemias and polycythemia vera. In Stein JE (ed): Internal Medicine (4th Ed). St. Louis, Mosby, 1994
6. Goldman JM: Chronic myelogenous leukemia. In Brain MC, Carbone PP (eds): Current Therapy in Hematology/Oncology (5th Ed). St. Louis, CV Mosby, 1995
7. Baer MR, Herzig GP, Bloomfield CD: Acute myeloid leukemia. In Brain MC, Carbone PP (eds): Current Therapy in Hematology-Oncology (5th Ed). St. Louis, CV Mosby, 1995
8. Appelbaum FR: Bone marrow failure. In Stein JE (ed): Internal Medicine (4th Ed). St. Louis, CV Mosby, 1994
9. Bush MT, Roy N: Hemophilia emergencies. Journal of Emergency Nursing 21:531–539, 1995
10. Kovachy RJ: Idiopathic thrombocytopenic purpura. In Wood ME, Bunn PA (eds): Hematology/Oncology Secrets. Philadelphia, Hanley & Belfus, 1994
11. Ellenberger BJ, Haas L, Cundiff L: Thrombotic thrombocytopenic purpura: Nursing during the acute phase. Dimensions in Critical Care Nursing 12:58–65, 1993
12. Paschall FE: Thrombotic thrombocytopenic purpura: The challenges of a complex disease process. AACN Clinical Issues in Critical Care Nursing 4:655–663, 1993
13. Kelton JG: Thrombotic thrombocytopenic purpura. In Brain MC, Carbone PP (eds): Current Therapy in Hematology/Oncology (5th Ed). St. Louis, CV Mosby, 1995

BIBLIOGRAPHY

Acevedo M: Blood dyscrasias: Polycythemias, idiopathic thrombocytopenic purpura, and thrombotic thrombocytopenic purpura. Journal of Intravenous Nursing 15:52–57, 1992

Bick R: Disseminated intravascular coagulation: Objective criteria for diagnosis and management. Med Clin North Am 73(3):511–543, 1994

Foley R, Brain MC: Anemia of chronic disease. In Brain MV, Carbone PP (eds): Current Therapy in Hematology/Oncology (5th Ed). St. Louis, CV Mosby, 1995

George JN, Kolodziej MA: Hemostasis and fibrinolysis. In Stein JH (ed): Internal Medicine (4th Ed). St. Louis, Mosby-Year Book, 1994

Holden JMC: An overview of common bleeding disorders. Journal of Intravenous Nursing 18:223–230, 1995

McCance K, Huether S: Pathophysiology: The Biologic Basis for Disease in Adults and Children (2nd Ed). St. Louis, CV Mosby, 1994

Rintel PB, Kenny RM, Crowley JP: Therapeutic support of the patient with thrombocytopenia. Hematology/Oncology Clinics of North America 8:1131–1155, 1994

Rohaly-Davis J, Johnston K: Hematological Emergencies in the Intensive Care Unit. Crit Care Nurs Q 18(4):35–43, 1995

Santosh-Kumar CR, Kolhouse JF: Aplastic anemia. In Wood ME, Bunn PA (eds): Hematology/Oncology Secrets. Philadelphia, Hanley & Belfus, 1994

Schafer AI: Thrombocytopenia and disorders of platelet function. In Stein JH (ed): Internal Medicine (4th Ed). St. Louis, Mosby-Year Book, 1994

Secor V: The inflammatory/immune response in critical illness: Role of the systemic inflammatory response syndrome. Crit Care Nurs Clin North Am 6(2):251–264, 1994

Sheuy K: Platelet-associated bleeding disorders. Semin-Oncol-Nurs 12(1):15–27, 1996

Wiley JS: Hereditary spherocytosis, elliptocytosis, and related disorders. In Brain MC, Carbone PP (eds): Current Therapy in Hematology/Oncology (5th Ed). St. Louis, CV Mosby, 1995

PART

V

Multisystem Dysfunction

49

Hypoperfusion States

OBJECTIVES

Based on the content in this chapter, the reader should be able to:

- Describe common pathophysiological processes involved in the generalized shock response.
- Compare and contrast the etiology and clinical manifestations of the major categories of shock.
- Differentiate between sepsis and systemic inflammatory response syndrome.
- Explain the anticipated medical management and rationale for treatment of the various shock states.
- Identify nursing management principles for patients experiencing shock.

▰▰ PATHOPHYSIOLOGY OF HYPOPERFUSION

Under normal conditions, the body provides sufficient oxygen to the cells to meet metabolic needs. Under stress, the body consumes its oxygen more rapidly, and compensatory mechanisms are initiated to restore oxygen and perfusion to cells. These compensatory mechanisms are the same, regardless of the clinical condition causing the cellular hypoperfusion. Clinical conditions that result in cellular hypoperfusions are often referred to as "shock states."

This chapter discusses various clinical conditions that create states of cellular hypoperfusion and alterations in oxygen delivery. These states include hypovolemia, cardiogenic shock, anaphylaxis, neurogenic shock, sepsis, and systemic inflammatory response syndrome (SIRS). Patients in critical care are at significant risk for developing any one of these compromised states of cellular hypoperfusion.

Oxygen Delivery and Consumption

Under normal conditions, oxygen consumption (VO_2) is independent of oxygen delivery (DaO_2). This means that when the cells need to consume additional oxygen to produce energy, cells can extract the necessary amount required to produce energy, adenosine triphosphate (ATP). During times of physiological stress, however, VO_2, becomes dependent on DaO_2. If additional oxygen is required, the cells cannot extract the oxygen and must convert to anaerobic metabolism to produce ATP. Anaerobic metabolism is not an efficient method of energy production. It creates an oxygen debt, which must be repaid once the body can meet all energy requirements through aerobic metabolism.

During shock states or poor perfusion, oxygen is consumed at a much greater rate than it is delivered, and it is difficult to predetermine the amount of oxygen the cells will consume. To meet the increased need for cellular VO_2, the body must compensate by increasing DaO_2. Although it is not possible to manipulate cellular VO_2 directly, DaO_2 can be manipulated and increased to the cells. The accompanying display summarizes the procedure for calculating oxygen parameters. The primary goal is to maximize DaO_2 to meet or exceed cellular oxygen requirements in an ongoing effort to prevent tissue and cell death and maintain end organ perfusion.

Compensatory Mechanisms

Cellular perfusion is dependent on the synergy of multiple physiological processes. The pulmonary and circulatory systems provide an intricate balance of oxygen exchange and delivery to the cells by generation of an adequate oxygenated blood supply and cardiac output (CO). The autonomic nervous system assists in the orchestration of this delicate balance.

During states of hypoxia, activated compensatory mechanisms increase the depth and rate of respirations. The cardiovascular system increases CO to enhance oxygen delivery to the cells. During states of low perfusion (low blood pressure) compensatory mechanisms are initiated and result in increases in heart rate (HR), systemic vascular resistance (SVR), preload, and cardiac contractility in an effort to restore appropriate circulatory volume. (Review Chapter 15 for a discussion of these terms.) The drop in systemic blood pressure activates a series of neurohormonal responses aimed at reestablishing sufficient CO and perfusion to vital organs. Baroreceptors respond to the fall in blood pressure by becoming less active; the result is an increase in sympathetic response (Fig. 49–1).

Subsequent vasoconstriction (SVR) attempts to increase the circulating volume and preload. Continued sympathetic stimulation causes an increased HR and contractile force. The kidneys respond by activating the renin–angiotensin

---

CLINICAL APPLICATION: Nursing Intervention Guidelines
Procedure for Calculating Oxygen Parameters

Calculated Oxygen Parameters	*Normal Parameters*
Fick Equation	
$CO = \dfrac{VO_2}{(Ca - v)O_2} \times 10$	Normal, 4–6 L/min
Oxygen Delivery	
$DaO_2 = CO \times Hbg \times SaO_2 \times 1.39 \times 10$	Normal, 800–1,200 L/min
$DaO_2I = \dfrac{DaO_2}{BSA}$	Normal range depends on patient's body surface area
Oxygen Consumption	
$VO_2 = CO \times (Ca - v)O_2 \times 10$	Normal, 180–250 L/min
$VO_2 = \dfrac{VO_2}{BSA}$	Normal range depends on patient's body surface area

Technique
1. Calculate the VO_2 to determine the cellular energy requirements of the patient with an oxygenation/perfusion problem.
2. Calculate the DaO_2.
3. Increase the DaO_2 by manipulating elements of the equation ($\uparrow$CO, $\uparrow$Hgb, $\uparrow$oxygenation) through titration of vasoactive and inotropic agents or fluids, administration of blood, maximized oxygenation, and ventilatory support. As DaO_2 is increased, VO_2 of the cellular energy needs will be met, maintaining aerobic metabolism.

CO, cardiac output; Ca − v, content of arterial oxygen (obtained from arterial blood gas) − content of venous oxygen (obtained from mixed venous blood gas); BSA, body surface area; I, indexed

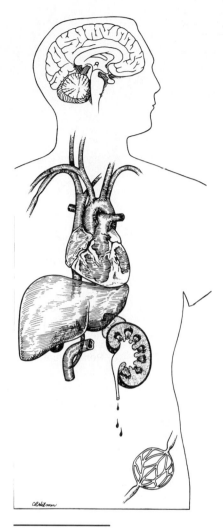

Brain
- Thirst
- Increased production and release ADH

Cardiovascular system
- Increased heart rate
- Increased force of contraction
- Increased peripheral resistance
- Constriction of blood flow to
  - Kidney
  - Gastrointestinal tract
  - Skin
  - Skeletal muscles
- Constriction of the veins

Adrenal gland
- Increased production and release of
  aldosterone by the adrenal cortex
- Increased production and release of
  the catecholamines (epinephrine and
  norepinephrine) by the adrenal medulla

Liver
- Constriction of veins and sinusoids
  with mobilization of blood stored in
  the liver

Kidney
- Increased retention of sodium and water
- Decreased urine output

Capillary bed
- Increased reabsorption of water into
  the capillary from the interstitial
  spaces due to constriction of the
  arterioles with a resultant decrease
  in capillary pressure

FIGURE 49-1

Compensatory mechanism in hypovolemic shock. Porth C: Pathophysiology: Concepts of altered health states (3rd Ed), p 392. Philadelphia, JB Lippincott, 1990.

system. Activation stimulates the release of aldosterone and causes the pituitary gland to release antidiuretic hormone, leading to water and sodium retention, all in an effort to increase thse circulating volume and CO (Fig. 49–2).

The patient's clinical presentation will depend on the initiating event of the shock state. Altered level of consciousness, tachypnea, tachycardia, hypotension, and decreased urine output are common disturbances found in all states of hypoperfusion.

CLASSIFICATION OF SHOCK

Shock states have historically been classified according to the causative failing organ or system. *Hypovolemic shock* results in a state of hypoperfusion because of a loss of circulation volume. A significant insult to the myocardium, resulting in the loss of the structural and mechanical function of the heart, will cause *cardiogenic shock. Anaphylactic shock* is the body's

overwhelming response to an antigen. The disruption of sympathetic tone causes the clinical state of *neurogenic shock.* Lastly, *septic shock* is a state of overwhelming infection and inflammatory response causing a maldistribution of the circulating blood volume resulting in organ hypoperfusion.

HYPOVOLEMIC SHOCK

Etiology

Hypovolemic shock is a result of inadequate circulating volume. Volume disorders in the critically ill patient may be classified as either depletion or expansion disorders and involve both intracellular and extracellular (EC) compartments. Acute fluid volume loss does not allow the normal compensatory mechanisms to conserve appropriate circulating volume. Hypovolemic shock most commonly is due to sudden blood loss and severe dehydration. Some injuries, such as burns, cause significant fluid shifts from the intravascular space to the interstitial space, resulting in hy-

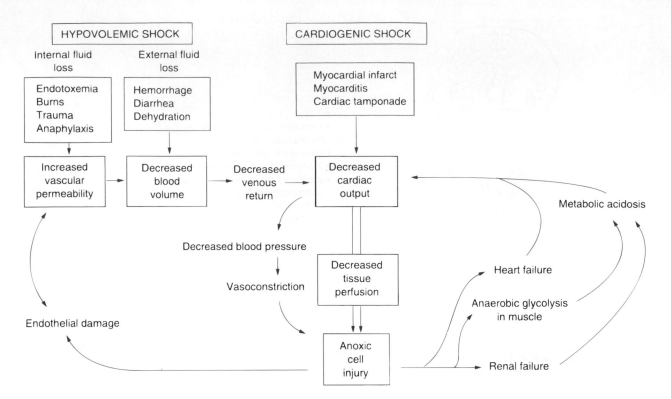

FIGURE 49-2

This flow chart shows the integration of many factors in the progression of shock. Shock is initiated by one of two principal events: pump failure of "cardiogenic shock," and loss of circulatory volume, or "hypovolemic shock." Hypovolemic shock follows internal fluid loss, such as that in endotoxemia, burns, trauma, and anaphylaxis, or external fluid loss, such as that caused by hemorrhage, diarrhea, and dehydration. The effects of both events are increased cardiac output and decreased tissue perfusion. The resulting cell injury prompts several vicious circles. Metabolic acidosis (renal failure, anaerobic glycolysis) and heart failure lead to further decline in cardiac output. Endothelial damage increased vascular permeability and decreases effective blood volume, reducing venous return and decreasing cardiac output. From Bullock: Pathophysiology (4th Ed.), p 257. Philadelphia, Lippincott-Raven 1996

povolemia (see Chapter 51). If left untreated, hypovolemia can lead to a variety of secondary complications, such as hypotension, electrolyte and acid–base disturbances, and organ dysfunction due to hypoperfusion.

Pathophysiological Principles

A sudden loss of EC volume decreases venous return to the heart and results in a reduction in CO. Compensatory mechanisms are initiated to increase the circulating volume through the activation of the sympathetic nervous system and neurohormonal responses. If the condition persists, existing blood volume is shunted to the vital organs (heart, lungs, and brain), causing hypoperfusion to such organs as the liver, gut, and kidneys. As the body continues to compensate for a decrease in circulating volume, if volume is not replaced, compensatory mechanisms eventually become ineffective. The failure of the compensatory mechanisms to restore adequate circulating volume causes cellular hypoperfusion and the inability to meet cellular VO_2 requirements. The cells must convert to anaerobic metabolism in an effort to meet their ATP requirements, resulting in a worsening of the acidotic state.

Failed compensatory mechanisms, which were initiated to restore CO, cause the myocardium to fatigue. Attempts to alter preload by increasing HR and SVR escalate the heart's workload. The heart beats too rapidly and must eject against a greater vascular resistance, a situation requiring more oxygen and energy production. Such stress on the heart causes an increase in myocardial oxygen consumption (MvO_2). The continued lack of circulating volume prevents appropriate oxygen delivery to the heart. A vicious cycle is created. Inability of the circulatory system to provide end organ perfusion and oxygen will force the body to convert to anaerobic metabolism to meet cellular metabolic needs. Ischemic damage will ensue. The organ systems will continue to attempt to compensate until they fail.

Assessment

Clinical findings are directly related to the severity and acuteness of the volume loss (Table 49–1). Some patients, especially older patients or those who have chronic diseases, will have more subtle compensatory responses, which may be overlooked. Trending physical assessment findings is essential to treat the patient and prevent vascular collapse.

TABLE 49-1

Correlation of Clinical Findings Associated With Volume Loss in Hemorrhagic Shock

Estimated Blood Loss	Clinical Findings
<500 mL	None
500–1,000 mL	• Tachycardia (↑HR >20% of patient's baseline) • Hypotension (↓SBP >10% of patient's baseline) • ↓Urine output • Pulses weaker • Skin and extremities cool to touch • Hemodynamics: within normal limits CO, ↑SVR
1,000–2,000 mL	• Tachycardia (↑HR >20%–30% of patient's baseline) • Hypotension (↓SBP >10%–20% of patient's baseline) • Tachypnea (↑RR >10% of patient's baseline) • Oxygen saturation may not be altered dependent on the percentage of exogenous oxygen the patient is receiving • S$\bar{\text{v}}$O$_2$ <60% • ↓Urine output (<30 mL/h) • Altered level of consciousness: restlessness, agitation, confusion, or obtunded • Cool, diaphoretic skin • Poor peripheral pulses • Hemodynamics: ↓CO, ↑SVR
2,000–3,000 mL	• Tachycardia (↑HR >20%–30% of patient's baseline) • Hypotension (↓SBP >10%–20% of patient's baseline) • Tachypnea (↑RR >10%–20% of patient's baseline) • ↓Oxygen saturation • S$\bar{\text{v}}$O$_2$ <55%–60% • Oliguria → anuria • Mental stupor • Marked peripheral vasoconstriction: cold extremities, poor peripheral pulses, pallor • Hemodynamics: ↓CO, ↑SVR

SBP, systolic blood pressure; SVR, systemic vascular resistance; CO, cardiac output; RR, respirations; HR, heart rate

HISTORY

A thorough history of the patient's presenting problem will provide a high degree of suspicion for hypovolemic shock. Patients experiencing significant blood loss due to gastric hemorrhage or liver or splenic rupture from trauma must have a rapid replacement of circulating blood volume to prevent the consequences of hypovolemia. Very young and older patients are at greater risk of hypovolemia due to dehydration.

CLINICAL MANIFESTATIONS

Patients with hypovolemic shock will demonstrate the following signs and symptoms due to poor organ perfusion: Mentation becomes altered, ranging from lethargy to unresponsiveness. Respirations will be rapid and deep, gradually becoming labored and more shallow as the patient's condition deteriorates. The skin will be cool and clammy with weak and thready pulses. Tachycardia will be present as the body attempts to increase the CO. Urine output will be de-

creased, dark, and concentrated. Helpful laboratory tests include a hemoglobin and hematocrit reflective of the severity of blood loss or hemoconcentration due to dehydration. Serum lactate level and arterial pH will assist in assessment of the severity of the patient's acidosis and can be used to measure the effectiveness of fluid replacement therapy.

Management

Management focuses on restoring circulating volume and resolving the cause of volume loss. Composition of volume replacement therapy depends on what was lost. Crystalloid solutions are used primarily as first-line therapy. Isotonic solutions, such as lactated Ringer's solution or 0.9% normal saline solution, are preferred over hypotonic solutions (5% dextrose solution). Blood products and other colloid solutions (albumin and synthetic volume expanders) are often used to assist in the resuscitation process, especially if blood loss is the primary cause. The use of packed red blood cells is of utmost importance if hypotension is due to hemorrhage.

Nursing management of the patient with hypovolemic shock focuses on the restoration of circulating volume through fluid and colloid administration. Care must be taken to administer fluids as rapidly as possible without compromising the pulmonary system. Fluids given too rapidly may cause pulmonary congestion, further exacerbating the oxygen debt. Placing the patient in Trendelenburg position may assist in elevating the blood pressure during early fluid resuscitation. Obtaining and maintaining adequate intravenous (IV) access is essential. Ideally, large IV catheters are inserted in the antecubital space or central venous system to assist with the rapid infusion of fluids. Continued assessment of IV access and patency is required. Documentation of vital signs, pulses, respiratory rate, depth, oxygen saturation, urine output, and mentation is crucial.

Complications

Complications associated with hypovolemic shock are dependent on the length of time and severity of the hypotensive crisis. Complications may range from renal damage to cerebral anoxia and death.

▇ CARDIOGENIC SHOCK

Etiology

Cardiogenic shock is a result of the loss of critical contractile function of the heart. Usually it is diagnosed by the presence of systemic and pulmonary hemodynamic alterations, which result in an inadequate CO and tissue perfusion. Typically, this occurs when greater than 40% of ventricular mass is damaged. The most common cause of this shock is an extensive left ventricular myocardial infarction (MI). The reported incidence of cardiogenic shock due to MI ranges from 5% to 15%. It is believed that this rate has decreased since the introduction of rapid invasive monitoring and revascularization procedures.[1] Although cardiogenic shock can develop within a few hours after the onset of MI symptoms, it often occurs after hospitalization. Other causes include papillary muscle rupture, free wall rupture, and ventricular septal rupture, all of which are mechanical complications of MI.

The display on risk factors shows independent predictors for developing cardiogenic shock. Patients with all five risk factors have a 54% chance of developing cardiogenic shock. Research indicates that mortality rates for patients presenting with cardiogenic shock versus those who develop it in the hospital are similarly high. Identifying patients at risk for developing cardiogenic shock to formulate strategies for prevention is extremely important.

Pathophysiological Principles

Because of the loss of ventricular contractile force, there is a decrease in CO. Compensatory mechanisms are activated in an effort to restore adequate CO. Cardiogenic shock and

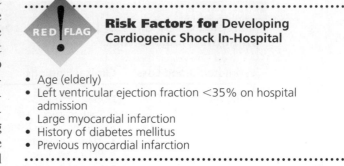

RED FLAG

Risk Factors for Developing Cardiogenic Shock In-Hospital

- Age (elderly)
- Left ventricular ejection fraction <35% on hospital admission
- Large myocardial infarction
- History of diabetes mellitus
- Previous myocardial infarction

the response of compensatory mechanisms cause a vicious cycle that can lead to progressive deterioration.

Adding to an already tenuous state of myocardial functioning is a decrease in coronary perfusion pressure caused by the profound hypotension. This decreased coronary perfusion pressure further exacerbates the decrease in oxygen delivery, high oxygen extraction, and increased lactate production, resulting in a decreased contractile state that continues to drop the CO.

Assessment

Patients admitted with the diagnosis of MI require close monitoring. Trending of assessment findings allows the nurse to pick up the subtle changes that signal the beginning of cardiogenic shock.

HISTORY

A thorough history provides the information necessary to predict patients at risk for developing cardiogenic shock. Cardiogenic shock frequently occurs in individuals who have suffered a large MI, have an admission ejection fraction of less than 35%, have diabetes mellitus, or are older. These patients in particular bear close monitoring. These predisposing factors should alert the clinician to assess for the initial phases of shock, allowing for rapid, life-saving intervention. It is important to rule out other causes of decreased CO prior to initiating therapy. Some complications associated with MI may require further intervention, including surgery.

CLINICAL MANIFESTATIONS

Clinical manifestations associated with cardiogenic shock are outlined in the display. In addition to the signs and symptoms mentioned in the table, patients who develop cardiogenic shock will often experience recurrent chest pain, suggestive of infarct extension. Other clinical findings are directly related to the decrease in CO.

Laboratory findings suggestive of persistent myocardial tissue death reveal a continuous release of creatine kinase and myocardial bands into the circulation. This prolonged elevation, associated with delayed peaking or additional enzyme rise, accompanied by progressive hemodynamic compromise and clinical deterioration, is often the hallmark of extensive myocardial necrosis often seen with cardiogenic shock.

Management

The goal of management is to correct reversible problems, protect the ischemic myocardium, and improve tissue perfusion. Early treatment is imperative. Reversing the hypoxemia, acidosis, hypoglycemia, and hypocalcemia that may exist can improve the patient's ability to respond to other therapies. Treatment is aimed at increasing myocardial oxygen delivery, maximizing CO, and decreasing left ventricular workload.

Nursing management for the patient with cardiogenic shock is centered on the conservation of myocardial energy and decreasing the workload of the heart. The use of narcotic analgesics and sedatives to minimize the sympathetic nervous response is helpful, but the nurse will need to assist patients with much of their physical care. Patient care should be given between periods of rest to minimize myocardial energy expenditure.

Increasing oxygen concentrations of inspired air is a simple but important step and may require initiation of mechanical ventilation. Also, the administration of narcotic analgesics, such as morphine sulfate, can increase venous capitance.

Maximizing CO requires sophistication and caution. Dysrhythmias often occur with acute MI, ischemia, or acid–base imbalances and can further drop CO. Correcting these problems with antiarrhythmic agents, cardioversion, or pacing can help restore a stable heart rhythm and enhance CO.

Adequate filling pressures will assist in restoration of CO but must be achieved cautiously. Generally, a preload (left ventricular end diastolic pressure, LVEDP) of 14 to 18 mmHg should be maintained (see Chapter 17). Fluids can be used to achieve this goal but must be stopped when filling pressures increase without a subsequent rise in CO. The critical care nurse must obtain, trend, and carefully interpret the patient's hemodynamic parameters so that the goal of increasing CO is met without other poor outcomes. If the goal is overshot, symptoms of pulmonary edema will appear, and diuretics may be needed.

Pharmacological agents can be used to augment CO, but they too must be used cautiously. Many agents can increase MVO₂ without having an appreciable effect on the CO. Decisions to use some pharmacological agents are based on an overall cost-benefit ratio. Drugs such as sympathomimetic amines (eg, isoproterenol hydrochloride and epinephrine hydrochloride) can enhance CO but have serious side effects that often prove deleterious to the patient. Agents with positive inotropic effects, such as dopamine hydrochloride, dobutamine hydrochloride, amrinone lactate, and milrinone, are used more frequently and with more favorable results.

There are two ways to decrease the workload of the left ventricle—vasodilators and mechanical support devices. Vasodilators, such as sodium nitroprusside, reduce the LVEDP and SVR, resulting in a rise in the CO and improved left ventricular function. These drugs can also be used in combination with peripheral vasodilators to provide a balanced effect. Mechanical support for the failing ventricle includes the intra-aortic balloon pump and a left ventricular assist device. Both devices reduce the workload of the left ventricle.

New therapies are designed to expedite revascularization through invasive cardiac procedures, such as percutaneous translumenal coronary angioplasty, thrombolytic therapy, stent placement, and rotoblade therapy. The earlier these procedures are performed, the greater the survival rate. (See Chapter 17 for discussion of these management modalities.)

■ ANAPHYLACTIC SHOCK

Etiology

Anaphylactic shock is a type of distributive shock resulting from exposure to a specific allergen that evokes a life-threatening hypersensitivity response. If left untreated, decreased tissue perfusion and vascular collapse will occur. Prompt intervention is critical. Predisposing factors, such as age, sex, race, occupation, allergic tendencies, or geographical location, do not seem to have a role in development of anaphylactic shock.

Antigens, the substances that elicit the response, can be introduced into the body through injection, ingestion, skin, or the respiratory tract. Substances capable of evoking an anaphylactic reaction in humans include a multitude of factors as outlined in Table 49–2.

Anaphylactic reactions can be either immunoglobulin E (IgE) or non-IgE mediated. Non–IgE responses occur without the presence of IgE antibodies and are called *anaphylactoid reactions*. It is thought that direct activation of mediators causes the response, but it may be that these reactions have not been investigated thoroughly enough as yet. Examples of such reactions are commonly associated with nonsteroidal anti-inflammatory agents and aspirin. Patients who have this type of response should be followed and instructed to avoid subsequent exposure to the precipitating antigen because the second exposure may elicit an anaphylactic reaction.

IgE-mediated reactions occur as a result of the immune response. The first time the immune system is exposed to an antigen, a very specific antibody IgE is formed. This highly specialized antibody is then stored in mast cells and basophils. When a second exposure to this antigen occurs, the antigen binds to IgE, thus triggering the release of histamine and other biochemical mediators that initiate anaphylactic shock.

Pathophysiological Principles

The antibody–antigen reaction causes antibody-specific mast cells and basophils to rupture or secrete substances, such as histamine, leukotrienes, eosinophil chemotactic substance, heparin, prostaglandins, neutrophil chemotactic substance, and platelet-activating factors.[2] These substances, in particular histamine, cause systemic vasodilation, increased capillary permeability, bronchoconstriction,

coronary vasoconstriction, and cutaneous reactions. Other substances precipitate a continued downward spiral by causing myocardial depression, inflammation, excessive mucus secretion, and peripheral vasodilation. This diffuse peripheral vasodilation creates a maldistribution of blood volume to tissues. As the reaction continues, peripheral vasodilation results in decreased venous return, coupled with increased capillary permeability, which leads to a loss of vascular volume. This causes a drop in CO and subsequent impaired tissue perfusion. While the patient initially experiences itching, hives, and some difficulty breathing, death can occur within minutes or hours.

Assessment

Because there may not be any predisposing factors that precipitate anaphylactic shock, it is important to recognize the various clinical expressions the patient may exhibit. Prevention is usually the best way to safeguard against anaphylactic shock. The nurse must obtain a thorough history of allergies and responses to drugs, foods, blood product, or anesthetic agents.

CLINICAL MANIFESTATIONS

Regardless of the etiology of the reaction, the treatment will depend on the patient's clinical symptoms. The earlier the symptoms appear, the more severe the response. The patient will develop generalized erythema, urticaria, pruritus, and subsequent angioedema. By now, the patient may begin to experience anxiety and restlessness and complain of dyspnea, feeling warm, and even pain. As the episode progresses, respiratory manifestations, such as laryngeal edema, bronchoconstriction, and stridor, may develop. Hy-

Table 49-2 Agents Commonly Implicated in Anaphylactic and Anaphylactoid Reactions

Antibiotics	Penicillin and its synthetics, cephalosporins, erythromycin, streptomycin, tetracyclines
Anti-inflammatory agents	Salicylates, aminopyrine
Narcotic analgesics	Morphine, codeine, meprobamate
Other medications	Protamine, chlorpropamide, parenteral iron, iodides, thiazide diuretics
Anesthetics	Procaine, lidocaine, cocaine, thiopental
Anesthetic adjuncts	Succinylcholine, tubocurarine
Blood products	Red blood cell, white blood cell, and platelet transfusions; gamma globulin
Immune sera	Rabies, tetanus, diphtheria antitoxin, snake and spider antivenom
Diagnostic agents	Iodinated radiocontrast agents
Venoms	Bees, wasps, hornets, spiders, snakes, jellyfish
Hormones	Insulin, corticotropin, pituitary extract
Enzymes and other biologicals	Acetylcysteine, pancreatic enzyme supplements
Extracts used in desensitization	Food, pollen, venoms
Foods	Eggs, fish, shellfish, milk, nuts, legumes

potension from vasodilation will soon occur. As circulatory collapse progresses, the patient's level of consciousness will deteriorate to unresponsiveness.

Management

Early recognition and treatment of anaphylactic shock is essential. Therapeutic goals include removal of the offending antigen, reversal of the effects of the biochemical mediators, and restoration of adequate tissue perfusion. If the symptoms are mild, immediate therapy includes oxygen and subcutaneous or IV administration of epinephrine (Adrenaline). Adrenaline dosage is given in the display. Other pharmacotherapy includes diphenhydramine, corticosteroids, and if necessary, vasoconstrictors and positive inotropic agents.

Nursing care revolves around maintaining an adequate airway and monitoring patient response to the antigen. The nurse will also monitor respirations, HR, level of anxiety, and blood pressure and institute comfort measures related to the dermatological manifestations. Patient education regarding prevention and treatment is critical for any person who experiences a significant antibody–antigen reaction.

NEUROGENIC SHOCK

Neurogenic shock results from loss or disruption of sympathetic tone, which causes peripheral vasodilation and subsequent decreased tissue perfusion. The disturbance of sympathetic tone can be caused by any event that disrupts the sympathetic nervous system. The most common cause of neurogenic shock is a spinal cord injury above the level of T6, but it may also be the result of spinal analgesia, emotional stress, pain, drugs, or other central nervous system problems. (The reader is referred to Chapter 36 for a thorough discussion on spinal cord injury and neurogenic shock.)

CLINICAL APPLICATION: Drug Therapy
Adrenaline Dosage in Anaphylaxis

- Adults—0.5 mL of a 1:1,000 solution intramuscularly or 3–5 mL of a 1:10,000 solution intramuscularly or slowly intravenously
- Children—0.01 mL of a 1:1,000 solution per kg intramuscularly or 0.1 mL of a 1:10,000 solution per kg intravenously

The dosage is not one ampoule

Fisher M: Treatment of acute anaphylaxis. Br Med J 311:731–734, 1995 (used with permission)

SYSTEMIC INFLAMMATORY RESPONSE SYNDROME AND SEPTIC SHOCK

The cause of SIRS, a recently defined state, is an overwhelming injury that activates the inflammatory/immune response (IIR) and causes an uncontrolled cascade of mediator responses. Septic shock is triggered by an invading microbe and more importantly, by the body's immune responses. Both may progress to states of hypoperfusion resulting in cell, tissue, and organ death. A patient with SIRS will have the same clinical presentation as a patient with sepsis, except all cultures will be negative. Sepsis, severe sepsis, and septic shock represent the same syndrome but at progressive stages of illness (Fig. 49–3).

In 1991, the Society of Critical Care Medicine and the American College of Chest Physicians established universal definitions for the term sepsis and other associated clinical conditions.[3] Their goals were to promote earlier detection and intervention of these states, improve outcomes, and standardize terminology used in research protocols so that the information derived would be easier to disseminate and apply to practice. The accompanying display summarizes these definitions.

Etiology

There are approximately 500,000 new episodes of sepsis each year in the United States with an associated 35% mortality rate.[4] Moreover, among hospitalized patients in noncoronary intensive care units (ICUs), sepsis has been reported to be the most common cause of death and is the 13th leading cause of death overall.[4] The same factors that place the patient at risk for developing states of hypoperfusion and the use of certain therapies may increase the risk for developing septic shock (see display). The high incidence of sepsis may reflect an increased number of chronically ill or immunocompromised patients who live longer because of improved medical therapy but have greater risk for sepsis because of invasive medical procedures and devices.

Pathophysiological Principles

According to Secor,[5] when the body receives an insult, whether mechanical, ischemic, chemical, or microbial, multiple elements of the IIR are activated to protect the body from invading pathogens, limit the extent of injury, and promote rapid healing of involved tissues. The IIR represents one of the body's most exquisite and complicated homeostatic mechanisms, spanning all levels of physiological interaction from the molecular to the systemic through numerous humoral, cellular, and biochemical pathways.[5] Normally the IIR is an essential, tightly regulated, and controlled protective mechanism. In some patients, however,

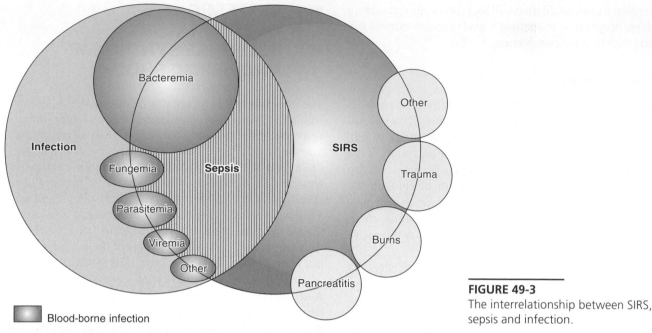

Blood-borne infection

FIGURE 49-3
The interrelationship between SIRS, sepsis and infection.

the regulation and control are lost. The result is an overwhelming IIR response that initiates pathophysiological changes, tissue destruction, and organ death.

Typically, septic shock is initiated by gram-negative bacteria (*Escherichia coli, Klebsiella, Pseudomonas, Bacteroides,* and *Proteus*). It may also be caused by gram-positive organisms (staphylococci, streptococci, and pneu-

mococci), fungi, and viruses.[6] In many patients, multiple causative organisms are identified. Bacteria may be introduced by invasive catheters or may translocate across an impaired gut mucosal barrier. This introduction of bacteria is associated with release of endotoxin and mediators of inflammation, resulting in the hemodynamic and metabolic responses of the septic cascade.

Clinical Terminology: Sepsis and Organ Failure

Definitions Developed by the Consensus Conference of Society of Critical Care Medicine and American College of Chest Physicians

Infection: Microbial phenomenon characterized by an inflammatory response to the presence of microorganisms or the invasion of normally sterile host tissue by those organisms

Bacteremia: The presence of viable bacteria in the blood

Systemic inflammatory response syndrome: The systemic inflammatory response to a variety of severe clinical insults. The response is manifested by two or more of the following conditions:

> Temperature >38°C or <36°C (100.4°F or 96.8°F)
> Heart rate >90 beats/min
> Respiratory rate >20 breaths/min or PaCO₂ <32 mmHg (<4.3 kPa)
> WBC >12,000 cell/mm³, <4,000 cells/mm³, or >10% immature (band) forms

Sepsis: The systemic response to infection. This systemic response is manifested by two or more of the following conditions as a result of infection:

> Temperature >38°C or <36°C

> Heart rate >90 beats/min
> Respiratory rate >20 breaths/min or PaCO₂ <32 mmHg (<4.3 kPa)
> WBC >12,000 cell/mm³, <4,000 cells/mm³, or >10% immature (band) forms

Severe sepsis: Sepsis associated with organ dysfunction, hypoperfusion, or hypotension. Hypoperfusion and perfusion abnormalities may include, but are not limited to, lactic acidosis, oliguria, or an acute alteration in mental status.

Septic shock: Sepsis with hypotension, despite adequate fluid resuscitation, along with the presence of perfusion abnormalities that may include, but are not limited to, lactic acidosis, oliguria, or an acute alteration in mental status. Patients who are on inotropic or vasopressor agents may not be hypotensive at the time that perfusion abnormalities are measured.

Hypotension: A systolic BP of <90 mmHg or a reduction of >40 mmHg from baseline in the absence of other causes for hypotension

Multiple organ dysfunction syndrome: Presence of altered organ function in an acutely ill patient such that homeostasis cannot be maintained without intervention

---

Bone RC: Definitions for sepsis and organ failure and guidelines for the use of innovative therapies in sepsis. Chest 101:1644–1653, 1992 (used with permission)

Risk Factors for Hypoperfused States

Host Factors	Treatment-Related Factors
Extremes of age	Use of invasive catheters
Malnutrition	Surgical procedures
General debilitation	Traumatic or thermal wounds
Chronic debilitation	Invasive diagnostic procedures
Chronic illness	Drugs (antibiotics, cytotoxic agents,
Drug or alcohol abuse	steroids)
Neutropenia	
Splenectomy	
Multiple organ failure	

Endotoxin is a component of the gram-negative cell wall. It is a lipopolysaccharide with an inner layer of lipid A, the substance considered most responsible for endotoxin activity.[6] The endotoxin's damage is most likely related to its ability to trigger the complement and coagulation cascades, along with multiple inflammatory mediators, causing increased microvascular permeability, vasodilation, and the microthrombi seen in septic patients.

Events surrounding the complex interactions of the mediators of IIR remain an ongoing area of research. Several mediators are believed to play a key role in the maldistribution of blood flow and oxygen delivery–consumption imbalance associated with SIRS and sepsis. Table 49–3 lists these key mediators and summarizes their activity.

PERFUSION IMBALANCE

Vasodilation resulting in low SVR is a predominant effect of the IIR. Increased capillary permeability sequesters fluid and proteins in the interstitial space, thus decreasing the effective intravascular circulating volume. In response to the deceased SVR and circulating volume, the CO may be high but inadequate to maintain tissue and end organ perfusion.

In conjunction with vasodilation, the mediators also cause tissue edema, vascular vasoconstriction, and microthrombi formation, which obstructs blood flow to the microvasculature, tissues, and organs. The net effects are adequate blood flow to some tissues with inadequate or poor blood flow in other tissue beds. This results in regions of tissue hypoxia and concomitant organ damage.

The inability of the circulatory system to meet cellular oxygen demands causes the cells to resort to anaerobic metabolism for energy production. The end product of anaerobic metabolism, lactic acid, is measured clinically to evaluate the effectiveness of end organ tissue perfusion.

MYOCARDIAL ALTERATIONS

Although maldistribution of blood flow is certainly one of the major abnormalities associated with septic shock, there is evidence that depressed myocardial performance, in the form of decreased ventricular ejection fraction and impaired con-

tractility, also is involved.[7] Myocardial depressant factor, thought to originate from ischemic pancreatic tissue, is one proposed causative agent.[8] Other studies suggest that impaired coronary perfusion is at fault or that other mediators, including tumor necrosis factor and IL-1, may also depress cardiac contractility.[7] The presence of lactic acidosis, which decreases myocardial responsiveness to catecholamines, may provide another explanation. Whatever the mechanism, the heart demonstrates impaired contractility and ventricular performance in the presence of septic shock. Figure 49–4 summarizes the cardiovascular pathophysiological events known to occur in the presence of septic shock.

Two different patterns of cardiac dysfunction are evident in septic shock. One form is characterized by high CO and low SVR, and the second form is hypodynamic, characterized by low CO and increased SVR. It is appropriate to view these processes as a continuum rather than distinct forms, with the hyperdynamic response denoting early shock and the hypodynamic phase indicative of late shock.

PULMONARY ALTERATIONS

The events initiated by endotoxin, IIR, and its mediators affect the lung both directly and indirectly. The initial pulmonary response is bronchoconstriction, resulting in pulmonary hypertension and increased respiratory work. Neutrophils are activated and infiltrate the pulmonary vasculature and tissue, causing an accumulation of extravascular lung water. Activated neutrophils are known to produce other substances that alter the integrity of the pulmonary parenchymal cells, resulting in increased permeability. As

---

Insights Into Clinical Research

Sasse K, Nauenberg E, et al: Long term survival after intensive care unit admission with sepsis. Crit Care Med 23(6):1040–1047, 1995

The purpose of this prospective study was to assess factors predictive of long-term survival in patients critically ill with sepsis.

Using the criteria developed by the American College of Chest Physicians and the Society of Critical Care Medicine, 153 patients met the definition of sepsis. Models were developed to predict the length of survival and the probability of survival at discharge, 1 month, 6 months, and 1 year. Discharge mortality rate was 51%. Other mortality rates were: 1 month, 40.5%; 6 months, 64.7%; and 1 year after discharge, 71.9%. Thirty-three patients survived past the 1-year study period.

Age was not associated with long- or short-term survival. The acute physiological score (APACHE II) was a major predictor of survival after discharge, as was the etiological organism of the sepsis. The highest rates of survival were associated with *Escherichia coli*, *Streptococcus pneumoniae*, and *Staphylococcus epidermidis*. Concomitant malignancy and human immunodeficiency virus infection contributed to significantly poorer outcomes.

TABLE 49-3
Mediators of the Inflammatory/Immune Responses (IIR)

Mediator	Description of Activity	Clinical Response
Endotoxin	• Activates complement system and coagulation cascades • Activates macrophages, which release TNF and IL-1	• Increased microvascular permeability, vasodilation, third-spacing, microthrombi formation • Inflammatory response
Tumor necrosis factor (TNF)	• Released by monocyte–macrophage system as a part of the IIR • Multiple effects locally and systemically • Stimulates other mediator activity	• Hypotension, tachycardia, myocardial depression, tachypnea, hyperglycemia, metabolic acidosis, third spacing, fever, microvascular vasoconstriction
Interleukin-1 (IL-1)	• Released by monocyte–macrophage system as part of the IIR • Stimulates leukocytosis • Triggers production of acute phase proteins and release of amino acids from skeletal muscle • Activates procoagulant activity • Decreases vascular responsiveness to catecholamines	• Increased white blood cells • High urinary nitrogen excretion and muscle wasting • Elevated coagulation laboratory values • Decreased SVR, which is not as responsive to low dosages of vasopressor or synthetic catecholamine agents
Complement cascade	• Inflammatory process • Opsonization and lysis of foreign particles and cells • Stimulates neutrophils (and oxygen radicals) and IL-1 • Degranulation of mast cells and basophils	• Edema formation, vasodilation, vascular permeability, third spacing • All effects of IL-1
Platelet aggregating factor (PAF)	• Released by mast cells, basophils, macrophages, neutrophils, platelets, and damaged endothelium • Increases platelet aggregation • Increases neutrophil adhesion • Increases vascular permeability and bronchoconstriction • Negative inotropic effects on the heart	• Microthrombi formation interfering with perfusion • Third spacing • Bronchoconstriction, rhonchi and wheezes, increased pulmonary airway pressures • Decreased heart contractility and force, which is not as responsive to low dosages of vasopressor and inotropic agents
Arachidonic acid metabolites (AA)	• Stimulation of AA causes the release of metabolites prostaglandins (PG), thromboxanes (TX), and leukotrienes (LT) • PGF and TXA_2 cause pulmonary hypertension, vasoconstriction, and platelet activation and aggregation • PGE, PGD, and prostacyclin cause vasodilation and decreased platelet aggregation • Leukotrienes increase neutrophil chemotaxis, vascular constriction, and increased vascular permeability • Increases gastric permeability to gram-negative bacteria	• Oxygenation and ventilation difficulties, increased airway resistance, wheezing • Third spacing and edema formation • Gram-negative bacteria translocation into the bloodstream, initiating endotoxin release
Oxygen radicals	• Generate metabolites (O_2^-, H_2O_2, OH^-) during the respiratory burst of the neutrophils • Damage cell structure and interfere with cell activities • Damage endothelial cells, which stimulate the coagulation system • Increase permeability	• Inflammatory response, edema formation, fever • Microthrombi formation • Third spacing

fluid collects in the interstitium, pulmonary compliance is reduced, gas exchange is impaired, and hypoxemia results.

Adult respiratory distress syndrome (ARDS) frequently is associated with septic shock. Forty to 60% of all patients with septic shock are at risk for development of ARDS. All vasoactive mediators discussed previously have been implicated in the development of ARDS secondary to increased capillary permeability and microthrombi formation, resulting in pulmonary edema and areas of poor pulmonary perfusion.

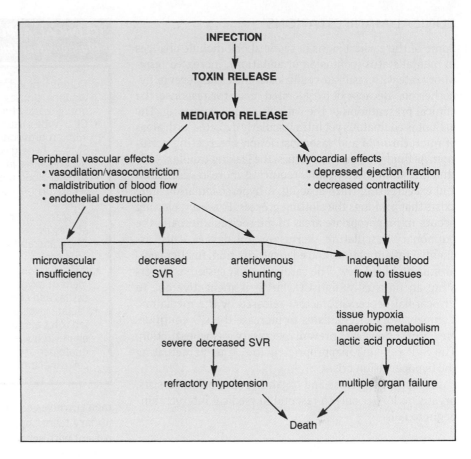

FIGURE 49-4

Pathophysiological cardiovascular events that occur in the presence of septic shock. (Reproduced with permission from Parillo JE (moderator): Septic shock in humans: Advances in understanding of pathogenesis, cardiovascular dysfunction, and therapy. Ann Intern Med 113: 227–242, 1990)

HEMATOLOGICAL ALTERATIONS

Bacteria or their toxins cause complement activations. Because sepsis involves a global inflammation response, overreactive complement activation may contribute to responses that eventually become detrimental rather than protective. Complement causes mast cells to release histamine, which stimulates vasodilation and increased capillary permeability. These actions further contribute to the circulatory alterations in volume distribution and the development of interstitial edema.

Platelet abnormalities also occur in septic shock because endotoxin indirectly causes platelet aggregation and subsequent release of more vasoactive substances (serotonin and TXA_2). Circulating platelet aggregates have been identified in the microvasculature, causing blood flow obstruction and compromised cellular metabolism. In addition, endotoxin or the bacterial infectious process itself activates the coagulation system. Over time, as clotting factors are depleted, a coagulopathy results, with the potential of progressing to disseminated intravascular coagulation.

METABOLIC ALTERATIONS

Widespread metabolic disturbances are seen with septic shock. The body manifests a progressive inability to use glucose, protein, and fat as energy sources. Hyperglycemia is a frequent finding in early shock. It is caused by increased gluconeogenesis and insulin resistance, which prevents the uptake of glucose into the cell. As shock progresses, hypo-

glycemia results as glycogen stores are depleted and peripheral supplies of proteins and fats are insufficient to meet the body's metabolic demands.

Protein breakdown occurs in septic shock. It is evidenced by high urinary nitrogen excretion. Muscle protein is broken down to amino acids, some of which are used for oxidation. Others are transported to the liver for use in gluconeogenesis. In later stages of shock, the liver is unable to use the amino acids due to its own metabolic dysfunction. Amino acids then accumulate in the bloodstream.

As the shock state progresses, adipose tissue is broken down (lipolysis) to furnish the liver with lipids for energy production. Lipid metabolism produces ketones, which then are used in the Krebs cycle. As liver function decreases, however, triglycerides begin forming that collect in the mitochondria and inhibit the Krebs cycle (oxidative metabolism). Increased lactate production is the result.

The net effect of these metabolic derangements is that the cell becomes energy starved. This energy deficit is implicated in the emergence of multiple organ failure that frequently develops regardless of the ability to support the circulatory and organ systems.

Assessment

A thorough understanding of the mediator responses that occur during SIRS and sepsis will help the critical care nurse assess the patient and evaluate the patient's response to management therapies.

CLINICAL MANIFESTATIONS

Some of the earliest signs of septic shock include changes in mental status (confusion or agitation), increased respiratory rate with respiratory alkalosis, and either fever or hypothermia. Because of exaggerated mediator response, the clinical presentation of the patient is often confusing. The patient is edematous yet intravascularly depleted with areas of microthrombi and vasoconstriction obstructing perfusion. As fluid replacement occurs, the leaking capillary beds shift the fluid interstitially, requiring more resuscitation and exacerbating third-spacing. A hypercoagulation state exists that prolongs the clotting process. However, clotting occurs in inappropriate areas of microcirculation and the pulmonary vasculature. Perfusion imbalances cause ischemia, inflammation, and edema formation, further compromising blood flow. The cardiovascular system is generating an unusually high CO, but it is ineffective due to myocardial depressant factors released by the mediators. Compensatory mechanisms to increase the CO continue. Mediators, however, prevent necessary vasoconstriction. The SVR remains inappropriately low, thus perpetuating the hypoperfusion crisis.

As sepsis progresses and organ hypoperfusion persists, organs no longer able to respond to medical interventions begin to fail.

DIAGNOSTIC STUDIES

Diagnostic studies that may be helpful in the identification of sepsis are summarized in the display. Despite the use of such testing, the early diagnosis of sepsis and septic shock is usually made on the basis of clinical findings.

Management

Patients with septic shock require prompt and aggressive monitoring and management in the ICU. Because septic shock is a complex and generalized process, its manage-

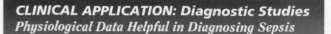

CLINICAL APPLICATION: Diagnostic Studies
Physiological Data Helpful in Diagnosing Sepsis

- Cultures: blood, sputum, urine, surgical or nonsurgical wounds, sinuses, and invasive lines; positive results are not necessary for diagnosis.
- CBC: WBCs usually will be elevated and may decrease with progression of shock.
- SMA-7: hyperglycemia may be evident, followed by hypoglycemia in later stages.
- Arterial blood gases: respiratory alkalosis is present in sepsis (pH >7.456, PCO_2 <35), with mild hypoxemia (PO_2 <80)
- CT scan may be needed to identify sites of potential abscesses.
- Chest and abdominal radiographs may reveal infectious processes.
- $S\overline{V}O_2$ pulmonary artery catheter will assist in the assessment of oxygen delivery and consumption needs of the tissues and cells.
- Lactate level: decreasing levels of lactate in the serum indicates aerobic metabolism is able to meet cellular energy requirements. Elevated levels indicate inadequate perfusion and anaerobic metabolism to meet cellular energy requirements.

ment involves all organ systems and requires a multidisciplinary team approach. The primary goals in treating the patient with septic shock are to provide supportive therapy and maximize oxygen delivery above the cellular oxygen consumption requirements in an effort to halt the exaggerated IIR and mediator response. A collaborative care guide outlines some of the care given in septic shock.

PREVENTION

Because diagnosis of sepsis is so complex and mortality from septic shock so high, it is imperative that preventive infection control measures be in place. The critically ill patient with impaired defense mechanisms must be protected from hospital-acquired (nosocomial) infections. Nosoco-

---

COLLABORATIVE CARE GUIDE
for the Patient in Septic Shock

OUTCOMES	INTERVENTIONS
Oxygenation/Ventilation	
Patent airway is maintained. Lungs are clear on auscultation.	• Auscultate breath sounds q2–4h and PRN. • Suction endotracheal airway when appropriate (see Collaborative Care Guide for Patient on a Ventilator, Chapter 24). • Hyperoxygenate and hyperventilate before and after each suction pass.
Arterial blood gases are within normal limits.	• Monitor pulse oximetry and end tidal CO_2. • Monitor arterial blood gases as indicated by changes in noninvasive parameters. • Monitor intrapulmonary shunt ($\dot{Q}s/\dot{Q}t$ and PaO_2/FiO_2)
Peak, mean, and plateau pressures are within normal limits.	• Monitor airway pressures q1–2h.

(continued)

COLLABORATIVE CARE GUIDE
for the Patient in Septic Shock (Continued)

OUTCOMES	INTERVENTIONS
There is no evidence of atelectasis or infiltrates.	• Turn side to side q2h.
	• Consider kinetic therapy or prone positioning.
There is no evidence of adult respiratory distress syndrome (ARDS).	• Do daily chest x-ray (see Collaborative Care Guide for Patient with ARDS, Chapter 26).
Circulation/Perfusion	
Blood pressure, heart rate, CVP, and pulmonary artery pressures are within normal limits.	• Assess vital signs q1h.
	• Assess hemodynamic pressures q1h if patient has pulmonary artery catheter.
	• Administer intravascular volume as ordered to maintain preload.
Vascular resistance is within normal limits.	• Assess SVR and PVR q6–12 h.
	• Administer intravascular volume and vasopressors as ordered.
Oxygen delivery is >600 mL O_2/m^2 and oxygen consumption is >150 mL O_2/m^2.	• Monitor cardiac output, DaO_2, and VO_2 q6–12h.
	• Administer red blood cells, positive inotropic agents, colloid infusion as ordered to increase oxygen delivery.
	• Consider monitoring gastric mucosal pH as a guide to systemic perfusion.
Serum lactate will be within normal limits.	• Monitor serum lactate qd until it is within normal limits.
Fluids/Electrolytes	
Urine output is >30 mL/h (or >0.5 mL/kg/h).	• Monitor intake and output q1h.
	• Administer fluids and diuretics to maintain intravascular volume and renal function, per order.
There is no evidence of electrolyte imbalance or renal dysfunction.	• Monitor electrolytes daily and PRN.
	• Replace electrolytes as ordered.
	• Monitor BUN, creatinine, serum osmolality, and urine electrolytes daily.
Mobility/Safety	
There is no evidence of complications related to bed rest and immobility.	• Initiate deep vein thrombosis prophylaxis.
	• Reposition frequently.
	• Mobilize to chair when acute phase is past, and hemodynamic stability and hemostasis are achieved.
	• Consult physical therapist.
	• Conduct range-of-motion and strengthening exercises.
Normalization of temperature and WBC and negative blood cultures as evidence that source and microorganisms causing sepsis are obliterated.	• Identify source of infection: obtain urine, sputum, and blood cultures; central vascular line tip cultures; wound cultures.
	• Administer antibiotics as directed by culture results.
	• Monitor serum antibiotic levels.
	• Obtain infectious disease consult.
	• Monitor systemic inflammatory response syndrome criteria: increased WBCs, increased temperature, tachypnea, tachycardia.
There is no evidence of new infection.	• Use strict aseptic technique during procedures, and monitor technique of others.
	• Maintain sterility of invasive catheters and tubes.
	• Per hospital protocol, change chest tube and other dressings and invasive catheters.
Skin Integrity	
Skin will remain intact.	• Assess skin q4h and each time patient is repositioned.
	• Turn q2h.
	• Consider pressure relief/reduction mattress.
	• Use Braden Scale to assess risk of skin breakdown.

(continued)

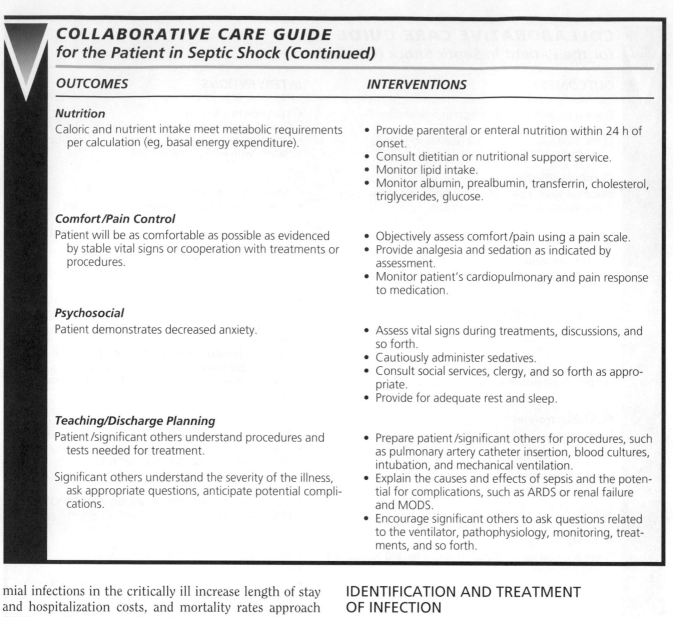

COLLABORATIVE CARE GUIDE
for the Patient in Septic Shock (Continued)

OUTCOMES	INTERVENTIONS
Nutrition	
Caloric and nutrient intake meet metabolic requirements per calculation (eg, basal energy expenditure).	• Provide parenteral or enteral nutrition within 24 h of onset. • Consult dietitian or nutritional support service. • Monitor lipid intake. • Monitor albumin, prealbumin, transferrin, cholesterol, triglycerides, glucose.
Comfort/Pain Control	
Patient will be as comfortable as possible as evidenced by stable vital signs or cooperation with treatments or procedures.	• Objectively assess comfort/pain using a pain scale. • Provide analgesia and sedation as indicated by assessment. • Monitor patient's cardiopulmonary and pain response to medication.
Psychosocial	
Patient demonstrates decreased anxiety.	• Assess vital signs during treatments, discussions, and so forth. • Cautiously administer sedatives. • Consult social services, clergy, and so forth as appropriate. • Provide for adequate rest and sleep.
Teaching/Discharge Planning	
Patient/significant others understand procedures and tests needed for treatment. Significant others understand the severity of the illness, ask appropriate questions, anticipate potential complications.	• Prepare patient/significant others for procedures, such as pulmonary artery catheter insertion, blood cultures, intubation, and mechanical ventilation. • Explain the causes and effects of sepsis and the potential for complications, such as ARDS or renal failure and MODS. • Encourage significant others to ask questions related to the ventilator, pathophysiology, monitoring, treatments, and so forth.

mial infections in the critically ill increase length of stay and hospitalization costs, and mortality rates approach 35%[9]. A critical aspect of nursing care involves adherence to aseptic techniques, thorough handwashing, and a continuing awareness of multiple sites and causes of infection in the critically ill patient. Sources of equipment-related infections are listed in the display.

RED FLAG   **Equipment-Related Sources of Infections**

Intravascular catheters
Endotracheal/tracheostomy tubes
Indwelling urinary catheters
Surgical wound drains
Intracranial monitoring devices and catheters
Orthopedic hardware
Nasogastric tubes
Gastrointestinal tubes

IDENTIFICATION AND TREATMENT OF INFECTION

Identification and eradication of the infection's source is of utmost concern. Before the source or type of organism has been ascertained, empiric antibiotic therapy is initiated. Patients will require multiple antibiotics to provide broad-spectrum coverage against gram-negative and gram-positive bacteria and anaerobes. Many clinicians empirically use broad-spectrum antibiotics, such as third-generation cephalosporins or aminoglycosides. Other definitive measures to isolate and alleviate the cause of sepsis include resection or drainage of purulent tissues or secretions.

Removing the cause of sepsis is not sufficient to treat the generalized system reactions seen with septic shock. The patient needs supportive measures to establish and maintain adequate tissue perfusion, in addition to other therapies aimed at blocking or interfering with the action of the various mediators implicated in the shock process. Aspects of supportive care include the following:

• Restoring intravascular volume
• Maintaining an adequate CO

- Ensuring adequate ventilation and oxygenation
- Providing an appropriate metabolic environment[7]

RESTORATION OF INTRAVASCULAR VOLUME

Adequate volume replacement is important for reversing hypotension. Patients may require several liters or more of fluid because of the mediator-induced vasodilation. Fluid replacement should be guided by the hemodynamic parameters and urine output; therefore, patients will usually require pulmonary artery and arterial catheterization for close monitoring. A downward trend in the serum lactate level is a good indicator of improving tissue perfusion.

There is some controversy as to whether crystalloid or colloid fluids should be used for volume replacement.[7] The patient's underlying condition and response will guide this decision. Blood products may be administered in the absence of bleeding to enhance the delivery of oxygen to cells. Administering the fluid and closely monitoring the patient's response to fluid therapy are important nursing responsibilities.

MAINTENANCE OF ADEQUATE CARDIAC OUTPUT

In the early phase of septic shock, CO may be either normal or elevated. Because of decreased SVR and peripheral vasodilation, nevertheless, it is not adequate to maintain tissue oxygenation and perfusion. As septic shock progresses, CO begins to drop because of cardiac dysfunction. Therefore, enhancing CO is an essential therapeutic goal. Current research suggests that to enhance survival of the septic patient, one must maximize the CO and DaO2 in an effort to surpass the VO2 needs. Consequently, a cardiac index (CI) greater than 5.5 L/min/m², DaO2 > 1,000 mL/min/m², and VO2 >190 mL/min/m² may enhance survival.[10]

If adequate volume replacement does not improve tissue perfusion, vasoactive drugs will be administered to support circulation. Dopamine, which increases SVR and improves renal and mesenteric blood flow, is a preferred agent. Dobutamine may be added for its inotropic effects on the heart. Other vasoactive drugs frequently used include levarterenol (Levophed), epinephrine, phenylephrine, and the vasodilator nitroprusside (Nipride). Some patients with low CO and high SVR may benefit from the use of vasodilators to redistribute blood flow and improve perfusion.[7] Many times, no single drug can achieve the desired hemodynamic effects. In these situations, various combinations of drugs are individualized to the patient's response. The nurse's role in this therapy is to administer the drugs, usually titrating the dosage to a desired response or effect, and closely monitoring the patient for response and potentially harmful side effects.

MAINTENANCE OF ADEQUATE VENTILATION AND OXYGENATION

Maintaining a patent airway, augmenting ventilation, and ensuring adequate oxygenation in the patient with septic shock usually requires endotracheal intubation and mechanical ventilation. Positive end-expiratory pressure frequently is needed to aid oxygenation (for nursing management issues on ventilation, see Chapter 24).

An essential element in the assessment of circulatory support, ventilation, and oxygenation is frequent evaluation of the patient's DaO2 and VO2 needs. The goal is to maximize DaO2 to supranormal limits to ensure that VO2 remains independent of DaO2. Through the delivery of adequate oxygen to the cells, aerobic metabolism will be maintained, and hopefully tissue energy needs will be met.

MAINTENANCE OF APPROPRIATE METABOLIC ENVIRONMENT

The many and varied metabolic derangements associated with septic shock necessitate frequent monitoring of hematological, renal, and liver function. Concurrently, nutritional stores are depleted in shock, and the patient will need supplemental nutrition to prevent malnutrition and to optimize cellular function. Enteral nutrition (EN) is the preferred route of nutritional support because it maintains the integrity of the gastrointestinal tract,[11] decreasing the probability of gut ischemia and translocation of bacteria into the bloodstream. EN feeding intolerance may necessitate the use of total parenteral nutrition (TPN), but ideally, a small amount of nutrition through the gut can still be delivered. Recent research suggests that specific nutrients typically found in EN and some in TPN may assist with support of the immune system during states of stress. Essential nutrients for immune support include arginine, glutamine, nucleotidase, omega-3 fatty acids, branch-chain amino acids, and antioxidant vitamins[11] (see Chapter 39 for discussion of nutritional support).

INVESTIGATIONAL THERAPIES

Although antibiotics and supportive therapy are the mainstays of treatment for septic shock, certain investigational drugs and therapies may be used. These drugs are aimed directly at the bacterial toxins and the mediators implicated in the immunological response seen with sepsis and SIRS. The complexity of this response leads many investigators to believe that it is unlikely that any one agent will prove to be effective. Multiple therapies tailored to individual circumstances most likely will be needed. Treatment of septic shock and SIRS is summarized in the display.

Complications

Multisystem organ dysfunction syndrome (MODS) may be a consequence of inability to maintain end organ perfusion in patients with shock states. The mortality rate associated with MODS ranges from 40% to 90%. When one or two systems are involved, the mortality rate varies from 41% to 67%; however, when three or more organs begin to dysfunction, the mortality rate jumps to 60% to 100%.[10]

NURSING PERSPECTIVE
Summary of Management Highlights for Septic Shock

Definitive Therapies

- Identify and eliminate the source of infection.
- Use multiple broad-spectrum antibiotics.

Supportive Therapies

- Restore intravascular volume.
- Maximize cardiac output.
- Maximize oxygen delivery to meet oxygen consumption needs.
- Provide appropriate metabolic environment.

Investigational Therapies

- Antihistamines
- Monoclonal antibodies/antagonists to
  endotoxin
  TNF
  lipid A
  IL-1
  C5a
  Cyclooxygenase inhibitors
  Lipoxygenase inhibitors
  Leukotriene antagonists
  Thromboxane A inhibitors
  Nitric oxide synthase inhibitors
- Nonsteroidal agents: ibuprofen, indomethacin
- Naloxone
- Neutrophil inhibitors
- Corticosteroids

Typically, the first organs to manifest signs of dysfunction are the lungs and kidneys. Hepatic failure tends to occur later in the progression of MODS due to the liver's amazing compensatory capacity. The ability to maintain end organ perfusion and adequate oxygen delivery is necessary to prevent the development of MODS.

CLINICAL APPLICATION: Patient Care Study

Mrs. Cox, a 50-year-old woman, presented to the clinic with complaints of abdominal pain with nausea and vomiting for 3 days and one episode of lower GI bleeding. Past medical history includes chronic renal failure, dialysis three times a week, kidney transplant 1.5 years ago, and rejection and transplant nephrectomy 2 months ago. She reported feeling weak and tired.

On physical examination, Mrs. Cox was an obese woman with abdominal tenderness in the epigastric region, with no rebound or guarding. She had a peritoneal dialysis catheter in place with redness and swelling noted at the insertion site. Her vital signs were HR, 116; RR, 30; BP, 140/90; T, 38.5°C (101.3°F).

Laboratory Values

Hgb, 5 g/dL
Hct, 15%
WBC, 19.4
Glucose, 140 mg/dL
Sodium, 135 mEq/L
Potassium, 4.1 mEq/L
Chloride, 102 mEq/L
CO_2, 19 mEq/L
BUN, 36 mg/dL
Creatinine, 6.0 mg/dL
Amylase, 140 U/L
AST/SGOT and ALT/SGPT, within normal limits

Mrs. Cox was admitted to the hospital for abdominal pain workup and anemia. She was transfused with 2 U of packed red blood cells; her hematocrit increased to 26%, her skin color improved, and she reported less weakness. Two days after admission, she had an increase in WBCs to 26.1, her temperature was 39.8°C (103.6°F), and colonoscopy findings suggested ischemic bowel versus intra-abdominal infection (perhaps secondary to an infected peritoneal dialysis catheter). Surgery was scheduled for later that day. Blood cultures were drawn, and Mrs. Cox received preoperative antibiotics. She had an arterial line and pulmonary artery catheter inserted. Initial parameters were cardiac output (CO), 8.0 L/min; cardiac index (CI), 5.2 L/min/m²; pulmonary artery wedge pressure (PAWP), 6 mmHg; SVR, 800 dynes/s/cm⁻⁵; BP, 100/60; mean arterial pressure (MAP), 73 mmHg; HR, 132. Arterial blood gases (ABGs) revealed respiratory alkalosis with pH, 7.50; PCO_2, 20 mmHg; PO_2, 68 mmHg; HCO_3, 17 mEq/L. Mrs. Cox received 4 L of IV fluid and was started on dopamine to maintain her MAP >60 mmHg.

Operating Room Findings

Mrs. Cox had pancreatitis with a collection of inflamed tissue and pus drained, and 6 ft of necrotic small bowel resected. Her abdominal incision was only partially closed; she was hemodynamically unstable, remained intubated and on the ventilator, and was transported to the surgical intensive care unit (SICU).

On postoperative day 1, Mrs. Cox remained hemodynamically unstable: T, 39.3°C; HR, 140–150; BP, 110/90 on 12 μg/kg/min of dobutamine. Pulmonary artery readings were hyperdynamic: CO, 9.2 L/min; CI, 5.8 L/min/m²; PCW, 18 mmHg; SVR, 480 dynes/second/cm^{-5}. She required large amounts of fluid resuscitation (6–8 L in the first 24 hours postop) and was given 0.9% normal saline and blood products for a persistently low hematocrit (25%). Her ABGs revealed a metabolic acidosis and a serum lactate level of 5.8 mmol/L. WBCs dropped to 8.6, and her preoperative blood cultures were positive for *Proteus*. Mrs. Cox was responsive to pain, unable to follow commands, and was being medicated with intermittent doses of midazolam and morphine.

On postoperative day 2, the patient's hemodynamic status was not improved. Epinephrine at .05 μg/kg/min was added to help maintain her MAP greater than 60 mmHg. Her lactate level was 9.0 mmol/L, WBCs dropped to 2.3, and coagulation parameters were showing evidence of a coagulopathy: PT, >15 seconds; PTT, 40 seconds; platelets, 60,000. Liver function tests were elevated, and Mrs. Cox was showing signs of scleral jaundice. She remained on the ventilator with PEEP at 12 cm H₂O to improve oxygenation. Her mental status fluctuated between being obtunded yet responsive to pain, to awake and agitated. The SICU care was focused on supportive and monitoring issues. Triple antibiotics were being administered (metronidazole, vancomycin, gentamicin), and she had no change in blood culture results. Her wound remained open without any signs of infection, and she was started on total parenteral nutrition.

The large fluid requirements combined with her chronic renal failure and septic shock produced significant peripheral edema, especially in her face and extremities. Because of the potential for skin breakdown, the nurses placed her on a specialty bed designed to prevent skin breakdown and improve pulmonary status.

By postoperative day 5, Mrs. Cox began showing signs of improvement. Her BP was stabilizing, and the vasoactive drugs were being weaned. Her hemodynamic parameters were normalizing (CO, 7.7 L/min, CI, 5.0 L/min/m²; PCW, 11–16 mmHg; SVR, 1,100 dynes/s/cm^{-5}). Her lactate levels were decreasing. Coagulation parameters were within normal limits, WCBs remained low but improving, and her blood cultures were negative. Mrs. Cox's mental status was clearing, and although she had brief episodes of confusion, she was able to communicate and interact with her family. Her skin remained intact, and her wound was showing signs of granulation.

By postoperative day 8, Mrs. Cox was extubated, off all vasoactive drugs, and had only a central line in place for central venous pressure monitoring. Over the next 2 weeks, she continued to improve, resumed dialysis, and eventually was transferred to the medical/surgical unit, with eventual discharge home.

■ CONCLUSION

Complex intertwining physiological processes are initiated by the body during states of stress and hypoperfusion. Appropriate medical and nursing interventions are essential to reverse the shock state and support body systems. Attention to the patient's history of illness, risk factors, VO₂, and trending of vital signs and neurological status often provide key information that may allow earlier intervention and prevention of prolonged states of hypoperfusion and organ failure.

Clinical Applicability Challenges

Self-Challenge: Critical Thinking

1. Compare and contrast medical and nursing management interventions for the various types of clinical shock states.

2. Early detection and prevention of shock are primary nursing responsibilities in the critical care setting. Develop an assessment plan that will help you identify these clinical situations.

Study Questions

1. Hypovolemic shock is frequently the result of
   a. a disruption in sympathetic tone.
   b. hemorrhage or the fluid shifts associated with burn injuries.
   c. the sudden loss of intracellular fluid.
   d. All of the above

2. Initial treatment priorities for care of the patient in cardiogenic shock include
   a. oxygenation, antiarrhythmics, fluids, and vasopressors.
   b. oxygenation, steroids, fluids, and surgery.
   c. oxygenation, antibiotics, vasopressors, and transplantation.
   d. None of the above

3. During the initial treatment for septic shock, the nurse would expect to
   a. limit IV fluids to keep open rate, give antibiotics pending culture results, administer vasopressors to increase the blood pressure.
   b. administer many liters of IV fluids, give antibiotics before culture results, titrate vasopressors according to blood pressure response.
   c. closely monitor the patient, pending treatment until definitive culture results are obtained.
   d. assist with intubation and ventilation, monitor vital signs, and prepare the patient for surgery.

4. The difference between SIRS and sepsis is
   a. SIRS will not progress into shock, while sepsis may.
   b. SIRS has no identifiable causative organism and sepsis does.
   c. SIRS has a higher mortality rate than sepsis.
   d. Sepsis has no identifiable causative organism and SIRS does.

5. Which signs and symptoms best describe the patient in early septic shock?
   a. Confused, hyperthermic, hypotensive, and in metabolic acidosis
   b. Obtunded, hyperthermic, hypotensive, and in metabolic alkalosis
   c. Agitated, normothermic, hypotensive, and in respiratory acidosis
   d. Confused, hypothermic, hypotensive, and in respiratory alkalosis

REFERENCES

1. Moscuscci M, Bates E: Cardiogenic shock. Cardiology Clinics 13: 391–405, 1995
2. Guyton A, Hall J: Textbook of Medical Physiology (9th Ed), p 454. Philadelphia, WB Saunders, 1996

3. Ackerman MH: The systemic inflammatory response, sepsis, and multiple organ dysfunction; new definitions for an old problem. Critical Care Nursing Clinics of North America 6:243–250, 1994

4. Rangel-Fraust MS, Pittet D, Costigan M: The natural history of the systemic inflammatory response syndrome: A prospective study. JAMA 273:117–123, 1995

5. Secor VH: The inflammatory/immune response in critical illness. Critical Care Nursing Clinics of North America 6:251–262, 1994

6. Colletti RC, Dew RB, Goulart AE: Antiendotoxin therapy in sepsis. Critical Care Nursing Clinics of North America 5:345–353, 1993

7. Parrillo JE: Septic shock in humans: Clinical evaluation, pathogenesis, and therapeutic approach. In Shoemaker WC (ed): Textbook of Critical Care (3rd Ed). Philadelphia, WB Saunders, 1995

8. Secor VH: The systemic inflammatory response syndrome: Role of inflammatory mediators in multiple organ dysfunction syndrome. In Secor VH (ed): Multiple Organ Dysfunction and Failure, pp 47–72. St. Louis, Mosby, 1996

9. Pittet D, Tarara D, Wenzel R: Nosocomial bloodstream infection in critically ill patients: Excess length of stay, extra costs, and attributable mortality. JAMA 271(20):1598–1601, 1994

10. Shoemaker WC, Appel PL, Kram HB, et al: Sequence of physiologic patterns in surgical septic shock. Crit Care Med 21:1876–1888, 1993

11. Bagley SM: Nutritional needs of the acutely ill with acute wounds. Critical Care Nursing Clinics of North America 8:159–168, 1996

BIBLIOGRAPHY

Bone RC: Definitions for sepsis and organ failure and guidelines for the use of innovative therapies in sepsis. Chest 101:1644–1653, 1992

Brass NJ: Predisposition to multiple organ dysfunction. Crit Care Nurs Q 16:1–7, 1994

Fisher M: Treatment of acute anaphylaxis. Br Med J 311:731–734, 1995

Graham P, Brass NJ: Multiple organ dysfunctions: Pathophysiology and therapeutic modalities. Crit Care Nurs Q 16:8–15, 1994

Hazinski MF: Mediator-specific therapies for the systemic inflammatory response syndrome, sepsis, severe sepsis, and septic shock. Critical Care Nursing Clinics of North America 6(2):303–319, 1994

Holmes DR, Bates ER, Kleiman NS, et al: Contemporary reperfusion therapy for cardiogenic shock. The GUSTO-1 trial experience. J Am Coll Cardiol 26(3):668–674, 1995

Isselbacher K, Braunwald E, Wilson HD: Harrison's Principles of Internal Medicine (2nd Ed), pp 1632–1634. New York, McGraw-Hill, 1994

Lynn WA, Cohen J: Adjunctive therapy for septic shock: A review of experimental approaches. Clinical Infectious Diseases 20:143–158, 1995

McMahon K: Multiple organ failure: The final complication of critical illness. Crit Care Nurse 15:20–28, 1995

Metrangolo L, Fiorillo M, Friedman G, et al: Early hemodynamic course of septic shock. Crit Care Med 23:1971–1975, 1995

Society of Critical Care Medicine: American College of Chest Physicians/Society of Critical Care Medicine Consensus Conference: Definitions for sepsis and organ failure and guidelines for the use on innovative therapies in sepsis. Crit Care Med 20:864–873, 1992

50

Trauma

OBJECTIVES

Based on the content in this chapter, the reader should be able to:

- Outline phases of initial assessment and related care of the trauma patient.
- Discuss the treatment of and nursing actions associated with trauma to the chest and heart.
- Contrast the response of solid and hollow abdominal organs to trauma.
- Use nursing actions related to abdominal trauma.
- Explain nursing responsibilities associated with trauma to the extremities.
- Discuss disorders involved in multiple organ failure.

*T*rauma is the leading cause of death in people between the ages of 1 and 44 years. In people over 44 years, trauma is surpassed only by cancer and cardiovascular disease. The cost of trauma in terms of potential lost years of productive life, however, exceeds that of both cancer and cardiovascular disease.[1] Trauma is also a major cause of disability. Trauma can be accidental (eg, motor vehicle accidents, falls, hunting accidents), self-inflicted (eg, suicidal jumps or gunshot wounds), or the result of violence (eg, firearm injuries, stabbings, assaults, domestic abuse). As a major cause of death and disability, trauma has become a significant health and social problem.

Many advances in the care of traumatized patients have been made in the last several decades. The development of trauma centers has decreased mortality and morbidity among trauma victims. Improved prehospital care and transportation have resulted in an increasing number of critically injured people reaching hospitals alive. Consequently, traumatized patients arriving in today's intensive care units (ICUs) tend to have serious injuries involving multiple organs, and they often require extensive and complex nursing care.

PATHOPHYSIOLOGICAL PRINCIPLES

Mechanical, or kinetic, energy injury accounts for the majority of traumatic injuries and is the only type of injury addressed in this chapter. Mechanical trauma can be caused by a blunt or penetrating force. Information related to the pattern or mechanism of injury is helpful in diagnosis of potential disorders.

Blunt Trauma

Blunt trauma most often occurs in motor vehicle accidents (MVAs) but can also result from a fall, assault, crush, or sports injury. Rapid deceleration during an MVA or fall can cause shearing forces. As the body comes to an abrupt stop, organs or structures continue to move forward leading to tearing of tissues and mobile organs. For instance, the heart can tear away from adjacent anchoring great vessels. Likewise, abdominal organs may tear away from the mesentery. Another mechanism of blunt injury involves compression caused by severe crushing forces. In such cases, the heart can be compressed between the sternum and spine. The liver, spleen, and pancreas are also often compressed against the spine. Solid organs are more susceptible to injury caused by crushing forces. Encapsulated organs (kidney, liver, spleen) may fragment or rupture when compressed. Crush injuries frequently cause internal damage with few external signs of trauma.

Generally, the greater the speed involved in the accident, the greater the injury. In an automobile accident, the vehicle offers some protection and absorbs energy from the collision. The unrestrained driver or passenger, however, can be ejected from the car and receive additional injuries on impact. Motorcyclists have minimal protection and frequently sustain severe injuries when thrown. Likewise, pedestrians struck by an automobile tend to suffer severe injuries, as shown in Figure 50–1.

Penetrating Trauma

Gunshot wounds and stab wounds account for most penetrating injuries. Death due to firearms is predicted to surpass MVA-caused deaths within the next decade.[2]

GUNSHOT WOUNDS

Severity of injury following gunshot wounds is related to the amount of kinetic energy transferred from the missile (bullet) to the tissues. The extent of damage depends on the size and speed of the bullet, distance from which the bullet is fired, and the type of tissue affected. For instance, elastic tissue like that of the bowel wall is more resistant to permanent damage, whereas inelastic tissue like that of the liver or brain is more likely to sustain damage that is permanent. Figure 50–2 shows the results of gunshot wounds at various distances from the body, including the entry and exit wounds.

As a missile enters the body, tissue is displaced, thus forming a tract or cavity. This is called cavitation. With low-velocity weapons (eg, .22 caliber handguns) cavitation is minimal. High-velocity weapons (eg, rifles, military weapons) cause greater injury due to increased cavitation. High-velocity missiles can produce a cavity many times

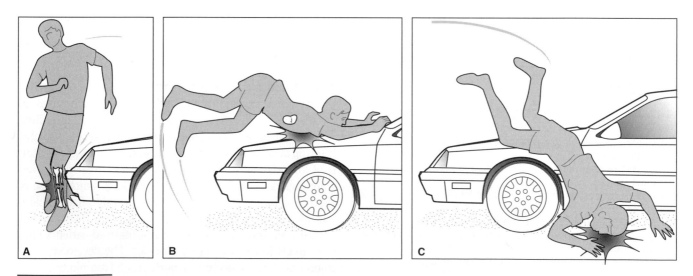

FIGURE 50-1
Pedestrians may be hurt critically when hit by a moving vehicle. (**A**) A common injury is the fracture of the tibia and fibula at the time of imact, (**B**) Impact when the pedestrian strikes the hood of the car may cause fractured ribs and a ruptured spleen, (**C**) Injuries to the head and additional fractures of the extremities may occur as the pedestrian rolls off the braking car or is thrown by the impact.

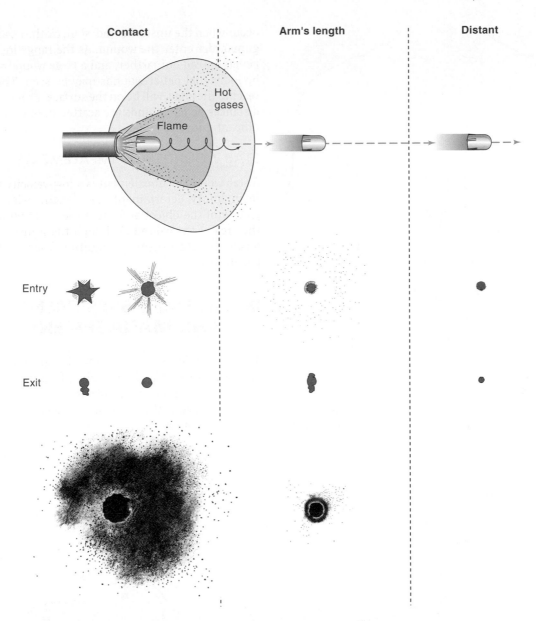

FIGURE 50-2
Diagrammatic views of the effects of gunshot wounds on the body surface. Kinetic energy is dependent on the distance from which the weapon is fired and the tissue involved. Entry and exit wounds are shown when in direct contact, at arm's reach, and at a distance. The bottom illustrations show entry wounds of a .22 rifle at 5-cm range (*left*) and at 20-cm range (*right*). The drilled in entry wound and faint powder markings are indicated.

their diameter, thus damaging structures outside the direct path. This is known as the "blast effect." The entire tract or cavity is subject to tissue devitalization and contamination.

Bullets can also fragment, ricochet, or tumble, resulting in additional injuries. Some bullets (eg, hollow-point) are designed to expand on impact, thus increasing the amount of kinetic energy dissipated. Internal bleeding, organ perforation, and fractures can all be caused by gunshot wounds. Possible organ damage is shown in Figure 50–3.

SHOTGUN WOUNDS

A shotgun discharges a shell containing multiple pellets, gunpowder, and a paper or plastic wad that separates the pellets from the gunpowder. The pellets spread out as they leave the gun barrel. The distance from which the shotgun was fired and pellet spread are the major factors determining severity of injury (Fig. 50–4). At closer than 6 ft, the pellets are still tightly grouped, causing a single entrance wound. Significant damage and contamination occur when the unsterile wad, skin, clothing, and burning gunpowder enter the wound. As the range increases, the pellets spread out farther, and a large wound surrounded by individual pellet wounds may be seen. The wad, if it reaches the body, will be on the surface. From even greater distances pellet wounds are scattered, often without significant injury.

STAB WOUNDS AND IMPALEMENTS

A stab wound or impalement is a low-velocity injury. The main injury determinants are length, width, and trajectory of the object and the presence of vital organs in the area of the wound. Although the injuries tend to be localized, deep organs and multiple body cavities can be penetrated.

▰ INITIAL ASSESSMENT AND MANAGEMENT

The severely injured person must be assessed quickly and efficiently. Criteria and protocols to facilitate initial assessment, intervention, and triage of the trauma victim have been developed by the American College of Surgeons, Committee on Trauma.

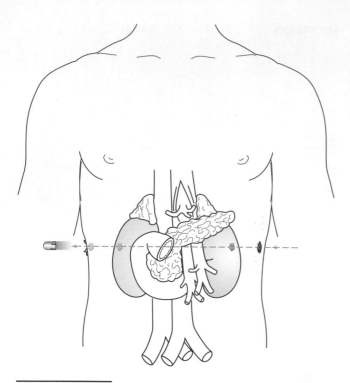

FIGURE 50-3
Internal organs may sustain extensive damage from gunshot wounds. Damage may be fatal if several organs are damaged.

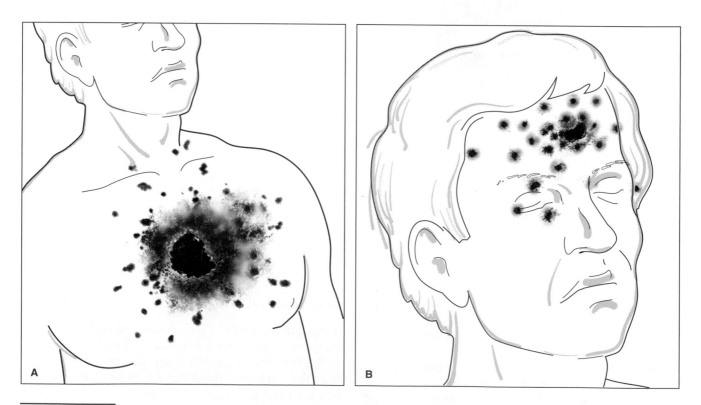

FIGURE 50-4
Damage caused by shotguns at two different distances. (**A**) At close range, opening is extensive and is surrounded by blood spatters and powder burns. (**B**) At medium range (8–10 ft), the larger entry wound is surrounded by individual pellet wounds.

Prehospital Management

Initial management often determines the final outcome. Assessment and management of the trauma patient begins at the accident scene with the ABCs:

ABCs

    A = airway
    B = breathing
    C = circulation

After an airway is established, breathing and circulation are evaluated and supported. Initial circulatory resuscitation includes control of external hemorrhage, initiation of intravenous fluid therapy, and occasionally the application of a pneumatic antishock garment (PASG). The cervical spine and injured extremities are immobilized. Neurological status is noted, and the patient is transported to an appropriate hospital as quickly and safely as possible.

Inhospital Management

Assessment and care performed on arrival at the hospital can be divided into four phases: primary evaluation, resuscitation, secondary assessment, and definitive care.

PRIMARY EVALUATION

The primary evaluation begins with another assessment of the ABCs. Information about the accident scene (eg, bent steering wheel) can provide clues about possible serious injuries. Full exposure of the patient (removal of all clothing) is necessary to detect all external signs of injury. Abrasions and contusions should not be overlooked; they may increase suspicion of internal injury. The primary survey should always include a neurological examination. The accompanying display outlines assessments and interventions in the initial hospital examination.

RESUSCITATION

Resuscitation for life-threatening conditions frequently begins during the primary evaluation. The patient may require endotracheal intubation or cricothyrotomy, administration of oxygen, intravenous fluid therapy (using large-bore catheters or a central line), blood transfusion, and control of hemorrhage. Life-threatening conditions, such as tension or open pneumothorax, massive hemothorax, and cardiac tamponade, are treated quickly. Blood samples may be obtained for type and cross-match and other laboratory tests. Arterial blood gases should be assessed and hemodynamic stability monitored continuously. Unless contraindicated, a urinary catheter and nasogastric tube are inserted.

Initial Assessment and Intervention of the Trauma Patient

Airway
  Assessment
    • Air exchange
    • Airway patency
  Interventions
    • Jaw thrust, chin lift
    • Removal of foreign bodies
    • Suctioning
    • Oropharyngeal or nasopharyngeal airway
    • Endotracheal intubation (orally or nasally)
    • Cricothyrotomy

Breathing
  Assessment
    • Respirations (rate, depth, effort)
    • Color
    • Breath sounds
    • Chest wall movement and integrity
    • Position of trachea
  Interventions
    • Oxygen through nonrebreather mask
    • Ventilation with bag–valve device
    • Treatment of life-threatening conditions (eg, tension pneumothorax)

Circulation
  Assessment
    • Pulse, blood pressure
    • Capillary refill
    • Obvious external bleeding
    • Electrocardiogram
  Interventions
    • Hemorrhage control: Direct pressure, elevate extremity, pneumatic antishock garment
    • Intravenous therapy: blood transfusion
    • Treatment of life-threatening conditions (eg, cardiac tamponade)
    • Cardiopulmonary resuscitation

Disability
  Assessment
    • Level of consciousness
    • Pupils

Exposure
  Assessment
    • Inspection of entire body for injuries

SECONDARY ASSESSMENT

After the patient's condition is stabilized, a complete medical history must be obtained and a thorough physical examination performed. Information about the mechanism of injury often aids in diagnosis of additional injuries. For instance, following a high-velocity gunshot wound, structures in the vicinity of the wound tract may also have sustained injury due to cavitation and blast effect. In the case of an MVA, information about the vehicle can aid in injury detection. A head-on collision producing a damaged windshield or dashboard indicates possible head, facial, tracheal, or cervical spine trauma. Whereas a broken steering wheel increases suspicion of injury to the chest, ribs, heart, trachea, spine, and abdomen. Frontal impacts, illustrated in Figure 50–5, are also associated with trauma of the lower extremities. Thoracic, abdominal, and pelvic injuries are often seen after a lateral impact. Collisions damaging the side of the vehicle can be associated with multiple injuries.

An assault victim is most likely to have head, chest, and abdominal injuries. If assessment of the patient following assault reveals multiple injuries of varying ages, domestic abuse should be suspected and reported. Secondary assessment also includes an electrocardiogram (ECG), various laboratory tests, and radiological studies (Table 50–1). If abdominal injuries are suspected, a diagnostic peritoneal lavage (DPL) also may be necessary. The patient's condition must be monitored continuously, and emotional support should be provided to the patient and family.

DEFINITIVE CARE

The trauma patient has a higher chance of a positive outcome if definitive care is initiated within the first hour after injury. Although treatment begins in the emergency department or operating room, definitive care occurs mostly

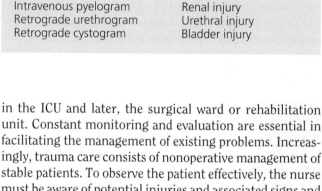

TABLE 50-1	
Radiological Procedures Indicated in Trauma	
Procedure	**Suspected Injury**
Radiograph	
Chest	Pneumothorax
	Hemothorax
	Fractured ribs
	Pulmonary contusion
	Tracheobronchial injury
	Great vessel injury
Pelvis	Fracture
Extremities	Fracture
Angiogram	Great vessel injury
	Renal injury
	Vascular injury of the pelvis
	Vascular injury of the extremities
Computed tomography	Abdominal injury
	Retroperitoneal injury
	Thoracic injury
	Renal injury
	Pelvic fracture
Gastrografin upper GI series	Duodenal hematoma or laceration
Intravenous pyelogram	Renal injury
Retrograde urethrogram	Urethral injury
Retrograde cystogram	Bladder injury

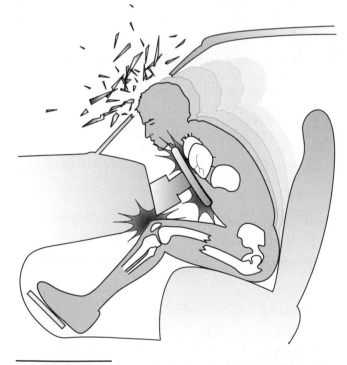

FIGURE 50-5

In a motor vehicle accident, if the driver is not wearing a seatbelt, damage may occur in various sections of the body. Common injuries occur to the skull, scalp, face, sternum, ribs, heart, liver, or spleen. Bones of the pelvis and lower extremities also may be damaged.

in the ICU and later, the surgical ward or rehabilitation unit. Constant monitoring and evaluation are essential in facilitating the management of existing problems. Increasingly, trauma care consists of nonoperative management of stable patients. To observe the patient effectively, the nurse must be aware of potential injuries and associated signs and symptoms. Other important elements of definitive care include the management of preexisting medical conditions and the identification of injuries missed during treatment of life-threatening problems. Once again, knowledge regarding the mechanism of injury is necessary. Psychosocial problems are also addressed during this phase. Finally, the patient is monitored for the development of complications.

Death caused by trauma can be divided into three phases: immediate (within minutes), early (within hours), and late (days to weeks after the injury). Most immediate and early deaths are caused by central nervous system injury or hemorrhage, whereas late deaths are mostly due to sepsis and multiple organ failure (MOF). The critical care nurse must be aware of these phases and related risk factors. Certain situations, such as prolonged extrication, prolonged hypothermia, respiratory or cardiac arrest, massive fluid resuscitation, or massive blood transfusions, lead one to suspect an increased likelihood of severe injuries and greater chance of complications and death following trauma.

ASSESSMENT AND MANAGEMENT OF SPECIFIC INJURIES

Thoracic Trauma

Approximately 25% of trauma deaths are due to thoracic injury.[3] Automobile accidents account for the majority of blunt trauma. Thoracic injuries from falls are also a common cause of hospitalization. Although not as frequent as stab wounds to the chest, gunshot wounds are associated with a significantly higher mortality rate.

Diagnosis of chest injuries begins with a physical examination and a chest radiograph. Specific injuries noted on the radiograph increase the likelihood of more serious underlying problems. For instance, rib fractures (especially of the first or second ribs) indicate a strong force of impact and are frequently associated with injury to the lung or great vessels. Likewise, great vessel injury or cardiac contusion may accompany a sternal fracture. Scapular fractures are often indicative of pulmonary contusion. Many potentially life-threatening injuries to the thorax, such as tension or open pneumothorax, massive hemothorax, flail chest, and cardiac tamponade, can be managed quickly and easily, often without major surgery. Untreated, they can be life threatening.

PNEUMOTHORAX AND HEMOTHORAX

Blunt and penetrating trauma can cause pneumothorax or hemothorax. The patient usually exhibits dyspnea, decreased or absent breath sounds on the affected side, and signs and symptoms of impaired gas exchange. Following severe injuries, hemodynamic instability is often present.

Physical examination and chest radiograph usually provide the diagnosis. Frequently, the only treatment needed is the placement of a chest tube. A massive hemothorax (>1,500 mL initially or >200 mL/h) may require a thoracotomy, whereas chest tube reexpansion of the lung often is sufficient to tamponade most smaller sources of bleeding. Surgical intervention also may be necessary in the case of an open pneumothorax (sucking chest wound) or uncontrolled air leak. Effectiveness of treatment is evaluated with chest radiographs, arterial blood gases, and physical examination.

In addition to providing routine postoperative care (spirometry, coughing, and deep-breathing exercises), the critical care nurse should assess respiratory and hemodynamic function carefully. The patient with lung injuries has an increased risk for development of pulmonary complications, such as atelectasis, pneumonia, and empyema. Chest tubes must be assessed for patency and function and the physician notified if drainage is excessive. For large blood loss from chest tubes, autotransfusion may be initiated (see Chapter 17).

FLAIL CHEST

A flail chest occurs when blunt trauma causes multiple rib fractures, leading to instability of the chest wall. Flail chest can be associated with pneumothorax, hemothorax, pulmonary contusion, or myocardial contusion. In flail chest injuries, chest wall movement is asymmetric, resulting in symptoms of dyspnea and tachypnea. The severity of hypoxia varies in relation to associated injuries and size of the flail segment. Diagnosis is made with a chest radiograph.

The main goal of treatment for flail chest is promotion of adequate ventilation and oxygenation. If the respiratory

---

Insights into Clinical Research

Luchette F, Radafsher S, et al: Prospective evaluation of epidural versus intrapleural catheters for analgesia in chest wall trauma. J Trauma 36(6):865–869, 1994

The purpose of this study was to evaluate the effectiveness of epidural versus intrapleural bupivacaine in controlling pain and improving pulmonary function in patients with severe chest wall trauma. Patients were randomized into two groups that either received epidural bupivacaine or intrapleural bupivacaine, each method started within 72 hours of injury. Pain was assessed at rest and with movement or coughing, and patients subjectively evaluated their pain. Tidal volume, vital capacity, minute volume, FiO2, negative inspiratory force, and respiratory rate were measured q12h for 72 hours. In the epidural group, pain was significantly less at rest and with movement, and the use of parenteral narcotics was significantly reduced. Pulmonary function tests were unchanged for both groups except for tidal volume and negative inspiratory force, which were significantly improved in the epidural group by the third day.

status is compromised or surgery for an associated injury is necessary, intubation and mechanical ventilation are indicated. Positive end-expiratory pressure (PEEP) may also be used. In some instances, operative stabilization with wires or staples may be performed. Rib fractures are not taped or splinted because this only further decreases pulmonary function.

Rib fractures often are associated with severe pain. Adequate pain control promotes lung expansion without the need for lengthy mechanical ventilation. Parenteral, intramuscular, or patient-controlled analgesia often is ordered. Systemic analgesics, however, may not be potent enough to relieve the pain of a flail chest, necessitating other methods of pain relief, such as intercostal blocks, intrapleural administration of narcotics, or epidural analgesia.

Nursing care of the patient with a flail chest is aimed at pain assessment and control, along with the promotion of adequate oxygenation and gas exchange. Hypoventilation due to pain increases the risk for respiratory complications, including atelectasis and pneumonia. Adult respiratory distress syndrome (ARDS) is a common complication of flail chest. Various interventions to improve respiratory function may be indicated, including coughing and deep breathing, spirometry, postural drainage and clapping, mucolytics, bronchodilators, intermittent positive pressure breathing, mechanical ventilation, endotracheal or nasotracheal suctioning, and therapeutic bronchoscopy.

Serial pulmonary assessments, including chest x-rays, arterial blood gases, physical examinations, and occasionally oximetric monitoring, are essential.

PULMONARY CONTUSION

A pulmonary contusion is a bruising of the lung parenchyma, often caused by blunt trauma. This disorder may not be diagnosed on the initial chest x-ray; however, the presence of a scapular fracture, rib fractures, or a flail chest should lead to the suspicion of a possible pulmonary contusion.

Pulmonary contusion occurs when rapid deceleration ruptures capillary cell walls, causing hemorrhage and extravasation of plasma and protein into alveolar and interstitial spaces. This results in atelectasis and consolidation, leading to intrapulmonary shunting and hypoxemia. Presenting signs and symptoms include dyspnea, rales, hemoptysis, and tachypnea. Severe contusions also will result in increasing peak airway pressures, hypoxemia, and respiratory acidosis. Pulmonary contusion may mimic ARDS; both are poorly responsive to high inspired oxygen fractions (FIO_2). Table 50–2 lists the differences between ARDS and pulmonary contusion. See Chapter 26 for a discussion of ARDS.

Treatment of pulmonary contusion is supportive, and the patient with a mild contusion requires close observation. Frequent arterial blood gas (ABG) measurements or pulse oximetry often are necessary. Additional nursing interventions include frequent respiratory assessment, pulmonary care, and pain control. Chest physiotherapy and continuous epidural analgesia also may be beneficial. Severe pulmonary contusion may require ventilatory support

TABLE 50-2
Differences Between Pulmonary Contusion and ARDS

Pulmonary Contusion	ARDS
Gradual onset of respiratory failure	Sudden onset of respiratory failure
Radiograph changes can be immediate	Radiograph changes frequently delayed 2–3 d after symptoms appear
Focal infiltrates	Diffuse infiltrates
Can lead to cavitation and lung abscess	Can lead to chronic pulmonary fibrosis

with PEEP. An oximetric pulmonary artery catheter (oximetric Swan-Ganz) and arterial line usually are placed to facilitate monitoring of ABGs, hemodynamics, and respiratory parameters (oxygen delivery, oxygen consumption, intrapulmonary shunt). Although alveolar ventilation improves as PEEP is added, blood flow to alveoli may diminish, leading to an increased intrapulmonary shunt. To optimize tissue perfusion and oxygenation, each change in PEEP requires assessment of the status of the shunt, oxygen delivery, and other indicators of tissue perfusion (cardiac output, blood pressure, urine output). Adequate pain control is necessary and may require epidural or intrapleural infusions or intracostal block. In severe cases of respiratory compromise, increased sedation or paralysis may be indicated to decrease energy expenditure and oxygen requirements. A rotation bed, such as the Roto-Rest (Kinetic Concepts, Inc., San Antonio, TX) also should be considered. Positioning the patient with the injured side up is beneficial in the case of a severe unilateral contusion. In rare instances, when the patient is not responding to traditional mechanical ventilation, dual lung ventilation (simultaneous independent lung ventilation) is instituted.[4]

Fluid management also is important. Intake and output, daily weights, central venous pressure, and pulmonary capillary wedge pressure should be monitored. Concentration of medications may be needed to diminish excess intake, and diuretics may be required periodically. Severe fluid restriction is not indicated. Instead, fluid balance should be maintained at a near-normal level to support optimal cardiac output and oxygen delivery. The contused lung should show radiographic signs of improvement within 72 hours. The presence of persistent infiltrates may indicate complications. Pneumonia and superimposed ARDS are common complications. Long-term sequelae include prolonged reduced functional residual capacity, dyspnea, and fibrosis.

TRACHEOBRONCHIAL INJURY

Injuries to the trachea or bronchi can be caused by blunt or penetrating trauma and frequently are accompanied by esophageal and vascular damage. Ruptured bronchi often are present in association with upper rib fractures or pneumothorax. Severe tracheobronchial injury has a high mortality rate; however, with continued improvements in pre-hospital care and transport, more of these patients are surviving.

Airway injuries often are subtle. Presenting signs include dyspnea (occasionally the only sign), hemoptysis, cough, and subcutaneous emphysema. A chest x-ray can alert the physician to a possible injury; however, diagnosis usually is made with bronchoscopy or during surgery. Tracheobronchial injury should be considered whenever a persistent air leak accompanies a pneumothorax.

Small lung lacerations or pleural tears can be managed conservatively with mechanical ventilation by endotracheal tube or tracheostomy. Larger injuries may require surgical repair. Simultaneous independent lung ventilation may also be used.

Nursing care involves the assessment of oxygenation and gas exchange, along with appropriate pulmonary care. During the first few days, the physician may perform a bronchoscopy to visualize the repair site and to provide more effective suctioning. Pneumonia is a potential short-term complication, whereas tracheal stenosis may occur later.

MYOCARDIAL CONTUSION

Bruising of the myocardium is caused most often by the impact of the chest against the steering column or dashboard during an MVA. Rapid deceleration causes the mobile heart to strike the anterior chest wall. The right ventricle, due to its anterior location, is affected most commonly. A contusion also can result as the heart is compressed between the sternum and spine.

Symptoms of cardiac contusion vary from none (common) to severe congestive heart failure and cardiogenic shock. Complaints of chest pain must be evaluated carefully after trauma. Nonspecific ECG changes are seen frequently and can include any type of dysrhythmia. Atrial dysrhythmias and conduction disturbances may be seen with injuries to the right side of the heart; ventricular disturbances are more likely following a left-sided cardiac injury.

Diagnosis of cardiac injury can be difficult. Therefore, because of the poor predictive value of traditional tests (serial ECGs and serial myocardial isoenzymes) and after a baseline ECG has been obtained, cardiac monitoring and close observation of high-risk patients is necessary.[5,6] Symptomatic dysrhythmias are treated. Oxygenation, hemodynamics, and activity tolerance should be monitored. If a tachycardia develops, alternative causes (eg, pain, volume depletion) should be considered. An echocardiogram may be ordered if the patient is experiencing persistent unexplained hemodynamic instability. Deterioration of the patient's hemodynamic status may also indicate possible cardiac tamponade. Inotropic support may be necessary with a severe myocardial contusion.

PENETRATING CARDIAC INJURY

In a majority of cases, a penetrating injury to the heart results in prehospital death. In the remainder of patients, hemorrhage and shock are common presenting signs. The right ventricle is injured most often, because of its anterior location. Occasionally, small stab wounds to the ventricles seal themselves owing to the thick ventricular musculature. Treatment of hemodynamically stable patients remains controversial. In some instances, monitoring the patient with serial computed tomography (CT) scanning is recommended.[7] In other cases, surgery to create a subxiphoid pericardial window may be necessary to aid in diagnosis.[8] In the presence of ongoing hemorrhage and shock, lost blood volume is replaced, and the patient is immediately transported to the operating room for a median sternotomy and exploration. In severe cases, a thoracotomy in the emergency department may be required as a life-saving measure.

After surgical repair, a pulmonary artery catheter (Swan-Ganz) and arterial line are placed to facilitate careful hemodynamic monitoring. Vasopressors or inotropic agents may be necessary to maintain adequate blood pressure and cardiac output. Fluid and electrolyte balance, along with cardiac rhythm, must be monitored closely. Heart sounds should be assessed for murmurs, indicating valvular or septal defects, and for signs of congestive heart failure. Chest and mediastinal tube drainage are recorded frequently. Fresh frozen plasma and platelets are administered, as indicated, to correct coagulopathies. Complications include continued hemorrhage and postcardiotomy syndrome. In the event of massive blood transfusions, the risk of ARDS and disseminated intravascular coagulation (DIC) is heightened. Other complications are listed in the display. An extended period of hypotension increases the possibility of renal failure.

CARDIAC TAMPONADE

Cardiac tamponade can result from both penetrating and blunt trauma. Blood fills the pericardium and compresses the heart, causing decreased cardiac filling, which leads to reduced cardiac output and eventually shock. Only a small amount of pericardial blood is necessary to produce shock. Initial signs may include decreased blood pressure and increased central venous pressure as manifested by distended neck veins and muffled heart sounds. Because these signs may be obscured in the hypovolemic trauma victim, pa-

RED! FLAG

Complications Related to Massive Blood Transfusions

- ARDS
- Coagulopathy
- DIC
- Hyperkalemia
- Hypocalcemia (citrate toxicity)
- Metabolic acidosis
- Hypothermia
- Volume overload
- Transfusion reaction
- Transmission of infection

tients with a history of precordial trauma must be treated with a high index of suspicion. A pericardiocentesis may be diagnostic and therapeutic; however, thoracotomy often is necessary to identify and repair the source of bleeding. Postoperative nursing care is similar to that for a penetrating cardiac injury.

INJURY TO THE GREAT VESSELS

Most patients with a transection or tear of the aorta exsanguinate before reaching a hospital. Rapid deceleration causes shearing forces between the aortic arch and the tethered descending aorta. The most common site of injury is near the ligamentum arteriosum. Distal to this point, the aorta is closely applied to the thoracic spine, whereas proximal to this point, it is freely movable. Immediate death is prevented if the hemorrhage is contained within the aortic adventitia. This "false aneurysm" can rupture at any time, however, and thus requires prompt diagnosis and treatment.

Suspicion of an aortic or other great vessel injury is increased with fractures of the first and second ribs, high sternal fracture, or a massive left hemothorax. A widened mediastinum on an upright chest x-ray frequently is indicative of aortic injury, necessitating further evaluation. The role of CT versus aortogram in the diagnosis of aortic injury is still debated. Most of the time the decision is based on the degree of suspicion for injury. A low-risk patient with a worrisome chest x-ray may undergo CT scanning to evaluate the entire thorax. Aortography would be used in high-risk patients or patients with an abnormal CT scan (Fig. 50–6). Additional diagnostic signs, although not always present, include hypertensive upper extremities with reduced pulses or neurological deficit of the lower extremities. Injuries to the subclavian or innominate arteries may cause decreased pulses in the upper extremities.

A positive aortogram indicates the need for surgical repair. The torn aorta requires end-to-end anastomosis or, more commonly, the placement of a synthetic graft. Cardiopulmonary bypass may be necessary for repair of the ascending aorta or the aortic arch. However, repair of the descending thoracic aorta is usually accomplished during aortic cross-clamping. Because this maneuver occludes distal blood flow, it is imperative that the cross-clamp time be as short as possible (less than 30 minutes). To prevent leakage from the repair site, postoperative vasodilators may be administered to reduce afterload. A vasopressor may be added to prevent hypotension. Nursing care focuses on hemodynamic monitoring with a Swan-Ganz catheter and titrating medications to maintain optimal blood pressure. Autotransfusion also may be necessary.

Complications are related to the level of the tear and the extent of altered perfusion. Hypoperfusion and resulting damage to organs below the level of the laceration can result from the injury itself or from prolonged cross-clamping during repair. Serious complications include renal failure, bowel ischemia, lower extremity weakness, or

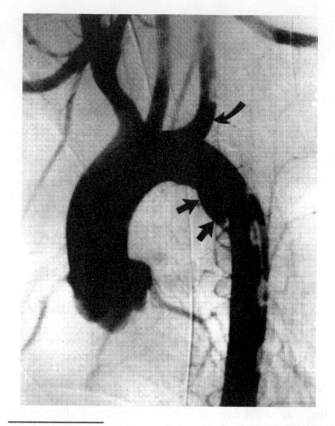

FIGURE 50-6

Arch aortogram demonstrates laceration of descending aorta (*straight arrows*) just distal to origin of left subclavian artery (*curved arrow*). Extravasated contrast material is contained by aortic adventitia. (Courtesy of Michael Mestek, MD, Denver General Hospital, Denver, CO)

permanent paralysis of the lower extremities. Other sequelae, such as ARDS or DIC, can be a consequence of multiple blood transfusions.

Abdominal Trauma

The abdominal cavity contains solid and hollow organs. Blunt trauma is likely to cause serious damage to solid organs, and penetrating trauma most often injures the hollow organs. The compression and deceleration of blunt trauma lead to fractures of solid organ capsules and parenchyma, whereas the hollow organ can collapse and absorb the force. The bowel, however, which occupies most of the abdominal cavity, is prone to injury by penetrating trauma. In general, solid organs respond to trauma with bleeding. Hollow organs rupture and release their contents into the peritoneal cavity, causing inflammation and infection.

Most gunshot wounds and stab wounds penetrating deep fascia are surgically explored, though some conservative management techniques are under investigation. Nonoperative management of select patients with penetrating abdominal injuries has been used by some trauma centers.[9,10] Hemodynamically unstable blunt trauma patients undergo a DPL. The procedure for DPL is outlined in the accompanying display. A positive DPL necessitates surgical exploration. Stable blunt trauma victims will have a CT scan. Depending on the extent of injury identified with CT, surgical repair or nonoperative management (ie, observation) will be prescribed. Diagnostic laparoscopy as an adjunct to DPL and CT, following blunt trauma, is still investigational.[11,12]

Because DPL and CT are not 100% accurate and conservative management is gaining popularity, the critical care nurse must use astute assessment skills and awareness of mechanism of injury to assist in injury identification. Frequent abdominal assessments are crucial. The nurse must look for signs and symptoms of an acute abdomen: distention, rigidity, and rebound tenderness. Additional signs that can indicate injury include subcutaneous emphysema over the abdomen (ruptured bowel), Grey Turner's sign (retroperitoneal bleeding from pancreas, duodenum, kidneys, vena cava, or aorta), and Cullen's sign (peritoneal bleeding from liver or spleen). Serial amylase and hematocrit levels are often ordered. Surgical exploration may be necessary with the onset of signs or symptoms indicating injury.

CLINICAL APPLICATION: Diagnostic Studies
Procedure for Diagnostic Peritoneal Lavage (DPL)

Purpose: To detect intraperitoneal bleeding

Indications
- Blunt abdominal injury with:
    Altered pain response
    Decreased: head or spinal cord injury; presence of alcohol or drugs
    Increased: pelvic, lumbar spine or lower rib fractures
    Unexplained hypovolemia in multiple trauma victim
- Penetrating abdominal trauma (if exploration not indicated)

Possible Contraindications
- History of multiple abdominal operations
- Immediate laparotomy needed
- Advanced cirrhosis of the liver
- Morbid obesity
- Known history of coagulopathy

Technique
1. Insert lavage catheter into peritoneal cavity through 1–2 cm incision.
2. Attempt to aspirate peritoneal fluid.
3. Infuse normal saline or Ringer's lactate by gravity.
4. Turn patient from side to side (unless contraindicated).
5. Allow fluid to run back into bag by gravity.
6. Send specimens to laboratory.

Positive Results
- 10–20 mL gross blood on initial aspirate
- Greater than 100,000 RBCs/mm³
- Greater than 500 WBCs/mm³
- Elevated amylase level
- Presence of bile, bacteria, or fecal matter

STOMACH AND SMALL BOWEL TRAUMA

Significant gastric injury is rare; however, the small bowel is more commonly injured. Although frequently damaged by penetrating trauma, blunt trauma also can cause the small bowel to burst. The multiple convolutions occasionally form a closed loop that is subject to rupture with increased pressure from impact with a steering wheel or seat belt. The bowel's mobility around fixed points (such as the ligament of Treitz) predisposes it to shearing injuries with deceleration.

Blunt small bowel or gastric injury can present with blood in the nasogastric aspirate or hematemesis. Physical signs often are absent, and CT findings may be subtle and nonspecific. Close observation is required; often diagnosis is not made until peritonitis develops. Penetrating injuries usually cause a positive DPL. Although a mild bowel contusion can be managed conservatively (gastric decompression and withholding oral intake), surgery usually is necessary to repair penetrating wounds.

Postoperative decompression, either with a nasogastric or gastric tube, is maintained until bowel function returns. In most cases, a feeding jejunostomy tube is placed distal to the repair site. Tube feedings can be initiated early in the postoperative course. As the concentration and rate of feedings are advanced slowly, frequent assessment for signs of intolerance (distention, vomiting) is essential. Because the stomach and small bowel contain an insignificant amount of bacteria, the risk of sepsis is small. On the other hand, the acidic gastric juice is irritating to the peritoneum and may cause peritonitis. Other potential complications are listed in the accompanying display. Some of these conditions may necessitate additional surgical procedures. Malabsorption syndrome is rare unless more than 200 cm of bowel has been removed.

DUODENUM AND PANCREAS TRAUMA

The pancreas and duodenum are discussed together because they both are retroperitoneal organs and are closely related anatomically and physiologically. A great deal of force is necessary to injure these organs, because they are well protected deep in the abdomen. Injuries to adjacent organs almost always are present. The retroperitoneal location makes these injuries difficult to diagnose with DPL. An

**Complications Related to
Stomach and Small Bowel Trauma**

- Intolerance to tube feedings
- Peritonitis
- Postoperative bleeding
- Hypovolemia caused by "third spacing"
- Development of a fistula or obstruction

abdominal CT scan is very useful in this instance. Signs and symptoms may include an acute abdomen, increased serum amylase levels, epigastric pain radiating to the back, nausea, and vomiting.

Small lacerations or contusions may require only the placement of drains, whereas larger wounds need surgical repair. Most pancreatic injuries will require closed suction drainage postoperatively to prevent fistula formation. A distal pancreatectomy and Roux-en-Y anastomosis are two procedures commonly performed for injuries to the body and tail of the pancreas. Occasionally, the spleen also must be removed owing to its multiple vascular attachments. Damage to the head of the pancreas is associated with duodenal injury and severe hemorrhage because of the close proximity of vascular structures. Surgical procedures used in these cases include pancreaticoduodenectomy, Roux-en-Y anastomosis, and on rare occasions, total pancreatectomy.

Postoperative nursing assessment and care are similar for the various procedures. Patency of drains must be maintained, and the patient must be monitored for the development of fistulas, the most common complication. Skin protection is important if a cutaneous fistula does develop, because of the high enzyme content of pancreatic fluid. Assessment of fluid and electrolyte balance is important because a pancreatic fistula results in fluid loss, along with potassium and bicarbonate. Pancreatic stimulation can be decreased by administering parenteral hyperalimentation or jejunal feedings instead of an oral diet. The onset of diabetes mellitus is rare unless a total pancreatectomy is performed.

Complications related to duodenum or pancreas trauma are listed in the display.

Primary repair or resection with reanastamosis is sufficient to manage most penetrating duodenal injuries. A duodenostomy tube may be placed for decompression and a jejunostomy tube for feeding. Blunt trauma to the duodenum can cause an intramural hematoma, which may lead to duodenal obstruction. The diagnosis is made with a diatrizoate (Gastrografin) upper gastrointestinal study. A complete obstruction generally requires surgical drainage of the hematoma.

Complications Related to
Duodenum or Pancreas Trauma

- Onset of diabetes mellitus (rare unless total pancreatectomy performed)
- Bleeding from a fistula eroding into vessels
- Peritonitis
- Intra-abdominal or systemic sepsis
- Pancreatitis
- Pseudocyst
- Mechanical bowel obstruction

COLON TRAUMA

Usually colon injury is a result of penetrating trauma. The nature of the injury most often dictates surgical exploration. Primary repair is the treatment of choice for lacerations of the colon.[13] In some situations, such as injury to the left colon or massive blood transfusion, an exteriorized repair or colostomy is required. A cecostomy tube may be placed for decompression. The subcutaneous tissue and skin of the incision site are often left open to decrease the chance of wound infection. The colon has a high bacterial count; spillage of the contents will predispose to intra-abdominal sepsis and abscess formation.

Postoperative nursing care focuses on the prevention of infection. Dressing changes are necessary for the open incision, and prophylactic antibiotics may be used. In the case of an exteriorized colon repair, an end-to-end anastomosis is performed, and the repair site is exteriorized to facilitate identification of a leak. The exteriorized colon must be kept moist and covered with a nonadhering dressing or bag to protect the integrity of the sutures. Because sepsis is a major complication of colon injuries, a series of radiographic and surgical procedures may be required to locate and drain abscesses.

HEPATIC TRAUMA

After the spleen, the liver is the most commonly injured abdominal organ. Both blunt and penetrating trauma can cause injuries (Fig. 50–7). Fractures of the right lower ribs should increase suspicion of a liver injury. Presenting signs and symptoms range from right upper quadrant pain, rebound tenderness, hypoactive to absent bowel sounds, or signs of hypovolemic shock. Hemodynamically stable patients may be managed nonoperatively with serial CT scans. In many cases, however, the patient's clinical condition will dictate the need for surgery. Hepatic trauma can cause a large blood loss into the peritoneum, but bleeding may stop spontaneously. In some instances, vessels may be ligated or embolized. Small lacerations are repaired, whereas larger injuries may require segmental resection or débridement. In the case of uncontrollable hemorrhage, the liver is packed. After packing, the abdomen may be closed or simply covered with mesh. An additional surgical procedure is required within the next few days to remove the packing and repair the laceration. Large liver injuries also need postoperative drainage of bile and blood with closed suction drains.

After surgery, hypovolemic shock and coagulopathies may be present. Incomplete hemostasis also is a possibility and must be differentiated from coagulopathy-induced bleeding. Severe bleeding resulting from incomplete hemostasis requires clot removal, packing, and additional repair. With a coagulopathy, bleeding arises from numerous sites, whereas with incomplete hemostasis, the bleeding is mainly from the surgical site. Nursing care includes the replacement of blood products while monitoring the hematocrit and coagulation studies. Assessment of the type and

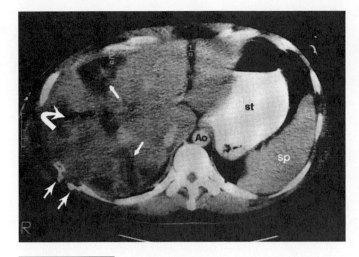

FIGURE 50-7

Cross-section from abdominal computed tomography scan shows multiple liver lacerations that contain blood (*small straight arrows*) and air (*large curved arrows*). Rib fractures are present posteriorly on the right (*large straight arrows*). Note normal aorta (*Ao*) and spleen (*sp*). Stomach (*st*) contains oral contrast material. (Courtesy of Winfield M. Craven, MD, Fort Collins Radiologic Associates, Fort Collins, CO)

amount of tube drainage, along with fluid balance, also is essential. Potential complications of liver injury include hepatic or perihepatic abscess, biliary obstruction or leak, sepsis, ARDS, and DIC.

SPLENIC TRAUMA

The spleen is the most commonly injured abdominal organ, usually as a result of blunt trauma. The presence of left lower rib fractures should increase suspicion of a splenic injury. Presenting signs and symptoms include left upper quadrant pain radiating to the left shoulder (Kehr's sign), hypovolemic shock, and the nonspecific finding of an increased white blood cell count. The DPL or abdominal CT scan usually are necessary for diagnosis.

Adults with minor injuries and most children are treated nonoperatively with observation (serial abdominal examinations, serial hematocrits) and nasogastric decompression. Because the spleen and stomach are both in the left upper quadrant, decompression of the stomach reduces pressure on the injured spleen. Preferred surgical treatment is splenorrhaphy, although in some cases, splenectomy is necessary. Splenic autotransplantation, a fairly new procedure, which consists of implanting splenic fragments into pockets of omentum, may be performed after severe injuries.[14]

Early complications include recurrent bleeding, subphrenic abscess, and pancreatitis resulting from surgical trauma. Late complications consist of thrombocytosis and overwhelming postsplenectomy sepsis (OPSS). Because the spleen plays an important role in the body's response to infection, a splenectomy predisposes the patient to an in-

creased risk for infection. This risk is especially high among children and highest in those younger than 2 years. *Pneumococcus*, an encapsulated microorganism resistant to phagocytosis, is the organism that most often infects patients after splenectomy. Therefore, pneumococcal pneumonia frequently is the initial presentation of OPSS, often resulting in a fulminant sepsis. Postsplenectomy patients can increase their immunity toward pneumococcal pneumonia with polyvalent pneumococcal vaccine (Pneumovax). Complications of OPSS include adrenal insufficiency and DIC. This syndrome has a high incidence and mortality rate, especially within the first year after surgery. Teaching should focus on detection of signs and symptoms of infection. Splenic autotransplantation may prove beneficial in decreasing the incidence of OPSS.

RENAL TRAUMA

Penetrating injury to the kidney may lead to a "free" hemorrhage, contained hematoma, or the development of an intravascular thrombus. A sudden deceleration injury can cause avulsion of smaller vessels or tear the renal artery intima, which also may lead to thrombosis of the vessel. Blunt and penetrating trauma can also cause a laceration or contusion of the renal parenchyma or rupture of the collecting system. Lower rib fractures should raise suspicion of an associated renal injury. Signs and symptoms, when present, consist of hematuria, pain, a flank mass, or ecchymosis over the flank. Because the bleeding is retroperitoneal, it can be difficult to detect. A CT scan, intravenous pyelogram, or angiogram usually provide the diagnosis. Many injuries can be managed conservatively with observation and bed rest until gross hematuria resolves. However, in some instances (mainly for vascular injury), surgical repair or nephrectomy is necessary.

Postoperative assessment and support of renal function are imperative. Low-dose dopamine may be ordered, and optimal fluid balance must be maintained to ensure renal perfusion. The major complications consist of arterial or venous thrombosis and acute renal failure. Other complications include bleeding, perinephric abscess, the development of a urinary fistula, and late onset of hypertension.

BLADDER TRAUMA

The bladder can be lacerated or ruptured, most often as the consequence of blunt trauma. Bladder injuries frequently

 Considerations for the Pediatric Patient
Trauma to the Spleen

- Splenectomy increases the risk of infection, especially in children.
- Risk of infection is highest in patients younger than 2 years.

are associated with pelvic fractures. The presence of blood at the urethral meatus, a scrotal hematoma, or a displaced prostate gland requires examination for urethral injuries with a retrograde urethrogram and cystogram before the insertion of a urinary catheter.

A bladder injury can cause intraperitoneal or extraperitoneal urine extravasation. Extraperitoneal extravasation often can be managed with urinary catheter drainage. Intraperitoneal extravasation, however, requires surgery. A suprapubic cystostomy tube may be placed. Complications are infrequent, but infection due to the urinary catheter or sepsis from extravasation of infected urine can occur.

PELVIC FRACTURE

Complex pelvic fractures are associated with a high mortality. Secondary hemorrhage is the most frequent cause of early death, whereas sepsis causes most delayed mortality. Because significant force is required to fracture the pelvic ring, associated intra-abdominal or urogenital injuries are common. Pelvic fractures are most often caused by high-speed car accidents with ejection, automobile–pedestrian collisions, motorcycle accidents, or severe fall or crush injuries. Radiographs and a CT scan can confirm the presence and define the extent of pelvic fractures. A pelvic fracture often causes the laceration of small vessels that bleed into soft tissue in the retroperitoneal space. This area extends from the diaphragm to midthigh and will accommodate several liters of blood before tamponade occurs. An angiogram often is necessary to localize and embolize the source of bleeding.

Hemorrhage control is of primary concern. The PASG may be applied in the prehospital phase or in the emergency department but is used infrequently in the ICU. It splints the pelvis and tamponades the hemorrhage. Because the PASG decreases tidal volume, ventilatory support may be necessary. Internal or external fixation is more effective in stabilizing the fracture and controlling the bleeding. In addition, early fixation reduces pain and facilitates earlier ambulation. Early fracture stabilization may be associated with decreased mortality.[15] Surgical packing also may be necessary to control the hemorrhage. A diverting colostomy is indicated to decrease the risk of contamination following an open pelvic fracture.

The critical care nurse's primary concern is to prevent hemorrhagic shock. Multiple transfusions and hemodynamic monitoring are necessary in the case of a significant hemorrhage. Adequate oxygen delivery must be maintained. The nurse must also promote pain control and assess the patient for signs and symptoms of infection. A pelvic hematoma can be a source of sepsis and may require percutaneous or surgical drainage. In addition to sepsis and multiple organ failure, other complications of pelvic fractures include pelvic nerve involvement and pulmonary emboli. Prolonged physical therapy and rehabilitation frequently are necessary.

Extremity Trauma

Trauma to the extremities is often associated with other serious injuries. Extremity injuries can result from blunt or penetrating insults and may affect bone, soft tissue, nerve, muscles, or blood vessels. Mechanisms of injury include auto accidents, falls, and assaults (including child abuse and domestic violence). Underlying bone disease, often present in the older person, increases the risk of injury following a fall. Domestic abuse can also result in extremity trauma. Suspicion should be heightened if the degree or type of injury is inconsistent with the accident history. Although rarely life threatening, extremity injuries can be permanently disabling. Timely management helps reduce the risk of disability and death.

FRACTURES

Fractures occur often in blunt trauma and less frequently in penetrating trauma. Fractures are occasionally missed on the initial assessment, but subsequent pain, swelling, deformity, and instability may indicate the presence of a fracture. Once a radiograph confirms the fracture, stabilization or repair is undertaken. Because orthopedic procedures can be time consuming, other life-threatening injuries often take precedence, and surgical repair may be postponed until a later date. Internal fixation of fractures often allows earlier ambulation in patients with multiple injuries in whom complications of prolonged bed rest (decubitus ulcers, pulmonary embolus, muscle wasting) otherwise may develop. Fracture management also may be accomplished with external fixation or skeletal traction. Open fractures may require surgical débridement.

Nursing responsibilities include assessment of neurovascular status, along with wound and pin care. Open fractures have an increased risk of infection. Other potential complications are fat emboli from long bone fractures and compartment syndrome. Nursing care must be directed toward the prevention and early detection of these problems. The nurse must work closely with the physical therapist also to promote strengthening and early mobilization.

VASCULAR INJURIES

Vascular injuries frequently result in bleeding or thrombosis of a vessel. They usually result from penetrating trauma and less often are the consequence of fractures. An expanding hematoma or signs and symptoms of abnormal distal perfusion can indicate vascular trauma. Doppler ultrasonography often is used to diagnose peripheral vascular injury. An angiogram also may be performed to locate the site of injury and identify arteriovenous fistulas, pseudoaneurysms, and intimal flaps. Some arteriovenous fistulas or pseudoaneurysms may be amenable to catheter-directed embolization. Primary surgical repair, ligation, or vascular grafting may also be undertaken.

In the immediate postoperative period, there is a risk for continued bleeding or thrombotic occlusion of the vessel.

Both require a return to the operating room. The nurse must assess distal pulses, color, sensation, movement, and temperature of the involved extremity. Ankle-brachial indices (ABIs) often are helpful in detecting the development of an occlusion after lower extremity trauma. To calculate an ABI, the systolic blood pressure of the ankle is divided by the systolic blood pressure of the arm. Decreasing ABIs suggest worsening obstruction of a lower extremity vessel. This method provides more objective data than simply palpating pulses. The nurse also must watch for the development of compartment syndrome, which may require fasciotomy. Other complications include pulmonary embolus, deep vein thrombosis, and venous claudication.

COMPLICATIONS OF MULTIPLE TRAUMA

Causes of death following multiple trauma can be divided into three phases: immediate, early, and late.

Immediate Complications

Immediate deaths occur at the scene and within minutes of the accident. Most common causes of immediate deaths are brain stem or high spinal cord laceration, cardiac rupture, transection of the great vessels, and airway obstruction.

Early Complications

Severe head injuries (eg, intracranial hematoma) and hemorrhage are responsible for most early deaths. These deaths tend to occur within hours of the injury, most often in the emergency department or operating room. Often death at this stage can be prevented with quick assessment, resuscitation, and management of injuries. (Management of head injuries is discussed in Chapter 34.)

To prevent exsanguination, hemorrhage must be controlled and volume resuscitation begun with the infusion of crystalloids and blood. Patients may require surgical ligation or packing, and embolization by angiography. Massive intra-abdominal hemorrhage complicated by hypothermia, metabolic acidosis, and coagulopathy is highly lethal. To increase the likelihood of survival, the abdomen may be packed and the patient transferred to the ICU for warming and replacement of clotting factors. A return to the operating room is then necessary within 48 hours for removal of packing and definitive closure of the abdomen.[16]

Late Complications

Continued hemorrhage because of incomplete hemostasis or an undiagnosed injury can lead to hypovolemic shock and eventually decreased organ perfusion. The various organs respond differently to the decrease in perfusion caused by hypovolemia, as listed in the accompanying display. Multiple blood transfusions are often necessary, further increasing the likelihood of ARDS and MOF.

Another frequent and potentially serious complication of multiple trauma is infection. This can range from a minor wound infection to fulminant sepsis syndrome and septic shock. The release of toxins causes dilation of vessels, leading to venous pooling that results in a decrease in venous return. Initially, cardiac output rises to compensate for decreased systemic vascular resistance. Eventually, the compensatory mechanisms are overcome, and cardiac output falls along with blood pressure and organ perfusion (ie, septic shock). The risk of infection is increased following close-

RED FLAG

Complications of Hypovolemia **on Different Organ Systems**

Cardiac System
- Tachycardia
- Decreased systolic blood pressure
- Narrowing of pulse pressure
- Eventual cardiac failure

Skin
- Cool, clammy, pale, cyanotic

Central Nervous System
- Anxiety, restlessness
- Confusion, altered sensorium
- Decreased level of consciousness

Renal System
- Decreased urine output
- Decreased glomerular filtration (increased BUN, serum creatinine)
- Acute or chronic renal failure

Pulmonary System
- Tachypnea
- Increased pulmonary capillary permeability (ARDS)

Hepatic System
- Decreased manufacture of clotting factors
- Impaired drug metabolism
- Decreased synthesis of plasma proteins (decreased serum albumin)
- Reduced serum glucose levels
- Decreased elimination of ammonia (increased BUN)
- Decreased phagocytosis

Gastrointestinal System
- Adynamic ileus
- Ulceration
- Decreased absorption of nutrients
- Increase in toxins passing from lumen into bloodstream

Vascular System
- DIC

Cellular System
- Anaerobic metabolism (lactic acidosis)

range shotgun blasts, high-velocity penetrating injuries, penetrating wounds to the colon, prolonged surgery, multiple blood transfusions, and injury to multiple organs. Other risk factors include age, underlying immunosuppression, and history of diabetes mellitus.

The source of infection must be found and eradicated to treat sepsis effectively. The critical care nurse must watch for the sometimes subtle indicators of sepsis. Hyperthermia or hypothermia and altered mental status often are present early in the septic process and should prompt further assessment to detect a possible infectious source.

When sepsis is suspected, antibiotics are prescribed, cultures obtained, radiological studies begun, and exploratory surgery frequently is performed. Intra-abdominal abscess is a frequent cause of sepsis. Some abscesses can be drained percutaneously, whereas others require surgery. After the surgical drainage of an abdominal abscess, the incision is left open with drains in place to allow healing and prevent recurrence. Other sources of infection are invasive lines, urinary tract, and lungs.

Pneumonia is a common cause of sepsis in trauma patients. Causative factors include age, underlying pulmonary disease, thoracic or abdominal surgery, and prolonged intubation. Hemodynamics are altered, and metabolic demands are increased during sepsis. The typical patient will exhibit elevated cardiac output, decreased systemic vascular resistance, and increased oxygen consumption. Hemodynamics must be supported and a balance between oxygen delivery and oxygen consumption maintained.

Sepsis may predispose the patient to ARDS. In addition to sepsis, specific injuries (eg, head trauma, pulmonary contusion, multiple major fractures), massive blood transfusions, aspiration, and pneumonia can also increase the likelihood of ARDS. With a mortality rate of about 50% to 70%, ARDS is characterized by hypoxemia with shunting, decreased lung compliance, tachypnea, dyspnea, and the appearance of diffuse bilateral pulmonary infiltrates. The syndrome requires intensive ventilatory support with PEEP.[17] Oxygen delivery is assessed and supported (see Chapter 26).

More than 10% of critically injured patients will develop MOF.[18,19] Many factors have been associated with the development of MOF, including hemorrhage, massive blood transfusion, hypovolemic shock, and sepsis. Characterized by the failure of two or more organs, MOF accounts for more than 50% of late deaths in trauma patients.[20]

Usually the lungs are the first organs to fail (heralded by the onset of ARDS), followed by the liver, gastrointestinal tract, and kidneys.

Liver failure can result from initial damage, vascular compromise, shock, and sepsis. Jaundice is a common indicator of deteriorating liver function, although other causes, such as posttraumatic biliary obstruction, must be ruled out. Liver function tests are diagnostic. Liver failure can lead to a decreased level of consciousness, abnormal clotting studies, and hypoglycemia (see Chapter 40).

Gastrointestinal failure manifests with hemorrhage from stress ulcers requiring blood transfusion. Prophylactic neutralization of gastric acid can minimize the risk of bleeding (see Chapter 40).

Renal failure can be precipitated by a renal injury, ischemia, radiographic contrast material, hypovolemia (due to hemorrhage, third spacing), or sepsis. Initial signs include a rising blood urea nitrogen and serum creatinine. Renal failure may be polyuric or oliguric. Dialysis often is necessary (see Chapter 30).

Cardiovascular failure, DIC, metabolic changes (eg, hyperglycemia, metabolic acidosis), and central nervous system changes, ranging from confusion to obtundation, also may be evident in MOF (see Chapter 48 for a discussion of DIC).

Research suggests that early nutritional support decreases the development of sepsis and MOF. Enteral feeding should be used whenever possible, because it is associated with a lower incidence of sepsis than total parenteral nutrition. A jejunostomy tube is often placed during initial laparotomy and feeding begun the day of surgery.[21,22]

Complications associated with multiple trauma are numerous (see accompanying display). Because most trauma patients are in the ICU when these complications develop, the critical care nurse plays an essential role in detecting and preventing these sequelae.

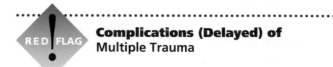

Complications (Delayed) of Multiple Trauma

Hematologic
- Hemorrhage, coagulopathy, DIC

Cardiac
- Dysrhythmia, heart failure, ventricular aneurysm

Pulmonary
- Atelectasis, pneumonia, emboli (fat or thrombotic), ARDS

Gastrointestinal
- Peritonitis, adynamic ileus, mechanical bowel obstruction, acalculous cholecystitis, anastomotic leak, fistula, bleeding

Hepatic
- Liver abscess, liver failure

Renal
- Hypertension, myoglobinuria, renal failure

Orthopedic
- Compartment syndrome

Skin
- Wound infection, dehiscence, skin breakdown

Systemic
- Sepsis

The unexpected nature of trauma tends to amplify fear and anxiety. Therefore, nursing care also must provide psychosocial support for the seriously injured patient and his or her family through a multidisciplinary approach that recognizes concerns and offers frequent explanations.

CLINICAL APPLICATION: Patient Care Study

A 31-year-old heavy equipment operator sustained blunt trauma when an industrial tire exploded and threw him 10 feet. He arrived unconscious in the emergency department with a blood pressure of 80/palpable and heart rate of 135 beats/min. Multiple radiological studies, a diagnostic peritoneal lavage, and exploratory surgery were performed. The following injuries were identified: epidural hematoma, multiple bilateral rib fractures (flail chest), right hemothorax, left pneumothorax, severe liver lacerations, bilateral forearm fracture, and an open fracture of the left tibia and fibula. Bilateral chest tubes were placed, and the patient underwent surgery for evacuation of the epidural hematoma, packing of liver lacerations, and débridement of the open fracture. All fractures were externally stabilized.

After surgery, he was maintained on a mechanical ventilator with an FiO_2 of 0.40 to 0.45 and positive end-expiratory pressure of 5 cm. Mechanical ventilation with PEEP promoted adequate lung expansion and stabilization of the flail chest. Parenteral nutritional support was initiated. Repeated blood transfusions were administered; however, the hematocrit and systolic blood pressure remained low (Hct = 20%–25%; SBP = 90 mm Hg). Continued internal bleeding necessitated a return to the operating room for débridement and repacking of the liver. By the next day, the bleeding had resolved. The packing was then removed, liver lacerations repaired, and drains placed.

The next day, signs and symptoms of sepsis developed in the patient. They included elevated temperature and white blood cell count, tachycardia, tachypnea, increased cardiac output, decreased systemic vascular resistance, and decreased level of consciousness. Cultures were obtained and antibiotics begun. Adult respiratory distress syndrome and acute renal failure developed, requiring increased ventilatory support and hemodialysis.

Intensive nursing care was necessary to manage the existing disorders and prevent further complications. Psychosocial support for the patient and his family also was provided.

After a third surgical procedure to débride necrotic tissue and drain a perihepatic abscess, the patient finally began to improve. Several weeks later, dialysis and ventilatory support were discontinued. Two months after admission, the patient was transferred out of the intensive care unit and 3 weeks later discharged home.

CONCLUSION

Caring for the multiply injured person is challenging. Many trauma patients have injuries to more than one body system, and most present with a unique combination of injuries. The critical care nurse must be able to integrate knowledge of organ systems and consider how they interrelate. Aggressive and knowledgeable nursing care plays a crucial role in decreasing mortality and morbidity in seriously injured patients.

Clinical Applicability Challenges

Self-Challenge: Critical Thinking

1. Compare and contrast assessment and management of blunt chest trauma with those of penetrating abdominal trauma.

2. Explore the relationship of hemorrhage (eg, after major hepatic trauma) with the development of MOF.

Study Questions

1. A 31-year-old man arrives in the emergency department with multiple injuries, including a massive right hemothorax. During which phase of care should chest tubes be inserted to treat the hemothorax?
   a. Primary evaluation
   b. Resuscitation
   c. Secondary assessment
   d. Definitive care

2. Nursing care of the patient with a flail chest may include all of the following actions except
   a. assisting the patient to cough and deep breathe.
   b. administering pain medication.
   c. taping rib fractures.
   d. assessing oxygenation and gas exchange.

3. Hemorrhage is most likely to occur after injury to
   a. the liver.
   b. the small bowel.
   c. the colon.
   d. the stomach.

4. A multiple-trauma patient is in the ICU after repair of severe liver lacerations. The nurse should monitor the patient for
   a. incomplete hemostasis.
   b. development of sepsis.
   c. signs and symptoms of DIC.
   d. All of the above

5. Nursing responsibilities when caring for the multiple-trauma patient with a fracture may include
   a. maintaining skeletal traction.
   b. wound and pin care.
   c. assessment for signs and symptoms of compartment syndrome.
   d. All of the above

6. The first manifestation of MOF usually is
   a. congestive heart failure.
   b. ARDS.
   c. DIC.
   d. gastrointestinal bleeding.

REFERENCES

1. American College of Surgeons Committee on Trauma: Advanced Trauma Life Support. Chicago, American College of Surgeons, 1993
2. Deaths resulting from firearm and motor vehicle related injuries—United States, 1968–1991. MMWR 43(3):37–42, 1994
3. Bridges KG, Welch G, Silver M, et al: CT detection of occult pneumothorax in multiple trauma patients. J Emerg Med 11(2):179–186, 1993
4. Cohn S: Pulmonary contusion. Trauma Quarterly 11(3):196–208, 1994

5. Grindlinger GA: Myocardial contusion: A review. Trauma Quarterly 11(3):223–236, 1994
6. Daleiden A: Clinical manifestations of blunt cardiac injury: A challenge to the critical care practitioner. Crit Care Nurse Q 17(2):13–23, 1994
7. Renz BM, Felicianco DV: Gunshot wounds to the right thoracoabdomen: A prospective study of nonoperative management. J Trauma 37(5):737–744, 1994
8. Andrade-Aleggre R, Mon L: Subxiphoid pericardial window in the diagnosis of penetrating cardiac trauma. Annals of Thoracic Surgery 58(4):1139–1141, 1994
9. Rosemary AS II, Albrink MH, Olson SM, et al: Abdominal stab wound protocol: Prospective study documents applicability for widespread use. Am Surg 61(2):112–116, 1995
10. Chmielewski GW, Nicholas JM, Dulchavsky SA, et al: Nonoperative management of gunshot wounds of the abdomen. Am Surg 61(8):665–668, 1995
11. Smith RS, Fry WR, Morabito DJ, et al: Therapeutic laparoscopy in trauma. Am J Surg 170(6):632–636, 1995
12. Townsend MC, Flancbaum L, Chobon PS, et al: Diagnostic laparoscopy as an adjunct to selective conservative management of solid organ injuries after blunt abdominal trauma. J Trauma 35(4):647–651, 1993
13. Taheri PA, Ferrara JJ, Johnson CE, et al: A convincing case for primary repair of penetrating colon injuries. Am J Surg 166(1):39–44, 1993
14. Pisters PW, Pachter HL: Autologous splenic transplantation for splenic trauma. Ann Surg 219(3):225–235, 1994
15. Bone LB, McNamara K, Shine B, et al: Mortality in multiple trauma patients with fractures. J Trauma 37(2):262–264, 1994
16. Richardson RR, Mattox KL: Hemorrhage. In Mattox KL (ed): Complications of Trauma, pp 1–13. New York, Churchill Livingstone, 1994
17. Schwab CW, Angood PB, Hanson CW III : Respiratory Failure. In Mattox KL (ed): Complications of Trauma, pp 15–40. New York, Churchill Livingstone, 1994
18. Regel G, Lobenhoffer P, Grotz M, et al: Treatment results of patients with multiple trauma: An analysis of 3406 cases treated between 1972 and 1991 at a German level 1 trauma center. J Trauma 38(1):70–78, 1995
19. Moore FA, Sauaia A, Moore EE, et al: Postinjury multiple organ failure: A bimodal phenomenon. J Trauma 40(4):501–510, 1996
20. Sauaia A, Moore A, Moore EE, et al: Epidemiology of trauma deaths: A reassessment. J Trauma 38(2):185–193, 1995
21. Barone JE: Multiple organ failure. In Mattox KL (ed): Complications of Trauma, pp 81–100. New York, Churchill Livingstone, 1994
22. Dent D, Kudsk KA, Minard G, et al: Risk of abdominal septic complications after feeding jejunostomy placement in patients undergoing splenectomy for trauma. Am J Surg 166(6):686–689, 1993

BIBLIOGRAPHY

Cardona VP, Hurn PD, Mason PJB, et al: Trauma Nursing From Resuscitation Through Rehabilitation (2nd Ed). Philadelphia, WB Saunders, 1994

Mattox KL (ed): Complications of Trauma. New York, Churchill Livingstone, 1994

Trauma Nursing Core Course Revision Task Force: Trauma Nursing Core Course (4th Ed). Park ridge, IL, Emergency Nurses Association, 1995

51

Burns

OBJECTIVES

Based on the content in this chapter, the reader should be able to:

- Examine the major pathophysiological changes associated with burn injury.
- Analyze the rationale for specific management of major clinical problems in each phase of recovery after burn injury.
- Assess the major psychosocial issues associated with burn injury.
- Explore the nursing role in assessing, managing, and evaluating a plan of care for the patient after a burn injury.

*B*urns represent the fourth leading cause of accidental death in the United States. People who suffer burn injury present a health care crisis. A person who is well can rapidly become a person with extensive burns. Concomitant with dramatic physiological alterations is the emotional impact of burn injury. Not only is the burn victim affected, but the family is affected emotionally also.

PATHOPHYSIOLOGICAL PRINCIPLES

Burn injury affects all organs and systems. The magnitude of this pathophysiological response is proportional to the extent of burn injury and reaches a plateau when approximately 60% of the total body surface is burned.[1] Cardiovascular dynamics are affected significantly by burn injury, which can result in hypovolemic shock.

Hypovolemic Shock

The person with a major burn injury experiences a form of hypovolemic shock known as burn shock (Fig. 51–1). Within minutes of thermal injury, a marked increase in capillary hydrostatic pressure occurs in the injured tissue, accompanied by an increase in capillary permeability. This results in a rapid shift of plasma fluid from the intravascular compartment across heat-damaged capillaries, into interstitial areas (resulting in edema) and to the burn wound it-

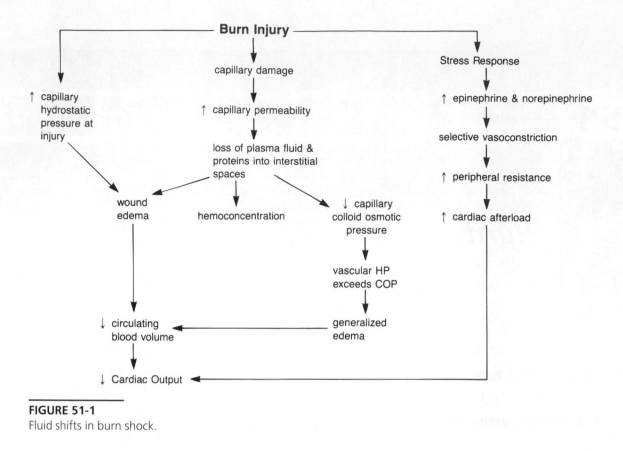

FIGURE 51-1
Fluid shifts in burn shock.

self. The loss of plasma fluid and proteins results in a decreased colloid osmotic pressure in the vascular compartment. As a result, fluid and electrolytes continue to leak from the vascular compartment, resulting in additional edema formation in the burned tissue and throughout the body.

This "leak," which consists of sodium, water, and plasma proteins, is followed by a decrease in cardiac output, hemoconcentration of red blood cells, diminished perfusion to major organs, and generalized body edema. The pathophysiological response after burn injury is biphasic. In the early postinjury phase, generalized organ hypofunction (ebb phase) develops as a consequence of decreased cardiac output. Peripheral vascular resistance increases as a result of the neurohumoral stress response after trauma. This increases cardiac afterload, resulting in a further decrease in cardiac output. The increase in peripheral vascular resistance (selective vasoconstriction) and the hemoconcentration resulting from plasma fluid loss may cause the blood pressure to appear normal at first. If fluid replacement is inadequate, however, and plasma protein loss continues, hypovolemic shock soon occurs.

In patients receiving adequate fluid resuscitation, the cardiac output usually returns to normal in the latter part of the first 24 hours after burn injury. As plasma volume is replenished during the second 24 hours, the cardiac output increases to hypermetabolic levels (hyperfunction phase)

and slowly returns to more normal levels as the burn wounds are closed.[2,3]

In some instances, with burns exceeding 60% total body surface area (TBSA), depressed cardiac output does not respond to aggressive volume resuscitation. A myocardial depressant factor capable of depressing ventricular contractility by 60% has been identified. Myocardial depression in the early postburn period also may be the result of reduced coronary blood flow.[3]

The response of the pulmonary vasculature is like that of the peripheral circulation. Pulmonary vascular resistance, however, is greater and lasts longer. Immediately after burn injury, the patient may experience a mild, transient pulmonary hypertension. A decrease in oxygen tension and lung compliance also may be evident.

The loss of fluid throughout the body's intravascular space results in a thickened, sluggish flow of the remaining circulatory blood volume. The effects reach all body systems. This slowing of circulation permits bacteria and cellular material to settle in the lower portions of blood vessels, especially in the capillaries, resulting in sludging.

The antigen–antibody reaction to burned tissue adds to circulatory congestion by the clumping or agglutination of cells. Coagulation problems occur as a result of the release of thromboplastin by the injury itself and the release of fibrinogen from injured platelets. If thrombi occur, they may cause ischemia of the affected part and lead to necrosis. The increased coagulation process may develop into disseminated intravascular coagulation. Because this is a widespread occurrence, any organ in the body may be involved, and organ failure may occur.

Metabolic Response

The stress response elicited by burn injury promotes a set of physiological responses characterized by increased energy expenditure and elevated nutritional requirements. Hypermetabolism, increased glucose flow, and severe protein and fat wasting are characteristic responses to trauma and infection. In no other disease state is this response as severe as it is after thermal injury (see Metabolic Response to Injury in Chapter 39). The metabolic rate of people with burns covering more than 40% TBSA often is twice normal. This hypermetabolic state peaks between days 7 and 17 postburn. Increased oxygen consumption, metabolic rate, urinary excretion, fat breakdown, and steady erosion of body mass are related directly to burn size and return to normal as the burn wound heals or is covered.

■ CLASSIFICATION OF BURN INJURY

The skin is the largest organ of the body. A cross-section of skin is shown in Figure 51–2. Several complex functions are performed by the skin. It is the body's first line of defense against invasion by microorganisms and environmental ra-

diation. It prevents loss of body fluids, controls body temperature, functions as an excretory and sensory organ, produces vitamin D, and influences body image. Burn injuries are described by depth, causative agent, and severity; a discussion of these follows.

Burn Depth

Damage to the skin frequently is described according to the depth of injury and is defined in terms of partial-thickness and full-thickness injuries, which correspond to the various layers of the skin (Table 51–1; also see Fig. 51–2).

Partial-thickness burns are differentiated into superficial and deep partial-thickness burns. *Superficial partial-thickness burns* (ie, first-degree burns) damage the epidermis, which is the thin layer of epithelial cells that is replaced continuously. This keratinized layer provides a protective wall between the host and the environment. A sunburn is a familiar example of a superficial partial-thickness injury. It feels painful at first and later itches due to the stimulation of sensory receptors. Because of the continued replacement of epithelial cells of the epidermis, this type of injury will heal spontaneously without scarring.

Deep partial-thickness injuries (ie, second-degree burns) involve varying degrees of the dermal layer. The dermis contains structures essential to normal skin function: sweat and sebaceous glands, sensory and motor nerves, capillaries, and hair follicles. A deep partial-thickness burn will be pinkish-red and painful, and it will form blisters and subcutaneous edema. Depending on the depth, these wounds will heal spontaneously in 3 to 35 days as the epidermal el-

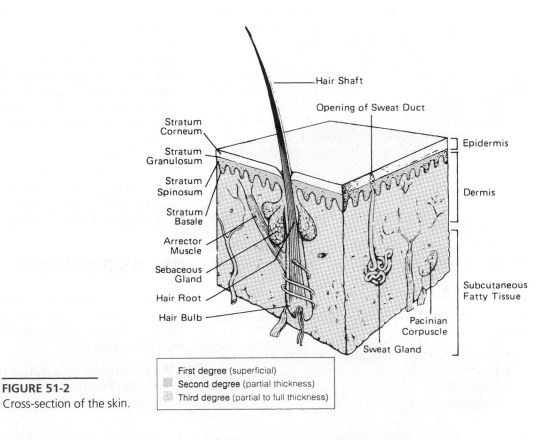

FIGURE 51-2
Cross-section of the skin.

TABLE 51-1
Characteristics of Burns of Various Depths

Depth	Tissues Involved	Usual Cause	Characteristics	Pain	Healing
Superficial partial-thickness (first degree)	Minimal epithelial damage	Sun	Dry Blisters after 24 h Pinkish red Blanches with pressure	Painful	About 5 d No scarring
Superficial partial-thickness (second degree)	Epidermis, minimal dermis	Flash Hot liquids	Moist Pinkish or mottled red Blisters Some blanching	Pain Hyperesthetic	21–28 d Minimal scarring
Deep dermal partial-thickness (second degree)	Entire epidermis, part of dermis: epidermal-lined hair and sweat glands intact	Above plus hot solids, flame, and intense radiant injury	Dry, pale, waxy No blanching	Sensitive to pressure	30 d–months Late hypertrophic scarring; marked contracture formation
Full-thickness (third degree)	All of above, and portion of subcutaneous fat; may involve connective tissue, muscle, bone	Sustained flame, electrical, chemical, and steam	Leathery, cracked avascular, white, cherry red, or black	Little pain	Cannot self-regenerate; needs grafting

ements germinate and migrate until the epidermal surface is restored. If the wound becomes infected or traumatized or if the blood supply is compromised, these burns will develop into full-thickness burns.

Full-thickness burns (ie, third-degree burns) expose the fat layer, which is composed of poorly vascularized adipose tissue. This layer contains the roots of the sweat glands and hair follicles. All epidermal elements are destroyed. These burns may appear white, red, brown, or black. Reddened areas do not blanch in response to pressure because the underlying blood supply has been interrupted. Brownish streaks are evidence of thrombosed blood vessels.

These burns are completely anesthetic because the sensory receptors have been totally destroyed. In addition, they may appear sunken because of the loss of underlying fat and muscle.

A small wound (< 4 cm) may be allowed to heal by granulation and migration of healthy epithelium from the wound margins. Extensive, open full-thickness wounds, however, leave the patient highly susceptible to overwhelming infection and malnutrition. Wound closure by skin grafting restores the integrity of the skin.

Causative Agent

Burns may be classified according to the agent causing the injury:

- Thermal (scald, contact, and flame injuries)
- Electrical
- Chemical
- Radiation

The extent and depth of burn injury are related to the intensity and duration of exposure to the causative agent.

Burn Severity

A burn injury may range from a small blister to massive third-degree burns. Recognizing the need for a clear description of terms, the American Burn Association developed the Injury Severity Grading System, which is used to determine the magnitude of the burn injury and to provide optimal criteria for hospital resources for patient care. Burn injury has been categorized into minor, moderate, and major burns, as outlined in the accompanying display.

Minor burn injuries can be treated in the emergency department with outpatient follow-up every 48 hours, until the risk of infection is reduced and wound healing is underway. Moderate uncomplicated burn injuries may be treated in the average hospital; patients with major burns should be cared for in a burn center.

ASSESSMENT

The extent and depth of the burn and the causative agent, time, and circumstances surrounding the burn injury are vital data. To assess the severity of the burn, several factors must be considered:

- Percentage of body surface area burned
- Depth of the burn
- Anatomical location of the burn

Minor burn injury
- Second-degree burn of <15% total body surface area (TBSA) burn in adults or <10% TBSA in children
- Third-degree burn of <2% TBSA not involving special care areas (eyes, ears, face, hands, feet, perineum, joints)
- Excludes electrical injury, inhalation injury, concurrent trauma, all poor-risk patients (ie, extremes of age, intercurrent disease)

Moderate, uncomplicated burn injury
- Second-degree burns of 15%–25% TBSA in adults or 10%–20% in children
- Third-degree burns of <10% TBSA not involving special care areas
- Excludes electrical injury, inhalation injury, concurrent trauma, all poor-risk patients (ie, extremes of age, intercurrent disease)

Major burn injury
- Second-degree burns of >25% TBSA in adults or 20% in children
- All third-degree burns of ≥10% TBSA
- All burns involving eyes, ears, face, hands, feet, perineum, joints
- All inhalation injury, electrical injury, concurrent trauma, all poor-risk patients

- Inhalation injury
- Age of the person
- Medical history
- Concomitant injury

Physical Examination

BURN AREA SIZE

Several methods using percentages of TBSA may be used in estimating the extent of a burn. The "rule of nines" divides the body parts into multiples of 9%, as shown in Figure 51–3. The head is considered to account for 9% of TBSA; each arm, 9%; each leg, 18%; the anterior trunk, 18%; the posterior trunk, 18%; and the perineum, 1%, making a total of 100%. Burns may be circumferential or may involve only one surface of a body part. A circumferential burn of an arm is 9%, whereas if only the anterior surface were burned, the value would be 4.5%.

The rule of nines is the most common method used for estimating burn area size. Berkow's method is more accurate, particularly for infants and children, because it accounts for proportionate growth. The extent of small scattered burns can be estimated by comparing the size of the nurse's hand to the patient's hand. Allowing for differences, the comparison will indicate that the palmar surface of an adult's hand equals approximately 1% of an adult's TBSA.

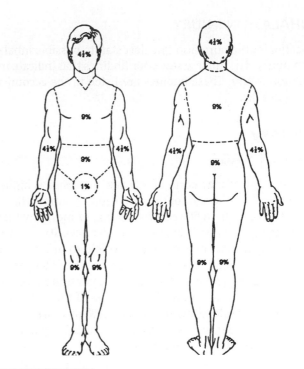

FIGURE 51-3
The "rule of nines" method for determining percentage of body area with burn injury.

BURN DEPTH

Burn classifications are based on the tissues involved (as discussed previously in this chapter) or classified as first-, second- (superficial or deep), and third-degree burns (see Table 51–1).

ANATOMICAL LOCATION

Location of the burn is important to healing and general rehabilitation. Burns of the face, head, neck, hands, feet, and genitalia create particular problems. Although they may be limited in surface area, these burns usually require hospitalization of the injured person and special care because they are important areas where rapid, uninfected healing with minimal scarring is desired.

Facial burns may involve edema and present problems with airway management. Burns of the head that involve the external ear and burns of the hands that involve the distal phalanges are particularly difficult to heal because these structures are primarily composed of cartilage, which lacks a good blood supply.

Perineal burns are difficult, if not impossible, to keep from becoming infected. Edema can be a problem also, and patients with perineal burns need to be catheterized as soon as possible.

If burns in any of these special areas do not heal well, serious psychosocial and economic problems related to appearance, self-concept, manual dexterity, and locomotion can occur.

INHALATION INJURY

Location of the burn also can alert staff to possible inhalation injury. The nurse assesses for findings that indicate inhalation injury. These findings are listed in the accompanying display.

History

PATIENT'S AGE

Although burns may occur at any age, incidence is higher at both ends of the age continuum. People younger than 2 years and older than 60 years have a higher mortality than other age groups with burns of similar severity. A child younger than 2 years is more susceptible to infection because of the immature immune response. The older person may have degenerative processes that complicate recovery and that may be aggravated by the stress of the burn. As a general rule, children with burns of 10% or more and all adults whose injuries account for 12% to 15% or more of TBSA will require hospitalization.

MEDICAL HISTORY

The nurse assesses to determine whether the patient has a disease that compromises the ability to manage fluid shifts and resist infection (eg, diabetes mellitus, congestive heart failure, cirrhosis) or if renal, respiratory, or gastrointestinal problems are present. Some problems, such as diabetes and renal failure, may become acute during the burn process. If inhalation injury has occurred in the presence of cardiopulmonary disease (eg, congestive heart failure, emphysema), the respiratory status is compromised tremendously.

Concomitant Injuries

Concurrent injuries may be observed while the nurse obtains a brief history from the patient. Usually burn patients are awake and alert, so any changes in neurological status usually indicate other injury, such as anoxia, head injury, drug use or intoxication, hypoglycemia, or myocardial infarction. Because burn wounds do not bleed, any external bleeding indicates lacerations of deeper structures. Extremities are assessed for fractures.

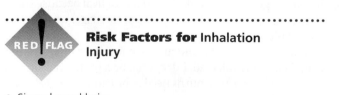

RED FLAG **Risk Factors for** Inhalation Injury

- Singed nasal hairs
- Burns of the oral or pharyngeal mucous membranes
- Burns in the perioral area or neck
- Coughing up of soot or change in voice
- Occurrence of burn in a confined area

Clinical Manifestations and Diagnostic Studies

INHALATION INJURY

If the burn was caused by a flame or if the person was burned in a confined area, the nurse assesses for signs of carbon monoxide poisoning, smoke inhalation, and accompanying signs of respiratory distress and pulmonary injury.

Carbon Monoxide Poisoning

Often the burn patient was trapped in a burning building and has inhaled significant amounts of carbon monoxide. Usually characteristic physical signs of carbon monoxide poisoning are not present. The hallmark cherry red skin color hardly ever is observed in burn patients. Diagnosis is made by direct determination of carboxyhemoglobin levels by spectrophotometry. Carboxyhemoglobin concentrations should be measured in all fire victims.

Central nervous system manifestations of carbon monoxide poisoning may range from headache to coma to death (see Table 52–3). It must not be taken for granted that central nervous system abnormalities are caused by carbon monoxide poisoning, however. Sometimes other potentially fatal diseases are present in thermally injured people, and these must be investigated. Conditions clinically similar to carbon monoxide poisoning in thermally injured people include acute drug overdose, uncontrolled diabetes, acute alcohol intoxication, acute head injury, acute psychotic reaction, insulin overdose, and hypovolemic or septic shock.

Respiratory Distress

Decreased arterial oxygenation often is seen after burn injury. Although the exact mechanism is unknown, restoration of cardiac output improves oxygenation. Hence, this decreased oxygenation may be related to poor tissue perfusion and shock rather than airway obstruction. Therefore, a falling arterial PO_2 may indicate either an airway obstruction or declining left heart output.

The immediate cause of respiratory distress often is laryngeal edema or spasm and the accumulation of mucus. Because actual signs of obstruction may not become apparent for several hours, it is necessary to monitor the patient

---

CLINICAL APPLICATION:
Assessment Parameters
Findings Following a Burn Injury

↑Hematocrit
↓Red blood cells
↑Leukocytes
↓Thrombocytes
↑K
↑Blood urea nitrogen
↑Urinary output
Myobloginuria

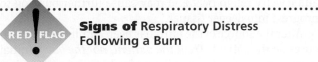

Signs of Respiratory Distress
Following a Burn

- Hoarseness
- Drooling
- Inability to handle secretions
- Rapid or labored breathing
- Crackles
- Stridor
- Hacking cough

continuously for hoarseness, drooling, or inability to handle secretions. Hoarseness indicates a significant decrease in the diameter of the airway. The edema may continue to develop for 72 hours, and endotracheal intubation or tracheostomy may be indicated. Because airway obstruction due to laryngeal edema subsides within 3 to 5 days, endotracheal or nasotracheal intubation is preferable to a tracheostomy.

Pulmonary Injury

Inhalation injury usually appears within the first 24 to 48 hours postburn and is secondary to the inhalation of combustible products. It is not the result of thermal injury because most heat is dissipated at the level of the distal trachea. Most commonly, especially in closed-space injuries, inhalation of the products of incomplete combustion results in a chemical pneumonitis. Inflammatory changes occur during the first 24 hours postburn. The pulmonary tree becomes irritated and edematous. Changes may not become apparent, however, until the second 24 hours. Pulmonary edema is a possibility any time from the first few hours to 7 days after the injury. The patient may be irrational or even unconscious, depending on the degree of hypoxia.

Serial arterial blood gases will show a falling PO_2. Usually, the admission chest film will appear normal because changes are not reflected until 24 to 48 hours postburn. A sputum specimen should be obtained for culture and sensitivity studies. Laryngoscopy and bronchoscopy may be of value in determining the presence of extramucosal carbonaceous material (the most reliable sign of inhalation injury) and the state of the mucosa (blistering, edema, erythema), which may have an effect on bronchospasm, atelectasis, hypoxemia, and pulmonary edema.

More specific confirmation of inhalation injury is achieved with the use of fiberoptic bronchoscopy, which permits direct examination of the proximal airway, and xenon-133 scintigraphy. Xenon-133 ventilation–perfusion scanning is helpful in establishing a diagnosis of injury to small airways and lung parenchyma.

Pulmonary damage, primarily as a result of inhalation, accounts for 20% to 84% of burn mortality. Three stages of injury have been described:

1. Acute pulmonary insufficiency may occur during the first 36 hours.
2. Pulmonary edema occurs in 5% to 30% of burn patients between 6 and 72 hours after burn.
3. Bronchopneumonia appears in 15% to 60% of burn patients 3 to 10 days after burn.

HEMATOLOGICAL MANIFESTATIONS

Hematological signs associated with major thermal injury vary. Initially, the hematocrit increases secondary to capillary leak and loss of circulating plasma volume. The hematocrit usually reaches 50% to 70% and remains elevated until plasma volume is restored.

During the initial burn period, 8% to 19% of the circulating red blood cells are hemolyzed by the effects of heat as they pass through the burned area at the time of injury. The survival time of other red cells is shortened by the burn injury, resulting in an additional 10% to 25% loss of circulating red blood cells. Still other red cells are trapped in engorged capillaries and are unavailable to the general circulation. Some small amount of blood loss occurs initially at the burn site; additional blood loss is slow and constant as débridements proceed. A unit of blood is lost every 3 to 4 days in adults with more than 40% TBSA burns. The burn-injured patient therefore needs frequent transfusions to maintain blood volume, correct anemia, and maintain hematocrit between 35% and 40%.

The leukocyte count may be high initially, due to hemoconcentration. If leukocytosis persists after 1 week, it usually indicates infection by a gram-positive organism, often *Staphylococcus aureus*.

During the resuscitative phase, platelet destruction is accelerated, resulting in a progressive thrombocytopenia. After the fifth day postburn, platelet levels return to normal or elevated levels.

As a result of increased platelet adhesiveness, increased blood viscosity, and the release of thromboplastin and fibrinogen, clotting factors V and VIII are elevated, and thrombin times are prolonged.

ELECTROLYTE IMBALANCE

Electrolyte concentrations are altered not only from the leaking process but also from direct injury to burned cells. Chemical changes are due to shifts in the composition of various fluids as they move from one body compartment to another. At first, electrolyte studies show an increase in serum potassium because of intracellular potassium release secondary to cell injury. The intracellular potassium is replaced by sodium; therefore, normal cellular function is impaired.

After approximately 48 hours, the capillary walls have healed sufficiently to stop the fluid shift from the vascular tree. Fluid is then drawn back into the blood vessels, edema subsides, the plasma volume expands, and diuresis begins. At this time, large amounts of potassium are lost, and replacement may be necessary. In severe burns, the alterations in potassium levels must be monitored carefully to avoid cardiac failure.

The plasma level of sodium and chloride is normal or slightly elevated at first but increases rapidly as excessive interstitial fluid is reabsorbed. The blood urea nitrogen may be elevated if excessive protein catabolism occurred. Blood glucose levels may be increased temporarily as a result of the action of epinephrine, which is released in reaction to the stress of the burn injury. The epinephrine acts on amino acids to produce glucose (gluconeogenesis), which the patient requires to meet the body's demands during stress.

RENAL PROBLEMS

Urinary output decreases due to hypotension, decreased renal blood flow, and secretion of antidiuretic hormone and aldosterone. Unless fluid resuscitation measures are taken promptly and appropriately, poor tissue perfusion can result in renal shutdown. Erythrocytes damaged by thermal injury release free hemoglobin, and damaged muscle tissue releases myoglobin. As the free hemoglobin and myoglobin pass through the kidney, they are excreted into the urine. If these substances block the nephrons, renal failure may develop.

Specialized protocols for treatment of myoglobinuria have been developed. The common features of these formulas are maintaining a high urine output and alkalinization of the urine to avoid precipitation of myoglobin or hemochromogens and subsequent acute renal failure. Myoglobinuria in the thermally injured patient cannot be treated in isolation. Overall volume deficits must be corrected and renal perfusion optimized before osmotic or loop diuretics are given.

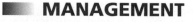

MANAGEMENT

Burn management requires multidisciplinary cooperation. It may be divided into various phases based on the patient's condition. Terms used in this chapter for these phases are resuscitative, acute, and rehabilitative.

The Resuscitative Phase

Some of the information in this section covers initial treatment before the burn patient reaches the intensive care unit (ICU). The critical care nurse considers care given at the scene of the fire and in the emergency department as he or she continues to provide multidisciplinary care.

INITIAL CARE AT THE SCENE

The first priority at the scene of injury is to stop the burning process and prevent further injury. Removing the source of burning is the first consideration. In the event of an electrical injury, the person should be removed from the current with a nonconducting object to ensure safety of the rescuer. If the patient has a chemical burn, all clothing should be removed, and the wound should be flushed with copious amounts of water.

Flames should be extinguished with water or smothered with a blanket, or the victim should be rolled on the ground. Smoldering clothing, constricting clothing, belts, and jewelry should be removed before swelling begins. Clothing and jewelry retain heat and may cause further burning to progress into deeper tissues.

After the source of the burn has been eliminated, care focuses on the patient: *Treat the patient, not the burn.* Initial management of patients with major burn injury requires airway support, fluid resuscitation, treatment for associated trauma and preexisting medical conditions, and initial wound treatment.

CARE IN THE EMERGENCY DEPARTMENT

Usually burn patients are awake, alert, and oriented immediately after burn injury. If the patient is conscious, maintaining an airway should not be a problem. If the patient is unconscious, standard cardiopulmonary life support measures should be used to establish an airway. If the patient was in an enclosed area with smoke, oxygen at 2 to 4 L/flow/min or 40% humidified oxygen should be administered until arterial blood gases are obtained. When in doubt, the nurse starts oxygen therapy; it can do no harm. If the patient has a major scald injury involving the face and neck, edema may form within 4 to 6 hours. Early prophylactic intubation is indicated. The nasotracheal tube should be secured with cotton twill tape, which can be loosened as edema progresses.[4]

If intravenous cannulation was not initiated in the field, a large-bore cannula should be inserted in a peripheral vein, or a central line should be started. All patients with burns greater than 20% to 30% TBSA should have an indwelling catheter inserted for accurate urinary output measurements. A nasogastric tube should be inserted in all patients at risk for adynamic ileus (burns greater than 25% TBSA). If inhalation injury or carbon monoxide poisoning is suspected, humidified 100% oxygen should be administered.

A tetanus toxoid booster should be administered if the patient has been immunized previously but has not received tetanus toxoid within the last 5 years. If a tetanus immunization history is unknown, the patient should receive 250 U of human tetanus-immune globulin and the first of a series of active immunizations with tetanus toxoid.

The patient should be covered with a nonadherent, nonfuzzy cover. Additional blankets can be added as needed to provide warmth and prevent hypothermia. Burn patients chill easily because they have lost their skin's protection against temperature changes. Covers also guard the wound against contamination and ease the pain caused by air currents. Cool, sterile water or saline may be applied to the burn to ease the pain; however, it is important to guard against hypothermia and tissue damage. Ice or ice water should not be used because extreme cold can cause further tissue damage.

Nursing responsibilities in the emergency department include monitoring for inhalation injury, monitoring fluid resuscitation, assessing the burn wound, monitoring vital signs, obtaining an accurate history, and carrying out emergency measures.

CARE IN THE INTENSIVE CARE UNIT

The critical care nurse plays an essential role in caring for the burn patient and family. The Collaborative Care Guide outlines multidisciplinary care given the burn patient and family.

COLLABORATIVE CARE GUIDE
for the Patient With a Burn

OUTCOMES	INTERVENTIONS
Oxygenation/Ventilation	
Patent airway is maintained. Lung is clear on auscultation.	• Auscultate breath sounds q2–4h and PRN. • Assess for inhalation injury, and anticipate intubation. • Assess quantity and color of tracheal secretions. • Suction endotracheal airway when appropriate (see Collaborative Care Guide for Patient on Ventilator). • Hyperoxygenate and hyperventilate before and after each suction pass.
Peak, mean, and plateau pressures are within normal limits for a patient on a ventilator.	• Monitor airway pressures q1–2 h. • Monitor lung compliance q8h (see Chapter 24). • Administer bronchodilators and mucolytics. • Perform chest physiotherapy q4h. • Monitor airway pressures and lung compliance for improvement after interventions.
There is no evidence of atelectasis or infiltrates.	• Turn side to side q2h. • Consider kinetic therapy or prone positioning. • Take daily chest x-ray.
Arterial blood gases are within normal limits.	• Monitor carboxyhemoglobin and carbon monoxide levels. • Monitor arterial blood gases using cooximeter analysis of arterial saturation. (Pulse oximeter and calculated SaO_2 are inaccurate measures in the presence of carbon monoxide.) • Provide humidified oxygen. • Consider hyperbaric therapy.
Circulation/Perfusion	
Blood pressure, heart rate, CVP, and pulmonary artery pressures are within normal limits.	• Assess vital signs q1h. • Assess hemodynamic pressures q1h if patient has PA catheter. • Administer intravascular volume as ordered to maintain preload (see below).
Temperature is within normal limits.	• Monitor temperature q1h. • Maintain a warm environment, and use warming lights or blankets to prevent hypothermia. • Treat fever with antipyretics and cooling blankets.
Perfusion to extremities is maintained; pulses are intact.	• Monitor perfusion using pulse oximetry, Doppler, palpation q1h. • Elevate burned extremities. • Prepare for escharotomy or fasciotomy.
Fluids/Electrolytes	

Restore and maintain fluid balance:
    Urine output 30–70 mL/h or 0.5 mL/kg.
    CVP, 8–12 mmHg; PAWP, 12–18 mmHg; blood pressure, WNL; heart rate, <120 bpm.
	• Assess intake and output q1h.
	• Give lactated Ringer's 4 mL/kg/% burn, divided into first 24 h postburn.
	• Monitor for spontaneous diuresis, and reduce IV infusion rate as indicated.
	• Take daily weight.

Electrolytes, mineral, and renal function values are within normal limits.	• Monitor and replace minerals and electrolytes. • Monitor BUN, creatinine, myoglobin, and urine electrolytes and glucose. • Monitor neurological status. • Monitor and treat dysrhythmias.
Mobility/Safety	
Patient is free of joint contractures.	• Provide passive and active range-of-motion exercises q1–2h. • Apply positioning splints as needed.

(continued)

COLLABORATIVE CARE GUIDE
for the Patient With a Burn (Continued)

OUTCOMES	INTERVENTIONS
There is no evidence of complications related to immobility. There is no evidence of infection.	• Turn and reposition q2h. • Consider kinetic therapy. • Consider DVT prophylaxis. • Maintain strict sterile technique, and monitor technique of others. • Maintain sterility of invasive catheters and tubes. • Per hospital protocol, change dressings and invasive catheters. Culture wounds, blood, urine, as necessary. • Monitor systemic inflammatory response syndrome criteria: increased WBC, increased temperature, tachypnea, tachycardia.
Skin Integrity Unburned skin will remain intact. Burns begin healing without complications.	• Assess skin q4h and each time patient is repositioned. • Turn q2h. • Consider pressure relief/reduction mattress. • Treat burns per hospital protocol; apply topical medications and débride as indicated. • Monitor skin graft viability. • Protect grafted areas (eg, bed cradle, dressings). • Consider air fluidized bed to enhance healing and relieve pressure from burned surface.
Nutrition Caloric and nutrient intake meets metabolic requirements per calculation (eg, Basal Energy Expenditure).	• Provide parenteral or enteral nutrition within 24 h of injury. • Consult dietitian or nutritional support service to assess nutritional requirements with team. • Monitor protein and calorie intake. • Monitor albumin, prealbumin, transferrin, cholesterol, triglycerides, glucose.
Comfort/Pain Control Patient will have minimal pain, <5 on pain scale, and discomfort.	• Assess pain and discomfort using objective pain scale q4h, PRN, and following administration of pain medication. • Administer analgesics prior to procedures, and monitor patient response. • Use nonpharmacological pain management techniques (eg, music, distraction, touch).
Psychosocial Patient demonstrates decreased anxiety.	• Assess vital signs during treatments, discussions, and so forth. • Administer sedatives prior to treatments/procedures. • Consult social services, clergy, and so forth as appropriate. • Provide for adequate rest and sleep. • Encourage discussion regarding long-term effects of burns, available resources, and coping strategies.
Teaching/Discharge Planning Patient/significant others understand procedures and tests needed for treatment. Significant others understand the severity of the illness, ask appropriate questions, anticipate potential complications.	• Prepare patient/significant others for procedures, such as débridement, escharotomy, fasciotomy, intubation, and mechanical ventilation. • Explain the potential effects of burns and the potential for complications, such as infection, respiratory or renal failure. • Encourage significant others to ask questions related to the management of burns, disfigurement, coping, and so forth.

Fluid Resuscitation

Therapy for burn shock is aimed at supporting the patient through the period of hypovolemic shock until capillary integrity is restored. Fluid resuscitation is the primary intervention in the resuscitative phase in the ICU. Goals in fluid resuscitation are as follows:

- Correct fluid, electrolyte, and protein deficits.
- Replace continuing losses, and maintain fluid balance.
- Prevent excessive edema formation.
- Maintain a urine output in adults of 30 to 70 mL/h.

Formulas for Fluid Administration. Numerous formulas have been developed for fluid resuscitation (Table 51–2). Each has advantages and disadvantages. They differ primarily in terms of recommended volume administration and salt content.

In general, lost crystalloid and colloid solutions must be replaced rigorously. Free water, given as 5% dextrose/water (D_5W) with or without added electrolytes, is regulated so that insensible fluid loss is covered. Ringer's lactate is used as the crystalloid solution because it is a balanced salt solution that closely approximates the composition of extracellular fluid. In addition, it has large molecules, which expand the circulating plasma volume.

The Parkland formula is the most commonly used resuscitation regimen in the United States. This formula requires 4 mL of Ringer's lactate per kilogram of body weight per percent TBSA burn. This amount is administered in the

TABLE 51-2
Formulas for Fluid Replacement/Resuscitation

	First 24 Hours			Second 24 Hours		
	Electrolyte	*Colloid*	*Glucose in Water*	*Electrolyte*	*Colloid*	*Glucose in Water*
Burn budget of F.D. Moore	1,000–4,000 mL lactated Ringer's and 1,200 mL 0.5N saline	7.5% of body weight	1,500–5,000 mL	1,000–4,000 mL lactated Ringer's and 1,200 mL 0.5N saline	2.5% of body weight	1,500–5,000 mL
Evans	Normal saline, 1 mL/kg/% burn	1.0 mL/kg/% burn	2,000 mL	One half of first–24-h requirement	One half of first-hour requirement	2,000 mL
Brooke	Lactated Ringer's, 1.5 mL/kg/% burn	0.5 mL/kg/% burn	2,000 mL	One half to three quarters of first–24-h requirement	One half to three quarters of first–24-h requirement	2,000 mL
Parkland	Lactated Ringer's 4 mL/kg/% burn				20%–60% of calculated plasma volume	As necessary to maintain urinary output
Hypertonic sodium solution	Volume of hypertonic lactated saline (HLS) to maintain urine output at 30 mL/h (fluid contains 250 mEq Na/L)			0.6 mL HLS/kg/% burn plus oral Haldane's solution to replace insensible water loss or one third of salt solution orally, up to 3,500 mL limit		
Modified Brooke	Lactated Ringer's 2 mL/kg/% burn				0.3–0.5 mL/kg/% burn	Goal: maintain adequate urinary output
Burnett Burn Center	Isotonic or hypertonic alkaline sodium solution/% burn/kg			$n_{51/4}$ NS maintenance	Colloid 0.5 mL/% burn/kg	D_5W (% burn) (TBSAm^2)

first 24 hours postinjury. One half is given in the first 8 hours postinjury, and the remainder is administered over the subsequent 16 hours postburn. The Parkland formula and other fluid resuscitation formulas are guidelines, and individual patients may require more or less than the 4 mL/kg/%TBSA during the first 24 hours. Other formulas contain various amounts of colloid or hypertonic saline. The argument against colloid administration in the first 12 hours postburn is that there is a diffuse postburn capillary leak that allows colloids to extravasate through endothelial junctions, thereby not producing any demonstrable oncotic benefit over administration of a crystalloid. Hypertonic saline resuscitation lowers the amount of fluid that needs to be given to selected patients but can cause severe hypernatremia and must be used cautiously.

The following example may help illustrate the very large amounts of fluid required. The Baxter, or Parkland, formula for a patient weighing 75 kg who received burns over 50% of the body would be stated as follows:

$$4 \text{ mL} \times 75 \text{ kg} \times 50\% = 15,000 \text{ mL}$$

Of this, 7,500 mL is to be administered during the first 8 hours, and 3,750 mL is to be administered in the second and third 8-hour periods. Hence, it is extremely difficult to avoid fluid overload and pulmonary edema when it is necessary to infuse fluids so rapidly. Consequently, digoxin may be given to severely burned patients to induce maximal function of the left ventricle and to minimize the chances of transient increases in left atrial pressure. Isoproterenol infusions may be used for symptoms of decreased cardiac output.

The time postinjury at which capillary integrity is restored varies among individuals but usually is between 12 and 14 hours. Many physicians administer colloids at this point to restore albumin levels to 2.0 to 3.0 mg/dL. Controversy exists over the type of colloid to be administered, with some centers using salt-poor albumin and others using fresh frozen plasma.

Nonprotein collagens may be used in burn shock resuscitation. Dextran and hetastarch are high–molecular-weight solutions that generate colloid osmotic pressure when given intravascularly. Allergic responses have been reported with dextran, but the risk virtually is eliminated by pretreatment with Promit, a very low–molecular-weight dextran.

After the first 24 hours postinjury, replacing the massive evaporative water loss is a major consideration in fluid management. The primary solution given at this time is D_5W, with the goal of keeping the patient's sodium concentration at 140 mEq/L.

Monitoring Fluid Replacement. The volume necessary to resuscitate burn patients depends on severity of injury, age, physiological status, and associated injury. Consequently, the volume recommended by a resuscitation formula must be modified according to the individual's response to therapy (Fig. 51–4). Urine output is the single best indicator of fluid resuscitation in patients with previously normal renal function. Other indications of adequate fluid replacement are listed in the display. Central lines and Swan-

Ganz catheters are not inserted routinely because of the danger of sepsis; however, they are used in selected instances.

Adequacy of fluid replacement is judged clinically for adults by a urinary output of 30 to 70 mL/h, pulse rate below 120, blood pressure in normal to high ranges, central venous pressure readings less than 12 cm H_2O or a pulmonary capillary wedge pressure reading below 18 mmHg, clear sensorium and clear lung sounds, and the absence of intestinal symptoms, such as nausea and paralytic ileus. Patients usually are weighed daily. A gain of 15% of admission weight may be expected. Intake and output must be monitored meticulously.

The onset of spontaneous diuresis is a hallmark indicating the end of the resuscitative phase. Infusion rates can be decreased by 25% for 1 hour if the urine output is satisfactory and can be maintained for 2 hours; the reduction then can be repeated. It is essential that urinary outputs be maintained in normal limits (50–70 mL/h).

Patients who sustain deep muscle injury (ie, second- or third-degree burns) are at risk for development of acute renal insufficiency. This renal dysfunction may be the result of inadequate fluid resuscitation or it may be the consequence of the liberation of the myoglobin and hemoglobin from damaged cells. These compounds, sometimes called hemochromogens, may precipitate in renal tubules, resulting in acute tubular necrosis. Hemochromogens produce a clear reddish-brown color in the urine. Should hemochromogens appear in the urine, acidosis should be corrected promptly and intravenous fluids increased to maintain a brisk urine output until the urine returns to its normal clear yellow.

Respiratory Support

Inhalation injury is the leading cause of death in the first 24 hours following burn injury and increases the mortality by 20 to 60% when combined with pneumonia.[5] Goals in treating inhalation injury follow:

- Improve oxygenation.
- Decrease interstitial edema and airway occlusion.

The conventional treatment of inhalation injury is largely supportive. Humidified oxygen is administered to prevent drying and sloughing of the mucosa. Upper airway edema peaks at 24 to 48 hours after injury. If the injury is mild or moderately severe, administration of aerosolized racemic epinephrine along with high Fowler's position may be sufficient to limit further edema formation. Severe upper airway obstruction may require endotracheal intubation to protect the airway until the edema subsides.

In patients with mild tracheobronchial injury, atelectasis may be prevented by frequent pulmonary toilet, including a high Fowler's position, coughing and deep breathing, chest physiotherapy, repositioning, frequent tracheal suctioning, and incentive spirometry. More severe inhalation injury requires more frequent suctioning and possible bronchoscopic removal of debris. These patients usually require endotracheal intubation and mechanical ventilatory support. The objective of ventilatory support is to provide adequate gas exchange at the lowest possible inspired oxygen concentration and airway pressure in an attempt to re-

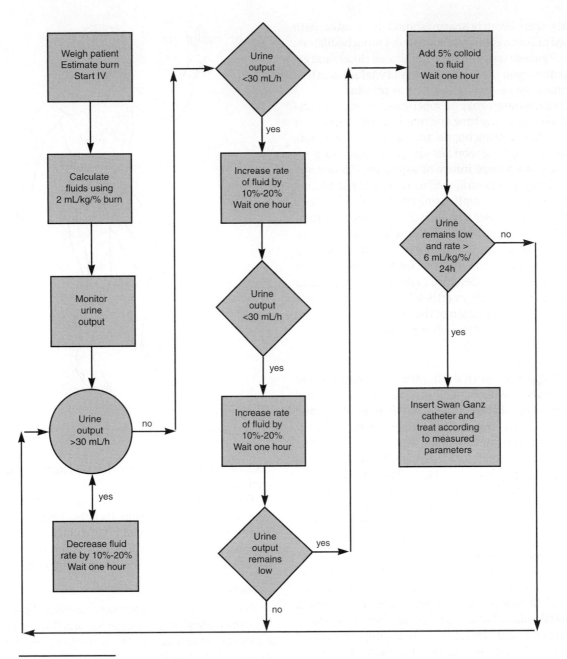

FIGURE 51-4
Initial 24-hour fluid management. (From Rue LW, Cioffi WG: Resuscitation of thermally injured patients. Critical Care Nursing Clinics of North America 3[2]:186, 1991)

duce the incidence of oxygen toxicity and pulmonary barotrauma. Recent studies[5,6] support the use of volumetric diffusive respiration (VDR), which appears to offer advantages over conventional mechanical ventilation. VDR involves the progressive accumulation of subtidal volume breaths that build to a set airway pressure, followed by passive exhalation. During inspiration, high-frequency pulsations of air are continuously injected into the patient. This method of inspiration seems to aid in ventilation and recruitment of partially obstructed alveoli. The provision of adequate gas exchange at lower airway pressures theoretically decreases the likelihood of pulmonary barotrauma (ie, lung injury due to excessive airway pressure).

CLINICAL APPLICATION:
Assessment Parameters
Indications of Adequate Fluid Replacement

Blood pressure	Normal to high ranges
Pulse rate	<120
CVP	<12 cm H_2O
PAWP	<18 mmHg
Urinary output	30–70 mL/h
Lungs	Clear
Sensorium	Clear
GI tract	Absence of nausea and adynamic ileus

Patients with bronchospasm should be treated with aerosolized or intravenously administered bronchodilators. Respiratory parameters should be monitored closely and extreme attention paid to breath sounds and vital signs so that fluid overload can be detected as early as possible.

Bronchopneumonia may be superimposed on other respiratory problems at any time and may be hematogenous or airborne. Airborne bronchopneumonia is most common, with an onset occurring soon after injury. It often is associated with a lower airway injury or aspiration. Hematogenous, or miliary, pneumonia begins as a bacterial abscess secondary to another septic source, usually the burn wound. The time of onset usually is 2 weeks after injury.

Prophylactic antibiotics and steroids have not been demonstrated to prevent the common complications of infection encountered in patients with inhalation injury. New avenues of investigation, designed to decrease the incidence of nosocomial pneumonia in critically ill patients, include the selective decontamination of the orodigestive tract and the use of sucralfate for stress ulcer prophylaxis.

Tissue Perfusion

Another area of concern during the resuscitative phase is tissue perfusion. With tissue injury, vessels are damaged and thrombosed. Adjacent intact vessels soon dilate, and platelets and leukocytes adhere to the vascular endothelium, resulting in eschar formation. The underlying tissues swell, but the area of a circumferential full-thickness burn is inelastic and remains contracted. The area acts like a tourniquet. An unyielding eschar contributes to a compromised vascular state with ischemic necrosis, which may eventually necessitate amputation. It is vital, therefore, that the nurse monitor tissue perfusion hourly by checking for capillary refill, numbness and tingling, loss of motor function and sensation, deep throbbing or aching pain, temperature and color of the skin, and the presence of peripheral pulses. An ultrasonic flowmeter often is useful in assessing for peripheral pulses. Pulse oximetry may be used to monitor the vascular status of extremities to identify the need for escharotomy. Extremities should be elevated and put through passive range of motion for at least 5 minutes each hour to prevent edema and mobilize what does accumulate.

Escharotomy. Although elevation decreases the edema, escharotomy often is necessary. An escharotomy is an incision through the entire thickness of the eschar that allows underlying viable edematous tissues to expand, thereby restoring adequate tissue perfusion. Escharotomy must be performed after some circulatory compromise has occurred, but before tissue hypoxia exists. If performed too soon, massive blood loss will occur from normal vasculature. If escharotomy is performed too late, tissue death results, hence the necessity for careful assessment of tissue perfusion by the nurse.

An escharotomy is made in the midlateral or midmedial line of the involved extremity (Fig. 51–5). The procedure is performed at the bedside and does not require local anesthesia. The escharotomy site is covered with a topical agent

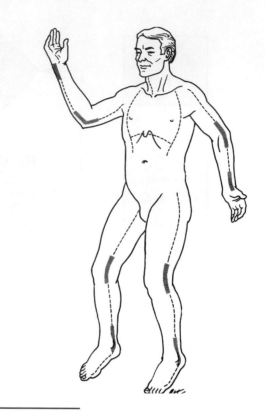

FIGURE 51-5
Preferred sites of escharotomy incisions.

because viable tissue is exposed, and a light dressing may be applied.

Fasciotomy. Only rarely are fasciotomies necessary to restore peripheral perfusion. Usually, this procedure is necessary only in the setting of high-voltage electrical current of concomitant crush injury. Fasciotomies would be undertaken in the operating room under general anesthesia.

Nutrition

Because of the risk of adynamic ileus and gastric distention, the patient should receive no oral fluid or nutrition. If a nasogastric tube is not already in place, one should be inserted if distention or nausea occurs. Gastric drainage initially may contain some blood. Therefore, observe the amount and type of drainage to ensure that the quantity of blood subsides.

The formation of gastroduodenal ulcers, also known as Curling's ulcers, used to be a major complication in burn patients. This complication now is preventable with the prophylactic administration of H_2 histamine receptor antagonists and antacids. H_2 histamine receptor antagonists (eg, cimetidine) are given orally or intravenously every 4 hours. Antacids are administered every 2 hours to titrate the gastric pH above 5.

Body Alignment and Pressure Relief

Because the burn victim is particularly susceptible to the hazards of immobility, proper body alignment and pressure relief are essential. Pressure ulcers may develop quickly. Therefore, the patient may be placed on a pressure-relief mattress or in a special pressure-relief bed. Endotracheal and nasogastric tubes should be secured midline in the nares to prevent erosion of the nasal septum or alae. Range-of-motion exercises should be performed for 5 minutes every hour to prevent contractures and reduce edema.

Wound Care

After hemodynamic and pulmonary stability have been achieved, attention is directed toward initial care of the burn wound. The wound should be cleaned with a surgical detergent disinfectant and gently débrided. Body hair is shaved from the wound and around the wound periphery. The wound then is covered with a topical antimicrobial agent. Isolation measures should be instituted to protect the patient. Wound care is discussed in the next section dealing with the acute phase of management.

Pain Control

Burn injuries are one of the most painful forms of trauma a person can experience. The degree of pain experienced by patients in both the resuscitative and acute phases of care is influenced by the depth of the injury, the patient's anxiety level, and the number of invasive monitoring and wound care procedures required.

Insights Into Clinical Research

Everett JJ, Patterson D, Marvin J, et al: Pain assessment from patients with burns and their nurses. J Burn Care Rehabil 15(2): 194–198, 1994

The primary objective of this study was to determine whether nurses could accurately assess levels of pain expressed by patients with burns. The investigators were also interested in elucidating any variables relating to accuracy of pain estimation. This study examined the distribution of pain scores for burn procedures, the relationships among nurse and patient pain ratings, and the relationship of different patient variables (eg, age, sex, TBSA) and nurse variables (eg, years of nursing experience, educational status) related to pain reports and accuracy of nurses' estimates of pain. Forty-nine adult patients with burns and 27 nurses submitted 123 pairs of visual analog scale pain ratings for burn wound débridements. While patients' overall visual analog scale pain scores were found to be evenly distributed, worst pain scores yielded a bimodal distribution with groups centered around means of 2.0 (low pain group) and 7.0 (high pain group). Low and high pain groups did not differ in age, sex, or TBSA. Patient and nurse pain ratings were found to be highly correlated. Nurses accurately assessed patients' pain approximately 54% of the time. Underestimation of pain occurred 12.2% of the time, while overestimation occurred 34.7% of the time. Accuracy of nurses' ratings was unrelated to nursing experience or educational level. Future strategies are presented for comparing high and low pain groups and increasing nurse pain rating accuracy.

When protective layers of the epidermis are damaged, nerve endings of pain fibers are exposed first to the atmosphere and later to fluid exudate. Air currents moving across exposed nerve endings cause extreme discomfort. Covering wounds with a clean sheet during transfer thus will decrease pain. Careful positioning and use of pressure-relieving beds or mattresses avoid pressure on injured tissue and promote comfort. Occlusive dressings provide relief from discomfort and reduce the family's fear when first seeing or touching the patient.

As exudate accumulates in the injured area, potassium, prostanoids, and substance P irritate exposed nerve endings, contributing even greater pain sensations. During the resuscitative phase, pain control may be achieved by frequent administration of small doses of intravenous morphine sulfate (3–5 mg for adults) or meperidine (30–50 mg).

Continuous intravenous infusion also may be used, with dosage titrated to the patient's response. Intramuscular and subcutaneous injections should be avoided. Because hypovolemia impairs soft tissue circulation, these agents will be sequestered with virtually no therapeutic effect until the patient becomes hemodynamically stable. As circulation is restored, intramuscular and subcutaneous medications would be reabsorbed, with the total circulatory dose unknown. When patients are hemodynamically stable (ie, acute phase), medications can be administered safely intravenously, intramuscularly, or orally.

The pain experience is a complex phenomenon, involving physiological, psychological, and cognitive processes. Physiological pain (ie, burn injury) can be influenced by anxiety, fear, cultural background, and life history patterns.

Because so many factors influence pain perception, a variety of techniques other than narcotics may be useful in alleviating pain. These methods include relaxation therapy, guided imagery techniques, biofeedback, hypnosis, patient-controlled analgesia, anxiolytic or antidepressant drug therapy, anesthesia, and transcutaneous electronic nerve stimulation. Because the pain experience is unique to each individual, the nurse must be resourceful and flexible in determining the best pain control approach for each patient (see Chapter 5).

Patient and Family Support

Providing psychological support for the newly admitted burn patient and family is not the least of the many tasks facing the critical care nurse. The patient most often is awake and alert, although anxious and overwhelmed by the suddenness and magnitude of injuries.

The overriding concern at this time is whether the patient will live or die. This should be handled as gently, tactfully, and honestly as possible. This often is the all-important basis for establishing a trusting relationship for the long months of rehabilitation ahead. The trusting relationship that is established initially provides a strong base for patient and family teaching and rehabilitation in the months to follow.

Patient Needs. Burn patients are under severe, long-term stress, and they nearly always manifest personality variants. Four of the most common are depression, regression, paranoia, and schizophrenia.

Burn patients often become depressed and withdrawn, asking to be left alone and not to be made uncomfortable. The nurse should respond by making certain *expectations* clear—expecting the patient to feed himself or herself, go to the bathroom, or do as much as the physical condition permits, communicating to the patient that the condition is not hopeless and that recovery is expected.

The best way to handle regression in a burn patient is to acknowledge it. First, the nurse must accept the fact that the patient may be unable to cope on an adult level and that the patient may be unstable emotionally and physically. Second, the nurse must devise ways to help the patient cope on an appropriate level. Interventions that usually help include following a regular schedule so that the patient knows what is expected, rewarding the patient for adult behavior, and permitting the patient as much control and choice as possible.

It is not uncommon for severely burned patients to transfer their fears to a specific caregiver (physician, nurse, therapist) and to complain that they are being treated unjustly or unkindly. Working with a psychiatric liaison nurse may help the burn victim recognize and deal with his or her fears more effectively and help the caregiver support the patient by responding therapeutically.

Hallucinations, confusion, and combativeness are common in severely burned patients for physical and mental reasons. Exhaustion, pain, and medications may distort reality and produce schizophrenic behavior.

The four personality variants are temporary. Schizophrenia and paranoia almost always disappear by the time the patient is discharged from the hospital. Regression and depression may continue into the rehabilitation period.

Family Needs. With high anxiety levels and lack of knowledge pertaining to burns, the family approaches the burn unit with fear, hesitancy, and sometimes hysteria. The physical appearance of the patient and the high-technology atmosphere of the burn unit are frightening. Preparing the family for the initial visit by explaining what to expect and escorting them to the bedside is extremely important. Visitors often are overwhelmed on the first visit and stand silently with feelings of anxiety and hopelessness growing. It may be helpful for the nurse to suggest that the family members leave and return when they feel stronger.

Although the patient tends to concentrate on the present, the family members look to the future and want to know what to expect. Information about the patient's condition and treatments should be shared with them. An honest and open approach should be used.

The Acute Phase: Managing the Burn Wound

Attention can be directed toward the burn itself after the patient's general condition has stabilized. Goals of topical burn care follow:

- Promote healing.
- Control infection.
- Help alleviate pain.

(See the Collaborative Care Guide earlier in the chapter.)

INFECTION CONTROL

The most significant complication in the acute phase of injury is sepsis. Because a major function of viable skin is to prevent infection, when skin integrity is impaired, the patient is susceptible to infection from a variety of organisms. Infection may arise from the burn wound itself or from pneumonia, suppurative thrombophlebitis, urinary tract infection or other infection in the body, invasive procedures, and invasive monitoring devices. The burn wound is the most frequent source of infection, caused by a variety of organisms. Early after the injury, the organisms tend to be gram positive; after the first week, the organisms tend to be gram negative.

Septic shock, seen most often in patients with extensive full-thickness burns, is caused by invading bacteria from the wound entering the bloodstream. Clinically, the signs listed in the accompanying display are expected in septic shock.

The nonviable and frequently necrotic burn wound eschar and granulating surfaces present a constant potential reservoir for contamination. Burn wound surfaces provide a warm, moist, protein-laden growth medium for microorganisms. General consensus is that it is unrealistic to maintain the burn wound sterile; however, control of the microbial flora is realistic and achievable. Systemic antibiotics are of little value in controlling this bacterial population because they are unable to reach the injured tissue due to impaired circulation. The best method of limiting bacterial proliferation in the burn eschar is the use of topical antimicrobial agents.

WOUND CARE

Management of wound healing entails the following:

- Providing daily hydrotherapy and débridement techniques
- Maintaining adequate nutrition
- Preventing hypothermia

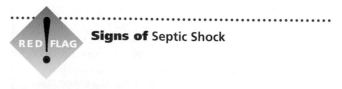

RED FLAG   **Signs of** Septic Shock

Temperature (varies)
Pulse (140–170—sinus tachycardia)
Decreased blood pressure
Adynamic ileus
Petechiae
Frank bleeding from wounds
Disorientation

- Controlling pain
- Maintaining joint mobility
- Adhering to infection-control procedures
- Performing astute wound assessment and monitoring

All burned areas should be cleaned once or twice a day with an antimicrobial liquid detergent (eg, chlorhexidine). After daily hydrotherapy, the burn wound is covered with a topical antimicrobial agent.

Hydrotherapy

Some centers immerse patients in a Hubbard tank to loosen exudates, clean and assess the wound, and provide range-of-motion exercises. Bath solutions vary, and may contain salt, povidone-iodine solutions, and bleaches. Because baths usually are painful, patients should receive an analgesic 20 to 30 minutes before. In addition, the patient should receive a complete explanation of and assistance with pain-controlling techniques (eg, imagery). Additional verbal support should be offered by ongoing explanations of what is to be done and why and by permitting the patient to participate in care as much as possible. Limiting the time the procedure takes is important to the patient's pain tolerance and temperature control. Hydrotherapy should be limited to 20 minutes to prevent extreme chilling, which increases metabolic demand.

Care must be taken to avoid cross-contamination of wounds during bathing procedures. For this reason, many centers no longer immerse patients in Hubbard tanks. Clean or healing wounds should be cleaned separately from contaminated ones.

Topical Antimicrobial Agents

The choice of topical agents depends on wound depth, location, condition, and presence of specific organisms. Common antimicrobial agents used from time of admission to a burn unit include 0.5% silver nitrate, mafenide acetate (Sulfamylon), nitrofurazone, povidone-iodine, silver sulfadiazine, gentamycin, and nystatin. No single agent is totally effective against *all* burn wound infections. Treatment is guided by in vitro testing or in vivo results. Eschar and granulating wound surfaces may be biopsied three times weekly to identify contaminating organisms and determine antibiotic sensitivity.

Silver sulfadiazine is the primary topical agent of choice on admission. The most common adverse reaction is leukopenia; therefore, serial complete blood counts must be monitored. If the white blood count falls below 3,000, the physician probably will change to another topical agent. When the leukocyte count returns to normal (4,000–5,000), silver sulfadiazone may be reinstituted.

If the colony counts increase, the topical agent of choice usually is mafenide acetate cream, an effective broad-spectrum bacteriostatic agent. Mafenide acetate diffuses through third-degree eschar to the burn wound margin within 3 hours after application. It inhibits carbonic anhydrase, resulting in metabolic acidosis. This acidosis initially is compensated for by hyperventilation. Oral administration of sodium citrate dihydrate (Bicitra) or intra-venous sodium bicarbonate usually corrects this acid–base imbalance.

The application of topical antimicrobial agents inhibits the rate of wound epithelialization and may increase the metabolic rate. Electrolyte imbalances (eg, sodium leaching by silver nitrate) and acid–base abnormalities may occur. The best topical agents are water soluble because they will not hold in heat and macerate the wound. With the application of any topical agent, it is important to use sterile technique. The nurse may apply the topical agent as indicated in Table 51–3.

Débridement of the Burn Wound

Eschar will cover the burn wound until it is excised or has separated spontaneously. In theory, burn wound management is simple. It calls for débridement of the eschar and skin graft closure before the eschar becomes infected. The sometimes serious systemic complications of burn injury, such as hypovolemia and sepsis, however, may delay this course of action significantly.

Mechanical Débridement. Mechanical débridement may be accomplished using forceps and scissors to lift gently and trim loose necrotic tissue. Another form of mechanical débridement is dressing the wound with coarse gauze in the form of wet-to-dry or wet-to-wet dressings.

Wet-to-dry dressings consist of layers of moistened coarse mesh gauze. As the inner layer dries, it adheres to the wound, entrapping exudate and wound debris. The dressing should be removed at a 90-degree angle, and every effort should be made to avoid damaging fragile, newly granulating tissue.

As the wound forms increasing amounts of granulation tissue, wet-to-wet dressings may be used to prevent desiccation and trauma. These dressings remain moist until the next dressing change. The dressing should be removed by first gently lifting from the edges toward the center of the wound, and then removed at a 180-degree angle. This procedure prevents detachment of newly formed epithelial tissue.

Enzymatic Débridement. Enzymatic débridement involves the application of a proteolytic substance to burn wounds to shorten the time of eschar separation. Travase and Elase are the most commonly used agents. The wound is first cleaned and débrided of any loose necrotic material, and the agent is applied directly to the wound bed and covered with a layer of fine mesh gauze. A topical antimicrobial agent is then applied, and the entire area is covered with saline-soaked gauze. The dressing is changed two to four times per day.

Enzymatic débridement has the advantage of eliminating the need for surgical excision; however, certain complications must be considered. Hypovolemia may occur as a result of excessive fluid loss through the wound. Hence, no more than 20% TBSA should be treated in this manner. Cellulitis and maceration of normal skin may occur around the wound periphery, and patients often complain of a burning sensation lasting 30 to 60 minutes after enzyme application.

TABLE 51-3   CLINICAL APPLICATION: Drug Therapy
Topical Antimicrobial Agents for Burn Wound Management

Agent	Indications	Nursing Considerations
Mafenide acetate (Sulfamylon)	Active agent against most gram-positive and gram-negative wound pathogens; drug of choice for electrical and ear burns Advantages: Excellent penetration of tissue and cartilage Disadvantages: Painful; 10% allergic rate; metabolic acidosis	Apply once or twice daily with sterile glove; do not use dressings that reduce effectiveness and cause maceration; monitor respiratory rate, electrolyte values, and arterial pH for evidence of metabolic acidosis; painful on application to partial-thickness burns for about 30 min.
Silver nitrate	Effective against wide spectrum of common wound pathogens and candidal infections; used in patients with sulfa allergy or toxic epidermal necrolysis; poor penetration of eschar Advantages: No allergic reactions; painless	Apply 0.5% solution wet dressings twice or three times a day; ensure that dressings remain moist by wetting every 2 hours; preserve solution in a light-resistant container; protect walls, floors, and so forth with plastic to prevent staining; monitor for hyponatremia and hypochloremia.
Silver sulfadiazine	Active against a wide spectrum of microbial pathogens; caution in patients with impaired renal or hepatic function Advantages: Painless; minimal sensitivity	Apply once or twice daily with a sterile gloved hand; leave wounds exposed or wrap lightly with gauze dressings; painless.

Surgical Excision. In surgical excision, the wound is excised to viable bleeding points while minimizing the loss of viable tissue. Early excision has contributed significantly to the survival of major burn victims. The open burn causes hypermetabolism and a stress response that will not be corrected until wound closure occurs. Surgical excision should be done as soon as the patient is hemodynamically stable, usually within 72 hours.

After excision is complete, hemostasis must be achieved. This may be accomplished by topical thrombin sprayed on the wound or application sponges soaked in a 1:10,000 epinephrine solution. After removal of necrotic tissue, the exposed underlying structures must be dressed with a temporary or permanent covering to provide protection and prevent infection.

Grafting

The ideal substitute for lost skin is an autograft of similar color, texture, and thickness from a close location on the body. Sheets of the patient's epidermis and a partial layer of the dermis are harvested from unburned locations using a dermatome. These grafts are referred to as split thickness and can be applied to the wound as a sheet or in a meshed form. They are called *sheet grafts*. The graft must be inspected frequently for collections of fluid under the graft. Fluid accumulation is prevented by rolling the graft with a cotton-tipped applicator. *Mesh grafts* are those in which the harvested skin is slit to allow it to expand and then placed on the burn site. This allows for greater coverage and drainage and is draped more easily over uneven surfaces. Over exposed areas, such as the face and hands, sheet grafts give a more natural appearance than do mesh grafts.

Mesh grafts frequently have to be expanded to get maximum coverage from each piece of autograft. An expansion rate of 1:3 or 1:4 often is practical. Sometimes ratios such as 1:6 or 1:7 are used to cover large burns. With these larger ratios, the expanded autograft is covered with either cadaver skin allografts or synthetic skin (Biobrane; Winthrop Pharmaceuticals). In addition to physically stabilizing the fragile mesh, the cover decreases evaporation, heat loss, and bacterial contamination.

Dressings are used postoperatively to immobilize the grafted area and prevent shearing and dislodging of the graft. Postoperative dressings also provide a degree of compression to minimize hematoma and seroma formation but may be a source of vascular compression in the extremities. Pulse checks distal to the dressings should be documented every 4 hours for 24 hours postoperatively. Autografts treated in an open method require immobilization of the grafted area.

The donor site is covered intraoperatively with a single layer of fine mesh gauze. Usually the gauze layer is removed and the site treated by exposure. A heat lamp may be used to hasten drying of the donor site. Positioning to prevent pressure on the site is important. Daily inspection of the donor site is essential to detect early signs of infection or cellulitis.

A new technique that involves the growth and subsequent graft placement of cultured epithelial autographs has become an important adjunct to permanent coverage of extensive burn wounds. Biopsies are taken from unburned skin and cells cultured in the laboratory. Sheets of cultured epithelial cells are attached to petroleum jelly gauze and applied to the wound. After 7 to 10 days, the petroleum jelly gauze is removed, and a nonadherent dressing is applied to prevent mechanical trauma.

Biological Dressings. Biological dressings used in the management of burn wounds include homograft skin (allograft) or heterograft skin (xenograft). Homograft skin is obtained from living or deceased human donors, usually the latter. Amniotic membranes have been used in the past, but are not used commonly at present. It is possible to transmit disease through the use of homograft skin; thus, it is important to test donor skin for human immunodeficiency virus, hepatitis B, and syphilis before use.

Because the demand for homograft skin exceeds the supply, heterografts have been used to achieve temporary wound closure. Porcine skin is the most commonly used substance.

Synthetic Dressings. Synthetic dressings are being developed in an attempt to overcome the pitfalls of biological dressings, namely disease transmission, storage problems, and limited supply.

Biobrane is a collagen-based substance that adheres to the wound surface within 48 hours after application. The membrane forms an occlusive barrier to protect against bacterial infection and fluid losses while permitting drainage of exudate and penetration of topical antimicrobial agents. The membrane is translucent, permitting direct visualization of the wound bed. Other synthetic substitutes used in small, clean, temporary wound closures are polyurethane films.

THERMOREGULATION

Hypothermia is a potential problem for the extensively burned patient, especially during hydrotherapy and immediately after surgery. Heat is lost through the open burn wounds by means of radiation and evaporation. Body temperature should be maintained at 99° to 101°F by maintaining environmental temperatures at 82° to 91°F with heat lamps or shields, foil blankets, and temperature-controlled air beds, if used, and by limiting body surface areas exposed at any one time.

NUTRITION

The precise energy requirements needed to achieve weight and nitrogen balance and energy equilibrium depend on variables such as burn size, patient age, and other coexisting medical conditions. This requirement has been found to be approximately 25 kcal/kg + 40 kcal ÷ % TBSA burn/24 hours. In some cases, this caloric load can exceed 5,000 kcal/d. Approximately 50 g of nitrogen a day are needed in addition to some polyunsaturated fats to prevent essential

fatty acid deficiency. The precise protein requirements for each person are modified based on nitrogen balance studies and serum urea nitrogen values. Multivitamins and increased amounts of vitamin C, potassium, zinc, and magnesium also are required.

A burn patient's appetite seldom exceeds preburn levels, and voluntary eating rarely meets protein, fat, and caloric requirements in patients with large burns. High caloric supplements between meals may be sufficient in patients with moderate burns, but those with large burns require constant interval feedings through feeding tubes. With around-the-clock administration, caloric loads of 5,000 kcal/d can be tolerated. Diarrhea may occur and can be treated with kaolin-pectin, Metamucil, or bran.

In some instances (ie, prolonged adynamic ileus, malnutrition before injury, failure to gain weight), parenteral nutrition may be required. When peripheral or central parenteral nutrition is required, absolute aseptic technique for line insertion and alteration of intravenous sites every 3 days are essential to prevent septic thrombophlebitis. Insulin supplementation may be necessary; frequent serum and urine glucose determinations and serial liver function tests are required for patients on parenteral nutrition (see Chapter 39).

Failure to reach the large caloric loads required for weight maintenance, nitrogen balance, and energy equilibrium results in delayed and abnormal wound healing.

The Rehabilitative Phase

Patients with extensive burns require many months for recovery and rehabilitation. Physical and psychological rehabilitation measures are begun in the ICU and continued through the recovery period.

PHYSICAL REHABILITATION

Two important physical measures are nutrition and prevention of scarring and contractures.

Nutrition

The diet should remain high in protein until all wounds have healed. As healing takes place, the diet should be tapered to meet normal caloric requirements. Burn patients may become accustomed to eating frequently and in large amounts. After healing is complete, metabolism returns to normal, and weight will be gained if eating habits are not controlled properly.

Prevention of Scarring and Contractures

Once regarded as inevitable, hypertrophic scarring and joint contractures now largely are preventable. Preventive measures start when the person is admitted to the hospital and continue for at least 12 months or until the scar is fully mature.

These preventive measures—positioning the body and helping the patient perform range-of-motion exercises—

are not new to the nurse. Positioning the body with extremities extended is extremely important. Although tightly flexed positions are preferred by patients for comfort, they will result in severe contractures. The range-of-motion exercises should be carried out with each dressing change or more often if indicated. Special splints are used to maintain arm, legs, and hands in extended yet functional positions. Later, when the wounds have healed sufficiently, the person is custom-fitted for a special pressure garment. The garment, by applying continuous uniform pressure over the entire area of the burn, prevents hypertrophic scarring and must be worn 24 hours a day for approximately 1 year. The smooth elastic garment forms a shield that permits the person to wear normal clothing and resume ordinary activities much sooner.

Healed and grafted skin will be dry and tight. Itching is a major patient complaint as healing occurs. A mild, nonirritating lotion massaged to the healed skin provides lubrication and aids in range of motion.

PSYCHOLOGICAL REHABILITATION

Psychological care of the burn patient is extremely difficult; the patient may, in the course of therapy, run the full gamut of behavioral responses. Initially, the combination of physical pain and emotional disturbance may lead to abnormal behavior, as discussed under Care in the Intensive Care Unit. Guilt is another response. It may be particularly severe if the patient feels that his or her carelessness was the cause of injuries to others, especially if others died as a result of the accident.

If burns involve the face, eyes, or hands, additional emotional support will be needed because damage to these structures will have a long-term affect on the patient's life and livelihood.

A consistent, truthful team approach that includes the patient and family is necessary. Several supportive measures will allow the patient time to assimilate what has happened and to grow in the ability to cope. Such guidelines are summarized in the accompanying display.

Staff Support

In addition to emotional support of the patient and family, support for the nursing staff is advisable. Faced with long and arduous care of burn patients, where progress is slow and setbacks are common, staff may quickly develop "burnout" unless some of their emotional reactions and problems can be aired and solved. Stress and coping behaviors for critical care nurses are discussed in Chapter 9.

▆ CONCLUSION

The skin serves multiple physiological functions that render it indispensable to life. When a large area of skin surface is destroyed, severe systemic reactions occur.

The burn victim goes through phases of recovery, each with its own special problems. The resuscitative phase begins with the burn injury and lasts until diuresis occurs (1–5 days). The major problems for the patient at this time are maintenance of an airway and adequate tissue perfusion. After diuresis, the patient enters the acute phase, during which the major problem is sepsis. Burn wound management is essential during this phase. Rehabilitation focuses on adequate nutrition and prevention of scarring and contractures. Psychological support is essential throughout the entire experience. A firm, compassionate team approach is essential throughout recovery.

CLINICAL APPLICATION:
Nursing Intervention Guidelines
Supportive Measures in Psychological Rehabilitation

- Stabilize staff as much as possible so that they become familiar with the patient's needs and so that a sense of identification between patient and nurse is established.
- Incorporate family members into the overall plan of care.
- Instruct family members in selected procedures.
- Encourage diversional therapy (ie, reading, watching television, listening to music) as soon as possible in recovery period.
- Begin occupational therapy as soon as the patient is able to participate.

Clinical Applicability Challenges

Self-Challenge: Critical Thinking

1. Distinguish between hypovolemic shock due to hemorrhage and burn shock.

2. Relate the rationale for fluid resuscitation to the pathophysiology of burn shock.

3. Prioritize the clinical problems in each phase of recovery following burn injury. Defend your list.

4. Develop criteria for assessing respiratory status in the burn patient. Relate the assessment to the type of burn injury.

Study Questions

1. Mr. John Frye is a victim of a house fire. He sustains burns that damage the epidermis, dermis, and subcutaneous tissue. Which of the following classifications of burns best describes his injuries?
   a. Second-degree burns
   b. Third-degree burns
   c. Superficial burns
   d. Partial-thickness burns

2. Which of the following statements best describe the development of burn shock?
   a. Increased capillary permeability causes an increase in vascular colloid osmotic pressure and a decrease in hydrostatic pressure.
   b. Release of epinephrine produces increased heart rate, but it is ineffective, and cardiogenic shock occurs.
   c. Increased capillary permeability results in decreased vascular colloid osmotic pressure and increased hydrostatic pressure.
   d. the stress response (epinephrine and norepinephrine) causes selective vasoconstriction, resulting in shock.

3. Mr. Frye complains of headache, nausea, and vertigo. What might these symptoms indicate?
   a. Smoke inhalation
   b. Carbon monoxide poisoning
   c. Cerebral edema
   d. Overhydration

4. Mr. Frye has sustained burns to his entire right arm and his anterior trunk. Using the "rule of nines" method, what is the percentage of his burn injury?
   a. 48%
   b. 27%
   c. 18%
   d. 9%

5. During the resuscitative phase, an elevated serum potassium may occur. This is primarily the result of
   a. cellular injury.
   b. fluid volume loss.
   c. increased capillary permeability.
   d. interstitial edema.

6. Intramuscular injection of analgesics during the resuscitative phase is not recommended because
   a. narcotics can severely depress the respiratory system.
   b. narcotics can further decrease the blood pressure.
   c. inadequate peripheral perfusion results in uneven absorption of the medication.
   d. tolerance to pain medication develops easily.

7. Silver sulfadiazine is the topical antimicrobial agent selected for Mr. Frye. Which of the following nursing actions is appropriate when using the drug?
   a. Premedicate Mr. Frye for pain before application.
   b. Monitor acid–base balance.
   c. Monitor white blood cell count.
   d. Observe for signs of hepatotoxicity.

REFERENCES

1. Rue LW, Cloffl WG: Resuscitation of thermally injured patients. Critical Care Nursing Clinics of North America 3:181–189, 1991
2. Shaw A, Anderson J, Hayward A, Parkhouse N: Pathophysiological basis of pain management. Br J Hosp Med 52(11):583–587, Dec. 1994–Jan. 1995
3. Carleton SC, Tomassoni AJ, Alexander J: Cardiac problems associated with burns. Cardiol Clin 3(2):257–262, 1995
4. Falmo L, Krantz M: Management of acute burns and burn shock resuscitation. AACN Clinical Issues in Critical Care Nursing 4(2):351–366, 1993
5. Rue LW, Cioffi WG, Mason AD, McManus WF, Pruitt BA: The risk of pneumonia in thermally injured patients requiring ventilatory support. J Burn Care Rehabil 16(3 part 1):262–268, 1995
6. Rodeberg DA, Housinger TA, Greenhalgh DG, Maschinot NE, Warden GD: Improved ventilatory function in burn patients using volumetric diffusive respiration. Journal of American College of Surgeons 179(5):518–522, 1994

BIBLIOGRAPHY

Byers JF, Flynn, MB: Acute burn injury: A trauma case report. Critical Care Nurse 16(4):55–66, 1996
Everett JJ, Patterson R, Martin JA, Montgomery B, Ordoney N, Campbell K: Pain assessment from patients with burns and their nurses. J Burn Care Rehabil 15(2):194–198, 1994
Fowler A: Nursing management of a patient with burns. British Journal of Nursing 3(21):1105–1111, 1994
Milner SM, Rylah LT, Bennett JD: The burn wheel: A practical guide to fluid resuscitation. Burns 21(4):288–290, 1995
Orr J, Hain T: Burn wound management: An overview. Professional Nurse 10(3):153–156, 1994
Walter PH: Burn wound management. AACN Clinical Issues in Critical Care Nursing 4(2):378–387, 1993
Weber JM, Tompkins DM: Improving survival: Infection control and burns. AACN Clinical Issues on Critical Care Nursing 4(2):414–423, 1993

52

Drug Overdose and Poisoning

THE POISONED OR OVERDOSED PATIENT
Poisoning
Substance Abuse
Therapy
ASSESSMENT
Triage
History Taking
Identification of the Toxidrome(s)
MANAGEMENT
Stabilization
Initial Decontamination
   Ocular Exposure

Dermal Exposure
Inhalation Exposure
Ingestions
Gastrointestinal Decontamination
   Emetics
   Gastric Lavage
   Adsorbents
   Cathartics
Elimination of the Drug or Toxin
   Multiple-Dose Activated Charcoal
   Whole-Bowel Irrigation
   Urine Alkalinization
   Hemodialysis
   Hemoperfusion

Hyperbaric Oxygenation Therapy
Exchange Transfusion
Antagonists
   Ineffective Universal Antidote
   Antivenin
   Antitoxin
Care in Commonly Occurring Poisoning
   and Overdose
Continuous Patient Monitoring
Prevention and Patient Teaching
CONCLUSION

OBJECTIVES

Based on the content in this chapter, the reader should be able to:

- Explain initial assessment and management for acutely poisoned patients.
- Compare and contrast similarities and differences of methods used to prevent absorption and enhance elimination in managing the acutely poisoned patient.
- Describe the groups of symptoms, or toxidromes, that may assist in identifying the drug(s) or toxin(s) to which the patient may have been exposed.
- Formulate a plan of care for the poisoned patient.

*I*n 1995, more than 2 million exposures were reported to the American Association of Poison Control Centers. Of these exposures, 724 resulted in death. The largest age group of human exposures (52.8%) was children younger than 6 years; however, the largest age group for fatalities was adults (90.9%).[1] The types of toxic exposures reported to poison control centers are diverse, including herbal remedies purchased at health food stores, snake and spider envenomations, substance abuse, occupational exposures, suicide attempts, accidental pediatric exposures, fumes emitted by faulty furnaces, plant ingestions, and exposures resulting from industrial hazardous material spills or releases.

Because of clinical experience and new research information, therapy for toxic exposure changes rapidly. Health care professionals may find it challenging to keep abreast of the most advanced therapy. Fortunately, poison control centers offer rapid access to this information by phone consultation in most parts of the country. The services of a local poison control center are a useful resource for the health care professional and the public.

This chapter presents general guidelines for assessment and management of the acutely poisoned or overdosed patient. It contains a table of commonly observed poisonings and a collaborative care guide for the patient with cocaine toxicity. The chapter ends with a section on prevention through patient teaching.

■ THE POISONED
OR OVERDOSED PATIENT

Poisonings and drug overdoses will cause quick physical and emotional changes in a person. Bystanders usually are the ones who have to initiate care and call a poison control center or emergency number. Commonly observed poisonings or drug overdoses are caused by the following: acetaminophen, amphetamines, benzodiazepines, carbon monoxide, cocaine, fluorinated hydrocarbons, LSD, methanol, salicylates, and tricyclic antidepressants. These particular substances and care in the toxic patient are described later in the chapter in Table 52–3.

Poisoning

Poisoning can occur in three ways: ingestion, inhalation, and absorption. Toxic chemical reactions compromise cardiovascular, respiratory, central nervous, hepatic, gastrointestinal (GI), or renal systems.

Poisoning in the home usually occurs by children's ingesting household cleaners or medicines. Improper storage of these items contributes to poisoning accidents. Plants, pesticides, and paint products are potential household poisons. Because of mental or visual impairment, illiteracy, or a language barrier, older adults may ingest incorrect amounts of medications. Poisoning may occur in the health care environment when medications are administered improperly. Cardiac medications, narcotics, cancer chemotherapy, and intravenous (IV) medications are potentially lethal.

Most exposures to toxic fumes occur in the home. Poisoning may result from improper mixing of household substances, prolonged use of strong cleaning products, or malfunctioning household appliances that release carbon monoxide. Gas, oil, coal, and kerosene heaters produce carbon monoxide that can be lethal. Carbon monoxide gas is colorless, odorless, tasteless, and nonirritating, which makes it especially dangerous. Prevention and patient teaching are discussed at the end of this chapter.

Substance Abuse

Excessive use of prescription and "street" drugs has become a major threat to society. Drug abuse has become a way of escaping stress for some. Many children and young people use substances as a means of being accepted by their peers. The results are addiction, dependency, physical and emotional consequences, more stress, and death. IV drug users suffer from frequent infections, hepatitis, and possibly acquired immunodeficiency syndrome.

Family dynamics are altered by substance abuse. Economic failure may become a major problem because of the high cost of drugs or inability to maintain a job because of

---

Insights Into Clinical Research

Heyman EN, LoCastro DE, Gouse LH, Morris DL, Lombardo BA, Montenegro HD, Takacs M: Intentional drug overdose: Predictors of clinical course in the intensive care unit. Heart Lung 25(3):246–252, 1996

Some people who are admitted to the intensive care unit (ICU) as the result of an intentional overdose may not need to be there. Instead, they require a less intense level of care as they recover. What, then, are the characteristics of patients with intentional overdose who require ICU care and those who do not? The purpose of this study was to describe these characteristics and determine the data that best predicted their clinical course.

Researchers collected data by retrospectively reviewing records of 43 patients who had been in the ICU in 1991 because of intentional overdose. Ages ranged from 16 to 95 years with a mean age of 33 years. There were twice as many women as men in the sample. Data included demographics, medical history, types of substances taken, results of the Acute Physiology and Chronic Health Evaluation (APACHE) II and Glasgow coma scales, cardiac rhythms and the presence of seizures, and interventions and outcomes.

Findings showed that 21 (49%) had medical illnesses and 24 (56%) overdosed with more than one substance. APACHE II scores ranged from 1 to 29 with a mean of 8. Glasgow Coma scores ranged from 3 to 15 with a mean of 12.6. Thirteen (39%) had a score of 15, while five (15%) had a score of 8.

None of the patients who survived (95%) had APACHE II scores higher than 21 or were comatose with a Glasgow Coma score above 5. The two patients who died had the highest APACHE II scores (29 and 21) and the lowest Glasgow Coma scores (3 and 5).

These data indicated that the Glasgow Coma score was the best predictor of complications. The study design and small sample size limit the generalizability of the findings. However, the findings imply that patients with high APACHE II and low Glasgow Coma scores (indicating a high risk of death and neurological impairment) require ICU care. They are also more likely to require intensive interventions, such as intubation, and treatment for seizures and cardiac dysrhythmias. Patients with a Glasgow Coma score higher than 6 who are not intubated may not need admission to ICU.

addiction. Drug abusers may turn to criminal acts to raise money for their habits. Parents may be unable to care for their children or may become abusive in their relationships. Children fail in school. The family may become isolated from community support. Arrest and incarceration may completely disrupt the family unit.

Commonly abused substances are nicotine, alcohol, marijuana, amphetamines, and cocaine. Some children and adolescents turn to common household substances because they are readily available.

People who exhibit stress through substance abuse require a comprehensive treatment program to address their coping and adaptation problems.

Therapy

Immediate care for the poisoned or overdosed patient requires evaluation and maintenance of airway, breathing, and circulation (ABCs). The patient's condition must be stabilized. Rapid measures are taken to prevent further absorption of the substance and to enhance elimination of the drug. These steps continue in the emergency department and intensive care unit (ICU).

ASSESSMENT

A systematic approach to the poisoned or overdosed patient in the health care facility includes triage, stabilization, history taking, identification of the toxidrome (eg, syndrome), and management.

Triage

The goal of immediate treatment in poisoning or drug overdose is patient stabilization. (Stabilization is discussed under Management later in this chapter.) Initial life-threatening problems are the ABCs. Although some type of triage probably was performed at the scene or by an emergency team, triage is the first step performed in the emergency department.

Triage Evaluation

- Is patient's life in immediate danger?
- Is patient's life in potential danger?
- Is patient's life in no immediate danger?

History Taking

History of the exposure provides a framework for managing the poisoning or overdose. Key points are to identify the drug(s) or toxin(s), the time and duration of the exposure, first aid treatment given before hospital arrival, allergies, and disease processes. An example of an assessment tool is the Rumack-Matthew Nomogram given in Figure 52–1. It is used in acetaminophen poisoning.

Information related to the poisoning or overdose may be obtained from the patient, family members, friends, res-

cuers, or bystanders. In some cases, the family or police may have to search the home for clues. Clothing and personal effects may supply additional information.

Identification of the Toxidrome(s)

A toxidrome is a group (syndrome) of signs and symptoms associated with overdose or exposure to a particular category of drugs and toxins. Recognizing the presence of a toxidrome may help identify the toxin(s) or drugs(s) to which the patient was exposed. Table 52–1 lists four common toxidromes with their signs and symptoms and common causes.

MANAGEMENT

Management in poisoning and drug overdose is aimed at preventing absorption and further exposure to the agent. Following triage to determine the ABCs, the patient must be stabilized. Treatment begins with first aid and continues in the emergency department and often the ICU.

Advanced general management involves further steps to prevent absorption and enhance elimination of the agent. Antidotes, antitoxins, or antivenins are administered. The nurse further supports vital functions and monitors and treats multisystem effects. This section begins with stabilization.

Stabilization

Stabilization includes the steps summarized in the accompanying display and discussed here.

Airway. Nasotracheal or endotracheal intubation may be necessary to maintain and protect the airway.

Respiratory Effort. Mechanical ventilation may be necessary to support the patient. Many drugs or toxin exposures, such as codeine overdose, depress the respiratory drive and require ventilator assistance until the drugs or toxins are eliminated from the body.

Adequate Circulation. Complications range from shock due to fluid loss, to fluid overload and are often related to the patient's hydration status and the ability of the cardiovascular system to adjust to drug- or toxin-induced changes. For example, rattlesnake envenomations often cause third-spacing of fluid into the area of the bite, leading to intravascular hypovolemia. As a consequence, the patient may develop hypotension, which usually responds to aggressive IV fluid therapy. Some toxic drug ingestions impair myocardial contractility, and fluid overload may be due to the heart's inability to pump effectively. In these cases, IV fluids need to be carefully controlled, and drug therapy may be necessary to prevent or minimize complications, such as pulmonary edema.

Cardiac Function. Many drugs and toxins cause cardiac conduction delays and dysrhythmias. The history of the drug(s) or toxin(s) involved may not be reliable or even known, especially when patients are "found down" or have attempted suicide. Therefore, continuous cardiac monitoring and 12-lead electrocardiograms help detect cardiotoxic effects.

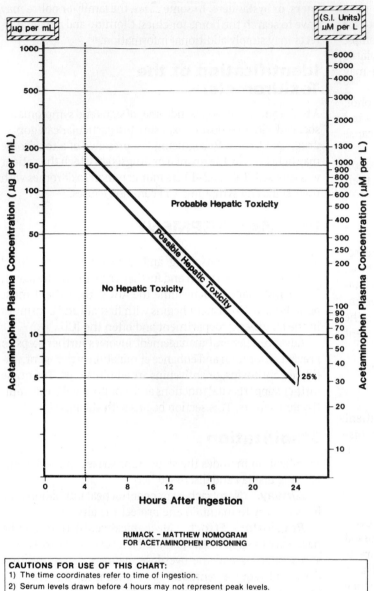

RUMACK – MATTHEW NOMOGRAM
FOR ACETAMINOPHEN POISONING

CAUTIONS FOR USE OF THIS CHART:
1) The time coordinates refer to time of ingestion.
2) Serum levels drawn before 4 hours may not represent peak levels.
3) The graph should be used only in relation to a single acute ingestion.
4) The lower solid line 25% below the standard nomogram is included to allow for possible errors in acetaminophen plasma assays and estimated time from ingestion of an overdose.

FIGURE 52-1

Semilogarithmic plot of plasma acetaminophen levels versus time. (With permission, from Rumack, BH, Matthew HJ: Acetaminophen poisoning and toxicity. Pediatrics 55:871–876, 1975)

Acid–Base Balance and Electrolyte Homeostasis.
Electrolyte abnormalities and metabolic acidosis frequently occur and may require serial electrolytes, arterial blood gases (ABGs), and other specific laboratory tests. For example, serial electrolytes and ABGs are a means of evaluating aspirin toxicity. Aspirin, in large ingestions, may form a solid mass in the GI tract called a concretion. Because absorption occurs from the outer layer of the concretion, absorption is delayed, so the development of toxic effects, such as hypokalemia, metabolic acidosis, and respiratory alkalosis, may not be fully observed for many hours. The course of salicylate toxicity is easily monitored by serial electrolytes, ABGs, and salicylate levels.

Mentation.   Several factors can affect the patient's mental status. Hypoglycemia or hypoxemia are two that can be life threatening but easily addressed by administering oxygen and IV dextrose until laboratory results are available. People with chronic alcoholism also have a special risk called Wernicke-Korsakoff syndrome. This syndrome is characterized by ataxia and altered mentation. Early administration of thiamine (vitamin B_1) given intravenously or intramuscularly may prevent exacerbation of the syndrome.

Naloxone (Narcan) is a narcotic antagonist that reverses narcotic-induced central nervous system (CNS) and respiratory depression. It is often initially given to comatose people. It must be given cautiously because it can precipitate withdrawal in narcotic-dependent individuals.

Injuries and Disease Processes Associated With Toxic Exposure.   Injuries associated with toxic exposure and other disease processes are identified by the examiner. For example, the street drug phencyclidine (also known as PCP or angel dust) may provoke violent, agi-

TABLE 52-1
Toxidromes

Toxidrome	Signs/Symptoms	Common Causes
Anticholinergic	Delirium; dry, flushed skin; dilated pupils; elevated temperature; decreased bowel sounds; urinary retention; tachycardia	Antihistamines, atropine, Jimson weed
Cholinergic	Excessive salivation, lacrimation, urination, diarrhea, and emesis; diaphoresis, bronchorrhea, bradycardia, fasciculations, central nervous system depression, constricted pupils	Organophosphate insecticides (eg, Malathion, Diazinon); carbamate insecticide (eg, carbaryl, propoxur)
Opioid	Central nervous system depression, respiratory depression, constricted pupils, hypotension, hypothermia	Opiates (eg, codeine, morphine, propoxyphene, heroin), diphenoxylate (eg, diphenoxylate [Lomotil])
Sympathomimetic	Agitation, tachycardia, hypertension, seizures, metabolic acidosis	Amphetamines, cocaine, theophylline, caffeine

tated, or bizarre behavior, leading to trauma during the acute toxic phase. The person with ischemic heart disease may not be able to tolerate hypoxemia associated with carbon monoxide poisoning as well as a young, healthy person.

Vital Signs and Temperature. Vital signs and temperature are measured frequently in the critical or potentially critical patient to track changes that would indicate additional problems in the patient.

Initial Decontamination

First aid may be given in the home by a family member who called a poison control center, by an emergency team, in the place of employment, or in the emergency department. The physiochemical properties of the agent and the amount, route, and exposure time help determine the type and extent of management required. Decontamination methods for ocular, dermal, inhalation, and ingestion exposures follow.

CLINICAL APPLICATION:
Nursing Intervention Guidelines
Stabilization of the Overdosed or Poisoned Patient

1. Assess, establish, and maintain the airway.
2. Evaluate respiratory effort.
3. Maintain adequate circulation.
4. Monitor cardiac function.
5. Maintain or correct acid–base balance and electrolyte homeostasis.
6. Assess mentation.
7. Identify injuries and disease processes that increase risk.
8. Measure vital signs and temperature frequently to track changes.

OCULAR EXPOSURE

Chemicals may accidentally splash in the eyes. The eyes must be flushed to remove the agent. The eyes are irrigated immediately with lukewarm water or normal saline. Continuous flooding of the eyes with a large glass or low pressure shower is used for 15 to 30 minutes. The patient blinks the eyes open and closed during the irrigation. The nurse tests the pH of the tears and continues irrigating until the pH returns to normal. An eye examination is needed when ocular irritation or visual disturbance persists after irrigation.

DERMAL EXPOSURE

When dermal exposure occurs, the patient floods the skin with lukewarm water for 15 to 30 minutes. Most companies who produce or use chemical agents have showers for that purpose. The person should remove clothing while running to the shower or can remove clothing while under the running water. After standing under the running water for the allotted time, the patient washes the area gently with soap and water and rinses thoroughly. Some toxins may require further decontamination. For example, three separate soap and water washings or showers are recommended to decontaminate the organophosphate pesticides (eg, Malathion or Diazinon). The health care provider should wear protective covering to reduce the risk for toxicity while handling contaminated clothing or assisting with skin decontamination.

Neutralization is the reaction between an acid and a base, in which the H+ of the acid and the OH− of the base react to produce H_2O (water). Neutralizing the skin is not recommended because it may result in a thermal burn.

INHALATION EXPOSURE

The responder moves the victim to fresh air while also protecting himself or herself from the airborne toxin. The next steps are to establish a patent airway, assess respiratory status, and administer artificial breathing if the victim does not breathe spontaneously. If respiratory failure continues, someone is sent to call for emergency backup. Further evaluation is needed for respiratory irritation or shortness of breath.

INGESTION

Milk or water will dilute ingested irritants or caustics. Adults are given one glass of milk or water and children are given 2 to 8 oz based on their size. Further evaluation is necessary if after dilution there is mucosal irritation or burns. Ingestions should not be diluted when they are accompanied by seizures, depressed mental status, or loss of the gag reflex because of the risk of aspiration. Solutions to neutralize the agent are not used because this can result in a burn.

Gastrointestinal Decontamination

Emetics, gastric lavage, adsorbents, and cathartics are used to prevent absorption and forestall toxicity from almost all drugs and a variety of toxins, such as long-acting anticoagulant rodenticides and poisonous mushrooms.

EMETICS

Giving an emetic to induce emesis is one method of GI decontamination. Syrup of ipecac is a common emetic that partially empties the stomach when given immediately after a drug or toxin is ingested. This over-the-counter medication may be used beneficially in the home under the supervision of a physician or poison control center for minor overdoses in children. The value of emesis is limited for two reasons:

- It may not completely empty the stomach.
- Vomiting may delay activated charcoal (AC) administration (see Adsorbents section, later).

Syrup of ipecac may be given to adults and children 6 months and older. To avoid aspiration of vomitus, it is best when given to children 6 to 12 months under the guidance of a health care provider. The syrup is administered as soon as possible after the ingestion (within 30 minutes) and followed with water and increased patient physical activity. If the initial dose fails to produce results in 20 to 30 minutes, one repeat dose may be given. Once the emesis is clear, food and fluids are withheld for 1 to 2 hours to settle the stomach. Adverse effects of syrup of ipecac include protracted vomiting, lethargy, and diarrhea. Rare complications include Mallory-Weiss syndrome (hemorrhage from a tear in the upper GI tract), pneumomediastinum (air or gas in the mediastinal tissues), and retropneumoperitoneum (gas or air in the space behind the peritoneum.[2,3]

To avoid aspiration of vomitus, emesis should not be induced when the following are present: depressed mental status, absent gag reflex, seizures, and ingestion of an agent that may produce rapid onset of CNS depression. If caustic agents have been ingested, an emetic is not used; reexposure and further injury to the GI tract must be prevented.

Other emetics such as apomorphine, cupric sulfate, and salt have been suggested but are not advisable. Apomorphine may cause CNS depression. Salt water used as an emetic has produced fatal hypernatremia.[4-6] Death from toxicity has been reported with use of cupric sulfate as an emetic.[7]

GASTRIC LAVAGE

Gastric lavage is another common method of gastric emptying. Fluid such as normal saline is introduced into the stomach through a large-bore orogastric or nasogastric tube and then removed in an attempt to reclaim part of the ingested agent before it is absorbed. During lavage, gastric contents can be collected for toxin or drug identification. Gastric lavage is suggested for patients in whom syrup of ipecac has failed to produce emesis and for those with a depressed mental status or absent gag reflex. Nasotracheal or endotracheal intubation may be necessary to protect the airway.

A large orogastric tube should be used to evacuate particulate matter effectively, including whole capsules or tablets. The orogastric tube size in an adult or adolescent is 36 to 40 Fr and in children, 16 to 28 Fr. Standard nasogastric tubes do not work well because of their small size. Large nasogastric tubes may be used but may cause mucosal trauma and epistaxis.

For the lavage, the patient is positioned in the left lateral decubitus position, with the head lower than the feet. The procedure entails attaching a funnel (or a catheter-tip syringe) to the end of the orogastric tube and instilling 150 to 200 mL of water or saline solution (50–100 mL in children) into the stomach. Lowering the funnel and tube below the patient will allow the fluid to return by gravity. This procedure is repeated until clear fluid returns or a minimum of 2 L of fluid has been used.

Complications of gastric lavage include esophageal perforation,[8] pulmonary aspiration, electrolyte imbalance, tension pneumothorax, and hypothermia in small children when cold lavage solutions are used.

Lavage is contraindicated because of risk of esophageal perforation when caustics have been ingested. It is contraindicated also in patients with uncontrolled seizures because of the risk of trauma and aspiration.

ADSORBENTS

An adsorbent is a solid substance that has the ability to attract and hold another substance to its surface ("to adsorb"). Activated charcoal (AC) is an effective nonspecific adsorbent of many drugs and toxins. AC adsorbs or traps the drug or toxin to its large surface area and prevents absorption from the GI tract. The accompanying display identifies both drugs or toxins that are adsorbed effectively by AC and those not adsorbed effectively.

Activated charcoal is a fine, black powder that is given as slurry with water, either orally or by nasogastric or orogastric tube, as soon as possible after the ingestion. Commercially available AC products may be mixed with 70% sorbitol to decrease grittiness, increase palatability, and serve as a cathartic. AC is used cautiously in patients with diminished bowel sounds and is contraindicated in patients with bowel obstruction.

Adsorbents

Charcoal-Adsorbed Drugs and Substances

Acetaminophen
Amitriptyline
Amphetamines
Carbamazepine
Codeine
Morphine
Pentobarbital
Phenytoin
Propoxyphene
Salicylates
Strychnine
Theophylline

Drugs and Substances Not Well Adsorbed by Charcoal

Acids
Alkalis
Ethanol
Iron
Lithium
Potassium chloride

CATHARTICS

Cathartics decrease absorption of drugs and toxins by speeding their passage through the GI tract, thereby limiting their contact with mucosal surfaces. The cathartic is administered along with the first dose of AC. Magnesium citrate, magnesium sulfate, sodium sulfate, and sorbitol 70% are often used.

Cathartics are given orally or by nasogastric or orogastric tube in all overdoses or poisonings in which AC is indicated, except in small children. In children younger then 1 year, the cathartic is omitted to avoid dehydration. The safety of more than one dose of cathartic has not been established. Hypermagnesemia has been reported after patients were given repeated doses of magnesium-containing cathartics.[9,10]

Elimination of the Drug or Toxin

The pharmacological characteristics of a drug or toxin greatly influence the severity and length of the clinical course in the acutely poisoned patient. These properties—absorption rate, body distribution, and elimination rate—must be considered when choosing ways to eliminate the drug or toxin from the body. There are seven methods of enhanced elimination:

- Multiple-dose AC
- Whole-bowel irrigation
- Alteration of urine pH
- Hemodialysis
- Hemoperfusion
- Hyperbaric oxygenation therapy (HBO)
- Exchange transfusion

MULTIPLE-DOSE ACTIVATED CHARCOAL

Administering multiple doses of AC may result in greater adsorption of many drugs or toxins. Adequate adsorption does not always occur with a single dose of AC because food interferes with binding, the substance has poor binding characteristics, or the drug is a sustained-release preparation.

Because drugs enter the GI tract through other routes, GI adsorption also helps the systematic clearance of drugs. For example, drugs enter the GI tract by diffusing from the systemic circulation into the GI lumen. This occurs when the concentration gradient created by some membrane-permeable drugs fosters diffusion. In addition, drugs or their active metabolites are excreted with bile into the GI tract. Multiple doses of AC inhibit diffusion back into the systemic circulation by reducing the concentration of the drug in the GI lumen.[11,12] It also prevents reabsorption of the drug by propelling it through the intestines and into the feces.

Multiple-dose AC given orally or by nasogastric or orogastric tube every 2 to 6 hours helps clear theophylline and aspirin. Complications of multiple-dose AC include aspiration and bowel obstruction.

WHOLE-BOWEL IRRIGATION

The goal of this procedure is to give large volumes of a balanced electrolyte solution rapidly to flush the bowel mechanically without creating electrolyte disturbances. Used as a bowel preparation for colonoscopy, it is also successful as a GI decontamination procedure for zinc sulfate, cocaine body packer, and modified release pharmaceuticals.[13–15]

Commercial products used in whole-bowel irrigation include Golytely and Colyte. Both products are dispensed as powders and are given after adding water. Whole-bowel irrigation is contraindicated in the patient with bowel obstruction or perforation.

URINE ALKALINIZATION

Alkalinizing the urine enhances excretion of drugs that are weak acids by increasing the amount of ionized drug in the urine. This form of enhanced elimination is also termed "iontrapping." The urine is alkalinized by administering a continuous IV infusion of 1 to 3 ampules of sodium bicarbonate per liter of fluid. Urine alkalinization is used in salicylate overdose.

Urine acidification, once also done, is no longer recommended due to the low drug clearance and risk of complications. Complications, such as cerebral and pulmonary edema and electrolyte imbalance, may also occur with urine alkalinization.

HEMODIALYSIS

Hemodialysis is the process of altering the solute composition of the blood by diffusion across a semipermeable membrane between blood and a salt solution. It is used in moderate to severe intoxications to remove a drug or toxin rapidly when more conservative methods (eg, gastric emptying, AC, antidotes) have failed. Low molecular weight, low protein binding, and water solubility are factors that make a toxin or drug suitable for hemodialysis. Toxins that may be removed by hemodialysis include methanol, ethylene glycol, theophylline, and salicylates.

HEMOPERFUSION

Hemoperfusion removes drugs and toxins from the blood by pumping the blood through a cartridge of adsorbent material, such as AC. An advantage of hemoperfusion over hemodialysis is that the total surface area of the dialyzing membrane is much greater with the hemoperfusion cartridges. As in hemodialysis, drugs that have high tissue-binding characteristics and a large volume distributed outside the circulation are not good candidates for hemoperfusion because little drug is available in the blood.

Although seldom used, hemoperfusion has been used successfully in theophylline overdose.

HYPERBARIC OXYGENATION THERAPY

With HBO, oxygen is administered to a patient in an enclosed chamber at a pressure greater than the pressure at sea level (eg, 1 atmosphere absolute). It has been used in carbon monoxide and methylene chloride poisonings. (Methylene chloride is metabolized to CO in the body after it is absorbed through inhalation.)

With HBO, the half-life ($t_{1/2}$) of CO is reduced, thereby enhancing elimination. For example, the $t_{1/2}$ of CO in room air is 5 to 6 hours, but in 100% oxygen, it is 90 minutes. The $t_{1/2}$ is reduced further to 20 minutes with HBO.[16] The small number of HBO chambers limits the wide use of this therapy.

Complications of HBO include pressure-related otalgia, sinus pain, tooth pain, and tympanic membrane rupture. Confinement anxiety, convulsion, and tension pneumothorax also have been observed in patients receiving HBO.

EXCHANGE TRANSFUSION

Exchange transfusion is a little-used technique of removing a portion of the patient's blood and replacing it with whole fresh blood. Toxicological literature reports its effective use in an iatrogenic caffeine overdose in a newborn,[17] an accidental analine poisoning of a 4½-year-old girl in whom persistent methemoglobinemia developed,[18] and a preterm infant with iatrogenic theophylline poisoning. In the latter case, exchange transfusion was implemented because hemodialysis or hemoperfusion were considered impractical because of the infant's size and hemodynamic status.[19]

Antagonists

An antagonist in the field of drugs is a substance that counteracts the action of another drug. Following a discussion of the universal antidote, this section continues with antivenin and antitoxin.

INEFFECTIVE UNIVERSAL ANTIDOTE

Although the universal antidote has been touted as the treatment for poisonings, it has no clinical significance. It consists of the following:

- 2 parts burnt toast = AC
- 1 part milk of magnesium = cathartic
- 1 part strong tea = tannic acid

The antidote is not effective in part because burnt toast is not AC.

Although commonly believed there is an antidote for every toxin, the opposite is closer to the truth. There are, in fact, very few antidotes. Antidotes for specific intoxications are listed in Table 52–2.

ANTIVENIN

Antivenins are antitoxins that neutralize the venom of the offending snake or spider. Antivenin (*Crotalidae*) polyvalent (equine) is active against snake venoms of members of the family *Crotalidae*, native to North, Central, and South America. Antivenin (*Latrodectus mactans*; equine) is available for black widow spider bites and antivenin (*Micrurus fulvius*; Equine) is available for envenomations by the eastern coral snake and the Texas coral snake.

Current research in the development of a new rattlesnake antivenin involves the concept of antibody therapy. It is similar to the concept used to develop digoxin-specific antibody fragments (Digibind) for digoxin toxicity.[20,21]

ANTITOXIN

Antitoxins neutralize a toxin, such as that of botulism. Botulism Antitoxin Trivalent (equine) is available through the Centers for Disease Control and Prevention, Atlanta, GA.

Care in Commonly Occurring Poisoning and Overdose

Care in 10 of the most common poisonings and overdoses is summarized in Table 52–3. Nursing assessments, clinical manifestations, and interventions are included in the table.

(text continues on page 1025)

TABLE 52-2
Antidotes

Drug/Toxin	Antidote
Acetaminophen	Acetylcysteine (Mucomyst)
Anticholinergics	Physostigmine (Antilirium)
Benzodiazepines	Flumazenil (Romazicon)
Beta-blocking agents	Glucagon
Calcium channel blockers	Calcium chloride
Carbon monoxide	Oxygen
Cyanide	Amyl nitrite, sodium nitrite, and sodium thiosulfate (Lilly Cyanide Antidote Kit)
Digoxin, cardiac glycosides	Digoxin-specific antibody Fab fragments (Digibind)
Ethylene glycol	Ethanol
Methanol	Ethanol
Nitrites	Methylene blue
Opiates	Naloxone (Narcan)
Organophosphate insecticides	Atropine, protopam

TABLE 52-3 CLINICAL APPLICATION: Nursing Intervention Guidelines
Commonly Observed Poisonings and Overdoses

Drug/Substance	Nursing Assessment/ Clinical Presentation	Intervention

Acetaminophen:
Common over-the-counter antipyretic and analgesic
Often sold as a component of combination drugs for pain or cough and colds
Examples: Tylenol, Tylenol Extended Relief, Tempra 3 Chewable Tablets, Children's Panadol, and Liquiprin Infant's Drops
Combination drugs: oxycodone hydrochloride and acetaminophen (Percocet), codeine and acetaminophen (Tylenol #3), hydrocodone bitartrate and acetaminophen (Lortab), decongestant, antihistamine, cough suppressant, and acetaminophen (Nyquil Nighttime Cold/Flu Medication), and diphenhydramine and acetaminophen (Unisom With Pain Relief)
Acetaminophen toxicity: hepatotoxicity and occasionally renal dysfunction, 1–3 d postingestion
	• Phase 1 (up to 24 h postingestion): anorexia, nausea, vomiting, malaise
	• Phase 2 (24–48 h postingestion): clinical picture improves; increase in AST, ALT, and total bilirubin; prolongation of prothrombin time
	• Phase 3 (72–96 h postingestion): peak hepatotoxicity usually observed
	• Coagulopathies
	• Jaundice
	• AST and ALT may rise into the 10,000–20,000 IU/L range and return to normal without the patient experiencing long-term sequelae
	• Chronic toxicity not well described in the medical literature
		Prevention of absorption:
		• Syrup of ipecac or gastric lavage
		• Activated charcoal
		• Cathartic
		Laboratory:
		• Draw acetaminophen level at 4 h (or later, if patient presents late to the health care facility); plot level on the Rumack-Matthew Nomogram (Fig. 52–1) to determine if antidote is indicated.
		• Monitor daily AST, ALT, total bilirubin, BUN, Cr, and prothrombin time in patients with a toxic acetaminophen level.
		Treatment:
		1. Antidote: N-acetylcysteine (NAC, Mucomyst)
		  a. Loading dose: 140 mg/kg orally
		  b. Maintenance doses: 70 mg/kg orally every 4 h for a total of 17 maintenance doses
		  c. Dilute NAC (20% solution) 3:1 with soft drink or juice
		  d. Repeat any dose not retained 1 h; may need large doses of antiemetics to control vomiting
		  Note: IV NAC is investigational
		2. Supportive care

Amphetamines: Group of drugs used therapeutically for narcolepsy, short-term treatment of obesity, and attention-deficit disorder in children As drugs of abuse, used for ability to stimulate central nervous system to combat fatigue or produce a "high" Prescription amphetamines and related agents: methylphenidate (Ritalin), dextroamphetamine sulfate (Dexedrine), pemoline (Cylert), and phenteramine (Fastin) Street names: MDA, Ecstasy, Love drug, Adam, MDM, EVE, Ice (smokeable methamphetamine), crystal meth, black beauties, bennies, speed, and uppers	• Restlessness • Talkativeness • Irritability • Confusion • Panic • Seizures • Intracranial hemorrhage • Hypertension • Tachycardia • Chest pain • Myocardial infarction • Cardiac dysrhythmias • Palpitations • Peripheral vasoconstriction • Nausea • Vomiting • Chronic amphetamine toxicity may lead to the development of paranoia with hallucinations. • Intravenous drug users may also develop complications such as hepatitis, sepsis, abscesses, and acquired immunodeficiency syndrome (AIDS)	Prevention of absorption: • Gastric lavage • Activated charcoal • Cathartic Laboratory: • Monitor electrolytes and acid–base status. • Urine drug screen may detect amphetamines. Treatment: 1. External cooling measures for hyperthermia 2. Benzodiazepines to control agitation 3. Severe hypertension controlled with intravenous nitroprusside (Nipride); other drugs suggested 4. Supportive care
Benzodiazepines: Antianxiety agents, anticonvulsants, muscle relaxants, and sedatives Examples: Aprazolam (Xanax), chlorazepate (Tranxene), chlordiazepoxide (Librium), diazepam	• Confusion • Lethargy • Slurred speech • Ataxia • Coma	Prevention of absorption: • Gastric lavage • Activated charcoal • Cathartic

(continued)

TABLE 52-3   CLINICAL APPLICATION: Nursing Intervention Guidelines
Commonly Observed Poisonings and Overdoses (Continued)

Drug/Substance	Nursing Assessment/ Clinical Presentation	Intervention
Benzodiazepines (continued): (Valium), flunitrazepam* (Rohypnol), flurazepam (Dalmane), midazolam (Versed), and triazolam (Halcion) Street names: yellow eggs and jelly babies Primarily cause respiratory and central nervous system depression Due to their low order of toxicity, fatalities unlikely unless ingested with other central nervous system depressants	• Respiratory depression • Hypotension	Laboratory • Urine drug screen may detect benzodiazepines. Treatment: 1. Flumazenil reverses central nervous system and respiratory depression. (Note: The half-life of flumazenil is shorter than several benzodiazepines; therefore, its use in management of an overdose is limited; due to the risk of unmasking controlled seizures, flumazenil is contraindicated in the face of simultaneous tricyclic antidepressant overdose.) 2. Supportive care
Carbon monoxide: Colorless, odorless gas that is a component of automobile exhaust, natural gas or propane furnaces and wood stove emissions, cigarette smoke, and pollution Methylene chloride, a component found in some floor strippers, is metabolized in the body to carbon monoxide after inhaled or ingested Displaces oxygen from the hemoglobin, leading to hypoxia Absorbed rapidly by inhalation and combines readily with the hemoglobin due to a greater affinity than oxygen Fetal carboxyhemoglobin levels possibly 10%–15% greater than the maternal carboxyhemoglobin level	• Flulike symptoms • Headache • Nausea • Vomiting • Syncope • Fatigue • Weakness • Lack of concentration • Irritability • Chest pain, especially in people with underlying cardiovascular disease • Occasionally, irreversible changes in memory and personality • Fetotoxicity • People usually report feeling better when not in the area of the carbon monoxide; for example, if the exposure is occurring at home due to a faulty furnace, the person will often report decrease or resolution of symptoms when away from the home.	Prevention of absorption: • Fresh air Laboratory: • Carboxyhemoglobin levels Treatment: 1. 100% oxygen until all signs and symptoms resolve 2. Thorough neurological examination 3. Hyperbaric oxygen therapy (HBO) to decrease half-life; however, due to lack of available HBO chambers, use limited; efficacy not well documented by research 4. Supportive care
Cocaine: Common street drug that produces a temporary feeling of well-being for the user Routes of exposure: intravenous administration, inhalation (eg, smoking), insufflation (eg, snorting), rectal or intravaginal insertion, or ingestion Therapeutically used as a local anesthetic and vasoconstrictor for ear, nose, and throat surgery Street names: crack (smokeable cocaine), coke, snow, Dama Blanca, rock, white lady, toot, nose candy, gold dust, champagne, and speedball (combination of cocaine and heroin)	• Tachycardia • Hypertension • Cardiac dysrhythmias • Chest pain • Myocardial infarction • Aortic dissection • Bowel infarction • Hyperthermia • Anxiety • Seizures • Tactile hallucinations ("cocaine bugs") • Cerebral hemorrhage • Cerebral infarction • Rhabdomyolysis • Rapid onset of toxic effects • In pregnant women, abruptio placenta or abortion possible • Chronic snorting, nasal septal perforation	Prevention of absorption: • Gastric lavage* • Activated charcoal* • Cathartic Laboratory: • Urine drug screen to detect cocaine or its metabolite benzoylecgonine • Cardiac enzymes as indicated to rule out myocardial infarction Treatment: 1. Benzodiazepines such as diazepam (Valium) usually will control hyperactivity, hypertension, tachycardia, and anxiety. 2. Seizure activity may be controlled with diazepam, or if necessary, phenytoin (Dilantin) or phenobarbital may be used.

* Not available in the U.S. legally; also called "roofies"; touted as the "date rape" drug

* Oral exposures

TABLE 52-3   CLINICAL APPLICATION: Nursing Intervention Guidelines
Commonly Observed Poisonings and Overdoses (Continued)

Drug/Substance	Nursing Assessment/ Clinical Presentation	Intervention
Toxic effects related to the rapid onset of central nervous system and cardiac stimulation	• If clinical presentation is inconsistent with cocaine alone, possibly adulterants or substitutes—a number of either have been reported	3. Life-threatening hyperthermia may be reduced by external cooling measures. 4. Cardiac monitoring and serial 12-lead electrocardiogram are used to evaluate dysrhythmias and myocardial ischemia. 5. Monitor for other organ ischemia or infarction. 6. Provide supportive care.
Fluorinated hydrocarbons: Agents used as propellants and refrigerants Freon, dichlorodifluoromethane (Freon 12), and trichloromonofluoromethane (Freon 11) included in this category Exposures to leaking household air conditioners and refrigerators usually minor, causing transient eye, nose, and throat irritation; dizziness; and palpitations. More concentrated exposures as in industrial spills or deliberate abuse, possibly fatal ventricular dysrhythmias (due to a surge of catecholamines) and pulmonary edema	• Eyes, nose, and throat irritation • Cough • Dizziness • Disorientation • Palpitations • Bronchial constriction • Pulmonary edema • Ventricular dysrhythmias • Frostbite possible with dermal exposures	Prevention of absorption: • Fresh air Laboratory: • No specific laboratory tests Treatment: 1. Quiet environment 2. Cardiac monitoring 3. Frostbite: complete rewarming 4. Supportive care
LSD: Common name for psychedelic drug lysergic acid diethylamide Common drug of abuse since its rise in popularity by "flower children" in the 1960s Street drug: available in tablet, capsule, sugar cubes, or as a substance on blotting paper known as "blotter acid" or "postage stamps" Other street names: acid, California sunshine, window panes, and white lightning One source of LSD is ingestion of morning glory seeds In addition to the psychedelic experience, may result in physical effects and behavior-related trauma during acute toxic phase	• Anxiety • Impaired color perception • Impaired judgment • Paranoia or ideas of persecution • Time distortions • Synesthesias (eg, colors heard and music seen) • Visual distortions • Blood pressure normal • Tachycardia • Tachypnea • Slight temperature elevation • Flashbacks (transient recurrences of a psychedelic experience) possible after a period of abstinence; may recur for years • Trauma due to behavioral changes associated with LSD use	Prevention of absorption: • Activated charcoal • Cathartic Laboratory: • Urine drug screen Treatment: 1. Acute anxiety may be managed with intravenous or oral diazepam (Valium). 2. A quiet, nonstimulating environment may be useful while trying to "talk down" the patient who is experiencing a "bad trip." 3. Evaluate for evidence of trauma. 4. Provide supportive care.
Methanol: Highly toxic antifreeze and solvent Available forms: most windshield washer fluids, Sterno canned heat, and components of some paints, gasoline additives, and shellacs Toxic effects: life-threatening acidosis and irreversible blindness, caused by the toxic metabolite, not the methanol itself	• Blurred vision • Decreased visual acuity • Subjective description of vision as if walking in a snowstorm • Retinal edema • Hyperemia of the optic disk • Irreversible blindness • Headache • Vertigo • Lethargy • Confusion • Coma • Nausea	Prevention of absorption: • Syrup of ipecac or • Gastric lavage • Activated charcoal and cathartic little value Laboratory: • Methanol level drawn 1 h postingestion • Serial electrolytes • If using ethanol therapy, serial glucose and blood ethanol level monitored every hour initially

(continued)

TABLE 52-3 CLINICAL APPLICATION: Nursing Intervention Guidelines
Commonly Observed Poisonings and Overdoses (Continued)

Drug/Substance	Nursing Assessment/ Clinical Presentation	Intervention
Methanol (continued):	• Vomiting • Abdominal pain • Metabolic acidosis	Treatment: 1. Antidote: intravenous ethanol infusion to maintain blood ethanol level between 100–130 mg/dL (to impede metabolism of methanol to toxic metabolites by supplying ethanol to compete for certain enzyme systems) Note: 4-methylpyrazole (4-MP), investigational drug in human trials as an alternative therapy for ethanol 2. Hemodialysis usually indicated for methanol levels >50 mg/dL, visual changes, renal failure, or refractory acidosis 3. Folic acid administration (to assist the oxidation of the toxic metabolite formic acid to carbon dioxide) 4. Supportive care
Salicylates: Group of drugs used primarily for anti-inflammatory, antipyretic, and analgesic properties Common sources: aspirin, some formulations of Alka-Seltzer, Aspergum, PeptoBismol, sunscreens, liniments such as Icy Hot, and oil of wintergreen (methylsalicylate) Life-threatening metabolic acidosis, cerebral edema, and pulmonary edema from salicylism Aspirin ingestions difficult to manage due to the formation of a mass of aspirin in the gastrointestinal tract called a concretion Concretion formation, delayed absorption and therefore delayed toxicity Chronic salicylism more common in older adults and possibly misdiagnosed Higher salicylates tolerated with acute overdose as opposed to chronic toxicity	• Tinnitus • Tachypnea • Pulmonary edema • Confusion • Lethargy • Seizures • Cerebral edema • Respiratory alkalosis coupled with metabolic acidosis (initially) • Hypokalemia • Platelet dysfunction • Hypothrombinemia • Gastrointestinal hemorrhage • Nausea • Vomiting • Hyperthermia • Dehydration	Prevention of absorption: • Syrup of ipecac or • Gastric lavage • Multiple-dose activated charcoal • Single dose of cathartic Laboratory: • Serial salicylate levels • Serial electrolytes • Arterial blood gas as indicated • Hematological and coagulation studies Treatment: Note: Treatment is based on serial salicylate levels and clinical presentation; each case is individually assessed and managed. 1. Hydrate patient. 2. Urinary excretion is enhanced by urine alkalinization (urine pH = 7.5–8.0); intravenous fluid is usually D5W with 20–40 mEq KCl and 2–3 ampules of sodium bicarbonate per liter to infuse at a rate of 2–3 mL/kg/h to achieve equal urine output. Note: It is difficult to alkalinize the urine without a normal serum potassium level. 3. Potassium is replaced intravenously as needed. 4. Monitor onset of cerebral or pulmonary edema; chest radiograph is taken as needed. 5. Hemodialysis is indicated for renal failure, cerebral edema, pulmonary edema, refractory acidosis, chronic salicylate level >50 mg/dL, or acute salicylate level >100 mg/dL postingestion. 6. Provide supportive care.

TABLE 52-3 CLINICAL APPLICATION: Nursing Intervention Guidelines
Commonly Observed Poisonings and Overdoses (Continued)

Drug/Substance	Nursing Assessment/ Clinical Presentation	Intervention
Tricyclic antidepressants (TCA): Class of drugs prescribed for depression and chronic pain Examples: amitriptyline (Elavil), clomipramine (Anafranil), desipramine (Norpramin), doxepin (Adapin, Sinequan), Imipramine (Tofranil), nortriptyline (Pamelor, Aventyl), protriptyline (Vivactil), and trimipramine (Surmontil)	• Tachycardia • Ventricular dysrhythmias (including ventricular tachycardia and ventricular fibrillation) • Cardiac conduction delays (eg, QRS >100 ms) • Hypotension • Agitation • Sedation • Seizures • Coma • Dry, flushed skin • Decreased gastrointestinal motility • Urinary retention • Metabolic acidosis	Prevention of absorption: • Syrup of ipecac contraindicated due to the rapid onset of sedation or seizures • Gastric lavage • Activated charcoal • Cathartic Laboratory: • Serum TCA levels not clinically useful in managing overdoses • Urine drug screen for TCAs • Serial electrolytes and arterial blood gases as indicated Treatment: 1. Prepare for rapid onset of cardiovascular collapse. 2. Seizures may be treated initially with intravenous diazepam (Valium), and if necessary, phenytoin (Dilantin) and phenobarbital. 3. Ventricular dysrhythmias may initially be controlled with systemic alkalinization (keeping blood pH = 7.45–7.55 using intravenous boluses of sodium bicarbonate or intubation and hyperventilation); ventricular dysrhythmias not controlled with systemic alkalinization may be controlled with lidocaine or bretylium (Bretylol). Do not use procainamide (Pronestyl) or quinidine due to similar effects on cardiac conduction such as TCAs. 4. Cardiac conduction delays (eg, QRS >100 ms) also are treated with systemic alkalinization as outlined in #3. Conduction delays not responsive to systemic alkalinization may be treated with phenytoin. 5. Hypotension may be addressed initially with Trendelenburg position and intravenous fluids; if necessary, follow with dopamine infusion. Norepinephrine (Levophed) may be necessary. 6. Provide supportive care.

Continuous Patient Monitoring

Seriously poisoned or overdosed patients may require continued monitoring for hours or days after exposure. Diagnostic tools and clinical signs and symptoms will provide information about the patient's progress and direct medical and nursing management. Diagnostic tools are listed in the accompanying display and discussed here.

Electrocardiography. Electrocardiography may provide evidence of drugs causing dysrhythmias or conduction delays (eg, tricyclic antidepressants).

Radiology. Many substances are radiopaque (eg, heavy metals, button batteries, some enteric-coated tablets) and can be examined by radiology. Chest x-rays will provide evidence of aspiration and pulmonary edema also.

Electrolytes, Arterial Blood Gases, and Other Laboratory Tests. Acute poisoning can cause an imbalance in electrolyte levels, including sodium, potassium, chloride, CO_2 content, magnesium, and calcium. Signs of inadequate oxygenation include cyanosis, tachycardia, hypoventilation, intercostal retractions, and altered mental status. Signs of

---

CLINICAL APPLICATION: Diagnostic Studies
Monitoring Parameters Useful in Toxicology

- Electrocardiography
- Radiology
- Electrolytes, arterial blood gases, and other laboratory tests
- Anion gap
- Osmolal gap
- Toxicology screens

---

inadequate ventilation or oxygenation should be evaluated by ABG measurements. Seriously poisoned patients require routine screening of electrolytes, creatinine, and glucose; complete blood count; urinalysis; and ABGs.

Anion Gap. The anion gap (AG) is a simple, cost-effective tool that uses common serum measures, such as sodium, chloride, and bicarbonate, to help evaluate the poisoned patient for certain drugs or toxins. The AG represents the difference between unmeasured anions and cations in the blood. Using measured anions and a cation, the AG is calculated with the following formula:

$$[Na] - ([Cl] + [HCO_3]) = AG$$

The normal value for the AG is approximately 8 to 16 mEq/L. An AG that exceeds the upper normal value may indicate metabolic acidosis due to an accumulation of acids in the blood. Drugs or toxins that can produce an elevated AG include methanol (eg, windshield washer fluids), ethanol, ethylene glycol (eg, automobile radiator antifreeze and coolant), and salicylates (eg, aspirin). Although these substances may cause an elevated AG, a normal AG alone does not preclude a toxic exposure.

Osmolal Gap. The osmolal gap (OG) is the difference between the measured osmolality (using the freezing point depression method) and the calculated osmolality. The calculated osmolality is derived using laboratory values for the major osmotically active substances in the serum, such as the sodium, glucose, and blood urea nitrogen. Like the AG, it is a simple, cost-effective tool for evaluating the poisoned patient for certain drugs or toxins.

The calculated osmolality (using serum electrolyte values) is defined as follows:

$$2[Na] + \frac{glucose}{18} + \frac{BUN}{2.8} = \text{Calculated osmolality}$$

The OG is then calculated as follows:

Measured osmolality − Calculated osmolality = OG

An OG that exceeds 10 mOsm is abnormal. Toxins that can cause an elevated OG include ethylene glycol and methanol. Ethanol may also cause an elevated OG because it is often used to treat methanol and ethylene glycol poisonings. In addition, the patient may have ingested ethanol

prior to arrival to the health care facility. Therefore, ethanol must be included in the above formula for calculated osmolality. The formula is:

$$2[Na] + \frac{glucose}{18} + \frac{BUN}{2.8} + \frac{BAL}{4.6} = \text{Calculated osmolality}$$

where BAL is the blood ethanol level measured in mg%.

Toxicology Screens. A toxicology screen is a laboratory analysis of a body fluid or tissue to identify drugs or other toxins. Although saliva, spinal fluid, and hair may be analyzed, blood or urine samples are used more frequently. The number and type of drugs on toxicology screens vary. Each screen includes specific drugs or agents. For example, drug abuse screens usually identify several common street or prescription drugs, while a coma panel detects common drugs that cause CNS depression. Comprehensive screens include many drugs (ranging from antidepressants to cardiac drugs to alcohols) and are more expensive. A number of factors limit the role of toxicology screens in managing overdoses or poisonings. The test sample must be collected while the drug is in the body fluid or tissue used for testing. For example, a screen may occur before or after the drug is absorbed into the circulation or excreted in the urine. Sometimes, even when the drug is not identified in the sample because it was collected too late, the metabolite(s) may be detected. For example, cocaine is a rapidly metabolized drug; however, its metabolite benzoylecgonine can be detected in the urine for several hours after cocaine use. A negative toxicology screen does not necessarily mean that a drug or toxin is not present, but only that none of the drugs or toxins screened for are present.

The sample must also be properly collected, and there must be a laboratory near enough to obtain results quickly. For many smaller, rural laboratories, these tests are taken by a courier service or mailed to a larger laboratory, and the results are not available for days. In these situations, the value of the test for managing the immediate overdose or poisoning needs to be considered.

Management of the patient who is toxic with cocaine is summarized in the Collaborative Care Guide.

Prevention and Patient Teaching

One of the interventions the nurse can perform in the ICU is preventive teaching. All patients who have survived a toxic reaction and parents should be taught how to prevent such an incident from recurring. Parents of young children need information on child-proofing their home. Teaching related to prevention of childhood poisoning is given in the display on p. 1028. Parents need to be made aware of common substances that are lethal. For instance, some people do not realize that parts of many plants are poisonous. Proper storage of poisonous substances is essential. Families should keep the number for their local poison control center near their phone. The family teaching display offers advice to give parents related to poisoning.

COLLABORATIVE CARE GUIDE
for the Patient With Cocaine Toxicity

OUTCOMES	INTERVENTIONS

Oxygenation/Ventilation

Arterial blood gases are within normal limits.

- Monitor pulse oximetry and arterial blood gases.
- Validate significant changes in pulse oximetry with co-oximetry arterial saturation measurement.

Respiratory rate and depth are within normal limits.

- Monitor q15min, then q1h.
- Prepare for intubation and mechanical ventilation (see Collaborative Care Guide for the Patient on a Ventilator).

Circulation/Perfusion

Blood pressure, heart rate are within normal limits.
Patient is free of dysrhythmias.
There is no evidence of myocardial dysfunction, such as altered ECG or cardiac enzymes.

- Monitor vital signs q15min then q1h.
- Provide continuous ECG monitoring.
- Monitor 12-lead ECG qd and PRN.
- Monitor cardiac enzymes, magnesium, phosphorus, calcium, and potassium as ordered.
- Assess for chest pain.
- Monitor ECG for dysrhythmias and changes consistent with evolving MI.

Patient is euthermic.

- Assess temperature q15–30min, then q1h.
- Provide a cool environment, and institute cooling strategies (eg, hypothermia blanket, tepid sponge bath), as indicated.

Fluids/Electrolytes

Patient's urine output >30 mL/h (or >0.5 mL/kg/h).

- Take intake and output q1h.
- Administer fluids and diuretics to maintain intravascular volume and renal function per order.

There is no evidence of electrolyte imbalance or renal dysfunction.

- Monitor electrolytes daily and PRN.
- Replace electrolytes as ordered.
- Monitor BUN, creatinine, serum osmolality, and urine electrolytes daily.

Mobility/Safety

There is no evidence of seizure activity.

- Monitor for seizure activity.
- Administer anticonvulsants.
- Assess anticonvulsant levels qd if indicated.
- Maintain calm, quiet environment.
- Institute seizure precautions.
- Institute fall precautions.

Patient does not harm self.

- Assess need for physical or chemical restraint to protect from self-injury.
- Monitor agitation and administer sedation when appropriate.
- Evaluate risk for suicide and take measures to protect patient.

Skin Integrity

There is no evidence of skin breakdown.

- Document skin integrity q8h.
- Turn and reposition q2h.
- Use Braden Scale to assess risk of skin breakdown.

Nutrition

Caloric and nutrient intake meet metabolic requirements per calculation (eg, Basal Energy Expenditure).

- Provide parenteral or enteral nutrition if patient is NPO.
- Consult dietitian or nutritional support service.
- Monitor protein and calorie intake.
- Monitor albumin, prealbumin, transferrin, cholesterol, triglycerides, glucose.

(continued)

COLLABORATIVE CARE GUIDE
for the Patient With Cocaine Toxicity (Continued)

OUTCOMES	INTERVENTIONS
Comfort/Pain Control Patient will have minimal discomfort related to withdrawal from cocaine and other substances.	• Obtain toxicology screen to identify other substances used by the patient. • Treat drug withdrawal and overdose symptoms promptly and with appropriate intervention (eg, remove from circulation, administer antidote, administer methadone).
Psychosocial Patient and family acknowledge substance abuse.	• Assess patient and family response to overdose. • Support healthy coping behaviors. • Consult substance abuse counselor and social worker. • Encourage patient discussion regarding use of illegal drugs, support system, financial concerns, and readiness for substance abuse treatment.
Teaching/Discharge Planning Patient and family have information about treatment and self-help resources. Patient and family each have a plan for follow-up care.	• Assess patient and family knowledge and understanding of substance abuse. • Provide literature and explanations to patient and family regarding substance abuse, treatment, relapse, legal issues, and self-help groups. • Refer family to self-help resources. • If patient agrees, initiate referral for substance abuse rehabilitation. • Coordinate referral with patient, family, and social worker to address other possible issues (eg, housing, financial issues, long-term care planning).

Installation of carbon monoxide detectors will alert families to problems within their homes. Utility companies and local health authorities can help with identifying and removing sources of fumes.

Drug abuse needs to be addressed by parents' talking with their children about the danger of substance abuse. Parents need to advise their children early about the dangers of substance abuse. Such discussion should include risks and physical, psychosocial, and economic consequences. Children can be helped to prepare strategies for refusing substances offered to them or to avoid peer pressure.

FAMILY TEACHING
Prevention of Childhood Poisoning

- Keep all medications and toxic products in original containers in a locked cabinet out of the reach of children.
- Read labels carefully before using drugs or toxic products.
- Use toxic chemical products in a well-ventilated area.
- Do not mix common household cleaning products.
- Identify any poisonous houseplants, and keep seeds, bulbs, leaves, and fruits of such plants away from children.
- Do not treat medicines as candy.
- Measure and give medicine in well-lit areas to avoid error.
- Use childproof containers when available.
- Destroy all old medications in a safe way.
- Keep syrup of ipecac in the home for emergencies, but use only under directions of the Poison Control Center or the family physician.
- Keep Poison Control Center telephone numbers posted by the phone.

Considerations for the Older Patient
Poison Prevention

- Poison Control Centers receive many calls from or related to older adults regarding accidental poisonings.
- Telephone numbers for the health care provider and the Poison Control Center should be in a readily accessible place.
- The older population uses more medicine than any other age group.
- Older people may be more susceptible to the effects of drugs.
- When questions arise concerning drugs, a responsible adult should not hesitate to call a health care provider.
- Side effects of medications should be reported to the health care provider.
- The patient should not change the dose nor stop taking prescription drugs without first consulting the physician or nurse.
- It is not wise to double medication when a pill is forgotten. The patient should seek the physician's or nurse's advice.
- Medications and alcohol should not be mixed without first checking with the pharmacist.
- The pharmacist can provide large-print labels.
- A medication calendar or diary will help the older person keep track of the dosing schedule.
- Pill dispensers are helpful for the patient who has to take a variety of pills or who has trouble remembering the schedule.
- When a drug is discontinued, the remaining medication should be thrown away.

◼ CONCLUSION

Because there are so few antidotes, the care of the poisoned patient is directed at maintaining the ABCs and taking measures to prevent absorption and enhance elimination of the drug or toxin. Maintaining ABCs may entail the use of IV fluids, vasopressors, ventilators, cardiac monitoring, antiarrhythmics, and other measures specific to the abnormalities, such as external cooling. The nurse can also participate in preventive teaching.

Clinical Applicability Challenges

Self-Challenge: Critical Thinking

1. *Formulate a nursing plan of care for the patient who arrives at the emergency department with an amitriptyline overdose. The plan should include initial stabilization, assessment, and follow-up care provided in the ICU.*

2. *Debate the efficacy of the different methods of gastric emptying, and discuss why certain methods are preferable or contraindicated in the management of the poisoned patient.*

Study Questions

1. *All of the following are examples of gut decontamination except*
   a. *syrup of ipecac.*
   b. *activated charcoal.*
   c. *gastric lavage.*
   d. *exchange transfusion.*

2. *Urine alkalinization may increase renal clearance of*
   a. *all drugs.*
   b. *salicylates.*
   c. *cyclic antidepressants.*
   d. *acetaminophen.*

REFERENCES

1. Litovitz T, Felberg L, White S, Klein-Schwartz W: 1995 Annual report of the American Association of Poison Control Centers toxic exposure surveillance system. Am J Emerg Med 14(5):487–537, 1996
2. Timberlake G: Ipecac as a cause of the Mallory-Weiss syndrome. South Med J 77:804–805, 1984
3. Wolowodiuk O, McMicken D, O'Brien P: Pneumomediastinum and retropneumoperitoneum: As unusual complication of syrup-of ipecac-induced emesis. Ann Emerg Med 13:1148–1151, 1984
4. Robertson W: A further warning on the use of salt as an emetic agent. J Pediatr 79:877, 1971
5. Streat S: Fatal salt poisoning in a child. N Z Med J 706(95):285–286, 1982
6. Gresham G, Mashru M: Fatal poisoning with sodium chloride. Forensic Sci Int 20:87–88, 1982
7. Stein R, Jenkins D, Korns M: Death after use of cupric sulfate as emetic. JAMA 235:801, 1976
8. Askenasi R, Abramowicz M, Jeanmart J, Ansay J, Degaute J: Esophageal perforation: An unusual complication of gastric lavage. Ann Emerg Med 13:146, 1984
9. Smilkstein M, Smolinske S, Kulig K, Rumack B: Severe hypermagnesemia due to multiple-dose cathartic therapy. West J Med 148:208 211, 1988
10. Weber C, Santiago R: Hypermagnesemia, a potential complication during treatment of theophylline intoxication with oral activated charcoal and magnesium-containing cathartics. Chest 95:56–59, 1989
11. Levy G: Gastrointestinal clearance of drugs with activated charcoal. N Engl J Med 307:677, 1982
12. Chyka P: Multiple-dose activated charcoal and enhancement of systemic drug clearance: Summary of studies in animals and human volunteers. J Toxicol Clin Toxicol 33(5):399–405, 1995
13. Burkhart K, Kulig K, Rumack R: Whole-bowel irrigation as treatment for zinc sulfate overdose. Ann Emerg Med 19:1167–1170, 1990
14. Hoffman R, Smilkstein M, Goldfrank L: Whole bowel irrigation and the cocaine body packer: A new approach to a common problem. Am J Emerg Med 8:523–527, 1990
15. Kirshenbaum L, Mathews S, Sitar D, Tenebein M: Whole-bowel irrigation versus activated charcoal in sorbitol for the ingestion of modified-released pharmaceuticals. Clin Pharmacol Ther 46:264–271, 1989
16. Rakel R (ed): 1995 Conn's Current Therapy. Philadelphia, W.B. Saunders, 1995
17. Perrin C, Debruyne D, Lacolte J, Laloum D, Bonte J, Moulin M: Treatment of caffeine intoxication by exchange transfusion in a newborn. Acta Paediatr Scand 76:679–681, 1987
18. Mier R: Treatment of aniline poisoning with exchange transfusion. J Clin Toxicol Clin Toxicol 26(5–6):357–364, 1988
19. Shannon M, Wernovsky G, Morris C: Exchange transfusion in the treatment of severe theophylline poisoning. Pediatrics 89:145–147, 1992
20. Seifert S, Boyer L, Dart R, Porter R, Sjostrom L: Correlation of venom effects, antivenin levels and venom antigenemia in a patient with *Crotalus Atrox* envenomation treated with a Fab antivenin (Abstract). J Toxicol Clin Toxicol 34(5):593, 1996

21. Boyer L, Seifert S, Clark R, NcNally J, Williams S, Nordt S, Walter F, Dart R: Coagulopathy in Crotalid envenomation treated with a new Fab antivenin (Abstract). J Toxicol Clin Toxicol 34(5):593, 1996

BIBLIOGRAPHY

Bond G: Home use of Syrup of Ipecac is associated with a reduction in pediatric emergency department visits. Ann Emerg Med 25(3):338–343, 1995

Boyes A: Repetition of overdose: A retrospective 5 year study. J Adv Nursing 20:262–468, 1994

Chamberlain J: A comprehensive review of Naloxone for the emergency physician. Am J Emerg Med 12:650–660, 1994

Graves H, Smith E, Braen G, et al: Clinical policy for the initial approach to patients presenting with acute toxic ingestion or dermal or inhalation exposure. An Emerg Med 24:570–585, 1995

Krenzelok E: The use of poison prevention and education stratgies to enhance the awareness of the poison information center and to prevent accidental pediatric poisoning. J Toxicol Clin Toxicol 33(6):663–667, 1995

APPENDIX 1

ACLS Guidelines

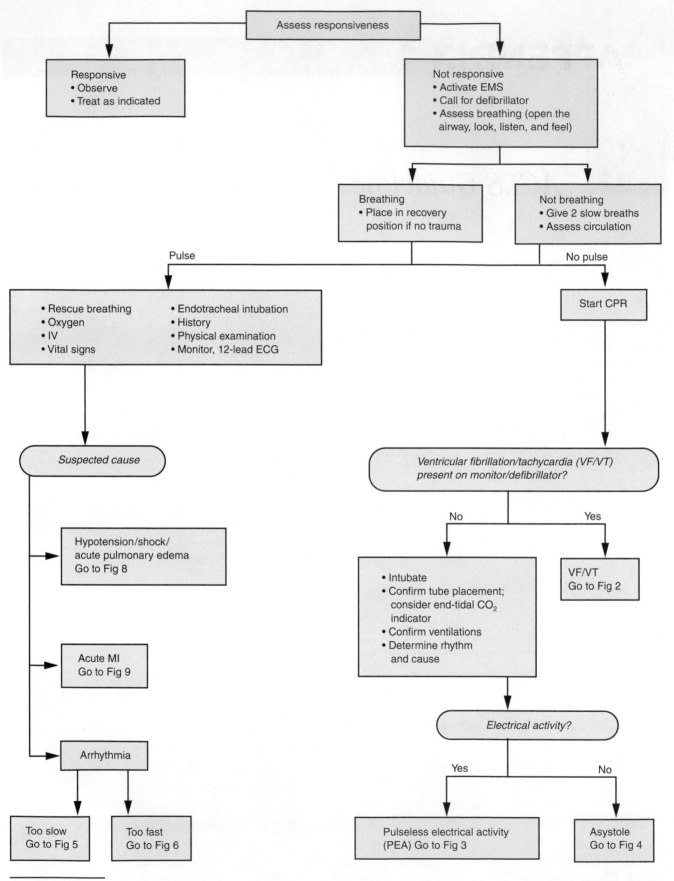

FIGURE 1

Universal algorithm for adult emergency cardiac care.

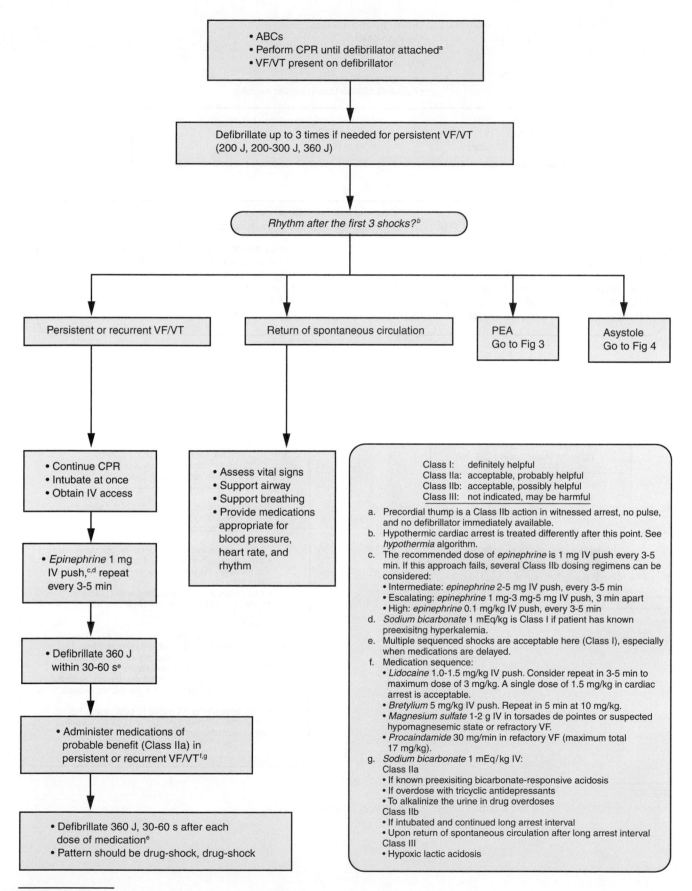

FIGURE 2

Ventricular fibrillation/pulseless ventricular tachycardia (VF/VT) algorithm.

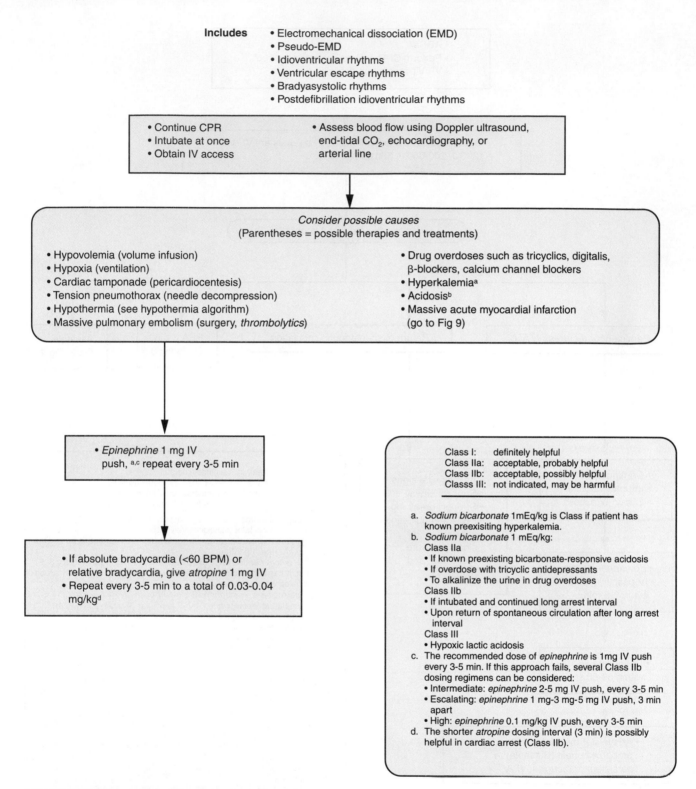

Includes
- Electromechanical dissociation (EMD)
- Pseudo-EMD
- Idioventricular rhythms
- Ventricular escape rhythms
- Bradyasystolic rhythms
- Postdefibrillation idioventricular rhythms

- Continue CPR
- Intubate at once
- Obtain IV access

- Assess blood flow using Doppler ultrasound, end-tidal CO_2, echocardiography, or arterial line

Consider possible causes
(Parentheses = possible therapies and treatments)

- Hypovolemia (volume infusion)
- Hypoxia (ventilation)
- Cardiac tamponade (pericardiocentesis)
- Tension pneumothorax (needle decompression)
- Hypothermia (see hypothermia algorithm)
- Massive pulmonary embolism (surgery, *thrombolytics*)

- Drug overdoses such as tricyclics, digitalis, β-blockers, calcium channel blockers
- Hyperkalemia[a]
- Acidosis[b]
- Massive acute myocardial infarction (go to Fig 9)

- *Epinephrine* 1 mg IV push, [a,c] repeat every 3-5 min

- If absolute bradycardia (<60 BPM) or relative bradycardia, give *atropine* 1 mg IV
- Repeat every 3-5 min to a total of 0.03-0.04 mg/kg[d]

Class I: definitely helpful
Class IIa: acceptable, probably helpful
Class IIb: acceptable, possibly helpful
Classs III: not indicated, may be harmful

a. *Sodium bicarbonate* 1mEq/kg is Class if patient has known preexisiting hyperkalemia.
b. *Sodium bicarbonate* 1 mEq/kg:
   Class IIa
   - If known preexisting bicarbonate-responsive acidosis
   - If overdose with tricyclic antidepressants
   - To alkalinize the urine in drug overdoses
   Class IIb
   - If intubated and continued long arrest interval
   - Upon return of spontaneous circulation after long arrest interval
   Class III
   - Hypoxic lactic acidosis
c. The recommended dose of *epinephrine* is 1mg IV push every 3-5 min. If this approach fails, several Class IIb dosing regimens can be considered:
   - Intermediate: *epinephrine* 2-5 mg IV push, every 3-5 min
   - Escalating: *epinephrine* 1 mg-3 mg-5 mg IV push, 3 min apart
   - High: *epinephrine* 0.1 mg/kg IV push, every 3-5 min
d. The shorter *atropine* dosing interval (3 min) is possibly helpful in cardiac arrest (Class IIb).

FIGURE 3

Pulseless electrical activity (PEA) algorithm (Electromechanical dissociation [EMD]).

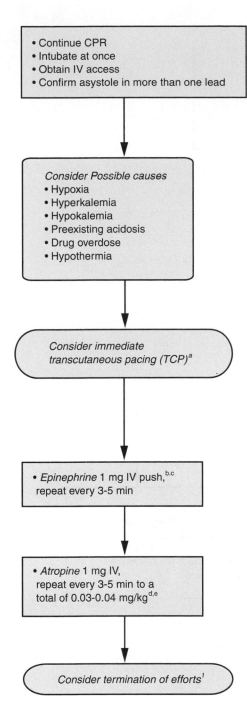

- Continue CPR
- Intubate at once
- Obtain IV access
- Confirm asystole in more than one lead

Consider Possible causes
- Hypoxia
- Hyperkalemia
- Hypokalemia
- Preexisting acidosis
- Drug overdose
- Hypothermia

Consider immediate transcutaneous pacing (TCP)[a]

- *Epinephrine* 1 mg IV push,[b,c] repeat every 3-5 min

- *Atropine* 1 mg IV, repeat every 3-5 min to a total of 0.03-0.04 mg/kg[d,e]

Consider termination of efforts[1]

Class I: definitely helpful
Class IIa: acceptable, probably helpful
Class IIb: acceptable, possibly helpful
Class III: not indicated, may be helpful

a. TCP is a Class IIb intervention. Lack of success may be due to delays in pacing. To be effective TCP must be performed early, simultaneously with drugs. Evidence does not support routine use of TCP for asystole.

b. The recommended dose of *epinephrine* is 1 mg IV push every 3-5 min. If this approach fails, several Class IIb dosing regimens can be considered:
- Intermediate: *epinephrine* 2-5 mg IV push, every 3-5 min
- Escalating: *epinephrine* 1 mg-3 mg-5 mg IV push, 3 min apart
- High: *epinephrine* 0.1 mg/kg IV push, every 3-5 min

c. *Sodium bicarbonate* 1mEq/kg is Class I if patient has known preexisting hyperkalemia.

d. The shorter *atropine* dosing interval (3 min) is Class IIb in asystolic arrest.

e. *Sodium bicarbonate* 1mEq/kg:
Class IIa
- If known preexisting bicarbonate-responsive acidosis
- If overdose with tricyclic antidepressants
- To alkalinize the urine in drug overdoses
Class IIb
- If intubated and continued long arrest interval
- Upon return of spontaneous circulation after long arrest interval
Class III
- Hypoxic lactic acidosis

f. If patient remains in asystole or other agonal rhythm after successful intubation and initial medications and no reversible causes are identified, consider termination of resuscitative efforts by a physician. Consider interval since arrest.

FIGURE 4
Asystole treatment algorithm.

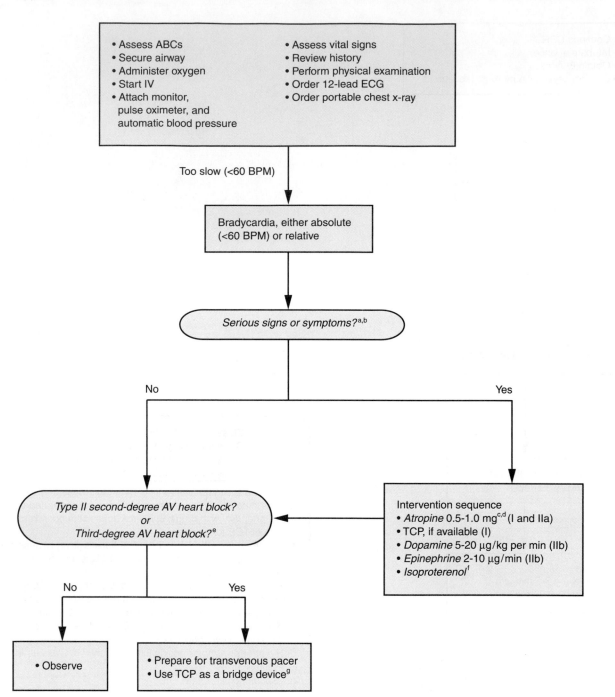

a. Serious signs or symptoms must be related to the slow rate. Clinical manifestations include
• Symptoms (chest pain, shortness of breath, decreased level of consciousness)
• Signs (low BP, shock, pulmonary congestion, CHF, acute MI)
b. Do not delay TCP while awaiting IV access or for *atropine* to take effect if patient is symptomatic.
c. Denervated transplanted hearts will not respond to *atropine.* Go at once to pacing, *catecholamine* infusion, or both.
d. *Atropine* should be given in repeat doses every 3-5 min up to total of 0.03-0.04 mg/kg. Use the shorter dosing interval (3 min) in several clinical conditions. It has been suggested that *atropine* should be used with caution in atrioventricular (AV) block at the His-Purkinje level (type II AV block and new third-degree block with wide QRS complexes) (Class IIb).
e. Never treat third-degree heart block plus ventricular escape beats with *lidocaine.*
f. *Isoproterenol* should be used, if at all, with extreme caution. At low doses it is Class IIb (possibly helpful); at higher doses it is Class III (harmful).
g. Verify patient tolerance and mechanical capture. Use analgesia and sedation as needed.

FIGURE 5
Bradycardia algorithm (Patient is not in cardiac arrest).

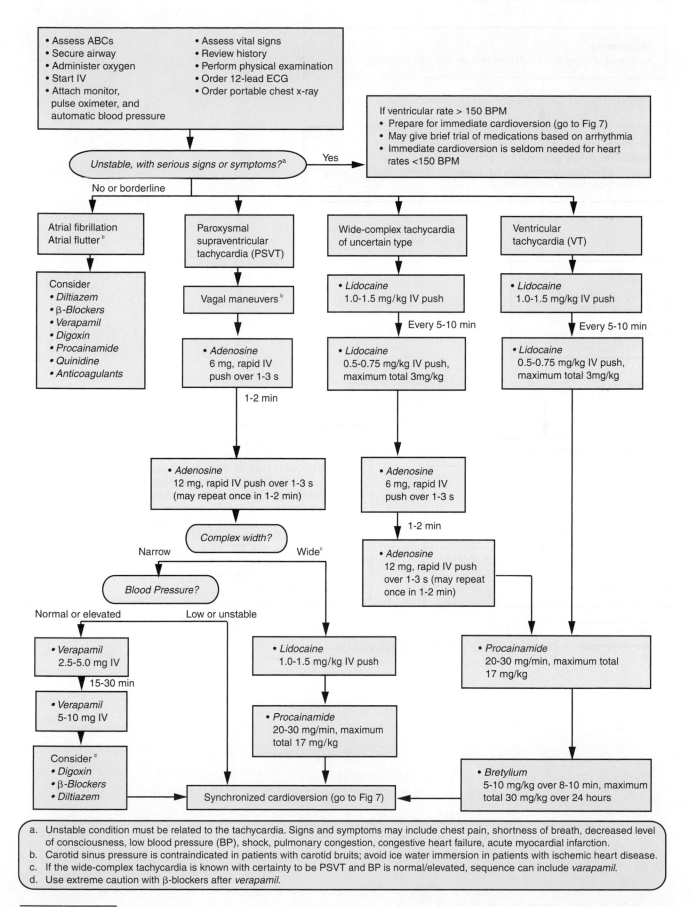

• Assess ABCs
• Secure airway
• Administer oxygen
• Start IV
• Attach monitor, pulse oximeter, and automatic blood pressure

• Assess vital signs
• Review history
• Perform physical examination
• Order 12-lead ECG
• Order portable chest x-ray

Unstable, with serious signs or symptoms?[a] → Yes

If ventricular rate > 150 BPM
• Prepare for immediate cardioversion (go to Fig 7)
• May give brief trial of medications based on arrhythmia
• Immediate cardioversion is seldom needed for heart rates <150 BPM

No or borderline

Atrial fibrillation Atrial flutter[b]

Consider
• *Diltiazem*
• β-*Blockers*
• *Verapamil*
• *Digoxin*
• *Procainamide*
• *Quinidine*
• *Anticoagulants*

Paroxysmal supraventricular tachycardia (PSVT)

Vagal maneuvers[b]

• *Adenosine* 6 mg, rapid IV push over 1-3 s

1-2 min

• *Adenosine* 12 mg, rapid IV push over 1-3 s (may repeat once in 1-2 min)

Complex width?

Narrow   Wide[c]

Blood Pressure?

Normal or elevated   Low or unstable

• *Verapamil* 2.5-5.0 mg IV

15-30 min

• *Verapamil* 5-10 mg IV

Consider[d]
• *Digoxin*
• β-*Blockers*
• *Diltiazem*

Wide-complex tachycardia of uncertain type

• *Lidocaine* 1.0-1.5 mg/kg IV push

Every 5-10 min

• *Lidocaine* 0.5-0.75 mg/kg IV push, maximum total 3mg/kg

• *Adenosine* 6 mg, rapid IV push over 1-3 s

1-2 min

• *Adenosine* 12 mg, rapid IV push over 1-3 s (may repeat once in 1-2 min)

Ventricular tachycardia (VT)

• *Lidocaine* 1.0-1.5 mg/kg IV push

Every 5-10 min

• *Lidocaine* 0.5-0.75 mg/kg IV push, maximum total 3mg/kg

• *Lidocaine* 1.0-1.5 mg/kg IV push

• *Procainamide* 20-30 mg/min, maximum total 17 mg/kg

• *Procainamide* 20-30 mg/min, maximum total 17 mg/kg

Synchronized cardioversion (go to Fig 7)

• *Bretylium* 5-10 mg/kg over 8-10 min, maximum total 30 mg/kg over 24 hours

a. Unstable condition must be related to the tachycardia. Signs and symptoms may include chest pain, shortness of breath, decreased level of consciousness, low blood pressure (BP), shock, pulmonary congestion, congestive heart failure, acute myocardial infarction.
b. Carotid sinus pressure is contraindicated in patients with carotid bruits; avoid ice water immersion in patients with ischemic heart disease.
c. If the wide-complex tachycardia is known with certainty to be PSVT and BP is normal/elevated, sequence can include *varapamil*.
d. Use extreme caution with β-blockers after *verapamil*.

FIGURE 6
Tachycardia algorithm.

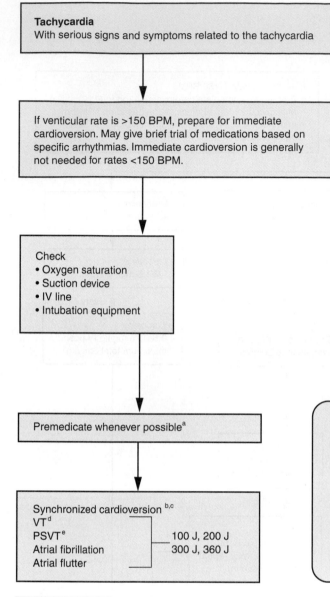

Tachycardia
With serious signs and symptoms related to the tachycardia

If venticular rate is >150 BPM, prepare for immediate cardioversion. May give brief trial of medications based on specific arrhythmias. Immediate cardioversion is generally not needed for rates <150 BPM.

Check
• Oxygen saturation
• Suction device
• IV line
• Intubation equipment

Premedicate whenever possible[a]

Synchronized cardioversion [b,c]
VT[d]
PSVT[e]   100 J, 200 J
Atrial fibrillation   300 J, 360 J
Atrial flutter

a. Effective regimens have included a seditive (eg, *diazepam, midazolam, barbiturates, etomidate, ketamine, methohexital)* with or without an analgesic agent (eg, *fentanyl, morphine, meperidine).* Many experts recommend anesthesia if service is reaily avaliable.
b. Note possible need to resynchronize after each cardioversion.
c. If delays in synchronization occur and clinical conditions are critical, go to immediate unsynchronized shocks.
d. Treat polymorphic VT (irregular form and rate) like VF:200 J, 200-300 J, 360 J.
e. PSVT and atrial flutter often respond to lower energy levels (start with 50 J.)

FIGURE 7
Electrical cardioversion algorithm (Patient is not in cardiac arrest).

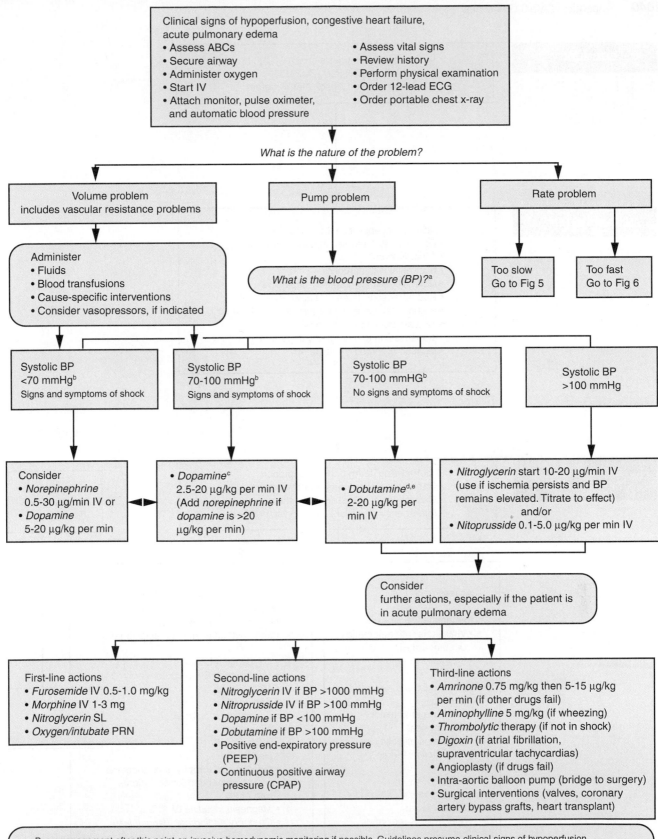

Clinical signs of hypoperfusion, congestive heart failure,
acute pulmonary edema
- Assess ABCs
- Secure airway
- Administer oxygen
- Start IV
- Attach monitor, pulse oximeter, and automatic blood pressure
- Assess vital signs
- Review history
- Perform physical examination
- Order 12-lead ECG
- Order portable chest x-ray

What is the nature of the problem?

Volume problem includes vascular resistance problems

Pump problem

Rate problem

Administer
- Fluids
- Blood transfusions
- Cause-specific interventions
- Consider vasopressors, if indicated

What is the blood pressure (BP)?[a]

Too slow
Go to Fig 5

Too fast
Go to Fig 6

Systolic BP <70 mmHg[b]
Signs and symptoms of shock

Systolic BP 70-100 mmHg[b]
Signs and symptoms of shock

Systolic BP 70-100 mmHG[b]
No signs and symptoms of shock

Systolic BP >100 mmHg

Consider
- *Norepinephrine* 0.5-30 μg/min IV or
- *Dopamine* 5-20 μg/kg per min

- *Dopamine*[c] 2.5-20 μg/kg per min IV (Add *norepinephrine* if *dopamine* is >20 μg/kg per min)

- *Dobutamine*[d,e] 2-20 μg/kg per min IV

- *Nitroglycerin* start 10-20 μg/min IV (use if ischemia persists and BP remains elevated. Titrate to effect) and/or
- *Nitoprusside* 0.1-5.0 μg/kg per min IV

Consider
further actions, especially if the patient is in acute pulmonary edema

First-line actions
- *Furosemide* IV 0.5-1.0 mg/kg
- *Morphine* IV 1-3 mg
- *Nitroglycerin* SL
- *Oxygen/intubate* PRN

Second-line actions
- *Nitroglycerin* IV if BP >1000 mmHg
- *Nitroprusside* IV if BP >100 mmHg
- *Dopamine* if BP <100 mmHg
- *Dobutamine* if BP >100 mmHg
- Positive end-expiratory pressure (PEEP)
- Continuous positive airway pressure (CPAP)

Third-line actions
- *Amrinone* 0.75 mg/kg then 5-15 μg/kg per min (if other drugs fail)
- *Aminophylline* 5 mg/kg (if wheezing)
- *Thrombolytic* therapy (if not in shock)
- *Digoxin* (if atrial fibrillation, supraventricular tachycardias)
- Angioplasty (if drugs fail)
- Intra-aortic balloon pump (bridge to surgery)
- Surgical interventions (valves, coronary artery bypass grafts, heart transplant)

a. Base management after this point on invasive hemodynamic monitoring if possible. Guidelines presume clinical signs of hypoperfusion.
b. Fluid bolus of 250-500 mL normal saline should be tried. If no response, consider sympathomimetics.
c. Move to *dopamine* and stop *norepinephrine* when BP improves. Avoid *dopamine* (consider *dobutamine*) if no signs of hypoperfusion.
d. Add *dopamine* (and avoid *dobutamine*) if systolic BP drops below 90 mm Hg.
e. Start with *nitroglycerin* if initial blood pressures are in this range.

FIGURE 8
Acute pulmonary edema/hypotension/shock algorithm.

Reproduced with permission. *Advanced Cardiac Life Support,*
Copyright © 1997, American Heart Association.

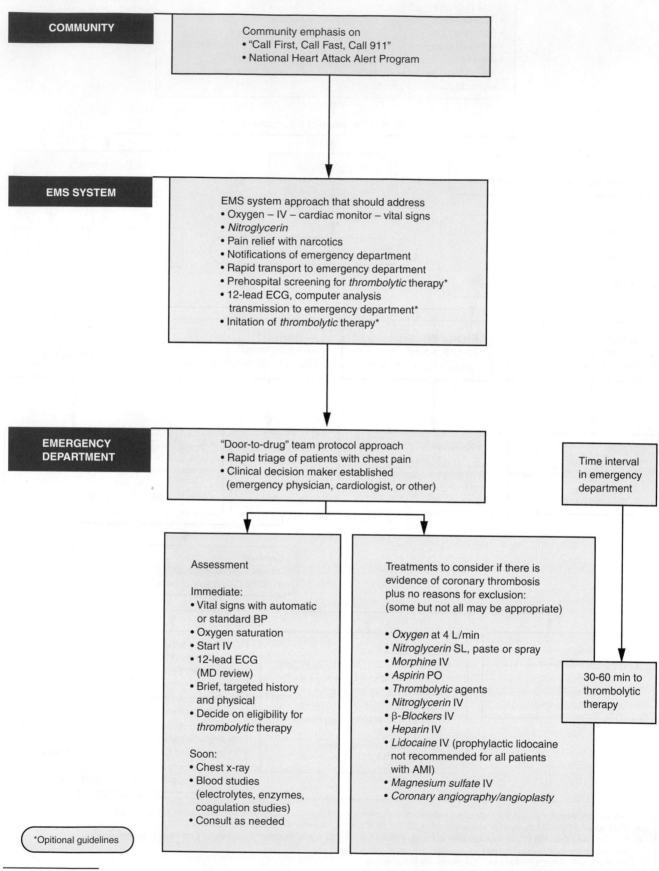

FIGURE 9

Acute myocardial infarction algorithm. Recommendations for early management of patients with chest pain and possible AMI.

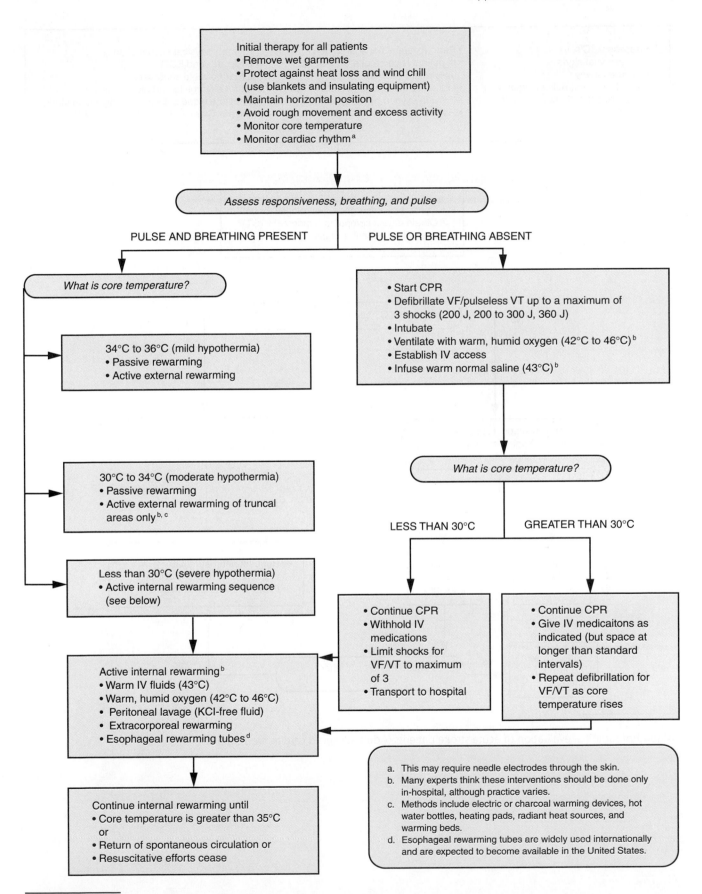

FIGURE 10

Hypothermia algorithm (Adult advanced cardiac life support).

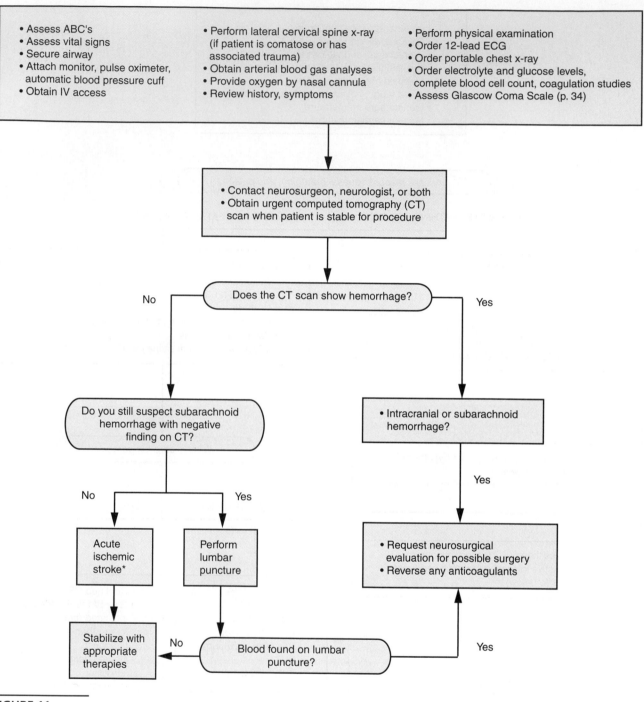

FIGURE 11

Algorithm for initial evaluation of acute stroke patients (Adult advanced cardiac life support).

APPENDIX 2

Clinical Applicability Challenges: Answer Key to Study Questions With Rationales

Chapter 2: The Patient's Experience With Critical Illness

1. d   Anxiety occurs whenever there is a threat to well-being. This includes anything that threatens the patient's sense of wholeness, security, and control.
2. b   Encouraging patients to discuss their fears and concerns and listening will let patients know they are important to and accepted by the nurse.
3. d   Order and predictability in routine and staff follow-through, offering choices, and having patients make as many decisions as possible about their care foster a sense of control.
4. a   In cognitive reappraisal, the patient clearly identifies the sources of stress and identifies his or her usual responses to the stimuli, then attempts to change these responses through the use of positive thinking.
5. d   Laughter produces all of the above effects.
6. b   Reassurance is useful for responding to exaggerated fears, calming a patient, and reducing an increased respiratory rate associated with anxiety. It should not stifle expression of feelings or emotions.
7. d   Denial occurs in the first stage of loss. This time helps the patient temporarily block out the loss and provides time to regroup energy. Stripping away the denial will increase the sense of helplessness.

Chapter 3: The Family's Experience With Critical Illness

1. c   Offering choices will help the family achieve a sense of control. It may also help lower their anxiety and enhance their problem-solving abilities.
2. d   Helping the family identify and define the problem increases their understanding of the problem, sets parameters for the problem, and gives the family a sense of cognitive mastery.
3. d   Conditions most likely to produce a crisis for the family include those that pose the threat of lasting consequences for the family, overwhelm their ability to problem solve and cope, and disrupt family homeostasis.

Chapter 4: Impact of the Critical Care Environment on the Patient

1. b   Sensory deprivation is related to a reduction in the amount and meaningfulness of sensory input. It can occur in people with normal defense mechanisms and to the critically ill within 24 hours of admission to an ICU.
2. c   Patients in the hospital environment are faced with unfamiliar sounds, routines, and people. They are also separated from their usual routine, environment, and interactions. This combination of sensory overload and deprivation is an added stress.
3. c   The onset of acute confusion is short and does not involve unconsciousness or affect recent memory.

Chapter 5: Relieving Pain and Providing Comfort

1. b   Hypertension is more commonly seen since vasoconstriction occurs due to the autonomic response to pain.
2. c   The patient's self-report always supercedes data obtained from observation and physiological parameters.
3. c   Reducing the dose is the best strategy because it is directed at the cause of the side effects and effective pain relief is still provided. With PRN dosing, fluctuating drug levels have a tendency to cause sedation and respiratory depression. Other medications given to treat the side effects may cause adverse effects of their own. Discontinuing the medication is a solution but there will be no pain relief.
4. b   Respiratory depression is the most serious complication related to epidural analgesia. Tachycardia is not associated with epidural anesthesia. The risk of pneumonia should be decreased if pain management is adequate. With an epidural catheter, activity is not restricted.
5. c   Naloxone (Narcan).

Chapter 6: Patient and Family Education in a Changing Health Care Environment

1. a   Learning readiness depends on the patient's anxiety level and the level of adaptation to illness. The best time to teach is when the anxiety level is mild and when physical and psychosocial adaptation to illness are congruent.
2. d   Intrinsic motivation involves the learner's attitudes, values, personality, and lifestyle. Lighting and noise are extrinsic factors.

Chapter 7: Ethical Issues in Critical Care

1. d   The Patient Self Determination Act of 1990 requires health care facilities to provide patients with information about their rights under state law to make decisions regarding medical care, including the right to accept or refuse care, and information about advance directives. The Act does not require advance directives (a), applies to all patients not just the terminally ill (b), and explains the DPA but does not do it automatically (c).
2. d   Ethics helps to clarify issues (a), examine responsibilities and obligations (b), and requires justification for decisions (c). Includes all of the above.
3. b   Nurses may object to care (a), support nonmaleficence (c), and exercise professional judgment (d). However, if they are opposed to and articulate their opposition to an aspect of care on moral grounds, they are still responsible to see that the patient is adequately cared for by another nurse. Anything less than this is abandonment of the patient and a violation of the promises made (ie, fidelity).
4. a   There is no morally significant difference between withdrawing and withholding treatment. In both cases, treatment should be offered if it has the potential of providing benefit to the patient, and the patient has agreed to it. Withdrawing or withholding treatment is usually done when the patient or surrogate withdraws consent or refuses the treatment.

Chapter 8: Legal Issues in Critical Care

1. c   *Respondeat superior* is translated "let the master answer for the sins of the servant" in which the employer is liable for the employees' negligent action when it is in the scope of their employment.
2. c   This act is designed to inform the public of their ability to communicate their health care wishes by way of advance directives applicable in their state.
3. a   A living will is only applicable when the person is incapacitated and terminally ill.

Chapter 9: Rewards and Challenges of Critical Care Nursing

1. c   Assertive persons value themselves, are aware of their needs, and speak up for themselves when their rights are openly violated. These behaviors help ease work-related stresses of over responsibility and selflessness.
2. b   Anxiety can interfere with problem-solving ability. Research has shown that the pressure associated with making many rapid patient care decisions creates stress for critical care nurses.
3. d   Companionship is a component of hardiness. Nurses who feel connected to others and have people with whom they can share feelings seem better able to handle critical care stresses.

Chapter 10: The Critically Ill Pediatric Patient

1. a   In the early stages of shock, vascular resistance increases in order to maintain blood pressure. One of the clinical signs of this compensation is increased capillary refill as peripheral perfusion is decreased.

2. b Based on the child's weight, a 4.5 mm endotracheal tube is the correct size.
3. d The infant has less ability to concentrate urine; therefore, the normal urine output is 2 mL/kg/hour.

Chapter 11: The Critically Ill Pregnant Woman

1. a Blood volume and CO increase to accommodate fetal circulation, BP and PVR decrease to allow for shunting of blood to uterus and placenta.
2. c Hydralazine, because of its vasodilating effect and it has been proven safe for mother and fetus.
3. d Abruptio placentae activates fibrinolytic and hemostasis systems concurrently, which consume coagulation factors; severe preeclampsia causes damage to endothelial linings of capillary beds, which stimulates the intrinsic pathway of the clotting cascade; sepsis when septic shock occurs; and fetal demise because thromboplastin is released into the maternal circulation, which activates the clotting cascade.

Chapter 12: The Critically Ill Older Patient

1. a There is a gradual loss of hearing with age and an impairment in the discrimination of sounds. Structural and functional changes of the eye occur that alter visual perception.
2. c Renal function is needed for drug excretion. Adequate hydration is needed for drug distribution. Drug interaction must be considered when administering medications.
3. b Mobilization and weight bearing are essential to slow the loss of bone mineral concentration, to promote lung expansion, and to maintain skin integrity.
4. d Abuse of the older person occurs in both homes and institutions. The abuse may be physical, psychological, or material.
5. c Cataracts form from a clouding of the lens of the eye. Glaucoma is an elevation in the pressure in the eye that causes nerve damage to the retina. Arcus senilis is a white or gray ring around the area where the cornea and sclera join. It may be caused by high blood levels of fatty substances. Retinal degeneration occurs in the elderly and distorts central vision.
6. b Differences in metabolism of alcohol in the older person may be related to the smaller volume of body water and the decrease in lean body tissue. Drug-alcohol interactions also place the older person at risk for alcohol-related problems.

Chapter 13: The Post-Anesthesia Patient

1. b Naloxone needs to be available to counteract the respiratory depression effects of the narcotic. Ephedrine is used to maintain the patient's blood pressure. With epidural anesthesia, hypotension is a frequent side effect so a vasoconstrictor needs to be available.
2. d Muscle rigidity occurs in about 75% of patients experiencing malignant hyperthermia. Elevated temperature, diaphoresis, and cyanosis are late signs of malignant hyperthermia. Cyanosis occurs because of intense vasoconstriction, which leads to skin mottling and cyanosis.
3. a Nondepolarizing muscle relaxants are pharmacologically reversed with anticholinesterases, which restore neuromuscular functioning by binding to the enzyme acetylcholinesterase and inactivating it, allowing levels of acetylcholine to rebuild. Acetylcholine ultimately displaces the nondepolarizing muscle relaxants, allowing for restoration of normal neuromuscular transmission.
4. c The depolarizing muscle relaxant, succinylcholine, mimics the action of acetylcholine. Succinylcholine binds to the cholinergic receptor sites on muscle cells causing depolarization of the cellular membranes. As long as the cell remains depolarized, it is incapable of responding to further stimulation of acetylcholine, resulting in neuromuscular blockade. Pancuronium, cistracurium, and atracurium, on the other hand, are nondepolarizing agents that compete with the acetylcholine at the cholinergic receptor site. Neuromuscular blockade occurs because of the high concentration of nondepolarizing muscular relaxant blocking the acetylcholine from reaching the motor end plate of the muscle cell.
5. b Aminophylline, physostigmine, and naloxone have all been used clinically for reversing benzodiazepine activity, but flumazenil exists as the only specific benzodiazepine antagonist. Flumazenil reverses the sedation, amnesia, muscle relaxation, anticonvulsant, and respiratory-depressant effects of benzodiazepines by working at the benzodiazepine receptor site.

Chapter 14: Interfacility Transport of the Critically Ill Patient

1. b As altitude increases, temperature decreases. Therefore, blankets are used to keep the patient warm.
2. a Maintenance of an airway is always the primary concern in any clinical situation.

Chapter 15: Anatomy and Physiology of the Cardiovascular System

1. c Preload refers to the degree of myocardial muscle fiber stretch just before contraction (systole). Preload is provided by venous return and is influenced by the volume of blood returning to the heart.
2. a Heart rate (beats per minute) times stroke volume (volume of blood in milliliters ejected during systole) is equal to volume of blood ejected per minute.
3. b The left anterior descending coronary artery supplies blood flow to the anterior two thirds of the ventricular septum, the anterior left ventricle, the apex, and most of the bundle branches.
4. d The pacemaker site for the heart is the sinoatrial node located in the wall of the right atrium.

Chapter 16: Patient Assessment: Cardiovascular System

Cardiac History and Physical Examination
1. c Cardiac pain is usually described as a squeezing, tightness, or heaviness in the chest. The pain often radiates to the neck, back, jaw, or left arm. The pain is not affected by movement of the chest or by taking a deep breath. The pain is sometimes relieved by lying down.
2. b S_1 represents the closure of the mitral and tricuspid valves at the beginning of ventricular systole.
3. c S_3 is a low frequency sound that occurs during the early, rapid-filling phase of ventricular diastole. A noncompliant or failing ventricle cannot distend to accept the rapid inflow of blood. This causes turbulent flow, resulting in the vibration of the AV valvular structures or the ventricles themselves producing a low-frequency sound.

Cardiac Laboratory Studies
1. c Myoglobin appears earlier in the serum than CK after the onset of symptoms and peaks before CK-MB. CK does not appear until approximately 2 hours after myocardial insult.
2. b When cardiac damage occurs, total CK rises and the percentage of the CK-MB is greater than 5%. In the presence of chest pain, a CK-MB greater than 5% is considered diagnostic for a myocardial infarction.
3. a LDH is found in many organs and therefore is evident in the serum for many disorders other than just cardiac injury. A rise in the serum level is not employed in the diagnosis of a myocardial infarction if the diagnosis can be confirmed by CK and CK-MB levels. In the face of nondiagnostic CK isoenzymes, there is no evidence that serial LDH or LDH isoenzymes sampling confirms the diagnosis of myocardial infarction.

Cardiovascular Diagnostic Procedures
1. b Dobutamine stress echocardiography (DSE) has been employed in patients who cannot tolerate physical exercise. Dobutamine pro-

vides both inotropic and chronotropic properties that mimic exercise, thus facilitating the opportunity to visualize blood flow using echocardiography.

2. **d** Radionuclide imaging provides information with regard to the presence of coronary artery disease and the quantity of myocardium at risk. Imaging studies can assist the practitioner in the selection of invasive or noninvasive treatment modalities.

3. **a** Ultrafast computed tomography has been shown to be of value in assessing myocardial blood flow when flow is normal or reduced, but is less accurate when flow is increased.

4. **c** Intravascular ultrasound (IVUS) can provide a circumferential assessment of the vessel with a 360-degree view. Routine angiography can only assess the diameter of the vessel in silhouette, while IVUS can determine cross-sectional dimensions, which can provide information on plaque composition and morphology.

Electrocardiographic Monitoring

1. **d** With a three-electrode monitoring system, only a modified version of a precordial lead can be obtained. To monitor an MCL_1 lead, the positive electrode is placed in a V_1 position (fourth intercostal space, right sternal border) and the negative electrode is placed under the left clavicle. The ground wire can be placed anywhere.

2. **b** With a three-electrode monitoring system, a lead II is obtained by placing the positive electrode below the level of the heart on the left side of the body and the negative electrode under the right clavicle. The placement is based on Einthoven's triangle. The ground wire can be placed anywhere.

3. **c** The most helpful leads in distinguishing ventricular ectopy from supraventricular rhythms with aberrancy are V_1 and V_6. Lead II is not a very helpful view in this situation.

Dysrhythmias and the Twelve Lead Electrocardiogram

1. **b** Intravenous atropine is the drug of choice for a sinus bradycardia that requires treatment. Atropine blocks vagal nerve impulses to the heart resulting in an increase in the heart rate.

2. **a** In atrial fibrillation, the atrial muscle merely quivers and does not contract normally. As a result, the atrial contraction (atrial kick) that contributes to cardiac output is lost.

3. **d** Premature ventricular contractions are a common dysrhythmia in persons with myocardial disease or with myocardial irritability. The irritability can be the result of hypokalemia, increased levels of catecholamines, or mechanical irritation with a catheter or wire.

4. **c** In a junctional rhythm the AV node is the pacemaker site. The stimulus from the AV node moves in a retrograde direction and depolarizes the atria before, with, or after the ventricles.

5. **b** In a complete heart block rhythm, also known as third degree heart block, stimulus from the atria are not conducted to the ventricles. The atria and ventricles function independently.

Effects of Serum Electrolyte Abnormalities on the Electrocardiogram

1. **c** Hypokalemia increases the sensitivity of the heart to digitalis and its accompanying dysrhythmias, even at normal levels of the drug. Untreated hypokalemia enhances instability in the myocardial cells.

2. **b** The major ECG finding associated with hypercalcemia is shortening of the QT interval. The shortened QT is mainly the result of shortening of the ST segment.

Hemodynamic Monitoring

1. **a** In the normal individual, PAWP is a 8–12 mmHg, which is the pressure at end-diastole of the left ventricle.

2. **a** When the PA catheter balloon is inflated, it creates a static column of blood during diastole from that point to the left ventricle, reflecting left ventricular end-diastolic pressure. The pressure in the ventricle at the end of diastole is a determinant of preload.

3. **c** Reduced intravascular volume, hypovolemia, decreases venous return and therefore the CVP.

4. **b** Generation of the cardiac output curve and computer calculation of cardiac output is based on a 4 second injection time.

5. **d** Cellular oxygen consumption is dependent on adequate oxygen supply and extraction of oxygen by the cells. When oxygen demand increases, oxygen delivery, extraction, and consumption also need to increase.

6. **c** Oxygen debt accumulation is caused by insufficient consumption of oxygen in relation to the demand. Insufficient oxygen consumption to meet oxygen demand may be due to inadequate oxygen delivery or oxygen extraction.

Chapter 17: Patient Management: Cardiovascular System

Pharmacological Therapy: Antiarrhythmic, Vasoactive, and Thrombolytic Agents

1. **a** Sotalol. The other three agents are all class III agents but only sotalol contains beta-blocking properties.

2. **c** Magnesium. The other three agents are proarrhythmic and can cause torsades de pointes.

3. **d** Increased contractility. Bronchoconstriction occurs as a result of beta 2 blockade. Decreased contractility and decreased heart rate occur as a result of beta 1 blockade.

4. **c** Bleeding. As thrombolytic agents lyse "pathologic clots" they also lyse "protective clots," creating an anticoagulant state in the body.

Percutaneous Transluminal Coronary Angioplasty and Percutaneous Balloon Valvuloplasty

1. **c** PTCA compares favorably to CABG in terms of morbidity, mortality, length of hospital stay and cost. Restenosis and acute closure are not issues associated with CABG.

2. **c** The definition of primary angioplasty is the dilation of an infarct-related coronary artery during the acute phase of a myocardial infarction *without* prior administration of thrombolytic therapy.

3. **a** A restenosis occurs when the coronary artery becomes blocked again. Choice b is the definition of valve stenosis, Choice c is the definition of atherectomy and choice d is the definition of a thrombolytic.

4. **d** Chest pain and back pain are not associated with an access site infection.

5. **c** Hyperlipidemia is a coronary risk factor, not a complication.

6. **b** ECG is a diagnostic modality, not a treatment. PTCA, stents, lasers, and directional coronary atherectomy are types of interventional cardiology procedures designed to open occluded coronary arteries.

Intra-Aortic Balloon Pump Counterpulsation and Ventricular Assist Devices

1. **b** The purpose of the intra-aortic balloon pump is to increase coronary artery perfusion during diastole. This is accomplished when the balloon inflates. The balloon pump also decreases afterload when the balloon deflates at the onset of systole.

2. **b** An intra-aortic balloon pump would not be used in patients with a terminal illness such as cancer. The pump is not used in a patient with an aortic aneurysm because of the risk of rupturing the aneurysm from the balloon inflation. The pump is not used in a patient with an incompetent aortic valve; blood would be forced back into the ventricle through an incompetent valve.

3. **b** Patients who are supported by ventricular assist devices have poor native ventricular function and are unable to generate an adequate cardiac output to sustain other vital organs. By using a ventricular assist device, the compromised ventricle is bypassed and the device assumes the workload of the failing ventricle with the intention of improving cardiac output, peripheral perfusion, and ultimately end-organ function. Answer a is incorrect because these devices are not always used to bridge a patient to transplantation. They may be used for short-term support after a surgical procedure or a myocardial infarction. Answer c is incorrect because with the implantable devices the goal is not to restrict activity but to rehabilitate these patients physically while awaiting heart transplantation. Answer d is incorrect because an assist device decreases ventricular workload by assuming the work of the native ventricle.

4. c Patients are often very frightened by the strange environment, the technology, and the interventions surrounding their care. Explaining procedures and activities relieves much anxiety for patients and family members. The remaining three answers (a, b, d) are incorrect because each may affect the orientation, sleep patterns, and social contact of the family of the patient. All three situations can contribute to increased patient anxiety and have a negative impact on the recovery process.

Autologous Blood Transfusion

1. a Characteristics of allogeneic blood include: decreased RBC wall integrity causing an increase in serum potassium; nonviable platelets within 24 hours of storage; anticoagulants; no 2,3-DPG after 10 days storage. Characteristics of autologous blood include: platelets remain viable with nearly normal platelet count and function; 2, 3-DPG is within normal levels.
2. b Although the incidence is small, coagulopathy associated with autologous blood collection and reinfusion techniques has been reported. Transfusion reaction, hepatitis, and HIV are risks associated with allogeneic blood.

Cardiopulmonary Resuscitation

1. a Epinephrine. The other three have not been cleared to administer in this way. The other agents that can be put down the ET tube are lidocaine and atropine. The dose is 2.5 times normal, diluted in 10cc of normal saline.
2. d Epinephrine. It raises coronary and cerebral perfusion pressures.
3. a The initial shock should be delivered at 200 joules by a trained member of the resuscitation team. Defibrillation should be performed as soon as possible after the VF arrest with at least 25 pounds of pressure to the paddles.

Management of Dysrhythmias

1. b The shock is synchronized with the R wave so that it is delivered during ventricular depolarization. The shock is never delivered during the vulnerable period of ventricular repolarization.
2. c The patient's signs and symptoms are possible indicators of cardiac perforation. The physician should be notified immediately of the patient's change in status.
3. b The ability of the pacer to detect the heart's intrinsic activity and respond appropriately is known as sensing. Capture is depolarization of the heart in response to a pacing stimulus. Telemetry is the communicating feature of some pacemakers. Output refers to the milliamperage (mA) of a pacemaker.
4. c A transcutaneous pacing system consists of external pacing electrodes (large patches) and an external pacing device.
5. b A DDDRO pacemaker paces and senses both the atria and the ventricle, responds to sensed activity by inhibiting or triggering pacing, and adjusts the pacing rate based on metabolic demand.
6. a Capture for a ventricular pacemaker is evidenced by a pacing stimulus followed by a QRS complex.
7. b The implantable cardioverter defibrillator is designed to treat ventricular tachydysrhythmias (ventricular tachycardia and ventricular fibrillation).
8. c Since his ventricular tachycardia is typically at a rate of 200 BPM, the ICD rate criteria would be set to 190 so that a rate above 190 BPM will initiate ICD therapy.
9. c Tiered therapy means the ICD has the ability to provide antitachycardia pacing, low energy cardioversion, defibrillation, and antibradycardia pacing.

Chapter 18: Common Cardiovascular Disorders

1. a Stress, infectious diseases, gout, and prior surgeries are not risk factors.
2. d This position may shift the pericardium from the diaphragm, making breathing less painful.
3. c Sudden stabbing pain is a classic description of acute aortic dissection. Pulses are unequal as a result of the dissection. Aortic insufficiency can develop if the dissection involves the aortic root.

Chapter 19: Heart Failure

1. b An early sympathetic response to decreased cardiac output and resultant tissue level hypoxia is tachycardia, which, of course, will decrease filling time.
2. a Tissue level acidosis is most likely to be caused by anaerobic metabolism.
3. a Dopamine is used to increase the renal perfusion and therefore diurese the body. Higher doses of dopamine will have adrenergic (dopaminergic) effects upon the patient.
4. c ACE inhibitors are vasodilator therapy to prolong life and decrease the symptoms of CHF.

Chapter 20: Acute Myocardial Infarction

1. c Approximately 33–50% of all patients with an inferior wall myocardial infarction also will have a right ventricular infarction. Both the inferior wall and the right ventricle receive their oxygenated blood supply from the right coronary artery.
2. b Patients with an anterior wall myocardial infarction are at high risk for cardiogenic shock if a significant amount of the left ventricle is infarcted. Evidence of shock is manifested by a systolic blood pressure < 85 mmHg, a mean arterial pressure < 65 mmHg, a cardiac index < 2.2 L/min/m², and a pulmonary artery wedge pressure > 25 mmHg.
3. d Mrs. Martin's heart rate, blood pressure, wedge pressure, cardiac index, and urine output are below normal. Low values indicate a low volume state.
4. c ST segment depressions and T wave inversions are seen with myocardial ischemia. ST segment elevations represent acute myocardial injury; Q waves with ST segment elevations represent an acute myocardial infarction; Q waves with normal ST segments represent a previous myocardial infarction.
5. a Hypertension has been classified by the American Heart Association as a major risk factor that can be altered. Hypertension is often known as the "silent killer." Obesity, diabetes mellitus, and stress are classified as contributing risk factors.

Chapter 21: Cardiac Surgery

1. c Because of the interface between blood and the nonphysiological surfaces of the bypass circuit, complement and platelets are activated and vasoactive substances are released, increasing capillary permeability. Damage to RBCs, hemodilution, and alterations in coagulation are also changes resulting from cardiopulmonary bypass.
2. b Research shows that biological valves have poor durability and many start deteriorating within 7 to 10 years post implant; therefore, mechanical valves are the valves of choice for younger individuals. Biological valves have a lower incidence of thromboembolism and may only require an initial period of anticoagulation until the valve surfaces are endothelialized.
3. d Postoperative bleeding can be treated by protamine to neutralize heparin "rebound," PEEP to increase intrathoracic pressure and decrease venous oozing, and autotransfusion to maintain normovolemia and hematocrit level.
4. d Increased afterload early after surgery usually results from vasoconstriction secondary to hypothermia. Blankets and radiant heat will increase body temperature causing vasodilation and decreased afterload. Answers a or c may also be considered as treatment for increased afterload, but only when the vasoconstriction occurs as compensation for hypovolemia. In this case, the PAWP would also be low.
5. c Pain perception varies from person to person and is an individual experience. The most reliable indicator of pain intensity is the patient's report. Patients may be able to sleep and may not exhibit physiological or nonverbal clues of pain yet report high pain scores.
6. a Cardiac muscle is fatigue resistant and can be stimulated to contract as a whole with one stimulus. Skeletal muscle is composed of separate motor units that contract separately and are easily fatigued. Therefore, conditioning of skeletal muscle is a gradual process with progressive stimulation by a pulse train over 7 to 8 weeks.

7. c   The facial nerve controls the ability to smile and frown. Since it traverses the surgical area, it can be traumatized during surgery. Vagus nerve damage would cause loss of gag reflex, difficulty swallowing, and hoarseness. Stroke would usually result in more generalized neurological deficits.

Chapter 22: Anatomy and Physiology of the Respiratory System

1. a   Conditions or situations that destroy lung tissue, cause it to become fibrotic, produce pulmonary edema, block alveoli, or in any way impede lung expansion and expansibility of the thoracic cage reduce lung compliance.
2. c   When an alveoli is adequately ventilated but not adequately perfused, dead space will develop and gas exchange cannot occur.
3. b   A shift of the curve to the right is caused by fever, acidosis, and an increased $PaCO_2$. As a result, more oxygen is released to the tissues.
4. d   The aortic and carotid bodies respond to hypercapnia and low pH by increasing ventilation. Their response is weak compared to medullary actions. The increased ventilation helps to eliminate CO_2 from the body.

Chapter 23: Patient Assessment: Respiratory System

1. c   Vesicular breath sounds are heard over the periphery of the lung. Bronchial breath sounds are heard over the trachea, and bronchovesicular breath sounds are heard over the major airways.
2. a   Normally mixed venous saturation of oxygen is 60–80%. The arterial oxygen saturation is normally 93–99%.
3. d   The pH is less than 7.40, representing acidosis. The $PaCO_2$ is elevated above 35–45 mmHg, indicating a respiratory acidosis. The HCO_3 is within normal limits. The oxygen level is normal for sea level. This represents uncompensated respiratory acidosis.
4. a   By definition *respiratory* alkalosis will be a dysfunction in the $PaCO_2$, the respiratory parameter. By definition, *alkalosis* in the respiratory parameter occurs from low levels of $PaCO_2$.
5. c   Hypothermia decreases oxygen demand, thus allowing more oxygen to return to the venous side. Pain, anxiety, and hyperthermia increase oxygen demand, thus less oxygen is returned to the venous side. Anemia results in a decreased supply of oxygen and therefore causes a lowered SvO_2.

Chapter 24: Patient Management: Respiratory System

1. c   Patients with a unilateral lung process have improved oxygenation when positioned with the good lung down. A semi-reclining position would not facilitate gravity drainage from a lower lobe. If bronchodilators are being administered, the patient should be suctioned after the treatment.
2. b   The only proven efficacy of CPT is in patients with a lobar atelectasis or in those with large amounts of sputum production, especially cystic fibrosis and bronchiectasis.
3. c   If the patient is able to talk, it indicates a large cuff leak. Breath sounds over only the right lung can indicate right mainstem intubation. An incessant cough indicates that the ETT is stimulating the carina. Correct placement is 3–7 cm above the carina.
4. b   Oxygen saturation would be much lower in a patient with a tension pneumothorax. There would be a mediastinal shift. The electrolyte abnormalities have nothing at all to do with pneumothoraces. Tension pneumothorax can quickly lead to death because of the mediastinal shift; therefore "b" is the correct answer.
5. a   These are signs of pneumothorax. Bubbling is expected immediately after the chest tube is inserted, indicating that the pneumothorax is being successfully evacuated. Fluctuation in the water seal chamber is normal and indicates that the chest tube is patent. The water level will evaporate over time and does need to be refilled; however this is not an emergency.
6. d   Steroids have not been shown to be beneficial in the treatment of ARDS. All of the other choices are adverse effects of steroids that are normally seen.
7. c   Answer "a" is a correct fact, but it is not a reason for monitoring NMBA dosage. NMBA dosage should be maintained at the lowest effective dose. Answer "d" has nothing to do with NMBAs. Prolonged and profound weakness has been reported after NMBA use. That weakness would contribute to a prolonged recovery and rehabilitation time.
8. d   The incorrect choices are cardiac tamponade, multiple trauma, and DIC.
9. b   One sign of pneumothorax is an elevation in peak airway pressure, which would cause the high pressure alarm to sound. A disconnection would cause a low pressure alarm. A paralytic drug should make the high pressure alarm stop sounding. An FIO_2 left on 1.00 should make the FIO_2 alarm sound.

Chapter 25: Common Respiratory Disorders

1. c   Atelectasis often presents as hypoxia, with or without cyanosis, decreased breath sounds, tachycardia and tachypnea, decreased chest wall motion over the affected area, and activity intolerance due to shortness of breath. Atelectasis will cause coughing with deep breathing, but will not cause pain.
2. a   The normal ventilation perfusion mismatch can be decreased if the drive to breathe increases (ie, due to exercise) but will not be increased. Pulmonary emboli result in *decreased* perfusion to part of the vascular bed in the pulmonary system, not necessarily the pulmonary *capillary* bed.
3. a   Cor pulmonale is most commonly seen with emphysema.
4. d   Most sleep apnea occurs in middle aged men (40–60 years). Cheyne-Stokes respirations may be seen in men 60–70 years old.

Chapter 26: Adult Respiratory Distress Syndrome

1. d   Increased endothelial permeability allows fluid to move into the interstitial and alveolar spaces, causing interstitial and alveolar edema which also causes the lungs to be less distensible. SIRS mediators released with ARDS cause vasoconstriction of the pulmonary vascular bed, which would **increase** the pulmonary artery wedge pressure.
2. a   Ventilator modes, such as pressure control or airway pressure release ventilation, reduce airway pressure by limiting inspiratory pressures, therefore decreasing injury to the lung epithelium.
3. d   The pulmonary alterations seen in ARDs are directly related to a cascade of events initiated by the systemic inflammatory response syndrome (SIRS). SIRS initiates the release of multiple inflammatory mediators that cause increased microvascular permeability, pulmonary hypertension, and pulmonary endothelial damage.

Chapter 27: Anatomy and Physiology of the Renal System

1. b   In the glomerulus, water and solutes are filtered from the blood to form urine. Reabsorption of essential materials from the urine filtrate occurs in the tubules.
2. b   The active transport of sodium out of the tubular fluid (reabsorption by distal tubule cells) requires a hydrogen or potassium ion to be secreted into the tubular fluid. The choice of cation depends on the extracellular fluid concentrations of these ions.
3. b   The increase in the filtrate osmotic pressure (OP) promotes the movement of water and small permeable molecules from the plasma into Bowman's capsule. The increased filtrate OP also decreases the sodium and water reabsorption leading to diuresis.

Chapter 28: Patient Assessment: Renal System

1. c   Creatinine is a by-product of normal muscle metabolism and is excreted in the urine primarily as a result of glomerular filtration. The amount of creatinine excreted in the urine normally remains constant unless significant muscle wasting is present. Therefore, creatinine clearance is an excellent clinical indicator of renal function.
2. a   Patients with renal failure have elevated levels of potassium, phosphate, and magnesium because the impaired kidney is unable to excrete them adequately.
3. d   Hypocalcemia results in skeletal muscle cramps and tetany. Chvostek's and Trousseau's signs occur when muscles are irritable due to hypocalcemia. These tests involve tapping or constricting specific muscles and observing for muscle spasm.

Chapter 29: Patient Management: Renal System

1. b   Although heparin is useful as an anticoagulant, patients at high risk for bleeding may be managed with frequent saline flushes to keep the system from clotting.
2. c   Reduced ultrafiltration occurs as the pores in the fibers become blocked by clots. Clotting turns the filter and lines dark, and raises venous pressure because resistance in the lines and filter increase. The first action would be to try to flush saline to assess the extent of clotting. Giving heparin would not be the correct choice because it does not reverse clotting, which has already occurred and may endanger the patient.
3. a   Peritonitis is an emergency which must be treated right away. By sending the fluid for culture and cell count immediately, specific antibiotic coverage can be ordered. In the meantime, a broad-spectrum antibiotic is given to control symptoms.

Chapter 30: Common Renal Disorders

1. d   A diuretic will help Mr. O'Keefe eliminate the fluid overload.
2. d   Prerenal causes of azotemia include physiological events that result in decreased circulation (ischemia) to the kidneys. Most commonly these include hypovolemia and heart failure.
3. c   Intrarenal acute renal failure is caused by physiological events directly affecting kidney tissue and function. These often include events causing damage to the interstitium and the nephron tissue.
4. a   When renal underperfusion persists for a sufficient period of time, the kidneys may become damaged. Therefore restoration of renal circulation as soon as possible is essential.
5. b   Oliguric renal failure is defined as a urine volume of less than 400 ml/day. The most common complication is overhydration with resulting cardiac failure, pulmonary edema, and death.
6. d   During the diuretic phase, urinary volume may exceed 4 to 5 liters per day. As a result, it is essential to maintain proper fluid and electrolyte balance.
7. b   If prerenal acute renal failure is not corrected, progression to intrarenal failure will occur. The adverse effects of reduced perfusion will affect kidney function.

Chapter 31: Anatomy and Physiology of the Nervous System

1. b   Axons carry impulses away from the cell body, and dendrites conduct the impulses toward the cell body.
2. a   Withdrawal reflex is a cord reflex, triggered by the sensation of pain. Pain stimulates the sensory neurons, which stimulate central interneurons, which then stimulate motor fibers that contract the skeletal muscles.
3. d   Arterioles dilate in response to cholinergic impulses.

4. d   The brainstem controls the vegetative functions of respiration, cardiac rate and blood vessel diameter. "We live in the brainstem and play in the cortex."

Chapter 32: Patient Assessment: Nervous System

1. a   A stuporous patient may inconsistently follow simple commands but is very hard to arouse. A comatose patient may respond with reflexive posturing or no response at all. A lethargic patient is drowsy but follows simple commands when stimulated.
2. c   Opiates cause constricted pupils; the other examples cause dilated pupils.
3. d   The optic nerve is checked by testing gross visual acuity. The facial nerve does not control the eye. The sensory portion of the oculomotor nerve controls pupil size.
4. b   This is also called central vision, and is caused by lesions around the optic chiasm such as pituitary tumors or aneurysms of the anterior communicating artery.
5. c   The hypoglossal nerve controls tongue movement. Deviation due to damage to the nerve will be to the side of the lesion.

Chapter 33: Patient Management: Nervous System

1. d   Although no single management technique is appropriate for all patients, first tier therapy routinely includes ventricular CSF drainage, mannitol, and hyperventilation.
2. c   Nursing care activity can compound primary and secondary intracranial insults, contributing to rapid deterioration in the unstable patient who has lost intracranial compliance, autoregulation, and vasomotor tone. To reduce potential causes of intracranial hypertension, it is important for the nurse to assess and prevent extracranial causes of increase in ICP, such as emotionally related conversation; position of head, neck, and hips that reduce venous return; and abdominal distention.
3. a   The purpose of a continuous-flush device is to prevent vascular lines from clotting. A continuous-flush device is contraindicated with all ICP monitoring techniques because it is not done in vascular spaces and the introduction of the additional volume of flush solution into the intracranium may result in cerebral herniation and death.
4. d   Shivering is a compensatory mechanism to produce heat when the body senses heat loss. The aerobic muscle activity associated with shivering increases the metabolic demand for oxygen, increasing oxygen consumption and carbon dioxide production, while decreasing glycogen stores.

Chapter 34: Head Injury

1. d   A concussion results in temporary and reversible neurological dysfunction. There is usually loss of consciousness, but it may not be documentable.
2. b   The motor strip in the cerebral cortex regulates voluntary control over the muscles used in breathing. Cranial nerves IX and X carry impulses from the chemoreceptors and stretch receptors to the brainstem. The cervical and thoracic spinal nerves carry information to activate the diaphragm and expand the chest wall. It is the pons and midbrain, not the medulla, that regulate the automaticity of breathing.
3. b   Apneustic breathing has a long pause at full inspiration or expiration. Cluster breathing presents as gasping breaths with irregular pauses. Totally irregular breathing is characteristic of ataxic breathing.
4. c   When using longer sentences the patient may forget the beginning of the sentence before he hears the end of the sentence. Simple language appropriate to the patient's age, delivered in a normal tone of voice, and punctuated by natural gestures will help the dysphasic patient understand what is being said.

Chapter 35: Common Neurological Disorders

1. b   Unilateral headache is a common chief complaint with an AVM. Headache with a stroke or hydrocephalus would more likely be generalized, with no focal localizing sign.
2. c   Aneurysm-forming vessels usually lie in the space between the arachnoid and the brain, so the hemorrhage is into the subarachnoid space.
3. c   Because of the sudden loss of consciousness, violent jerking movements, and potential for complications such as tongue-biting, rhabdomyolysis, and aspiration, the generalized tonic–clonic status is most serious.
4. d   Tensilon improves muscle strength in myasthenic crisis. The patient requires more anticholinesterase drugs in this crisis.
5. a   Brain tumors act as space-occupying masses inside the rigid skull, which will eventually cause an increase in ICP.

Chapter 36: Spinal Cord Injury

1. b   Autonomic dysreflexia is caused by a sympathetic discharge that produces reflex vasoconstriction, causing hypertension and headache.
2. a   There is loss of reflex activity below the level of injury, so the blood vessels are vasodilated, causing the skin tone to be warm and pink.
3. c   An injury at C1, C2, or C3 level will paralyze the diaphragm as well as the intercostals. At the C4 level, the patient usually needs intermittent mechanical ventilation. At C5, after spinal shock has resolved, the diaphragm should function so no mechanical ventilation is needed.
4. d   Autonomic dysreflexia may be caused by constipation or impaction, so the program should begin even before spinal shock has resolved. Nupercainal ointment may be used with the bowel program to prevent AD.
5. b   Fluids should be forced with any indwelling catheter (Foley or suprapubic). Fluids should be restricted with an intermittent cath program to prevent high residuals over 500 cc, which may be harmful to upper renal structures.

Chapter 37: Anatomy and Physiology of the Gastrointestinal System

1. a   The pancreas secretes amylase and bicarbonate, in addition to multiple other substances. The stomach, not the pancreas, secretes hydrochloric acid. The small intestine, not the pancreas, secretes secretin. Secretin in turn stimulates pancreatic secretion.
2. c   The colon is a major site for the reabsorption of water and electrolytes; it is not a site for digestion, absorption, or for secretion of gastrointestinal hormones.
3. d   The liver is not a site for the synthesis of immunoglobulins.
4. d   Defecation is a cord reflex that can be initiated via rectal stretch, and inhibited via central impulses.

Chapter 38: Patient Assessment: Gastrointestinal System

1. a   Dull sounds are heard over solid organs, whereas hollow organs or empty spaces are tympanitic in nature. Therefore, hollow organs, gastric air bubbles, or an empty colon would not sound dull on percussion.
2. b   Endoscopy is the only test in this group that allows for direct visualization of the GI tract. Abdominal x-rays, ultrasonography, and CT scans provide information related to general structure, organization, and abnormal presentations of organs, as well as air/fluid levels.
3. b   Tests that require direct visualization of the GI tract must be completed before those tests that coat the tract; therefore, the barium examination should be last. Arteriography, colonoscopy, and endoscopy all require direct visualization of the tract for maximal diagnostic value.

Chapter 39: Patient Management: Gastrointestinal System

1. d   Catecholemines cause liver and muscle glycogen to be converted to glucose, while insulin release from the pancreas is suppressed. There is decreased uptake of glucose in the peripheral tissues.
2. a   Serum albumin is a visceral protein that reflects protein mass of the internal organs.
3. c   Checking gastric residuals is one method to determine tolerance of tube feedings. When gastric residuals are high, tube feedings are withheld to allow time for digestion and decreasing the volume in the stomach. This reduces the risk for aspiration.
4. d   Hypovolemia is the most common complication of total parenteral nutrition therapy, due to the increased glucose load.

Chapter 40: Common Gastrointestinal Disorders

1. c   The primary goal in the initial management of *active* gastrointestinal bleeding is to achieve hemodynamic stability. This allows the patient to be prepared for surgery and other treatment options. Vasopressin administration may be appropriate to control bleeding, but will usually follow volume replacement therapy. Pain control is important but secondary to hemodynamic stability.
2. b   Migration of the esophageal balloon up into the airway can lead to suffocation. Necrosis of the nares, tearing of the cardiac sphincter, and tracheoesophageal fistulas are related to constant pressure on sensitive pressure points, not sudden deflation of the gastric balloon.
3. c   Strangulation and potentially necrotic bowel must be removed immediately. Pain control, NGT suction, and irrigation are not appropriate treatments for this emergent disorder. Endoscopy is not a *treatment* option for these patients.
4. c   SGOT/SGPT (ALT/AST) are enzymes released when hepatocytes are damaged. PT/PTT is an indicator of the liver's ability to create clotting factors, whereas alkaline phosphatase and amylase are indicators of gallbladder and pancreatic dysfunction.
5. c   Increased ammonia levels are associated with the development of hepatic encephalopathy. Although the other indicators may be abnormal in the patient with hepatic encephalopathy, they are not directly related to the mentation difficulties.
6. d   All of these complications of pancreatitis are amenable to surgical intervention, although the pseudocyst may not require such aggressive intervention.
7. c   Further release of pancreatic enzymes leads to further damage to the pancreas or increased complications. Therefore, decreasing enzymatic release is a primary goal of both medical and nursing care.

Chapter 41: Anatomy and Physiology of the Endocrine System

1. c   Glucocorticoid (steroid) medications can trigger the development of Cushing's syndrome, which includes diabetes, protein-wasting, and osteoporosis. They also cause peptic ulcers and immunosuppression.
2. a   Major factors that decrease growth hormones are elevated blood glucose, fatty acids or cortisol, and rapid eye movement (dreaming). Major factors that stimulate growth hormone include fasting, low blood glucose levels, exercise, and stress.
3. a   Insulin lowers blood glucose levels, whereas glucagon and norepinephrine elevate blood glucose levels. Aldosterone does not affect blood sugar.

Chapter 42: Patient Assessment: Endocrine System

1. b   Weight is the least significant parameter initially because it is not immediately life threatening. The remaining parameters are more significant because a high temperature, tachyarrhythmia, and hypertension need more immediate treatment.

Chapter 43: Common Endocrine Disorders

1. a Aspirin is not recommended as an antipyretic in thyroid crisis because it increases free T_3 and T_4 levels.
2. d Thyroid crisis increases body metabolism. This results in fever, tachycardia, and neurologic dysfunction such as tremors, restlessness, emotional ability and depressed consciousness.
3. b Myxedema coma is characterized by all but tachycardia. Decreased thyroid hormone depresses body activity. The heart rate is slower and there is a risk for heart block.
4. a Illness, stress, and mismanagement of sick days are frequent precipitating events for DKA. Insulin deficiency rather than overinsulinization is the cause of DKA.
5. a Volume replacement with isotonic or hypotonic saline is the traditional therapy for all patients with DKA. Bolus bicarbonate is only given in cardiac arrest whereas some patients may need mechanical ventilation, not with a tracheotomy. Likewise, fluid and electrolyte correction are achieved by replacement, not hemodialysis.
6. c Patients with HHNC do not have ketonemia or ketoacidosis. As a result the anion gap and bicarbonate levels are not abnormal. The main sign is a very high glucose level.
7. d Dehydration is the underlying issue. Rehydration also decreases the hyperglycemia.

Chapter 44: Anatomy and Physiology of the Hematological and Immune Systems

1. b Albumin regulates the passage of water and solutes through the capillaries.
2. c See Figure 44-2, Sequence of coagulation to review the conversion of prothrombin to thrombin.
3. c This statement is true of general immunity rather than specific immunity.
4. a Autoimmune disorders reflect a hypersensitivity of the immune system to self.

Chapter 45: Patient Assessment: Hematological and Immune Systems

1. c In the presence of a normal platelet count, consider a disorder of platelet function due to a deficiency in von Willebrand's factor, uremia from renal failure, drugs, food or spices.
2. d Examining the bone marrow will reveal if malignant cells remain in the bone marrow following chemotherapy and provide information about precursor cells of peripheral blood components.
3. a Protective measures are usually instituted when the absolute neutrophil count is less than 1000/uL.
4. b Although neutropenia may be caused by decreased production from bone marrow injury, the ANC is usually a measure of the degree of immunosuppression. The nadir of the WBC count simply refers to the lowest point in white blood cell levels. A bone marrow biopsy is the most important test for determining bone marrow functioning.

Chapter 46: Organ and Hemopoietic Stem Cell Transplantation

1. c The ability to pay is determined separately and does not affect the process of determining the patient's physical condition and medical suitability for transplantation.
2. c Although matching is performed for other organ transplants, it is not as important as it is for kidney and bone marrow transplants.
3. b This describes the difference between organ rejection and graft-versus-host disease.
4. d These two drugs are administered based on drug levels.

Chapter 47: Common Immunological Disorders

1. b CD4 count, along with CD4 percentage, are the most widely used tests to assess disease progression. As the CD4 count drops, the incidence of opportunistic illnesses increases, which may lead to overwhelming infections.
2. b It takes the immune system 6 weeks to 3 months before it begins to produce antibodies against HIV. During this time, the individual's ELISA will be negative because the ELISA detects the presence of antibodies.
3. c Blood, semen, vaginal fluids, and breast milk are the only fluids that have been implicated in the transmission of HIV.
4. d Multiple myeloma by its nature destroys the bone marrow, which results in release of large amounts of calcium into the blood stream.
5. c High Fowler's promotes venous drainage from the head and neck and enhances the patient's respiratory effort.

Chapter 48: Common Hematological Disorders

1. b Part of the cause of anemia of chronic disease is the suppression of bone marrow production of RBCs and decreased levels of erythropoietin. Transfusion and recombinant erythropoietin can help to partially correct anemia from these causes.
2. c Drugs to stimulate bone marrow function are of no benefit in aplastic anemia.
3. d Bleeding episodes in hemophiliacs are often managed by self-administration of intravenous factor at home at the time the earliest symptoms appear.
4. c Tissue thromboplastin in the circulation causes activation of the extrinsic pathway through the activation of factor VII.
5. a Platelets are consumed in the initial hypercoagulable state to form platelet plugs and to initiate clotting via the intrinsic pathway through the release of platelet factor 3.
6. d Decreased plasminogen levels would result in decreased levels of plasmin. Plasmin is the lytic enzyme that acts to break down fibrin. Hence, decreased plasmin levels result in decreased clot break down, lessening the chance of bleeding and consumption of clotting factors.

Chapter 49: Hypoperfusion States

1. d Any loss of circulating volume due to a loss of sympathetic tone (vasodilation as in sepsis), blood loss with hemorrhage, intravascular fluid depletion with burn injury due to a lack of epidermal/dermal tissue or intracellular dehydration will cause hypovolemia. If the volume lost is not replaced, hypovolemic shock will ensue.
2. d Treatment priorities include: oxygenation to enhance oxygen carrying capacity to minimize ischemia; inotropic support to enhance myocardial contractility; vasodilation for afterload reduction which decreases left ventricular workload; antiarrhythmic agents as needed to control ischemic dysrhythmias and improve cardiac output; and judicious use of fluids to maximize filling pressure (LVEDP 14–18 mmHg).
3. b Administer many liters of fluid to compensate for the fluid shifts from the intervascular to extravascular space as a result of the inflammatory response which causes capillary leaking; administer vasopressor agents to enhance sympathetic tone (↑SVR) which will enhance blood pressure; give broad spectrum antibiotics before culture results in an effort to treat the infectious source.
4. b SIRS is an overwhelming inflammatory/immune response, and is not due to a causative organism. Sepsis, however, is the result of an invading microbe and the body's immune response.
5. a Confusion due to altered tissue perfusion related to vasodilation, hypovolemia, and hypotension; hyperthermic response is the result of the inflammatory reaction to the invading microbe; hypotension as a consequence of the systemic inflammatory vasodilator response; and metabolic acidosis is the net result of the catabolic state and anaerobic metabolism.

Chapter 50: Trauma

1. b A massive hemothorax is potentially lethal; therefore chest tubes should be inserted during the resuscitation phase. The resuscitation phase is often conducted simultaneously with primary evaluation and includes treatment of life-threatening injuries.
2. c Rib fractures should not be taped or splinted because this reduces lung expansion and can lead to respiratory complications.
3. a Solid organs (liver) respond to trauma with bleeding, whereas hollow organs (small bowel, colon, stomach) collapse or rupture and spill their contents.
4. d Incomplete hemostasis, sepsis, and DIC are all possible complications of a severe liver laceration. The risk of sepsis and DIC are further increased with massive blood transfusions (frequently necessary following severe liver injury).
5. d Fractures can be pinned or placed in skeletal traction. Compartment syndrome is a common complication.
6. b MOF usually begins with pulmonary failure, manifested as ARDS. DIC, congestive heart failure, and gastrointestinal bleeding may be seen later, as MOF continues to progress.

Chapter 51: Burns

1. b Injury includes all layers, including subcutaneous tissue.

2. c Capillary damage results in loss of plasma fluid and protein into interstitial spaces. Loss of plasma proteins results in a decreased capillary colloidal osmotic pressure.
3. b CNS manifestations of carbon monoxide poisoning may range from headache to coma.
4. b Arm—9%; Anterior trunk—18%; Total: 27%
5. a Cell injury results in release of intracellular potassium into the extracellular fluid.
6. c Due to hypovolemia and decreased cardiac function, peripheral circulation is decreased. Intramuscular medication will not be absorbed until volume and cardiac output are restored.
7. c Most common adverse reaction of silver sulfadiazine is leukopenia.

Chapter 52: Drug Overdose and Poisoning

1. d Exchange transfusion, little used, is a method of enhanced elimination in which a portion of the patient's blood is removed and replaced with whole fresh blood.
2. b Urine alkalinization may enhance excretion of drugs that are weak acids such as salicylates.

Index

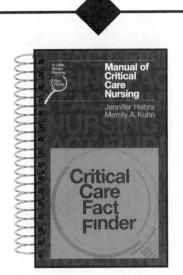
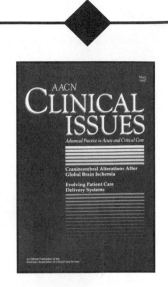